P9-ELO-876

MOSBY'S

Primary Care Consultant

MOSBY'S Primary Care Consultant

Sheila A. Dunn, RN, MSN, C-ANP

Nurse Practitioner,
John Cochran Veterans Administration
Medical Center;
Clinical Instructor,
St. Louis University,
St. Louis, Missouri

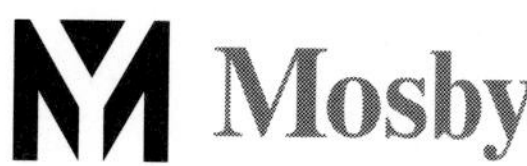

St. Louis Baltimore Boston Carlsbad Chicago Minneapolis New York Philadelphia Portland
London Milan Sydney Tokyo Toronto

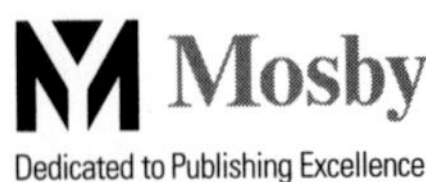

Dedicated to Publishing Excellence

A Times Mirror Company

Publisher: Nancy L. Coon
Editor: Barry Bowlus
Managing Editor: Lisa Potts
Developmental Editor: Jeanne Allison
Project Manager: Deborah L. Vogel
Senior Production Editor: Judith Bange
Production Editor: Karen L. Allman
Designer: Renée Duenow
Manufacturing Supervisor: Don Carlisle

Printed in the United States of America
Composition by Clarinda Company
Printing/binding by Maple-Vail Book Mfg Group

Mosby, Inc.
11830 Westline Industrial Drive
St. Louis, Missouri 63146

Library of Congress Cataloging in Publication Data

Dunn, Sheila A.
Mosby's primary care consultant / Sheila A. Dunn.
p. cm.
Includes bibliographical references and index.
ISBN 0-8151-2950-5
1. Physical diagnosis—Handbooks, manuals, etc. 2. Medical history taking—Handbooks, manuals, etc. 3. Primary care (Medicine—Handbooks, manuals, etc. 4. Nurse practitioners—Handbooks, manuals, etc. I. Title.
[DNLM: 1. Primary Health Care—handbooks. 2. Medical History Taking—handbooks. 3. Physical Examination—handbooks. W 49 D923m 1988]
RC76.D86 1998
616—dc21
DNLM/DLC
for Library of Congress 97-42363
CIP

98 99 00 01 02 / 9 8 7 6 5 4 3 2 1

REVIEWERS

Lucille A. Capo, MSN, RN-C, FNP
Family Nurse Practitioner,
Rural Outpatient Health Care,
Cass Medical Center,
Harrisonville, Missouri;
Nursing Faculty,
Graceland College
Independence, Missouri

Dorothy McDonnell Cook, RN, PhD
Associate Professor of Nursing,
School of Nursing,
St. Louis University,
St. Louis, Missouri

Susan Waldrop Donckers, RN, EdD, CS, FNP
Nurse Practitioner,
Lewis Gale Clinic,
Salem, Virginia

Jane A. Fox, EdD, PNP, RNCS
Clinical Associate Professor,
New York University School of Education,
Division of Nursing,
New York, New York;
Clinical Associate Professor,
SUNY at Stony Brook,
Stony Brook, New York

Pamela Hinthorn, PhD, FNP-C
Director,
Family Nurse Practitioner Program,
Fairfield University,
Fairfield, Connecticut

Ann H. Lewis, PhD, RN, C
Assistant Professor,
UAMS College of Nursing;
Director,
Family Nurse Practitioner Program;
University of Arkansas for Medical Sciences,
Little Rock, Arkansas

Margaret McAllister, RN, CS, FNP, PhD(C)
Coordinator,
Nurse Practitioner Programs,
University of Massachusetts at Boston,
Boston, Massachusetts

JoAnne Peach, RN, MSN, FNP
Assistant Professor of Nursing,
Nurse Practitioner Program,
University of Virginia School of Nursing,
Charlottesville, Virginia

Mary Ann Picone, RN, MSN
Instructor,
BSN Program,
Mississippi University for Women,
Columbus, Mississippi

Sophia Chu Rodgers, RN, MSN, FNP
Family Nurse Practitioner,
Lovelace Health Systems,
Albuquerque, New Mexico

Coralease C. Ruff, DNSc, RN, CFNP
Associate Professor and Assistant Dean,
College of Nursing,
Howard University,
Washington, D.C.

Suzanne M. Schroeder, MSN, RN, CS, FNP, COHN-S
Family Nurse Practitioner,
Kimberly-Clark Corporation,
Neenah, Wisconsin

Amy B. Sharron, MS, RN, CS, GNP
Breast Care Specialist/Educator,
Centre Community Hospital,
Comprehensive Breast Care Center,
State College, Pennsylvania

Susan R. Tussey, MSN, CRNP, NP-C
Family Nurse Practitioner,
Family Health Associates,
Lewistown, Pennsylvania

Joan D. Wentz, MSN, RN
Assistant Professor,
Jewish Hospital College of Nusing and Allied Health,
St. Louis, Missouri

To Tom and Ryan,
the loves of my life.

Thanks, guys!

PREFACE

Primary care plays an important and major role in the delivery of health care. The primary care provider has been defined as the gatekeeper for the entire health care system. Being able to provide quality health care in a timely manner challenges the primary care provider on a daily basis.

Mosby's Primary Care Consultant is designed as a quick reference for the busy primary care practitioner. It is directed primarily to the nurse practitioner or clinical nurse specialist providing primary care. However, any primary care practitioner may find the text useful.

Part One of the text is an alphabetical listing of conditions that may be encountered in the primary care clinic. To facilitate retrieval of the information, each condition is presented in either a two- or four-page format. The ICD-9 codes for each disorder are included on the top right corner of the right hand page. Disorder names are included when they differ from the names that appear in this book. Each condition has six major sections that are addressed—Overview, Assessment, Interventions, Evaluation, For Your Information, and Pharmacotherapeutics. Keeping the format the same in each section makes it easy for the user to find the information needed quickly. Each division is highlighted with an icon to depict what the section is about.

The Overview section gives the reader a short definition of the condition and describes its pathogenesis. The patient profile gives the reader the most common characteristics of the patients affected by the condition. The most common signs and symptoms and differential diagnosis are also included in the Overview section.

The Assessment section looks at important information to obtain during history taking, physical findings that may be encountered, and ancillary testing that may be beneficial. In every condition it is important to determine whether the patient has any underlying conditions such as diabetes or hypertension. When obtaining the patient's current medications, it is important to question the patient about the use of oral contraceptives, since many patients do not consider oral contraceptives to be medications. Also inquire about the use of over-the-counter medications and home remedies. The practitioner should ask female patients when their last menstrual cycle was. Physical findings are those findings that may be encountered during the physical assessment. It is important for the practitioner to keep in mind that not all patients will demonstrate the same physical findings. Commonly ordered laboratory tests, x-rays, and other helpful diagnostic tests are also listed.

The Interventions section provides the practitioner with the information needed to treat the specific condition. This section includes information on any office treatment that may need to be performed, lifestyle modifications, patient education, and referrals that may be needed.

The section on Evaluation provides the practitioner with outcomes that can be expected with proper treatment and any possible complications that could arise. It also addresses when follow-up care should occur and who should perform the follow-up care or examinations.

The For Your Information section provides a brief look at how the condition affects various age groups across the lifespan. Generally speaking, pediatrics is considered birth to 18 years and geriatrics is considered greater than 65 years. The miscellaneous section provides an area for important information that does not fit in any of the other sections. The reference section lists the main references used for a particular condition. For a complete list of references consult the bibliography.

The final section for each condition is the Pharmacotherapeutic section. This section is presented in a table format divided into the following four columns: Drug of Choice, Mechanism of Action, Prescribing Information, and Side Effects. The most commonly used medication is always listed first. In the section on prescribing information, the approximate cost of the medication is given. This cost reflects the average wholesale price of the drug. This is the cost to the pharmacist or pharmacy and not the cost to the patient. These dollar amounts are presented only as a guide to the practitioner to assist in providing the most cost-effective treatment.

Part Two, Patient History, is designed to provide the practitioner with a review of this important process. Whether you are a seasoned veteran or a new graduate, reviewing the history-taking process can only serve to enhance your expertise. This chapter includes a section on cultural variations and also a section with examples of health history forms that may be used to facilitate this process. Also included is a list of mnemonic devices helpful when taking a patient history.

Part Three, Physical Assessment, is designed to provide the practitioner with a review of the physical assessment process. It is designed primarily to provide the new practitioner with the information needed to become proficient in this area. The last section of this chapter provides an alphabetical listing of some of the more commonly performed assessment tests, how to perform each test, and interpretation of the results.

Two appendices are provided that include a list of drugs metabolized by the P450 system and also a list of computer sources available.

ACKNOWLEDGMENTS

First, I would like to thank all of the people at Mosby who have helped in any way with the production, publication, and distribution of this book. A special thank you goes to Jeanne Allison, whose patience and gentle prodding helped me keep focused and whose encouragement kept me working.

Second, I want to thank Dr. Sharon Lewis who helped me believe in myself and pushed me to reach out and try things that I never thought I could do.

Last, but certainly not least, I want to thank my husband and my son, Tom and Ryan. Without Tom's expert typing skills and gentle encouragement, my deadlines would have never been met. Ryan kept everything organized for me by keeping my filing system up to date, but most importantly they provided me with the encouragement, support, and above all else the love that kept me working on this project.

Sheila A. Dunn

CONTENTS

PART ONE
Primary Care Disorders, 1

MOSBY'S Primary Care Consultant

PART ONE

Primary Care Disorders

Acne Keloidalis

OVERVIEW

Acne keloidalis is chronic scarring of the hair follicles. It normally occurs over the posterior part of the neck and results in keloid formation (a thick scar of excessive growth of fibrous tissue).

Pathogenesis

- Cause—unknown
- Development of papules or pustules from hair follicles on back of neck
- Occurs at edge of hairline
- Papules or pustules grow together into firm plaques or nodules
- Inflammatory process can last for months or even years

Patient Profile

- Males—almost exclusively
- Most common age >18 years
- Most common in African-Americans

Signs and Symptoms

- Usually asymptomatic
- Group of hard papules on back of neck

Differential Diagnosis

- Hypertrophic scar formation
- Dermatofibroma
- Infiltrating basal cell carcinoma

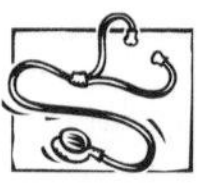

ASSESSMENT

History

Inquire about:

- Onset and duration of papules or pustules
- Treatments tried and results
- Underlying conditions
- Current medications

Physical Findings

- Hard, small, keloidal papules on back of neck at hairline
- May find soft pustules in same location
- Resembles acne vulgaris

Initial Workup

Laboratory: Usually none indicated (if pustules are present, a culture may be taken)
Radiology: None indicated

Further Workup

None indicated

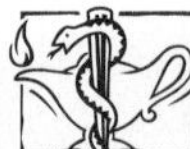

INTERVENTIONS

Office Treatment

None indicated

Lifestyle Modification

If possible, avoidance of protective headgear (hard hats)

Patient Education

Teach patient about:

- Condition and treatment
- Chronicity of condition
- Inflammatory process—may last months to years
- Use of intralesional steroid injections and antibiotics, and side effects (see Pharmacotherapeutics)

Referral

To dermatologist for intralesional injections

EVALUATION

Outcome

Control of inflammatory process with minimal keloid formation

Possible Complications

- Severe scarring
- Hair loss

Follow-up

Normally by dermatologist; if not, and if patient receiving long-term antibiotic therapy, follow-up every 2 weeks

FOR YOUR INFORMATION

Life Span

Pediatric: Not seen in this age group
Geriatric: Not seen in this age group
Pregnancy: N/A

Miscellaneous

Even though a bacterial etiology has never been proved in acne keloidalis, the condition usually responds to short- or long-term antibiotic use. It is necessary to have the infection under control before intralesional triamcinolone is used.

Reference

Habif TP: *Clinical dermatology: a color guide to diagnosis and therapy,* ed 3, St Louis, 1996, Mosby, p 251.

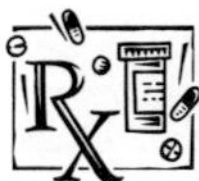

PHARMACOTHERAPEUTICS

All antibiotics should be tried for at least 3 weeks. If the patient is responsive, a trial without antibiotic is recommended. If the condition recurs, long-term antibiotic therapy may be necessary. Control may diminish over time, requiring a trial of another class of antibiotic.

Drug of Choice	Mechanism of Action	Prescribing Information	Side Effects
Erythromycin (E.E.S.), 500 mg PO bid or 250 mg PO qid	Macrolide; protein synthesis inhibitor; active against bacteria lacking cell walls, most gram-positive aerobes	*Contraindication:* Hypersensitivity *Cost:* 250-mg tab, 4/day × 10 days: $4 *Pregnancy category:* B	Nausea, vomiting, diarrhea, abdominal pain, anorexia, rash, urticaria, pseudomembranous colitis—rarely
Cephalexin (Keflex), 500 mg PO bid to qid	Cephalosporin; bactericidal cell wall inhibitor	*Contraindication:* Hypersensitivity *Cost:* 500-mg tab, 20 tabs: $5-$22 *Pregnancy category:* B	Headache, dizziness, weakness, nausea, vomiting, diarrhea, anorexia, pseudomembranous colitis, proteinuria, nephrotoxicity, leukopenia, thrombocytopenia, neutropenia, rash, urticaria, anaphylaxis
Trimethoprim sulfamethoxazole (Bactrim DS, Septra DS), 1 tab PO bid	Sulfamethoxazole (SMZ) interferes with biosynthesis of proteins; trimethoprim (TMP) blocks synthesis of tetrahydrofolic acid	*Contraindications:* Hypersensitivity; pregnancy at term; megaloblastic anemia; infants <2 months; creatinine clearance <15 ml/min; lactation *Cost:* 1-DS tab, 20 tabs: $3-$4 *Pregnancy category:* C	Headache, insomnia, hallucinations, depression, vertigo, allergic myocarditis, nausea, vomiting, abdominal pain, stomatitis, hepatitis, enterocolitis, renal failure, toxic nephrosis, leukopenia, neutropenia, thrombocytopenia, agranulocytosis, hemolytic anemia, Stevens-Johnson syndrome, erythema, photosensitivity, anaphylaxis
Dicloxacillin (Dynapen), 250 mg PO qid	Penicillin; bactericidal cell wall inhibitor; penicillinase resistant	*Contraindication:* Hypersensitivity *Cost:* 250-mg tab, 40 tabs: $20 *Pregnancy category:* B	Anemia, bone marrow depression, granulocytopenia, nausea, vomiting, diarrhea, pseudomembranous colitis, oliguria, proteinuria, hematuria, vaginitis, lethargy, hallucinations, anxiety, depression, coma, convulsions, anaphylaxis
Amoxicillin and clavulanate (Augmentin), 500 mg PO bid	Aminopenicillin/betalactamase inhibitor; bactericidal cell wall inhibitor; effective against gram-negative and gram-positive and beta-lactamase–producing organisms	*Contraindication:* Hypersensitivity to penicillin *Cost:* 500-mg tab, 20 tabs: $81 *Pregnancy category:* B	Anemia, bone marrow depression, granulocytopenia, nausea, vomiting, diarrhea, pseudomembranous colitis, oliguria, proteinuria, hematuria, vaginitis, lethargy, hallucinations, anxiety, depression, coma, convulsions, anaphylaxis

Acne Rosacea

OVERVIEW

Acne rosacea is a chronic inflammatory process of the face. There is flushing and dilation of the tiny blood vessels of the face.

Pathogenesis

- Cause—unknown; possibly impairment of venous flow, resulting in vasodilation, or increased hair follicle mites may cause inflammatory reaction
- Chronic disease with exacerbations and remissions
- 58% of patients develop ocular rosacea
- 20% of patients present with ocular rosacea before eruption of skin lesions
- Alcohol and hot drinks may accentuate flushing
- Sun exposure can precipitate acute episodes

Patient Profile

- Females > Males
- Most common age >30 years; rare over 60 years
- Most common in people of Celtic origin

Signs and Symptoms

- Erythema, edema, papules, pustules, and telangiectasia on face, nose, and cheeks
- May have one or all of the above signs and symptoms
- Irreversible hypertrophy of nose (rhinophyma)

Differential Diagnosis

- Acne vulgaris
- Cutaneous lupus erythematosus
- Drug eruptions
- Granulomas of skin
- Seborrheic dermatitis
- Carcinoid syndrome

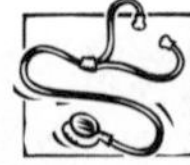

ASSESSMENT

History

Inquire about:

- Onset and duration of symptoms
- Factors that make condition better or worse
- Treatments tried and results
- Family history of acne rosacea
- Underlying conditions
- Current medications

Physical Findings

- Physical findings limited to face, primarily cheeks, nose, forehead, eyes
- Erythema, edema, papules, pustules
- Comedones rare; may have combination of acne rosacea and acne vulgaris
- Telangiectasia may be present
- May have granuloma formation
- Rhinophyma (hypertrophy of nose)

Initial Workup

Laboratory: Usually none indicated
Radiology: None indicated

Further Workup

If no response to conventional treatment and facial pustules are localized to one cheek, may want to do a potassium hydroxide preparation to look for mites or tinea

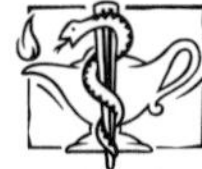

INTERVENTIONS

Office Treatment

None needed

Lifestyle Modification

Avoidance of products that increase facial flushing, such as hot drinks, alcohol, spicy foods

Patient Education

Teach patient about:

- Condition and treatment—treatment may consist of oral antibiotics, topical therapy, or isotretinoin
- Chronicity of disease
- Using sunscreen
- Avoiding oil-based cosmetics
- Medications used and side effects (see Pharmacotherapeutics)

Referral

To dermatologist or plastic surgeon for rhinophyma or telangiectatic vessels, or for treatment failure (isotretinoin should be used by someone experienced in its use)

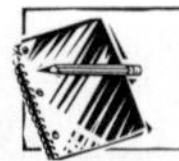

EVALUATION

Outcome

Response unpredictable; may have complete resolution of lesions in 2 to 4 weeks and remain free of symptoms for an extended period of time, or may require long-term antibiotic therapy; may never have complete resolution of lesions

Possible Complications

- Rhinophyma
- Conjunctivitis
- Blepharitis
- Keratitis

Follow-up

- Oral antibiotic or topical treatment—every 2 weeks × 2, then monthly
- Isotretinoin—every 2 weeks for duration of therapy

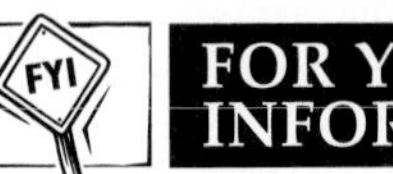

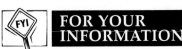

FOR YOUR INFORMATION

Life Span

Pediatric: Rare type found in children
Geriatric: Rare after 60 years
Pregnancy: Must be avoided if taking isotretinoin

Miscellaneous

Wilkin and DeWitt (1993) found that treatment with topical clindamycin was just as effective as treatment with oral tetracycline. In their study clindamycin applied twice daily in a lotion base was actually superior to oral tetracycline in the eradication of pustules. The authors concluded that topical clindamycin was a very safe and effective alternative to oral tetracycline.

References

Habif TP: *Clinical dermatology: a color guide to diagnosis and therapy,* ed 3, St Louis, 1996, Mosby, p 182.

Wilkin JK, DeWitt S: Treatment of rosacea: topical clindamycin versus oral tetracycline, *Int J Dermatol* 32(1):65-67, 1993.

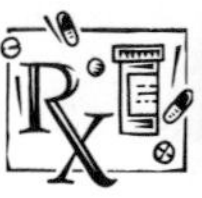

PHARMACOTHERAPEUTICS

Drug of Choice	Mechanism of Action	Prescribing Information	Side Effects
Topical metronidazole (Metrogel 0.75%), 45 g; apply to face bid after washing with gentle soap; use initially for mild cases or for maintenance after stopping oral antibiotic	Mechanism of action in rosacea is unknown, but may include antibacterial and/or antiinflammatory	***Contraindication:*** Hypersensitivity to metronidazole or paraben ***Cost:*** 45-g tube, 1 tube: $35 ***Pregnancy category:*** B	Avoid contact with eyes—causes tearing; local irritation can occur; use cautiously in patients with history of blood dyscrasias
Tetracycline, 500 mg PO bid or 250 mg PO qid until pustules clear; do *not* give with milk or milk products	Inhibits protein synthesis; bacteriostatic	***Contraindications:*** Hypersensitivity; children <8 years ***Cost:*** 500-mg tab, 100 tabs: $6-$20 ***Pregnancy category:*** D	Eosinophilia, neutropenia, thrombocytoenia, leukocytosis, hemolytic anemia, dysphagia, glossitis, oral candidiasis, anorexia, hepatotoxicity, rash, urticaria, photosensitivity, exfoliative dermatitis, angioedema
Erythromycin (E.E.S.), 500 mg PO bid until pustules clear	Macrolide; protein synthesis inhibitor; active against bacteria lacking cell walls, most gram-positive aerobes	***Contraindication:*** Hypersensitivity ***Cost:*** 250-mg tab, 40 tabs: $4 ***Pregnancy category:*** B	Nausea, vomiting, diarrhea, abdominal pain, anorexia, rash, urticaria, pseudomembranous colitis—rarely
Clindamycin lotion (Cleocin T 1%); apply thin film to face bid; has been shown to be as effective as oral tetracycline and is superior in eradication of pustules	Has been shown to have activity against *Propionibacterium acnes*	***Contraindications:*** Hypersensitivity; history of regional enteritis or colitis; history of antibiotic-associated colitis ***Cost:*** Topical gel—30-g tube: $20 ***Pregnancy category:*** B	Severe diarrhea, bloody diarrhea, pseudomembranous colitis, dryness, burning, erythema, abdominal pain, gram-negative folliculitis, stinging of eyes
Isotretinoin (Accutane), 0.5 mg/kg/day; use for severe refractory cases; use only as last resort in females of childbearing age; if used, 2 methods of birth control should be used and pregnancy test done at each visit; start medication 2nd or 3rd day of menses; monitor liver enzymes and lipids every 2 weeks; should only be used by someone experienced with drug; get consent form signed	Exact mechanism of action is unknown	***Contraindications:*** Hypersensitivity; pregnancy ***Cost:*** 10-mg tab, 100 tabs: $333 ***Pregnancy category:*** X	Dry skin, pruritus, cheilosis, joint pain, hair loss, photosensitivity, urticaria, bruising, hirsutism, petechiae, hyperostosis, arthralgia, chest pain, palpitations, tachycardia, nausea, vomiting, anorexia, increased liver enzymes, abdominal pain, eye irritation, conjunctivitis, epistaxis, hematuria, proteinuria, thrombocytopenia, lethargy, fatigue, Pseudotumor cerebri

Acne Vulgaris

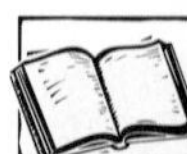

OVERVIEW

Acne vulgaris is an inflammatory disorder of the pilosebaceous glands of the face, chest, back, and upper outer arms. It consists of open and closed comedones, papules, pustules, and nodules. The disease may be mild, with only a few open and closed comedones, or it may be severe, with scarring nodules present.

Pathogenesis

- Sebum, the pathologic agent, is irritating and comedogenic
- Increased sebum production = comedo development
- Sebaceous glands are small during childhood; during puberty, testosterone is converted to dihydrotestosterone in the skin and acts directly on sebaceous glands, increasing their size
- *Propionibacterium acnes,* normal skin flora, proliferates in presence of sebum and produces substances that cause inflammation
- Substances attract neutrophils, which weaken follicle wall
- Wall thins until it ruptures, causing inflammatory reaction that results in acne pustules or cysts

Patient Profile

- Males = Females, but males tend to have more severe forms
- Most common age—puberty into 20s and 30s

Signs and Symptoms

- Closed comedones (whiteheads)
- Open comedones (blackheads)
- Papules, pustules, nodules, cysts
- Scarring from previous lesions
- Lesions may be present on face, chest, back, and upper arms

Differential Diagnosis

- Acne rosacea
- Molluscum contagiosum
- Steroid acne
- Folliculitis
- Occupational exposure to tars, oils, grease

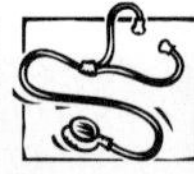

ASSESSMENT

History

Inquire about:

- Onset and duration of symptoms
- Type of lesions and where they are located
- Aggravating and alleviating factors
- Family history of acne
- Treatments tried and results
- Occupation
- Current medications, including use of anabolic steroids
- Underlying conditions

Physical Findings

- Examine skin for oiliness and scarring
- Determine types of lesions (papules, pustules, cysts) and severity of acne
- Use chart to record location and type of lesions present
- Examine face, chest, back, and upper arms
- Check for secondary infection

Initial Workup

Laboratory: Usually none indicated
Radiology: Usually none indicated

Further Workup

Usually none indicated

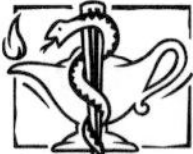

INTERVENTIONS

Office Treatment

Comedone removal

Lifestyle Modifications

- Well-balanced diet
- Avoidance of use of oil-based cosmetics, hair-styling mousse, and face creams
- Change in occupation, if possible, if work environment is aggravating factor

Patient Education

Teach patient about:

- Condition and treatment
- Length of time before results will be seen (could be 2 to 3 months)
- Using mild soaps for cleansing skin
- Not picking at lesions
- Keeping hair off skin
- Well-balanced diet
- Coping with this illness
- Medications used and side effects (see Pharmacotherapeutics)

Referral

To dermatologist for severe, cystic acne or for any acne resistant to treatment

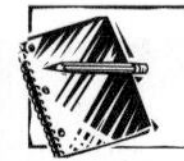

EVALUATION

Outcome

Lesions clear with no scarring or with as little scarring as possible

Possible Complications

- Acne conglobata
- Facial scarring
- Psychologic scarring

Follow-up

Every 3 weeks until there are signs of improvement; then every 3 months

FOR YOUR INFORMATION

Life Span

Pediatric: Mild acne can occur in neonates; usually resolves spontaneously
Geriatric: Not normally seen in this age group
Pregnancy: Best to use topical agents; isotretinoin should not be used

Miscellaneous

Males tend to have more severe cases of acne than females. This is thought to be because males produce about 10 times more androgen than do females. Studies have found that females with acne tend to have higher androgen levels than normal. It has also been found that females taking low-dose birth control pills have less acne.

References

Habif TP: *Clinical dermatology: a color guide to diagnosis and therapy,* ed 3, St Louis, 1996, Mosby, pp 148-161.

Uphold CR, Graham MV: *Clinical guidelines in adult health,* Gainesville, Fla, 1994, Barmarrae Books, pp 141-144.

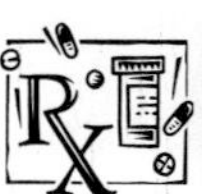

PHARMACOTHERAPEUTICS

Drug of Choice	Mechanism of Action	Prescribing Information	Side Effects
For mild acne, use topical agents.			
Benzoyl peroxide (many product names); start with 5% bid and increase strength as needed; apply after washing face with mild soap and water	Antibacterial agent effective against *Propionibacterium acnes*	***Contraindication:*** Hypersensitivity ***Cost:*** Gel, 45-g tube, 1 tube: $8 ***Pregnancy category:*** C	Irritation, contact dermatitis
Retinoic acid cream, gel (Retin-A), 0.025%, 0.05%, and 0.1%; start with low dose and use nightly; if patient unable to tolerate nightly applications, try using every other night; use in combination with benzoyl peroxide, using each once daily; very effective	Exact mechanism of action is unknown; decreases cohesiveness of follicular epithelial cells and decreases microcomedo formation; also stimulates mitotic activity	***Contraindication:*** Hypersensitivity ***Cost:*** 0.05%, 20-g tube, 1 tube: $27 ***Pregnancy category:*** C	Extreme redness of skin, edema, blistering, crusting, increased susceptibility to sunlight, hyperpigmentation or hypopigmentation
For moderate acne, use topical treatment as above and/or treatment below.			
Tetracycline, 500 mg bid for 3-6 weeks	Inhibits protein synthesis; bacteriostatic	***Contraindications:*** Hypersensitivity; children <8 years ***Cost:*** 500-mg tab, 100 tabs: $6-$20 ***Pregnancy category:*** D	Eosinophilia, neutropenia, thrombocytopenia, leukocytosis, hemolytic anemia, dysphagia, glossitis, oral candidiasis, anorexia, hepatotoxicity, rash, urticaria, photosensitivity, exfoliative dermatitis, angioedema
Erythromycin (E.E.S.), 500 mg bid for 3-6 weeks	Macrolide; protein synthesis inhibitor; active against bacteria lacking cell walls, most gram-positive aerobes	***Contraindication:*** Hypersensitivity ***Cost:*** 250-mg tab, 4 tabs/day × 10 days: $4 ***Pregnancy category:*** B	Nausea, vomiting, diarrhea, abdominal pain, anorexia, rash, urticaria, pseudomembranous colitis—rarely
Once improvement is seen, consider switching to one of the following topical antibiotics:			
Erythromycin 2% solution or gel (A/T/S); apply to clean skin bid	Macrolide; protein synthesis inhibitor; active against bacteria lacking cell walls, most gram-positive aerobes	***Contraindication:*** Hypersensitivity ***Cost:*** 2% gel, 30 g tube, 1 tube: $13-$18 ***Pregnancy category:*** B	Nausea, vomiting, diarrhea, abdominal pain, anorexia, rash, urticaria, pseudomembranous colitis—rarely
Clindamycin 1% solution, gel, or lotion (Cleocin T); apply a thin film bid	Has been shown to have activity against *Propionibacterium acnes*	***Contraindications:*** Hypersensitivity; history of regional enteritis or ulcerative colitis; history of antibiotic-associated colitis ***Cost:*** Topical gel, 30-g tube, 1 tube: $20 ***Pregnancy category:*** B	Severe diarrhea, bloody diarrhea, pseudomembranous colitis, dryness, burning, erythema, abdominal pain, gram-negative folliculitis, stinging of eyes
For severe acne:			
Isotretinoin (Accutane), 0.5-1 mg/kg/day in 2 divided doses; use for severe refractory cases; use only as last resort in females of child-bearing age; if used, 2 methods of birth control should be used, pregnancy test done at each visit; start medication 2nd or 3rd day of menses; monitor liver enzymes and lipids every 2 weeks; should only be used by someone experienced with drug; get consent form signed	Exact mechanism of action is unknown	***Contraindications:*** Hypersensitivity; pregnancy ***Cost:*** 10-mg tab, 100 tabs: $333 ***Pregnancy category:*** X	Dry skin, pruritus, cheilosis, joint pain, hair loss, photosensitivity, urticaria, bruising, hirsutism, petechiae, hyperostosis, arthralgia, chest pain, palpitations, tachycardia, nausea, vomiting, anorexia, increased liver enzymes, abdominal pain, eye irritation, conjunctivitis, epistaxis, hematuria, proteinuria, thrombocytopenia, lethargy, fatigue; pseudotumor cerebri

Addison's Disease

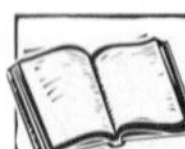

OVERVIEW

Addison's disease is defined as hypofunction of the adrenal glands, resulting in the reduction of mineralocorticoids, glucocorticoids, and androgens. Addisonian crisis, an acute, life-threatening complication of adrenal insufficiency, requires immediate emergency care.

Pathogenesis
- Cause: primary disease—autoimmunity, destruction of adrenal glands by antibodies
- Other causes—tuberculosis, hemorrhage, infarction, AIDS, metastatic cancer
- Iatrogenic causes—anticoagulant therapy, chemotherapy, bilateral adrenalectomy, ketoconazole treatment in AIDS

Patient Profile
- Females > Males
- Affects all ages
- Autoimmune disease—some hereditary predisposition

Signs and Symptoms
- Weakness
- Fatigue
- Weight loss
- Abdominal pain
- Muscle/joint aches
- Orthostatic hypotension
- Hyponatremia
- Hypoglycemia
- Hyperkalemia
- Hyperpigmentation of skin
- Anorexia
- Vomiting
- Diarrhea
- Decreased cold tolerance
- Dizziness
- Addisonian crisis—circulatory collapse, dehydration, nausea, vomiting, hypoglycemia

Differential Diagnosis
- Syndrome of inappropriate antidiuretic hormone
- Salt-losing nephritis
- Heavy metal ingestion
- Anorexia nervosa
- Sprue syndrome
- Hyper-parathyroidism

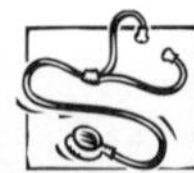

ASSESSMENT

History
Inquire about:
- Onset and duration of symptoms
- Family history of autoimmune disease
- Underlying conditions
- Current medications

Physical Findings
- Hyperpigmentation of skin—may be most striking objective finding
- Hypotension and orthostatic hypotension
- Weight loss

Initial Workup
Laboratory
- Chemistry panel—decreased sodium, increased potassium, increased BUN, decreased glucose
- Plasma cortisol level—decreased or fails to rise after administration of cortisol
- ACTH level—elevated
- CBC—may have moderate neutropenia

Radiology
- Chest film—may show adrenal calcification, decreased heart size
- CT scan of abdomen—adrenal glands may be abnormal in size or show calcification

Further Workup
Workup to determine cause (see Pathogenesis)

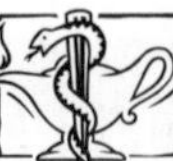

INTERVENTIONS

Office Treatment
None indicated

Lifestyle Modifications
- Stress reduction techniques and avoidance of infection
- Smoking cessation

Patient Education
Teach patient about:
- Condition and treatment
- Chronicity of disease
- Need for lifelong replacement therapy
- Signs and symptoms of infection and need for immediate medical intervention
- Stress reduction techniques—biofeedback, guided imagery, relaxation therapy
- Signs and symptoms of overdosage or underdosage of medications
- Times of increased stress requiring increased medication
- Obtaining a medical alert bracelet
- Administering IM injections (will need to teach family or significant other)
- Having 100 mg of IM hydrocortisone or 4 mg of dexamethasone phosphate available at all times
- Signs and symptoms of impending addisonian crisis
- Medications used and side effects (see Pharmacotherapeutics)

Referral
To endocrinologist

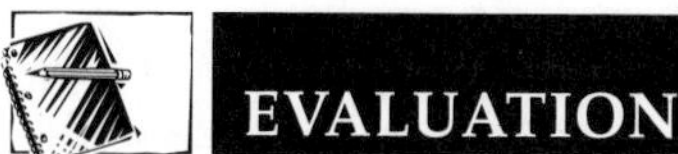

EVALUATION

Outcomes
- Control of disease with replacement therapy
- Prevention of complications, addisonian crisis
- Patient will adjust emotionally to chronicity of disease

Possible Complications
- Hyperpyrexia
- Psychotic reactions
- Addisonian crises

Follow-up
- Weekly, initially, to assess adequacy of therapy and patient's emotional status and coping ability, and to monitor BP, serum electrolytes, blood glucose level; then every 2 weeks; then monthly
- Patient will need lifelong monitoring
- Initially followed by endocrinologist; after stabilization, will probably be referred back to NP

FOR YOUR INFORMATION

Life Span
Pediatric: Lower medication dosage required

Geriatric: More likely to have addisonian crises

Pregnancy: Requires a specialist to manage

Miscellaneous
A good teaching plan is an important part of caring for a patient with Addison's disease. A well-educated and compliant patient can lead a very normal life with this disease. If the patient chooses not to follow the treatment plan, life will be a series of hospitalizations and life-threatening crises.

References

Gregerman RI: Selected endocrine problems: disorders of pituitary, adrenal, and parathyroid glands; pharmacological use of steroids; hypo and hypercalcemia; osteoporosis; water metabolism; hypoglycemia. In Barker LR, Burton JR, Zieve PD, editors: *Principles of ambulatory medicine,* ed 4, Baltimore, 1995, Williams & Wilkins, pp 1051-1053.

Haas LB: Endocrine problems. In Lewis SM, Collier IC, Heitkemper MM, editors: *Medical-surgical nursing: assessment and management of clinical problems,* ed 4, St Louis, 1996, Mosby, pp 1509-1510.

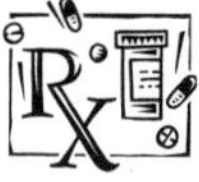

PHARMACOTHERAPEUTICS

Drug of Choice	Mechanism of Action	Prescribing Information	Side Effects
Hydrocortisone, 10 mg PO every morning and 5 mg PO every evening as starting dose; may need to adjust according to patient's symptoms; will need higher doses in times of increased stress; used with fludrocortisone; should have 100 mg of IM hydrocortisone available at all times	Replacement of glucocorticoids lost as a result of hypofunction of adrenal glands	*Contraindications:* Hypersensitivity; systemic fungal infections *Cost:* 10-mg tab, 100 tabs: $20; 100-mg vial, 1 vial: $2-$4 *Pregnancy category:* C	Sodium retention, fluid retention, congestive heart failure (CHF), hypokalemia, muscle weakness, osteoporosis, peptic ulcer, pancreatitis, abdominal distention, impaired wound healing, fragile skin, petechiae, ecchymosis, convulsions,vertigo, headache, cushingoid state; menstrual irregularities, diabetes mellitus, increased intraocular pressure, glaucoma
Fludrocortisone, 0.1-0.2 mg PO qd; used with hydrocortisone	Replaces mineralocorticoids	*Contraindications:* Hypersensitivity; systemic fungal infections *Cost:* 0.1-mg tab, 100 tabs: $45 *Pregnancy category:* C	Sodium retention, fluid retention, CHF, hypokalemia, muscle weakness, osteoporosis, peptic ulcer, pancreatitis, abdominal distention, impaired wound healing, fragile skin, petechiae, ecchymosis, convulsions, vertigo, headache, cushingoid state, menstrual irregularities, diabetes mellitus, increased intraocular pressure, glaucoma
Dexamethasone, 4 mg IM should be available at all times if IM hydrocortisone is not	Replaces glucocorticoids	*Contraindications:* Hypersensitivity; systemic fungal infections *Cost:* 8 mg/ml, 1 ml: $12 *Pregnancy category:* C	Sodium retention, fluid retention, CHF, hypokalemia, muscle weakness, osteoporosis, peptic ulcer, pancreatitis, abdominal distention, impaired wound healing, fragile skin, petechiae, ecchymosis, convulsions, vertigo, headache, cushingoid state, menstrual irregularities, diabetes mellitus, increased intraocular pressure, glaucoma

Adult Abuse

OVERVIEW

Adult abuse is a physical or verbal attack by an individual with close ties to the victim. With elderly victims the abuser is usually a relative who is a caregiver of the victim. With other adult victims the abuser is usually the spouse or a significant other with whom the victim has a close relationship.

Pathogenesis

- Usually results from ineffective coping skills and stress
- Frequently the abuser was either a witness to abuse or a victim of abuse
- Frequently the abuser uses recreational drugs, and attacks occur when the abuser has been using

Patient Profile

- Victim usually female
- Abuser usually male
- In elder abuse, victim usually female and abuser male or female
- Any age

Signs and Symptoms

- Anxiety
- Depression
- Poor self-esteem
- Malnutrition
- Skin dirty and smelly
- Withdrawal
- Skin markings—lacerations, bruises, burns, bites; fractures of facial bones, ribs; eye trauma, loss of teeth, ear trauma
- Frequent emergency room visits or office visits
- Overprotectiveness by abuser—insists on being in examination room; answers questions; victim looks to abuser for answers to questions
- Injuries to genitalia

Differential Diagnosis

Injuries due to other causes, such as bleeding disorders, metabolic diseases, gastrointestinal diseases, dementia, other mental illnesses

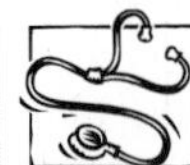

ASSESSMENT

History

- Inquire about:
    - When injury occurred
    - How it happened
    - Why it happened
    - Whether it could have been prevented
- May be difficult to get patient to admit being abused—need to put puzzle together
- May need to ask patient directly, "Who did this to you?"
- Patient may still not respond appropriately for fear of retaliation or loss of caregiver

Physical Findings

Depends on type of abuse:

- Verbal abuse—may be none or may demonstrate posturing indicative of depression, anxiety, poor self-esteem, timidity
- Physical abuse—bruising, lacerations, burns, bites, fractures; may be anywhere, but most common sites are head and face, chest, and genitalia

Initial Workup

Laboratory

- CBC
- Chemistry panel—to rule out pathophysiologic causes of problems
- Pregnancy test if patient was sexually assaulted

Radiology

- Films of suspected fractures
- If internal injuries suspected, may need CT scan or MRI of abdomen

Further Workup

Depends on results of initial workup

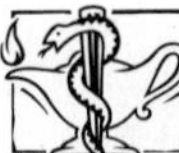

INTERVENTIONS

Office Treatment

- Suture minor lacerations
- Stabilize possible fracture sites
- Give Td booster
- May need to notify authorities and get patient into emergency shelter

Lifestyle Modifications

- Victim must be willing to make lifestyle modifications—if abuser is also victim's sole support and provides a home for victim, it may be difficult to get victim out of the situation
- Victim must be encouraged to remove himself or herself from the situation
- For the younger victim, this may mean learning a skill to find employment and caring for children alone
- For the elder victim, this may mean a retirement community or nursing home, which the victim may not be willing to accept

Patient Education

Teach patient about:

- Cycle of abuse
- Assistance available within the community
- Phone numbers for local authorities and crisis shelters
- Making a plan for escaping from the abusive environment
- Adult protective services (for elderly patient)
- Stress reduction techniques

Referrals

- To social worker
- To psychiatric NP
- To crises shelter and any other agencies available within community

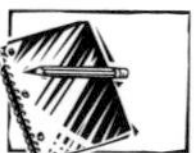

EVALUATION

Outcome

Patient will no longer be a victim of abuse

Follow-up

Every 2 weeks until situation has stabilized or patient is being followed by another professional trained in this area

FOR YOUR INFORMATION

Life Span

Pediatric: Important to question victim about presence of children in the home and to ascertain if children are in danger
Geriatric: May be difficult to get victim to admit abuse is occurring if victim fears being placed in a nursing home
Pregnancy: Often abuse begins in pregnancy; many abused women do not seek prenatal care until third trimester, which correlates with low birth-weight infants

Miscellaneous

The NP in primary care is often the first line of defense for the victim of domestic abuse. This is a widespread problem, and it is very important for the NP to carefully assess anyone who might be a victim. Prompt referral to the right agency may save someone's life.

References

Finucane TE, Burton JR: Geriatric medicine: special considerations. In Barker LR, Burton JR, Zieve PD, editors: *Principles of ambulatory medicine,* ed 4, Baltimore, 1995, Williams & Wilkins, p 77.

Harris N, Seimer B: Psychosocial health concerns. In Youngkin EQ, Davis MS, editors: *Women's health: a primary care clinical guide,* Norwalk, Conn, 1994, Appleton & Lange, pp 659-662.

McFarlane J, Parker B, Soeken K: Abuse during pregnancy: associations with maternal health and infant birth weight, *Nurs Res* 45 (1):37-42, 1996.

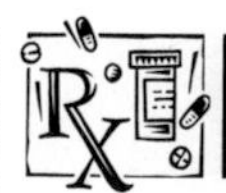

PHARMACOTHERAPEUTICS

There are no specific medications used for the treatment of abuse. Each case must be treated on an individual basis, with medications prescribed on the basis of the type of injury or medical problem that presents itself.

Alcoholism

OVERVIEW

Alcoholism is a chronic disease. The individual is physically and psychologically dependent on alcohol. The individual has impaired control over drinking, is preoccupied with alcohol, and has impaired thinking because of denial of the problem. Alcoholism can be a progressive and fatal disease.

Pathogenesis

- Multifactorial causes—physiologic, psychologic, and sociocultural factors involved
- There appears to be a predisposition to alcoholism that is inherited
- Many also have a preexisting mental condition

Patient Profile

- Males > Females (slightly)
- All ages; most predominant age group—18 to 29 years
- Risk factors—alcohol use; use of psychoactive drugs; family history of alcoholism; young, single male; consumption of 5 or more drinks at one sitting; getting drunk at least once per week; peer group pressure; family or sociocultural background promoting intoxication; easy accessibility to alcohol

Signs and Symptoms

Involves psychologic and physical symptoms

- Psychologic symptoms—social dysfunction, marital discord, anxiety, depression, insomnia, social isolation and frequent moves, either verbal or physical abuse, alcohol-related arrests or legal problems, financial difficulties, preoccupation with drinking, employment problems, repeated attempts to stop or reduce drinking, blackouts, complaints by family or friends about patient's drinking
- Physical symptoms—affects every body system
  - Dermatologic system—lacerations, abrasions, burns, spider angiomas, bruises, poor hygiene
  - Head, eyes, ears, nose, and throat (HEENT)—red-faced, parotid hypertrophy, poor oral hygiene, head and neck malignancies
  - Cardiovascular system—mild hypertension, arrhythmias or palpitations, cardiomyopathy
  - Respiratory system—aspiration pneumonia, bronchitis
  - Gastrointestinal system—anorexia, nausea, vomiting, abdominal pain, chronic liver disease, peptic ulcer disease, pancreatitis, gastric malignancies
  - Genitourinary system—impotence, menstrual irregularities, testicular atrophy
  - Endocrine system—hypercholesterolemia, hypertriglyceridemia, cushingoid appearance, gynecomastia
  - Musculoskeletal system—old fractures
  - Neurologic system—cognitive deficits, peripheral neuropathy, Wernicke-Korsakoff syndrome

Differential Diagnosis

Any of a variety of psychologic and physical disorders, including:

- Depression
- Anxiety
- Bipolar disease
- Manic-depression
- Essential hypertension
- Peptic ulcer disease
- Viral gastroenteritis
- Cholelithiasis
- Viral hepatitis
- Diabetes
- Pancreatitis
- Hyperlipidemia
- Sunburn
- Breast tumor
- Primary endocrine disorder
- Primary seizure disorder

ASSESSMENT

History

Inquire about:

- Onset and duration of symptoms
- Amount of alcohol consumed per day
- Age at first drink
- Family history of alcohol abuse, other substance abuse—nicotine, recreational drugs
- Underlying conditions
- Current medications, including OTC medications

Physical Findings

May be none in early stages; later may find:

- Red face
- Spider angiomas
- Numerous bruises
- Burns, scrapes
- Elevated BP
- Cardiac arrhythmia
- Adventitious breath sounds
- Abdominal pain
- Enlarged, tender liver
- Gynecomastia
- Testicular atrophy
- Perform CAGE questionnaire—positive response to one question is suspicious for alcoholism (see Assessment Tests in Part Three for the CAGE questionnaire).

Initial Workup

Laboratory

- Blood alcohol concentration is most diagnostic—>100 mg/dl (22 mmol/L) during an office visit; >150 mg/dl (33 mmol/L) without obvious signs of intoxication; >300 mg/dl (65 mmol/L) at any time
- Blood chemistry panel—the following are suggestive if increased: GGT, ALT, AST, alkaline phosphatase, LDH, bilirubin (total), amylase, uric acid, triglycerides, cholesterol, mean corpuscular volume, prothrombin time; the following are suggestive if decreased: calcium, phosphorus, magnesium, BUN, WBC count, platelet count, hematocrit, protein, coagulopathy

Radiology: As needed

Further Workup

May need liver biopsy, upper GI series

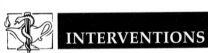

INTERVENTIONS

Office Treatment

None indicated

Lifestyle Modifications

- Well-balanced diet
- Cessation of alcohol intake
- Smoking cessation
- Major lifestyle modifications need to take place—may need a change in environment

Patient Education

Teach patient about:

- Disease and treatment
- Coping mechanisms
- Treatment programs available—inpatient and outpatient
- Indications for inpatient treatment—include symptoms of major withdrawal, failure to complete an outpatient program, associated medical problems, significant psychiatric symptoms, suicidal ideations, inadequate social support network
- Types of outpatient programs and support groups available—Alcoholics Anonymous is one of the most successful at dealing with alcoholism; usually has a phone number in local phone directory
- Needing to make a lifelong commitment to sobriety

- Importance of including family and friends in patient's attempt at sobriety
- Support groups available for family members—Al-Anon, Al-Ateen
- Well-balanced, nutritionally sound diet with vitamin supplement, particularly thiamine
- Medications used and side effects (see Pharmacotherapeutics)

Referral

To inpatient program or to psychiatric NP who deals with addictions

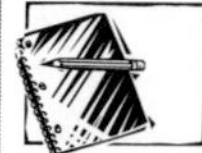

EVALUATION

Outcome

Abstinence from alcohol

Possible Complications

- Delirium tremens on initial withdrawal
- Relapse of drinking
- Wernicke-Korsakoff syndrome
- Alcoholic neuropathy
- Alcoholic dementia
- Increased susceptibility to infection
- Aseptic necrosis of hip
- Malignancies
- Cirrhosis
- Esophageal varices
- Cardiomyopathy

Follow-up

Initially, daily visits may be necessary; as patient stabilizes, weekly; then monthly

FOR YOUR INFORMATION

Life Span

Pediatric: Alcoholism is on the rise in children from grade school through high school
Geriatric: May be more difficult to diagnose, since effects of alcohol on the brain may be diagnosed as depression, anxiety, or dementia
Pregnancy: Alcohol usage is directly related to low-birth-weight infants and fetal alcohol syndrome

Miscellaneous

The Expected Treatment Outcome Scale is a new instrument to assess the severity of the disease and to evaluate the effectiveness of the treatment. It is currently undergoing vigorous testing to assess its reliability and validity. Perhaps in the near future, it will be a valuable instrument for those involved in the treatment of alcoholism.

References

Alemi F et al: A review of factors affecting treatment outcomes: expected treatment outcome scale, *Am J Drug Alcohol Abuse* 21 (4):483-509, 1995.

Fingerhood MI, Barker LR: Alcoholism and associated problems. In Barker LR, Burton JR, Zieve PD, editors: *Principles of ambulatory medicine,* ed 4, Baltimore, 1995, Williams & Wilkins, pp 222-242.

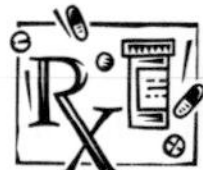

PHARMACOTHERAPEUTICS

There is no one drug used to promote sobriety. All the NP can do is treat the symptoms of withdrawal and assist the patient in abstinence.

Drug of Choice	Mechanism of Action	Prescribing Information	Side Effects
Disulfiram (Antabuse); never administer to a patient with alcohol in his or her system; initially, 500 mg PO daily for 1-2 weeks, then 250 mg PO daily; must abstain from alcohol for at least 12 hours before administration	Produces sensitivity to alcohol, which results in a highly unpleasant reaction to alcohol	***Contraindications:*** Hypersensitivity; severe myocardial disease or coronary occlusion; psychoses; patients who have received metronidazole, paraldehyde, alcohol, or alcohol containing products ***Cost:*** 500-mg tab, 50 tabs: $6-$19 ***Pregnancy category:*** Safe usage has not been established	Optic neuritis, peripheral neuritis, polyneuritis, hepatitis, skin eruptions, mild drowsiness, fatigability, impotence, headache, acne, allergic dermatitis, psychotic reactions
Benzodiazepines: • Chlordiazepoxide (Librium), 5-25 mg PO tid • Diazepam (Valium), 10 mg PO tid or qid for 24 hours, then 5 mg tid or qid • Lorazepam (Ativan), 2-6 mg PO every day in divided doses • Used for symptoms of alcohol withdrawal; CAUTION—may trade one addiction for another; for short-term use only; Schedule IV drugs	Wide range of selective CNS depression among the various members of this class; generally are muscle relaxant, antianxiety, anticonvulsant, and hypnotic agents	***Contraindications:*** Hypersensitivity; narrow-angle glaucoma; psychosis ***Cost:*** Chloriazepoxide, 5-mg tab, 100 tabs: $3-38; diazepam, 10-mg tab, 100 tabs: $3-$108; lorazepam, 2 mg tab, 100 tabs: $2-$131 ***Pregnancy category:*** D	Drowsiness, hiccups, lassitude, loss of dexterity, dry mouth, nausea, vomiting, headache, constipation, abdominal cramping, unsteadiness, dizziness, blurred vision, orthostatic hypotension, tachycardia, tinnitus, rash, dermatitis

Aldosteronism, Primary

OVERVIEW

Primary aldosteronism is a syndrome in which the patient has hypertension, hypokalemia, increased aldosterone secretion, and decreased renin activity. It is also called hyperaldosteronism.

Pathogenesis

Cause—most common form, unilateral aldosterone-producing adrenal adenoma; second most common form, idiopathic

Patient Profile

- Females > Males
- Most common age—20 to 50 years
- Rare condition

Signs and Symptoms

- May be asymptomatic
- Mild to severe hypertension
- Muscle weakness and cramping with marked hypokalemia
- Headaches
- Palpitations
- Polydipsia
- Polyuria
- Impaired glucose tolerance

Differential Diagnosis

- Diuretic use
- Renovascular hypertension
- Pheochromocytoma
- Renin-secreting tumor
- Malignant hypertension
- Congenital adrenal hyperplasia
- High-dose glucocorticoid therapy

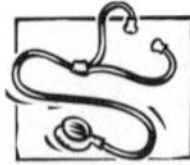

ASSESSMENT

History

Inquire about:

- Onset and duration of symptoms (if any present)
- Underlying conditions
- Current medications

Physical Findings

- May be none
- Mild to severe hypertension
- Fundoscopic examination—normal or grade 1 to 2 of retinal hypertension:
  - Grade 1—narrowing in terminal branches of vessels
  - Grade 2—general narrowing of vessels with severe local constriction

Initial Workup

Laboratory

- Chemistry profile—hypokalemia
- Urine or plasma aldosterone level increased before and after 2 L IV saline infusion
- Low plasma renin activity

Radiology: CT scan of adrenal glands

Further Workup

None indicated

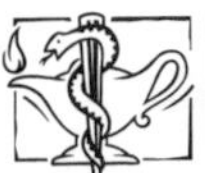

INTERVENTIONS

Office Treatment

None indicated

Lifestyle Modifications

- Low-sodium diet
- Smoking cessation

Patient Education

Teach patient about:

- Disease and treatment
  - If cause is unilateral adrenal adenoma, then surgical removal is treatment of choice; 70% cure of hypertension 1 to 4 months following removal
  - If cause is idiopathic or bilateral adrenal adenoma or patient is poor surgical candidate, then medication is treatment of choice
- Need for low-sodium diet
- Tips for smoking cessation
- Medications used and side effects (see Pharmacotherapeutics)

Referral

To endocrinologist or nephrologist

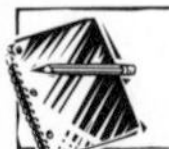

EVALUATION

Outcome

Adrenal adenoma removal—70% cured of hypertension in 1 to 4 months; other 30% and patients with idiopathic aldosteronism—stabilization of BP with medication

Possible Complication

Cardiac arrhythmia as a result of hypokalemia

Follow-up

Initially weekly until BP and potassium level stabilized; then every 2 weeks × 2; then monthly × 1; then every 3 to 6 months

FOR YOUR INFORMATION

Life Span

Pediatric: Most commonly will have bilateral adrenal hyperplasia
Geriatric: Less common than in general population
Pregnancy: Need to use drugs that are safe during pregnancy, such as methyldopa, to treat hypertension

Miscellaneous

Primary aldosteronism is a rather rare condition. It affects only 0.5% to 2% of the entire hypertensive population.

References

Haas LB: Endocrine problems. In Lewis SM, Collier IC, Heitkemper MM, editors: *Medical-surgical nursing: assessment and management of clinical problems,* ed 4, St Louis, 1996, Mosby, p 1514.

Rossiter KA: Hypokalemia. In Barker LR, Burton JR, Zieve PD, editors: *Principles of ambulatory medicine,* ed 4, Baltimore, 1995, Williams & Wilkins, p 541.

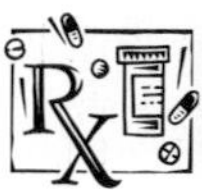

PHARMACOTHERAPEUTICS

Drug of Choice	Mechanism of Action	Prescribing Information	Side Effects
Spironolactone (Aldactone); can be used as a diagnostic test for aldosteronism; give patient 400 mg daily in divided doses for 3-4 weeks; if potassium level returns to normal and BP is controlled, yields presumptive diagnosis of aldosteronism; for long-term therapy, use lowest effective dose	Aldosterone antagonist; binds at receptor sites in distal convoluted tubules; increases sodium and water excretion and decreases potassium excretion	***Contraindications:*** Hypersensitivity; anuria; acute renal insufficiency; impaired renal function; hyperkalemia ***Cost:*** 100-mg tab, 100 tabs: $114 ***Pregnancy category:*** D	Gynecomastia, cramping and diarrhea, drowsiness, mental confusion, lethargy, impotence, irregular menses, hirsutism, headache
For treatment of hypertension if surgery is not an option, use one of the following:			
Hydrochlorothiazide (Hydrodiuril), 12.5-50 mg PO every day	Thiazide diuretic; acts on distal tubule and ascending limb of loop of Henle	***Contraindications:*** Hypersensitivity to thiazides or sulfonamides; anuria; renal decompensation; hypomagnesemia ***Cost:*** 25-mg tab, 100 tabs: $2-$12 ***Pregnancy category:*** B	Uremia, glucosuria, drowsiness, dizziness, fatigue, weakness, nausea, vomiting, anorexia, constipation, hepatitis, rash, urticaria, hyperglycemia, aplastic anemia, hemolytic anemia, leukopenia, agranulocytosis, thrombocytopenia, neutropenia, hypokalemia, orthostatic hypotension, hyponatremia, volume depletion
Calcium channel blocker: nifedepine (Procardia XL), 30-120 mg PO every day	Induces coronary artery vasodilation, which reduces myocardial O_2 requirements	***Contraindication:*** Hypersensitivity ***Cost:*** 30-mg tab, 100 tabs: $95 ***Pregnancy category:*** C	Headache, fatigue, drowsiness, dizziness, anxiety, depression, weakness, insomnia, tinnitus, dysrhythmias, edema, congestive heart failure (CHF), hypotension, pulmonary edema, nausea, vomiting, diarrhea, constipation, nocturia, polyuria, rash, pruritus, photosensitivity, flushing, sexual difficulties, fever, chills
Angiotensin-converting enzyme inhibitor: quinapril (Accupril), 10-80 mg PO every day	Prevents conversion of angiotensin I to angiotensin II, producing arterial dilation	***Contraindication:*** Hypersensitivity ***Cost:*** 5-mg tab, 100 tabs: $90 ***Pregnancy category:*** 1st trimester—C; 2nd and 3rd trimesters—D	Cough, hypotension, postural hypotension, syncope, decreased libido, impotence, increased BUN and creatinine, thrombocytopenia, agranulocytosis, angioedema, rash, sweating, photosensitivity, hyperkalemia, nausea, vomiting, gastritis, headache, dizziness, fatigue, somnolence, depression, malaise, back pain, arthralgias, arthritis
For treatment of pregnant patients:			
Methyldopa (Aldomet), 250-500 mg PO bid or tid; adjust q2d as needed; maximum 3 g per day in 2-4 divided doses	Centrally acting alpha-adrenergic inhibitor	***Contraindications:*** Hypersensitivity; active liver disease; blood dyscrasias ***Cost:*** 500-mg tab, 100 tabs: $12-$64 ***Pregnancy: category:*** B	Nausea, vomiting, diarrhea, liver dysfunction, orthostatic hypotension, bradycardia, drowsiness, weakness, dizziness, sedation, headache, leukopenia, thrombocytopenia, hemolytic anemia, positive Coombs test, impotence

Allergic Rhinitis

OVERVIEW

Allergic rhinitis is an immediate or delayed allergic reaction to airborne allergens. It is noninfectious and is either seasonal or perennial.

Pathogenesis

- Antigen-antibody response to offending substance
- Cascade of events occur in mast cells
- Ends in production of histamine, leukotrienes, prostaglandins, proteases, and platelet-activating factor
- Most common allergens: mold, dust, pollens, animal dander

Patient Profile

- Males = Females
- Usually begins before age 30

Signs and Symptoms

- Nasal congestion
- Watery eyes
- Itchy nose, eyes, ears, and palate
- Sneezing
- Fatigue
- Dry mouth—from mouth breathing
- Scratchy throat and voice
- Cough—from postnasal drip
- Dark circles under eyes (allergic shiners)
- Sensation of ears being plugged

Differential Diagnosis

- Nasal polyps
- Deviated nasal septum
- Chronic sinusitis
- Flu
- Upper respiratory tract infection
- Foreign body
- Medications—rebound from chronic use of decongestant nasal sprays or drops; chronic aspirin use

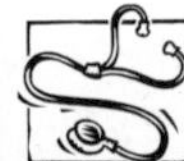

ASSESSMENT

History

Inquire about:

- Onset and duration of symptoms
- Exposure to known allergen
- Past history of allergic reactions
- Medications used (particularly nasal sprays)
- Past treatments tried and results
- Underlying conditions
- Current medications (ask about OTC medications—many available)

Physical Findings

- Nasal mucosa—pale, boggy, gray/bluish purple color
- Nasal polyps
- Conjunctiva injected
- Transverse nasal crease
- Nasal turbinates swollen
- Dark circles under eyes
- Clear postnasal drip
- Throat may be slightly red

Initial Workup

Laboratory

- CBC with differential—possible eosinophilia
- Nasal probe smear—eosinophils

Radiology: Sinuses—look for opacity, fluid level, and thickening

Further Workup

Skin testing to determine allergen

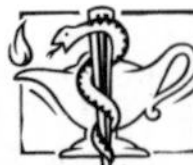

INTERVENTIONS

Office Treatment

None indicated

Lifestyle Modifications

Need to limit exposure to allergen:

- Staying indoors
- Air conditioning in home and car
- Smoking cessation
- Air filtration
- Removing carpeting and drapes from home
- Covering mattress with plastic
- Eliminating animals
- May need diet change
- May need employment change

Patient Education

Teach patient about:

- Disease process and treatment options
- Symptomatic treatment—antihistamines, decongestants, steroid nasal sprays, sympathomimetic nasal sprays
- Immunotherapy
- Lifestyle modifications
- Medications used and side effects (see Pharmacotherapeutics)

Referral

To allergist for testing

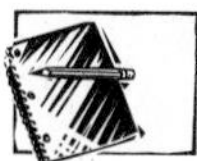

EVALUATION

Outcome
Control of symptoms

Possible Complications
- Sinusitis
- Otitis media
- Epistaxis
- Secondary infection
- Decreased pulmonary function

Follow-up
Every 2 weeks until symptom control achieved

FOR YOUR INFORMATION

Life Span
Pediatric: Need to educate parents and obtain their cooperation
Geriatric: Increased medication side effects
Pregnancy: Physiologic changes may aggravate allergic rhinitis

Miscellaneous
Ten percent of the population between the ages of 16 years and 64 years suffer from allergic rhinitis.

References

Bull TR: *Color atlas of E.N.T. diagnosis,* ed 3, London, 1995, Mosby-Wolfe, p 124.

Valentine MD: Allergy and related conditions. In Barker LR, Brown JR, Zieve PD, editors: *Principles of ambulatory medicine,* ed 4, Baltimore, 1995, Williams & Wilkins, pp 278-288.

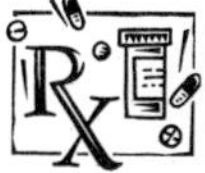

PHARMACOTHERAPEUTICS

Drug of Choice	Mechanism of Action	Prescribing Information	Side Effects
Antihistamines: • Diphenhydramine (Benadryl), 25-50 mg PO qid; children 6-12 years, 12.5-25 mg PO qid • Loratadine (Claritin), 10 mg 1 qd PO—do not use in children <6 years • Astemizole (Hismanal), 10 mg 1 qd PO—do not use in children <12 years • Fexofenadine (Allegra), 60 mg PO bid—do not use in children <12 years	Compete with histamine for cell receptor sites	***Contraindications:*** Coadministration of erythromycin, ketoconazole, or other drugs metabolized by P450 system with Hismanal; hypersensitivity ***Cost:*** Benadryl, 25-mg dose, 4/day × 30 days: $4; Claritin, 10-mg tab, 1/day × 30 days: $53; Hismanal, 10-mg tab, 1/day × 30 days: $53; Allegra, 60-mg tab, 2/day × 30 days: $50 ***Pregnancy category:*** Benadryl and Claritin—B; Hismanal and Allegra—C	Sedation—marked with Benadryl and lesser with the others; headache, fatigue, dizziness, nausea and vomiting, dry mouth, cough, rash, nervousness
Topical steroids: • Beclomethasone (Beconase AQ), 2 sprays each nostril bid; children 6-12 years, 1 spray each nostril daily—not for children <6 years • Flunisolide (Nasalide), 2 inhalations each nostril bid; children >6 years, 2 inhalations each nostril bid—do not use in children <6 years • Triamcinolone (Nasacort), 2 inhalations each nostril daily; may increase to 2 inhalations bid—for use in children 12 years and older	Potent glucocorticoids; antiinflammatory—mechanism for this is unknown	***Contraindication:*** Hypersensitivity ***Cost:*** Beconase AQ, 21 g:$31; Nasalide, 25 ml: $27; Nasacort, 10 g: $38 ***Pregnancy category:*** C	Use caution if patient is being transferred from oral steroids because could show signs of adrenal insufficiency; headache; nasal irritation; dry mucous membranes; throat discomfort
Oral decongestants: 130 different products listed in *PDR* for nonprescription drugs; many in combination with an antihistamine; most contain pseudoephedrine, phenylephrine, or phenylpropanolamine; see labels for dosage—do not exceed dosage	Sympathomimetics; cause nasal vasoconstriction, producing decongestion	***Contraindications:*** Hypersensitivity; hypertension (controversial); diabetes; heart or thyroid disease; prostate enlargement ***Cost:*** Varies with product ***Pregnancy category:*** Pseudoephedrine—B; phenylephrine and phenylpropanolamine—C	Drowsiness, dry mouth, insomnia, headache, nervousness, fatigue, irritability, disorientation, rash, palpitations, sore throat, cough

Alopecia

OVERVIEW

The term *alopecia* is defined as hair loss from any part of the body that would normally be expected to have hair. Alopecia is classified as scarring or nonscarring.

Pathogenesis

NONSCARRING ALOPECIA

- Hair follicle is not permanently damaged, and hair regrowth is possible
- Types include:
  - Androgenic alopecia—male and female hair loss due to increased levels of male hormones
  - Alopecia areata—common, asymptomatic disease—rapid onset of total hair loss in well-defined areas; etiology unknown; once thought to be stress induced, but recent research does not implicate stress
  - Telogen effluvium—loss of resting hair; can have many causes, including a high fever, severe physiologic or psychologic trauma, postpartum hair loss, and drugs, including aminosalicylic acid, amphetamines, bromocriptine, captopril, carbamazepine, cimetidine, coumadin, enalapril, levodopa, lithium, metoprolol, and propranolol
  - Anagen effluvium—abrupt hair loss from follicles in their growing phase; caused by an abrupt insult to metabolic and follicular reproductive apparatus by chemotherapeutic agents
  - Trichotillomania—act of manually removing hair, an irresistible urge to pull one's hair out
  - Tinea capitis—dermatophyte infection caused by a fungus
  - Systemic causes—thyroid disease, systemic lupus erythematosus, drug-induced hair loss, secondary syphilis

SCARRING ALOPECIA

- Hair follicle is destroyed
- Types include:
  - Kerion formation as a result of tinea capitis or discoid lupus erythematosus—usually no systemic disease is present; is thought to be caused by an autoantibody, although antinuclear antibodies are present only in small amounts
  - Lichen planus—inflammatory disease of unknown cause
  - Aplasia cutis congenita—small blister or eroded area that may be present at birth
  - Congenital absence of skin

Patient Profile

Profile will vary with cause:

- Androgenic alopecia:
  - Males = Females
  - Increases with age
- Alopecia areata:
  - Males = Females
  - Most common age—<40 years
- Telogen and anagen effluvium:
  - Males = Females
  - Any age
- Trichotillomania:
  - Females > Males
  - Most common age—children and adolescents, but seen in adults
- Tinea capitis:
  - Males = Females
  - More common in children and adolescents, but seen in adults
- Systemic diseases—see specific disease for patient profile

Signs and Symptoms

- Hair loss, pruritis, erythema, and scaling of scalp in tinea capitis
- Broken hairs in tinea capitis and in trichotillomania
- Patchy hair loss with well-defined borders, rapid onset, tapered hair at borders of patches of hair loss, and easily removable hair in alopecia areata

Differential Diagnosis

Diagnose type of hair loss and search for a reversible cause

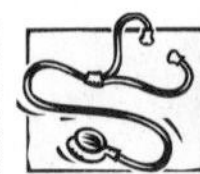

ASSESSMENT

History

Inquire about:

- Onset and duration of symptoms
- Location of hair loss
- In females, postpartum status
- Use of commercial hair products with strong chemicals, such as lye
- Systemic symptoms, such as weight loss or gain
- Arthritic symptoms
- Stressors
- Treatments tried and results
- Diet, including any severe diets tried recently or in the past
- Underlying conditions or trauma
- Family history of alopecia
- Current and past medications, including OTC medications

Physical Findings

- Depends on cause
- Examine scalp for erythema, scaling, scratch marks
- Examine hair shafts
- Assess length of hair that may or may not be present in bald areas
- Assess for follicular plugging
- Assess loss pattern
- Assess for scarring and inflammatory lesions
- May need to perform complete physical examination

Initial Workup

Laboratory

- Thyroid function tests
- CBC with differential
- Free testosterone and dehydroepiandrosterone sulfate (DHEA-S) in women
- Ferritin level
- VDRL or rapid plasma reagin (RPR) for syphilis
- Lymphocyte T- and B-cell counts, sometimes low in alopecia areata

Radiology: Usually none indicated unless secondary cause is being sought

Further Workup

- Light hair pull test (positive in alopecia areata)
- Direct microscopic examination of hair shaft
- Potassium hydroxide (KOH) preparation of scalp scale (positive for hyphae in tinea capitis)
- Fungal culture of scalp scale

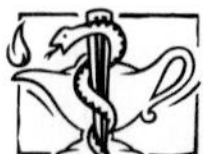

INTERVENTIONS

Office Treatment

For alopecia areata, intralesional steroid injections with triamcinolone—usually done by dermatologist

Lifestyle Modifications

- Good, well-balanced diet encouraged
- Counseling for trichotillomania
- Cessation of all nonessential medications

Patient Education

Teach patient about:

- Condition and cause (if known)
- Regrowth—possible with nonscarring alopecia; not possible with scarring alopecia
- Hair transplants, scalp reduction and flaps, and stores selling wigs and hairpieces
- Systemic illness and its treatment if found to be causative factor
- Well-balanced diet and need to avoid severe diets
- Medication (minoxidil) used and side effects (see Pharmacotherapeutics)

Referral

To dermatologist if unable to determine type and cause or for treatment failure, or to psychologist or psychiatrist if suspicion of trichotillomania

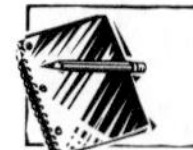

EVALUATION

Outcome

Hair regrowth or psychologic adaptation to hair loss

Possible Complication

Severe psychologic damage

Follow-up

- Tinea capitis—follow about every 2 weeks when patient taking griseofulvin (see section on tinea capitis)
- Others should be followed every 2 weeks × 2; then every 3 to 6 months

FOR YOUR INFORMATION

Life Span

Pediatric: Tinea capitis most common cause

Geriatric: Incidence of androgenic alopecia increases

Pregnancy: Postpartum hair loss due to physiologic changes

Miscellaneous

Recent research by Schmidt (1994) has demonstrated that androgenic hair loss in both men and women may be a result of multilayered interaction of both thyroid hormones and androgenic hormones. The research demonstrated a significant elevation of cortisol in both men and women. This research points to the fact that androgenic hair loss cannot be attributed to just an elevation of androgenic hormones, but is actually caused by a number of hormones.

References

Habif TP: *Clinical dermatology: a color guide to diagnosis and therapy,* ed 3, St Louis, 1996, Mosby, pp 742-756.

Schmidt JB: Hormonal basis of male and female androgenic alopecia: clinical relevance, *Skin Pharmacol* 7(1-2):61-66, 1994.

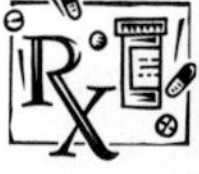

PHARMACOTHERAPEUTICS

Treatment of alopecia depends on the causative factor. For hair loss resulting from a systemic illness or from tinea capitis, consult the respective disease for further information on pharmacotherapeutics. The following discusses pharmacotherapeutics for androgenic alopecia, alopecia areata, and telogen and anagen effluvium, all of which are conditions that allow hair regrowth to occur.

Drug of Choice	Mechanism of Action	Prescribing Information	Side Effects
Minoxidil (Rogaine); used for treatment of androgenic alopecia, telogen and anagen effluvium alopecia, and alopecia areata; 2% or 5%, apply 1 ml to dry scalp twice daily; long time passes before results seen; ensure scalp is healthy, without abrasions or dermatitis; if use stopped, hair loss will resume	Stimulates hair regrowth; exact mechanism is unknown, but vasodilation probably plays a role	***Contraindication:*** Hypersensitivity ***Cost:*** 60 ml: $60 ***Pregnancy category:*** C	Eczema, local erythema, pruritus, dry skin, scalp flaking, sexual dysfunction, visual disturbances, increased hair loss; although rare, can develop systemic effects such as dizziness, faintness, increased/decreased blood pressure, edema, chest pain, palpitations

Alzheimer's Disease/Dementia of Alzheimer's Type (DAT)

OVERVIEW

Alzheimer's disease is a type of dementia. It is a severe, degenerative organic condition of the brain that affects the patient's mental status. It produces a progressive decline in intellectual functioning.

Pathogenesis

- No single cause known
- Theories—disordered immune function; slow virus; genetic factors—marker on chromosome 21

Patient Profile

- Females > Males
- 40 to 75 years of age
- 50% have positive family history

Signs and Symptoms

- Onset is very slow and insidious
- Early symptom is loss of short-term memory
- Progresses to profound short- and long-term memory loss
- Personal hygiene deteriorates
- Attention span deteriorates
- Communication is lost
- Ability to perform activities of daily living stops
- General deterioration continues until death

Differential Diagnosis

- Depression
- Vascular dementia
- Multiinfarct dementia
- Creutzfeldt-Jakob disease
- Brain tumor
- Subdural hematoma
- Metabolic dementia
- Drug reactions
- Toxicity from liver or kidney failure
- Nutritional deficiencies
- Alcoholism or drug addiction
- Hydrocephalus

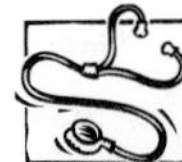

ASSESSMENT

History

Inquire about:

- Onset and duration of symptoms—question both patient and family members
- Loss of immediate, recent, or remote memory
- Ability to make sound judgments
- Diet and appetite
- Sleep-wake pattern
- Alcohol and/or drug abuse
- Underlying conditions
- Past history of head trauma
- Current medications

Physical Findings

- Depends on stage of disease
- Early stage:
  - May score 20 points or higher on mini–mental status examination
  - Slight inattention during examination
- As disease progresses:
  - Mini–mental status examination score falls
  - Restlessness, inattentiveness
  - Deteriorating hygiene
  - Shuffling or stumbling gait
  - Bowel and bladder incontinence
- Diagnosis based mainly on history—diagnosis of Alzheimer's disease is one of exclusion—need to look for physical findings for other causes of dementia, such as thyroid enlargement, cranial nerve dysfunction, carotid bruits

Initial Workup

Laboratory: To rule out other causes of dementia:

- CBC
- Chemistry panel
- Thyroid panel
- Folate and B_{12} level
- VDRL
- Urinalysis
- ECG

Radiology: CT scan or MRI of head to rule out tumors, subdural hematomas, cerebral infarcts, hydrocephalus

Further Workup

- EEG
- Only positive diagnosis is on autopsy

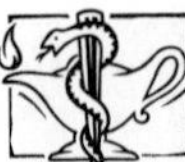

INTERVENTIONS

Office Treatment

Supportive environment for caregiver

Lifestyle Modifications

- Modification of home to prevent accidents as necessary
- Obtaining help for care of patient from home health agency
- Major life crisis that requires drastic lifestyle modifications

Patient Education

Teach patient/caregiver about:

- Disease progression and treatment options (no specific treatment—treat symptoms)
- Support groups available for caregiver
- Adult day care programs
- Visiting nurses
- Music therapy—has calming effect on agitated patient
- Nursing home, if necessary
- Exercises to reduce restlessness
- Using short sentences to communicate
- Giving one instruction at a time
- Getting patient's affairs in order; legal guardianship
- Medications used and side effects (see Pharmacotherapeutics)

Referrals

- To geriatrician or geriatric NP specializing in Alzheimer's care if possible
- To home health agency for nursing, physical therapy, occupational therapy, social work needs

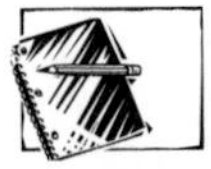

EVALUATION

Outcomes

- Patient maintained in home environment as long as possible
- Caregiver able to adjust and maintain a good quality of life

Possible Complications

- Progression to stage of uncontrollable hostile behavior and inability to communicate
- Survival time of 2 to 20 years

Follow-up

- Every 2 weeks × 3; then every 6 weeks
- If patient taking tacrine—ALT/SGPT done weekly × 6; then every 2 weeks × 16

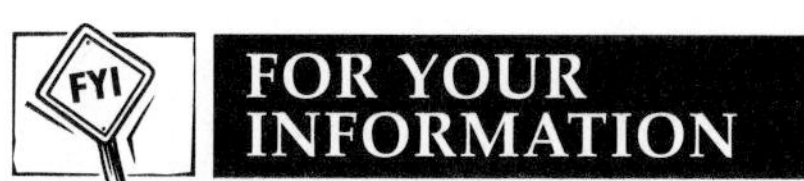

FOR YOUR INFORMATION

Life Span

Pediatric: Not a pediatric illness
Geriatric: Frequent and serious disorder for this age group
Pregnancy: N/A

Miscellaneous

Alzheimer's disease is devastating for both the patient and the family. The NP must provide the patient and family with as much support as possible.

References

Crandall L: Daily living with Alzheimer's disease. In Carnevali DL, Patrick M, editors: *Nursing management for the elderly,* ed 3, Philadelphia, 1993, JB Lippencott, pp 296-310.

Golden R: Dementia and Alzheimer's disease indications, diagnosis, and treatment, *Minn Med* 78(1):25-29, 1995.

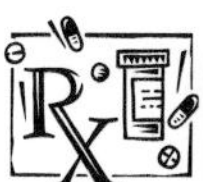

PHARMACOTHERAPEUTICS

There is no one specific drug to treat Alzheimer's disease. Medication therapy is only used to attempt to control secondary behavior problems. Use medications cautiously.

Drug of Choice	Mechanism of Action	Prescribing Information	Side Effects
For mild to moderate dementia of Alzeheimer's type			
Tacrine (Cognex), 10 mg PO qid for 6 weeks; ALT/SGPT should be checked weekly, initially; may increase dose up to 180 mg/day in divided doses qid; after initial 6 weeks, check ALT/SGPT every 2 weeks for 16 weeks (see package insert for dosage modifications based on lab results); appears to slightly improve cognition	Unsure, but appears to act by increasing acetylcholine	***Contraindications:*** Hypersensitivity; patients who developed treatment-associated jaundice; use with caution in patients with history of neuromuscular disease, abnormal liver function studies, seizures, or asthma ***Cost:*** 10-mg tab, 100 tabs: $120 ***Pregnancy category:*** C	Hepatoxicity, nausea, vomiting, diarrhea, dyspepsia, anorexia, headache, fatigue, chest pain, back pain, asthenia, myalgia, dizziness, confusion, ataxia, insomnia, somnolence, agitation, depression, anxiety, hallucinations, rhinitis, rash, urinary tract infection
Donepezil (Aricept), initially 5 mg PO q hs; may increase to 10 mg after 4-6 weeks	Reversible acetylcholinesterase inhibitor	***Contraindications:*** Hypersensitivity; use with caution in patients with asthma or siezures ***Cost:*** 5-mg tab × 30 days: $33 ***Pregnancy category:*** C	Nausea, diarrhea, GI bleeding, insomnia, vomiting, muscle, cramps, fatigue, anorexia
For anxiety:			
Buspirone (Buspar), 2.5-5.0 mg PO bid or tid	Anxiolytic; inhibits action of serotonin	***Contraindication:*** Hypersensitivity; children <18 years ***Cost:*** 5-mg tab, 3/day × 120 days: $210 ***Pregnancy category:*** B	Dizziness, headache, depression, insomnia, nervousness, numbness, nausea, dry mouth, diarrhea, tachycardia, palpitations, congestive heart failure (CHF), myocardial infarction (MI), sore throat, tinnitus, pain, cerebrovascular accident (CVA), weakness, rash, edema, sweating
Benzodiazepine; use one that is short-acting, such as lorazepam (Ativan), 0.25-0.5 mg PO bid or tid	Antianxiety; potentiates actions of gamma aminobutyric acid (GABA)	***Contraindications:*** Hypersensitivity; narrow-angle glaucoma; psychosis; pregnancy; children <12 years; history of drug abuse; chronic obstructive pulmonary disease (COPD) ***Cost:*** 1-mg tab, 2/day for 120 days: $6 ***Pregnancy category:*** D	Dizziness, drowsiness, confusion, hallucinations, constipation, dry mouth, rash, orthostatic hypotension, tachycardia, ECG changes, blurred vision
For nighttime irritability and insomnia:			
Haloperidol (Haldol); 0.25-1 mg PO 1 hour before bedtime	Antipsychotic; depresses cerebral cortex, hypothalamus, limbic system; blocks neurotransmission produced by dopamine; strong alpha adrenergic	***Contraindications:*** Hypersensitivity; blood dyscrasias; brain damage; bone marrow depression; alcohol and barbiturate withdrawal; Parkinson's disease; angina; epilepsy; urinary retention; narrow-angle glaucoma ***Cost:*** 0.5-mg tab, 100 tabs: $3-$15 ***Pregnancy category:*** C	Laryngospasm, respiratory depression, extrapyramidal symptoms, seizures, neuroleptic malignant syndrome, rash, dry mouth, nausea, vomiting, anorexia, constipation, ileus, hepatitis, orthostatic hypotension, cardiac arrest, tachycardia

Amblyopia

OVERVIEW

Amblyopia is a reduction in visual acuity in one eye. It cannot be corrected with eyeglasses or contact lenses and is not a result of a structural or pathologic abnormality in the eye.

Pathogenesis

Several different types and causes:

- Strabismus amblyopia—loss of visual acuity due to suppression of images in eye, which turns in or out
- Anisometric amblyopia—one eye has significantly different refractive error—leads to blurred vision
- Refractive amblyopia—uncorrected high refractive error—vision blurred in either one or both eyes
- Deprivation amblyopia—visual deprivation due to congenital abnormality

Patient Profile

- Males = Females
- Any age—may be present from birth
- Usually diagnosed in childhood

Signs and Symptoms

- Complaints of visual blurring
- Decreased vision in one eye
- Often diagnosed on preschool screening
- May not have any signs or symptoms

Differential Diagnosis

Organic lesion

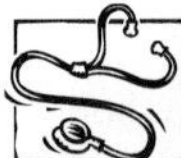

ASSESSMENT

History

Inquire about:

- Onset and duration of symptoms
- Last eye examination
- Underlying conditions
- Current medications

Physical Finding

May find one eye turning inward or outward

Initial Workup

Laboratory: None indicated
Radiology: None indicated

Further Workup

Done by ophthalmologist

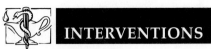

INTERVENTIONS

Office Treatment

None indicated

Lifestyle Modification

May need to wear eye patch on strong eye

Patient Education

Teach patient/parents about:

- Condition and that it will not correct itself
- Ophthalmologists available
- Possible treatment options—corrective lenses, patching strong eye, surgical correction
- No medications for condition

Referral

To ophthalmologist

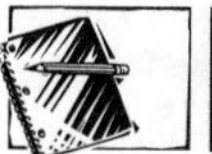

EVALUATION

Outcome
Vision is corrected

Possible Complication
Permanent and profound vision loss

Follow-up
By ophthalmologist

FOR YOUR INFORMATION

Life Span
Pediatric: Most commonly diagnosed in this age group
Geriatric: Diagnosis was usually made in childhood
Pregnancy: N/A

Miscellaneous
Therapy for amblyopia is usually not very effective after 12 years of age.

References
Fraser H: Amblyopia—or lazy eye, *Austr Fam Physician* 24(6):1021-1023, 1995.

Ludwig-Beymer P, Huether SE, Schoessler M: Pain, temperature regulation, sleep, and sensory function. In McCance KL, Huether SE, editors: *Pathophysiology: the biological basis for disease in adults and children,* ed 2, St Louis, 1994, Mosby, p 462.

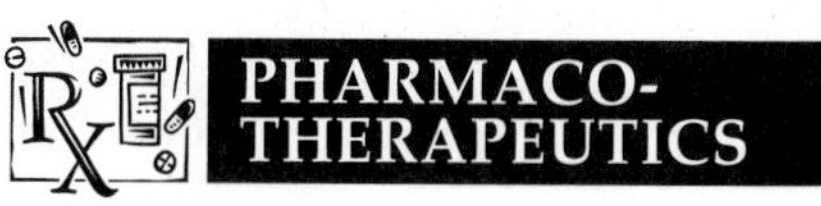

PHARMACO-THERAPEUTICS

No medications are available for treatment of this condition.

Amebiasis

OVERVIEW

Amebiasis is an infection of the intestinal tract caused by an intestinal protozoa.

Pathogenesis
Cause—*Entamoeba histolytica,* a protozoa; transmitted through contaminated food or water or person-to-person contact

Patient Profile
- Males = Females
- All ages

Signs and Symptoms
Depends on severity:
- Noninvasive amebiasis:
  - Asymptomatic
  - Mild diarrhea
  - Abdominal discomfort
- Intestinal invasion:
  - Abdominal pain and tenderness
  - Rectal pain
  - Diarrhea
  - Bloody stools
  - Fever
  - Systemic toxicity
- Infection outside intestine:
  - Fever
  - Systemic toxicity
  - Abdominal pain and tenderness—right upper quadrant
  - Nausea, vomiting
  - Diarrhea
- Vast majority of cases—noninvasive

Differential Diagnosis
- Shigellosis
- *Campylobacter* infection
- Pseudomembranous colitis
- Salmonella
- Ulcerative colitis
- Crohn's disease
- Ischemic colitis
- Hepatic amebiasis

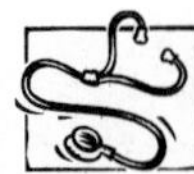

ASSESSMENT

History
Inquire about:
- Onset and duration of symptoms
- Recent travel to Mexico, South Africa, India
- Camping trip without sanitary facilities
- Where patient lives (institutional living is risk factor)
- Occupation (sanitation workers more at risk)
- Sexual preferences (male homosexuals at risk)
- Underlying conditions
- Current medications

Physical Findings
- Crampy abdominal pain
- Hyperactive bowel sounds
- Fever

Initial Workup
Laboratory
- Stool for ova and parasites
- Diarrheal stool should be examined for trophozoites immediately; if diarrhea severe, check serum electrolytes, glucose
- A commercial antigen detection kit will soon be available

Radiology: CT scan or MRI of liver if hepatic infection suspected

Further Workup
- Rectosigmoidoscopy
- Needle aspiration of hepatic lesions

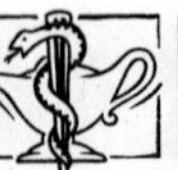

INTERVENTIONS

Office Treatment
None indicated

Lifestyle Modifications
- Avoidance of reinfection
- Good hand-washing technique

Patient Education
Teach patient about:
- Disease, mode of transmission, and treatment options—medication
- How to wash hands effectively and importance of frequent hand washing
- Need for increased fluid intake and bland diet
- How to avoid reexposure
- How to take medication and side effects (see Pharmacotherapeutics)

Referral
Usually none; to gastroenterologist if severe infection

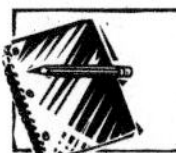

EVALUATION

Outcome
Resolves without sequelae; may have irritable bowel symptoms for several weeks after treatment

Possible Complications
- Toxic megacolon
- Rupture of hepatic abscess
- Peritonitis
- Can be fatal

Follow-up
Every 2 weeks × 2

FOR YOUR INFORMATION

Life Span
Pediatric: May be more severe; be alert for signs and symptoms of dehydration
Geriatric: Same as for pediatrics
Pregnancy: Difficult to treat because of teratogenic effect of medications

Miscellaneous
Incubation is a few days to months.

References

Bennett RG: Acute gastroenteritis and associated conditions. In Barker LR, Burton JR, Zieve PD, editors: *Principles of ambulatory medicine,* ed 4, Baltimore, 1995, Williams & Wilkins, pp 307-318.

Haque R et al: Rapid diagnosis of *Entamoeba* infection by using *Entamoeba* and *Entamoeba histolytica* stool antigen detection kits, *J Clin Microbiol* 33(10):2558-2561, 1995.

NOTES

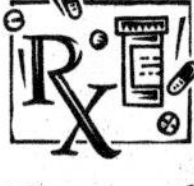

PHARMACOTHERAPEUTICS

Drug of Choice	Mechanism of Action	Prescribing Information	Side Effects
For noninvasive infection:			
Iodoquinol (Yodoxin); adults, 650 mg PO tid × 20 days; children, 40 mg/kg/day PO in divided doses × 20 days	Direct-acting amebicide	***Contraindications:*** Hypersensitivity to this drug or iodine; renal disease; severe thyroid disease; hepatic disease; preexisting optic neuropathy ***Cost:*** 650-mg tab, 100 tabs: $40 ***Pregnancy category:*** C	Agranulocytosis; rash; pruritus; discolored skin, hair, and nails; alopecia; malaise; headache; agitation; peripheral neuropathy; fever; chills; blurred vision; sore throat; retinal edema; anorexia; nausea; vomiting; diarrhea; epigastric distress; gastritis; abdominal cramps; rectal irritation; anal itch
For invasive infection:			
Metronidazole (Flagyl); adults, 750 mg PO tid × 10 days, followed by 20-day course of above drug; children, 35-50 mg/kg/day in 3 divided doses × 10 days, followed by 20-day course of above drug	Direct-acting amebicide	***Contraindications:*** Hypersensitivity; renal disease; hepatic disease; contracted visual or color fields; blood dyscrasias; pregnancy (1st trimester); lactation; CNS disorders ***Cost:*** 500-mg tab, 50 tabs: $5-$40; 250-mg tab, 100 tabs: $5-$110 ***Pregnancy category:*** B (2nd and 3rd trimesters)	Flat T-waves, headache, dizziness, irritability, restlessness, fatigue, drowsiness, convulsions, incoordinations, blurred vision, sore throat, retinal edema, dry mouth, metallic taste, furry tongue, nausea, vomiting, diarrhea, epigastric distress, anorexia, constipation, abdominal cramps, pseudomembranous colitis, darkened urine, vaginal dryness, albuminuria, neurotoxicity, leukopenia, bone marrow depression, aplasia, rash, pruritus, urticaria, flushing

Amenorrhea

OVERVIEW

Amenorrhea is the absence of menses. It is classified as either primary or secondary. Primary amenorrhea is the absence of menarche by age 16 or absence of menses and secondary sexual characteristics by age 14. Absence of menses for 3 cycles or 6 months in patients who previously menstruated is classified as secondary amenorrhea.

Pathogenesis

Many causes:

- Primary amenorrhea:
  - Imperforate hymen
  - Agenesis of uterus and upper two thirds of vagina
  - Turner's syndrome
  - Constitutional delay
- Secondary amenorrhea:
  - Pregnancy
  - Lactation
  - Menopause
  - Anatomic deviations
  - Stress
  - Severe weight loss
  - Untreated sexually transmitted diseases
  - Excessive exercise
  - Pituitary disease
  - Endocrine disease
  - Radiation therapy
  - Autoimmune diseases
  - Premature ovarian failure
  - Medications (oral contraceptives, danazol, systemic steroids)

Patient Profile

- Females only
- Ages 14 to 55 years

Signs and Symptoms

- Absence of menses as defined in Overview
- Galactorrhea
- Temperature intolerance
- Symptoms of early pregnancy
- Signs of androgen excess

Differential Diagnosis

- Any of the causes listed above
- Most common cause of secondary amenorrhea is pregnancy

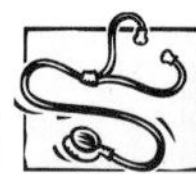

ASSESSMENT

History

- For primary amenorrhea, inquire about:
  - Growth and development
  - Occurrence of growth spurt
  - Family history of amenorrhea
  - Development of secondary sexual characteristics
  - Severe weight loss
  - Past illnesses
  - Excessive exercise
  - Sexual activity
  - Underlying conditions
  - Current medications
- For secondary amenorrhea, inquire about:
  - Age of menarche
  - Regularity of and interval between menses
  - Duration and characteristics of menstrual flow
  - Past medical history
  - Severe weight loss
  - Excessive exercise
  - Obstetric history
  - Sexual activity
  - Body changes, such as nipple discharge, hirsutism, hot flashes, insomnia, headaches
  - Underlying conditions
  - Current medications

Physical Findings

- Depends on cause
- Note general appearance; height and weight
- Note stage of development of secondary sex characteristics (use Tanner staging)
- Assess for gonadal dysgenesis—neck folds, setting of ears, chest configuration, fourth metacarpal short, cubitus, and valgus
- Assess thyroid for enlargement or nodules
- Assess breasts for development, nipple discharge
- Palpate abdomen for masses
- Look for hirsutism, clitorimegaly, or acne
- Assess appearance of genitalia, imperforate hymen, vaginal septum
- Perform speculum examination for presence of vagina and uterus; clear mucus in os indicates estrogen present
- Perform bimanual examination for masses

Initial Workup

Laboratory

- Pregnancy test
- TSH and T_4
- Serum prolactin
- Glucose
- FSH >40 mIU/ml = ovarian failure
- LH/FSH ratio >2.5 mIU/ml = polycystic ovaries

Radiology: With increased prolactin level >60 ng/dl, order coronal CT scan with contrast or MRI of head to rule out pituitary adenoma

Further Workup

- Total testosterone >200 ng/L = tumor
- Dehydroepiandrosterone sulfate >700 μg/dl = adrenal disorder or tumor
- Cortisol level increased >25 μg/dl in a morning specimen = adrenal hyperactivity

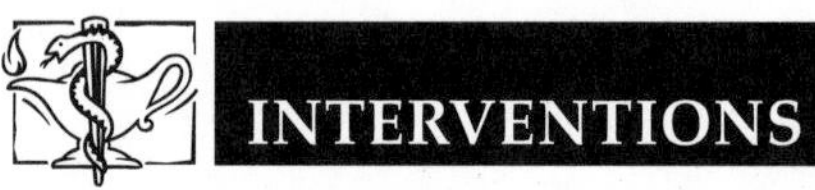

INTERVENTIONS

Office Treatment

None indicated

Lifestyle Modifications

- Depends on cause
- Nutritionally balanced diet to increase or decrease weight
- Moderate exercise program
- May need to adjust to infertility

Patient Education

Teach patient about:

- Condition and cause
- Possibility of infertility
- Importance of maintenance of appropriate weight
- Exercise and effects of excessive exercise
- For imperforate hymen, same day surgery
- Progesterone challenge test to establish diagnosis of anovulation, defective uterus, or outflow tract
- Hormone replacement therapy
- Medications used and side effects (see Pharmacotherapeutics)

Referral

For primary amenorrhea, refer to MD after initial history and physical; for secondary amenorrhea, consult with MD on treatment

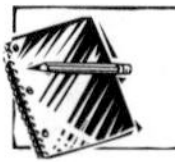

EVALUATION

Outcome
Depends on cause

Possible Complications
Decreased estrogen—hot flashes, vaginal dryness, osteoporosis

Follow-up
- Depends on cause
- Initially may need to follow every 2 weeks during workup; then every 3 months × 1; then annually

FOR YOUR INFORMATION

Life Span
Pediatric: May have primary or secondary amenorrhea in adolescence
Geriatric: Secondary amenorrhea due to menopause
Pregnancy: Primary cause of secondary amenorrhea

Miscellaneous
N/A

References
Aloi JA: Evaluation of amenorrhea, *Compr Ther* 21 (10):575-578, 1995.

Baker S: Menstruation and related problems and concerns. In Youngkin EQ, Davis MS, editors: *Women's health: a primary care clinical guide,* Norwalk, Conn, 1994, Appleton & Lange, pp 78-82.

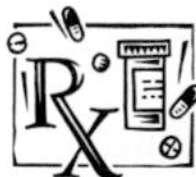

PHARMACOTHERAPEUTICS

Drug of Choice	Mechanism of Action	Prescribing Information	Side Effects
For progesterone challenge test:			
Progesterone in oil, 100-200 mg IM, or medroxyprogesterone acetate (Provera), 5-10 mg PO × 5-10 days; if no galactorrhea and bleeding starts 2-7 days after medication stopped, diagnosis is anovulation	Inhibits secretion of pituitary gonadotropins; stimulates growth of mammary tissue	***Contraindications:*** Hypersensitivity; breast cancer; thromboembolic disorders; reproductive cancer; undiagnosed vaginal bleeding; pregnancy ***Cost:*** 50 mg/ml, 10 ml: $9-30; 5-mg tab, 30 tabs: $16 ***Pregnancy category:*** X	Dizziness, headache, migraines, depression, hypotension, thrombophlebitis, thromboembolism, pulmonary embolism, myocardial infarction (MI), nausea, vomiting, cholestatic jaundice, weight gain, diplopia, cervical erosion, breakthrough bleeding, dysmenorrhea, vaginal candidiasis, spontaneous abortion, rash, urticaria, acne, hirsuitism, photosensitivity
If no bleeding with progesterone:			
Estrogen (Estrace), 2.5 mg PO × 21 days with medroxyprogesterone acetate, 10 mg PO days 16-21; if no bleeding after medications, repeat; if still no bleeding, indicates defective uterus or outflow tract	Affects release of pituitary gonadotropins; inhibits ovulation	***Contraindications:*** Hypersensitivity; breast cancer; thromboembolic disorders; reproductive cancer; undiagnosed vaginal bleeding; pregnancy ***Cost:*** 2.5-mg tab, 100 tabs: $50 ***Pregnancy category:*** X	Dizziness, headache, migraines, depression, hypotension, thrombophlebitis, thromboembolism, pulmonary embolism, MI, nausea, vomiting, cholestatic jaundice, weight gain, diplopia, cervical erosion, breakthrough bleeding, dysmenorrhea, vaginal candidiasis, spontaneous abortion, rash, urticaria, acne, hirsutism, photosensitivity
If bleeding occurs:			
Start patient on combination oral contraceptives (many brands available)—dosage and instructions vary for different types; see individual package insert for directions	Prevent ovulation by suppressing FSH and LH	***Contraindications:*** Hypersensitivity; breast cancer; thromboembolic disorders; reproductive cancer; undiagnosed vaginal bleeding; pregnancy; hepatic tumor/disease; women 40 years and over; cerebrovascular accident (CVA) ***Cost:*** Varies by brand; $20-$30/month ***Pregnancy category:*** X	Dizziness, headache, migraines, depression, hypotension, thrombophlebitis, thromboembolism, pulmonary embolism, MI, nausea, vomiting, cholestatic jaundice, weight gain, diplopia, cervical erosion, breakthrough bleeding, dysmenorrhea, vaginal candidiasis, spontaneous abortion, rash, urticaria, acne, hirsutism, photosensitivity
If estrogen is contraindicated:			
Give medroxyprogesterone acetate only on days 1-10, 1-14, or 16-26			

Anaphylaxis

OVERVIEW

Anaphylaxis is an acute immune hypersensitivity reaction to an antigen to which the patient has previously been sensitized.

Pathogenesis

- Exaggerated immune response to antigen exposure
- Majority are IgE mediated
- Antigen causes mast cell degranulation
- Common causes:
  - Antibiotics (penicillin; topical antibiotics)
  - Insect stings
  - Immunotherapy
  - Blood products
  - Foods (nuts, berries, beans, seafood, etc.)
  - Insulin
  - Dextran
  - Latex gloves
  - Exercise
  - Cold
  - Iodinated contrast media

Patient Profile

- Males = Females
- Any age

Signs and Symptoms

- Diffuse erythema of skin
- Pruritis
- Flushing
- Urticaria
- Angioedema
- Dyspnea
- Cough
- Wheezing
- Rhinorrhea
- Difficulty swallowing
- Nausea, vomiting
- Abdominal cramps
- Diarrhea
- Malaise
- Tachycardia
- Hypotension
- Shock

Differential Diagnosis

- Pheochromocytosis
- Carcinoid syndrome
- Serum sickness
- Globus hystericus

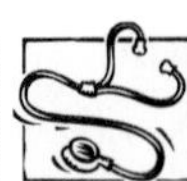

ASSESSMENT

History

Medical emergency—history should be taken quickly; inquire about:

- Onset and duration of symptoms
- Known exposure to antigen and what causative agent is
- Previous anaphylactic reactions
- Underlying conditions
- Current medications

Physical Findings

- Diffuse erythema of skin
- Respiratory distress with wheezing and rhonchi
- Hypotension
- Tachycardia
- Angioedema

Initial Workup

Laboratory: None diagnostic; obtain arterial blood gases
Radiology: None indicated

Further Workup

None indicated

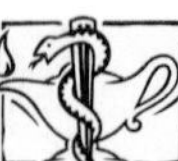

INTERVENTIONS

Office Treatment

- Apply tourniquet proximal to injection or sting site
- Maintain airway
- Provide oxygen
- Maintain supine position with legs elevated
- If possible, start IV
- Monitor vital signs frequently
- Administer epinephrine
- Transport immediately to emergency room if necessary

Lifestyle Modifications

- Avoidance of causative agent
- Need to carry or wear medical alert information at all times
- Need to carry emergency epinephrine kit

Patient Education

Teaching will need to occur after immediate emergent period; teach patient about:

- Condition and cause if known (if unknown, patient will need to be referred to allergy specialist)
- Desensitization therapy
- Obtaining an emergency epinephrine kit and how to use it
- Obtaining a medical alert card, bracelet, and/or necklace
- Avoiding specific causative agent
- Medications used and side effects (see Pharmacotherapeutics)

Referral

To allergy specialist

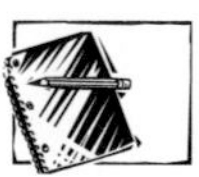

EVALUATION

Outcome
Prognosis is good if treated quickly

Possible Complications
- Hypoxemia
- Cardiac arrest
- Death

Follow-up
1 week after hospitalization if needed

FOR YOUR INFORMATION

Life Span
Pediatric: Treatment is the same
Geriatric: Treatment is the same; may have more difficult recovery because of concomitant illnesses
Pregnancy: Treatment is the same

Miscellaneous
N/A

References
Lewis SL: Nursing role in management: altered immune responses. In Lewis SM, Collier IC, Heitkemper MM, editors: *Medical-surgical nursing: assessment and management of clinical problems,* ed 4, St Louis, 1996, Mosby, pp 214-215.

Valentine MD: Allergy and related conditions. In Barker LR, Burton JR, Zieve PD, editors: *Principles of ambulatory medicine,* ed 4, Baltimore, 1995, Williams & Wilkins, pp 290-294.

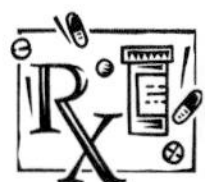

PHARMACOTHERAPEUTICS

There are many medications used for the patient suffering from anaphylaxis. This section covers those medications that may be available in the primary care clinic.

Drug of Choice	Mechanism of Action	Prescribing Information	Side Effects
• Epinephrine, *less severe reactions:* 0.3-0.5 mg (0.3-0.5 ml of 1:1000 solution) SQ or IM q20-30 min up to 3 doses • Epinephrine, *life-threatening reactions:* 0.5 mg (5 ml of 1:10,000 solution) given slowly IV and repeated every 5-10 minutes; if IV line not available, give intralingually or endotracheally	B_1 and B_2 agonist; produces bronchodilation and cardiac and CNS stimulation; large doses produce vasoconstriction; small doses produce vasodilation	***Contraindications:*** Hypersensitivity to sympathomimetics; narrow-angle glaucoma ***Cost:*** 0.1 mg/ml of 1:1000 solution; 10 ml: $12-$14 ***Pregnancy category:*** B	Urinary retention, tremors, anxiety, insomnia, headache, dizziness, cerebral hemorrhage, palpitations, tachycardia, hypertension, dysrhythmias, anorexia, nausea, vomiting, dyspnea
For severe reaction, give both H_1 and H_2 antihistamines.			
Diphenhydramine (H_1) (Benadryl), 25-50 mg IV, IM, or PO q6h × 24 hours	Blocks histamine at H_1 receptor sites	***Contraindications:*** Hypersensitivity; acute asthma attack ***Cost:*** 25-mg tab, 100 tabs: $2-$20; 50 mg/ml, 10 ml: $4-$17 ***Pregnancy category:*** B	Dizziness, drowsiness, fatigue, anxiety, euphoria, increased thick secretions, wheezing, chest tightness, thrombocytopenia, agranulocytosis, hemolytic anemia, dry mouth, nausea, anorexia, photosensitivity, urinary retention, dysuria, blurred vision, dilated pupils, tinnitus, nasal stuffiness, dry nose and/or throat
Cimetidine (H_2) (Tagamet), 300 mg IV over 3-5 minutes	Blocks histamine at H_2 receptor sites	***Contraindication:*** Hypersensitivity ***Cost:*** 300 mg/2 ml, 50 ml: $45-$100 ***Pregnancy category:*** B	Confusion, headache, depression, dizziness, anxiety, weakness, convulsions, bradycardia, tachycardia, diarrhea, paralytic ileus, jaundice, gynecomastia, agranulocytosis, thrombocytopenia, neutropenia, aplastic anemia, increased prothrombin time, urticaria, exfoliative dermatitis

Anemia, Iron Deficiency

OVERVIEW

Iron deficiency anemia occurs as a result of depletion of iron stores.

Pathogenesis

- Iron loss exceeds intake
- Stored iron is depleted
- Causes:
  - In adults, generally only as a result of bleeding
  - In infant, adolescent, and geriatric populations, may be dietary

Patient Profile

- Females > Males
- Any age
- Very common in menstruating females

Signs and Symptoms

- May be asymptomatic early
- Fatigue
- Dyspnea
- Headache
- Irritability
- Listlessness
- Poor concentration
- Pallor
- Spoon shaped, brittle nails
- Cheilitis
- Increased susceptibility to infections

Differential Diagnosis

- Anemia of chronic disease
- Any disease causing acute or chronic blood loss
- Defective iron utilization
- Defective iron reutilization
- Decreased erythropoietin production

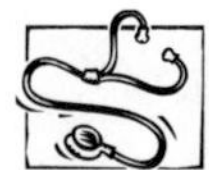

ASSESSMENT

History

Inquire about:

- Onset and duration of symptoms
- Past history of gastrointestinal (GI) bleeding
- GI complaints
- Color of stool
- Menstrual history—age at menarche, length of cycle, length of menses, number of pads or tampons used
- Recent surgery
- Underlying conditions
- Current medications, including use of aspirin and nonsteroidal antiinflammatory drugs

Physical Findings

- Pallor, particularly of conjunctivae
- Nails—spoon shaped, brittle
- Cheilosis
- Abdominal examination—tenderness and enlargement of spleen
- Physical examination may be within normal limits, with mild anemia

Initial Workup

Laboratory

- CBC—hemoglobin—13 g/dl or less (men), 12 g/dl or less (women); hematocrit—38% or less (men), 35% or less (women); RBC count—decreased; mean corpuscular volume (MCV)—low
- Serum ferritin (best noninvasive test)—decreased
- Serum iron—decreased and total iron-binding capacity—increased (less sensitive and less specific than ferritin)
- B_{12} and folate level within normal limits
- Stool for occult blood
- Reticulocyte count—decreased

Radiology: Upper and lower GI series or endoscopy

Further Workup

Bone marrow aspiration; must search for cause in men and nonmenstruating women

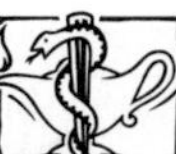

INTERVENTIONS

Office Treatment

None indicated

Lifestyle Modification

Diet rich in protein and iron-containing foods

Patient Education

Teach patient about:

- Condition and cause
- Treatment—must treat underlying cause
- Iron supplement
- Foods high in protein and iron
- Increasing dietary fiber to prevent constipation from iron
- Limiting milk to 1 pint per day for adults
- No milk or other dairy products, antacids, or tetracycline within 2 hours of iron supplement
- Medications used and side effects (see Pharmacotherapeutics)

Referral

To MD if unable to identify cause

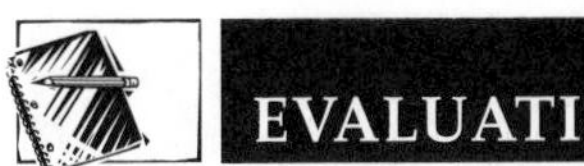

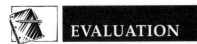

EVALUATION

Outcome
Underlying cause corrected; anemia reversed

Possible Complication
Severe hemorrhage from unidentified bleeding point

Follow-up
Every 2 weeks × 2; then monthly × 2; then every 3 to 6 months

FOR YOUR INFORMATION

Life Span
Pediatric: Infants frequently suffer from iron deficiency anemia, since their major source of nutrition is cow's milk
Geriatric: May be diet related but must rule out other causes of blood loss, such as chronic disease or medications
Pregnancy: Pregnant patient should take prenatal vitamins with iron

Miscellaneous
An iron overdose is extremely toxic. Iron tablets should be kept out of reach of children, and patients should be cautioned to take them only as directed.

References
Waterbury L: Anemia. In Barker LR, Burton JR, Zieve PD, editors: *Principles of ambulatory medicine,* ed 4, Baltimore, 1995, Williams & Wilkins, pp 595-596.

Whedon M, Daly L, Jennings B: Nursing assessment: hematologic system. In Lewis SM, Collier IC, Heitkemper MM, editors: *Medical-surgical nursing: assessment and management of clinical problems,* ed 4, St Louis, 1996, Mosby, pp 778-783.

NOTES

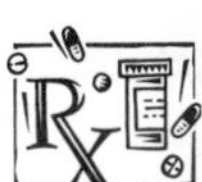

PHARMACOTHERAPEUTICS

Drug of Choice	Mechanism of Action	Prescribing Information	Side Effects
Ferrous sulfate, 300 mg PO tid 1 hour before meals; can be taken with meals but will reduce delivery of iron by up to 50%; children, 3 mg/kg/day in divided doses; do not administer concomitantly with antacids or tetracyclines	Replaces depleted iron stores	***Contraindications:*** Hypersensitivity; ulcerative colitis; Crohn's disease; hemosiderosis; hemochromatosis; peptic ulcer disease; hemolytic anemia; cirrhosis ***Cost:*** 300-mg tab, 100 tabs: $3-$7 ***Pregnancy category:*** A	Nausea, constipation, epigastric pain, black tarry stools, vomiting, diarrhea

Anemia, Pernicious

OVERVIEW

Pernicious anemia is a megaloblastic anemia caused by vitamin B_{12} deficiency.

Pathogenesis

- Autoimmune disease
- Intrinsic factor secretion by parietal cells of gastric mucosa fails because of gastric mucosal atrophy; leads to decreased B_{12} absorption in terminal ileum

Patient Profile

- Females > Males
- Older adults >60 years of age
- Most common in persons of Northern European ancestry and African-Americans

Signs and Symptoms

- Atrophic glossitis
- Sore tongue
- Anorexia
- Nausea
- Vomiting
- Abdominal pain
- Pallor
- Palpitations
- Weakness
- Paresthesias
- Ataxia
- Muscle weakness
- Confusion
- Dementia
- Exertional dyspnea
- Poor finger coordination
- Reduced vibratory sense
- Tachycardia
- Tinnitus
- Vertigo

Differential Diagnosis

- Alcoholism
- Hypothyroidism
- Drug effects
- Liver dysfunction
- Myelodysplasia
- Folic acid deficiency

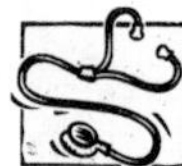

ASSESSMENT

History

Inquire about:

- Onset and duration of symptoms
- Alcohol intake
- Family history of B_{12} deficiency
- Diet—24-hour diet recall
- Underlying conditions
- Current medications

Physical Findings

- Red, shiny tongue
- Pallor
- Tachycardia
- Neurologic examination—poor finger coordination, decreased position sense, positive Romberg's sign, positive Babinski's sign
- Decreased vibration sense
- Weight loss
- Abdominal examination—hepatomegaly, splenomegaly
- Mental status examination—confusion, dementia

Initial Workup

Laboratory

- CBC with differential—decreased hemoglobin and hematocrit; mean corpuscular volume increased to 110 to 140
- Peripheral smear—poikilocytosis, anisocytosis, Howell-Jolly bodies, macrocytes, hypersegmented neutrophils
- Serum ferritin increased
- Serum B_{12} level < 100 pg/ml (<74 pmol/L)
- Direct bilirubin increased
- Schilling's test—decreased

Radiology: None indicated

Further Workup

Bone marrow aspiration

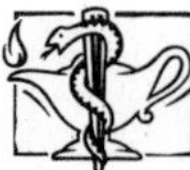

INTERVENTIONS

Office Treatment

None indicated

Lifestyle Modifications:

- Adjusting to chronic disease requiring treatment for life
- Diet high in meat, animal protein foods, legumes

Patient Education

Teach patient about

- Condition and treatment—vitamin B_{12} replacement for life
- Administering injection—may be given IM or deep subcutaneously; may need to teach a significant other to administer
- Diet high in meat, animal protein foods, legumes
- Medications used and side effects (see Pharmacotherapeutics)

Referrals

- To home health nurse for B_{12} administration
- To dietitian

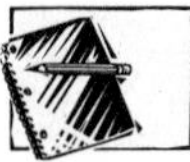

EVALUATION

Outcomes

- Anemia can be reversed
- Long-standing neurologic problems may improve but not reverse

Possible Complications

- Permanent, irreversible neurologic symptoms
- Stomach cancer
- Gastric polyps

Follow-up

In 2 weeks to evaluate response; then every 3 months

FOR YOUR INFORMATION

Life Span

Pediatric: Can have congenital pernicious anemia, which manifests itself before age 3, or juvenile pernicious anemia in older children
Geriatric: More common in this age group
Pregnancy: N/A

Miscellaneous

N/A

References

Mansen TJ, McCance KL, Parker-Cohen PD: Alterations of erythrocyte function. In McCance KL, Huether SE, editors: *Pathophysiology: the biological basis for diseases in adults and children,* ed 2, St Louis, 1994, Mosby, p 865.

Woolliscroft JO: *Current diagnosis and treatment: a quick reference for the general practitioner,* Philadelphia, 1996, Current Medicine, pp 24-25.

NOTES

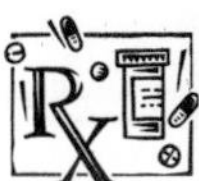

PHARMACOTHERAPEUTICS

Drug of Choice	Mechanism of Action	Prescribing Information	Side Effects
Cyanocobalamin (vitamin B_{12}), 100 μg IM or deep SQ × 7 days; if no improvement observed, give same amount every other day × 7 days, then every 3-4 days × 2-3 weeks, then 100 μg/month for life; may increase dose as needed to obtain normal hematologic values; maximum dose 1000 μg	Vitamin B_{12} replacement	***Contraindications:*** Hypersensitivity; optic nerve atrophy ***Cost:*** 100 μg/ml, 1 ml: $3 ***Pregnancy category:*** A	Flushing, optic nerve atrophy, diarrhea, congestive heart failure (CHF), peripheral vascular thrombosis, pulmonary edema, itching, rash, pain at injection site, hypokalemia, anaphylactic shock

Anemia, Sickle Cell

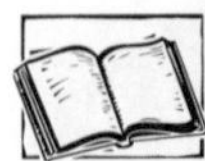

OVERVIEW

Sickle cell anemia is a severe, chronic hemoglobinopathy. It occurs in people who are homozygous for hemoglobin S and is marked by severe anemia, painful "crises," and infections. There is a heterozygous condition in which the patient has hemoglobin A/S; it is called sickle cell trait, and the patient is usually asymptomatic, with no anemia.

Pathogenesis

- Autosomal recessive genetic disorder
- Hemoglobin S develops because a valine amino acid is substituted for a glutamic acid → abnormal linking reaction → lowered O_2 tension → deformed, crescent-shaped RBCs
- Abnormally shaped cell cannot travel through small blood vessels → more oxygen deprivation → more sickling → more sluggish circulation
- Body hemolyzes abnormal cell → vaso-occlusive crises from tissue necrosis

Patient Profile

- Males = Females
- First symptoms after 6 months of age
- Predominantly African-Americans
- Can affect people from Mediterranean, Caribbean, South and Central America, Arabia, or East India

Signs and Symptoms

- Pallor
- Painful, symmetric swelling of hands and feet
- Failure to thrive
- Chronic hemolytic anemia
- Mild scleral icterus
- Painful crises in bones, joints, abdomen, back, viscera
- Infections
- Delayed physical/sexual development

Differential Diagnosis

- Sickle cell–beta thalassemia
- Other hemoglobinopathies
- Infections

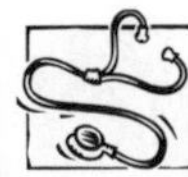

ASSESSMENT

History

Inquire about:

- Onset and duration of symptoms
- Family history of sickle cell anemia
- Previous medical treatment received
- Underlying conditions
- Current medications

Physical Findings

- Pallor
- Symmetric swelling of hands and feet
- Scleral icterus
- Delayed growth and development
- Failure to thrive

Initial Workup

Laboratory

- CBC with differential: hemoglobin—5 to 11 g/dl; indices usually normal; platelets—increased
- Peripheral smear—few sickled RBCs and nucleated RBCs
- Hemoglobin electrophoresis—Hgb S predominates, no Hgb A
- In sickle cell trait, Hgb S & A present
- Sickledex test
- Reticulocyte count—increased
- Serum bilirubin—mildly elevated

Radiology

- Skeletal x-ray films to rule out bone and joint deformities
- Bone scan to rule out osteomyelitis
- CT scan or MRI of head to rule out CVA

Further Workup

None indicated

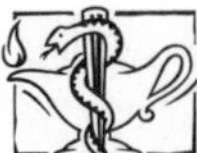

INTERVENTIONS

Office Treatment

If in severe, painful crises, immediate hospitalization

Lifestyle Modifications

- Adjustment to chronic disease
- Prevention of crises
- Wearing or carrying of medical alert tag at all times

Patient Education

Teach patient about:

- Disease and treatment—no cure for disease
- Prevention of crises—avoiding dehydration, high altitudes, viral or bacterial infections; seeking treatment at first sign or symptom (temperature >101° F [38.3° C]); avoiding emotional or physical stress or using stress reduction techniques (biofeedback, relaxation therapy, yoga); no smoking
- Fact that crises may occur spontaneously
- Obtaining a medical alert tag and wearing it at all times
- Pain management during crises—medications, guided imagery, relaxation techniques, therapeutic touch
- Mild cases—treat as outpatient, use acetaminophen or ibuprofen
- Severe cases—hospitalization required, treat with narcotic analgesics
- Medications used and side effects (see Pharmacotherapeutics)

Referral

To specialist in sickle cell disease

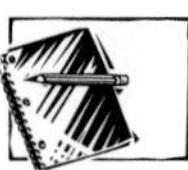

EVALUATION

Outcomes

- Minimize number of crises
- Live as normal a life as possible
- Rarely live past 50 years of age

Possible Complications

- Bone infarction
- Cerebrovascular accident
- Aseptic necrosis of femoral head
- Priapism
- Chronic leg ulcers
- Serious infections
- Cardiac enlargement

Follow-up

- Routine assessment of growth and development
- Regular immunizations, including yearly flu vaccine and pneumonia vaccine every 5 years
- Frequency of office visits depends on number and severity of crises
- Will probably be followed by specialist

FOR YOUR INFORMATION

Life Span

Pediatric: Usually diagnosed after 12 weeks of age; very difficult for child psychologically
Geriatric: Rarely live past 50 years
Pregnancy: Very complicated and hazardous; fetal mortality—35% to 40%

Miscellaneous

For contraception consider Depo-Provera. Women with sickle cell anemia should be encouraged to seek genetic counseling before getting pregnant.

References

Whedon MB: Nursing role in management: hematologic problems. In Lewis SM, Collier IC, Heitkemper MM, editors: *Medical-surgical nursing: assessment and management of clinical problems,* ed 4, St Louis, 1996, Mosby, pp 788-791.

Woolliscroft JO: *Current diagnosis and treatment: a quick reference for the general practitioner,* Philadelphia, 1996, Current Medicine, pp 362-363.

NOTES

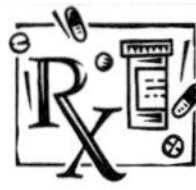

PHARMACOTHERAPEUTICS

The medications presented here are for mild cases. For severe cases, hospitalize and treat with parenteral narcotics—meperidine hydrochloride (Demerol) or morphine—and IV fluids to correct dehydration.

Drug of Choice	Mechanism of Action	Prescribing Information	Side Effects
Acetaminophen (Tylenol), 325 mg-650 mg PO every 4-6 hours; for children, use Children's Tylenol and follow label directions	Decreases fever through action on hypothalamic heat-regulating center of brain; analgesia by increasing pain threshold	***Contraindications:*** Hypersensitivity; bleeding disorders or anticoagulant therapy; last trimester of pregnancy; asthma; gastric ulcers ***Cost:*** OTC ***Pregnancy category:*** Not categorized	Rash; hepatic toxicity with alcohol ingestion or overdose
Ibuprofen (Motrin), 400 mg qid PO; children 6 mo to 12 yr, 5-10 mg/kg PO q6h	Not well understood; may be related to inhibition of prostaglandin synthesis	***Contraindications:*** Aspirin allergy; hypersensitivity; asthma; last trimester of pregnancy; gastric ulcer; bleeding disorders ***Cost:*** 400-mg tab, 4/day × 5 days: $3 ***Pregnancy category:*** Not categorized but not recommended	Nausea, heartburn, diarrhea, GI upset and bleeding, dizziness, headache, rash, tinnitus, edema, acute renal failure

Angina Pectoris

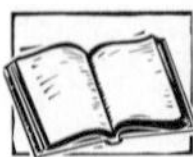

OVERVIEW

Angina pectoris is literally defined as pain (angina) in the chest (pectoris). It occurs as a result of myocardial ischemia and usually lasts only a short time. It typically occurs as a result of a precipitating event, such as exertion.

Pathogenesis

- Cause—myocardial ischemia due to myocardial O_2 demand exceeding the amount of O_2 the coronary arteries can supply, usually as a result of narrowing of coronary arteries
- Types of angina:
    - Stable angina—chest pain with same pattern of onset, duration, and severity—usually exercise induced
    - Unstable angina—increasing severity, frequency, and duration—often occurs at rest; may indicate impending myocardial infarction
    - Prinzmetal's angina—often occurs at rest; caused by coronary artery spasms

Patient Profile

- Males > Females
- Middle-aged and older men
- Postmenopausal women

Signs and Symptoms

- Chest pain, tightness, pressure, heaviness; may radiate to back, neck, arms
- Brought on by exercise, emotional stress, heavy meal
- Shortness of breath
- Nausea
- Diaphoresis
- Epigastric pain
- Weakness

Differential Diagnosis

- Esophageal spasm
- Peptic ulcer
- Gastritis
- Pericarditis
- Aortic dissection
- Mitral valve prolapse
- Pulmonary hypertension
- Costochondritis
- Pleurisy
- Pneumothorax
- Pulmonary embolism

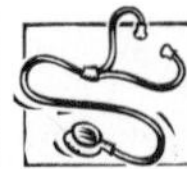

ASSESSMENT

History

Inquire about:

- Onset and duration of symptoms
- Precipitating factors
- Quality/intensity of pain
- Treatment tried and results
- Past history of heart problems
- Associated symptoms of nausea, shortness of breath
- Risk factors—smoking, hypertension, elevated cholesterol, family history
- Underlying conditions
- Current medications

Physical Findings

- Complete physical examination—may be within normal limits if not during an attack
- During attack:
    - General appearance—diaphoretic, pallor, apprehension, dyspnea
    - Increased BP, heart rate
    - Neck—look for jugular vein distention
    - Heart—third or fourth heart sound may be present
    - Assess peripheral pulses
    - Extremities—assess for edema
    - Lungs—assess for adventitious sounds

Initial Workup

Laboratory

- No test diagnostic for angina
- Cholesterol panel: total cholesterol—increased; HDL cholesterol—decreased; LDL cholesterol—increased
- Cardiac enzymes—should be within normal limits

Radiology

- Stress echocardiography
- Stress thallium
- Coronary angiography

Further Workup

- ECG—frequently within normal limits
- Exercise stress testing

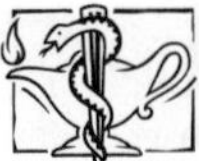

INTERVENTIONS

Office Treatment

If patient unstable (pain >20 minutes, pulmonary edema, mitral regurgitation murmur, ST segment changes, S3 or rales, or hypotension), transport to emergency room

Lifestyle Modifications

- Smoking cessation
- Stress reduction
- Moderate exercise program
- Low-cholesterol diet

Patient Education

Teach patient about:

- Condition and treatment
- Tips for smoking cessation
- Stress reduction—biofeedback, relaxation therapy, yoga
- Moderate exercise program, such as walking
- Low-cholesterol, low-fat diet
- Possible surgical procedures—coronary artery bypass grafting, percutaneous transluminal coronary angioplasty
- Medications used and side effects (see Pharmacotherapeutics)

Referral

To cardiologist for evaluation

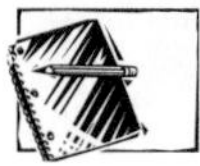

EVALUATION

Outcome
Depends on extent of coronary artery disease and willingness to make lifestyle modifications

Possible Complications
- Myocardial infarction
- Arrhythmias
- Cardiac arrest
- Congestive heart failure

Follow-up
For stable patient, every 3 to 6 months

FOR YOUR INFORMATION

Lifespan
Pediatric: In children with coronary artery disease, suspect hereditary lipid disorder
Geriatric: May not have typical chest pain; use medications cautiously and in lowest effective dose
Pregnancy: Should be under the care of an obstetrician and cardiologist

Miscellaneous
Risk factors for angina include hypertension, tobacco abuse, alcohol abuse, male gender, hypercholesterolemia, family history, obesity, and diabetes mellitus.

References
Braunwald E et al: *Diagnosing and managing unstable angina,* Quick Reference Guide for Clinicians No 10, AHCPR Pub No 94-0603, Rockville, Md, 1994, US Department of Health and Human Services, Public Health Service, Agency for Health Care Policy and Research and National Heart, Lung, and Blood Institute.
Massie BM: Heart. In Tierney LM Jr, McPhee SJ, Papadakis MA, editors: *Current medical diagnosis and treatment,* ed 34, Norwalk, Conn, Appleton & Lange, pp 309-315.
Uphold CR, Graham MV: *Clinical guidelines in adult health,* Gainesville, Fla, 1994, Barmarrae Books, pp 296-304.

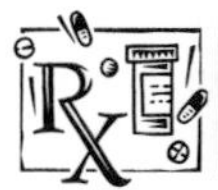

PHARMACOTHERAPEUTICS

Drug of Choice	Mechanism of Action	Prescribing Information	Side Effects
Nitroglycerin, 0.3-0.4 mg sublingually when attack begins; repeat q5min × 3; if no relief, seek emergency treatment; take 1 tab sublingually 5-10 minutes before activity; may also be used in the transdermal patch form or long-acting tabs	Dilates coronary arteries, which improves blood flow	***Contraindications:*** Hypersensitivity; severe anemia; increased intracranial pressure; cerebral hemorrhage ***Cost:*** 0.3-mg tab, 100 tabs: $7; sustained-release, 2.5-mg tab, 100 tabs: $5-$17; transdermal patch, 0.3 mg/hr, 30 disks: $46-$57 ***Pregnancy category:*** C	Postural hypotension, tachycardia, syncope, nausea, vomiting, pallor, sweating, rash, headache, flushing, dizziness
Aspirin, 80-325 mg PO qd	Decreases platelet aggregation	***Contraindications:*** Hypersensitivity; bleeding disorders or anticoagulant therapy; last trimester of pregnancy; asthma; gastric ulcers ***Cost:*** OTC ***Pregnancy category:*** Not categorized	Rash, anaphylactic reactions, GI upset and bleeding
Beta-blocker: propranolol (Inderal), 30-120 mg PO bid or tid or 160 mg PO qd extended-release; many other beta-blockers available, including atenolol, betaxolol, bisoprolol, esmolol, levobunolol, metoprolol, sotalol, and timolol—see manufacturer's insert for prescribing information	Reduces myocardial O_2 requirement by decreasing heart rate, myocardial contractility, and blood pressure	***Contraindications:*** Hypersensitivity; cardiac failure; cardiogenic shock; 2nd- or 3rd-degree heart block; bronchospastic disease; sinus bradycardia; (CHF) ***Cost:*** 40-mg tab, 100 tabs: $2-$40 ***Pregnancy category:*** C	Bronchospasm, dyspnea, bradycardia, hypotension, congestive heart failure (CHF), palpitations, atrioventricular (AV) block, agranulocytosis, thrombocytopenia, nausea, vomiting, diarrhea, constipation, impotence, decreased libido, joint pain, arthralgia, facial swelling, rash, pruritus, depression, hallucinations, dizziness, fatigue, lethargy, sore throat, laryngospasm, blurred vision
Calcium channel blocker: nifedipine (Procardia XL), 30-120 mg PO qd; may also use verapamil, diltiazem, nicardipine, and amlodipine	Induces coronary artery vasodilation, which reduces myocardial O_2 requirements	***Contraindication:*** Hypersensitivity ***Cost:*** 30-mg tab, 100 tabs: $95 ***Pregnancy category:*** C	Headache, fatigue, drowsiness, dizziness, anxiety, depression, weakness, insomnia, tinnitus, dysrhythmias, edema, CHF, hypotension, pulmonary edema, nausea, vomiting, diarrhea, constipation, nocturia, polyuria, rash, pruritus, photosensitivity, flushing, sexual difficulties, fever, chills

Animal Bites

OVERVIEW

Bite wounds to human beings may be caused by dogs, cats, or other mammals, including humans.

Pathogenesis

- Dog and cat bites fairly common
- Most dog and cat bites are from domestic animals—dog and cat bites usually occur as a result of an insult to the animal; animal lashes back at intruder
- Human bites are usually from someone hitting another person in the face with a fist
- Most bites occur to hands
- Bites allow introduction of bacteria into wound, resulting in wound infection

Patient Profile

- Males = Females
- Any age

Signs and Symptoms

- Tears
- Punctures
- Scratches
- Avulsion or crush injuries
- Erythema
- Bleeding and loose tissue possibly
- Dog bites—hands most common site bitten, followed by face, lower extremities, and very rarely the trunk
- Cat bites—more commonly puncture-type wounds; more common to hands, lower extremities, face, and trunk
- If infection present, may have pain, decreased range of motion (ROM) swelling, purulent drainage, fever

Differential Diagnosis

If appropriate history is obtained and skin wound present, diagnosis fairly straight forward

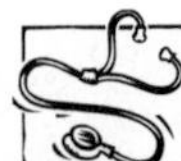

ASSESSMENT

History

Inquire about:

- When wound occurred—important to ascertain how much time has elapsed since wound occurred—delay in seeking treatment can mean bacteria have proliferated
- Whether animal was domestic or nondomestic
- Whether animal was being provoked or not—most animals with rabies bite when unprovoked
- Condition of the animal—did it appear ill?
- Where the animal is
- Immunizations of the animal—all up to date? (If unknown, local rabies control facility needs to be notified so that animal can be taken into custody. Check local guidelines for reporting procedures.)
- Tetanus immunization status and any prior rabies immunization
- Whether alcohol was involved
- OTC preparations that have been tried
- Underlying conditions
- Current medications

Physical Findings

- Check distal to wound for neurovascular compromise and motor function—check ROM and sensation
- May find a puncture, scratch, avulsion, or tear injury; check extent of tissue damage
- Check for tendon or bone damage
- May be some bleeding and erythema
- Look for any purulent drainage—may indicate infection is already present

Initial Workup

Laboratory

- Culture and sensitivity of wound—85% of all bite wounds have a positive culture
- If wound is more than 24 hours old, consider CBC with differential

Radiology: Plain radiograph of bone or joint if indicated

Further Workup

May need surgical exploration to assess extent of injury

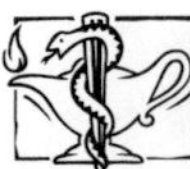

INTERVENTIONS

Lifestyle Modifications

- Alcohol rehabilitation if appropriate
- Caution patients against approaching unknown animals

Patient Education

Teach patient about:

- Ways of preventing recurrence
- Signs and symptoms of infection
- Changing dressing
- Elevating injured part to prevent swelling
- Medications used and side effects (see Pharmacotherapeutics).

Office Treatment

- Irrigate with copious amounts of saline under pressure, using a Water-Pik or large syringe and needle
- Scrub surrounding tissue with povidone-iodine and rinse with saline
- Debride wound and trim jagged edges
- Suture wound or use a Steri-Strip if clean and less than 12 hours old
- Do not suture wounds that are likely to get infected, such as hand bites, bites that are older than 12 hours old, deep or puncture bites, or bites with extensive injury
- Apply pressure dressing
- May apply topical antibiotic (controversial)
- Splint hand
- Use of antibiotic prophylaxis is controversial, but generally recommended
- Give tetanus toxoid if it has been 5 years or longer since immunization
- Consider antirabies therapy if serious concern that animal was rabid

Referral

To surgeon or plastic surgeon if wound involves tendons, joints, bone, or bites of ears, face, or genitalia

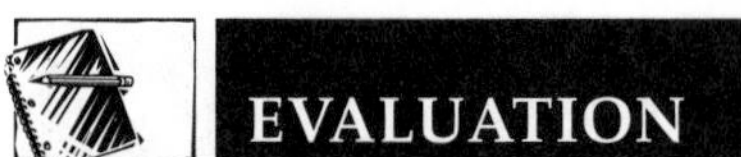

EVALUATION

Outcome
Wound heals without sequelae in 7 to 10 days

Possible Complications
- Septic arthritis
- Osteomyelitis
- Extensive soft tissue injury
- Sepsis
- Hemorrhage
- Gas gangrene
- Death

Follow-up
- If no signs of infection at initial visit, follow in 48 hours; then in 10 days
- If infection present, see daily until infection controlled

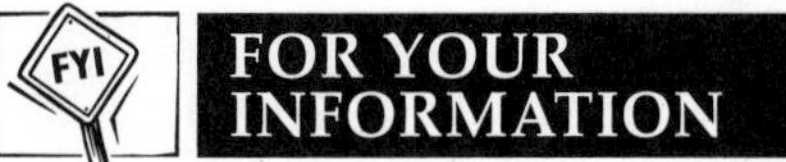

FOR YOUR INFORMATION

Life Span
Pediatric: Be alert to possibility of child abuse
Geriatric: Increased risk of infection; be alert to possibility of elder abuse
Pregnancy: Cautious use of medication

Miscellaneous
There is an increased risk of serious injury and infection in the elderly. The elderly may also be less forthcoming with information regarding the animal that caused the bite if it is their own pet. Elderly patients are very fond of their animals and may be afraid that you, as the provider, will cause them to lose the animal. It is important to question them carefully and avoid being judgmental in your query.

References
Habif TP: *Clinical dermatology: a color guide to diagnosis and therapy,* ed 3, St Louis, 1996, Mosby, p 477.

Uphold CR, Graham MV: *Clinical guidelines in adult health,* Gainesville, Fla, 1994, Barmarrae Books, pp 693-696.

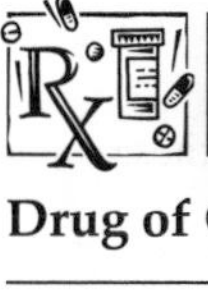

PHARMACOTHERAPEUTICS

Drug of Choice	Mechanism of Action	Prescribing Information	Side Effects
Amoxicillin/clavulanate (Augmentin), 500-875 mg PO bid for 3 days; may be used in established infection for 10 days; children, 25-45 mg/kg/day PO in 2 divided doses	Bactericidal; cell wall inhibitor; effective against beta-lactamase–producing organisms	***Contraindication:*** Hypersensitivity ***Cost:*** 500-mg tab, 20 tabs: $82 ***Pregnancy category:*** B	Diarrhea, nausea, vomiting, stomatitis, black hairy tongue, pseudomembranous colitis, candidiasis, rash, urticaria, angioedema, anaphylaxis, arthralgia, myalgia, anemia, thrombocytopenia, leukopenia, anxiety, insomnia, confusion
Penicillin VK, 500 mg PO qid for 3 days; children <12 years, 15-50 mg/kg/day PO in 4 divided doses × 3 days for prophylaxis	Bactericidal cell wall inhibitor; effective against gram-positive cocci, most anaerobes, and *Neisseria*	***Contraindication:*** Hypersensitivity ***Cost:*** 500-mg tab, 12 tabs: $4 ***Pregnancy category:*** B	Bone marrow depression, granulocytopenia, nausea, vomiting, diarrhea, oliguria, proteinuria, hematuria, moniliasis, glomerulonephritis, lethargy, depression, convulsions, anaphylaxis
Amoxicillin, 500 mg tid for 3 days; 20-40 mg/kg/day in 3 divided doses × 3 days for prophylaxis	Bactericidal; broad-spectrum; *not* effective against beta-lactamase–producing pathogens	***Contraindications:*** Hypersensitivity to penicillins ***Cost:*** 500-mg tabs, 9 tabs: $4 ***Pregnancy category:*** B	Anaphylactoid reaction, nausea, vomiting, diarrhea, rashes, Stevens-Johnson syndrome, pseudomembranous colitis
Erythromycin (E.E.S.), 500 mg PO bid for 10 days; children, 30-50 mg/kg/day in 4 divided doses × 10 days; may be used for prophylaxis or established infections	Macrolide; protein synthesis inhibitor; active against bacteria lacking cell walls, most gram-positive aerobes	***Contraindication:*** Hypersensitivity ***Cost:*** 250-mg tabs, 40 tabs: $4 ***Pregnancy category:*** B	Nausea, vomiting, diarrhea, abdominal pain, anorexia, rash, urticaria, pseudomembranous colitis—rarely

Ankylosing Spondylitis

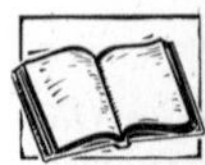

OVERVIEW

Ankylosing spondylitis is a chronic inflammatory disease of the joints of the axial skeleton. The hallmark of the disease is progressive morning stiffness of the low back and sacroiliac joint.

Pathogenesis

Cause—unknown; frequently familial

Patient Profile

- Males > Females
- Usually begins around 15 to 30 years of age

Signs and Symptoms

- Early-morning low-back stiffness (lasting >3 months)
- Bilateral sacroiliac tenderness
- Stiffness improves with activity, worsens with rest
- Joints involved are usually hips, shoulders, and/or knees; any other joint may be involved
- Pleuritic chest pain with decreased chest expansion on inhalation
- Anterior uveitis
- Aortic regurgitation murmur

Differential Diagnosis

- Reiter's syndrome
- Psoriatic arthritis
- Arthritis associated with inflammatory bowel disease
- Rheumatoid arthritis

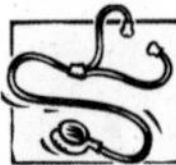

ASSESSMENT

History

Inquire about:

- Onset and duration of symptoms
- Family history of ankylosing spondylitis
- Underlying conditions
- Current medications

Physical Findings

- Decreased range of motion (ROM) in lumbar spine
- Bilateral sacroiliac tenderness
- Decreased chest expansion (<2 to 5 cm, measured at fourth intercostal space)
- Anterior uveitis
- Murmur of aortic regurgitation

Initial Workup

Laboratory

- Erythrocyte sedimentation rate—elevated
- CBC—mild hypochromic anemia
- HLA-B27 tissue antigen—present in 90% to 100% of cases

Radiology

- Films of sacroiliac joints and lumbar spine—bilateral sacroiliitis
- Squaring of vertebral bodies in lumbar spine gives appearance of bamboo

Further Workup

None indicated

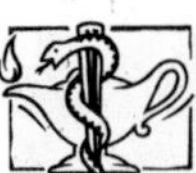

INTERVENTIONS

Office Treatment

None indicated

Lifestyle Modifications

- Smoking cessation
- Maintenance of active lifestyle

Patient Education

Teach patient about:

- Condition and treatment—nonsteroidal antiinflammatory medication
- Posture training—avoiding stooping, sitting erect
- ROM exercises
- Sleeping on a firm mattress or bed board; supine position; no pillows under knees
- Performing breathing exercises 2 to 3 times daily
- Importance of maintaining ideal body weight
- Swimming as excellent exercise
- Tips for smoking cessation
- Surgical options if disease progresses—hip arthroplasty (reankylosis may occur)
- Medications used and side effects (see Pharmacotherapeutics)

Referral

To orthopedist for severe cases or those resistant to treatment

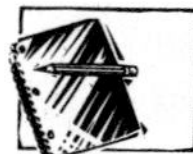

EVALUATION

Outcome
Very unpredictable—some resolve without sequelae; others result in progressive disability

Possible Complications
- Pseudoarthrosis
- Cervical spine fracture
- Restrictive lung disease
- Cardiac conduction defects

Follow-up
Initially every 2 weeks × 2; if stable, every 3 months

FOR YOUR INFORMATION

Life Span
Pediatric: May have onset in adolescence
Geriatric: Rare onset after age 40
Pregnancy: May pose problems for natural childbirth

Miscellaneous
N/A

References
Hellman DB: Arthritis and musculoskeletal disorders. In Tierney LM Jr, McPhee SJ, Papadakis MA, editors: *Current medical diagnosis and treatment,* ed 34, Norwalk, Conn, 1995, Appleton & Lange, pp 729-730.

Mercier LR: *Practical orthopedics,* ed 4, St Louis, 1995, Mosby, pp 160-163.

NOTES

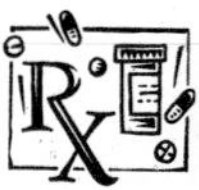

PHARMACOTHERAPEUTICS

Drug of Choice	Mechanism of Action	Prescribing Information	Side Effects
Aspirin, enteric coated, 1 g PO tid or qid; may increase by 300-600 mg/day each week until maximal response seen or toxicity occurs (tinnitus usually 1st symptom); if toxicity occurs, decrease by 600-900 mg/day every 3 days until symptoms resolve	Antiinflammatory action may be caused by inhibition of synthesis and release of prostaglandins	***Contraindications:*** Hypersensitivity; GI bleeding; bleeding disorders ***Cost:*** OTC ***Pregnancy category:*** Should not be used in 3rd trimester	Dyspepsia, thirst, nausea, vomiting, GI bleeding/ulceration, tinnitus, vertigo, reversible hearing loss, prolongation of bleeding time, leukopenia, thrombocytopenia, purpura, urticaria, angioedema, pruritus, asthma, anaphylaxis, mental confusion, drowsiness, dizziness, headache, fever
Nonsteroidal antiinflammatory drugs (NSAIDs): many different types currently marketed; consult manufacturer's package insert for specific dosing and prescribing information	Exact action unknown; may work by inhibition of synthesis of prostaglandins and arachidonic acid	***Contraindications:*** Hypersensitivity to NSAIDs, aspirin; severe hepatic failure; asthma ***Cost:*** Varies with type ***Pregnancy category:*** Depends on product	Stomach distress, flatulence, nausea, abdominal pain, constipation or diarrhea, dizziness, sedation, rash, urticaria, angioedema, anorexia, urinary frequency, increased blood pressure, insomnia, anxiety, visual disturbances, increased thirst, alopecia

Anorexia Nervosa

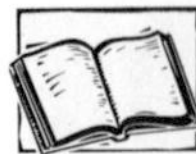

OVERVIEW

Anorexia nervosa is a psychiatric disorder in which patients are dissatisfied with their body and refuse to maintain >85% of their ideal body weight. Patients' eating habits are severely disturbed, and they will go to great lengths to hide their eating behavior from others. These patients have an intense fear of gaining weight and becoming fat, even though they are very thin.

Pathogenesis

Exact cause unknown; frequently stressors within family have occurred (divorce, death, change of location, etc.)

Patient Profile

- Females > Males
- Common age groups—adolescents and young adults

Signs and Symptoms

- Pronounced weight loss
- Claims of feeling fat
- Preoccupation with body size and weight
- Denial that a problem exists
- Refusal of food
- Extensive exercise
- Cracked/dry skin
- Sparse scalp hair
- Hypotension
- Bradycardia
- Hypothermia
- Peripheral edema
- Severe constipation
- Amenorrhea
- Breast atrophy
- Lanugo

Differential Diagnosis

- Other psychiatric illnesses—depressive disorder, food phobia, conversion disorder, schizophrenia, bulimia nervosa
- Other physical disorders causing eating difficulty—cancer, brain tumor, gastrointestinal disorders, malabsorption syndrome, Addison's disease, Crohn's disease

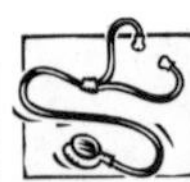

ASSESSMENT

History

Thorough history imperative; inquire about:

- Attitude toward weight
- Weight 6 months before visit
- Highest and lowest weights
- Use of recreational drugs and tobacco
- 24-hour diet record
- Frequency and type of exercise
- Menstrual history—date of last menstrual period
- Social history
- Recent stressors or changes in lifestyle
- Use of laxatives
- Use of syrup of ipecac
- Suicidal ideations
- Underlying medical conditions
- Current medications, including diuretics or appetite suppressants

Physical Findings

- Cachectic appearance
- Dry skin
- Poor skin turgor
- Lanugo
- Brittle nails
- Hair loss
- Buccal mucosa—erythematous from vomiting
- Atrophied breasts
- Peripheral edema
- Cardiac arrhythmias
- Hypoactive bowel sounds
- Hemorrhoids secondary to constipation
- Height, weight, body fat, and body mass below ideal (measure height and weight, and calculate ideal weight—women 100 pounds plus 5 pounds for every inch over 5 feet; men 110 pounds plus 5 pounds for every inch over 5 feet—measure percentage of body fat using calipers—women 22% and men 15% ideal—calculate body mass—weight in kilograms/height in centimeters squared)

Initial Workup

Laboratory

- Urinalysis—presence of ketones and protein indicate low carbohydrate metabolism
- Pregnancy test—if patient is amenorrheic
- CBC—anemia and neutropenia possibly
- Blood chemistry panel—decreased calcium, magnesium, chloride, sodium, albumin, BUN, and globulin may be seen, as well as decreased potassium (may cause cardiac arrhythmia)
- Liver function tests—to rule out other causes of weight loss; some values may be decreased as a result of malnutrition
- Endocrine tests—follicle-stimulating hormone and luteinizing hormone may be decreased; borderline low thyroid hormone levels
- ECG—arrhythmias may be present

Radiology: None indicated

Further Workup

Psychologic testing—Eating Attitudes Test, Diagnostic Survey for Eating Disorders, Eating Disorder Inventory, Bulimia Test

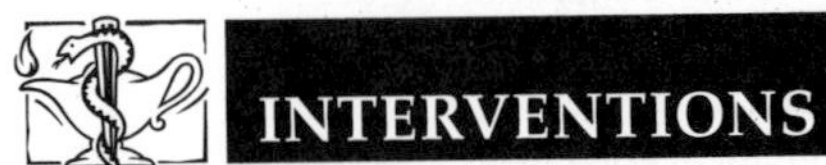

INTERVENTIONS

Office Treatment

- Build a trusting, nonjudgmental relationship with patient
- Negotiate contract with acceptable weight range, exercise plan, food intake, and follow-up

Lifestyle Modifications

- Adequate, nutritionally sound diet with consumption of three meals daily
- Cessation of use of laxatives and emetics
- Exercise in moderation
- Cessation of smoking, alcohol, or drugs if appropriate

Patient Education

Teach patient about:

- Disease process and possible end result
- Nutritionally sound diet
- Proper amount of exercise
- Need for extensive psychologic counseling
- Long-term treatment and commitment to change
- Keeping a food and exercise diary
- If any of the following are present—severe emaciation, decreased sodium and potassium levels, abnormal ECG, continuing weight loss, minimal food intake, severe depression, suicidal ideations, inability to function at school or home, etc.—need for inpatient treatment program
- Medications used and side effects (see Pharmacotherapeutics)

Referrals

- To support group
- To psychiatric NP or clinical nurse specialist specializing in eating disorders
- To psychiatrist or psychologist specializing in eating disorders

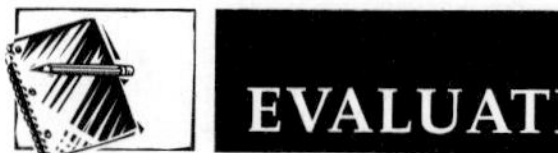

EVALUATION

Outcomes

- Improved nutritional status
- Rational attitude about weight
- Improved self-image
- Modest weight gain and moderate amounts of exercise
- Prognosis—variable; better if diagnosed at early age

Possible Complications

- Cardiac arrhythmias
- Cardiac arrest
- Exhaustion
- Collapse
- Nitrogen depletion
- Cardiomyopathy
- Congestive heart failure
- Convulsions
- Osteoporosis

Follow-Up

Monitor weight weekly until stable; then monthly

FOR YOUR INFORMATION

Life Span

Pediatric: Most commonly begins in adolescents, but is increasing in younger age group

Geriatric: May be difficult to diagnose; important to look for pathophysiologic cause

Pregnancy: Requires specialized care; high incidence of spontaneous abortions, low birth weight, and premature delivery

Miscellaneous

The mortality rate for anorexia nervosa is about 6%, with a substantial number of these patients committing suicide. It is imperative that the practitioner assess the patient's suicide potential at each visit.

References

Harris N, Seimer B: Psychosocial health concerns. In Youngkin EQ, Davis MS, editors: *Women's health: a primary care clinical guide,* Norwalk, Conn, 1994, Appleton & Lange, pp 680-684.

Scherzer LN: Adolescent patients: special considerations. In Barker LR, Burton JR, Zieve PD, editors: *Principles of ambulatory medicine,* ed 4, Baltimore, 1995, Williams & Wilkins, pp 59-61.

Westfall UE, Deters GE: Problems of nutrition. In Lewis SM, Collier IC, Heitkemper MM, editors: *Medical surgical nursing: assessment and management of clinical problems,* ed 4, St Louis, 1996, Mosby, pp 1106-1107.

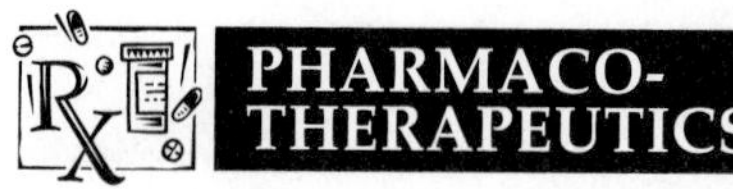

PHARMACOTHERAPEUTICS

Caution must be used when prescribing medications for a patient suffering from anorexia nervosa. Most authorities believe that medication should only be administered under the direct supervision of health care professionals while the patient is in an inpatient program. Because of the patient's poor nutritional status, medications must be started at lower-than-normal starting doses to prevent toxicity. Some of the more common medications used are benzodiazepines to decrease anxiety surrounding food and weight gain, antidepressants to treat depression, cyproheptadine to increase appetite, metoclopramide to decrease abdominal distention, and vitamin and mineral supplements. Medications should not be prescribed for more than 1 week at a time because of the potential risk of attempted suicide.

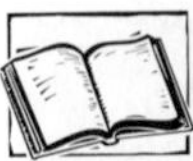

OVERVIEW

Anxiety can be defined as a psychophysiologic condition. It may be acute or chronic and is a relatively common condition. The most common characteristics of anxiety are fearful emotions, worry, nervousness, muscle tension, hyperactivity, and hypervigilance. Although it can be an adaptive response to danger, when excessive, anxiety can lead to distress and impaired functioning. There are several subtypes of anxiety:

- Acute situational anxiety—response to a recent stressful event, usually short term
- Adjustment disorder with anxiety—follows psychosocial stress and may last up to 6 months
- Generalized anxiety disorder—excessive anxiety and worry; a chronic condition
- Phobias—enduring fears of harmless objects, causing patients to go to great lengths to avoid the object or objects of their fear
- Panic disorder—recurrent or discrete attacks of intense fear and panic; may be associated with somatic symptoms or psychic symptoms of anxiety; may be with or without agoraphobia (fear of not being able to escape from a situation)
- Obsessive-compulsive disorder—persistent, recurrent, resisted thoughts and behaviors that interfere with daily life
- Posttraumatic stress disorder—intrusive recollections or dreams of a severe physical or emotional trauma; may be associated with autonomic symptoms

Pathogenesis

- Panic disorder and obsessive-compulsive disorder—genetic predisposition
- Other types may be caused by abnormalities of neurotransmitter systems, particularly serotonin and norepinephrine

Patient Profile

- Females > Males
- Most common age group—25 to 40 years
- Most common psychiatric illness

Signs and Symptoms

May vary with subtype; following is list of possible symptoms that might be seen:

- Excessive anxiety and worry
- Sense of impending doom
- Nervousness
- Tachycardia
- Palpitations
- Instability
- Hyperventilation
- Inability to swallow, with choking sensation
- Sighing respiration
- Paresthesia
- Diaphoresis
- Labile hypertension
- Dizziness or syncope
- Muscle tension
- Flushing
- Restlessness
- Headache
- Backaches
- Muscle spasm
- Chest tightness
- Recurrent nightmares
- Systolic click murmur

Differential Diagnosis

Any pathophysiologic problem that could cause above symptoms:

- Cardiovascular problems—ischemic heart disease, valvular heart disease, cardiomyopathies, myocarditis, arrhythmias, mitral valve prolapse
- Respiratory problems—asthma, emphysema, pulmonary embolism
- Central nervous system problems—transient cerebral insufficiency, psychomotor epilepsy, essential tremor
- Endocrine problems—hyperthyroidism, pheochromocytoma, adrenal insufficiency, Cushing's syndrome, hypokalemia, hypoglycemia, hyperparathyroidism
- Nutritional problems—thiamine, pyridoxine, or folate deficiency; iron deficiency anemia
- Drug abuse or withdrawal—caffeine, alcohol, cocaine, sympathomimetics, amphetamines

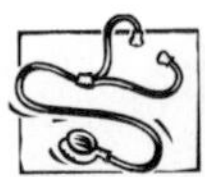

ASSESSMENT

History

Inquire about:

- Onset and duration of symptoms
- Past history of traumatic event
- Family history of anxiety disorder
- Underlying conditions
- Current medications

Physical Findings

- Anxious demeanor
- Tachycardia
- Systolic click murmur
- Hyperventilation
- Hypertension
- Abdominal pain

Initial Workup

Laboratory

- Base workup on presenting symptoms—must rule out physical causes for symptoms
- Minimum workup should include CBC with differential, chemistry panel, and thyroid function

Radiology: Chest x-ray film if indicated

Further Workup

Determined by initial workup and symptoms; consider EEG and ECG

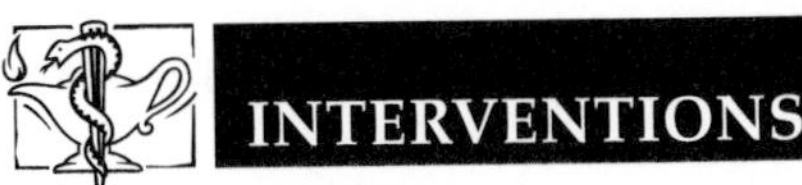

INTERVENTIONS

Office Treatment

None indicated

Lifestyle Modifications

- Cessation of alcohol or drug use
- Significantly decreased consumption or elimination of caffeine
- Nutritionally sound diet
- Regular exercise program

Patient Education

Teach patient about:

- Condition and treatment
- Relaxation techniques, such as biofeedback, muscle relaxation, diaphragmatic breathing, self-hypnosis, and meditation—can reduce autonomic activity and muscle tension
- Medications used and side effects (see Pharmacotherapeutics)

Referral

To psychiatric NP, clinical nurse specialist, psychologist, or psychiatrist as appropriate

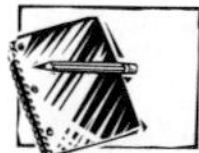

EVALUATION

Outcomes

- Control of anxiety and resumption of normal daily activities
- Obsessive-compulsive disorder and post-traumatic stress disorder—more difficult to treat, requiring long-term psychotherapy and medication

Possible Complications

- Impaired social/occupational functioning
- Medication side effects
- Dependence on benzodiazepines
- Cardiac arrhythmias with tricyclic antidepressants

Follow-up

Every 2 weeks until stable; then monthly

FOR YOUR INFORMATION

Life Span

Pediatric: Use medication cautiously and at a lower dose

Geriatric: Start medication at lower dose; monitor closely for side effects

Pregnancy: Attempt to control without medication; refer to specialist if medication needed

Miscellaneous

Many patients who suffer from anxiety also suffer from depression, which may be masked initially. Careful evaluation for depression should occur at each visit, and if depression is diagnosed, it should be treated with antidepressant medication.

Reference

Roca RP: Anxiety. In Barker LR, Burton JR, Zieve PD, editors: *Principles of ambulatory medicine,* ed 4, Baltimore, 1995, Williams & Wilkins, pp 139-152.

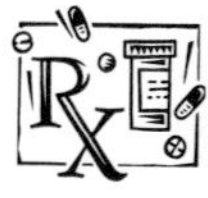

PHARMACOTHERAPEUTICS

There are many medications available for control of the various anxiety states. The following is a partial list of the most commonly used medications.

Drug of Choice	Mechanism of Action	Prescribing Information	Side Effects
Buspirone (Buspar), 5 mg PO bid-tid, maximum 60 mg daily; used for generalized anxiety disorder; not recommended for children <18 years; do not administer with monoamine oxidase inhibitors (MAOIs)	Unknown; anxiolytic	***Contraindication:*** Hypersensitivity ***Cost:*** 5-mg tab, 100 tabs: $60-$65 ***Pregnancy category:*** B	Dizziness, insomnia, nervousness, drowsiness and lightheadedness, nausea, vomiting, headache, fatigue
Benzodiazepines (alprazolam, lorazepam, diazepam)—dosage depends on drug used: • Alprazolam (Xanax), 0.5 mg PO bid-tid; not recommended for children <18 years • Lorazepam (Ativan), 1-3 mg PO bid-tid; not recommended for children <12 years • Diazepam (Valium), 2-10 mg PO tid-qid; children, 1-2.5 mg PO tid-qid • Controlled substances, Schedule IV	Antianxiety, anticonvulsant, and hypnotic effects; muscle relaxant	***Contraindications:*** Hypersensitivity; narrow-angle glaucoma; psychosis ***Cost:*** Alprazolam, 0.5-mg tab, 100 tabs: $7-$72; lorazepam, 1-mg tab, 100 tabs: $23; diazepam, 2-mg tab, 100 tabs: $2-$43 ***Pregnancy category:*** D	Drowsiness, hiccups, dizziness, loss of dexterity, constipation, confusion, nausea, decreased libido, vertigo, sleep disturbances, headaches, abdominal cramping, unsteadiness, blurred vision, addiction—all have high abuse potential
Imipramine (Tofranil), 10-25 mg PO hs, maximum dose 300 mg; used for panic disorder; for children, should only be used for nocturnal enuresis	Tricyclic antidepressant; blocks reuptake of norepinephrine	***Contraindications:*** Hypersensitivity; use of MAOIs; acute recovery phase of myocardial infarction (MI) ***Cost:*** 10-mg tab, 100 tabs: $2-$26 ***Pregnancy category:*** C	Agranulocytosis, thrombocytopenia, eosinophilia, leukopenia, dizziness, drowsiness, confusion, headache, anxiety, diarrhea, dry mouth, nausea, paralytic ileus, hepatitis, urinary retention, acute renal failure, orthostatic hypotension, tachycardia, palpitations, blurred vision
Fluvoxamine (Luvox), 50 mg PO hs, maximum dose 100-300 mg daily; used for obsessive-compulsive disorder; safety not established in children <18 years; drug potentiates or interacts with many other drugs; consult package insert for further details and before prescribing	5-Hydroxytryptamine (5-HT) reuptake inhibitor	***Contraindications:*** Coadministration of terfenadine, astemizole, or cisapride; hypersensitivity ***Cost:*** 50-mg tab, 100 tabs: $199 ***Pregnancy category:*** C	Headache, drowsiness, dizziness, convulsions, sleep disorders, nausea, anorexia, constipation, hepatotoxicity, vomiting, diarrhea, rash, sweating, decreased libido, dry mouth

Appendicitis

OVERVIEW

Appendicitis is an acute inflammation of the vermiform appendix.

Pathogenesis

Cause—obstruction of appendiceal lumen from:

- Fecaliths
- Lymphoid tissue hypertrophy
- Hardened barium
- Vegetable or fruit seeds or other foreign bodies
- Intestinal worms
- Strictures

Patient Profile

- Males > Females
- Any age, but more common from 10 to 30 years of age

Signs and Symptoms

- Gradual onset of symptoms
- Abdominal pain—starts around umbilicus and proceeds to right lower quadrant
- Constipation
- Nausea, vomiting (may be projectile)
- Muscle guarding
- Anorexia
- Slight fever
- Slight tachycardia

Differential Diagnosis

- Any condition that causes acute abdominal pain
- Acute pelvic inflammatory disease
- Twisted ovarian cyst
- Ruptured graafian follicle
- Acute gastroenteritis

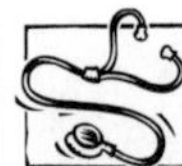

ASSESSMENT

History

Inquire about:

- Onset and duration of symptoms
- Location of pain
- Underlying conditions
- Current medications

Physical Findings

- Slight fever
- Slight tachycardia
- Muscle guarding
- Pain at McBurney's Point with rebound tenderness
- Positive obturator sign
- Positive psoas sign

Initial Workup

Laboratory

- CBC with differential—leukocytes (10,000 to 18,000), left shift
- Urinalysis—hematuria, pyuria, albuminuria

Radiology: If uncertain of diagnosis or to detect complications—KUB, barium enema, CT scan of abdomen

Further Workup

None indicated

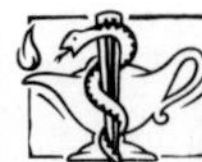

INTERVENTIONS

Office Treatment

Prompt referral to emergency room or direct hospital admission

Lifestyle Modifications

Restricted activity 4 to 6 weeks postoperatively—no heavy lifting, no driving, no pushing or pulling heavy objects

Patient Education

If time allows it, teach patient about:

- Condition and treatment options—surgical removal of appendix, either open or laparoscopic
- Turning, coughing, and deep breathing postoperatively
- Ambulation a couple of hours after surgery
- Return to regular diet after bowel sounds return (in 24 to 48 hours)
- Signs and symptoms of postoperative infection
- In uncomplicated appendicitis, one dose of antibiotic preoperatively
- In complicated appendicitis, antibiotic continued 7 days postoperatively
- Medications used and side effects (see Pharmacotherapeutics)

Referral

To surgeon

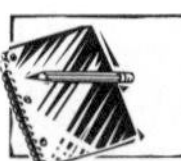

EVALUATION

Outcome
Patient recovers without sequelae

Possible Complications
- Wound infection
- Peritonitis with paralytic ileus
- Intestinal obstruction
- Incisional hernia

Follow-up
In 2 weeks and 4 weeks postoperatively

FOR YOUR INFORMATION

Life Span
Pediatric: Higher fever; more vomiting (projectile); rupture earlier; recover more quickly
Geriatric: More serious procedure in this age group; higher rate of rupture; takes longer to recover
Pregnancy: Uncommon; classic signs not present—pain in right upper quadrant or entire right side of abdomen

Miscellaneous
N/A

References
Heitkemper M, Sawchuck L: Nursing role in management: problems of absorption and elimination. In Lewis SM, Collier IC, Heitkemper MM, editors: *Medical-surgical nursing: assessment and management of clinical problems,* ed 4, St Louis, 1996, Mosby, pp 1220-1222.

Smith CW Jr: Surgical care. In Driscoll CE et al, editors: *The Family practice desk reference,* ed 3, St Louis, 1996, Mosby, pp 502-503.

NOTES

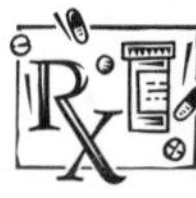

PHARMACOTHERAPEUTICS

The medications presented here are preoperative agents.

Drug of Choice	Mechanism of Action	Prescribing Information	Side Effects
Cefotetan (Cefotan), 1 g IV 1 hour before surgery—not recommended for children	Cephalosporin; broad-spectrum bactericidal	***Contraindications:*** Hypersensitivity to cephalosporins; children; use with caution in patients hypersensitive to penicillin ***Cost:*** 1 g/ml, 1 ml: $12 ***Pregnancy category:*** B	Headache; dizziness; weakness; nausea; vomiting; diarrhea; anorexia; pain; glossitis; bleeding; increased AST, ALT, and bilirubin; abdominal pain; nephrotoxicity; renal failure; leukopenia; thrombocytopenia; neutropenia; lymphocytosis; eosinophilia; pancytopenia; rash; dermatitis; anaphylaxis
Cefoxitin (Mefoxin), 1 g IV 1 hour before surgery; children, 80-160 mg/kg/day IV, 1 hour before surgery	Cephamycin; broad-spectrum bactericidal	***Contraindications:*** Hypersensitivity to cephalosporins; infants <3 months ***Cost:*** 1 mg/ml, 10 ml: $90 ***Pregnancy category:*** B	Headache, dizziness, weakness, nausea, vomiting, diarrhea, anorexia, pseudomembranous colitis, nephrotoxicity, renal failure, leukopenia, thrombocytopenia, agranulocytosis, neutropenia, lymphocytosis, eosinophilia, pancytopenia, rash, urticaria, anaphylaxis

Arteriosclerotic Heart Disease

OVERVIEW

Arteriosclerotic heart disease occurs as a result of thickening of the walls of the coronary arteries. This thickening of the walls and loss of elasticity occur in response to the aging process, as well as in response to elevated total serum cholesterol and low-density lipoprotein levels, which cause the formation of atheromas. It is a chronic, progressive process that normally occurs over many years.

Pathogenesis

Causes:

- Atheromas in subintima of large and medium vessels
- Narrowing of coronary arteries and loss of elasticity

Patient Profile

- Males > Females
- Most common ages: men—45 to 60 years; women—60 to 70 years

Signs and Symptoms

- May be asymptomatic
- Substernal chest pain
- Dyspnea on exertion
- Irregular heart beat
- Orthopnea
- Tachycardia
- Pedal edema

Differential Diagnosis

- Peptic ulcer disease
- Pericarditis
- Aortic dissection
- Gastritis
- Pulmonary hypertension
- Pneumothorax
- Pneumonia
- Cholecystitis

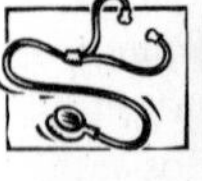

ASSESSMENT

History

Inquire about:

- Onset and duration of symptoms
- Precipitating factors
- Quality of pain
- Intensity of pain
- Treatment tried and results
- Past history of heart problems
- Associated symptoms of nausea, shortness of breath
- Risk factors—smoking, hypertension, elevated cholesterol, family history
- Underlying conditions
- Current medications

Physical Findings

- Complete physical examination—may be within normal limits
- If having chest pain, may appear anxious
- Pallor
- Increased heart rate
- Irregular heart rate
- Systolic murmur
- Increased respiratory rate
- Shortness of breath
- Pedal edema

Initial Workup

Laboratory

- Lipid panel—increased triglycerides, total cholesterol, low-density lipoproteins; decreased high-density lipoproteins
- Cardiac enzymes—within normal limits

Radiology

- Stress thallium test—positive
- Angiography—narrowed coronary arteries

Further Workup

- ECG—ST segment depression, inverted T waves
- Exercise stress test—positive

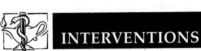

INTERVENTIONS

Office Treatment

None indicated

Lifestyle Modifications

- Smoking cessation
- Stress reduction
- Moderate exercise program
- Low-cholesterol diet

Patient Education

Teach patient about:

- Condition and treatment
- Tips for smoking cessation
- Stress reduction—biofeedback, relaxation therapy, yoga
- Moderate exercise program, such as walking
- Low-cholesterol, low-fat diet
- Medications used and side effects (see Pharmacotherapeutics)

Referrals

To dietitian, cardiologist if appropriate

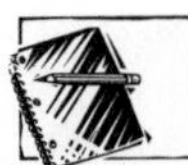

EVALUATION

Outcome

Depends on willingness to make lifestyle changes

Possible Complications

- Myocardial infarction
- Congestive heart failure
- Angina pectoris
- Sudden cardiac death

Follow-up

Frequent visits to monitor progress of lifestyle modifications and to provide support

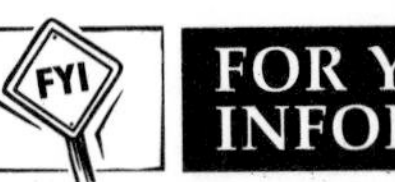

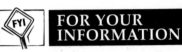

FOR YOUR INFORMATION

Life Span

Pediatric: Should be taught proper nutrition, benefits of exercise, and smoking avoidance

Geriatric: Common in this age group

Pregnancy: Extremely rare

Miscellaneous

N/A

References

Griego L, House-Fancher MA: Nursing role in management: coronary artery disease. In Lewis SM, Collier IC, Heitkemper MM, editors: *Medical-surgical nursing: assessment and management of clinical problems,* ed 4, St Louis, 1996, Mosby, pp 884-894.

Uphold CR, Graham MV: *Clinical guidelines in adult health,* Gainesville, Fla, 1994, Barmarrae Books, pp 296-304.

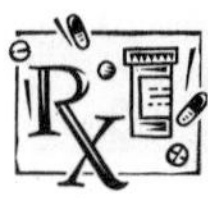

PHARMACOTHERAPEUTICS

Drug of Choice	Mechanism of Action	Prescribing Information	Side Effects
Aspirin, 80-325 mg PO qd	Decreases platelet aggregation	***Contraindications:*** Hypersensitivity; bleeding disorders or anticoagulant therapy; last trimester of pregnancy; asthma; gastric ulcers ***Cost:*** OTC ***Pregnancy category:*** Not categorized	Rash, anaphylactic reaction, GI upset/bleeding
Cholesterol-lowering agents:			
Bile acid–sequestering agent: cholestyramine or colestipol, 1-6 packets or scoopfuls or 4-24 tabs/day in single or multiple doses; powder must be mixed with fluid; at least 4 oz of water should follow every 4 tabs taken; start with low dose and increase as needed	Binds with bile acids in intestine, and complex is excreted in feces	***Contraindications:*** Hypersensitivity; patient with complete biliary obstruction; other drugs should be taken either 1 hour before or 4-6 hours after to avoid impeding absorption ***Cost:*** Powder, 378 g: $36 ***Pregnancy category:*** No studies done in pregnancy	Constipation, abdominal discomfort, flatulence, nausea, vomiting, dyspepsia, eructation, anorexia
Niacin or nicotinic acid (Nicolar), 500 mg to 3 g bid, tid, or qid; start with low dose and increase as needed	Interferes with synthesis of cholesterol and lipoproteins; decreases low-density lipoproteins (LDLs) and triglycerides	***Contraindication:*** Hypersensitivity ***Cost:*** 500-mg tab, 500 tabs: $12 ***Pregnancy category:*** C	Severe hepatic toxicity; generalized flushing—can block with an aspirin taken with niacin; atrial fibrillation and other cardiac arrhythmias can occur; dyspepsia; vomiting; diarrhea; peptic ulceration; decreased glucose tolerance; hyperuricemia
Lovastatin (Mevacor); patient should be on low-cholesterol, low-fat diet; starting dose is 20 mg/day; Mevacor should be administered with evening meal; many other drugs available for lowering cholesterol: pravastatin, atorvastatin, fluvastatin	HMG-CoA reductase inhibitor; effective at lowering both LDL and total cholesterol levels	***Contraindication:*** Hypersensitivity ***Cost:*** 20-mg tab, 60 tabs: $125 ***Pregnancy category:*** X	Chest pain, increased serum transaminase, acid regurgitation, dry mouth, vomiting, leg pain, shoulder pain, insomnia, eye irritation, alopecia, pruritus
For postmenopausal women, hormone replacement therapy:			
Estrogen (Premarin), 0.625 mg PO 1 tab daily; estrogen is available in pills, as a transdermal patch, or as a vaginal cream; method of administration should be decided on by the NP and patient together by determining which method best meets the patient's needs	Affects release of pituitary gonadotropins; inhibits ovulation	***Contraindications:*** Hypersensitivity; breast cancer; thromboembolic disorders; reproductive cancer; undiagnosed vaginal bleeding; pregnancy ***Cost:*** 0.625-mg tab, 100 tabs: $50; transdermal or topical estrogen per year: $107 ***Pregnancy category:*** X	Dizziness, headache, migraines, depression, hypotension, thrombophlebitis, thromboembolism, pulmonary embolism, myocardial infarction (MI), nausea, vomiting, cholestatic jaundice, weight gain, diplopia, amenorrhea, cervical erosion, breakthrough bleeding, dysmenorrhea, vaginal candidiasis, spontaneous abortion, rash, urticaria, acne, hirsutism, photosensitivity
If patient has intact uterus, add medroxyprogesterone acetate (Provera), 10 mg PO on days 1-12 or days 13-25; or give 2.5 mg PO daily; estrogen and medroxyprogesterone acetate are now available in 1 tab sold under the trade name Prempro	Inhibits secretion of pituitary gonadotropins; stimulates growth of mammary tissue	***Contraindications:*** Hypersensitivity; breast cancer; thromboembolic disorders; reproductive cancer; undiagnosed vaginal bleeding; pregnancy ***Cost:*** 5-mg tab, 30 tabs: $16 ***Pregnancy category:*** X	Dizziness, headache, migraines, depression, hypotension, thrombophlebitis, thromboembolism, pulmonary embolism, MI, nausea, vomiting, cholestatic jaundice, weight gain, diplopia, amenorrhea, cervical erosion, breakthrough bleeding, dysmenorrhea, vaginal candidiasis, spontaneous abortion, rash, urticaria, acne, hirsutism, photosensitivity

Arthritis, Septic/Bacterial Arthritis/Pyogenic Arthritis

OVERVIEW

Septic arthritis is usually a monarticular disease in which a joint is invaded by a microorganism. Large peripheral joints, such as the hip or knee, are more frequently involved. It is one of the few curable types of arthritis.

Pathogenesis

- Entrance to joint occurs by hematogenous seeding, direct penetration due to trauma, or joint injection
- Causes—50% *Neisseria gonorrhoeae, Staphylococcus aureus,* or *Haemophilus influenzae* (particularly in children); many other microorganisms can be causative
- In IV drug users, gram-negative rods frequently involved

Patient Profile

- *N. gonorrhoeae:*
  - Females > Males
  - Most common age group—15 to 40 years
- Non–*N. Gonorrhoeae:*
  - Males > Females
  - Any age

Signs and Symptoms

- Acute-onset monarticular joint pain (hip and knee most commonly)
- Limited movement
- Joint effusion, tenderness
- Joint warmth and redness
- Fever
- Chills
- Malaise

Differential Diagnosis

- Gout
- Pseudogout
- Rheumatoid arthritis
- Juvenile rheumatoid arthritis
- Reiter's syndrome
- Cellulitis

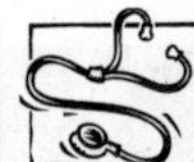

ASSESSMENT

History

Inquire about:

- Onset and duration of symptoms
- Recent infection elsewhere
- Previous joint damage
- Underlying conditions
- Current medications

Physical Findings

- Warm, red, tender joint
- Passive range of motion (ROM) extremely painful
- Swollen joint
- Fever

Initial Workup

Laboratory

- CBC—leukocytosis
- Joint aspiration—WBCs markedly increased
- Gram stain and culture of aspirate

Radiology: Plain film of joint—soft tissue swelling

Further Workup

Possibly CT scan or MRI

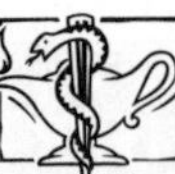

INTERVENTIONS

Office Treatment

None indicated

Lifestyle Modification

Safe sex practices

Patient Education

Teach patient about:

- Disease and treatment
- Need for hospitalization and parenteral antibiotic therapy based on culture results
- Using moist heat and traction to decrease pain
- Need for joint aspiration (may need to be repeated frequently)
- Possible need for surgical drainage
- Safe sex practices and use of condoms
- Medications used and side effects (see Pharmacotherapeutics)

Referral

To primary care physician or rheumatologist if NP does not have hospital privileges or is unable to perform joint aspiration

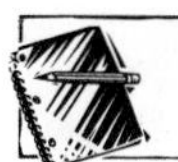

EVALUATION

Outcome
Infection resolved without sequelae

Possible Complications
- Limited joint ROM
- Septic necrosis
- Sinus formation
- Osteomyelitis
- Death

Follow-up
1 week after hospitalization; then 1 week after antibiotic stopped; then in 1 month

FOR YOUR INFORMATION

Life Span
Pediatric: Consult infectious disease specialist
Geriatric: Higher morbidity and mortality rate; consult infectious disease specialist
Pregnancy: Consult infectious disease specialist

Miscellaneous
N/A

References
Hellman DB: Arthritis and musculoskeletal disorders. In Tierney LM Jr, McPhee SJ, Papadakis MA, editors: *Current medical diagnosis and treatment,* ed 34, Norwalk, Conn, 1995, Appleton & Lange, pp. 732-734.

Mercier LR: *Practical orthopedics,* ed 4, St Louis, 1995, Mosby, pp 267-268.

NOTES

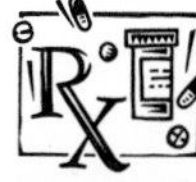

PHARMACOTHERAPEUTICS

Antibiotic therapy must be based on the results of the culture and sensitivity tests.

Drug of Choice	Mechanism of Action	Prescribing Information	Side Effects
Most commonly used antibiotic is aqueous penicillin G, 12 mil units/day IV in divided doses q4-6h; may be used for suspected *Neisseria gonorrheae* and many non-*Neisseria* infections; children, 25,000-300,000 IV units/day in divided doses	Interferes with cell wall replication	***Contraindications:*** Hypersensitivity; neonates ***Cost:*** 600,000 units/ml, 10 ml: $68 ***Pregnancy category:*** B	Bone marrow depression; granulocytopenia; nausea; vomiting; diarrhea; oliguria; proteinuria; hematuria; vaginitis; moniliasis; glomerulonephritis; lethargy; hallucinations; convulsions; coma, hyperkalemia/hypokalemia; local pain, tenderness, and erythema at injection site; anaphylaxis; hypersensitivity; rash; urticaria

Asbestosis

OVERVIEW

Asbestosis is a form of pneumoconiosis that develops from regular exposure to asbestos. It is characterized by interstitial fibrosis, thickened pleura, and calcified plaques.

Pathogenesis

Cause—exposure and inhalation of asbestos dust and fibers, resulting in macrophage-induced damage to lung parenchyma

Patient Profile

- Males > Females
- Most common age group—40 to 75 years

Signs and Symptoms

- Dyspnea or exertional dyspnea
- Cyanosis
- Chest discomfort
- Fatigue
- Nonproductive cough
- Clubbing of fingers

Differential Diagnosis

- Coal worker's pneumoconiosis
- Silicosis
- Siderosis

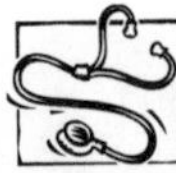

ASSESSMENT

History

Inquire about:

- Onset and duration of symptoms
- Past exposure to asbestos
- Smoking history
- Underlying conditions
- Current medications

Physical Findings

- Clubbing of fingers
- Cyanosis
- Lungs—inspiratory crackles

Initial Workup

Laboratory

- Blood gases—hypoxemia
- CBC—increased hemoglobin and hematocrit

Radiology: Chest film—interstitial fibrosis, calcified pleural plaques, pleural thickening, bilateral pleural effusion, honeycombed lungs

Further Workup

- Bronchoscopy
- Pulmonary function studies—decreased vital capacity, total lung capacity, and diffusing capacity

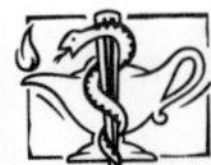

INTERVENTIONS

Office Treatment

None indicated

Lifestyle Modification

Smoking cessation

Patient Education

Teach patient about:

- Condition and treatment—no effective treatment
- Tips for smoking cessation (patient is at higher risk for lung cancer)
- Importance of physical activity to the extent allowed
- Signs and symptoms of infection and to report promptly
- Using supplemental oxygen if necessary
- Using inhaled bronchodilators
- Medications used and side effects (see Pharmacotherapeutics)

Referral

To pulmonologist if treatment fails

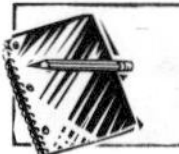

EVALUATION

Outcome

Disease is irreversible; severity depends on duration and intensity of exposure

Possible Complications

- Lung cancer
- Mesothelioma
- Asphyxiation

Follow-up

- Yearly chest x-ray
- Possibly annual pulmonary function tests

FOR YOUR INFORMATION

Life Span

Pediatric: Not seen in this age group
Geriatric: Most commonly seen in this age group
Pregnancy: N/A

Miscellaneous

Asbestos workers need a yearly physical examination with chest x-ray and pulmonary function studies. Encourage workers to use protective devices.

References

Mitchell JT: Nursing role in management: lower respiratory problems. In Lewis SM, Collier IC, Heitkemper MM, editors: *Medical-surgical nursing: assessment and management of clinical problems,* ed 4, St Louis, 1996, Mosby, pp 654-656.

Stauffer JL: Lung. In Tierney LM Jr, McPhee SJ, Papadakis MA, editors: *Medical diagnosis and treatment,* ed 34, Norwalk, Conn, 1995, Appleton & Lange, pp 263-264.

NOTES

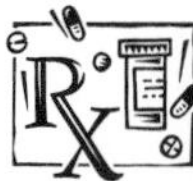

PHARMACOTHERAPEUTICS

Drug of Choice	Mechanism of Action	Prescribing Information	Side Effects
Albuterol (Proventil, Ventolin); inhaler, 2 puffs PO qid; tabs, 2 mg PO qid	Bronchodilator; B_2 agonist—increases cAMP, which relaxes smooth muscle, leading to bronchodilation and CNS and cardiac stimulation; increases diuresis and gastric acid secretion	***Contraindications:*** Hypersensitivity; tachydysrhythmias; severe cardiac disease ***Cost:*** Metered dose inhaler: \$13-\$22; tabs, 2-mg tab, 100 tabs: \$3-\$37 ***Pregnancy category:*** C	Tremors, anxiety, insomnia, headache, dizziness, stimulation, restlessness, hallucinations, flushing, dry nose, palpitations, tachycardia, hypertension, angina, heartburn, nausea, vomiting, muscle cramps
Or:			
Pirbuterol (Maxair), 2 inhalations PO qid	Bronchodilator; B_2 agonist—increases cAMP, which relaxes smooth muscle, leading to bronchodilation and CNS and cardiac stimulation; increases diuresis and gastric acid secretion	***Contraindications:*** Hypersensitivity; tachydysrhythmias; severe cardiac disease ***Cost:*** 14-g autoinhaler: \$34 ***Pregnancy category:*** C	Tremors, anxiety, insomnia, headache, dizziness, stimulation, restlessness, hallucinations, flushing, dry nose, palpitations, tachycardia, hypertension, angina, heartburn, nausea, vomiting, muscle cramps, gastritis, coughing

OVERVIEW

Ascites is an abnormal accumulation of serous fluid in the abdominal cavity. The fluid contains large amounts of protein and electrolytes. Ascites may occur in any condition that causes generalized edema.

Pathogenesis

Causes:

- Children—nephrotic syndrome, malignancy
- Adults—cirrhosis, heart failure, nephrotic syndrome, chronic peritonitis, spontaneous bacterial peritonitis
- Causes of exudate fluid—neoplasm, tuberculosis, pancreatitis, myxedema, biliary problem
- Causes of transudate fluid—congestive heart failure, constrictive peritonitis, inferior vena cava obstruction, cirrhosis, nephrotic syndrome, hypoalbuminemia

Patient Profile

- Males = Females
- Any age

Signs and Symptoms

- Abdominal pain
- Fullness
- Discomfort
- Distention
- Anorexia
- Nausea
- Weight gain
- Early satiety
- Shortness of breath
- Penile and scrotal edema
- Umbilical herniation
- Pedal edema
- Tachycardia
- Abdominal fluid wave

Differential Diagnosis

- Obesity
- Distended intestine from air or fluid

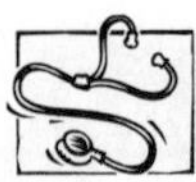

ASSESSMENT

History

Inquire about:

- Onset and duration of symptoms
- Alcohol intake
- Past history of heart problems or cancer
- Recent weight gain and appetite
- Underlying conditions
- Current medications

Physical Findings

- Abdominal distention
- Abdominal fluid wave
- Shifting dullness on percussion of flanks
- Rales
- Tachycardia
- Penile, scrotal, or pedal edema
- Weight gain
- Shortness of breath

Initial Workup

Laboratory

- Ascitic fluid (Table 1)—total protein, lactate dehydrogenase (LDH), WBC count, differential, amylase, acid-fast or fungal culture, cytology, triglycerides
- Blood tests—chemistry profile, total protein, amylase, CBC with differential

Radiology: CT scan or ultrasound of abdomen

Further Workup

Peritoneoscopy

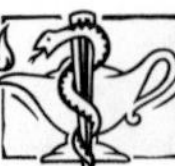

INTERVENTIONS

Office Treatment

Diagnostic paracentesis if NP trained to perform; otherwise refer to MD.

Lifestyle Modifications

- Depends on underlying cause
- All need sodium-restricted diet (<2 g daily)
- May need fluid restriction
- Bed rest if peripheral edema present
- Smoking cessation
- Alcohol cessation

Patient Education

Teach patient about:

- Underlying cause
- Treatment options for ascites—diuretics, low-sodium diet, fluid restriction
- How to record input and output
- What is considered a fluid (anything liquid at room temperature)
- How to keep track of weight
- If resistant to above treatment, may need paracentesis, peritoneovenous shunt, or transjugular intrahepatic shunt
- Medications used and side effects (see Pharmacotherapeutics)

Referral

To MD if NP untrained in paracentesis or for hospital admission

TABLE 1 *Laboratory Values for Ascitic Fluid*

	Exudate	Transudate
Protein	>2 g/dl	<2 g/dl
LDH	>200 IU/L	<200 IU/L
WBCs	>500 mm^3	<500 mm^3
Differential	>200 mm^3 Polymorphonuclear neutrophils	<200 mm^3 Polymorphonuclear neutrophils

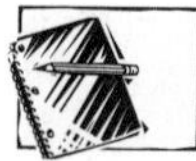

EVALUATION

Outcome
Prognosis depends on underlying cause

Possible Complications
- Hypokalemia secondary to overly aggressive diuresis
- Intravascular volume depletion
- Renal failure
- Spontaneous bacterial peritonitis
- Pleural effusion
- Inguinal, femoral, umbilical hernia
- Mesenteric venous thrombosis

Follow-up
Every 2 weeks

FOR YOUR INFORMATION

Life Span
Pediatric: Nephrotic syndrome and malignancy common cause
Geriatric: Start with half-normal starting dose of diuretics
Pregnancy: N/A

Miscellaneous
N/A

Reference
Woolliscroft JO: *Current diagnosis and treatment: a quick reference for the general practitioner,* Philadelphia, 1996, Current Medicine, pp 46-47.

NOTES

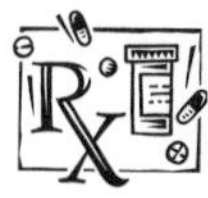

PHARMACOTHERAPEUTICS

Drug of Choice	Mechanism of Action	Prescribing Information	Side Effects
Spironolactone (Aldactone), 100-300 mg/day PO, single or divided doses; best for cirrhotic ascites; children, 3.3 mg/kg/day PO in single or divided doses	Competes with aldosterone at receptor sites in distal tubule, resulting in excretion of sodium chloride and water and retention of potassium and phosphate	*Contraindications:* Hypersensitivity; anuria; severe renal disease; hyperkalemia; pregnancy *Cost:* 25-mg tab, 100 tabs: \$5-\$15 *Pregnancy category:* D	Headache, confusion, drowsiness, diarrhea, cramps, bleeding, gastritis, vomiting, anorexia, dysrhythmias, rash, pruritus, urticaria, impotence, gynecomastia, decreased WBCs, platelets, hyperchloremic metabolic acidosis, hyperkalemia, hyponatremia
Furosemide (Lasix), 40-120 mg PO qd; best for all other etiologies; children, 2 mg/kg/day PO, increase to maximum of 6 mg/kg/day	Inhibits reabsorption of sodium and chloride at proximal and distal tubule and in the loop of Henle	*Contraindications:* Hypersensitivity to sulfonamides; anuria; hypovolemia; infants; lactation; electrolyte depletion *Cost:* 20-mg tab, 30 tabs: \$2 *Pregnancy category:* C	Headache, fatigue, weakness, orthostatic hypotension, chest pain, ECG changes, circulatory collapse, loss of hearing, ear pain, tinnitus, hypokalemia, hypochloremic alkalosis, hypomagnesemia, hyperuricemia, hypocalcemia, hyperglycemia, nausea, diarrhea, dry mouth, vomiting, polyuria, renal failure, thrombocytopenia, agranulocytosis, leukopenia, neutropenia, rash, pruritus, Stevens-Johnson syndrome, cramps

Aspergillosis

OVERVIEW

Aspergillosis is a disease that primarily affects the lungs. It is caused by a mold. There are different presentations of aspergillosis:

- Allergic aspergillosis—extrinsic allergic alveolitis or allergic bronchopulmonary aspergillosis
- Aspergillomas—colonization of preexisting pulmonary cavities
- Invasive aspergillosis—found in immunodeficient patients; affects lungs and other organs; frequently fatal

Pathogenesis

Cause—*Aspergillus fumigatus, Aspergillus flavus,* or *Aspergillus niger*

Patient Profile

- Males = Females
- Any age
- Risk factors—asthma, chronic obstructive pulmonary disease (COPD), bronchiectasis, tuberculosis, malignancy, immunodeficiency, corticosteroid therapy

Signs and Symptoms

- Allergic aspergillosis—cough, wheezing, pulmonary infiltrates, mucous plugs
- Aspergillomas—hemoptysis
- Invasive aspergillosis—fever, cough, gastrointestinal bleeding, adventitious breath sounds, CNS signs

Differential Diagnosis

- Allergic aspergillosis—other causes of asthma
- Aspergillomas—neoplasm, tuberculosis
- Invasive aspergillosis—pneumonia, malignancy

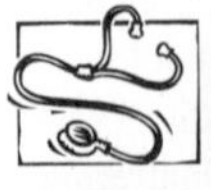

ASSESSMENT

History

Inquire about:

- Onset and duration of symptoms
- History of asthma
- Smoking history
- Underlying conditions
- Current medications

Physical Findings

- Depends on type
- Generally—cough, wheezing, rales, rhonchi, fever, hemoptysis

Initial Workup

Laboratory

- Allergic aspergillosis:
  - CBC with differential—eosinophilia; *Aspergillus* precipitins in blood
  - Skin test—positive reaction to *Aspergillus* antigen
- Invasive aspergillosis:
  - Sputum culture
  - Bronchial washing—culture

Radiology: Chest film—PA and lateral:

- Allergic aspergillosis—pulmonary infiltrates
- Aspergillomas—round intercavity mass
- Invasive aspergillosis—nodular or patchy infiltrates, diffuse consolidation, and cavitation

Further Workup

Lung biopsy

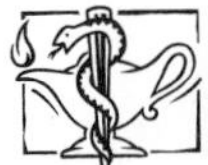

INTERVENTIONS

Office Treatment

None indicated

Lifestyle Modifications

- Smoking cessation
- Allergic aspergillosis—avoidance of exposure

Patient Education

Teach patient about:

- Condition and treatment
  - Allergic aspergillosis—using bronchodilators and steroids; tips for avoiding exposure
  - Aspergillomas—treating underlying condition (COPD, tuberculosis, malignancy)
  - Invasive aspergillosis—hospitalization; IV antifungal therapy; treating underlying cause of immunodeficiency; tips for smoking cessation
- Medications used and side effects (see Pharmacotherapeutics)

Referral

To specialist for invasive aspergillosis

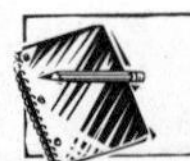

EVALUATION

Outcomes

- Allergic aspergillosis—with treatment, prognosis good
- Aspergillomas—prognosis depends on underlying disease
- Invasive aspergillosis—poor prognosis

Possible Complications

- Allergic aspergillosis—bronchiectasis, pulmonary fibrosis, obstructive lung disease
- Invasive aspergillosis—death

Follow-up

- Allergic aspergillosis—every week until stable
- Invasive aspergillosis—1 week after hospitalization

FOR YOUR INFORMATION

Life Span

Pediatric: More common to see allergic or invasive aspergillosis

Geriatric: More common to see aspergillomas because of chronic lung disease in this population

Pregnancy: N/A

Miscellaneous

N/A

References

Hollander H: Infectious diseases: mycotic. In Tierney LM Jr, McPhee SJ, Papadakis MA, editors: *Medical diagnosis and treatment,* ed 34, Norwalk, Conn, 1996, Appleton & Lange, pp 263-264.

Woolliscroft JO: *Current diagnosis and treatment: a quick reference for the general practitioner,* Philadelphia, 1996, Current Medicine, pp 142-143.

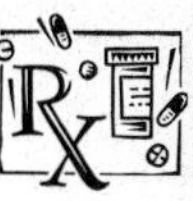

PHARMACOTHERAPEUTICS

Drug of Choice	Mechanism of Action	Prescribing Information	Side Effects
For allergic aspergillosis, start with one of the following:			
Albuterol (Proventil, Ventolin); inhaler—adults and children >4 years, 2 puffs PO qid; extended-release tabs—adults and children >12 years, 4-8 mg PO q12h; children 6-12 years, 2 mg PO q12h; syrup—children 2-6 years, 0.1 mg/kg/day in 3 divided doses	Bronchodilator; B_2 agonist—increases cAMP, which relaxes smooth muscle, leading to bronchodilation and CNS and cardiac stimulation; increases diuresis and gastric acid secretion	***Contraindications:*** Hypersensitivity; tachydysrhythmias; severe cardiac disease ***Cost:*** Metered dose inhaler: $13-$22; tabs, 2-mg tab, 100 tabs: $3-$37 ***Pregnancy category:*** C	Tremors, anxiety, insomnia, headache, dizziness, stimulation, restlessness, hallucinations, flushing, dry nose, palpitations, tachycardia, hypertension, angina, heartburn, nausea, vomiting, muscle cramps
Pirbuterol (Maxair); adults and children >12 years, 2 inhalations PO qid	Same as for albuterol	Same as for albuterol	Same as for albuterol plus gastritis, coughing
If patient is using above medication more than qid and on a daily basis, add one of the following:			
Inhaled corticosteroid: beclomethasone (Beclovent/Vanceril); adults and children >12 years, 2 puffs PO tid or qid, maximum 20 inhalations; children 6-12 years, 1-2 puffs tid or qid, maximum 10 inhalations; instruct patient to rinse mouth after using	Corticosteroid; decreases inflammation	***Contraindications:*** Hypersensitivity; status asthmaticus; nonasthmatic bronchial disease ***Cost:*** MDI 6.7 g, 1: $17 ***Pregnancy category:*** C	Bronchospasm, dry mouth, hoarseness, candidal infection, sore throat
Cromolyn (Intal); adults and children >5 years, 2 puffs PO qid; also available in gelatin capsules and capsules or solution for use in nebulizer	Mast cell stabilizer that prevents release of chemical mediators after an antigen-IgE interaction	***Contraindications:*** Hypersensitivity to this drug or lactose; status asthmaticus ***Cost:*** 112 sprays/bottle: $40 ***Pregnancy category:*** B	Throat irritation, cough, burning eyes, headache, dizziness, urinary frequency, dysuria, nausea, vomiting, anorexia, rash, urticaria, angioedema, joint pain/swelling
If symptoms persist, add a long-acting beta agonist, such as the following:			
Salmeterol (Serevent); adults and children >12 years, 2 puffs PO bid; ensure that patient understands that this is *not* a rescue drug for bronchospasm	Long-acting beta agonist; causes bronchodilation; prevents nocturnal symptoms	***Contraindications:*** Hypersensitivity; tachyarrhythmias; severe cardiac disease ***Cost:*** 13-g canister, $49 ***Pregnancy category:*** C	Tremors, anxiety, insomnia, headache, stimulation, restlessness, hallucinations, palpitations, tachycardia, hypertension, dysrhythmias, heartburn, muscle cramps, bronchospasm
If symptoms still persist, consider the following:			
Theophylline (Theo-Dur/Uniphyl), 100-200 mg PO q6h; children, 50-100 mg q6h; dose must be individualized; available in sustained-release form; take hs	Xanthine; relaxes smooth muscle, which causes bronchodilation	***Contraindications:*** Hypersensitivity; tachydysrhythmias ***Cost:*** 400-mg tab sustained-release, 100 tabs: $67 ***Pregnancy category:*** C	Anxiety; restlessness, insomnia, dizziness, convulsions, headache, palpitations, sinus tachycardia, hypotension, anorexia, diarrhea, dyspepsia, flushing, urticaria
For allergic bronchopulmonary aspergillosis, use the following:			
Prednisone, 60-120 mg PO qd, then taper over several days	Corticosteroid; decreases inflammation	***Contraindications:*** Hypersensitivity; psychosis; idiopathic thrombocytopenia; acute glomerulonephritis; amebiasis; AIDS; TB; children <2 years ***Cost:*** 15-mg tab, 100 tabs: $14-$35 ***Pregnancy category:*** C	Hypertension, circulatory collapse, thrombophlebitis, embolism, tachycardia, fungal infections, increased intraocular pressure, diarrhea, nausea, GI hemorrhage, thrombocytopenia, acne, poor wound healing, fractures, osteoporosis, weakness
For invasive aspergillosis, use the following:			
Amphotericin B, up to 1 mg/kg/day IV	Antifungal; increases cell membrane permeability; decreases potassium, sodium, and nutrients in cell	***Contraindications:*** Hypersensitivity; severe bone marrow depression ***Cost:*** 50 mg/15 ml, 1 vial: $21-$42 ***Pregnancy category:*** B	Tinnitus, deafness, dermatitis, rash, headache, fever, chills, convulsions, peripheral neuropathy, hypokalemia, azotemia, renal tubular acidosis, anuria, oliguria, anorexia, hemorrhagic gastroenteritis, acute liver failure, arthralgia, thrombocytopenia, agranulocytosis, leukopenia, eosinophilia, hypokalemia, hyponatremia

Asthma

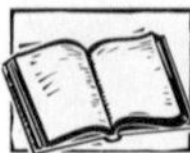

OVERVIEW

Asthma is a disorder of the tracheobronchial tree in which there is reversible airway obstruction, inflammation, and hyperresponsiveness.

Pathogenesis

- Recurrent bronchospasm or airway hyperreactivity in response to an inflammatory process
- Causes:
  - Allergic reaction
  - Smoke and other pollutants
  - Pharmacologic agents such as aspirin
  - Exercise
  - Gastroesophageal reflux

Patient Profile

- Children <10 years—Males > Females
- Puberty—Males = Females
- Adults—Females > Males
- Onset can occur at any age

Signs and Symptoms

- Wheezing
- Coughing
- Prolonged expiration
- Decreased breath sounds
- Chest tightness
- Tachycardia
- Nocturnal attacks
- Cyanosis
- Use of accessory respiratory muscles
- Symptoms usually occur episodically; may range from a few mild episodes to daily attacks

Differential Diagnosis

- Viral respiratory infection
- Chronic bronchitis
- Foreign body aspiration
- Cystic fibrosis
- Pneumonia
- Thyroid dysfunction
- Congestive heart failure
- Tuberculosis
- Cough secondary to medications

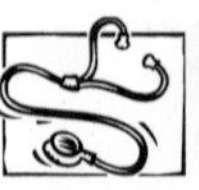

ASSESSMENT

History

Inquire about:

- Onset and duration of symptoms
- History of allergies, rhinitis, pneumonia, gastroesophageal reflux
- Precipitating events or aggravating factors, such as animals, mold, pollen, dust, exercise, medications
- When attacks occur
- Number of trips to emergency room
- Treatments tried and results
- Impact on lifestyle
- Underlying conditions
- Current medications

Physical Findings

- Physical examination findings may be normal
- Lungs—bilateral expiratory wheezes
- Use of accessory muscles to breathe
- Retractions, nasal flaring, cyanosis
- Assess for nasal polyps, postnasal drainage, allergic shiners

Initial Workup

Laboratory: CBC—normal unless infection present

Radiology: Chest film—PA and lateral—usually normal

Further Workup

- Pulmonary function tests—reversible airway obstruction
- Consider allergy testing and exercise tolerance testing
- PPD

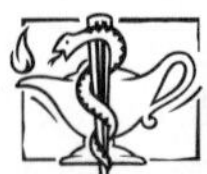

INTERVENTIONS

Office Treatment

If having an acute attack, may need nebulizer treatment with albuterol

Lifestyle Modifications

- Avoidance of known triggers
- Smoking cessation
- Use of medications as prescribed
- Home peak-flow-rate monitoring
- Living with a chronic illness
- Stress reduction

Patient Education

Teach patient about:

- Condition and treatment
- Using inhalers and/or spacers—have patient do return demonstration
- Using peak-flow meter—have patient perform twice daily × 2 weeks and determine personal best; set up guide for patient:

PEFR	Action
≥80% of personal best	Continue same treatment
50%-80% of personal best	Increase use of inhalers
<50% of personal best	Immediate bronchodilator; emergency treatment if still <50% of personal best after treatment

- Avoiding known triggers
- Tips for smoking cessation
- Avoiding aspirin and NSAIDs (will exacerbate asthma in 5% to 20% of patients)
- Importance of obtaining yearly flu vaccine and pneumonia vaccine every 5 years
- Avoiding overuse of inhalers
- Stress-reduction techniques—biofeedback, yoga, relaxation therapy
- Medications used and side effects (see Pharmacotherapeutics)

Referral

To pulmonologist if patient has severe, life-threatening asthma attacks, has uncertainty about diagnosis, or does not respond to treatment

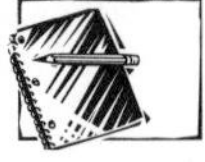

EVALUATION

Outcome

Chronic illness—prognosis good if treatment plan followed

Possible Complications

- Respiratory failure
- Atelectasis
- Death
- Side effects of medications

Follow-up

In 1 week × 2 when first initiating treatment; then every 2 weeks × 2; if stable, every 3 months

FOR YOUR INFORMATION

Life Span

Pediatric: 50% of new asthma diagnoses occur in children <10 years of age

Geriatric: Unusual for onset to occur in this age group, although it has been seen more in recent years

Pregnancy: 50% have no change; 25% improve; 25% get worse

Miscellaneous

Asthma is one of the leading causes of missed school days.

References

Barach EM: Asthma in ambulatory care: use of objective diagnostic criteria, *J Fam Pract* 38(2):161-165, 1994.

Wise RA, Liu MC: Obstructive airways diseases—asthma and chronic obstructive pulmonary disease. In Barker LR, Burton JR, Zieve PD, editors: *Principles of ambulatory medicine,* ed 4, Baltimore, 1995, Williams & Wilkins, pp 654-666.

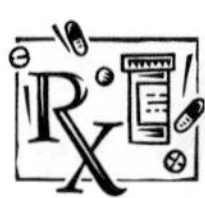

PHARMACOTHERAPEUTICS

Drug of Choice	Mechanism of Action	Prescribing Information	Side Effects
Start with one of the following:			
Albuterol (Proventil, Ventolin); inhaler—adults and children >4 years, 2 puffs PO qid; extended-release tabs—adults and children >12 years, 4-8 mg PO q12h; children 6-12 years, 2 mg PO q12h; syrup—children 2-6 years, 0.1 mg/kg/day in 3 divided doses	Bronchodilator; B_2 agonist—increases cAMP, which relaxes smooth muscle, leading to bronchodilation and CNS and cardiac stimulation; increases diuresis and gastric acid secretion	***Contraindications:*** Hypersensitivity; tachydysrhythmias; severe cardiac disease ***Cost:*** Metered dose inhaler: $13-$22; tabs, 2-mg tab, 100 tabs: $3-$37 ***Pregnancy category:*** C	Tremors, anxiety, insomnia, headache, dizziness, stimulation, restlessness, hallucinations, flushing, dry nose, palpitations, tachycardia, hypertension, angina, heartburn, nausea, vomiting, muscle cramps
Pirbuterol (Maxair), adults and children >12 years, 2 inhalations PO qid	Bronchodilator; B_2 agonist—increases cAMP, which relaxes smooth muscle, leading to bronchodilation and CNS and cardiac stimulation; increases diuresis and gastric acid secretion	***Contraindications:*** Hypersensitivity; tachydysrhythmias; severe cardiac disease ***Cost:*** 14-g autoinhaler: $34 ***Pregnancy category:*** C	Tremors, anxiety, insomnia, headache, dizziness, stimulation, restlessness, hallucinations, flushing, dry nose, palpitations, tachycardia, hypertension, angina, heartburn, nausea, vomiting, muscle cramps, gastritis, coughing
If patient is using above medications more than qid and on a daily basis, add one of the following:			
Inhaled corticosteroid: beclomethasone (Beclovent/Vanceril); adults and children >12 years, 2 puffs PO tid or qid, maximum 20 inhalations; children 6-12 years, 1-2 puffs tid or qid, maximum 10 inhalations; other types available include triamcinolone (Aristocort) and flunisolide (AeroBid); instruct patient to rinse mouth after using	Corticosteroid; decreases inflammation	***Contraindications:*** Hypersensitivity; status asthmaticus; nonasthmatic bronchial disease ***Cost:*** MDI 6.7 g, 1: $17 ***Pregnancy category:*** C	Bronchospasm, dry mouth, hoarseness, candidal infection, sore throat
Cromolyn (Intal); adults and children >5 years, 2 puffs PO qid; if patient has exercise-induced asthma, use 20 minutes before exercise; also available in gelatin capsules and capsules or solution for use in nebulizer	Mast cell stabilizer that prevents release of chemical mediators after an antigen-IgE interaction	***Contraindications:*** Hypersensitivity to this drug or lactose; status asthmaticus ***Cost:*** 112 sprays/bottle: $40 ***Pregnancy category:*** B	Throat irritation, cough, burning eyes, headache, dizziness, urinary frequency, dysuria, nausea, vomiting, anorexia, rash, urticaria, angioedema, joint pain/swelling
If symptoms persist, add a long-acting beta agonist, such as the following:			
Salmeterol (Serevent); adults and children >12 years, 2 puffs PO bid; ensure that patient understands that this is *not* a rescue drug	Long-acting beta agonist; causes bronchodilation; prevents nocturnal symptoms	***Contraindications:*** Hypersensitivity; tachyarrhythmias; severe cardiac disease ***Cost:*** 13-g canister, $49 ***Pregnancy category:*** C	Tremors, anxiety, insomnia, headache, stimulation, restlessness, hallucinations, palpitations, tachycardia, hypertension, dysrhythmias, heartburn, nausea, vomiting, muscle cramps, bronchospasm
If symptoms still persist, consider the following:			
Theophylline (Theo-Dur/Uniphyl), 100-200 mg PO q6h; children, 50-100 mg q6h; dose must be individualized; available in sustained-release form; take hs to prevent nocturnal symptoms	Xanthine; relaxes smooth muscle, which causes bronchodilation	***Contraindications:*** Hypersensitivity; tachydysrhythmias ***Cost:*** 40-mg tab sustained-release, 100 tabs: $67 ***Pregnancy category:*** C	Anxiety, restlessness, insomnia, dizziness, convulsions, headache, palpitations, sinus tachycardia, hypotension, nausea, vomiting, anorexia, diarrhea, dyspepsia, flushing, urticaria
For acute exacerbation:			
Nebulizer treatment with albuterol and short course of prednisone, 60-120 mg PO qd, then taper over several days	Corticosteroid; decreases inflammation	***Contraindications:*** Hypersensitivity; psychosis; idiopathic thrombocytopenia; acute glomerulonephritis; amebiasis; nonasthmatic bronchial disease; AIDS; TB; child <2 years old ***Cost:*** 15-mg tab, 100 tabs: $14-$35 ***Pregnancy category:*** C	Hypertension, circulatory collapse, thrombophlebitis, embolism, tachycardia, fungal infections, increased intraocular pressure, diarrhea, nausea, GI hemorrhage, thrombocytopenia, acne, poor wound healing, fractures, osteoporosis, weakness

Atelectasis

OVERVIEW

Atelectasis is an abnormal condition in which a portion of the lung has collapsed.

Pathogenesis
Several different events may occur:
- Increased alveolar surface tension from pulmonary edema, infection, or primary surfactant deficiency
- Obstruction of major airways and bronchioles
- Compression of lung from fluid or air in pleural space
- Compression of lung from tumor outside lung
- Restriction of chest wall from skeletal deformity and/or muscular weakness

Patient Profile
- Males = Females
- Any age

Signs and Symptoms
Depends on size of area affected:
- May be asymptomatic if small
- Large atelectasis—tachypnea, cough, hypoxia, dyspnea, absent breath sounds, wheezing

Differential Diagnosis
Look for underlying cause:
- Infection
- Mucus
- Tumor
- Foreign body
- Lobar emphysema
- Cardiomegaly
- Scoliosis
- Neuromuscular disease
- General anesthesia
- High oxygen concentration

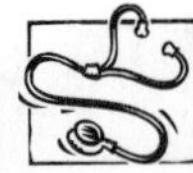

ASSESSMENT

History
Inquire about:
- Onset and duration of symptoms
- Smoking history
- Prior history of atelectasis
- Underlying conditions
- Current medications

Physical Findings
- Tachypnea
- Absent breath sounds
- Dullness to percussion over affected area
- Tracheal or point of maximal impulse (PMI) shift
- Cyanosis
- Increased heart rate
- Increased blood pressure

Initial Workup
Laboratory
- Arterial blood gases—hypoxia
- Other laboratory testing done according to possible cause

Radiology: Chest film—PA and lateral—demonstrates area of collapse

Further Workup
- Depends on cause
- Possibly—bronchoscopy, chest CT scan or MRI, echocardiogram, barium swallow

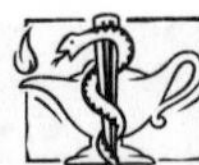

INTERVENTIONS

Office Treatment
If severe, direct hospital admission

Lifestyle Modifications
- Smoking cessation
- Weight loss if appropriate

Patient Education
Teach patient about:
- Condition and treatment
- Need for hospitalization if severe; possibly supplemental oxygen
- Chest physiotherapy—percussion and postural drainage (teach significant other how to perform)
- Using positive end-expiratory pressure mask or incentive spirometer
- Importance of remaining as active as possible
- Medications used and side effects (see Pharmacotherapeutics)

Referral
To MD for hospitalization if NP does not have privileges

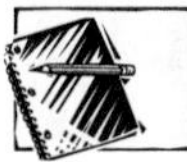

EVALUATION

Outcome

Resolves without sequelae, although recurrence is common, depending on cause

Possible Complications

Infection with chronic lung damage

Follow-up

- If outpatient, telephone contact in 48 hours; return visit in 1 week
- If hospitalized, follow-up within 1 week after hospitalization
- Monthly chest films until completely resolved

FOR YOUR INFORMATION

Life Span

Pediatric: Look for congenital abnormality
Geriatric: Most common cause—lung tumors
Pregnancy: Consult a specialist

Miscellaneous

Atelectasis is not a specific disease, but a symptom of a disease process. It is imperative that the NP uncover the underlying cause.

References

Smith PI, Britt EJ, Terry PB: Common pulmonary problems: cough, hemoptysis, dyspnea, chest pain, and the abnormal chest X-ray. In Barker LR, Burton JR, Zieve PD, editors: *Principles of ambulatory medicine,* ed 4, Baltimore, 1995, Williams & Wilkins, pp 643-644.

Stauffer JL: Lung. In Tierney LM Jr, McPhee SJ, Papadakis MA, editors: *Medical diagnosis and treatment,* ed 34, Norwalk, Conn, 1995, Appleton & Lange, pp 222-223.

NOTES

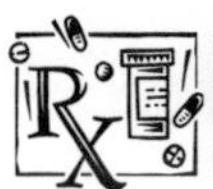

PHARMACOTHERAPEUTICS

Many medications may be used, depending on the cause. Refer to the specific condition for appropriate treatment. The medication presented here is used for most cases of atelectasis regardless of cause.

Drug of Choice	Mechanism of Action	Prescribing Information	Side Effects
Albuterol (Proventil/Ventolin); adults and children >4 years, metered dose inhaler—2 puffs qid or nebulizer treatment q4-6h	Bronchodilator; B_2 agonist—increases cAMP, which relaxes smooth muscle, leading to bronchodilation and CNS and cardiac stimulation; increases diuresis and gastric acid secretion	***Contraindications:*** Hypersensitivity; tachydysrhythmias; severe cardiac disease ***Cost:*** Metered dose inhaler: \$13-\$22; tabs, 2-mg tab, 100 tabs: \$3-\$37 ***Pregnancy category:*** C	Tremors, anxiety, insomnia, headache, dizziness, stimulation, restlessness, hallucinations, flushing, dry nose, palpitations, tachycardia, hypertension, angina, heartburn, nausea, vomiting, muscle cramps

Atherosclerotic Occlusive Disease/Peripheral Arterial Disease/Peripheral Vascular Disease

OVERVIEW

Atherosclerotic occlusive disease is a disorder of the larger arteries of the upper or, more commonly, lower extremities. It is due to narrowing or obstruction of the aorta or its major branches, which disrupts blood flow to either the feet and legs (most common) or the hands and arms.

Pathogenesis

- Cause—atherosclerotic lesions
- Start as fatty streaks and progress to fibrous plaques (elevated areas of intimal thickening) and finally become complicated lesions (calcified fibrous plaques)

Patient Profile

- Males > Females
- Middle and older adulthood

Signs and Symptoms

- Intermittent claudication (pain on exercise, relieved by rest)
  - Pain in buttock, hip, thigh = aortoiliac disease
  - Pain in calf = femoral-popliteal disease
- As disease progresses, pain at rest
- Impotence
- Decreased or absent pulses distal to obstruction
- Bruit over narrowed artery
- Muscle atrophy
- Hair loss
- Shiny skin
- Thickened nails
- Limb is cool and pale or develops rubor

Differential Diagnosis

- Raynaud's phenomenon
- Thromboangiitis obliterans

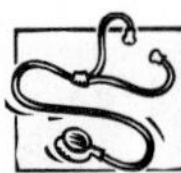

ASSESSMENT

History

Inquire about:

- Onset and duration of symptoms
- Occurrence of pain with exercise and/or at rest
- Location of pain
- Impotency
- Risk factors such as smoking, increased cholesterol, physical stress
- Underlying conditions
- Current medications

Physical Findings

- Diminished or absent pulses in affected extremity
- Limb may be cool, pale, with smooth, shiny skin or rubor
- Bruit (turbulent blood flow) over narrowed artery
- Examine skin for ischemic lesions

Initial Workup

Laboratory: None diagnostic
Radiology: Angiography

Further Workup

- Doppler ultrasound
- Ankle/brachial BP (<0.95 indicates occlusive disease)

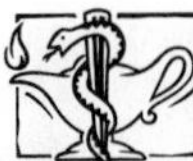

INTERVENTIONS

Office Treatment

None indicated

Lifestyle Modifications

- Cessation of use of any type of tobacco
- Weight loss
- Good foot hygiene

Patient Education

Teach patient about:

- Condition and treatment—surgery if patient is candidate
- Tips for stopping use of tobacco
- Weight loss diet
- Walking to the point of discomfort at least twice weekly (aim for daily)
- Proper foot care, including hygiene, nail maintenance, and care of cuts, sores, and lesions
- Seeking medical care for any open areas on feet or legs
- Importance of wearing well-fitting shoes
- Keeping feet warm
- Medications used and side effects (see Pharmacotherapeutics)

Referral

To surgeon if surgical candidate

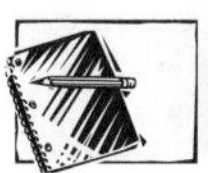

EVALUATION

Outcome
Depends on speed of progression; if slow and patient is willing to make lifestyle changes, long-term prognosis is good

Possible Complications
- Necrosis
- Gangrene
- Limb amputation

Follow-up
Depends on severity of symptoms; if stable with medication, every 3 months

FOR YOUR INFORMATION

Life Span
Pediatric: N/A
Geriatric: Most commonly seen in this age group
Pregnancy: N/A

Miscellaneous
N/A

References
Jones CE: Peripheral vascular disease and arterial aneurysms. In Barker LR, Burton JR, Zieve PD, editors: *Principles of ambulatory medicine,* ed 4, Baltimore, 1995, Williams & Wilkins, pp 1298-1305.

Uphold CR, Graham MV: *Clinical guidelines in adult health,* Gainesville, Fla, 1994, Barmarrae Books, pp 308-311.

NOTES

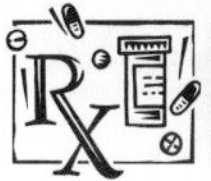

PHARMACOTHERAPEUTICS

Drug of Choice	Mechanism of Action	Prescribing Information	Side Effects
Pentoxifylline (Trental), 400 mg PO tid with meals	Reduces blood viscosity and increases RBC flexibility; reduces platelet aggregation; decreases fibrinogen concentration	***Contraindication:*** Hypersensitivity to this drug or xanthines ***Cost:*** 400-mg tab, 100 tabs: $58 ***Pregnancy category:*** C	Epistaxis, laryngitis, nausea, congestion, leukopenia, malaise, blurred vision, sore throat, headache, anxiety, tremors, dizziness, dyspepsia, nausea, vomiting, anorexia, bloating, belching, dry mouth, rash, pruritus, angina, dysrhythmias, palpitations, hypotension, chest pain, edema

Atopic Dermatitis

OVERVIEW

Atopic dermatitis is a condition characterized by eczematous eruptions that are itchy, recurrent, flexural, and symmetric. Intense pruritis is a hallmark of the disease. Most of the patients also have a history of one or more of the following: hay fever, asthma, very dry skin, and eczema.

Pathogenesis

- Generally begins early in life and follows periods of remission and exacerbation
- Exact pathogenesis of disease is unknown; appears to be a malfunction or an overfunctioning of the patient's immune system
- Associated with elevated T-lymphocyte activation, hyperstimulatory Langerhans' cells, defective cell-mediated immunity, and β-cell IgE overproduction

Patient Profile

- Males = Females
- Starts in early childhood after 2 months of age
- Normally resolves after age 30

Signs and Symptoms

- Intense pruritis
- Erythema
- Scaling and dryness of skin
- Infant phase (birth to 2 years):
  - Appears usually during winter
  - Erythema and scaling of cheeks; may have generalized eruption of papules
  - Oozing, weeping lesions are typical
- Childhood phase (2 to 12 years):
  - Inflammation in antecubital fossae, popliteal fossae, neck, wrists, and ankles (flexural areas); perspiration stimulates burning and itching
  - Starts with papules that coalesce into plaques, which become lichenified
  - Plaques are pale and slightly inflamed, or bright red and scaling; borders may be sharp or poorly defined
- Adult phase (12 years to adult):
  - Resurgence of inflammation, perhaps because of hormonal changes or stresses of adolescence
  - Flexural inflammation
  - Hand dermatitis is most common symptom in adults; redness and scaling of dorsal surface of hands and fingers; lichenification or oozing and crusting may occur
  - Inflammation around eyes may occur
  - Lichenification of anogenital area may occur

Differential Diagnosis

- Photosensitivity rashes
- Contact dermatitis
- Seborrheic dermatitis
- Scabies
- Psoriasis
- Lichen simplex chronicus

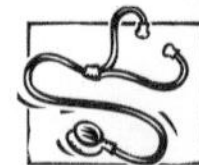

ASSESSMENT

History

Inquire about:

- Onset and duration of symptoms
- Itching
- Appearance of lesions and where located
- Family history of atopy, allergic rhinitis, and asthma
- Bath habits, such as how many times per day, type of soap, type of lotions, types of bubble bath or oils used
- Previous treatment tried and results
- Underlying conditions
- Current medications

Physical Findings

- Erythema
- Scaling
- Dry skin
- Lichenification
- Assess for signs and symptoms of secondary infection

Initial Workup

Laboratory: None indicated
Radiology: None indicated

Further Workup

None indicated

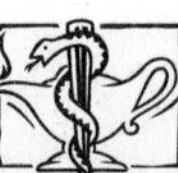

INTERVENTIONS

Office Treatment

- Phototherapy if available
- Psoralen and ultraviolet light therapy may be appropriate

Lifestyle Modifications

- Environment should be slightly cool and humidified
- Avoidance of frequent hand washing and bathing
- When bathing, use of nonperfumed soaps, such as Dove
- Stress reduction
- Diet free of alcohol, spices, and/or caffeine (may or may not be beneficial)

Patient Education

Teach patient/family about:

- Condition and treatment
- Stress reduction techniques, such as relaxation, biofeedback, guided imagery
- Chronicity of disease
- Lubricating skin 2 to 3 times daily with petrolatum
- Avoiding exposure to chemicals
- Wearing gloves when doing "wet" work
- Importance of not scratching
- Keeping fingernails trimmed
- Avoiding extreme temperature changes
- Avoiding commonly implicated foods, such as peanuts, eggs, milk, preservatives
- Medications used and side effects (see Pharmacotherapeutics)

Referral

To dermatologist for treatment failure

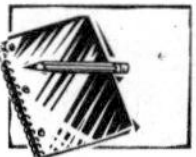

EVALUATION

Outcome
Control of the disease to prevent disability

Possible Complications
- Secondary skin infection with bacterial or viral organisms
- Side effects of topical steroids if overused or used on large areas of skin

Follow-up
In 1 week and then monthly until control is achieved

FOR YOUR INFORMATION

Lifespan
Pediatric: Starts in this age group
Geriatric: Very rare
Pregnancy: May experience remission or exacerbation

Miscellaneous
According to the European Task Force on atopic dermatitis, a scoring index has been designed to help evaluate the severity of a patient's atopic dermatitis. The tool is called SCORAD (Severity scoring, 1993).

References

Habif TP: *Clinical dermatology: a color guide to diagnosis and therapy,* ed 3, St Louis, 1996, Mosby, pp 100-121.

Severity scoring of atopic dermatitis: the SCORAD index: consensus report of the European task force on atopic dermatitis, *Dermatology,* 186(1):23-31, 1993.

Whitmore E: Common problems of the skin. In Barker LR, Burton JR, Zieve PD, editors: *Principles of ambulatory medicine,* ed 4, Baltimore, 1995, Williams & Wilkins, pp 1456-1458.

NOTES

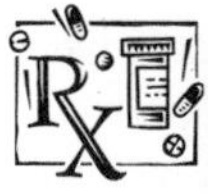

PHARMACOTHERAPEUTICS

Drug of Choice	Mechanism of Action	Prescribing Information	Side Effects
Topical corticosteroid: 1% hydrocortisone cream (Cortaid); apply to affected area bid up to qid; effective in 90% of cases; in adults, may need to prescribe one of the more potent topical steroids, such as mometasone furoate (Elocon cream) or betamethasone dipropionate (Diprolene cream); not for use in children <12 years; for lichenified plaques, apply cream and occlusive dressing for 10-14 days	Antiinflammatory, antipruritic, and vasoconstrictive	*Contraindication:* Hypersensitivity *Cost:* Some OTC; mometasone 0.1%, 15 g: $16; betamethasone 0.05%, 15 g: $3-$21 *Pregnancy category:* C	Burning, itching, irritation, dryness, folliculitis, acneiform eruptions, maceration of skin, secondary infection, skin atrophy; with overuse, systemic side effects could occur
For puritus:			
Hydroxyzine (Atarax), 10-25 mg PO qid; children 6-12 years, 50-100 mg/day PO in divided doses; children <6 years, 50 mg/day PO in divided doses	Antihistaminic	*Contraindications:* Hypersensitivity; pregnancy *Cost:* 10-mg tab, 100 tabs: $2-$49 *Pregnancy category:* See contraindications	Drowsiness, but usually transitory; dry mouth; tremors; rarely, convulsions (high doses)

Atrial Fibrillation

OVERVIEW

Atrial fibrillation is a supraventricular dysrhythmia in which there is chaotic electrical activity that replaces normal sinus rhythm. Because of the chaotic atrial activity, the ventricular response is rapid and irregular. Atrial fibrillation may be chronic (permanent fibrillation) or paroxysmal (episodic attacks).

Pathogenesis

- Multiple, rapid, atrial contractions (300 to 600/min) emit multifocal reentrant impulses
- AV node slows rate of conduction; therefore not all impulses conducted, resulting in irregular ventricular rate of 150 to 200
- Causes:
  - Ischemia
  - Myocardial infarction
  - Hypertension
  - Valvular disease
  - Rheumatic heart disease
  - Pulmonary embolism
  - Cardiomyopathy
  - Congestive heart failure
  - Coronary artery disease
  - Cardiothoracic surgery
  - Sick sinus syndrome
  - Alcohol withdrawal
  - Sepsis
  - Thyrotoxicosis
  - Idiopathic

Patient Profile

- Males = Females
- Incidence increases with age

Signs and Symptoms

- May be asymptomatic
- Irregular pulse
- Tachycardia
- Hypotension
- Light-headedness
- Fatigue
- Dyspnea
- Angina
- Poor exercise capacity
- Near syncope or syncope
- Stroke
- Embolism

Differential Diagnosis

- See causes under Pathogenesis
- Multifocal atrial tachycardia
- Sinus tachycardia with frequent premature atrial contractions
- Atrial flutter

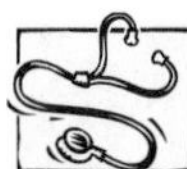

ASSESSMENT

History

Inquire about:

- Onset and duration of symptoms
- Chest pain
- Weight loss
- Mood change
- Tremor (hyperthyroidism)
- Number of previous attacks, treatment tried, and results
- Family history of heart problems
- Underlying conditions
- Current medications

Physical Findings

In chronic fibrillation or during an attack of paroxysmal fibrillation:

- Tachycardia
- Irregular pulse
- Hypotension
- Shortness of breath
- Diaphoresis

Initial Workup

Laboratory

- Thyroid function tests
- Electrolytes
- BUN and creatinine
- ECG—no clear P waves; irregular pattern of QRS complexes

Radiology

- Echocardiogram
- Chest film—PA and lateral

Further Workup

- Holter monitor for paroxysmal fibrillation
- Ventilation/perfusion scan if pulmonary embolism suspected

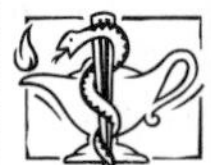

INTERVENTIONS

Office Treatment

None indicated

Lifestyle Modifications

Smoking, caffeine, and alcohol cessation

Patient Education

Teach patient about:

- Condition and treatment options
- Medication therapy—consists of anticoagulation, slowing of ventricular rate, conversion and maintenance of sinus rhythm using either cardioversion or medication
- Tips for smoking, caffeine, and alcohol cessation
- Activity—as tolerated
- Diet—depends on underlying cause of atrial fibrillation; if overweight, weight-reduction diet
- Possible surgical procedures—dual chamber pacing, ablation procedure
- Medications used and side effects (see Pharmacotherapeutics)

Referral

To MD/cardiologist if new diagnosis and/or hospitalization required

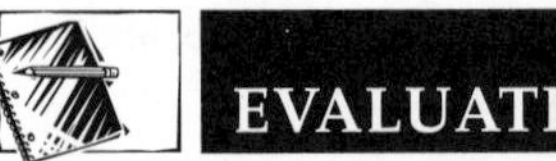

EVALUATION

Outcome

Depends on cause

Possible Complications

- Embolic stroke
- Medication complications

Follow-up

Initially every 2 weeks for prothrombin time

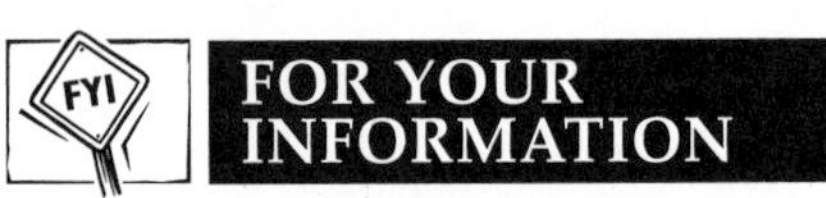

FOR YOUR INFORMATION

Life Span

Pediatric: May be seen with congenital heart problems

Geriatric: Increased incidence in this age group

Pregnancy: Should be handled by a specialist

Miscellaneous

Cardioversion may be attempted by either direct-current cardioversion or by chemical conversion. When antiarrhythmic therapy is initiated, the patient should be hospitalized and on a cardiac monitor.

References

Gottlieb SH: Arrhythmias. In Barker LR, Burton JR, Zieve PD, editors: *Principles of ambulatory medicine,* ed 4, Baltimore, 1995, Williams & Wilkins, pp 749-751.

Massie BM: Heart. In Tierney LM Jr, McPhee SJ, Papadakis MA, editors: *Current medical diagnosis and treatment,* ed 34, Norwalk, Conn, 1995, Appleton & Lange, pp 337-340.

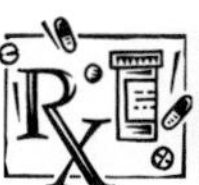

PHARMACOTHERAPEUTICS

Antiarrhythmic therapy should be initiated with the patient hospitalized and on a cardiac monitor. The continued use of antiarrhythmic medication, such as procainamide, quinidine, flecainide, sotalol, or amiodarone, after cardioversion is controversial; therefore these medications are not presented here. Consult an acute care text on the use of antiarrhythmic medications.

Drug of Choice	Mechanism of Action	Prescribing Information	Side Effects
For anticoagulation:			
Warfarin (Coumadin); usually start with 10-15 mg PO qd, then titrate to maintain prothrombin time INR between 2.0-3.0	Depresses synthesis of coagulation factors that are dependent on vitamin K (II, VII, IX, X)	***Contraindications:*** Hypersensitivity; hemophilia; peptic ulcer disease; thrombocytopenic purpura; severe hepatic disease; severe hypertension; subacute bacterial endocarditis; acute nephritis; blood dyscrasias; pregnancy ***Cost:*** 5-mg tab, 100 tabs: $30-$50 ***Pregnancy category:*** D	Diarrhea, nausea, vomiting, anorexia, stomatitis, cramps, hepatitis, hematuria, rash, dermatitis, fever, hemorrhage, agranulocytosis, leukopenia, eosinophilia
To control ventricular rate, use one of the following:			
Beta-blocker: propranolol (Inderal), 30-120 mg PO bid or tid or 160 mg PO qd extended-release; many other beta-blockers available (metoprolol, atenolol, nadolol, etc.)—see manufacturer's insert for prescribing information	Reduces myocardial O_2 requirement by decreasing heart rate, myocardial contractility, and BP	***Contraindications:*** Hypersensitivity; cardiac failure; cardiogenic shock; 2nd- or 3rd-degree heart block; bronchospastic disease; sinus bradycardia; congestive heart failure (CHF) ***Cost:*** 40-mg tab, 100 tabs: $2-$40 ***Pregnancy category:*** C	Bronchospasm, dyspnea, bradycardia, hypotension, CHF, palpitations, atrioventricular (AV) block, agranulocytosis, thrombocytopenia, nausea, vomiting, diarrhea, constipation, impotence, decreased libido, joint pain, arthralgia, facial swelling, rash, pruritus, depression, hallucinations, dizziness, fatigue, lethargy, sore throat, laryngospasm, blurred vision
Calcium channel blocker: nondihydropyridine diltiazem (Cardizem), 90-360 mg PO qd in either single dose for sustained-release or multiple doses; can also use verapamil	Inhibits calcium ion influx, causing relaxation of coronary vascular smooth muscle; dilates coronary arteries; slows sinoatrial (SA)/AV node conduction; dilates peripheral arteries	***Contraindications:*** Sick sinus syndrome; 2nd- or 3rd-degree heart block; hypotension; acute myocardial infarction (MI); pulmonary congestion ***Cost:*** 90-mg tab, 100 tabs: $80-$105 ***Pregnancy category:*** C	Dysrhythmia, edema, CHF, bradycardia, hypotension, palpitations, nausea, vomiting, diarrhea, gastric upset, nocturia, polyuria, acute renal failure, rash, pruritus, headache, fatigue, drowsiness, dizziness, depression, insomnia, weakness, tremor, paresthesia
Digoxin (Lanoxin), 0.125-0.5 mg PO qd; monitor therapeutic level q3-6 mos once stabilized on maintenance dose	Cardiac glycoside; increases cardiac output	***Contraindications:*** Hypersensitivity; ventricular fibrillation or tachycardia; carotid sinus syndrome; 2nd- or 3rd-degree heart block ***Cost:*** 0.25-mg tab, 100 tabs: $8-$16 ***Pregnancy category:*** C	Headache, drowsiness, apathy, confusion, fatigue, depression, dysrhythmia, hypotension, bradycardia, AV block, blurred vision, yellow-green halos, photophobia, nausea, vomiting, anorexia, abdominal pain, diarrhea

Attention Deficit Hyperactivity Disorder (ADHD)

OVERVIEW

Attention deficit hyperactivity disorder (ADHD) is a syndrome characterized by a short attention span, low frustration tolerance, impulsivity, distractibility, and usually hyperactivity.

Pathogenesis

Actual cause unknown—may be multifactorial; associated with:

- Poor prenatal health
- Learning disabilities
- Tourette's syndrome
- Mood disorders
- Oppositional defiant disorder
- Conduct disorder

Patient Profile

- Males > Females
- Predominant age—children <7 years
- Is being diagnosed more in adult population

Signs and Symptoms

- Easily distracted
- Can't wait turn
- Blurts out answers before question is complete
- Difficulty following instructions
- Difficulty remaining seated; fidgets
- Short attention span
- Talks excessively
- Interrupts others
- Difficulty playing quietly
- Antisocial behavior
- Poor academic performance
- Shifts from one uncompleted task to another

Differential Diagnosis

- Dysfunctional family situation
- Learning disability
- Hearing/vision disorder
- Oppositional/defiant disorder
- Lead poisoning
- Medication reaction
- Pervasive developmental delay
- Hyperthyroidism
- Absence seizures

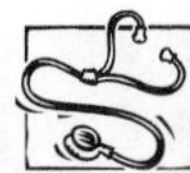

ASSESSMENT

History

Obtain a thorough history from either patient or patient's parents or teacher; inquire about:

- Onset and duration of symptoms
- Family history
- Behavior pattern
- School performance
- In adult, past performance in school and in workplace
- History of psychiatric or neurologic conditions
- Psychosocial evaluation of home environment
- Underlying medical conditions
- Current medications

Physical Findings

- Observe patient's behavior during visit
- Probably no physical abnormalities

Initial Workup

Laboratory: Rarely needed; may want to do chemistry panel, CBC, and lead level in children for screening purposes

Radiology: None needed

Further Workup

If concerned about seizures, may do EEG

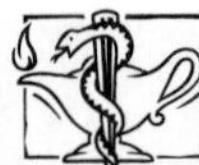

INTERVENTIONS

Office Treatment

None needed

Lifestyle Modifications

- Have definite routine in home, at school, or at work
- Take frequent breaks and only perform one task at a time
- Maintain nutritionally sound diet; may want to experiment with elimination of sugars, dyes, or additives (no dietary changes have been proved to help)

Patient Education

Teach patient and family about:

- Condition and treatment options—medications
- Lifestyle modifications
- Importance of reinforcing good behavior
- Making eye contact when talking to patient
- Stopping behavior before it escalates
- Support groups and educational material available
- Medications used and side effects (see Pharmacotherapeutics)

Referral

To psychiatric NP, psychologist, or psychiatrist specializing in ADHD, as appropriate

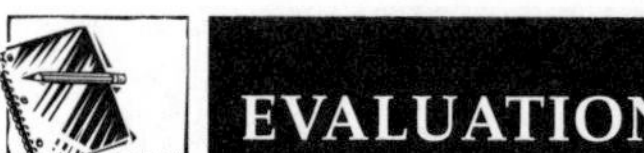

EVALUATION

Outcome
Improved performance at school or work

Possible Complications
Related to drug therapy—headaches, abdominal pain, growth delay

Follow-up
Reassess every 2 weeks × 2 months; then every 3 months; will probably be followed by specialist

FOR YOUR INFORMATION

Life Span
Pediatric: Most commonly seen in this age group
Geriatric: Normally not seen in this age group
Pregnancy: Generally, stimulants should not be used

Miscellaneous
Increasing attention is being paid to the diagnosis of ADHD in the adult. NPs working in college health need to be alert to the possibility that students may present for initial evaluation at the student health center. These patients may be treated with the same medications, but often considerably larger doses will be needed to obtain results.

References

Heiligenstein E, Keeling RP: Presentation of unrecognized attention deficit hyperactivity disorder in college students, *J Am Coll Health* 43(5):226-228, 1995.

Wilens TE et al: Pharmacotherapy of adult attention deficit/hyperactivity disorder: a review, *J Clin Psychopharmacol* 15(4):270-279, 1995.

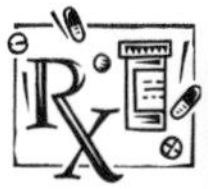

PHARMACOTHERAPEUTICS

Drug of Choice	Mechanism of Action	Prescribing Information	Side Effects
Methylphenidate (Ritalin); adults, initially 5 mg PO bid or tid; may increase weekly; maximum 60 mg daily; children >6 years, 5 mg PO bid before breakfast and lunch; may increase weekly; maximum 60 mg daily, controlled substance, Schedule II	Presumably activates the brainstem arousal system and cortex—produces stimulant effect	***Contraindications:*** Hypersensitivity; marked anxiety; tension; agitation; glaucoma; family history or diagnosis of Tourette's syndrome or motor tics ***Cost:*** 5-mg tab, 100 tabs: $25-$31 ***Pregnancy category:*** Should not be used in women of childbearing age	Nervousness, insomnia, skin rash, urticaria, arthralgia, exfoliative dermatitis, anorexia, nausea, dizziness, palpitations, headache, dyskinesia, drowsiness, increased or decreased BP and pulse, tachycardia, abdominal pain, weight loss; long-term use can lead to abuse and tolerance
Pemoline (Cylert); adults and children >6 years, 18.75 mg/day PO in 1 dose, maximum dose 112.5 mg/day PO; controlled substance, Schedule IV	CNS stimulant	***Contraindications:*** Hypersensitivity; impaired hepatic function ***Cost:*** 37.5-mg tab, 100 tabs: $129 ***Pregnancy category:*** B	May produce dependency, hepatic dysfunction, seizures, hallucinations, dyskinetic movements of tongue, insomnia, aplastic anemia, dizziness, headache, drowsiness, anorexia, weight loss, nausea, growth suppression
Dextroamphetamine (Dexedrine); adults, 5 mg PO bid, maximum 60 mg/day; children >6 years, 5 mg PO qd or bid, may increase weekly; children 3-5 years, 2.5 mg PO qd, may increase weekly; controlled substance, Schedule II	CNS stimulant	***Contraindications:*** Hypersensitivity; advanced arteriosclerosis; cardiovascular disease; hypertension—moderate to severe; hyperthyroidism; glaucoma; agitated states; history of drug abuse; monoamine oxidase inhibitors (MAOIs) ***Cost:*** 5-mg tab, 100 tabs: $18-20 ***Pregnancy category:*** C	Palpitations, tachycardia, increased BP, psychotic episodes, overstimulation, restlessness, dizziness, insomnia, euphoria, dysphasia, tremors, headache, dry mouth, unpleasant taste, diarrhea, constipation, anorexia, weight loss, urticaria, impotence

Bacterial Vaginosis/*Gardnerella* Vaginosis/Bacterial Vulvovaginitis

OVERVIEW

Bacterial vaginosis is an infection of the vagina and (rarely) the vulva.

Pathogenesis
- Exact cause unknown
- Associated with *Gardnerella vaginalis, Mobiluncus* species, *Mycoplasma hominis, Peptostreptococcus,* and other organisms
- Associated with sexual activity, but not considered exclusively a sexually transmitted disease (STD)

Patient Profile
- Females
- Any age after puberty

Signs and Symptoms
- 50% asymptomatic
- Gray-white vaginal discharge—scant or profuse; adheres to vaginal walls; musty or fishy odor
- Vaginal/vulvar irritation

Differential Diagnosis
- *Neisseria gonorrhoeae*
- *Chlamydia trachomatis*
- Trichomoniasis
- Candidiasis

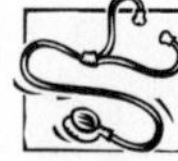

ASSESSMENT

History
Inquire about:
- Onset and duration of symptoms
- Past history of bacterial vaginosis
- Underlying conditions
- Current medications

Physical Findings
Pelvic examination:
- Gray-white discharge coating vaginal walls
- Musty or fishy odor to discharge
- Vaginal fluid pH >4.5

Initial Workup
Laboratory
- Wet mount—presence of clue cells
- Whiff test—10% KOH added to discharge produces fishy or amine odor
- If concerned about STDs—gonorrhea and *Chlamydia* cultures, rapid plasma reagin (RPR), HIV screen

Radiology: None indicated

Further Workup
None indicated

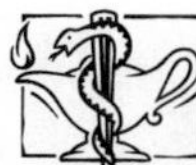

INTERVENTIONS

Office Treatment
None indicated

Lifestyle Modification
Safe sex practices

Patient Education
Teach patient about:
- Condition and treatment—antibiotics
- Condition not exclusively sexually transmitted, but safe sex should still be practiced (limit number of partners; use condoms)
- Male partners do not need treatment
- Proper perineal hygiene
- Recurrence rates are high
- Medications used and side effects (see Pharmacotherapeutics)

Referral
None indicated

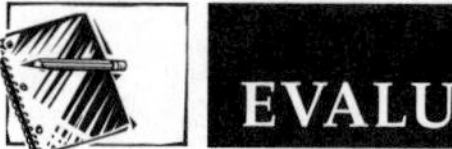

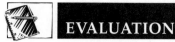

EVALUATION

Outcome
Resolves without sequelae

Possible Complications
Uncommon, but may include:
- Intrauterine infections
- Pelvic inflammatory disease
- Adnexal tenderness
- Pelvic abscess
- Preterm labor
- Premature rupture of membranes

Follow-up
None indicated unless symptoms persist

FOR YOUR INFORMATION

Life Span
Pediatric: Rare in females who are not sexually active; consider sexual abuse if young child
Geriatric: Treatment is the same
Pregnancy: Metronidazole should not be used during first trimester, but can be used during second and third; clindamycin, 2% cream intravaginally qhs can be used during first trimester; need for treatment during pregnancy controversial

Miscellaneous
In recurrent cases, the clinician may wish to consider treatment of the partner.

References
Bennett EC: Vaginitis and sexually transmitted diseases. In Youngkin EQ, Davis MS, editors: *Women's health: a primary care clinical guide,* Norwalk, Conn, 1994, Appleton & Lange, pp 208-210.

Reed BD, Eyler A: Practical therapeutics: vaginal infections: diagnosis and management, *Am Fam Physician* 47(8):1805-1816, 1993.

NOTES

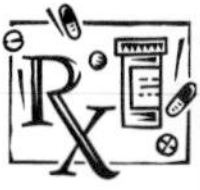

PHARMACOTHERAPEUTICS

Drug of Choice	Mechanism of Action	Prescribing Information	Side Effects
Metronidazole (Flagyl), 500 mg PO bid × 7 days *or* 2 g PO × 1 dose *or* 0.75% vaginal gel, 1 applicator full intravaginally bid × 5 days; children, 35-50 mg/kg/day in 3 divided doses	Direct-acting amebicide/ trichomonacide	***Contraindications:*** Hypersensitivity; 1st trimester pregnancy; CNS disorders ***Cost:*** 500-mg tab, 14 tabs: $3 ***Pregnancy category:*** B in 2nd and 3rd trimesters	Flat T waves, headache, confusion, irritability, depression, fatigue, insomnia, convulsions, blurred vision, sore throat, retinal edema, nausea, vomiting, diarrhea, anorexia, abdominal cramps, pseudomembranous colitis, dark urine, albuminuria, dysuria, neurotoxicity, leukopenia, bone marrow depression, aplasia, rash, pruritus, flushing
Clindamycin (Cleocin), 300 mg PO bid × 7 days *or* 2% cream intravaginally hs × 7 days; cream can be used in 1st trimester of pregnancy; children, 8-25 mg/kg/day PO in divided doses q8h	Suppresses protein synthesis in organism	***Contraindications:*** Hypersensitivity; ulcerative colitis/ enteritis; infants < 1 month ***Cost:*** 2% cream, 40-g tube: $30; tabs, 150-mg tab, 100 tabs: $85-$114 ***Pregnancy category:*** B	Leukopenia; eosinophilia; agranulocytosis; thrombocytopenia; polyarthritis; nausea, vomiting, abdominal pain, diarrhea, pseudomembranous colitis; anorexia; weight loss; increased AST, ALT, bilirubin, alkaline phosphatase; jaundice; vaginitis; rash; urticaria; pruritus

Balanitis

OVERVIEW

Balanitis is an inflammation of the glans penis. It most commonly occurs in uncircumcised males, but it can occur in circumcised males.

Pathogenesis

Causes:

- Idiopathic—allergic reaction (latex condom, contraceptive jelly)
- Fungal infection *(Candida albicans)*
- Bacterial infection
- Fixed drug eruption
- Plasma cell infiltration (Zoon's balanitis)
- Often occurs with posthitis

Patient Profile

- Males
- Adolescence through adulthood
- Higher risk in uncircumcised and diabetic patients

Signs and Symptoms

- Penile pain
- Dysuria
- Erythema
- Phimosis
- Plaques
- Drainage from site
- Ulcers

Differential Diagnosis

- Psoriasis
- Reiter's syndrome
- Leukoplakia
- Lichen planus
- Primary syphilis
- Genital herpes

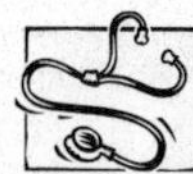

ASSESSMENT

History

Inquire about:

- Onset and duration of symptoms
- Circumcised versus uncircumcised
- Use of condoms or contraceptive jellies, foams, or creams
- Underlying conditions
- Current medications

Physical Findings

All of the following are found on glans penis:

- *C. albicans*—red erosions; may also have white drainage
- Erythema
- Ulcers
- Plaque
- Drainage from lesion

Initial Workup

Laboratory

- Culture of drainage
- Wet mount
- Rapid plasma reagin (RPR)
- Serum glucose

Radiology: None indicated

Further Workup

Biopsy if symptoms persist

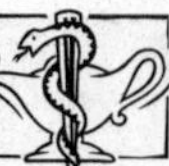

INTERVENTIONS

Office Treatment

None indicated

Lifestyle Modifications

- Improved hygiene
- Avoidance of allergens

Patient Education

Teach patient about:

- Condition, cause (if known), and treatment—topical ointments; oral antibiotic if indicated
- Warm saline compresses or sitz baths for comfort
- Proper hygiene—daily, pull foreskin back, clean with mild soap and rinse with water, pat dry, replace foreskin
- Avoidance of allergens
- Possible need for circumcision after inflammation resolves
- Medications used and side effects (see Pharmacotherapeutics)

Referral

To urologist if treatment fails or for circumcision

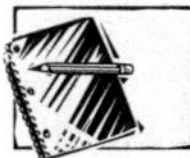

EVALUATION

Outcome
Resolves without sequelae

Possible Complications
- Phimosis
- Meatal stenosis
- Premalignant changes from chronic irritation
- Urinary tract infections
- Commonly recurs

Follow-up
In 1 week × 2

FOR YOUR INFORMATION

Life Span
Pediatric: PO antibiotics and diaper rash predispose infants to balanitis
Geriatric: Use of condom catheters can predispose to balanitis
Pregnancy: N/A

Miscellaneous
N/A

References
Edwards S: Balanitis and balanoposthitis: a review, *Genitourinary Med* 72(3):155-159, 1996.

Robinson KM, McCance KL, Gray DP: In McCance KL, Huether SE, editors: *Pathophysiology: the biologic basis for disease in adults and children,* ed 2, St Louis, 1994, Mosby, pp 771-772.

NOTES

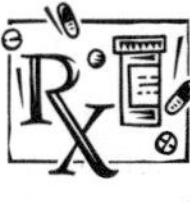

PHARMACOTHERAPEUTICS

Drug of Choice	Mechanism of Action	Prescribing Information	Side Effects
For fungal infection, use one of the following:			
Clotrimazole 1% cream (Lotrimin); apply bid to affected area	Fungicidal; interferes with DNA replication	***Contraindication:*** Hypersensitivity ***Cost:*** 15-g tube: $7-$10 ***Pregnancy category:*** B	Rash, urticaria, stinging, burning, peeling, blistering, skin fissures, erythema, general irritation
Nystatin (Mycostatin); apply bid to qid to affected area	Fungicidal; interferes with DNA replication	***Contraindication:*** Hypersensitivity ***Cost:*** 100,000 units/g, 15-g tube: $2-$11 ***Pregnancy category:*** B	Rash, stinging, urticaria, burning, general irritation
For bacterial infection, use one of the following. May also need PO antibiotics based on culture results.			
Bacitracin; apply to affected area bid to qid	Antibacterial; interferes with protein synthesis	***Contraindication:*** Hypersensitivity ***Cost:*** OTC ***Pregnancy category:*** C	Rash, urticaria, stinging, burning, contact dermatitis
Mupirocin 2% (Bactroban); apply small amount to area tid	Inhibits bacterial protein synthesis	***Contraindication:*** Hypersensitivity ***Cost:*** 15-g tube: $5-$7 ***Pregnancy category:*** B	Burning, stinging, itching, rash, dry skin, swelling, contact dermatitis, erythema, tenderness, increased exudate
For dermatitis and Zoon's balanitis:			
Topical steroid cream: 1%-2.5% hydrocortisone cream; apply to affected area qid	Antiinflammatory, antipruritic, and vasoconstrictive	***Contraindications:*** Hypersensitivity; fungal infections ***Cost:*** 1% 5-g tube: $2 ***Pregnancy category:*** C	Burning, dryness, itching, irritation, secondary infection

Barotitis Media/Middle Ear Barotrauma/Ear Block

OVERVIEW

Barotitis media (ear block) is a condition of the middle ear produced by sudden pressure differences between the middle ear and the surrounding atmosphere.

Pathogenesis
- Inability of eustachian tube to equilibrate middle ear pressure with atmospheric air
- Atmospheric air pressure changes rapidly when flying or scuba diving
- Tympanic membrane retracts and protracts, resulting in inflammation

Patient Profile
- Males = Females
- All ages
- High prevalence among scuba divers
- Risk factors—upper respiratory infections, allergic rhinitis, nasal polyps

Signs and Symptoms
- Ear pain with abrupt onset—usually occurs on descent when flying or diving
- Feeling of fullness in ear
- Conductive hearing loss
- Dizziness
- Vertigo
- Tinnitus
- Nausea and vomiting

Differential Diagnosis
- Acute or chronic otitis media
- Serous otitis media
- External otitis

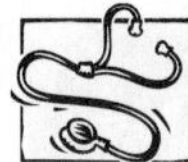

ASSESSMENT

History
Inquire about:
- Onset and duration of symptoms
- Recent flying or scuba diving
- Past history of ear problems or surgeries
- Treatments tried and results
- Underlying medical conditions
- Current medications

Physical Findings
- Patient may be anxious and in pain
- Tympanic membrane—retracted or protracted; injected; edematous
- Conductive hearing loss

Initial Workup
Laboratory: None indicated
Radiology: To rule out sinusitis or tumor, if uncertain about diagnosis

Further Workup
None indicated

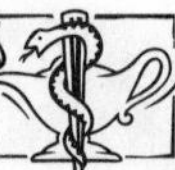

INTERVENTIONS

Office Treatment
- Have patient perform Valsalva maneuver (inhale, pinch nose shut, exhale with mouth closed)
- If unsuccessful, use nasal decongestant and Valsalva maneuver again
- If unsuccessful in office, take oral decongestants and repeat Valsalva maneuver at home

Lifestyle Modifications
- No flying or diving until completely resolved
- Allergies—avoidance of allergens
- Smoking cessation
- Diet—avoidance of food allergens

Patient Education
Teach patient about:
- Condition and treatment (see Office Treatment)
- Possible complications
- How to avoid recurrence—avoid flying or diving with upper respiratory infection or allergic rhinitis; take decongestants before diving or flying, slowed ascent or descent when flying or diving
- If treatment fails, return to higher altitude if possible and perform Valsalva maneuver or refer to otolaryngologist for politzerization
- Medications used and side effects (see Pharmacotherapeutics)

Referral
To otolaryngologist if necessary

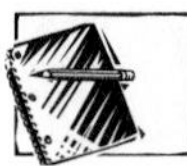

EVALUATION

Outcome

Ear block clears without difficulty, and patient has no further problems

Possible Complications

- Permanent hearing loss
- Ruptured tympanic membrane
- Serous otitis media

Follow-up

- If ear unblocked in office, follow-up in 1 week
- If ear not unblocked, follow-up in 72 hours

FOR YOUR INFORMATION

Life Span

Pediatric: Allowing small children to cry or suck on bottle/pacifier when changing altitude will auto-inflate their eustachian tube
Geriatric: More prone to vertigo that is disabling
Pregnancy: Increased nasal congestion makes patient more prone to barotitis media

Miscellaneous

Barotrauma can also occur in the sinuses. The patient with chronic sinusitis should avoid diving or flying. If diving or flying is absolutely necessary, an oral decongestant should be used before the event.

Reference

Niparko JK: Hearing loss and associated problems. In Barker LR, Burton JR, Zieve PD, editors: *Principles of ambulatory medicine,* ed 4, Baltimore, 1995, William & Wilkins, p 1410.

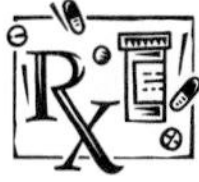

PHARMACOTHERAPEUTICS

Drug of Choice	Mechanism of Action	Prescribing Information	Side Effects
Topical decongestant: Oxymetazoline (Afrin, Neo-Synephrine); children 6 years and up, 2 sprays each nostril bid	Sympathomimetic; causes vasoconstriction, which decreases congestion	***Contraindications:*** Hypersensitivity; hypertension; diabetes; heart disease; thyroid disease; difficulty urinating because of enlarged prostate ***Cost:*** OTC: \$3-\$5 ***Pregnancy category:*** C	Do not use for >3-4 days or exceed dosing because rebound congestion may occur; habituation; stinging of nasal mucosa; dry membranes
Oral decongestants: 130 different products listed in *PDR* for nonprescription drugs; many in combination with an antihistamine; most contain pseudoephedrine, phenylephrine, or phenylpropanolamine; see labels for dosage—do not exceed dosage	Sympathomimetics; cause nasal vasoconstriction, producing decongestion	***Contraindications:*** Hypersensitivity; hypertension—controversial diabetes; heart or thyroid disease; prostate enlargement ***Cost:*** Varies with product ***Pregnancy category:*** Pseudoephedrine—B; phenylephrine and phenylpropanolamine—C	Drowsiness, dry mouth, insomnia, headache, nervousness, fatigue, irritability, disorientation, rash, palpitations, sore throat, cough
Antihistamines: • Diphenhydramine (Benadryl), 25-50 mg qid PO; children 6-12 years, 12.5-25 mg PO qid • Loratadine (Claritin), 10 mg 1 qd PO—do not use in children <12 years • Astemizole (Hismanal), 10 mg, 1 qd PO—do not use in children <12 years • Fexofenadine (Allegra), 60 mg PO bid—do not use in children <12 years	Compete with histamine for cell receptor sites	***Contraindications:*** Coadministration of erythromycin, ketoconazole, or other drugs metabolized by P450 system with Hismanal hypersensitivity ***Cost:*** Benadryl, 25-mg dose, 4/day × 30 days: \$4; Claritin, 10-mg tab, 1/day × 30 days: \$53; Hismanal, 10-mg tab, 1/day × 30 days: \$53; Allegra, 60-mg tab, 2/day × 30 days: \$50 ***Pregnancy category:*** Benadryl and Claritin—B; Hismanal and Allegra—C	Sedation—marked with Benadryl and lesser with the others; headache; fatigue; dizziness; nausea, vomiting; dry mouth; cough; rash; nervousness

Basal Cell Carcinoma (BCC)

OVERVIEW

Basal cell carcinoma (BCC) is a malignant skin tumor that arises from the basal cells of the epidermis. The most common skin cancer, it rarely metastasizes.

Pathogenesis
- Usually occurs at site of previous injury, such as a scar or thermal burn
- Rises from basal keratinocytes of epidermis, hair follicles, and eccrine sweat ducts
- Grows by direct extension and appears to require surrounding stroma to support growth
- Is induced by ultraviolet B radiation
- Cells are not capable of metastasizing through blood and lymphatics
- 85% occur on head and neck, with 20% to 30% occurring on nose
- Untreated, can destroy whole side of face and invade bone and brain

Patient Profile
- Males > Females
- Any age, but dramatically increases after age 40
- Fair skinned > dark skinned; rare in African-Americans
- Excessive sun exposure is predisposing factor
- Increased use of tanning salons—increased incidence in the young
- Increased incidence in persons living in sunny climates, working outdoors, and with increased age

Signs and Symptoms
- Patient complains of a sore that bleeds, heals, and then recurs
- Tumor takes many forms—nodular, noduloulcerative, pigmented, superficial, sclerosing, or cystic

Differential Diagnosis
- Actinic keratosis
- Leukoplakia
- Common nevus
- Seborrheic keratosis
- Solar lentigo
- Molluscum contagiosum

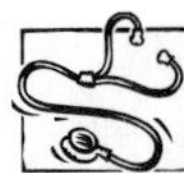

ASSESSMENT

History
Inquire about:
- Onset and duration of symptoms
- Family or personal history of skin cancers and treatment
- Exposure and overexposure to sun or use of tanning salons
- Prior radiation or thermal injury
- Any sores that heal and recur
- Underlying conditions
- Current medications

Physical Findings
- Inspect entire skin surface and evaluate all pigmented skin lesions carefully, looking for sores that are bleeding or scabbed
- Nodular form (most common)—appears as pearly colored nodule with fine telangiectasia over surface; may have depressed center or rolled edge
- Noduloulcerative—lesions appear same as nodular but may be ulcerated and crusted
- Pigmented nodular—contains brown or black pigment
- Superficial—resembles psoriasis or eczema
- Sclerosing—flat, yellow, or skin-colored lesion
- Cystic—translucent, cystic nodule

Initial Workup
Laboratory: Pathologic examination of removed lesion to confirm diagnosis
Radiology: None indicated

Further Workup
None indicated

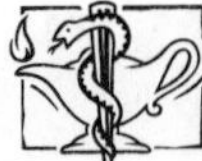

INTERVENTIONS

Office Treatment
- None in primary care office
- Dermatology or surgeon's office—electrodesiccation and curettage for nodular BCCs <6 mm in diameter
- Excision surgery preferred for large tumors with well-defined borders
- Cryosurgery—liquid nitrogen—for nodular and superficial types
- Mohs' micrographic surgery for tumors with poorly defined margins

Lifestyle Modification
Reduce exposure to ultraviolet B

Patient Education
Teach patient about:
- Condition and treatment—various surgical procedures may be used
- Using sunscreen with SPF rating of 25 or higher
- Wearing protective clothing, such as wide-brimmed hat
- Performing skin self-examination (see below)
- Importance of regular follow-up visits and prompt treatment if another lesion appears

How to perform a skin self-examination

Remember, you are looking for any new lesions or changes in old lesions.

1. Remove all clothing, examine both sides of the hands and arms.
2. Stand in front of a mirror, raise arms, and examine underarms.
3. Stand facing a full-length mirror and examine entire front of body.
4. Stand with the back to a full-length mirror and examine entire back of body. This may be done by turning the head to look in the mirror or by using a hand-held mirror to see reflection. Be sure to examine the skin behind the ears by gently pulling the ears forward.
5. Use a hand-held mirror to examine top of head. Move hair away from scalp to see skin.
6. Use a hand-held mirror to examine backs of both legs and bottoms of both feet while sitting down.
7. Inspect the skin between the toes of both feet.

Referral
To dermatologist or surgeon

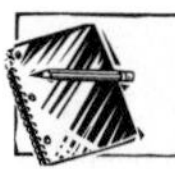

EVALUATION

Outcome

- If lesion is fully excised, no recurrence
- If recurrence, most will recur within 5 years

Possible Complications

- Local recurrence
- Rarely—metastasis

Follow-up

By dermatologist

FOR YOUR INFORMATION

Life Span

Pediatric: Rare in children; educate on use of sunscreen
Geriatric: More common in this age group; educate on use of sunscreen
Pregnancy: N/A

Miscellaneous

According to Marghoob et al. (1995), patients with BCC are at an increased risk of developing malignant melanoma. These authors recommend lifelong total cutaneous examinations of these patients to detect early, curable malignant melanomas.

References

Habif TP: *Clinical dermatology: a color guide to diagnosis and therapy,* ed 3, St Louis, 1996, Mosby, pp 649-659.

Kuflik AS, Janniger CK: Basal cell carcinoma, *Am Fam Physician* 48(7):1273-1276, 1993.

Marghoob AA et al: Basal cell and squamous cell carcinomas are important risk factors for cutaneous malignant melanoma: screening implications, *Cancer* 75:707-714, 1995.

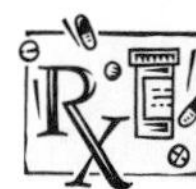

PHARMACOTHERAPEUTICS

Usually no medications will be prescribed by the NP. If the patient comes to the clinic with an infection after excision, the NP may need to order systemic antibiotics or topical antibiotics.

Bell's Palsy

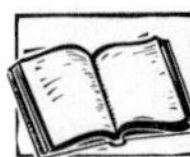

OVERVIEW

Bell's palsy is paralysis or weakness of the facial muscles due to inflammation of the seventh cranial nerve (facial nerve). It is usually unilateral.

Pathogenesis

- Cause—unknown
- Current theory—possibly caused by herpes simplex virus causing inflammation and demyelination of nerve (onset often accompanied by herpes vesicles around or in ear)
- May also be associated with Lyme disease and AIDS

Patient Profile

- Males = Females
- Affects all ages; most common over age 30

Signs and Symptoms

- Sudden onset of flaccidity of one side of face
- Drooping of mouth
- Drooling
- Unilateral loss of taste
- Inability to smile, frown, or whistle
- May have loss of tearing or excessive tearing
- Pain behind ear on affected side

Differential Diagnosis

- Cerebrovascular accident (CVA)
- Lyme disease
- Guillain-Barré syndrome
- Tumor
- Meningitis—all types
- Trauma
- Multiple sclerosis

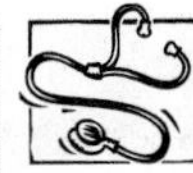

ASSESSMENT

History

Inquire about:

- Onset and duration of symptoms
- History of other neurologic symptoms
- Recent outbreak of herpes around ear on affected side
- Cerebrovascular and cardiac risk factors
- Recent infection
- History of trauma
- Underlying conditions
- Current medications

Physical Findings

- Unilateral, total, or partial paralysis of face
- Inability to frown, smile, or whistle
- May find evidence of herpes lesions around affected ear
- Pain on palpation around ear
- Flat nasolabial fold
- Affected eyeball rolls up, but lid does not close
- Possibly parotid gland swelling

Initial Workup

Laboratory

- Usually none needed, unless uncertain about diagnosis
- Lyme titer possibly

Radiology: CT scan or MRI of head to rule out tumor or CVA, if history and physical examination warrant it

Further Workup

May include the following, but usually not necessary:

- Electromyography
- Nerve conduction studies
- Spinal tap

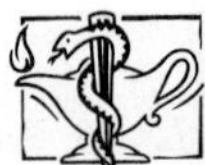

INTERVENTIONS

Office Treatment

None indicated

Lifestyle Modifications

- Smoking cessation
- May need to patch affected eye, which will affect visual ability
- May need to eat softer foods if difficulty chewing is present
- May have impact on patient's employment because of appearance or speaking ability

Patient Education

Teach patient about:

- Disease process and treatment options—oral steroids if diagnosed within 4 days of onset
- Eye drops for lubrication and how to apply
- How to tape eye shut at night
- Physical therapy—heat therapy, electrical stimulation, massage, facial exercises
- No specific treatment for Bell's palsy; usually resolves within 6 weeks
- Medications used and side effects (see Pharmacotherapeutics).

Referrals

- To physical therapist
- To MD if symptoms worsen or do not resolve

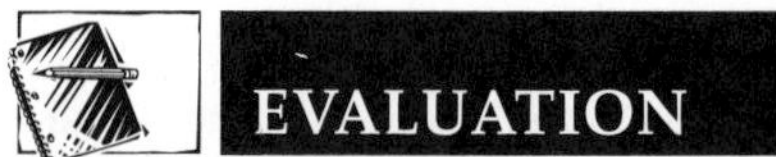

EVALUATION

Outcome
Complete resolution within 6 weeks

Possible Complications
- Corneal abrasion or ulcer
- Hemifacial spasms with total denervation

Follow-up
In 3 to 4 days for moderate to severe symptoms; for others, every 2 weeks until resolution

FOR YOUR INFORMATION

Life Span
Pediatric: Rare in children
Geriatric: Need to reassure patient frequently that this is not a CVA and that full recovery can be obtained
Pregnancy: Consult with obstetrician before using steroids

Miscellaneous
Be alert to the possibility that the use of steroids may mask subclinical infections.

References
Bull TR: *Color atlas of E.N.T. diagnosis,* ed 3, London, 1995, Mosby-Wolfe, p 91.
Michalec DH, Walleck CA: Nursing role in management: peripheral nerve and spinal cord problems. In Lewis SM, Collier IC, Heitkemper MM, editors: *Medical-surgical nursing: assessment and management of clinical problems,* ed 4, St Louis, 1996, Mosby, pp 1795-1796.

NOTES

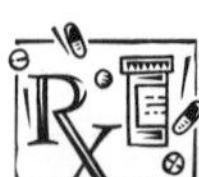

PHARMACOTHERAPEUTICS

Drug of Choice	Mechanism of Action	Prescribing Information	Side Effects
Hydroxypropyl methylcellulose (Tears Naturale II), 1-2 gtt to affected eye as needed	Replaces natural eye lubricant; methylcellulose is viscous solution to extend eye contact time	***Contraindication:*** Hypersensitivity ***Cost:*** 15 ml: $5 ***Pregnancy category:*** Not categorized	Rare side effects: burning, stinging, irritation
Prednisone (Deltasone); 2 methods of dosing: 60 mg PO/day × 3 days; 50 mg PO/day × 3 days; 40 mg PO/day × 2 days; 30 mg PO/ day × 1 day; 20 mg PO/day × 1 day; 10 mg PO/day × 1 day; *or* 20 mg PO qid × 5 days; 20 mg PO tid × 1 day; 20 mg PO bid × 1 day; 20 mg PO qd × 1 day; 10 mg PO qd × 1 day	Potent antiinflammatory agent	***Contraindications:*** Systemic fungal infections; psychosis; hypersensitivity; idiopathic thrombocytopenia; acute glomerulonephritis; amebiasis; AIDS; tuberculosis ***Cost:*** 10 mg tab, 100 tabs: $4-$12 ***Pregnancy category:*** C	Depression, flushing, hypertension, circulatory collapse, thrombophlebitis, embolism, diarrhea, nausea, GI hemorrhage, thrombocytopenia, poor wound healing, acne, ecchymosis

Benign Prostatic Hyperplasia (BPH)

OVERVIEW

Benign prostatic hyperplasia (BPH) is enlargement of the prostate gland. Enlargement of the prostate may result in bladder outlet obstruction.

Pathogenesis

Exact cause unknown; evidence points to systemic hormonal alteration, which may or may not act with growth factors, increasing stromal or glandular hyperplasia

Patient Profile

- Males only
- Most common age >50 years; rarely <40 years

Signs and Symptoms

- Obstructive symptoms—weak urinary stream, hesitancy, postvoid dribbling, straining to void, inability to voluntarily stop stream, incomplete bladder emptying, urinary retention
- Irritative symptoms—frequency, nocturia, urgency, back pain
- Other—increased postvoid residual, prostate enlargement

Differential Diagnosis

- Other causes of bladder outlet obstruction—prostate cancer, urethral stricture, bladder neck contracture
- Nonobstructive causes—neurogenic, myogenic, or psychogenic impairment of detrusor muscle
- Inflammatory disorders—prostatitis, cystitis, urethritis
- Medication such as anticholinergic and sympathomimetics

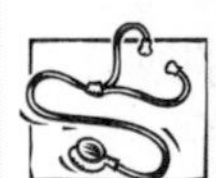

ASSESSMENT

History

- Inquire about:
  - Onset and duration of symptoms
  - Number of times patient urinates during the day and at night
  - Urinary stream (difficulty starting/stopping; weak; dribbling)
  - Pain or discomfort on urination
  - Back pain or blood in urine
  - Underlying conditions
  - Current medications
- Have patient fill out the American Urological Association (AUA) Symptom Index (Table 2)

Physical Findings

- Abdominal examination—distended bladder, renal tenderness, mass
- Rectal examination—normal prostate 2.5 × 3 cm; median sulcus can be palpated midline
- BPH—enlarged, smooth, rubbery, no median sulcus
- Prostate cancer—asymmetric, nodular, with hard, fixed mass

Initial Workup

Laboratory

- Urinalysis and serum creatinine
- Prostate specific antigen (PSA)—should be drawn before manipulation of prostate; may be elevated but usually <10 μg/L
- CBC
- Chemistry profile to include electrolytes (optional)
- BUN and serum acid phosphatase (optional)

Radiology

- Transrectal ultrasonography (best at estimating prostate size)
- IVP (optional)

Further Workup

- Postvoid residual urine by either ultrasound or catheterization
- Prostate biopsy
- Uroflow studies
- Cystometrogram (optional)

TABLE 2 *AUA Symptom Index*

	Not at all	Less than 1 time in 5	Less than half the time	About half the time	More than half the time	Almost always
1. Over the past month, have you had a sensation of not emptying your bladder completely after you finished urinating?	0	1	2	3	4	5
2. Over the past month, how often have you had to urinate again less than 2 hours after you finished urinating?	0	1	2	3	4	5
3. Over the past month, how often have you found you stopped and started again several times when you urinated?	0	1	2	3	4	5
4. Over the past month, how often have you found it difficult to postpone urination?	0	1	2	3	4	5
5. Over the past month, how often have you had a weak urinary stream?	0	1	2	3	4	5
6. Over the past month, how often have you had to push or strain to begin urination?	0	1	2	3	4	5
7. Over the past month, how many times did you most typically get up to urinate from the time you went to bed at night until the time you got up in the morning?	0	1	2	3	4	5

From Barry MJ et al: The American Urological Association Symptoms Index for benign prostatic hyperplasia, *J Urol 11*(148):1549-1557, 1992.
The sum of the 7 circled numbers is the AUA Symptom Score. Interpretation of AUA Symptom Index: mild symptoms—0-7; moderate symptoms—8-19; severe symptoms—20-35.

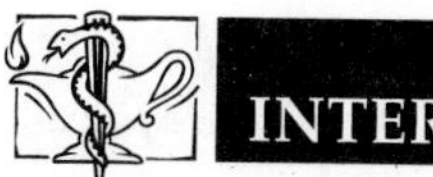

INTERVENTIONS

Office Treatment
None indicated

Lifestyle Modifications
- Frequent urination
- Avoidance of large amounts of fluids after evening meal
- Avoidance of sympathomimetic or anticholinergic medications (cold preparations)

Patient Education
Teach patient about:
- Condition, cause, and treatment (appears to be part of aging process)
- Necessity of voiding frequently
- Avoiding large amounts of fluid
- Avoiding sympathomimetic and anticholinergic medications
- Prostate massage after intercourse
- Avoiding caffeine and alcohol, which cause sudden diuresis
- Treatment options based on AUA Index score:
  - Mild symptoms—watchful waiting, will often stabilize
  - Moderate to severe symptoms—medications, balloon dilation, surgery
- Medications used and side effects (see Pharmacotherapeutics)

Referral
To urologist or surgeon if above treatment fails

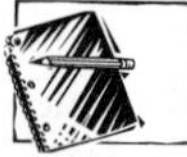

EVALUATION

Outcome
Symptoms improve or stabilize with or without medication

Possible Complications
- Urinary tract infections
- Bladder stones
- Prostatitis
- Renal failure
- Prostate cancer; up to 30% of patients with BPH have occult cancer

Follow-up
- Every 2 weeks to monitor symptoms until stabilized; then every 6 months for urinalysis and serum creatinine
- Yearly digital examination and PSA

FOR YOUR INFORMATION

Life Span
Pediatric: N/A
Geriatric: 80% of men >70 years have BPH
Pregnancy: N/A

Miscellaneous
Procedures used to treat BPH:
- Transurethral resection of prostate (TURP)
- Transurethral incision of prostate
- Open prostatectomy
- Transurethral dilation of prostate
- Transurethral microwave thermotherapy
- Transrectal prostatic hyperthermia
- Transurethral laser-induced prostatectomy

References
McConnell JD et al: *Benign prostatic hyperplasia: diagnosis and treatment,* Clinical Practice Guideline No 8, AHCPR Pub No 94-0582, Rockville, Md, 1994, US Department of Health and Human Services, Public Health Service, Agency for Health Care Policy and Research.

Stutzman RE: Bladder outlet obstruction. In Barker LR, Burton JR, Zieve PD, editors: *Principles of ambulatory medicine,* ed 4, Baltimore, 1995, Williams & Wilkins, pp 579-586.

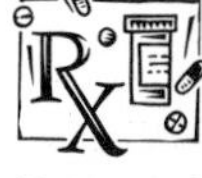

PHARMACOTHERAPEUTICS

Drug of Choice	Mechanism of Action	Prescribing Information	Side Effects
Finasteride (Proscar), 5 mg PO qd	5-Alpha-reductase inhibitor; decreases size of prostate	***Contraindication:*** Hypersensitivity; children; women ***Cost:*** 5-mg tab, 30 tabs: $57 ***Pregnancy category:*** X; crushed tablet should not be handled by pregnant female, nor should she come in contact with semen from someone taking this drug	Impotence, decreased libido, decreased volume of ejaculate
Terazosin (Hytrin), 1 mg PO hs; increase dosage slowly to maximum of 10 mg	Relaxation of smooth muscle resulting from blockade of alpha-1 adrenoceptors in the bladder neck and prostate	***Contraindication:*** Hypersensitivity ***Cost:*** 5-mg tab, 100 tabs: $123 ***Pregnancy category:*** C	Palpitations, orthostatic hypotension, tachycardia, edema, dizziness, headache, drowsiness, anxiety, depression, vertigo, nausea, vomiting, diarrhea, urinary frequency, incontinence, impotence, blurred vision, epistaxis, dry mouth, dyspnea

Blepharitis

OVERVIEW

Blepharitis is an inflammation of the eyelid. It is usually either seborrheic or staphylococcal, or the two types may coexist.

Pathogenesis

- Seborrheic blepharitis—accelerated skin shedding with sebaceous gland dysfunction; caused by seborrheic dermatitis of scalp and eyelids
- Staphylococcal blepharitis—caused by staphylococcal bacteria

Patient Profile

- Males = Females
- Predominant age—adult, but may be seen in children

Signs and Symptoms

- Seborrheic blepharitis:
  - Erythema of lid margin
  - Dry flakes, oily secretions on lid margins
  - Seborrheic dermatitis of scalp and eyebrows
- Staphylococcal blepharitis:
  - Itching
  - Burning
  - Tearing
  - Crusting after sleeping
  - Photophobia
  - Recurrent stye
  - Recurrent inflammation of meibomian gland
- Mixed type—combination of above symptoms

Differential Diagnosis

- Squamous cell cancer
- Basal cell carcinoma
- Sebaceous cell cancer

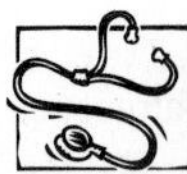

ASSESSMENT

History

Inquire about:

- Onset and duration of symptoms
- Past history of blepharitis, and treatment tried and results
- Eye pain, tearing, or visual disturbances
- History of seborrheic dermatitis
- Underlying conditions
- Current medications

Physical Findings

- Erythematous lid margin (seborrheic)
- Dry flakes on lid margin or eyelashes (seborrheic)
- Ulcerations at base of eyelashes (staphylococcal)
- Photophobia (staphylococcal)

Initial Workup

Laboratory: None indicated
Radiology: None indicated

Further Workup

If does not resolve within 1 month, culture and biopsy for carcinoma

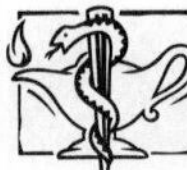

INTERVENTIONS

Office Treatment

None indicated

Lifestyle Modification

Discontinue contact lens use

Patient Education

Teach patient about:

- Disease process and treatment
- Eyelid cleansing
- Seborrheic blepharitis—use of antiseborrheic shampoos (pyrithione zinc; see section on seborrheic dermatitis) on scalp and eyebrows, cleansing eyelid margins with baby shampoo
- Staphylococcal blepharitis—use and side effects of antibacterial eye ointments (see Pharmacotherapeutics)

Referral

To ophthalmologist if resistant to treatment

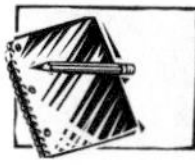

EVALUATION

Outcome
Will probably require long-term eyelid hygiene to control

Possible Complications
- Hordeolum
- Scarring of eyelid margin
- Corneal infection

Follow-up
Every 2 weeks × 1 month; then monthly until controlled

FOR YOUR INFORMATION

Life Span
Pediatric: Children often have a prior history of cradle cap
Geriatric: Usually have history of seborrheic dermatitis
Pregnancy: Cautious use of medications

Miscellaneous
If swelling or inflammation of the eyelid does not resolve in 1 month, the patient must be referred for biopsy. Squamous cell, basal cell, and sebaceous cell cancers can masquerade as blepharitis, styes, or chalazions. This is known as "masquerade syndrome."

References
Goldblum K, Collier IC: Nursing assessment: vision and hearing. In Lewis SM, Cox IC, Heitkemper MM, editors: *Medical-surgical nursing: assessment and management of clinical problems,* ed 4, St Louis, 1996, Mosby, p 447.

Schachat AD: The red eye. In Barker LR, Burton JR, Zieve PD, editors: *Principles of ambulatory medicine,* ed 4, Baltimore, 1995, Williams & Wilkins, p 1435.

NOTES

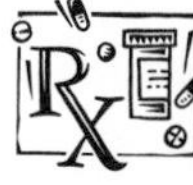

PHARMACOTHERAPEUTICS

Drug of Choice	Mechanism of Action	Prescribing Information	Side Effects
For staphylococcal blepharitis, use one of the following:			
Bacitracin ophthalmic ointment (Ocutracin); adults and children, apply to eyelid nightly for mild cases, up to qid for severe cases	Bactericidal against gram-positive organisms	***Contraindication:*** Hypersensitivity ***Cost:*** 3.5-g tube: $4 ***Pregnancy category:*** Not categorized	Irritation, sensitivity, burning, itching, increased inflammation, discontinue if above symptoms occur
Erythromycin ophthalmic ointment; adults and children, apply bid to lid margin	Inhibits protein synthesis in organism	***Contraindication:*** Hypersensitivity ***Cost:*** 3.5-g tube: $4 ***Pregnancy category:*** B	Irritation, sensitivity, burning, itching, increased inflammation, discontinue if any of above occur
For severe cases:			
Tetracycline (Achromycin), 250 mg PO qid × 4 weeks; then 250 mg/day × 2 months; children >8 years, 25-50 mg/kg/day—do not use in children <8 years; take 1 hour before or 2 hours after meals	Bacteriostatic; inhibits protein synthesis; active against gram-negative and gram-positive organisms	***Contraindications:*** Hypersensitivity; pregnancy; nursing mothers; children <8 years ***Cost:*** 250-mg tabs, 4/day × 10 days: $2 ***Pregnancy category:*** D	May increase digoxin levels; monitor prothrombin time in patients taking coumadin; anorexia; nausea; vomiting; diarrhea; glossitis; enterocolitis; inflammatory lesions; rash; photosensitivity; increased BUN; urticaria; hemolytic anemia; thrombocytopenia; neutropenia

Breast Abscess

OVERVIEW

A breast abscess is a localized collection of pus. It is frequently associated with lactation, but it may be associated with fistulous tracts, which may be a result of squamous epithelial neoplasia or duct occlusion.

Pathogenesis

- Formed as a result of suppuration in a localized infection; may be due to a blocked lactiferous duct
- Cavity containing pus, surrounded by inflamed tissue
- Usual pathogen is staphylococcus but can have a sterile abscess

Patient Profile

- Female
- Any age after puberty
- Risk factors:
  - Mastitis
  - Diabetes
  - Rheumatoid arthritis
  - Steroids
  - Silicone implants
  - Lumpectomy with radiation
  - Heavy cigarette smoking

Signs and Symptoms

- Tender, fluctuant breast lump
- Erythema
- Purulent drainage
- Local edema
- Malaise
- Fever
- Nipple and skin retraction
- Proximal lymphadenopathy

Differential Diagnosis

- Inflammatory carcinoma
- Tuberculosis
- Actinomycosis
- Typhoid
- Sarcoid
- Syphilis
- Hydatid cyst
- Sebaceous cyst
- Mastitis

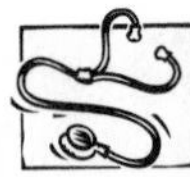

ASSESSMENT

History

Inquire about:

- Onset and duration of symptoms
- Family history of breast cancer
- Lactation
- Silicone implants
- Recent treatment for mastitis
- Smoking history
- Underlying conditions such as diabetes or rheumatoid arthritis
- Current medications

Physical Findings

- Tender breast lump with erythema and edema
- Fluctuance
- Fever
- Purulent drainage
- Fissured nipple

Initial Workup

Laboratory

- Culture and sensitivity of drainage
- CBC with differential—leukocytosis and left shift possible
- Sample of drainage for pathology
- Rapid plasma reagin (RPR) and purified protein derivative (PPD) (nonpuerperal associated with syphilis and tuberculosis)

Radiology: Ultrasound and/or mammogram

Further Workup

None

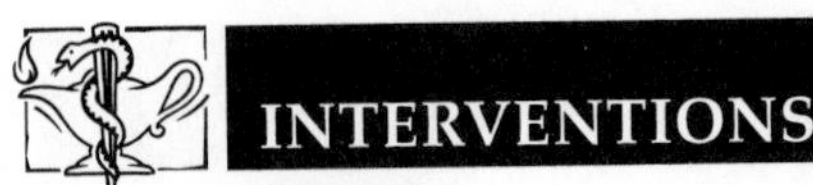

INTERVENTIONS

Office Treatment

- Fine-needle aspiration to remove fluid
- Incision and drainage, making sure to open all sinus tracts

Lifestyle Modifications

- If breast-feeding, may need to express milk and discard
- May need to stop breast-feeding
- Smoking cessation

Patient Education

Teach patient about:

- Condition and treatment
- Needle aspiration, incision and drainage, antibiotics
- Care of wound following needle aspiration or incision and drainage
- Cold compresses and expression of milk to help relieve pain
- Using nipple shield if nipple is fissured and painful
- Medications used and side effects (see Pharmacotherapeutics)

Referral

To surgeon if NP unable to perform procedures

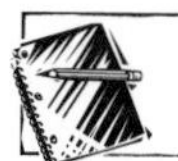

EVALUATION

Outcomes

- Abscess heals without sequelae
- Healing normally occurs in 8 to 10 days

Possible Complications

- Fistula formation
- Systemic infection

Follow-up

48 hours after incision and drainage and then again in 2 weeks, either by surgeon or NP

FOR YOUR INFORMATION

Life Span

Pediatric: May be seen anytime after puberty; treatment the same
Geriatric: More common to see subareolar abscess
Pregnancy: Most commonly seen in postpartum lactation

Miscellaneous

Bundred et al. (1992) discovered a significant correlation between cigarette smoking and nonlactational breast abscesses. These authors also found that cigarette smoking may predispose the patient to anaerobic breast infections and the development of mammillary fistulas.

References

Bundred NJ et al: Breast abscesses and cigarette smoking, *Br J Surg* 79(1):58-59, 1992.
Driscoll CE: Pregnancy. In Driscoll CE et al, editors: *The family practice desk reference,* ed 3, St Louis, 1996, Mosby, p 221.
Vorpahl CL: Breast disorders. In Lewis SM, Collier IC, Heitkemper MM, editors: *Medical-surgical nursing: assessment and management of clinical problems,* ed 4, St Louis, 1996, Mosby, pp 1545-1546.

NOTES

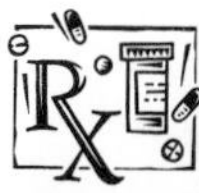

PHARMACOTHERAPEUTICS

Drug of Choice	Mechanism of Action	Prescribing Information	Side Effects
Amoxicillin/clavulanate (Augmentin), 500-875 mg PO bid for 10 days; children, 25-45 mg/kg/day PO in 2 divided doses	Bactericidal; cell wall inhibitor; effective against beta-lactamase–producing organisms	***Contraindication:*** Hypersensitivity ***Cost:*** 500-mg tab, 30 tabs: $82 ***Pregnancy category:*** B	Diarrhea, nausea, vomiting, stomatitis, black hairy tongue, pseudomembranous colitis, candidiasis, rash, urticaria, angioedema, anaphylaxis, arthralgia, myalgia, anemia, thrombocytopenia, leukopenia, anxiety, insomnia, confusion
Erythromycin (E.E.S.), 500 mg PO bid for 10 days; children, 30-50 mg/kg/day in 4 divided doses	Macrolide; protein synthesis inhibitor; active against bacteria lacking cell walls, most gram-positive aerobes	***Contraindication:*** Hypersensitivity ***Cost:*** 250-mg tabs, 4/day × 10 days: $4 ***Pregnancy category:*** B	Nausea, vomiting, diarrhea, abdominal pain, anorexia, rash, urticaria, pseudomembranous colitis—rarely

Breast Cancer

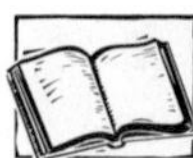

OVERVIEW

Breast cancer is an overgrowth of neoplastic cells of the breast. It may be classified as invasive or noninvasive, with about 70% to 80% being invasive (Table 3).

Pathogenesis

Exact cause unknown

Patient Profile

- Females > Males; males account for only 1% of cases
- Rare <30 years of age; usually between 30 and 80 years; peak incidence between 45 and 65 years; two-thirds >50 years
- High-risk factors:
  - Previous history of breast cancer
  - Atypical hyperplasia on previous biopsy
  - Mother or sister with breast cancer
- Moderate risk factors:
  - Advancing age
  - Menarche before 12 years or menopause after 55 years
  - Nulliparity
  - First child born after age 30
  - Obesity
  - Current or past oral contraceptive use
  - Postmenopausal estrogen therapy
  - Alcohol use

Signs and Symptoms

- Palpable breast mass
- Dimpling
- Nipple retraction
- Nipple discharge
- Nipple ulceration
- Recent onset of breast pain
- Color change with skin changes (peau d' orange)
- Breast enlargement
- Lymph node enlargement

Differential Diagnosis

- Benign diseases—abscesses, hematomas, or fibroadenomas
- Proliferative diseases—fibrocystic changes, ductal and lobular hyperplasia, or sclerosing adenosis
- Various types of malignancies

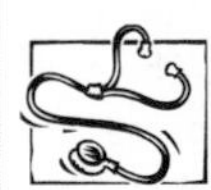

ASSESSMENT

History

Inquire about

- Onset and duration of symptoms; location; mobility; size; single or multiple masses
- Pain
- Nipple discharge—bloody, serous, clear, milky
- Family history
- Diet
- Previous breast cancer
- Previous breast biopsies and diagnosis
- Age of menarche
- If appropriate—age of menopause
- Age when first full-term pregnancy occurred
- Last menstrual period
- Use of birth control pills or hormone replacement therapy
- Last mammogram and results
- Underlying conditions
- Current medications

Physical Findings

- Examine patient sitting:
  - Inspect for symmetry, contour, vascular pattern
  - Inspect skin for color, retraction, dimpling, edema
  - Have patient raise arms above head and inspect for same
  - Have patient place hands on hips and push, and inspect for same
  - Palpate axillary, supraclavicular, and intraclavicular areas
- Examine patient supine:
  - Palpate breast tissue, supraclavicular region, chest wall
  - Dominant area—measure size with fingers; assess opposite breast for similar area; draw picture in chart of abnormal areas

Initial Workup

Laboratory: Consider CBC and liver enzymes and bone function studies
Radiology: Mammogram and/or ultrasound

Further Workup

- Fine-needle biopsy; excisional or incisional biopsy for definitive diagnosis; normally done by surgeon
- Once diagnosis is made—Chest film, bone scan, and liver imaging; estrogen and progesterone receptor assay; usually done by oncologist

TABLE 3 *Types of Breast Cancer*

Type	% of Diagnosed breast cancers	Facts	Prognosis
Invasive ductal carcinoma	70	Can rapidly spread to lymph nodes	80%-90% 5-year survival with negative nodes
Medullary carcinoma	7	Grows in a capsule; less frequent metastasis	80% 5-year survival
Comedocarcinoma	5	Grows in mammary duct; usually does not metastasize	Good
Mucinous carcinoma	3	Slow-growing, ductal cancer; less frequent metastasis	Good
Tubular ductal carcinoma	2 or less	Invasive cancer, but cells arranged in tubules; metastasis uncommon	Better than for invasive
Invasive lobular carcinoma	3	Originates in lobules; metastasis common	Poor
Inflammatory breast cancer	1	Usually wide-spread at time of diagnosis	Poor
Paget's disease	1-4	Cancer of nipple; usually associated with intraductal carcinoma	Varies, but generally poor

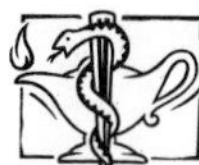

INTERVENTIONS

Office Treatment

Fine-needle aspiration if trained in this procedure; usually none

Lifestyle Modifications

- Decrease in consumption of dietary fat and alcohol—controversial
- Smoking cessation

Patient Education

Teach patient about:

- Condition and treatment options—surgery: lumpectomy or modified radical mastectomy; radiation therapy; chemotherapy; hormonal therapy
- Choosing a surgeon
- Postmastectomy concerns:
  - Prevention of lymphedema
  - Psychologic and physical difficulties
  - Exercises
  - Prosthesis selection
  - Support groups
  - Importance of breast self-examination
  - Importance of yearly mammograms
- Medications used and side effects (see Pharmacotherapeutics)

Referrals

- To surgeon
- To oncologist

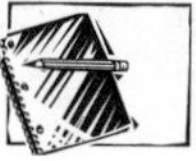

EVALUATION

Outcomes

- Cancer is removed
- Psychologic adaptation

Possible Complications

- Immediate postoperative period—wound infection, lymphedema
- Side effects of chemotherapy—nausea, vomiting, anorexia, alopecia, leukopenia, stomatitis, skin rashes, etc.
- Side effects of radiation therapy—skin irritation, pulmonary fibrosis, arm edema, etc.
- Recurrence of cancer
- Death

Follow-up

- By surgeon in immediate postoperative period
- By oncologist as necessary
- By NP as needed

FOR YOUR INFORMATION

Life Span

Pediatric: Occurs rarely in children; adolescents should be taught breast self-examination

Geriatric: Increased incidence; may have more difficulty tolerating chemotherapy or radiation therapy

Pregnancy: Diagnosis is infrequent; requires difficult decisions regarding treatment; will need to be handled by a specialist

Miscellaneous

Early detection is the key to a good outcome. In women over 50, mammography screening can decrease the mortality rate by 30%. All women over the age of 35 should have a baseline mammogram. Women 40 to 49 years old should have mammograms every 1 to 3 years, and women over 50 should have mammograms yearly. All females from adolescents on should be taught breast self-examination.

References

Branch LG: Breast health. In Youngkin EQ, Davis MS, editors: *Women's health: a primary care clinical guide,* Norwalk, Conn, Appleton & Lange, pp 296-302.

Conry C: Evaluation of a breast complaint: is it cancer? *Am Fam Physician* 49(2):445-450, 1994.

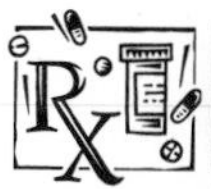

PHARMACOTHERAPEUTICS

There are more than 50 chemotherapeutic agents that may be used in the treatment of breast cancer. The following is a list of the five most commonly used agents. These agents are usually given in combinations of two. There are also several hormonal agents that may be used, but only the most commonly used agent is listed here.

Drug of Choice	Mechanism of Action	Prescribing Information	Side Effects
Doxorubicin (Adriamycin), cyclophosphamide (Cytoxan), methotrexate (Abitrexate), fluorouracil (Adrucil), vincristine (Oncovin); dosage individualized for each patient; given intravenously	Doxorubicin—probably binds to DNA and inhibits nucleic acid synthesis; cyclophosphamide—cross-linking of tumor cell DNA; methotrexate—interferes with DNA synthesis, repair, and replication; fluorouracil—interferes with synthesis of DNA and inhibits RNA; vincristine—arrests dividing cells	***Contraindications:*** Hypersensitivity; pregnancy ***Cost:*** Doxorubicin, 2 mg/ml, 10-ml vial: $97; cyclophosphamide, 2-g vial: $86; methotrexate, 2.5-mg tab, 20 tabs: $58-$71; fluorouracil, 50 mg/ml, 10 ml: $38; vincristine, 1 mg/ml, 1 ml: $15-$30 ***Pregnancy category:*** D	Myelosuppression, impairment of fertility, mutagenic effects, cardiotoxicity, reversible alopecia, acute severe nausea and vomiting, stomatitis, anorexia, diarrhea, hypersensitivity
Tamoxifen (Nolvadex), 10 mg, 1-2 tabs PO bid; used for tumors that are estrogen receptor positive	Nonsteroidal agent; potent antiestrogen; competes for estrogen-binding sites	***Contraindications:*** Hypersensitivity; pregnancy ***Cost:*** 10-mg tab, 60 tabs: $85-$90 ***Pregnancy category:*** D	Hot flushes, nausea and vomiting, menstrual irregularities, skin rash, weight gain, fluid retention, impaired fertility

Bronchiectasis

OVERVIEW

Bronchiectasis is a condition in which there is abnormal dilation of the bronchi. It is irreversible and may be congenital or acquired. It is usually accompanied by infection.

Pathogenesis

Causes:

- Cystic fibrosis (50%)
- Alpha-1–anti-trypsin deficiency
- Aspergillosis
- Tuberculosis
- Lung abscess
- Pneumonia
- Humoral immunodeficiency
- Foreign body
- Tumor
- Hypogammaglobulinemia

Patient Profile

- Males = Females
- Any age; most often begins in childhood

Signs and Symptoms

- Chronic cough
- Copious amounts of foul-smelling, mucopurulent sputum
- Hemoptysis
- Wheezing
- Cyanosis
- Dyspnea
- Weight loss
- Fatigue
- Fever
- Recurrent pneumonia
- Pallor
- Tachycardia
- Tachypnea

Differential Diagnosis

- Cystic fibrosis
- Chronic bronchitis
- Chronic obstructive pulmonary disease (COPD)
- Tuberculosis
- Asthma

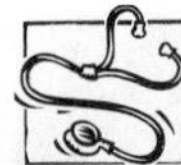

ASSESSMENT

History

Inquire about:

- Onset and duration of symptoms
- History of pneumonia
- Family history of cystic fibrosis
- Underlying conditions
- Current medications

Physical Findings

- General—pallor, fever, halitosis, emaciation, barrel chest, cyanosis
- Lungs—wheezes, coarse/moist crackles, decreased breath sounds, tachypnea
- Copious amounts of foul-smelling, mucopurulent sputum

Initial Workup

Laboratory

- CBC with differential—anemia; leukocytosis possible with left shift
- Sputum culture—(+) (*Haemophilus influenzae, Streptococcus pneumoniae,* staphylococci, or anaerobes)
- Serum immunoglobulins—hypogammaglobulinemia

Radiology: Chest film—PA and lateral—may be normal or coarse lung markings, cystic lesions

Further Workup

- Sweat test—positive in cystic fibrosis
- Bronchoscopy
- Chest CT scan
- Pulmonary function test

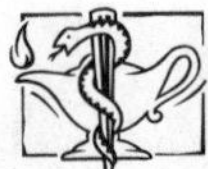

INTERVENTIONS

Office Treatment

None indicated

Lifestyle Modifications

- Smoking cessation
- Adequate hydration
- Learning to live with a chronic illness

Patient Education

Teach patient about:

- Condition and treatment
- Chest percussion and postural drainage (will need to train significant other)
- Using bronchodilators and/or positive expiratory pressure
- Tips for smoking cessation
- Reporting signs and symptoms of infection promptly
- Reporting severe hemoptysis promptly (may require lung resection)
- Strategies for living with a chronic illness
- Medications used and side effects (see Pharmacotherapeutics)

Referrals

- To pulmonologist or surgeon for bronchoscopy
- To social worker
- To home health care

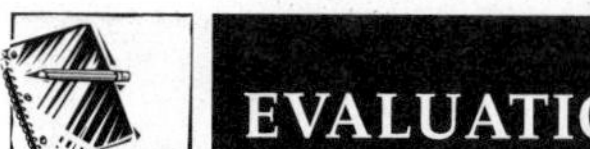

EVALUATION

Outcome
Chronic course; if disease is localized, surgical lung resection may be curative

Possible Complications
- Recurrent pulmonary infections
- Pulmonary hypertension
- Secondary amyloidosis
- Cor pulmonale
- Brain abscess

Follow-up
Depends on severity of disease; initially, every 2 weeks

FOR YOUR INFORMATION

Life Span
Pediatric: Must rule out cystic fibrosis
Geriatric: Higher morbidity and mortality; need to discuss patient's wishes regarding cardiopulmonary resuscitation (CPR) and mechanical ventilation
Pregnancy: Should be handled by a specialist

Miscellaneous
Bronchiectasis is much less common than it once was because of more effective treatment of childhood respiratory infections.

References
Stauffer JL: Lung. In Tierney LM, Jr, McPhee SJ, Papadakis MA, editors: *Medical diagnosis and treatment,* ed 34, Norwalk, Conn, Appleton & Lange, pp. 223-224.

Woolliscroft JO: *Current diagnosis & treatment: a quick reference for the general practitioner,* Philadelphia, 1996, Current Medicine, pp 58-59.

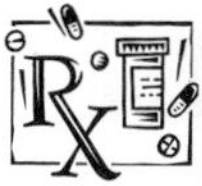

PHARMACOTHERAPEUTICS

Drug of Choice	Mechanism of Action	Prescribing Information	Side Effects
Albuterol (Proventil, Ventolin); inhaler—adults and children >4 years, 2 puffs PO qid; extended-release tabs—adults and children >12 years, 4-8 mg PO q12h; children 6-12 years, 2 mg PO q12h; syrup—children 2-6 years, 0.1 mg/kg/day in 3 divided doses	Bronchodilator; B_2 agonist—increases cAMP, which relaxes smooth muscle, leading to bronchodilation and CNS and cardiac stimulation; increases diuresis and gastric acid secretion	***Contraindications:*** Hypersensitivity; tachydysrhythmias; severe cardiac disease ***Cost:*** Metered dose inhaler: \$13-\$22; tabs, 2-mg tab, 100 tabs: \$3-\$37 ***Pregnancy category:*** C	Tremors, anxiety, insomnia, headache, dizziness, stimulation, restlessness, hallucinations, flushing, dry nose, palpitations, tachycardia, hypertension, angina, heartburn, nausea, vomiting, muscle cramps
Pirbuterol (Maxair); adults and children >12 years, 2 inhalations PO qid	Bronchodilator; B_2 agonist—increases cAMP, which relaxes smooth muscle, leading to bronchodilation and CNS and cardiac stimulation; increases diuresis and gastric acid secretion	***Contraindications:*** Hypersensitivity; tachydysrhythmias; severe cardiac disease ***Cost:*** 14-g autoinhaler: \$34 ***Pregnancy category:*** C	Tremors, anxiety, insomnia, headache, dizziness, stimulation, restlessness, hallucinations, flushing, dry nose, palpitations, tachycardia, hypertension, angina, heartburn, nausea, vomiting, muscle cramps, gastritis, coughing

Antibiotic therapy should be based on the results of the sputum culture and sensitivity tests. The patient may be treated empirically with one of the following:

Drug of Choice	Mechanism of Action	Prescribing Information	Side Effects
Ampicillin, 250-500 mg PO q6h; children, 50-100 mg/kg/day PO in divided doses q6h	Interferes with cell wall replication	***Contraindication:*** Hypersensitivity ***Cost:*** 500-mg tab, 40 tabs: \$5-\$13 ***Pregnancy category:*** B	Rash, urticaria, anemia, bone marrow depression, granulocytopenia, nausea, vomiting, diarrhea, moniliasis, glomerulonephritis, lethargy, hallucinations, depression, convulsions
Tetracycline (Achromycin), 250-500 mg PO q6h; children >8 years, 25-50 mg/kg/day PO in divided doses q6h	Inhibits protein synthesis and phosphorylation in microorganisms	***Contraindications:*** Hypersensitivity; children <8 years; lactation ***Cost:*** 500-mg tab, 40 tabs: \$4-\$15 ***Pregnancy category:*** D	Eosinophilia, neutropenia, thrombocytopenia, leukocytosis, hemolytic anemia, dysphagia, glossitis, oral candidiasis, nausea, abdominal pain, vomiting, diarrhea, hepatotoxicity, flatulence, abdominal cramps, rash, urticaria, photosensitivity, exfoliative dermatitis, angioedema

Bronchitis, Acute

OVERVIEW

Acute bronchitis is an inflammatory condition of the tracheobronchial tree that is a result of a respiratory tract infection.

Pathogenesis

Many causes:
- Adenovirus
- Influenza
- *Mycoplasma pneumoniae*
- *Chlamydia pneumoniae*
- *Moraxella catarrhalis*
- Coxsackie virus
- *Haemophilus influenzae*
- Rhinovirus
- Secondary bacterial infection

Patient Profile

- Males = Females
- Any age

Signs and Symptoms

- Report of upper respiratory tract infection
- Cough—nonproductive early/productive late
- Fever
- Fatigue
- Hemoptysis
- Chest burning
- Dyspnea
- Adventitious breath sounds

Differential Diagnosis

- Pneumonia
- Pertussis
- Influenza
- Asthma
- Aspiration

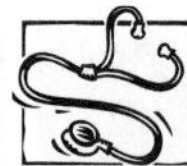

ASSESSMENT

History

Inquire about:
- Onset and duration of symptoms
- Preceding upper respiratory tract symptoms
- Smoking history
- Underlying conditions
- Current medications

Physical Findings

- May or may not have fever
- Lungs—may be clear; may have coarse sounds, rales, rhonchi, or wheezes

Initial Workup

Laboratory
- Bronchitis is diagnosis of exclusion; no laboratory test is diagnostic
- CBC—leukocytosis if bacterial

Radiology: Chest film—PA and lateral—usually normal in bronchitis

Further Workup

Usually none needed

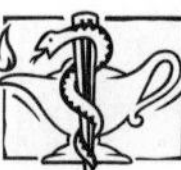

INTERVENTIONS

Office Treatment

None indicated

Lifestyle Modification

Smoking cessation

Patient Education

Teach patient about:
- Condition and treatment
- Cause—most viral (treat symptomatically); if suspect bacterial cause, treat with antibiotics
- Increasing fluids
- Using cool-mist or steam vaporizer
- Tips for smoking cessation
- Obtaining adequate amount of rest
- Avoiding irritants and air pollutants
- Medications used and side effects (see Pharmacotherapeutics)

Referral

To MD if treatment fails and symptoms persist

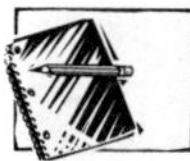

EVALUATION

Outcome
Usually resolves without sequelae

Possible Complications
- Pneumonia
- Postbronchitic reactive airway disease
- Acute respiratory failure

Follow-up
If symptoms persist longer than 2 weeks or if symptoms worsen

FOR YOUR INFORMATION

Life Span
Pediatric: With repeated attacks, evaluate child for congenital defects of respiratory tract
Geriatric: Higher morbidity and mortality
Pregnancy: Cautious use of medications

Miscellaneous
Acute bronchitis is a very common condition seen in the primary care setting

References
Koster FT, Barker LR: Respiratory tract infections. In Barker LR, Burton JR, Zieve PD, editors: *Principles of ambulatory medicine,* ed 4, Baltimore, 1995, Williams & Wilkins, pp 340-341.

Uphold CR, Graham MV: *Clinical guidelines in adult health,* Gainesville, Fla, 1994, Barmarrae Books, pp 330-332.

NOTES

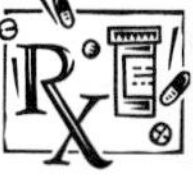

PHARMACOTHERAPEUTICS

Drug of Choice	Mechanism of Action	Prescribing Information	Side Effects
For fever and myalgia:			
Acetaminophen (Tylenol), 325-650 mg PO q4-6h; for children, use Children's Tylenol—follow label directions	Blocks pain impulse by inhibition of prostaglandins; decreases fever by inhibition of prostaglandins in hypothalamic heat-regulating center	***Contraindication:*** Hypersensitivity ***Cost:*** OTC ***Pregnancy category:*** Not categorized	Rash, hepatic toxicity with alcohol ingestion or overdose, leukopenia, neutropenia, hemolytic anemia, thrombocytopenia, nausea, vomiting, rash, angioedema, toxicity
When there is a secondary bacterial infection, use one of the following:			
Erythromycin (E-Mycin), 250-500 mg PO qid; children, 30-50 mg/kg/day in divided doses q6h	Inhibits protein synthesis	***Contraindication:*** Hypersensitivity ***Cost:*** 250-mg tabs, 4/day × 10 days: $4 ***Pregnancy category:*** B	Nausea, vomiting, diarrhea, abdominal pain, anorexia, rash, urticaria, pseudomembranous colitis—rarely
Sulfamethoxazole (SMZ) and trimethoprin (TMP) DS (Bactrim DS), 1 DS tab PO bid; children, 8 mg/kg TMP and 40 mg/kg SMZ qd in 2 divided doses	Blocks 2 consecutive steps in bacterial synthesis of nucleic acids and protein	***Contraindications:*** Hypersensitivity to TMP or sulfonamides; term pregnancy; lactation; megaloblastic anemia; infants <2 months; creatinine clearance <15 ml/min ***Cost:*** DS tab × 14 days: $3 ***Pregnancy category:*** C	Anaphylaxis/hypersensitivity, Stevens-Johnson syndrome, allergic myocarditis, nausea, vomiting, abdominal pain, hepatitis, enterocolitis, renal failure, toxic nephrosis, leukopenia, thrombocytopenia, hemolytic anemia
Ampicillin, 250-500 mg PO q6h; children 50-100 mg/kg/day PO in divided doses q6h	Interferes with cell wall replication	***Contraindication:*** Hypersensitivity ***Cost:*** 500-mg tab, 40 tabs: $5-$13 ***Pregnancy category:*** B	Rash, urticaria, anemia, bone marrow depression, granulocytopenia, nausea, vomiting, diarrhea, moniliasis, glomerulonephritis, lethargy, hallucinations, depression, convulsions

Bulimia Nervosa

OVERVIEW

Bulimia nervosa is a chronic eating disorder. It is characterized by eating a large amount of food in a 2-hour period and feeling a lack of control over the behavior. To compensate for this behavior, the patient then engages in behaviors to prevent weight gain. These behaviors include self-induced vomiting; abuse of laxatives, diuretics, or other medications; fasting; or excessive exercise. This cycle will occur 2 or more times weekly. Bulimia nervosa may be seen with anorexia nervosa, and one third to one half of patients suffer from major depressive syndrome.

Pathogenesis

Cause unknown; thought to be psychologic or emotional

Patient Profile

- Females > Males, except perhaps in athletes
- Predominant age group—adolescents and young adults

Signs and Symptoms

- Average weight or slightly overweight
- Drug and/or alcohol abuse, particularly diet pills, diuretics, laxatives, ipecac, thyroid medications
- Dental problems from vomiting
- Swollen glands and salivary gland hypertrophy
- Pharyngitis
- Facial puffiness
- Chronic indigestion
- Irregular menses
- Electrolyte imbalances
- Abdominal pain
- Depression
- Stress fractures from excessive exercise
- Preoccupation with weight control
- Denial that a problem exists
- Patient strictly suffering from bulimia may have few or no signs or symptoms

Differential Diagnosis

- Anorexia nervosa (many times concomitant)
- Gastrointestinal disorder
- Psychogenic vomiting
- Hypothalamic brain tumor
- Epileptic equivalent seizures
- Schizophrenic disorder

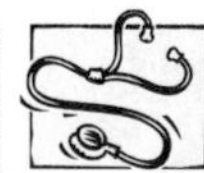

ASSESSMENT

History

Inquire about:

- Onset and duration of symptoms
- Weight history
- Eating pattern
- Use of drugs to control weight
- Exercise history
- Past history or current feelings of depression
- Suicidal ideation
- Participation in competitive sports
- Underlying conditions
- Current medications

Physical Findings

- Weight—may be normal or slightly overweight
- Skin lesions on back of hands over metacarpophalangeal joint—called Russell's sign—from repeated trauma to skin from self-induced vomiting
- Dental caries
- Swollen neck glands and salivary gland hypertrophy
- Red, irritated throat
- Facial puffiness
- Poor skin turgor
- Cardiac arrhythmias
- Decreased gag reflex

Initial Workup

Laboratory

- Chemistry panel—hypokalemia, hypochloremia, elevated BUN, metabolic alkalosis
- Urinalysis—positive ketones, proteinuria
- Check thyroid, liver, and renal function

Radiology: None indicated

Further Workup

- ECG
- Drug screen or alcohol level if indicated

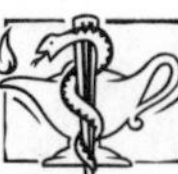

INTERVENTIONS

Office Treatment

None indicated

Lifestyle Modifications

- Nutritionally sound diet—3 meals daily
- Moderate exercise program
- Abstinence from laxatives, diuretics, weight control medications
- Attendance at support group meetings
- May need extensive inpatient treatment program, which will disrupt normal activities

Patient Education

Teach patient about:

- Bulimia and possible physical problems that could develop if bulimia continues
- Treatment options—inpatient programs, outpatient support groups, psychotherapy, antidepressants for those severely depressed
- Childbearing and harm that poor nutritional status can cause to unborn child
- Nutritionally sound diet and importance of eating 3 meals per day
- Appropriate amount of exercise
- Hazards of abusing laxatives, diuretics, diet pills
- Maintaining a food diary and setting goals
- Making a lifelong commitment to changing previous habits
- Medications used and side effects (see Pharmacotherapeutics)

Referral

Depends on severity—to inpatient treatment program and/or specialist in field of eating disorders

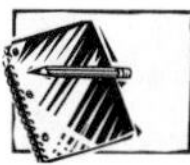

EVALUATION

Outcomes

- Patient obtains and maintains appropriate weight
- Improvement of physical signs and symptoms
- Improvement of laboratory tests

Possible Complications

- Suicide
- Potassium depletion with subsequent cardiac arrhythmia and cardiac arrest

Follow-up

- Weekly until stable as demonstrated by laboratory values returning to normal; then every 2 weeks for 2 months; then monthly
- Will probably be followed by specialist

FOR YOUR INFORMATION

Life Span

Pediatric: Most common in adolescents, but may be seen in younger children
Geriatric: N/A
Pregnancy: Low-birth-weight infants, spontaneous abortions, and preterm labor more common

Miscellaneous

It is thought that the incidence of bulimia is increasing, that it is even more common than anorexia, and that it is frequently misdiagnosed.

References

Depression Guideline Panel: *Depression in primary care,* vol 1, *Detection and diagnosis: clinical practice guideline, No 5,* AHCPR Pub No 93-0550, Rockville, Md, 1993 US Department of Health and Human Services, Public Health Service, Agency for Health Care Policy and Research.

Westfall UE, Deters GE: Problems of nutrition. In Lewis SM, Collier IC, Heitkemper MM, editors; *Medical-surgical nursing: assessment and management of clinical problems,* ed 4, St Louis, 1996, Mosby, p 1107.

NOTES

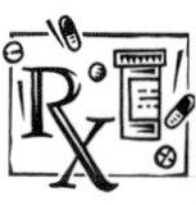

PHARMACOTHERAPEUTICS

Medication should be used with caution, particularly in those patients who have been abusing medications. Antidepressant medication and psychotherapy have been found to be effective in patients who have bulimia with or without major depression.

Drug of Choice	Mechanism of Action	Prescribing Information	Side Effects
Fluoxetine (Prozac), 20 mg PO qd; increase at 2-week intervals as needed, maximum dose 80 mg qd in divided doses bid; safety in children not established	Inhibits reuptake of serotonin	***Contraindications:*** Hypersensitivity; with or within 14 days of monoamine oxidase inhibitors (MAOIs) ***Cost:*** 20-mg tab 30 tabs: $67 ***Pregnancy category:*** B	Anxiety, nervousness, insomnia, weight loss, decreased appetite, seizures, suicide, headache, decreased libido, impotence, nausea, diarrhea, abdominal pain, rash, urticaria, hot flushes, palpitations
Imipramine (Tofranil); adults, 75 mg PO hs; may increase in 2 weeks, maximum dose 200 mg/day; adolescents, 30-40 mg PO hs; may increase in 2 weeks, maximum dose 100 mg PO qd	Tricyclic antidepressant; blocks reuptake of norepinephrine	***Contraindications:*** Hypersensitivity; acute recovery phase of myocardial infarction (MI); with or within 14 days of MAOIs ***Cost:*** 25-mg tab, 100 tabs: $2-$50 ***Pregnancy category:*** C	Orthostatic hypotension, hypertension, tachycardia, palpitation, MI, hallucinations, anxiety, restlessness, agitation, insomnia and nightmares, extrapyramidal symptoms, dry mouth, constipation, skin rash, urticaria, nausea, vomiting, anorexia, diarrhea, bone marrow depression, impotence, drowsiness, dizziness

OVERVIEW

Burns are a result of injury to the tissue from application of heat, chemicals, electricity, or irradiation. First- and second-degree burns are classified as partial-thickness burns. Third-degree burns are classified as full-thickness burns.

Pathogenesis

- First-degree burns (partial-thickness—superficial)—superficial layers of epidermis affected
- Second-degree burns (partial-thickness—deep)—epidermis (with blisters) and part of dermis
- Third-degree burns (full-thickness)—epidermis, dermis, fat layer, and into or including muscle layer; coagulation necrosis present
- Many causes:
  - Excessive sun exposure
  - Open flame
  - Hot liquid
  - Careless cigarette smoking
  - Chemicals and acids (may take several days for signs and symptoms to show)
  - Electricity (may have little damage to overlying skin but extensive internal injury)

Patient Profile

- Males = Females
- Any age—leading cause of accidental death in infants; very young and elderly much more susceptible to injury

Signs and Symptoms

- First-degree burns—erythema; skin blanches with pressure; skin tenderness; painful
- Second-degree burns—erythema with blisters; skin very tender; painful
- Third-degree burns—skin charred, dry, leathery; may be white; no pain

Differential Diagnosis

Staphylococcal scalded skin syndrome or Ritter's disease

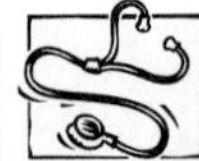

ASSESSMENT

History

Inquire about:

- Onset and duration of symptoms
- Causative agent and how burn occurred
- Treatments tried
- Status of tetanus immunization
- Underlying conditions
- Current medications

Physical Findings

- Red skin
- Blisters (second-degree burns)
- Assess nose for singed nasal hair
- Pain
- If electrical, look for entry and exit points
- Use rule of nines to determine body surface area burned:
  - Each upper extremity—adult and child 9%
  - Each lower extremity—adult 18%; child 14%
  - Anterior trunk—adult and child 18%
  - Posterior trunk—adult and child 18%
  - Head and neck—adult 10%; child 18%

Initial Workup

Laboratory

- If indicated, base decision on age of patient and extent of burn
- CBC
- Electrolytes
- BUN and creatinine
- Urinalysis

Radiology: Chest film—PA and lateral (if concerned about inhalation)

Further Workup

Usually none

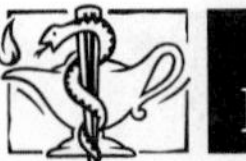

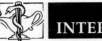

INTERVENTIONS

Office Treatment

- Administer pain medication—depends on severity of wound
- Apply cold compresses if burn just occurred
- Clean wound thoroughly with antiseptic soap such as povidone iodine scrub
- Rinse area with sterile saline
- Debride wound as necessary using aseptic technique
- Leave blisters intact
- Apply topical antimicrobial agent and cover
- Administer tetanus booster

Lifestyle Modifications

- Turn down hot water heaters
- If occupation outdoors, need to keep area covered
- Smoking cessation
- Alcohol cessation

Patient Education

Teach patient about:

- Condition and treatment—pain medication and topical antimicrobials
- Using sunscreens
- Isolating household chemicals
- Smoke detectors in home and workplace
- Proper storage and use of flammable substances
- Having evacuation plan
- Caring for wound and dressing changes as needed
- Medications used and side effects (see Pharmacotherapeutics)

Referral

To tertiary care center

- Electrical or inhalation injury
- Immunocompromised patients
- Children and elderly if at increased risk of complications
- All third-degree (full-thickness) burns
- Second-degree (partial-thickness) burns >18% in adult or >12% in child or involving face, hands, feet, eyes, perineum, or ears
- If not responding to outpatient treatment

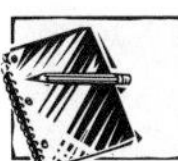

EVALUATION

Outcomes

- No wound infection develops
- Wound heals with little or no scarring

Possible Complications

- Wound infection
- Scarring
- Curling's ulcer
- Sepsis

Follow-up

48 hours after initial injury; then weekly until healed

FOR YOUR INFORMATION

Life Span

Pediatric: Possibility of child abuse
Geriatric: Higher morbidity and mortality; possibility of elder abuse
Pregnancy: Cautious use of medications

Miscellaneous

Smoke inhalation syndrome occurs within 72 hours. Suspect an inhalation burn if the burn occurred in an enclosed space.

References

Smith CW: Surgical care. In Driscoll CE et al, editors: *The family practice desk reference,* ed 3, St Louis, 1996, Mosby, pp 484-486.

Solotkin KC, Knipe CJ: Burn patient. In Lewis SM, Collier IC, Heitkemper MM, editors: *Medical-surgical nursing: assessment and management of clinical problems,* ed 4, St Louis, 1996, Mosby, pp 533-543.

NOTES

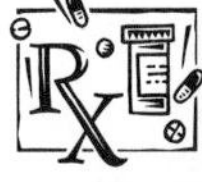

PHARMACOTHERAPEUTICS

Drug of Choice	Mechanism of Action	Prescribing Information	Side Effects
For pain control, use one of the following:			
Meperidine hydrochloride (Demerol); adults, 50-100 mg IM or PO; children, 1 mg/kg IM or PO; give in office before cleaning and debriding; controlled substance, Schedule II; ensure that patient has transportation home	Narcotic analgesic with multiple actions; depresses pain impulse at spinal cord level	***Contraindications:*** Hypersensitivity; with or within 14 days of monoamine oxidase inhibitors (MAOIs) ***Cost:*** 75 mg/ml, 10 ml: \$6-\$11 ***Pregnancy category:*** B	Respiratory depression, circulatory depression, dizziness, confusion, headache, increased intracranial pressure, nausea, vomiting, anorexia, constipation, urinary retention, rash
Tramadol hydrochloride (Ultram), 50 mg PO 1-2 tabs q4-6h; prn pain relief	Centrally acting analgesic effect	***Contraindications:*** Hypersensitivity; acute intoxication with alcohol, hypnotics, centrally acting analgesics; opiates, psychotropic drugs ***Cost:*** 50-mg tab, 100 tabs: \$60-\$66 ***Pregnancy category:*** C	Seizures, dizziness, vertigo, somnolence, nausea, vomiting, pruritus, CNS stimulation, sweating, dyspepsia, diarrhea, dry mouth, has abuse and dependence potential
Silver sulfadiazine (Silvadene); apply to burned area once or twice daily	Topical antimicrobial; bactericidal; effective against gram-negative and gram-positive organisms and yeast	***Contraindications:*** Hypersensitivity; pregnant women approaching term; premature infant; infant <2 months ***Cost:*** 1% cream, 50 g: \$4-\$8 ***Pregnancy category:*** B; not used in women approaching term	Transient leukopenia, skin necrosis, erythema multiforme, skin discoloration, burning sensation, rash

Other, less potent, pain medications can be used for less severe injuries. These include, but are not limited to, the nonsteroidal antiinflammatory medications and acetaminophen.

Bursitis

OVERVIEW

Bursitis is an inflammation of the bursa. Bursae are the fluid-filled sacs that are found wherever muscles or tendons move over bony prominences. They lubricate the area with synovial fluid. The most common sites of bursitis are the knee, shoulder, elbow, and hip.

Pathogenesis

- May be acute or chronic
- Cause:
  - Trauma (most common cause)
  - Commonly associated with overuse activity or infectious, inflammatory, gouty conditions
  - Associated with rheumatoid arthritis

Patient Profile

- Males > Females
- Any age
- Most common in adults

Signs and Symptoms

- Pain, often after repetitive activity
- Tenderness
- Swelling over affected bursa
- Erythema and warmth
- Decreased range of motion (ROM)
- Occasionally crepitus present
- Insidious onset

Differential Diagnosis

- Gout
- Pseudogout
- Rheumatoid arthritis
- Osteoarthritis
- Tendinitis
- Strains and sprains
- Stress fracture
- Degenerative joint disease
- Septic bursitis (infection in bursa; exquisitely painful; erythematous and hot)

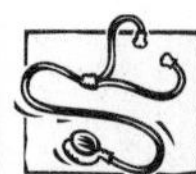

ASSESSMENT

History

Inquire about:

- Onset and duration of symptoms
- Repetitive movement (playing tennis/racquetball) or position (kneeling—housemaid's knees)
- Known trauma
- Underlying conditions
- Current medications

Physical Findings

- Localized pain and tenderness to palpation
- Erythema, swelling
- Decreased ROM

Initial Workup

Laboratory

- May wish to rule out rheumatic and connective tissue disease
- CBC, erythrocyte sedimentation rate
- Rheumatoid factor
- Serum uric acid
- Most cases of bursitis do not require laboratory testing

Radiology: Plain films of joint—may show calcification or bone spur formation; not done routinely

Further Workup

Joint aspiration by orthopedist

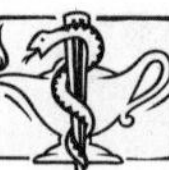

INTERVENTIONS

Office Treatment

None indicated

Lifestyle Modifications

- Avoidance of overuse
- Appropriate warm-up and cool-down period when exercising

Patient Education

Teach patient about:

- Condition and treatment:
  - Rest, moist heat, immobilization, elevation
  - Nonsteroidal antiinflammatory drugs
  - Steroid and lidocaine injected into joint, done by orthopedist
- Importance of adequately resting injured joint
- Restarting exercise program—starting slowly; performing warm-up and stretching exercises before vigorous routines
- Avoiding overuse
- Medications used and side effects (see Pharmacotherapeutics)

Referral

To orthopedist if conservative treatment fails and joint aspiration and injection are required

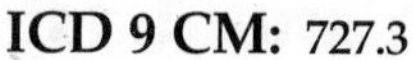

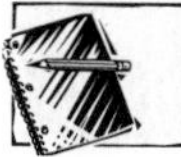

EVALUATION

Outcomes

- Resolves without sequelae
- Repeated acute bursitis may lead to chronic bursitis

Possible Complications

- Chronic bursitis
- Limited ROM

Follow-up

In 2 weeks to evaluate treatment

FOR YOUR INFORMATION

Life Span

Pediatric: Most common after skeletal maturity is reached

Geriatric: Should be considered in differential diagnosis if patient complains of arthritis

Pregnancy: Cautious use of medication

Miscellaneous

N/A

References

Hellman DB: Arthritis and musculoskeletal disorders. In Tierney LM Jr, McPhee SJ, Papadakis MA, editors: *Current medical diagnosis and treatment,* ed 34, Norwalk, Conn, 1995, Appleton & Lange, pp 710-711.

Mercier LR: *Practical orthopedics,* ed 4, St Louis, 1995, Mosby, pp 226-227.

NOTES

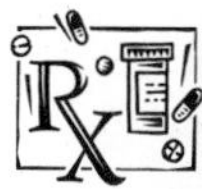

PHARMACOTHERAPEUTICS

Drug of Choice	Mechanism of Action	Prescribing Information	Side Effects
Aspirin, enteric-coated, 1 g PO tid or qid; may increase by 300-600 mg/day each week until maximal response seen or toxicity occurs (tinnitus usually 1st symptom); if toxicity occurs, decrease by 600-900 mg/day every 3 days until symptoms resolve	Antiinflammatory action may result from inhibition of synthesis and release of prostaglandins	***Contraindications:*** Hypersensitivity; GI bleeding; bleeding disorders ***Cost:*** OTC ***Pregnancy category:*** Should not be used in 3rd trimester	Dyspepsia, thirst, nausea, vomiting, GI bleeding/ulceration, tinnitus, vertigo, reversible hearing loss, prolongation of bleeding time, leukopenia, thrombocytopenia, purpura, urticaria, angioedema, pruritus, asthma, anaphylaxis, mental confusion, drowsiness, dizziness, headache, fever
Nonsteroidal antiinflammatory drugs (NSAIDs): many different types currently marketed; consult manufacturer's package insert for specific dosing and prescribing information	Exact action unknown; may result from inhibition of synthesis of prostaglandins and arachidonic acid	***Contraindications:*** Hypersensitivity to NSAIDs, aspirin; severe hepatic failure; asthma ***Cost:*** Varies with type ***Pregnancy category:*** Depends on product	Stomach distress, flatulence, nausea, abdominal pain, constipation or diarrhea, dizziness, sedation, rash, urticaria, angioedema, anorexia, urinary frequency, increased BP, insomnia, anxiety, visual disturbances, increased thirst, alopecia

Candidiasis

OVERVIEW

Candidiasis is an infection of the skin and mucous membranes caused by the yeastlike fungus *Candida albicans.*

Pathogenesis

- *C. albicans* is part of normal flora
- Epidermis is invaded when moisture, warmth, and breaks allow overgrowth
- May be consequence of antibiotic therapy, diabetes, or being immunocompromised
- Areas commonly affected include
  - Oral cavity—can spread to angles of mouth, trachea, esophagus
  - Intertriginous areas
  - Female genitalia—vagina and vulva
  - Male genitalia—Glans and shaft of penis, occasionally scrotum
  - Nails

Patient Profile

- Females > Males
- Any age
- Very common
- More common in obese individuals and individuals with undiagnosed diabetes

Signs and Symptoms

Depends on location:

- Oral cavity—white plaque on erythematous base, usually on tongue (thrush)
- Intertriginous areas—red, moist, glistening plaque or moist red papules and pustules
- Female genitalia—cheesy discharge with white plaques on erythematous base of vagina; vulva red and swollen
- Male genitalia—multiple, round, red erosions on glans, shaft, and maybe scrotum
- Nails—erythema and swelling at nail margin; nontender

Differential Diagnosis

- Oral cavity—geographic tongue, aphthous stomatitis, leukoplakia
- Intertriginous areas—miliaria, bacterial infection
- Female genitalia—bacterial vaginosis, trichomonas, allergic contact dermatitis, pediculosis pubis
- Male genitalia—bacterial infection, psoriasis, tinea
- Nails—bacterial infection, tinea

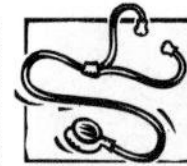

ASSESSMENT

History

Inquire about:

- Onset and duration of symptoms
- Location of lesions
- Associated symptoms—drainage or discharge; itching; pain
- Underlying chronic conditions (diabetes or family history of diabetes)
- Current medication (inhaled or oral steroids, antibiotics)

Physical Findings

Depends on location—examine skin, mucous membranes, and nails:

- Oral cavity—white plaques on erythematous base; easily removed with tongue blade
- Intertriginous—red, moist plaques or moist papules and pustules
- Vagina—cheesy discharge with white plaques on erythematous base
- Penis—red erosions on glans, shaft, maybe scrotum
- Nails—erythema of nail margin
- Check for lymph node enlargement

Initial Workup

Laboratory: Potassium hydroxide (KOH) preparation to test for pseudohyphae and budding spores

Radiology: None indicated

Further Workup

Consider workup for diabetes and HIV if indicated

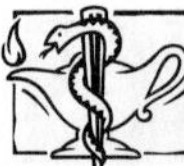

INTERVENTIONS

Office Treatment

None indicated

Lifestyle Modifications

Depends on type and if underlying chronic condition present:

- Nails—need to be kept dry; may need a change in occupation or may need to use gloves
- Intertriginous areas—weight loss may help problem
- Vagina—wear cotton underwear, no tight slacks or nylons; use mild soaps; no douching.

Patient Education

Teach patient about:

- Condition and treatment
- Prevention of recurrence through lifestyle modifications (see above)
- Any chronic condition uncovered (diabetes, HIV, etc.)
- Medications used and side effects (see Pharmacotherapeutics)

Referrals

- Usually none
- To physician if resistant case or if disseminated to esophagus or trachea

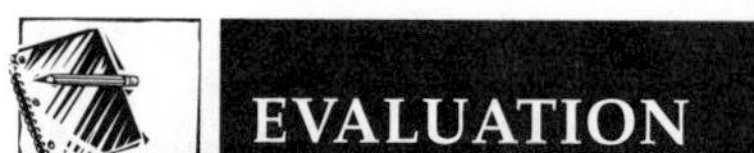

EVALUATION

Outcome
Usually resolves without sequelae

Possible Complications
Usually none, but can disseminate and cause pyelonephritis, endocarditis, myocarditis, pneumonitis, arthritis, or CNS infection

Follow-up
- Usually none
- In 2 weeks if no improvement
- Disseminated candidiasis is followed by physician

FOR YOUR INFORMATION

Life Span
Pediatric: Vaginal—consider child abuse
Geriatric: Evaluate carefully for underlying chronic condition
Pregnancy: Attempt to control infection before labor; if active, baby could be born with thrush

Miscellaneous
N/A

References
Bull TR: *Color atlas of E.N.T. diagnosis,* ed 3, London, 1995, Mosby-Wolfe, pp 190-191.

Habif TP: Superficial fungal infections. In *A color guide to diagnosis and therapy: clinical dermatology,* ed 3, St Louis, 1996, Mosby, pp 391-401.

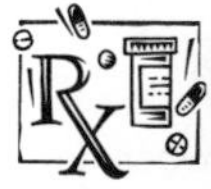

PHARMACOTHERAPEUTICS

Drug of Choice	Mechanism of Action	Prescribing Information	Side Effects
Fluconazole (Diflucan), 150 mg 1 time for vaginal candidiasis; oral and esophageal, 200 mg on day 1 and 100 mg daily for 2 weeks; children, 3-6 mg/kg/day PO	Highly selective inhibitor of fungal cytochrome P450 sterol and C-14 alpha-demethylation; fungistatic	***Contraindication:*** Hypersensitivity ***Cost:*** 100-mg tab, 30 tabs: $174 ***Pregnancy category:*** C	May cause severe hypoglycemia in patients on oral hypoglycemic agents; other drug interactions possible (see manufacturer's insert); also nausea, headache, vomiting, diarrhea, hepatotoxicity, anaphylaxis, seizures, Stevens-Johnson syndrome, leukopenia, thrombocytopenia, hypercholesterolemia
Miconazole (Monistat 2% cream); adults and children, 1 applicator or suppository intravaginally hs × 7 days; *or* apply dermatologic cream to affected area bid	Fungicidal activity	***Contraindication:*** Hypersensitivity ***Cost:*** Topical kit (nails): $14; topical kit (vaginal): $27; topical dermatologic cream, 15 g: $2-$13 ***Pregnancy category:*** C	Irritation, burning, maceration, allergic contact dermatitis
Clotrimazole (Gyne-Lotrimin, Mycelex); adults and children, 1% cream, 1 applicator-full intravaginally hs × 6-7 days, or apply to affected area bid; intravaginal suppositories, 100 mg HS × 6-7 days or 200 mg HS × 3 days; oral, 10-mg troches, slowly dissolve in mouth 5 times per day	Broad-spectrum antifungal; action is against dividing and growing organisms	***Contraindication:*** Hypersensitivity ***Cost:*** 1% cream, 15 g: $9-$12; vaginal tube, 45 g: $14 ***Pregnancy category:*** B	Irritation, burning, contact dermatitis
Nystatin oral suspension (Mycostatin); adults and children, swish and swallow 5-10 ml over 20 minutes 4-5 times per day; cream, apply to affected area bid × 2 weeks; vaginal tab, 1 daily × 2 weeks; safety in children not established for vaginal tabs	Binds to sterols in cell membrane; allows leakage of cellular components	***Contraindication:*** Hypersensitivity ***Cost:*** Cream, 15 g: $1-$12; suspension, 60 ml: $3-$22; vaginal tabs, 15 tabs: $4-$13 ***Pregnancy category:*** Vaginal tabs—C	Diarrhea, nausea, vomiting, rash, irritation

Carpal Tunnel Syndrome

OVERVIEW

Carpal tunnel syndrome is an entrapment neuropathy that results from compression of the median nerve of the wrist by surrounding anatomic structures.

Pathogenesis

- Carpal tunnel (rigid compartment in wrist) contains median nerve and nine tendons—any decrease in size of tunnel, enlargement of nerve, or increase in size of other structures within tunnel may cause compression of median nerve
- Often no cause found
- Common causative factors:
  - Trauma
  - Hypothyroidism
  - Rheumatoid and gouty arthritis
  - Degenerative joint disease
  - Ganglion cyst
  - Acromegaly
  - Renal failure
  - Congestive heart failure
  - Tumor

Patient Profile

- Females > Males
- Common age—40 to 60 years, although any age can be affected
- Predisposing factors:
  - Repetitive activity involving upper extremity
  - Pregnancy
  - Prolonged improper positioning

Signs and Symptoms

- Tingling or prickling sensation of fingers, usually index and long fingers
- Dull, aching pain in hand; pain increases at night
- Weakness or clumsiness when using hand
- Symptoms abate if wrist is rubbed or shook

Differential Diagnosis

- DeQuervain's disease
- Cervical radiculopathy
- Generalized peripheral neuropathy
- Brachial plexus lesion

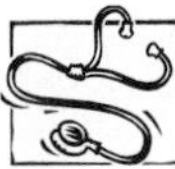

ASSESSMENT

History

Inquire about:

- Onset and duration of symptoms
- History of trauma
- Occupation
- Hobbies
- Whether pain is worse at night and relieved by shaking
- Underlying conditions
- Current medications, including OTC medications for pain relief

Physical Findings

- Dry skin on thumb, index, and middle finger
- Atrophy of thenar muscle
- Positive Tinel's sign
- Positive Phalen's maneuver

Initial Workup

Laboratory: No laboratory test that is diagnostic; may do laboratory tests such as chemistry panel and thyroid function studies to rule out other associated conditions

Radiology: If indicated:

- Wrist film—for old fractures, bone deformity, joint disease, local tumor
- Cervical spine film—radiculopathy
- Chest film—thoracic outlet syndrome

Further Workup

Confirmation of diagnosis—nerve conduction studies and electromyographic needle examination—delayed conduction across wrist

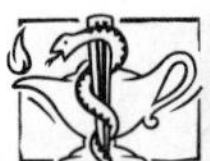

INTERVENTIONS

Office Treatment

Application of wrist splint

Lifestyle Modifications

If repetitive movement is cause, need to eliminate—may necessitate job change or adapting to use of wrist brace or giving up a hobby

Patient Education

Teach patient about:

- Condition, possible causes, and treatment options—wrist splint, nonsteroidal antiinflammatory medication, injection of carpal tunnel with steroids, surgery
- Need to eliminate cause:
  - Avoiding extremes of wrist position
  - Taking a break once per hour when doing repetitive hand work
- Medications used and side effects (see Pharmacotherapeutics)

Referral

If conservative treatment fails, to orthopedic surgeon or neurosurgeon for either injection or surgery

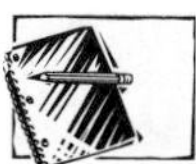

EVALUATION

Outcome
Symptoms relieved and patient able to resume normal activities

Possible Complication
Untreated—permanent loss of function

Follow-up
In 2 weeks × 1; then monthly to assess effectiveness of treatment

FOR YOUR INFORMATION

Life Span
Pediatric: Uncommon
Geriatric: Use medications with caution and monitor for gastrointestinal problems
Pregnancy: Commonly occurs in third trimester (may spontaneously resolve after delivery)

Miscellaneous
Carpal tunnel syndrome is a common occupational condition, particularly in people using computers.

References
Katz RT: Carpel tunnel syndrome: a practical review, *Am Fam Physician* 49(6):1371-1379, 1994.

Mercier LR: *Practical orthopedics,* ed 4, St Louis, 1995, Mosby, pp 101-103.

NOTES

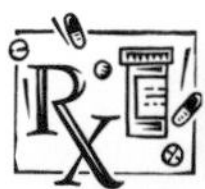

PHARMACOTHERAPEUTICS

Drug of Choice	Mechanism of Action	Prescribing Information	Side Effects
Nonsteroidal antiinflammatory drugs (NSAIDs): • Ibuprofen, 400 mg 1 PO tid or qid; children, 20-40 mg/kg/day in 3-4 divided doses • Ketoprofen (Orudis), 50 mg 1 PO tid, maximum dose 300 mg/day; not recommended for children • Several newer formulations that only require once-daily dosing; for elderly, start with half recommended dosage	Inhibit prostaglandin synthesis by decreasing enzyme needed for biosynthesis; analgesics; antiinflammatory agents; antipyretics	***Contraindications:*** Hypersensitivity; asthma, urticaria, or angioedema produced by aspirin; cautious use in severe renal disease; severe hepatic disease; ulcer disease ***Cost:*** Ibuprofen: 400-mg tab, 3/day for 365 days: $42; ketoprofen: 50-mg tab, 100 tabs: $80-$90 ***Pregnancy category:*** B	Nausea, anorexia, vomiting, diarrhea, cholestatic hepatitis, dizziness, drowsiness, tachycardia, nephrotoxicity, dysuria, hematuria, tinnitus, hearing loss, hypersensitivity

OVERVIEW

A cataract is an opacity of the lens of the eye. It can affect one or both eyes. There are several types: age-related cataracts, congenital cataracts, cataracts associated with systemic disease, and cataracts caused by trauma.

Pathogenesis

- Age-related cataracts:
  - Addition of fibrous lens layers creates hard, dehydrated lens
  - Aging alters chemical and osmotic balance necessary for clarity
- Congenital cataracts—baby born with cataracts may be result of:
  - Drugs or infection in first trimester
  - Diabetes in mother
  - Maternal malnutrition
- Other types—Biochemical/osmotic imbalance disrupts lens clarity

Patient Profile

- Males = Females
- 90% of cataracts are age related—92% of 75- to 85-year-olds have some cataract formation
- Risk factors for non-age-related/noncongenital cataracts:
  - Ultraviolet-B radiation
  - Diabetes
  - Drugs—steroids, diuretics, phenothiazines, chlorpromazine
  - Smoking; alcohol
  - Decreased antioxidant vitamins

Signs and Symptoms

- Age-related cataracts:
  - Blurred vision, distortion, fog over the eye, decreased visual acuity (particularly in bright lights or night driving)
  - May see rings or halos
  - Falls or accidents
- Congenital cataracts:
  - Parents notice visual inattention or strabismus
  - Lens opacity at birth or within 3 months
  - Visual acuity test abnormal
- Other types—decreased visual acuity

Differential Diagnosis

- Age-related cataracts:
  - Scarring
  - Tumor
  - Retinal detachment
  - Gliotic retinal scar
  - Macular degeneration
- Congenital cataracts:
  - Tumor
  - Nerve glioma
  - Retinopathy of prematurity

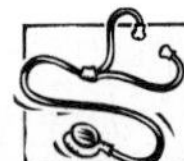

ASSESSMENT

History

Inquire about:

- Onset and duration of symptoms
- History of trauma (heat, electrical shock, radiation, concussion, perforating eye injuries)
- Ability to perform everyday activities
- Ability to participate in hobbies
- Ability to work
- Underlying conditions
- Current medications

Physical Findings

- Lens opacity
- Visual acuity decreased with Snellen chart

Initial Workup

Laboratory: None indicated
Radiology: None indicated

Further Workup

NP may do presurgical workup:

- CBC
- Chemistry panel that includes electrolytes
- ECG
- Chest x-ray film

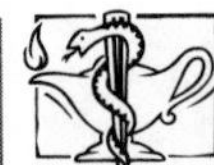

INTERVENTIONS

Office Treatment

None indicated

Lifestyle Modifications

- Smoking cessation
- Need to wear hat and dark glasses when in sun
- If opting for surgery, may need assistance at home because of eye shield and no bending or lifting

Patient Education

Teach patient about:

- Disease process and treatment options—surgery
- Use of strong bifocals or magnification
- Possible slowing of progression by decreasing amount of sun exposure
- Need for cataract removal only if activities are limited
- Surgery—same day: use of eye shield; no bending or lifting for a few weeks; eye drops; risks versus benefits (risks—glaucoma, intraocular hemorrhage, dislocated lens, loss of vision, double vision; benefits—improved vision, ability to resume previous activities)
- Tips for smoking cessation
- Increasing antioxidant vitamin intake

Referral

To ophthalmologist who specializes in cataract care

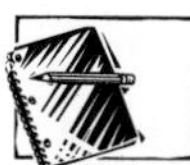

EVALUATION

Outcomes

- Patient will be able to maintain activity level
- Congenital cataracts—prognosis is poor because of high risk of amblyopia

Possible Complication

Blindness

Follow-up

By ophthalmologist

FOR YOUR INFORMATION

Life Span

Pediatric: Must always rule out tumor—early detection of retinoblastoma may be lifesaving

Geriatric: Most common age group with cataracts

Pregnancy: Early prenatal care is imperative in prevention of congenital cataracts

Miscellaneous

It is important for the NP to ensure that the patient understands that surgery is only necessary if activities are limited.

References

Cataract Management Guideline Panel: *Cataract in adults: management of functional impairment,* Clinical Practice Guideline No 4, AHCPR Pub No 93-0542, Rockville, Md, 1993, US Department of Health and Human Services, Public Health Service, Agency for Health Care Policy and Research.

Uphold CR, Graham MV: Clinical guidelines in adult health, Gainesville, Fla, 1994, Barmarrae Books, pp 195-197.

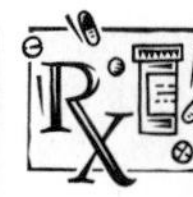

PHARMACOTHERAPEUTICS

There is no medication presently available to prevent, slow the progression of, or cure cataracts. Some authors believe that taking antioxidant vitamins may help slow the progression of cataracts, but more research is needed in this area.

Cellulitis

OVERVIEW

Cellulitis is an acute, diffuse infection of the dermis and subcutaneous structures. Erysipelas is a type of superficial cellulitis. See Erysipelas section for further information.

Pathogenesis

- Bacteria invade dermis and subcutaneous fat, with subsequent spread through lymphatics
- Causes:
  - Group A beta-hemolytic streptococci
  - Non–Group A beta-hemolytic streptococci
  - *Haemophilus influenzae* type B
  - *Staphylococcus aureus*
  - *Streptococcus pyogenes*
  - Anaerobes
  - Fungi
  - Atypical mycobacterium
  - Usually occurs secondary to skin trauma, such as lacerations, bites, scratches, anything that causes an opening in skin surface

Patient Profile

- Males = Females
- No specific age; may be more common in elderly because of fragility of skin

Signs and Symptoms

- Erythema
- Edema
- Pain
- Fever
- Malaise
- Lymphadenopathy
- Skin warm to touch

Differential Diagnosis

- Acute gout
- Ruptured Baker's cyst
- Thrombophlebitis
- Osteomyelitis
- Pressure erythema
- Pseudogout

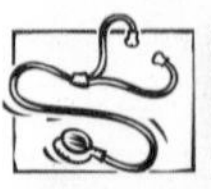

ASSESSMENT

History

Inquire about:

- Onset and duration of symptoms
- Pain
- Wound to the area
- Fever
- Chills
- Malaise
- Status of tetanus immunization
- Underlying conditions
- Current medications

Physical Findings

- Erythema
- Edema
- Pain
- Fever
- Chills
- Malaise
- Lymphadenopathy
- Emergent conditions:
  - Infected extremity—swollen/cool with diminished arterial pulses
  - Presence of necrosis
  - Immunocompromised or diabetic patient
  - Periorbital cellulitis
  - Cellulitis of central triangle of hand
  - Cellulitis of perineal area
  - Septicemia

Initial Workup

Laboratory

- Culture and sensitivity with Gram stain from wound
- CBC
- Blood cultures if concerned about septicemia

Radiology: Usually none indicated

Further Workup

Usually none indicated

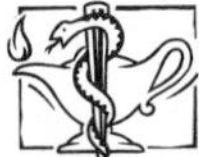

INTERVENTIONS

Office Treatment

- Application of moist heat
- Possibly IV antibiotic

Lifestyle Modifications

- Smoking cessation
- Good skin hygiene
- Care of skin abrasions

Patient Education

Teach patient about:

- Condition and treatment—antibiotics, moist heat, elevation of extremity, immobilization
- Tips for smoking cessation
- Importance of keeping abrasions clean to prevent cellulitis
- Wearing support stockings for peripheral edema
- Medications used and side effects (see Pharmacotherapeutics)

Referrals

- To MD for recurrent cases
- To emergency room for emergent cases
- May need referral to home health for IV antibiotics

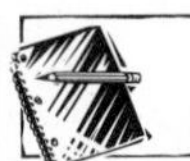

EVALUATION

Outcome

Resolves without sequelae; no recurrence

Possible Complications

- Bacteremia
- Thrombophlebitis
- Superinfection
- Osteomyelitis
- Scarring
- Meningitis
- Gangrene
- Amputation
- Death

Follow-up

In 48 hours; then in 2 weeks; then in 1 month

FOR YOUR INFORMATION

Life Span

Pediatric: Perianal cellulitis primarily seen in this age group.

Geriatric: More prone to development of complications; higher morbidity and mortality

Pregnancy: Intrauterine infection can cause newborn to have periorbital cellulitis

Miscellaneous

N/A

References

Habif TP: *Clinical dermatology: a color guide to diagnosis and therapy,* ed 3, St Louis, 1996, Mosby, pp 242-243.

Pierce NF: Bacterial infections of the skin. In Barker LR, Burton JR, Zieve PD, editors: *Principles of ambulatory medicine,* ed 4, Baltimore, 1995, Williams & Wilkins, pp 304-305.

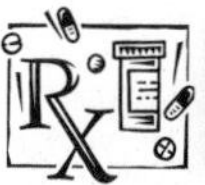

PHARMACOTHERAPEUTICS

Many types of antibiotics may be used. The following is a list of the most commonly recommended antibiotics.

Drug of Choice	Mechanism of Action	Prescribing Information	Side Effects
For mild infections:			
Penicillin VK, 250-500 mg PO qid for 10 days; children <12 years, 15-50 mg/kg/day in divided doses q6h	Bactericidal cell wall inhibitors; effective against gram-positive cocci, most anaerobes, and *Neisseria*	***Contraindication:*** Hypersensitivity ***Cost:*** 500-mg tab, 40 tabs: $4 ***Pregnancy category:*** B	Bone marrow depression, granulocytopenia, nausea, vomiting, diarrhea, oliguria, proteinuria, hematuria, moniliasis, glomerulonephritis, lethargy, depression, convulsions, anaphylaxis
If cellulitis is caused by animal or human bite, use one of the following:			
Amoxicillin/clavulanic acid, 500-875 mg PO bid × 10 days; children, 25-45 mg/kg/day PO in 2 divided doses	Bactericidal; cell wall inhibitor; effective against beta-lactamase–producing organisms	***Contraindication:*** Hypersensitivity ***Cost:*** 500-mg tab, 30 tabs: $82 ***Pregnancy category:*** B	Diarrhea, nausea, vomiting, stomatitis, black hairy tongue, pseudomembranous colitis, candidiasis, rash, urticaria, angioedema, anaphylaxis, arthralgia, myalgia, anemia, thrombocytopenia, leukopenia, anxiety, insomnia, confusion
Dicloxacillin, 250-500 mg PO qid; children <40 kg, 12.5 mg/kg/day in divided doses q6h × 10 days for mild infections	Bactericidal cell wall inhibitor; effective against gram-positive cocci except enterococci	***Contraindication:*** Hypersensitivity to penicillins ***Cost:*** 500-mg tab, 50 tabs: $19-$88 ***Pregnancy category:*** B	Bone marrow depression, granulocytopenia, nausea, vomiting, diarrhea, oliguria, proteinuria, hematuria, moniliasis, glomerulonephritis, lethargy, depression, convulsions, anaphylaxis
For mild infections in patients with penicillin allergy:			
Erythromycin (E.E.S.), 500 mg PO bid for 10 days; children, 30-50 mg/kg/day in 4 divided doses × 10 days; may be used for prophylaxis or established infections	Macrolide; protein synthesis inhibitor; active against bacteria lacking cell walls, most gram-positive aerobes	***Contraindication:*** Hypersensitivity ***Cost:*** 250-mg tabs, 4/day × 10 days: $4 ***Pregnancy category:*** B	Nausea, vomiting, diarrhea, abdominal pain, anorexia, rash, urticaria, pseudomembranous colitis—rarely
For more severe infection:			
Ceftriaxone (Rocephin), 250-500 mg IM initially and then 10 days of one of above antibiotics	Cephalosporin; inhibits bacterial cell wall synthesis	***Contraindication:*** Hypersensitivity to cephalosporins ***Cost:*** 250-mg vial: $11 ***Pregnancy category:*** B	Headache; dizziness; weakness; paresthesias; nausea, vomiting; diarrhea; anorexia; increased AST, ALT, bilirubin, LDH, alkaline phosphatase; pseudomembranous colitis; proteinuria; nephrotoxicity; leukopenia; thrombocytopenia; agranulocytosis; neutropenia; hemolytic anemia; rash; urticaria; anaphylaxis
For severe infection, use one of the following:			
Ampicillin/sulbactam (Unasyn), 1.5-3.0 g IV q6h—not recommended for children <12 years; length of treatment depends on response	Bactericidal; cell wall inhibitor; beta-lactamase inhibitor	***Contraindication:*** Hypersensitivity to penicillin ***Cost:*** 15-g vial: $55 ***Pregnancy category:*** B	Bone marrow depression, granulocytopenia, nausea, vomiting, diarrhea, oliguria, proteinuria, hematuria, moniliasis, glomerulonephritis, lethargy, depression, convulsions, anaphylaxis
Clindamycin (Cleocin), 600-900 mg IV q6h; children, 15-40 mg/kg/day IV in divided doses q6h	Lincomycin derivative; suppresses protein synthesis	***Contraindications:*** Hypersensitivity; infants <1 month ***Cost:*** 150 mg/ml, 6 ml: $26 ***Pregnancy category:*** B	Leukopenia, eosinophilia, agranulocytosis, nausea, vomiting, abdominal pain, diarrhea, pseudomembranous colitis, vaginitis, rash, urticaria, pruritus

Cerebrovascular Accident (CVA)

OVERVIEW

A cerebrovascular accident (CVA) has occurred when there is a sudden onset of neurologic deficits as a result of infarction or hemorrhage in the brain.

Pathogenesis

Many causes; most common:

- Lack of blood or ischemia caused by thrombosis or emboli due to either atherosclerotic plaque within vessels of brain or cardiac dysfunction, such as atrial fibrillation, acute myocardial infarction, prosthetic heart valves, endocarditis
- Hemorrhage caused by chronic hypertension, generalized bleeding problems, trauma, syphilis, meningitis, drug abuse (cocaine, amphetamines), excessive anticoagulation therapy

Patient Profile

- Males > Females
- Most common >45 years of age, but can occur in any age group, particularly from trauma
- Highest incidence in patients >70 years old

Signs and Symptoms

- Carotid artery occlusion:
  - Hemiplegia
  - Expressive and receptive aphasia
  - Visual field defects
  - May neglect affected side of body
  - Amnesia, confusion
  - Maybe headaches
  - Seizures
- Vertibrobasilar occlusion (brainstem or cerebellar):
  - Diplopia
  - Dysarthria
  - Vertigo
  - Ataxia
  - Tinnitus
  - Motor and sensory deficits on both sides of body
  - Dysphagia
  - Extraocular movement (EOM) dysfunction
  - Nausea, vomiting
  - Impaired level of consciousness
  - Headache
  - Facial weakness
- Hemorrhagic events:
  - Sudden, severe headache
  - Fever, sweating
  - Tachycardia
  - Altered level of consciousness
  - Nausea, vomiting
  - Can be minor bleed resulting in minimal problems to severe bleed leading to coma

Differential Diagnosis

- Tumors
- Subdural hematoma
- Multiple sclerosis
- Bell's palsy
- Hypoglycemia
- Focal seizures

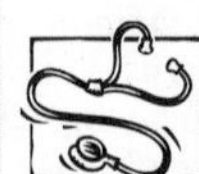

ASSESSMENT

History

Inquire about:

- Onset and duration of symptoms
- Double vision
- Nausea, vomiting
- Difficulty swallowing and speaking
- Trauma
- Dizziness
- May need to include family in history-taking process
- Visual difficulties
- Limb weakness
- Underlying conditions (hypertension)
- Current medications

Physical Findings

- Carotid occlusion:
  - Hemiplegia
  - Expressive and receptive aphasia
  - Amnesia
  - Confusion
  - Carotid artery bruit on auscultation
- Vertibrobasilar occlusion:
  - Diplopia
  - Dysarthria
  - Ataxia
  - Tinnitus
  - Bilateral motor and sensory deficits
  - EOMs abnormal
- Hemorrhage:
  - Altered level of consciousness
  - Fever, sweating
  - Tachycardia
  - Increased BP—needs immediate referral to emergency department

Initial Workup

Laboratory

- CBC
- Chemistry panel—hypoglycemia
- Rapid plasma reagin (RPR)
- Urinalysis
- ECG
- Lipid panel

Radiology: CT scan of head with and without contrast or MRI to distinguish ischemia, hemorrhage, tumor

Further Workup

- Carotid Doppler studies if carotid bruit present
- Holter monitor if arrhythmia suspected

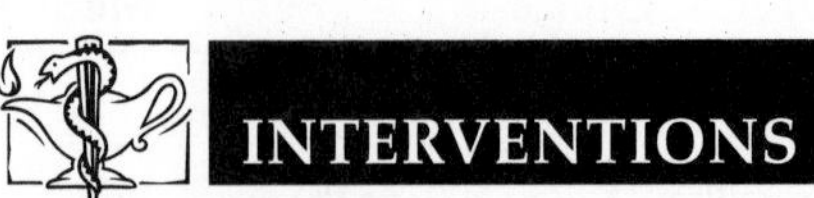

INTERVENTIONS

Office Treatment

None indicated

Lifestyle Modifications

- Smoking cessation
- No added salt and low-fat/low-cholesterol diet
- Depending on severity, may cause major disability with resultant loss of employment

Patient Education

Teach patient about:

- Disease process and treatment options:
  - Acute phase requires hospitalization
  - Carotid endarterectomy if carotid partially blocked and patient is a surgical candidate
- Posthospitalization:
  - Medication
  - Importance of controlling hypertension, blood glucose level
  - Tips for smoking cessation
  - Limiting alcohol intake
  - Nutritionally sound diet
  - Rehabilitation and importance of following exercise plan
- Medications used and side effects (see Pharmacotherapeutics)

Referrals

- During acute phase, consult with MD regarding hospitalization
- To vascular surgeon if indicated
- Posthospitalization—to home health agency for nursing, physical, and/or occupational therapy

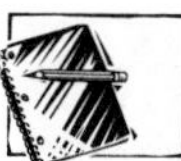

EVALUATION

Outcome
Patient will be able to resume previous activities or will adjust to limitations

Possible Complications
- Muscle atrophy and wasting or muscle spasticity
- Depression
- Sympathetic dystrophy
- Total disability
- Death

Follow-up
Within 1 week of hospital discharge, then every 2 weeks × 1; then monthly × 2; then every 3 months for 1 year

FOR YOUR INFORMATION

Life Span
Pediatric: Cardiac abnormalities are major causative factor
Geriatric: Rehabilitation may be more difficult and take longer; may need placement in extended-care facility
Pregnancy: Increased risk at time of delivery for aneurysm rupture or embolism from amniotic fluid

Miscellaneous
A CVA can be devastating for both the patient and his or her family. The recuperation period can be lengthy, and the patient and family alike need a great deal of support and encouragement.

Reference
Johnson CJ: Cerebrovascular disease. In Barker LR, Burton JR, Zieve PD, editors: *Principles of ambulatory medicine,* ed 4, Baltimore, 1995, Williams & Wilkins, pp 1229-1239.
Wooliscroft JO: *Current diagnosis and treatment: a quick reference for the general practitioner,* Philadelphia, 1996, Current Medicine, pp 374-375.

NOTES

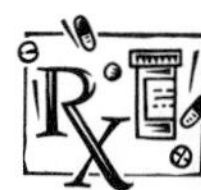

PHARMACOTHERAPEUTICS

Drug of Choice	Mechanism of Action	Prescribing Information	Side Effects
Aspirin, enteric-coated, 650 mg, 1 PO bid	Decreases platelet aggregation	***Contraindications:*** Hypersensitivity to salicylates, tartrazine; GI bleeding; bleeding disorders; children <12 years; pregnancy; lactation; vitamin K deficiency; peptic ulcer ***Cost:*** OTC ***Pregnancy category:*** D	Thrombocytopenia, agranulocytosis, leukopenia, hemolytic anemia, convulsion, confusion, dizziness, nausea, vomiting, GI bleeding, hepatitis, anorexia, rash, tinnitus, rapid pulse, pulmonary edema, wheezing, hypoglycemia, hyponatremia, hypokalemia
Ticlopidine (Ticlid), 250 mg PO bid—not recommended for children <18 years	Inhibits platelet aggregation	***Contraindications:*** Hypersensitivity; active liver disease; blood dyscrasias ***Cost:*** 250-mg tab, 30 tabs: $41 ***Pregnancy category:*** B	Rash, pruritis, nausea, vomiting, diarrhea, cholestatic jaundice, hepatitis, bleeding, agranulocytosis, neutropenia, thrombocytopenia

Cervical Cancer

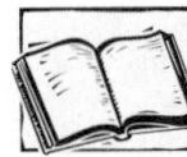

OVERVIEW

Cervical cancer is a malignancy of the cervix of the uterus.

Pathogenesis

Cause—relatively unknown; may be related to viral infections, particularly human papilloma virus

Patient Profile

- Females
- 30 to 50 years of age
- Increased incidence in African-American and Hispanic women
- Risk factors:
  - Infection with or exposure to human papilloma virus
  - Smoking
  - Early age at first coitus
  - Multiple sexual partners
  - History of sexually transmitted diseases (STDs)
  - Exposure to DES in utero

Signs and Symptoms

- Early disease asymptomatic
- As disease progresses:
  - Irregular vaginal bleeding—postcoital and intermenstrual
  - Dark, foul-smelling discharge
  - Dyspareunia
- Late symptoms:
  - Pain
  - Weight loss
  - Hematuria
  - Anemia

Differential Diagnosis

- Cervicitis
- Cervical polyp
- Carcinoma of endometrium with cervical extension
- Metastatic carcinoma

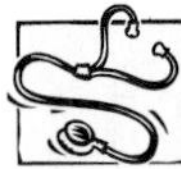

ASSESSMENT

History

Inquire about:

- Onset and duration of symptoms
- Menstrual history, including age of menarche, time between cycles, duration of bleeding
- Obstetric history
- Age of first coitus
- Maternal use of DES
- History of STDs
- Underlying conditions
- Current medications

Physical Findings

- Possibly orthostatic hypotension
- Speculum examination—enlarged cervix; may or may not be friable
- Bimanual examination—may or may not elicit pain

Initial Workup

Laboratory

- CBC—anemia
- Pap smear—abnormal

Radiology: For advanced disease, CT scan of abdomen and pelvis

Further Workup

- Colposcopy and endocervical sampling
- Cervical cone biopsy

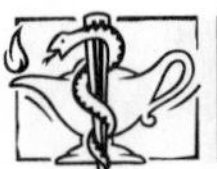

INTERVENTIONS

Office Treatment

None indicated, or possibly colposcopy

Lifestyle Modifications

- Smoking cessation
- Prevention through decreased exposure to STDs

Patient Education

Teach patient about:

- Condition and treatment—depends on Pap smear results: within normal limits, repeat Pap smear in 1 year
- Importance of regular Pap smears every 1 to 3 years, depending on age of patient and risk factors
- With any Pap smear with suspicious atypia or squamous intraepithelial lesion, colposcopy and biopsy should be done
- Results of biopsy and further treatment necessary (Table 4)
- Possible need for hysterectomy and/or radiation/chemotherapy (will depend on results of biopsy)
- Need for referral to someone experienced in colposcopy and biopsy

Referral

To gynecologist

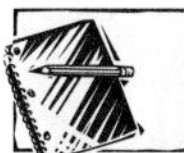

EVALUATION

Outcome
Depends on stage of cancer:

Stage	% Survival at 5 years
0	95-100
1	75-85
2	50-75
3	20-30
4	1-10

Possible Complications
- Ureteral fistula
- Metastatic cancer
- Hydronephrosis
- Uremia
- Death

Follow-up
By gynecologist

FOR YOUR INFORMATION

Life Span
Pediatric: N/A
Geriatric: Longer recuperation time
Pregnancy: Choice of therapy and need for therapeutic abortion based on stage of cancer and gestational age of fetus

Miscellaneous
The role of the primary care NP is to diagnose and make an appropriate referral for patients with cervical cancer.

References

Clinical Guidelines: Cancer detection by physical examination: breast and pelvic organ examination, *Nurse Pract* 19(10):20-24, 1994.

Clinical Guidelines: Papanicolaou smear, *Nurse Pract* 19(12):74-77, 1994.

Forrest DE: Common gynecologic pelvic disorders. In Youngkin EQ, Davis MS, editors: *Women's health: a primary care clinical guide,* Norwalk, Conn, 1994, Appleton & Lange, pp 274-275.

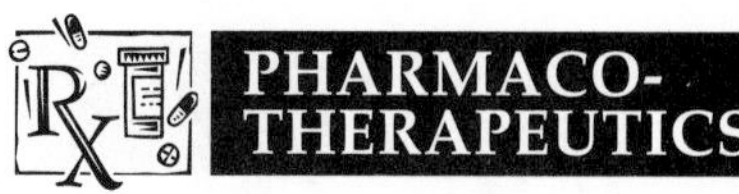

PHARMACO-THERAPEUTICS

There are many different chemotherapeutic agents used with radiation. The type of therapy done will be determined by the pathology reports and the oncologist.

TABLE 4 *International Classification of Clinical Stages of Carcinoma of the Cervix*

Stage	Extent	Treatment
0	In situ, intraepithelial	Cervical conization, total hysterectomy, cryosurgery, laser surgery
I	Strict confinement to cervix (no consideration of extension to corpus)	
I A	Microinvasive (early stromal invasion)	Radiation or surgery
I B	All other cases of Stage I	Radiation, Wertheim's hysterectomy
II	Extension beyond cervix, but not to pelvic wall; involvement of vagina, but not as far as lower third	
II A	No obvious parametrial involvement	Radiation, Wertheim's hysterectomy
II B	Obvious parametrial involvement	Radiation; if this fails, pelvic exenteration may be required
III	Extension to pelvic wall; no cancer-free space between tumor and pelvic wall on rectal examination; involvement of lower third of vagina; hydronephrosis or nonfunctioning kidney	Radiation
III A	No extension to pelvic wall	
III B	Extension to pelvic wall or hydronephrosis or nonfunctioning kidney	
IV	Extension beyond true pelvis or cervical involvement of mucosa of bladder or rectum; no Stage IV classification with bullous edema alone	Radiation, pelvic exenteration
IV A	Spread to adjacent organs	
IV B	Spread to distant organs	

Modified from Patterson KA, Carnago L: Nursing role in management: female reproductive problems. In Lewis SM, Collier IC, Heitkemper MM, editors: *Medical-surgical nursing: assessment and management of clinical problems,* ed 4, St Louis, Mosby, p 1613.

Cervical Polyps

OVERVIEW

Cervical polyps are benign, pedunculated lesions that protrude from the cervix. They may vary in size and be either singular or multiple.

Pathogenesis
Cause—unknown; may result from chronic inflammation

Patient Profile
- Females
- Multiparous women in their 30s and 40s

Signs and Symptoms
- Usually asymptomatic
- May have postcoital spotting
- Leukorrhea
- Intermenstrual bleeding
- Postmenopausal bleeding
- Mucopurulent or blood-tinged discharge

Differential Diagnosis
- Cervical malignancy
- Endometrial polyps
- Prolapsed myomas
- Nabothian cysts

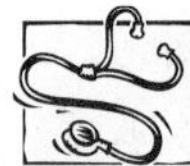

ASSESSMENT

History
Inquire about:
- Onset and duration of symptoms if present
- Underlying conditions
- Current medications

Physical Findings
- Speculum examination—pear-shaped lesions protruding from cervix—smooth, reddish-purple to cherry red; bleed easily when touched

Initial Workup
Laboratory
- Pap smear before treatment
- Polyps sent for pathology

Radiology: None indicated

Further Workup
None indicated

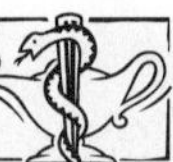

INTERVENTIONS

Office Treatment
- Polyp removal (special training required)—procedure:
  - Paint cervix with povidone-iodine
  - Grasp polyp at base with ring forceps and twist to remove
  - Apply silver nitrate or Monsel's solution to site to stop bleeding
  - Send specimens to laboratory

Lifestyle Modifications
No sexual intercourse or douching until after postoperative follow-up

Patient Education
Teach patient about:
- Condition and treatment—removal of polyps (see above)
- Need to rest pelvis following removal—no sexual intercourse or douching until postoperative follow-up visit (at 1 week)
- Need to call or return to clinic immediately for excessive bleeding or vaginal discharge
- Need to remove very large polyps in operating room
- Need for regular Pap smears and gynecologic examinations

Referral
If not trained in polyp removal, to OB/GYN NP or MD who can perform procedure

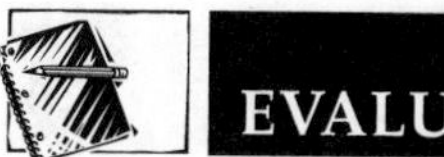

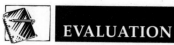

EVALUATION

Outcomes

- Uneventful postoperative recovery
- Polyps almost always benign

Possible Complications

- Bleeding
- Discharge
- Pain
- Infection
- Dysplasia or malignancy in polyp

Follow-up

In 1 week; recheck in 6 weeks

FOR YOUR INFORMATION

Life Span

Pediatric: Rarely seen
Geriatric: Rare
Pregnancy: Removal should be delayed until after delivery

Miscellaneous

Cervical polyps are the most common benign gynecologic condition. They occur in 4% of all women.

References

Forrest DE: Common gynecologic pelvic disorders. In Youngkin EQ, Davis MS, editors: *Women's health: a primary care clinical guide,* Norwalk, Conn, 1994, Appleton & Lange, pp 273-274.

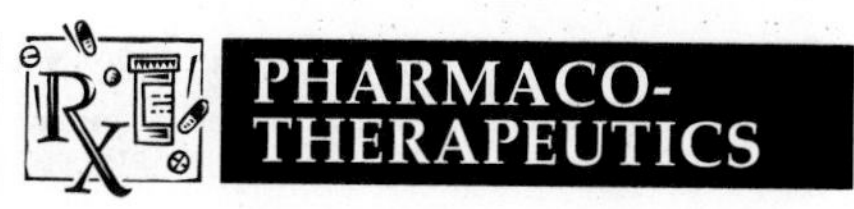

PHARMACOTHERAPEUTICS

No medications are required for treatment.

Chancroid

OVERVIEW

Chancroid is a painful ulceration of the genitals and is accompanied by inguinal adenopathy. It is a sexually transmitted disease.

Pathogenesis

Cause—gram-negative bacterial infection with *Haemophilus ducreyi*

Patient Profile

- Males > Females
- Any age if sexually active
- Uncommon in United States
- Incubation is 4 to 7 days
- More common in uncircumcised males

Signs and Symptoms

- Painful papule on genitals—ulcerates in 24 hours
- Men—ulcer occurs on shaft of penis, glans, or meatus
- Women—ulcer occurs on labia majora, labia minora, perineum, thigh, or cervix
- Women may have dysuria, vaginal discharge, dyspareunia, or be asymptomatic
- Both may have painful inguinal adenopathy with abscess formation (bubo)

Differential Diagnosis

- Syphilis
- Herpes simplex
- Lymphogranuloma venereum
- Granuloma inguinale

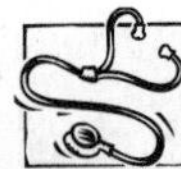

ASSESSMENT

History

Inquire about:

- Onset and duration of symptoms
- Known contact with infected partner
- Sexual history and practices, including number of partners
- Travel to developing countries
- Underlying conditions
- Current medications

Physical Findings

- Ulcerated genital lesion
- Inguinal adenopathy with erythema; painful on palpation—may spontaneously rupture

Initial Workup

Laboratory

- Serologic test for antibody; culture of lesion (antibody test and culture medium not widely available in United States)
- Gram stain; rapid plasma reagin (RPR); herpes culture; HIV screen (presumptive diagnosis of chancroid made if syphilis and herpes ruled out)

Radiology: None indicated

Further Workup

None indicated

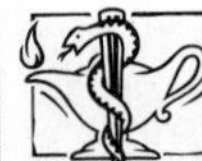

INTERVENTIONS

Office Treatment

Aspiration of bubo >5 cm

Lifestyle Modifications

- No sexual intercourse until treatment complete and ulcer heals completely
- Safe sex practices

Patient Education

Teach patient about:

- Disease and treatment—antimicrobials
- Keeping ulcer clean
- Need for treatment of all partners in last 10 days
- No sexual intercourse until ulcer completely resolved
- Prevention—avoiding multiple partners; use of condoms with every partner
- Medications used and side effects (see Pharmacotherapeutics)

Referrals

Usually none

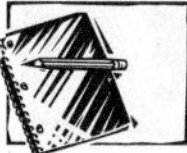

EVALUATION

Outcome
Resolves without sequelae

Possible Complications
- Phimosis
- Balanoposthitis
- Rupture of buboes
- May increase risk of HIV

Follow-up
- In 1 week to assess ulcer and bubo healing
- HIV testing 3 months after treatment

FOR YOUR INFORMATION

Life Span
Pediatric: Consider sexual abuse
Geriatric: Treatment is the same
Pregnancy: Cautious use of medication; mother-to-infant transmission not reported

Miscellaneous
Chancroid has been shown to be a risk factor for acquiring HIV.

References
Bartlett JG: *Pocket book of infectious disease therapy,* ed 7, Baltimore, 1996, Williams & Wilkins, p 308.

Bennett EC: Vaginitis and sexually transmitted diseases. In Youngkin EQ, Davis MS, editors: *Women's health: a primary care clinical guide,* Norwalk, Conn, 1994, Appleton & Lange, pp 213-214.

NOTES

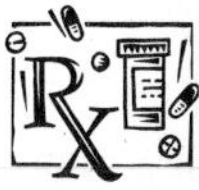

PHARMACOTHERAPEUTICS

Drug of Choice	Mechanism of Action	Prescribing Information	Side Effects
Ceftriaxone (Rocephin), 250 mg IM × 1 dose; children, 50-75 mg/kg IM × 1 dose	Cephalosporin; inhibits bacterial cell wall synthesis	***Contraindication:*** Hypersensitivity to cephalosporins ***Cost:*** 250-mg vial: $11 ***Pregnancy category:*** B	Headache; dizziness; nausea; vomiting; diarrhea; anorexia; glossitis; increased AST, ALT, bilirubin, LDH, alkaline phosphatase; proteinuria; nephrotoxicity; renal failure; leukopenia; thrombocytopenia; agranulocytosis; neutropenia; hemolytic anemia; rash; urticaria; pseudomembranous colitis; anaphylaxis
Azithromycin (Zithromax), 1 g PO × 1 dose	Macrolide; suppresses protein synthesis	***Contraindication:*** Hypersensitivity ***Cost:*** 250-mg tab, 18 tabs: $147 ***Pregnancy category:*** B	Rash, urticaria, pruritus, dizziness, headache, vertigo, diarrhea, hepatotoxicity, abdominal pain, cholestatic jaundice, flatulence, vaginitis, moniliasis
Erythromycin (E-Base), 500 mg PO bid × 7 days; children, 30-50 mg/kg/day in divided doses q12h	Macrolide; suppresses protein synthesis	***Contraindication:*** Hypersensitivity ***Cost:*** 500-mg tab, 100 tabs: $17 ***Pregnancy category:*** B	Rash, urticaria, pruritus, nausea, vomiting, diarrhea, hepatotoxicity, abdominal pain, stomatitis, heartburn, vaginitis, moniliasis

Chickenpox/Varicella

OVERVIEW

Chickenpox is a highly contagious viral disease that is more commonly seen in children.

Pathogenesis

- Causative organism—varicella-zoster virus, a herpesvirus
- Spread by direct contact or respiratory droplets
- After infection, herpesvirus becomes dormant in sensory ganglia of spinal cord and cranial nerves
- Incubation period—14 to 16 days
- Infectious period—from 48 hours before rash appears to when lesions crust

Patient Profile

- Males = Females
- Usually seen in children, preadolescents
- Peak age—5 to 9 years, but may occur at any age

Signs and Symptoms

- Prodromal period—fever, malaise, anorexia, mild headache
- Rash develops—teardrop vesicles on erythematous base, present in crops
- Usually starts on trunk and spreads
- Vesicles progress from macules to papules to vesicles, then crust
- Pruritic

Differential Diagnosis

- Herpes simplex
- Herpes zoster
- Impetigo
- Coxsackie virus infection
- Papular urticaria
- Scabies
- Dermatitis herpetiformis
- Drug rash

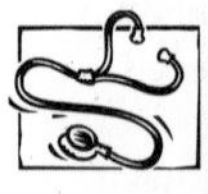

ASSESSMENT

History

Inquire about:

- Onset and duration of symptoms
- Pruritis
- Exposure to person with known chickenpox
- History of varicella vaccine
- Underlying conditions
- Current medications

Physical Findings

Examine all skin surfaces thoroughly; look for:

- Erythematous macular lesions, initially usually on trunk, then spread to face and extremities
- Papules or vesicles on erythematous base
- Fever

Initial Workup

Laboratory

- CBC if possibility of secondary infection (vesicles become very large and moist, with purulent drainage; painful)
- Tzanck smear from scrapings if unsure of diagnosis—multinucleated giant cells confirm diagnosis

Radiology: Usually none

Further Workup

Usually none

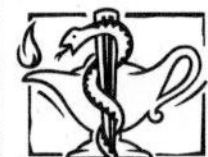

INTERVENTIONS

Office Treatment

None

Lifestyle Modifications

For both children and adults:

- Stay at home until all lesions crusted
- Keep isolated from others who have not had disease or been vaccinated
- Keep nails trimmed

Patient Education

Teach patient/family about:

- Condition and treatment
- Not scratching lesions (scarring and infection may occur) and keeping nails trimmed
- Using oatmeal bath and calamine lotion to control pruritis
- Increasing fluid intake
- Using acetaminophen or ibuprofen for fever control in children—NO ASPIRIN!
- Importance of proper vaccinations to prevent disease
- Medications used and side effects (see Pharmacotherapeutics)

Referrals

Usually none; to MD if complications arise

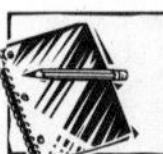

EVALUATION

Outcome

Resolves without sequelae in approximately 14 days—may be as short as 5 days or as long as 20 days

Possible Complications

- Skin infections
- Neurologic—Reye's syndrome; encephalitis
- Pneumonia
- Hepatitis

Follow-up

Usually none

FOR YOUR INFORMATION

Life Span

Pediatric

- Most common in this age group
- Varicella vaccine—<13 years, 1 dose; >13 years, 2 doses separated by 4 to 8 weeks

Geriatric: Rare in this group; higher morbidity and mortality

Pregnancy: Avoid exposure if possible; if exposed, give varicella immune globulin; DO NOT give vaccine during pregnancy!

Miscellaneous

The immunocompromised patient with chickenpox is at an increased risk for serious complications. Aggressive therapy with IV acyclovir and hospitalization may help prevent more serious complications.

References

Bartlett JG: *Pocket book of infectious disease therapy,* ed 7, Baltimore, 1996, Williams & Wilkins, pp 101, 103, 113, 182.

Habif TP: *Clinical dermatology: a color guide to diagnosis and therapy,* ed 3, St Louis, 1996, Mosby, pp 345-349.

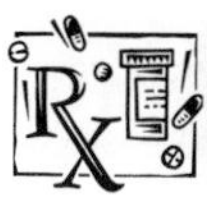

PHARMACOTHERAPEUTICS

Drug of Choice	Mechanism of Action	Prescribing Information	Side Effects
Acetaminophen (Tylenol), 325-650 mg PO every 4-6 hours for fever or myalgia; for children, use Children's Tylenol—follow label directions	Blocks pain impulse by inhibition of prostaglandin; decreases fever by inhibition of prostaglandins in hypothalamic heat-regulating center	***Contraindication:*** Hypersensitivity ***Cost:*** OTC ***Pregnancy category:*** Not categorized	Rash; hepatic toxicity with alcohol ingestion or overdose; leukopenia; neutropenia; hemolytic anemia; thrombocytopenia; nausea, vomiting; angioedema
Aspirin; adults only, 325-650 mg q4-6h; PO for fever and myalgia	Decreases platelet aggregation	***Contraindications:*** Hypersensitivity; bleeding disorders or anticoagulant therapy; last trimester of pregnancy; asthma; gastric ulcers ***Cost:*** OTC ***Pregnancy category:*** Not categorized	Rash, anaphylactic reaction, GI upset and bleeding
Ibuprofen (Motrin, Advil); adult, 200-400 mg PO q4-6h prn; children 6 months-12 years, fever <102.5° F (39.1° C), 5 mg/kg PO q6h; fever >102.5° F, 10 mg/kg PO q6h	Not well understood, but may be related to inhibition of prostaglandin synthesis	***Contraindication:*** Hypersensitivity to ibuprofen or aspirin ***Cost:*** 400-mg tab, 100 tabs: $3-$22; available OTC ***Pregnancy category:*** B	Tachycardia, peripheral edema, hypertension, dizziness, drowsiness, fatigue, tremors, confusion, tinnitus, hearing loss, nausea, anorexia, vomiting, jaundice, peptic ulcer, cholestatic hepatitis, nephrotoxicity, blood dyscrasias, rash, pruritus
Diphenhydramine (Benadryl); antihistamine to control itching; adults, 25-50 mg PO tid or qid; children >20 lb, 12.5-25 mg PO tid or qid; warn patient not to operate automobiles or heavy machinery	Appears to compete with histamine for cell receptor sites	***Contraindications:*** Hypersensitivity; newborn or premature infants; nursing mothers; should not be used as local anesthetic ***Cost:*** 25-mg tab, 100 tabs: $2-$23; available OTC ***Pregnancy category:*** B	Sedation; sleepiness; dizziness; incoordination; confusion; rash; dryness of mouth, nose, and throat; epigastric distress; hypotension; urinary retention; chest tightness; nausea; vomiting; vertigo
Acyclovir (Zovirax); adults, 800 mg PO 5×/day, 7-10 days; children, 20 mg/kg/dose PO q6h × 5 days, maximum 800 mg/dose; for immunocompromised, may need IV treatment; must treat within 24 hours; appears to lessen number of lesions and shorten course	Synthetic purine nucleoside analogue; inhibits human herpes viruses	***Contraindication:*** Hypersensitivity ***Cost:*** 400-mg tab, 100 tabs: $189 ***Pregnancy category:*** C	Side effects of short-term therapy: nausea, vomiting, headache, diarrhea, dizziness, anorexia, fatigue, edema, rash, leg pain, inguinal adenopathy, sore throat
Varicella-zoster immune globulin (VZIG), 125 units/10 kg, 625 units maximum for patients over 50 kg; give IM; used in immunocompromised and pregnant patients	Gamma globulin that activates the immune system; provides passive immunity for up to 3 weeks	***Contraindication:*** Hypersensitivity ***Cost:*** Information not available ***Pregnancy category:*** Not categorized	Slight fever, sore injection site, minor rash, severe side effects—encephalitis and convulsions
Varicella vaccine (Varivax); adults and children >13 years, 0.5 ml SQ × 2 doses, 2nd dose 4-8 weeks after first; children 12 months-12 years, 0.5 ml SQ × 1 dose; if patient given immune globulin, must wait 5 weeks before giving vaccine	Live attenuated virus causes body to produce antibodies to varicella-zoster virus	***Contraindications:*** Hypersensitivity; history of anaphylactoid reaction to neomycin; blood dyscrasias; leukemia; lymphoma; other bone marrow or lymphatic malignancy; immunosuppressed individuals; acquired immunodeficiency states; family history of congenital or hereditary immunodeficiency; untreated, active TB; any febrile illness; pregnancy ***Cost:*** 1 dose: $50 ***Pregnancy category:*** C	Fever, rash, painful injection site, cough, irritability/nervousness, fatigue, diarrhea, loss of appetite, vomiting, headache, malaise, abdominal pain, nausea, myalgia

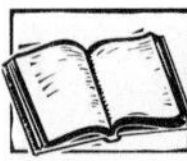

OVERVIEW

Chlamydia pneumoniae is an obligate intracellular bacterium that can cause infection in the upper and lower respiratory tract.

Pathogenesis
Cause—*C. pneumoniae*

Patient Profile
- Males > Females
- Any age

Signs and Symptoms
- Infection may be asymptomatic
- Clinical presentation:
  - Atypical pneumonia similar to *Mycoplasma pneumoniae*
  - Sore throat and hoarseness (may precede cough by a week or more)
  - Cough
  - Fever (early in illness)
  - Rhinitis
  - Headache
  - Malaise
  - Sinus congestion
  - Adventitious breath sounds
  - Sinus tenderness

Differential Diagnosis
Other causes of pneumonia—*Streptococcus, Haemophilus, Klebsiella, Mycoplasma, Legionella*

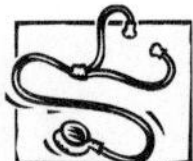

ASSESSMENT

History
Inquire about:
- Onset and duration of symptoms
- Sore throat and hoarseness 1 week or more before presentation
- Underlying conditions
- Current medications

Physical Findings
- Fever
- Lungs—rales, rhonchi, or wheezing
- Throat—erythematous
- Sinuses—tender on palpation

Initial Workup
Laboratory
- CBC—leukocytes normal or low
- Serologic tests specific for *C. pneumoniae*—not widely available and costly

Radiology: Chest film—PA and lateral—infiltrates

Further Workup
None indicated

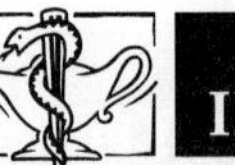

INTERVENTIONS

Office Treatment
None indicated

Lifestyle Modifications
- Smoking cessation
- Good hand-washing technique

Patient Education
Teach patient about:
- Condition and treatment—antimicrobial therapy
- Tips for smoking cessation
- Proper hand-washing technique to prevent spread of infection
- Proper disposal of soiled tissues
- Medications used and side effects (see Pharmacotherapeutics)

Referral
To MD if treatment fails

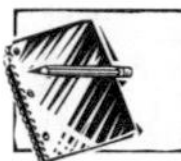

EVALUATION

Outcome

Resolves without sequelae; cough and malaise may require several weeks to resolve

Possible Complications

- Asthma
- Erythema nodosum
- Endocarditis
- Myocarditis
- Pericarditis

Follow-up

Every week until resolved

FOR YOUR INFORMATION

Life Span

Pediatric: Uncommon in children <5 years
Geriatric: Higher morbidity and mortality
Pregnancy: Cautious use of medication

Miscellaneous

N/A

References

Chambers HF: Infectious diseases: bacterial and chlamydial. In Tierney LM Jr, McPhee SJ, Papadakis MA, editors: *Current medical diagnosis and treatment,* ed 34, Norwalk, Conn, Appleton & Lange, p 1196.

Koster FT, Barker LR: Respiratory tract infections. In Barker LR, Burton JR, Zieve PD, editors: *Principles of ambulatory medicine,* ed 4, Baltimore, 1995, Williams & Wilkins, pp 342-344.

NOTES

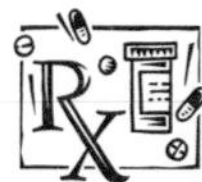

PHARMACOTHERAPEUTICS

Drug of Choice	Mechanism of Action	Prescribing Information	Side Effects
Doxycycline (Doryx), 100 mg PO bid × 14 days; children >8 years, 4.4 mg/kg/day divided q12h × 14 days	Tetracycline; inhibits protein synthesis	***Contraindications:*** Hypersensitivity; children <8 years ***Cost:*** 100-mg tab, 20 tabs: $5 ***Pregnancy category:*** D	Eosinophilia, neutropenia, thrombocytopenia, hemolytic anemia, dysphagia, glossitis, nausea, abdominal pain, vomiting, diarrhea, anorexia, hepatotoxicity, flatulence, abdominal cramps, gastritis, pericarditis, rash, urticaria, exfoliative dermatitis, angioedema
Azithromycin (Zithromax), 500 mg PO qd on day 1, then 250 mg PO qd on days 2-5; children, 10 mg/kg qd × 1 day, then 5 mg/kg qd × 4 days	Macrolide; suppresses protein synthesis	***Contraindication:*** Hypersensitivity ***Cost:*** 250-mg tab, 18 tabs: $147 ***Pregnancy category:*** B	Rash, urticaria, pruritus, dizziness, headache, vertigo, diarrhea, hepatotoxicity, abdominal pain, cholestatic jaundice, flatulence, vaginitis, moniliasis
Erythromycin (E-Mycin), 500 mg PO qid × 14-21 days; children, 30-50 mg/kg/day PO in divided doses qid × 14-21 days	Inhibits protein synthesis	***Contraindication:*** Hypersensitivity ***Cost:*** 250-mg tab, 4/day × 10 days: $4 ***Pregnancy category:*** B	Nausea, vomiting, diarrhea, abdominal pain, anorexia, rash, urticaria, pseudomembranous colitis—rarely

OVERVIEW

Chlamydia trachomatis is the microorganism responsible for the most common sexually transmitted disease (STD) in the United States.

Pathogenesis

Cause—*C. trachomatis:*

- Obligate intracellular parasite
- Displays properties of gram-negative bacteria
- Considered specialized bacterium

Patient Profile

- Males = Females
- Adolescence to young adulthood most common age, but can affect any age

Signs and Symptoms

- Males:
  - Urethritis
  - Epididymitis
  - Proctitis
- Females:
  - Many asymptomatic
  - Cervicitis
  - Urethral syndrome
  - Vaginal discharge
  - Pelvic pain
  - Fever
  - Dysuria
  - Salpingitis

Differential Diagnosis

- *Neisseria gonorrhoeae*
- Salpingitis
- Urethritis
- Pelvic inflammatory disease (PID)

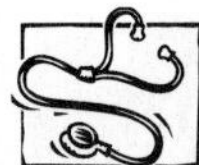

ASSESSMENT

History

Inquire about:

- Onset and duration of symptoms
- Known contact with infected partner
- Sexual history and practices
- Underlying conditions
- Current medications

Physical Findings

- Males:
  - May have discharge from penis
  - Epididymitis—scrotal tenderness, swelling
- Females:
  - Speculum examination—may be normal or show mucopurulent discharge, friable cervix; check for cervical motion tenderness (indicates PID)
  - Obtain specimen with either cytology brush or Dacron-tipped swab; insert 1 to 2 cm into endocervix and rotate

Initial Workup

Laboratory

- Chlamydial culture—expensive; takes 2 to 6 days for results
- Direct immunofluorescence assay
- Polymerase chain reaction and ligase chain reaction—low cost, fast

Radiology: None indicated

Further Workup

None indicated

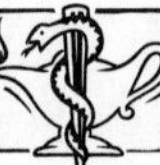

INTERVENTIONS

Office Treatment

None indicated

Lifestyle Modifications

- No sexual intercourse for 24 hours after treatment completed
- Safe sex practices

Patient Education

Teach patient about:

- Condition and treatment—antimicrobials
- Abstinence from sexual intercourse for 24 hours after treatment completed and for 24 hours after partner has completed treatment and symptoms have resolved
- Importance of finishing all medication
- In females, possibility of infection causing infertility
- Prevention—limit number of partners; use condoms
- Importance of having partner(s) treated
- Medications used and side effects (see Pharmacotherapeutics)

Referrals

Usually none

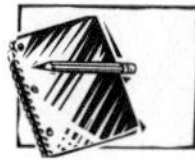

EVALUATION

Outcome

Resolves without sequelae

Possible Complications

- Males:
  - Transient oligospermia
  - Postepididymitis urethral stricture
- Females:
  - Tubal infertility
  - Tubal pregnancy
  - Chronic pelvic pain

Follow-up

None unless symptoms persist

FOR YOUR INFORMATION

Life Span

Pediatric: Consider sexual abuse
Geriatric: Treatment is the same
Pregnancy: Newborns of infected mothers may develop conjunctivitis or pneumonitis

Miscellaneous

Twenty percent of all patients visiting STD clinics and 3% to 5% of the general population have chlamydial infection. There are more than 4 million cases per year in the United States.

References

Bartlett JG: *Pocket book of infectious disease therapy,* ed 7, Baltimore, 1996, Williams & Wilkins, pp 304-306.

Bennett EC: Vaginitis and sexually transmitted diseases. In Youngkin EQ, Davis MS, editors: *Women's health: a primary care clinical guide,* Norwalk, Conn, 1994, Appleton & Lange, pp 214-217.

NOTES

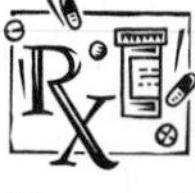

PHARMACOTHERAPEUTICS

Drug of Choice	Mechanism of Action	Prescribing Information	Side Effects
Doxycycline (Doryx), 100 mg PO bid × 7 days; children >8 years, 4.4 mg/kg/day divided q12h × 7 days	Tetracycline; inhibits protein synthesis	***Contraindications:*** Hypersensitivity; children <8 years ***Cost:*** 100-mg tab, 20 tabs: $5 ***Pregnancy category:*** D	Eosinophilia, neutropenia, thrombocytopenia, hemolytic anemia, dysphagia, glossitis, nausea, abdominal pain, vomiting, diarrhea, anorexia, hepatotoxicity, flatulence, abdominal cramps, gastritis, pericarditis, rash, urticaria, exfoliative dermatitis, angioedema
Azithromycin (Zithromax), 1 g PO × 1 dose	Macrolide; suppresses protein synthesis	***Contraindication:*** Hypersensitivity ***Cost:*** 250-mg tab, 18 tabs: $147 ***Pregnancy category:*** B	Rash, urticaria, pruritus, dizziness, headache, vertigo, diarrhea, hepatotoxicity, abdominal pain, cholestatic jaundice, flatulence, vaginitis, moniliasis
Erythromycin (E-Base), 500 mg PO qid × 7 days; children, 30-50 mg/kg/day in divided doses q12h × 7 days	Macrolide; suppresses protein synthesis	***Contraindication:*** Hypersensitivity ***Cost:*** 500-mg tab, 100 tabs: $17 ***Pregnancy category:*** B	Rash, urticaria, pruritus, nausea, vomiting, diarrhea, hepatotoxicity, abdominal pain, stomatitis, heartburn, vaginitis, moniliasis

Cholecystitis

OVERVIEW

Cholecystitis is an acute or chronic inflammation of the gallbladder.

Pathogenesis

Both forms—acute and chronic—generally caused by gallstones

Patient Profile

- Females > Males
- Middle-aged
- Often obese
- Increased incidence in Caucasians and Native Americans

Signs and Symptoms

- Acute cholecystitis:
  - Often precipitated by large, fatty meals
  - Severe (R) upper quadrant pain or epigastric pain; may radiate to (R) shoulder or subscapular area
  - Nausea
  - Vomiting
  - Fever
  - Muscle guarding
  - Rebound pain
  - Eructation
- Chronic cholecystitis—often asymptomatic, mild dyspepsia following fatty meals
- Stone in common bile duct:
  - Jaundice
  - Fever
  - Chills
  - Biliary colic
  - Pruritis
  - Light-colored, loose bowel movements
  - Abdominal distention
  - Mild tenderness
  - Hepatomegaly

Differential Diagnosis

- Ulcer
- Hepatitis
- Acute pancreatitis
- Diverticulitis
- Pyelonephritis
- Irritable bowel disease
- Bowel obstruction
- Appendicitis

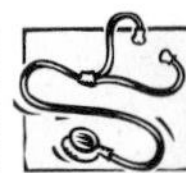

ASSESSMENT

History

Inquire about:

- Onset and duration of symptoms
- Location and radiation of pain
- Nausea
- Vomiting
- Anorexia
- Whether pain is precipitated by fatty meal
- Prior history of dyspepsia
- Underlying conditions
- Current medications

Physical Findings

- (R) upper quadrant abdominal tenderness
- Positive Murphy's sign
- Elevated temperature
- Elevated BP due to pain
- Hepatomegaly
- Possibly palpable gallbladder

Initial Workup

Laboratory: Acute:

- CBC—leukocytosis, possibly with left shift on differential
- Liver function tests—ALT, AST slightly elevated
- Bilirubin—elevated with common duct stone
- Alkaline phosphatase—slightly elevated

Radiology: Gallbladder ultrasound; if equivocal, consider oral cholecystogram

Further Workup

Usually none indicated

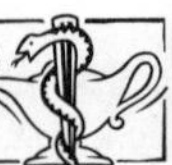

INTERVENTIONS

Office Treatment

None indicated

Lifestyle Modification

Off work for surgery and postoperative recuperation

Patient Education

Teach patient about:

- Condition and treatment options—surgical removal of gallbladder, either laparoscopically (preferred method) or by laparotomy:
  - Laparoscopic procedure—patient home either day of surgery or following day; may return to work 3 days postoperatively
  - Laparotomy—hospitalized 4 to 5 days and up to 4 weeks before return to work
- About hospital procedures and what to expect postoperatively
- Gallstones and the possibility that they can recur in bile ducts following cholecystectomy

Referral

To primary care physician or surgeon

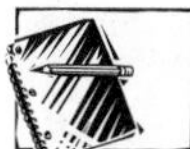

EVALUATION

Outcome
Full recovery

Possible Complications
- Perforation
- Abscess formation
- Fistula formation
- Gangrene
- Empyema
- Cholangitis
- Hepatitis
- Pancreatitis
- Postoperative wound infection
- Gallstones

Follow-up
By surgeon

FOR YOUR INFORMATION

Life Span
Pediatric: N/A
Geriatric: Signs and symptoms may be more subtle; recuperation may take longer
Pregnancy: Thought to contribute to development of gallstones

Miscellaneous
Risk factors for gallbladder disease include multiparity, use of estrogen, obesity, rapid weight loss, high-fat diet, Crohn's disease, ulcerative colitis, cirrhosis, diabetes, high cholesterol level, and family history.

References
Frielman LS: Liver, biliary tract, and pancreas. In Tierney LM Jr, McPhee SJ, Papadakis MA, editors: *Current medical diagnosis and treatment, 1995,* ed 34, Norwalk, Conn, 1995, Appleton & Lange, pp 580-583.

Uphold CR, Graham MV: *Clinical guidelines in adult health,* Gainesville, Fla, 1994, Barmarrae Books, pp 372-373.

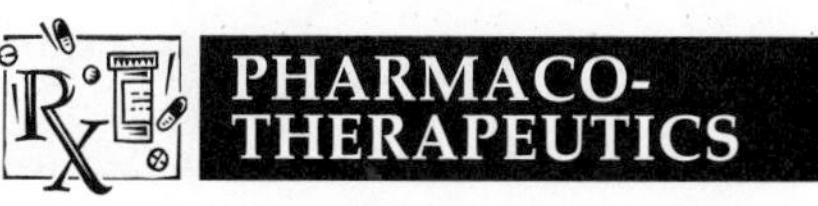

PHARMACOTHERAPEUTICS

The surgeon may use antibiotics preoperatively and possibly postoperatively. This will be decided by the surgeon based on the extent of infection present.

Cholelithiasis

OVERVIEW

Cholelithiasis is the presence of gallstones in the gallbladder. The stones may be from cholesterol, bile salts, or calcium deposits.

Pathogenesis

- Cholesterol, bile salts, or calcium precipitate out of solution
- Cause—infection or disturbance in metabolism of cholesterol

Patient Profile

- Females > Males
- Peak incidence during fifth and sixth decades
- Increased incidence in Caucasians and Native Americans

Signs and Symptoms

- Most asymptomatic
- Episodic (R) upper quadrant or epigastric pain
- Nausea
- Vomiting
- Indigestion
- Fatty food intolerance

Differential Diagnosis

- Coronary artery disease
- Peptic ulcer
- Hepatitis
- Pancreatitis
- Pneumonia
- Gallbladder cancer
- Renal stones
- Appendicitis

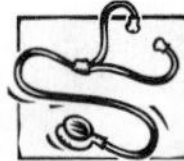

ASSESSMENT

History

Inquire about:

- Onset and duration of symptoms
- Location, intensity, and timing of pain
- Precipitating factors such as fatty meal
- Nausea, vomiting
- Underlying conditions
- Current medications

Physical Findings

- May be none if between attacks
- (R) upper quadrant pain on palpation
- Positive Murphy's sign if cholecystitis present

Initial Workup

Laboratory

- CBC with differential—within normal limits; if cholecystitis present, leukocytosis with left shift
- Chemistry profile, including liver function tests—within normal limits; if cholecystitis present, liver enzymes may be slightly elevated

Radiology: Gallbladder ultrasound; if equivocal, oral cholecystogram

Further Workup

None indicated

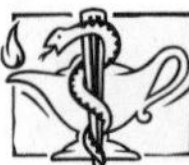

INTERVENTIONS

Office Treatment

None indicated

Lifestyle Modification

Low-fat diet may be helpful

Patient Education

Teach patient about:

- Presence of stones
- Treatment options:
  - Asymptomatic—observation and low-fat diet
  - Symptomatic—surgical removal of gallbladder (preferred treatment; may be laparoscopic or open; with laparoscopic removal, home same day or following day; with open method, 4 to 5 days in hospital and up to 4 weeks recuperation time)
- Oral dissolution of stones if surgery not an option
- Extracorporeal shockwave lithotripsy (investigational; not FDA approved)
- Medications used and side effects (see Pharmacotherapeutics)

Referral

To surgeon

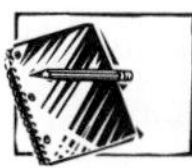

EVALUATION

Outcome

Fewer than half of patients with gallstones become symptomatic; postoperative prognosis good

Possible Complications

- Acute cholecystitis
- Gallstone pancreatitis
- Acute cholangitis
- Gallstone ileus
- Liver abscess
- Peritonitis
- Gallbladder cancer

Follow-up

- If patient taking oral dissolution agents, every 2 weeks initially; then monthly
- Monitor liver enzymes, cholesterol, gallbladder ultrasound in 6 months

FOR YOUR INFORMATION

Life Span

Pediatric: Rare before 10 years of age
Geriatric: More common in this age group
Pregnancy: Conservative therapy if possible

Miscellaneous

Oral dissolution is only effective if stones are radiolucent.

References

Friedman LS: Liver, biliary tract, and pancreas. In Tierney LM Jr, McPhee SJ, Papadakis MA, editors: *Current medical diagnosis and treatment, 1995,* ed 34, Norwalk, Conn, Appleton & Lange, pp 580-583.

Wooliscroft JO: *Current diagnoses and treatment: a quick reference for the general practitioner,* Philadelphia, 1996, Current Medicine, pp 146-147.

NOTES

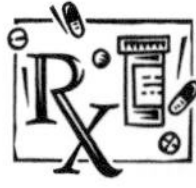

PHARMACOTHERAPEUTICS

Drug of Choice	Mechanism of Action	Prescribing Information	Side Effects
Ursodeoxycholic acid (Actigall), 8-10 mg/kg/day PO bid or tid	Suppresses hepatic synthesis, secretion of cholesterol; inhibits intestinal absorption of cholesterol	***Contraindications:*** Calcified cholesterol stones; radiopaque stones; radiolucent bile pigment stones; chronic liver disease; hypersensitivity ***Cost:*** 300-mg tab, 100 tabs: $200 ***Pregnancy category:*** B	Diarrhea, nausea, vomiting, abdominal pain, constipation, stomatitis, flatulence, pruritus, rash, urticaria, dry skin, headache, anxiety, depression, arthralgia, myalgia, cough, rhinitis
Chenodiol (Chenix), 250 mg PO bid × 2 weeks, then increase by 250 mg/day until reaching 13-16 mg/kg/day	Suppresses synthesis of cholesterol, choleic acid, replacing choleic acid with drug metabolite, which leads to degradation of gallstones	***Contraindications:*** Hypersensitivity; hepatic disease; bile duct obstruction; biliary GI fistula; pregnancy ***Cost:*** 250-mg tab, 100 tabs: $108 ***Pregnancy category:*** X	Leukopenia; diarrhea; fecal urgency; heartburn; nausea; cramps; increased ALT, AST, LDH; vomiting; hepatotoxicity; flatulence; dyspepsia

Chronic Fatigue Syndrome

OVERVIEW

Chronic fatigue syndrome is a condition that is characterized by debilitating fatigue. The fatigue is so severe as to reduce or impair daily activities. It is accompanied by a number of systemic and neuropsychiatric symptoms.

Pathogenesis

Cause—unknown; many theories postulated:
- Dysfunction of hypothalamus-pituitary-adrenal axis
- Viruses may precipitate syndrome; herpesvirus and retroviruses have been implicated
- Alterations in immune function
- May be reduced production of corticotropin-releasing hormone
- 70% suffer from depression; unsure whether depression is causative factor or if chronic fatigue syndrome causes depression, or if they are just associated

Patient Profile

- Females > Males, but only slightly
- Predominant age—adolescence and young adulthood

Signs and Symptoms

- Fatigue—in many is severe and debilitating
- Can identify a flulike illness or severe stressor before onset
- General muscle weakness and pain—unexplainable
- Joint aches and pains
- Forgetfulness and inability to concentrate
- Emotional lability—may be related to inability to cure illness
- Confusion and mood swings
- Low-grade fever
- Irritability
- Headaches
- Photophobia
- Difficulty sleeping
- Allergies
- Vertigo
- Adenopathy and painful lymph nodes
- Shortness of breath
- Chest pain
- Nausea
- Weight loss
- Palpitations
- Gastrointestinal complaints
- Rash

Differential Diagnosis

- Malignancy
- Autoimmune disease
- Localized infection
- Subacute or chronic bacterial disease
- Lyme disease
- Fungal disease
- Endocrine disorder
- HIV infection
- Psychiatric disease
- Chronic viral disease
- Drug dependency or abuse
- Fibromyalgia
- Side effects of medication or toxic agent exposure

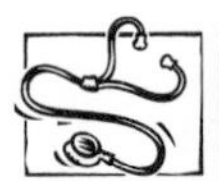

ASSESSMENT

History

Inquire about:
- Onset and duration of symptoms
- Other family members having similar symptoms
- Flulike illness before onset of symptoms
- Stressors present before onset of symptoms
- Prior history of autoimmune diseases, heart disease, fungal disease, parasitic disease, endocrine disorder, exposure to toxic agents or drug abuse, chronic viral illnesses
- Past history of psychiatric illness
- Depression and suicidal ideations
- Underlying conditions
- Current medications

Physical Findings

- May not find any physical abnormalities, since most of the symptoms are subjective in nature
- Patient often appears gaunt, frustrated, depressed, and fatigued
- The Centers for Disease Control has established the following criteria for diagnosing chronic fatigue syndrome; both major criteria *must* be present, along with (1) at least 6 symptoms plus at least 2 of 3 physical findings or (2) at least 8 symptoms
  - Major criteria—(1) new-onset fatigue lasting longer than 6 months, with a 50% reduction in activity, and (2) no other medical or psychiatric conditions that could cause symptoms
  - Symptoms—low-grade fever, sore throat, painful cervical or axillary adenopathy, generalized muscle weakness, myalgias, headaches, migratory arthralgias, sleep disturbances (hypersomnia or insomnia), neuropsychologic complaints (photophobia, visual scotomas, forgetfulness, irritability, confusion, difficulty concentrating, depression), prolonged generalized fatigue following exercise; onset of symptoms, either acute or subacute, as described by patient
  - Physical signs—low-grade fever, nonexudative pharyngitis, cervical or axillary adenopathy

Initial Workup

Laboratory
- No test specifically for chronic fatigue syndrome
- Extensive workup to rule out other causes is necessary—chemistry panel, CBC with differential, urinalysis, thyroid function, erythrocyte sedimentation rate (ESR), antinuclear antibody assay (ANA), rheumatoid factor, purified protein derivative (PPD), HIV screen, protein electrophoresis, Epstein-Barr serology, rapid plasma reagin (RPR)

Radiology: None indicated

Further Workup

Usually none indicated

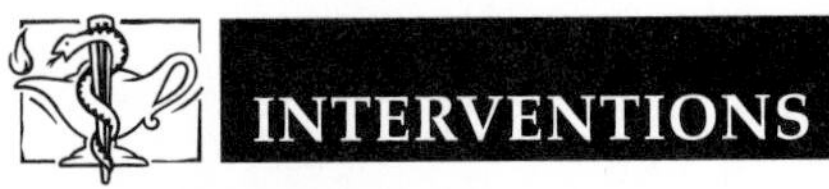

INTERVENTIONS

Office Treatment

None indicated

Lifestyle Modifications

- Can be debilitating condition
- Nutritionally sound diet
- Exercise as tolerated
- Work and school schedules may need to be modified or terminated

Patient Education

Teach patient about:
- Condition and treatment—no specific treatment available
- Need for supportive therapy
- Support group meetings
- Antidepressants—may provide some benefit
- Alternative therapies, such as chiropractic, homeopathy, and acupuncture, may be helpful, but no proven efficacy
- Coping strategies, such as biofeedback, relaxation techniques, yoga
- Nutritionally sound diet
- Exercise as tolerated—important to prevent muscle wasting, but patient should be aware that strenuous exercise may exacerbate symptoms
- Convincing family that condition is real—offer to talk with family members
- Medications used and side effects (see Pharmacotherapeutics)

Referrals

- To support groups
- To specialist in chronic fatigue syndrome if avilable

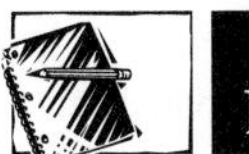

EVALUATION

Outcomes

- Most improve over time (months to years)
- May suffer substantial occupational and psychosocial impairment
- Condition tends to wax and wane

Possible Complications

- Severe depression
- Muscle wasting
- Increased susceptibility to infections

Follow-up

Every 2 weeks initially; then monthly

FOR YOUR INFORMATION

Life Span

Pediatric: Rare before adolescence, but has been reported
Geriatric: Rare; monitor nutritional status closely; use low dosages with medications
Pregnancy: Will need more frequent prenatal visits and close monitoring of nutritional status

Miscellaneous

There has been a great deal of controversy surrounding this condition. Since it was first recognized in the early 1980s, several investigators have tried to find the causative agent; however, at this point it has not been identified. Many, both in and out of the medical community, believe that the condition is strictly psychologic in nature. Patients are often made to feel as though they are just lazy or crazy. It is the NP's job to support the patient through this debilitating condition.

References

Lewis SL: Altered immune responses. In Lewis SM, Collier IC, Heitkemper MM, editors: *Medical-surgical nursing: assessment and management of clinical problems,* ed 4, St Louis, 1996, Mosby, pp 231-232.

US Department of Health and Human Services, Public Health Service, National Institutes of Health: *Chronic fatigue syndrome,* Jan 1997, America Online.

Waterbury L, Zieve PD: Selected illnesses affecting lymphocytes: mononucleosis, chronic lymphocytic leukemia and the undiagnosed patient with lymphadenopathy. In Barker LR, Burton JR, Zieve PD, editors: *Principles of ambulatory medicine,* ed 4, Baltimore, 1995, Williams & Wilkins, pp 627-628.

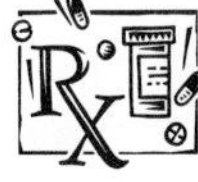

PHARMACOTHERAPEUTICS

There is no specific treatment for chronic fatigue syndrome. Supportive therapy may be needed.

Drug of Choice	Mechanism of Action	Prescribing Information	Side Effects
Buspirone (Buspar), 5 mg PO bid-tid, maximum 60 mg daily; used for generalized anxiety disorder; not recommended for children <18 years—do not administer with monoamine oxidase inhibitors (MAOIs)	Unknown; anxiolytic	***Contraindication:*** Hypersensitivity ***Cost:*** 5-mg tab, 100 tabs: $60-$65 ***Pregnancy category:*** B	Dizziness, insomnia, nervousness, drowsiness and lightheadedness, nausea, vomiting, headache, fatigue
Fluoxetine (Prozac), 40-80 mg/day; start with 20 mg and increase as needed—not dosed for children	Inhibits reuptake of serotonin	***Contraindications:*** Hypersensitivity; with or within 14 days of MAOIs ***Cost:*** 20-mg tab, 30 tabs: $67 ***Pregnancy category:*** B	Anxiety, nervousness, insomnia, weight loss, decreased appetite, seizures, suicide, headache, decreased libido, impotence, nausea, diarrhea, abdominal pain, rash, urticaria, hot flushes, palpitations
Ibuprofen (Motrin, Advil); adult, 200-400 mg PO q4-6h PRN; child, 6 months-12 years, fever <102.5° F (39.1° C), 5 mg/kg PO q6h; fever >102.5° F, 10 mg/kg PO q6h	Not well understood, but may be related to inhibition of prostaglandin synthesis	***Contraindication:*** Hypersensitivity to ibuprofen or aspirin ***Cost:*** 400-mg tab, 100 tabs: $3-$22; available OTC ***Pregnancy category:*** B	Tachycardia, peripheral edema, hypertension, dizziness, drowsiness, fatigue, tremors, confusion, tinnitus, hearing loss, nausea, anorexia, vomiting, jaundice, peptic ulcer, cholestatic hepatitis, nephrotoxicity, blood dyscrasias, rash, pruritus

Chronic Obstructive Pulmonary Disease (COPD)

OVERVIEW

Chronic obstructive pulmonary disease (COPD) is a syndrome in which there is a combination of the components of emphysema and chronic bronchitis, with one being predominant. Emphysema is a condition in which there is permanent dilation and destruction of the alveolar ducts. Chronic bronchitis is characterized by a cough with sputum production that occurs almost daily for at least 3 months during 2 consecutive years.

Pathogenesis

- Emphysema
  - Airway obstruction and hyperinflation
  - Loss of lung elasticity
  - Alveoli enlarged—septa lost
- Chronic bronchitis
  - Bronchial walls and mucous glands—hypertrophied
  - Mucosal inflammation
  - Increased mucus production
- Causes:
  - Most often, cigarette smoking
  - Recurrent or chronic respiratory tract infections
  - Occupational and environmental exposure to respiratory irritants
  - $Alpha_1$-antitrypsin deficiency

Patient Profile

- Males > Females
- Most common age group—>40 years
- $Alpha_1$-antitrypsin deficiency presents in patients in their 20s

Signs and Symptoms

EMPHYSEMA
- Minimal cough
- Weight loss
- Scant sputum
- Barrel chest
- Pursed-lip breathing
- Use of accessory muscles for breathing

CHRONIC BRONCHITIS
- Cough
- Frequent respiratory tract infections
- Sputum production
- Pedal edema
- Dyspnea on exertion
- Wheezing
- Weight gain

Differential Diagnosis

- Acute bronchitis
- Asthma
- Bronchiectasis
- Bronchogenic carcinoma
- Acute viral infection

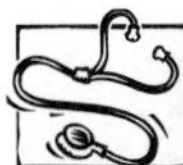

ASSESSMENT

History

Inquire about:
- Onset and duration of symptoms
- How far patient can walk before becoming short of breath
- Dyspnea at rest
- Depression and fatigue
- Cough and amount and color of sputum
- Changes in weight
- Smoking history
- Occupational history
- Underlying conditions
- Current medications

Physical Findings

- General—note appearance, color, respiratory effort, clubbing of fingers
- Weight increase or decrease
- Chest—use of accessory muscles, increased anteroposterior diameter
- Lungs—diminished breath sounds; crackles that clear with cough; wheezes and rhonchi
- Pedal edema
- Jugular vein distention
- Hepatomegaly

Initial Workup

Laboratory
- CBC—polycythemia
- Arterial blood gases—decreased PO_2, increased PCO_2
- If young patient, serum $alpha_1$-antitrypsin testing

Radiology: Chest film—PA and lateral:
- Increased bronchovascular markings and cardiomegaly—chronic bronchitis
- Small heart—hyperinflation; flat diaphragm—emphysema

Further Workup

Pulmonary function tests—decreased FEV_1; decreased FEV_1/FVC ratio; normal or increased total lung capacity; increased residual volume

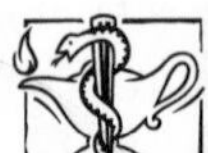

INTERVENTIONS

Office Treatment

None indicated

Lifestyle Modifications

- Smoking cessation
- Regular health maintenance

Patient Education

Teach patient about:
- Condition and treatment
- Tips for smoking cessation
- Signs and symptoms of infection and importance of reporting promptly
- Pursed-lip breathing
- Remaining as active as possible, with routine exercise program
- Using inhalers
- Importance of regular health maintenance with annual flu vaccine and pneumonia vaccine every 5 years
- Pulmonary rehabilitation programs
- Using home oxygen, if necessary, with attention to safety
- Medications used and side effects (see Pharmacotherapeutics)

Referrals

- To pulmonologist for severe disease
- To respiratory therapist for pulmonary rehabilitation
- To social worker
- To home health agency

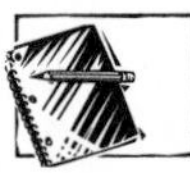

EVALUATION

Outcome

Irreversible, but with smoking cessation and treatment program, prognosis is fairly good

Possible Complications

- Frequent infections
- Malnutrition
- Cor pulmonale
- Polycythemia
- Pulmonary hypertension

Follow-up

- Depends on severity
- Initially every 2 weeks to reinforce teaching, encourage smoking cessation, and assess status

FOR YOUR INFORMATION

Life Span

Pediatric: If onset in adolescence, consider $alpha_1$-antitrypsin deficiency
Geriatric: Most commonly seen in this age group
Pregnancy: Should be handled by specialist

Miscellaneous

Not only is it important for the patient to stop smoking, but also, those individuals who reside with the patient need to stop smoking. Secondhand smoke can be just as harmful to the patient.

References

Johannsen JM: Chronic obstructive pulmonary disease: current comprehensive care for emphysema and bronchitis, *Nurse Pract* 19(1):59-67, 1994.

Wise RA, Liu MC: Obstructive airway diseases: asthma and chronic obstructive pulmonary disease. In Barker LR, Burton JR, Zieve PD, editors: *Principles of ambulatory medicine,* ed 4, Baltimore, 1995, Williams & Wilkins, pp 666-675.

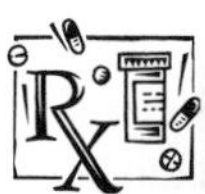

PHARMACOTHERAPEUTICS

Drug of Choice	Mechanism of Action	Prescribing Information	Side Effects
Start with the following:			
Ipratropium (Atrovent), 2 inhalations PO q4h, not to exceed 12 in 24 hours; or 500 μg PO qid by nebulizer	Anticholinergic; inhibits acetylcholine at receptor site on bronchial smooth muscle, resulting in bronchodilation	***Contraindication:*** Hypersensitivity to this drug, atropine, soya lecithin ***Cost:*** 18 μg/actuation, 1: $23 ***Pregnancy category:*** B	Nausea, vomiting, cramps, dry mouth, blurred vision, anxiety, headache, dizziness, nervousness, cough, worsening of symptoms, bronchospasms, rash, palpitation
If patient improves but improvement is suboptimal, add one of the following:			
Albuterol (Proventil, Ventolin), inhaler, 2 puffs PO qid or tabs, 2 mg PO qid	Bronchodilator; B_2 agonist—increases cAMP, which relaxes smooth muscle, leading to bronchodilation and CNS and cardiac stimulation; increases diuresis and gastric acid secretion	***Contraindications:*** Hypersensitivity; tachydysrhythmias; severe cardiac disease ***Cost:*** Metered dose inhaler: $13-$22; tabs, 2-mg tab, 100 tabs: $3-$37 ***Pregnancy category:*** C	Tremors, anxiety, insomnia, headache, dizziness, stimulation, restlessness, hallucinations, flushing, dry nose, palpitations, tachycardia, hypertension, angina, heartburn, nausea, vomiting, muscle cramps
Pirbuterol (Maxair), 2 inhalations PO qid	Bronchodilator; B_2 agonist—increases cAMP, which relaxes smooth muscle, leading to bronchodilation and CNS and cardiac stimulation; increases diuresis and gastric acid secretion	***Contraindications:*** Hypersensitivity; tachydysrhythmias; severe cardiac disease ***Cost:*** 14-g autoinhaler: $34 ***Pregnancy category:*** C	Tremors, anxiety, insomnia, headache, dizziness, stimulation, restlessness, hallucinations, flushing, dry nose, palpitations, tachycardia, hypertension, angina, heartburn, nausea, vomiting, muscle cramps, gastritis, coughing
If improvement is still suboptimal, discontinue beta agonist and add the following:			
Theophylline (Theo-Dur, Slo-Bid, Uniphyl), 400 mg/day PO in divided doses; dosing depends on brand used; some are long-acting; drug level needs to be checked to maintain therapeutic levels	Xanthine; blocks phosphodiesterase, which increases cAMP, causing smooth muscle relaxation	***Contraindications:*** Hypersensitivity; tachyarrhythmias ***Cost:*** 200-mg tab, 100 tabs: $30 ***Pregnancy category:*** C	Anxiety, restlessness, dizziness, convulsions, headache, lightheadedness, palpitations, sinus tachycardia, hypotension, nausea, vomiting, anorexia, diarrhea, bitter taste, dyspepsia, increased respiratory rate, flushing, urticaria
For advanced disease or exacerbations, use the following:			
Prednisone, 40 mg PO qd × 14 days, then taper to lowest effective dose or wean off completely	Corticosteroid; decreases inflammation	***Contraindications:*** Hypersensitivity; psychosis; idiopathic thrombocytopenia; acute glomerulonephritis; amebiasis; nonasthmatic bronchial disease; AIDS; TB; children <2 years ***Cost:*** 15-mg tab, 100 tabs: $14-$35 ***Pregnancy category:*** C	Hypertension, circulatory collapse, thrombophlebitis, embolism, tachycardia, fungal infections, increased intraocular pressure, diarrhea, nausea, GI hemorrhage, thrombocytopenia, acne, poor wound healing, fractures, osteoporosis, weakness

Cirrhosis of Liver

OVERVIEW

Cirrhosis of the liver is a chronic, degenerative disease in which the lobes are covered with fibrous tissue, the parenchyma degenerates, and the lobules are infiltrated with fat.

Pathogenesis

- Many causes:
  - Alcoholic cirrhosis (most common)
  - Chronic viral hepatitis
  - Wilson's disease
  - Hemochromatosis
  - Alpha$_1$-antitrypsin deficiency
  - Cystic fibrosis
  - Autoimmune chronic active hepatitis
  - Primary biliary cirrhosis
  - Secondary biliary cirrhosis
  - Primary sclerosing cholangitis
  - Cardiac cirrhosis
  - Drug induced
- Infancy and childhood, inherited causes:
  - Glycogen storage disease
  - Galactosemia
  - Fructose intolerance
  - Tyrosinemia
  - Acid cholesterol ester hydrolase deficiency
- Signs and symptoms occur as a result of hepatic cell dysfunction, portosystemic shunting, and portal hypertension

Patient Profile

- Males = Females
- Any age—see pathogenesis

Signs and Symptoms

- Insidious onset—fatigue, anorexia, nausea, abdominal discomfort, weakness, malaise
- As disease progresses—hematemesis, encephalopathy, jaundice, splenomegaly, ascites, gynecomastia, testicular atrophy, spider angiomas, esophageal varices, infections

Differential Diagnosis

Depends on signs and/or symptoms:

- Ascites—increased (R) heart pressure, hepatic vein thrombosis, peritoneal infection, malignant tumor, pancreatic disease, thyroid disease
- Hematemesis—ulcer, esophageal varices
- Encephalopathy—renal failure, cardiopulmonary encephalopathy, drugs

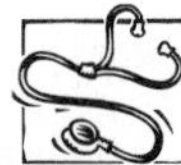

ASSESSMENT

History

Inquire about:

- Onset and duration of symptoms
- History of alcohol abuse
- Detailed past medical history
- Family history of cirrhosis
- Underlying conditions
- Current medications

Physical Findings

- Liver palpable and enlarged
- Spider nevi
- Palmar erythema
- Glossitis
- Cheilosis (vitamin deficiency)
- Weight loss (or weight gain if ascites present)
- Jaundice
- Peripheral edema
- Bruises
- Loss of axillary and pubic hair

Initial Workup

Laboratory

- Liver function tests—increased AST, increased ALT, and increased alkaline phosphatase mean liver injury
- Increased bilirubin, decreased albumin, and increased globulin mean functional impairment of liver
- Electrolytes—decreased potassium and decreased sodium (possibly)
- Prolonged prothrombin time means function of liver abnormal
- Run screening tests for cause of cirrhosis if not apparent:
  - Alpha-fetoprotein (hepatocellular cancer)
  - Hepatitis screen
  - Serum protein electrophoresis—increased IgG with any liver disease; increased IgM with primary biliary cirrhosis
- CBC with differential—anemia, slight leukopenia, moderate thrombocytopenia

Radiology: Ultrasound—bile duct dilation and space-occupying lesions

Further Workup

Liver biopsy—confirms diagnosis

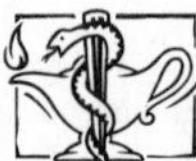

INTERVENTIONS

Office Treatment

None indicated

Lifestyle Modifications

- Alcohol cessation
- Diet with adequate calories and protein; salt restriction if ascites present
- May need fluid restriction if hyponatremic
- May have extensive disability

Patient Education

Teach patient about:

- Disease process and treatment options—no cure; treatment is to alleviate symptoms, prevent further liver damage, remove or alleviate underlying cause, and prevent complications
- Tips, support groups for alcohol cessation
- Diet with adequate calories and protein; if encephalopathy present, protein restriction; if ascites present, sodium restriction; if hyponatremia present, fluid restriction
- How to record intake and output
- Keeping record of weight—weigh same time each day, on same scale, with same clothes
- Medications used and side effects (see Pharmacotherapeutics)

Referral

Consult with MD concerning treatment approach

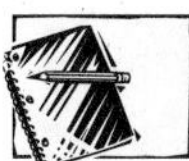

EVALUATION

Outcome

If treatable cause is identified and liver destruction stopped, prognosis may be good; otherwise, prognosis is poor

Possible Complications

- Ascites
- Hepatic encephalopathy
- Bleeding esophageal varices
- Liver failure

Follow-up

Every 2 weeks

FOR YOUR INFORMATION

Life Span

Pediatric: Usually an inherited disorder is causative factor
Geriatric: One of the leading causes of death in patients over 65 years
Pregnancy: N/A

Miscellaneous

Possible surgical procedures include the following: ligation of varices, splenectomy, splenorenal or portacaval anastomosis, and a liver transplant.

References

Friedman LS: Liver, biliary tract, and pancreas. In Tierney LM Jr, McPhee SJ, Papadakis MA, editors: *Current medical diagnosis and treatment,* ed 34, Norwalk, Conn, 1995, Appleton & Lange, pp 568-572.

Menzey E: Diseases of the liver. In Barker LR, Burton JR, Zieve PR, editors: *Principles of ambulatory medicine,* ed 4, Baltimore, 1995, Williams & Wilkins, pp 515-517.

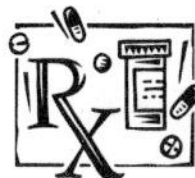

PHARMACOTHERAPEUTICS

Drug of Choice	Mechanism of Action	Prescribing Information	Side Effects
For ascites:			
Spironolactone (Aldactone), 100-300 mg/day PO single or divided doses; best for cirrhotic ascites; children, 3.3 mg/kg/day PO in single or divided doses	Competes with aldosterone at receptor sites in distal tubule, resulting in excretion of sodium chloride and water, retention of potassium and phosphate	***Contraindications:*** Hypersensitivity; anuria; severe renal disease; hyperkalemia; pregnancy ***Cost:*** 25-mg tab, 100 tabs: $5-$15 ***Pregnancy category:*** D	Headache, confusion, drowsiness, diarrhea, cramps, bleeding, gastritis, vomiting, anorexia, dysrhythmias, rash, pruritus, urticaria, impotence, gynecomastia, decreased WBCs, platelets, hyperchloremic metabolic acidosis, hyperkalemia, hyponatremia
Furosemide (Lasix), 40-120 mg PO qd; best for all other etiologies; children, 2 mg/kg/day PO, increase to maximum of 6 mg/kg/day	Inhibits reabsorption of sodium and chloride at proximal and distal tubule and in the loop of Henle	***Contraindications:*** Hypersensitivity to sulfonamides; anuria; hypovolemia; infants; lactation; electrolyte depletion ***Cost:*** 20-mg tab, 30 tabs: $2 ***Pregnancy category:*** C	Headache, fatigue, weakness, orthostatic hypotension, chest pain, ECG changes, circulatory collapse, loss of hearing, ear pain, tinnitus, hypokalemia, hypochloremic alkalosis, hypomagnesemia, hyperuricemia, hypocalcemia, hyperglycemia, nausea, diarrhea, dry mouth, vomiting, polyuria, renal failure, thrombocytopenia, agranulocytosis, leukopenia, neutropenia, rash, pruritus, Stevens-Johnson syndrome, cramps
For encephalopathy:			
Lactulose (Cephulac), 15-60 ml PO qd to produce 2-3 soft stools per day	Prevents absorption of ammonia in colon; increases water in stool	***Contraindications:*** Hypersensitivity; low-galactose diet ***Cost:*** 10 g/15 ml, 240 ml: $10-$15 ***Pregnancy category:*** C	Nausea, vomiting, anorexia, abdominal cramps, diarrhea, flatulence, distention, belching

Consult with MD regarding other treatment that may be necessary.

Coccidioidomycosis

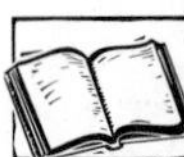

OVERVIEW

Coccidioidomycosis is a fungal infection that predominantly affects the lungs. The disease can become progressive and involve other sites, including the bones, central nervous system, and skin.

Pathogenesis

- Results from inhaled spores from disturbed soil
- Cause—*Coccidioides immitis*
- Incubation period—1 to 4 weeks

Patient Profile

- Males = Females
- Any age
- Endemic to Southwestern United States, Mexico, Central and South America
- Common opportunistic infection in HIV-infected patients
- At high risk for progressive disease—immunocompromised (HIV-positive) patients, pregnant women, African-Americans, Filipinos, diabetics

Signs and Symptoms

- Over 50% asymptomatic
- Fever and chills
- Pleuritic pain
- Nasopharyngitis
- Rash (1-2 days after onset)
- Arthralgias
- Swelling of knees and ankles
- Erythema nodosum
- Fatigue
- Malaise
- Cough (dry, nonproductive)
- Headache
- Night sweats
- Weight loss

Differential Diagnosis

- Tuberculosis
- Pneumonia
- Sarcoidosis
- Lung abscess
- Lymphoma
- Lung cancer

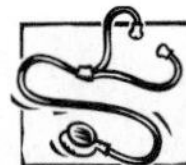

ASSESSMENT

History

Inquire about:

- Onset and duration of symptoms
- Residing in endemic area
- Working in the soil
- Underlying conditions
- Current medications

Physical Findings

- General—fever, weight loss, cyanosis, dyspnea
- Lungs—normal or crackles, wheezes, pleural friction rub
- Throat—erythematous
- Heart—tachycardia
- Abdomen—splenomegaly, hepatomegaly
- Skin—rash, erythema nodosum
- Joints—edema, pain with movement, crepitus

Initial Workup

Laboratory

- CBC with differential—moderate leukocytosis, eosinophilia
- Erythrocyte sedimentation rate—elevated; if it remains elevated or rises, consider progressive disease
- Skin test—positive after 3 weeks; typically negative in progressive disease
- Serologic testing—immunodiffusion test and precipitin test
- Fungal cultures of sputum, joint aspirate

Radiology: Chest film—PA and lateral—normal, infiltrate, nodule, cavity, mediastinal adenopathy, pleural effusion

Further Workup

Biopsy of affected tissue if unable to make diagnosis from above tests

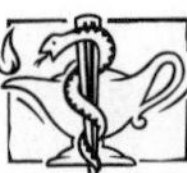

INTERVENTIONS

Office Treatment

None indicated

Lifestyle Modifications

- Smoking cessation
- Avoidance of high-risk activities (digging, construction, spelunking) by high-risk population

Patient Education

Teach patient about:

- Condition, how contracted, and treatment—if progressive or immunocompromised, possible hospitalization and IV amphotericin B
- Using a cool-mist humidifier
- Increasing fluid intake
- Obtaining adequate rest
- Activities to avoid
- Medications used and side effects (see Pharmacotherapeutics)

Referral

To pulmonologist or infectious disease specialist for severe, progressive disease or for immunocompromised patient

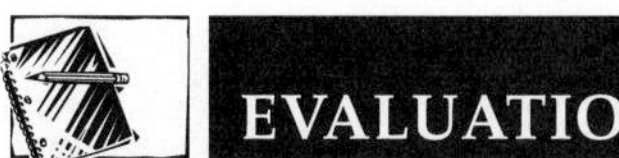

EVALUATION

Outcomes

- Most resolve without sequelae in a few months
- Relapse can occur

Possible Complications

- Destruction of lung tissue
- Severe cases can be fatal

Follow-up

- Every 2 weeks for serology titers; follow until titers are dropping and patient is improving
- Patient with progressive disease or immunocompromised patient will probably be followed by specialist

FOR YOUR INFORMATION

Life Span

Pediatric: Treatment is the same
Geriatric: Higher morbidity and mortality rate if disease is progressive
Pregnancy: More likely to develop progressive disease

Miscellaneous

The NP should consider this diagnosis when the patient presents with rather obscure symptoms and has lived in or visited an endemic area. Coccidioidomycosis is sometimes referred to as the "great imitator."

References

Bartlett JG: *Pocket book of infectious disease therapy,* ed 7; Baltimore, 1996, Williams & Wilkins, p 208.

Hollander H: Infectious diseases: mycotic. In Tierney LM Jr, McPhee SJ, Papadakis MA, editors: *Current medical diagnosis and treatment,* ed 34, Norwalk, Conn, 1995, Appleton & Lange, pp 1278-1279.

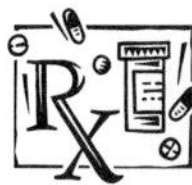

PHARMACOTHERAPEUTICS

Drug of Choice	Mechanism of Action	Prescribing Information	Side Effects
For cough:			
Dextromethorphan (Vicks Formula); available in many strengths; 10 mg/5 ml; adult, 10-20 mg PO q4h; children, 6-12 years, 5-10 mg PO q4h; children 2-6 years, 2.5-5 mg PO q4h; consult label for proper dosing	Antitussive; directly suppresses cough center in medulla	***Contraindications:*** Hypersensitivity; asthma; emphysema; productive cough ***Cost:*** 480-ml bottle: $5-$10; available OTC ***Pregnancy category:*** C	Dizziness, nausea
For pleuritic pain:			
Nonsteroidal antiinflammatory drugs (NSAIDs): many different types currently marketed; consult manufacturer's package insert for specific dosing and prescribing information	Exact action unknown; may result from inhibition of synthesis of prostaglandins and arachidonic acid	***Contraindications:*** Hypersensitivity to NSAIDs, aspirin; severe hepatic failure; asthma ***Cost:*** Varies with type ***Pregnancy category:*** Depends on product	Stomach distress, flatulence, nausea, abdominal pain, constipation or diarrhea, dizziness, sedation, rash, urticaria, angioedema, anorexia, urinary frequency, increased BP, insomnia, anxiety, visual disturbances, increased thirst, alopecia
For progressive disease or immunocompromised patient (HIV-positive):			
Amphotericin B, 0.5-1.0 mg/kg/day IV × 8 weeks or more; protect from light during infusion; use inline filter and infusion pump: may need 1 mg/kg/week for maintenance	Antifungal; increases cell membrane permeability; decreases sodium, potassium, and nutrients in cell	***Contraindications:*** Hypersensitivity; should only be used if condition is life-threatening and amphotericin B is only effective alternative ***Cost:*** 50-mg/15-ml vial: $22 ***Pregnancy category:*** B	Has serious side effects: fever, shaking, chills, hypotension, hypokalemia, shock, arrhythmias, anorexia, nausea, vomiting, necrosis at injection site, convulsions, anuria, oliguria, renal tubular acidosis, azotemia, hemorrhagic gastroenteritis, acute liver failure, arthralgia, myalgia, agranulocytosis, leukopenia, cardiorespiratory arrest
Alternative for initial treatment or for maintenance or prophylaxis:			
Fluconazole (Diflucan); for initial treatment, 400 mg PO qd; for maintenance or prophylaxis, 200 mg PO qd; interacts with several drugs—consult manufacturer's package insert	Antifungal; direct damage to membrane phospholipids	***Contraindication:*** Hypersensitivity ***Cost:*** 200-mg tab, 100 tabs: $947 ***Pregnancy category:*** C	Nausea, vomiting, diarrhea, cramping, hepatotoxicity, headache, Stevens-Johnson syndrome

Colorectal Cancer

OVERVIEW

Colorectal cancer is a malignant tumor of the colon, rectum, or anus. Adenocarcinoma is by far the most common type of colorectal cancer. The other types, carcinoid, squamous cell, and melanoma, are uncommon and are not discussed here.

Pathogenesis

- Cause remains unclear
- Adenocarcinoma arises from adenomatous polyps and spreads through walls of intestine into lymphatic system

Patient Profile

- Males = Females
- Age >50 years
- Genetic predisposition
- Risk factors:
  - High fat, low-fiber diet
  - Ulcerative colitis
  - Familial polyposis

Signs and Symptoms

Varies with location:

- (R) sided:
  - Anemia
  - Pain and/or mass in (R) lower abdominal quadrant
  - Occult blood in stool
  - Change in appearance of stool
- (L) sided:
  - Alternating constipation and diarrhea
  - Change in stool caliber (narrow, ribbon-like)
  - Red blood mixed in with stool
- Rectal:
  - Bright red blood
  - Spasms of rectum

Differential Diagnosis

- Neoplasms from other primary site
- Infections/inflammatory lesions
- Extrinsic masses

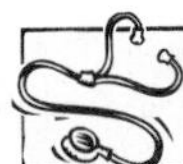

ASSESSMENT

History

Inquire about:

- Onset and duration of symptoms
- Character and quality of stools
- Family history of polyposis or ulcerative colitis
- Underlying conditions such as ulcerative colitis, colon polyps
- Current medications

Physical Findings

- Stool positive for occult blood
- (R) sided—pain and/or mass palpated in (R) lower quadrant of abdomen
- Rectal—mass palpated on digital examination

Initial Workup

Laboratory

- CBC—decreased hemoglobin and hematocrit
- Carcinoembryonic antigen (CEA)—increased

Radiology: Barium enema (air-contrast type best)

Further Workup

Colonoscopy—usually most diagnostic

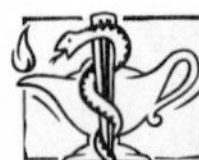

INTERVENTIONS

Office Treatment

None indicated

Lifestyle Modifications

- Depends on stage of cancer and location
- Patient may need radiation therapy and chemotherapy, with long recuperation period and interruption in lifestyle
- May need to adjust to stoma

Patient Education

Teach patient about:

- Disease process and treatment options—surgery, radiation therapy, chemotherapy
- Possibility of stoma
- Referral to surgeon
- Possible chemotherapeutic agents and side effects (see Pharmacotherapeutics)

Referral

To surgeon

TABLE 5 *Five-Year Survival of Colorectal Cancer by Stage*

Duke's stage	Extent of tumor	5-year survival (%)
A	Mucosal involvement with or without submucosal extension	95
B1	To muscularis propria but not through serosa	85-90
B2	Extends beyond serosa	60-70
C	Regional lymph nodes involved	15-25
D	Distant metastases (lung, liver)	5

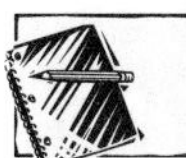

EVALUATION

Outcomes

- Prognosis depends on stage of tumor
- Overall 5-year survival is 55%; see Table 5 for 5-year survival by stage

Possible Complications

- Preoperatively:
  - Obstruction
  - Perforation
  - Acute hemorrhage
  - Fistula formation
- Postoperatively:
  - Mortality
  - Wound infection
  - Anastomotic stricture/leak/abscess
  - Pneumonia
  - Urinary tract infection
- With chemotherapy or radiation:
  - Stomatitis
  - Proctitis
  - Diarrhea
  - Temporary loss of hair

Follow-up

By surgeon

FOR YOUR INFORMATION

Life Span

Pediatric: Rare—prognosis poor
Geriatric: Longer recuperation time
Pregnancy: Rare; decision concerning fetus must be made

Miscellaneous

Primary prevention includes a low-fat, high-fiber diet and early removal of colon polyps. According to the U.S. Department of Health and Human Services (1994), everyone over 50 should have a stool examination for occult blood performed yearly and a sigmoidoscopy done every 1 to 3 years.

References

Heitkemper M, Sawchuck L: Nursing role in management: problems of absorption and elimination. In Lewis SM, Collier IC, Heitkemper MM, editors: *Medical-surgical nursing: assessment and management of clinical problems,* ed 4, St Louis, 1996, Mosby, pp 1240-1242.

U.S. Department of Health and Human Services, Public Health Service: *Clinician's handbook of preventive services: put prevention into practice,* Washington, DC, 1994, US Government Printing Office.

Wooliscroft JO, editor: *Current diagnosis and treatment: a quick reference for the general practitioner,* Philadelphia, 1996, Current Medicine, pp 82-83.

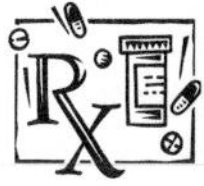

PHARMACOTHERAPEUTICS

Drug of Choice	Mechanism of Action	Prescribing Information	Side Effects
For carcinoma of anus and Duke's stage C:			
5-Fluorouracil (5-FU), 12 mg/kg/day IV × 4 days; may repeat 6 mg/kg on days 6, 8, 10, 12; maintenance, 10-15 mg/kg/week as single dose	Antineoplastic; inhibits DNA synthesis; interferes with cell replication	***Contraindications:*** Hypersensitivity; myelosuppression; pregnancy; poor nutritional status; serious infections ***Cost:*** 50 mg/ml, 10 ml: \$16-\$37 ***Pregnancy category:*** D	Myocardial ischemia, angina, thrombocytopenia, leukopenia, myelosuppression, anemia, agranulocytosis, anorexia, stomatitis, diarrhea, nausea, vomiting, hemorrhage, renal failure, epistaxis, rash, fever, lethargy, malaise, weakness
For carcinoma of anus:			
Combine with 5-FU, mitomycin C (Mutamycin), 2 mg/m^2/day IV × 5 days; skip 2 days, then repeat cycle	Antineoplastic; inhibits DNA synthesis	***Contraindications:*** Hypersensitivity; pregnancy—1st trimester; as a single agent; thrombocytopenia; coagulation disorders ***Cost:*** 20-mg vial: \$418 ***Pregnancy category:*** D—1st trimester	Thrombocytopenia, anemia, leukopenia, nausea, vomiting, anorexia, stomatitis, hepatotoxicity, urinary retention, renal failure, edema, rash, alopecia, extravasation, fibrosis, pulmonary infiltrate, dyspnea, fever, headache, confusion, drowsiness, syncope, fatigue

Common Cold

OVERVIEW

The common cold is a viral infection or acute upper respiratory tract infection that is mild and self-limiting. It can predispose the patient to bacterial infections.

Pathogenesis

- Spread by airborne droplets and through hand-to-hand contact
- There are several different types of viruses:
    - Rhinovirus—15% to 40% of cases; peaks in early fall and midspring
    - Coronavirus—10% to 15% of cases; peaks in midwinter
    - Influenza, parainfluenza, respiratory syncytial viruses, and adenoviruses—10% to 15% of cases; cause unknown in 30% to 50% of cases

Patient Profile

- Females > Males
- Adults average 2 to 4 colds per year
- Children 1 to 5 years of age average 7 to 8 colds per year
- Older children average 2 to 7 colds per year

Signs and Symptoms

- Incubation period—48 to 72 hours
- General malaise with low-grade or no fever
- Rhinorrhea and sneezing
- Pharyngitis
- Watery eyes
- Headache
- Muscle aches and pains
- Hoarseness and cough

Differential Diagnosis

- Allergic rhinitis
- Sinusitis
- Otitis media
- Pneumonia
- Foreign body in nose
- Streptococcal infection
- Measles (early stage before rash)

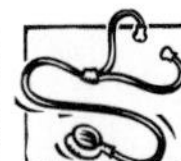

ASSESSMENT

History

Inquire about:

- Onset and duration of symptoms
- Fever and chills
- Color of sputum (normally white; may change to yellow in late stages)
- Appetite (usually decreased)
- Nausea and vomiting
- Diarrhea
- Color of nasal drainage (normally white; may change to yellow in late stages)
- Underlying conditions
- Current medications, including OTC medications

Physical Findings

- Temperature may or may not be slightly elevated
- Nasal mucosa swollen and red
- Conjunctivae may be slightly red
- Throat may be slightly red
- Cervical lymph nodes may be enlarged

Initial Workup

Laboratory

- Usually none
- CBC if concerned about bacterial infection
- Throat culture or rapid strep test if indicated

Radiology: Usually none; sinus films or chest film if indicated

Further Workup

None indicated

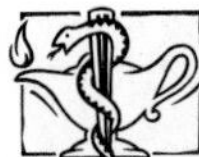

INTERVENTIONS

Office Treatment

None indicated

Lifestyle Modifications

- Smoking cessation
- Adequate rest
- Increased fluid intake
- Nutritionally sound diet—chicken soup loosens nasal mucus

Patient Education

Teach patient about:

- Course of disease (self-limiting; resolves in 5 to 7 days; may last 2 to 26 days)
- Use of OTC saline nasal spray or topical decongestant—topical decongestant should not be used for longer than 4 days
- Use of hard candy to soothe throat (not for children)
- Antibiotics—will not cure cold
- Importance of and technique for proper hand washing
- Use of steam/cool-mist vaporizer
- Use of vitamin C (never proved effective, but many authors feel that it is; overuse can cause diarrhea, precipitation of urate, oxalate, and cystine stones, and decrease effect of certain medications, such as warfarin)
- Proper disposal of soiled tissues
- Not sharing eating utensils or drinking glasses
- Medications used and side effects (see Pharmacotherapeutics)

Referrals

None indicated

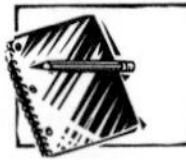

EVALUATION

Outcome

Resolves without sequelae, normally in 7 to 10 days

Possible Complications

- Bacterial infections of sinuses and middle ears
- Rarely, serious bacterial infections:
    - Osteomyelitis
    - Cavernous sinus thrombophlebitis
    - Brain abscess
- Herpes simplex of face, nose, lips

Follow-up

If symptoms worsen

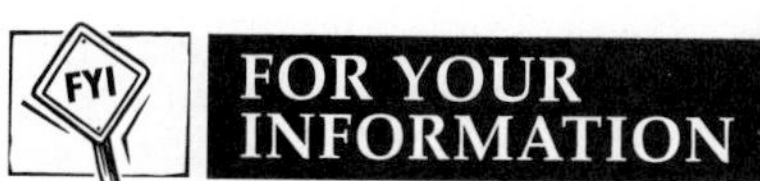

Life Span

Pediatric: 1- to 5-year-olds have highest frequency of colds; more likely to develop otitis media

Geriatric: Have additive adverse effects to medications

Pregnancy: Increased nasal congestion

Miscellaneous

According to Hilding (1994), there has been little to no progress in the fight against the common cold in the last century. Koster and Barker (1995) state that Americans spend between 500 to 700 million dollars on OTC cold remedies annually.

References

Hilding DA: Literature review: the common cold, *Ear Nose Throat J* 73:639-643, 646-647, 1994.

Koster FT, Barker LR: Respiratory Tract Infections. In Barker LR, Burton JR, Zieve PD, editors: *Principles of ambulatory medicine,* ed 4, Baltimore, 1995, Williams & Wilkins, pp 329-331.

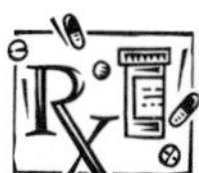

PHARMACOTHERAPEUTICS

Drug of Choice	Mechanism of Action	Prescribing Information	Side Effects
Acetaminophen (Tylenol), 325-650 mg PO q4-6h for fever or myalgia; for children, use Children's Tylenol—follow label directions; caution patient against use of alcohol	Decreases fever through action on hypothalamic heat-regulating center of brain; produces analgesia by increasing pain threshold	***Contraindication:*** Hypersensitivity ***Cost:*** OTC ***Pregnancy category:*** Not categorized	Anaphylaxis, leukopenia, neutropenia, drowsiness, nausea, vomiting, hepatotoxicity, rash, angioedema, urticaria, toxicity
Aspirin, 325-650 mg PO q4-6h for fever and myalgia—do not use in children and adolescents because of risk of Reye's syndrome	Analgesia via peripheral and central nervous systems—may inhibit prostaglandins; antipyretic via action on hypothalamic system	***Contraindications:*** Hypersensitivity; bleeding disorders or anticoagulant therapy; last trimester of pregnancy; asthma; gastric ulcers ***Cost:*** OTC ***Pregnancy category:*** D	Rash, anaphylactic reaction, GI upset and bleeding, Reye's syndrome in children and adolescents, nausea, vomiting, hepatitis, tinnitus, hearing loss, wheezing, pulmonary edema
Ibuprofen (Motrin), 400 mg qid PO for fever and myalgias; children 6 months to 12 years, 5 mg/kg q6h if temperature <102.5° F (39.1° C); 10 mg/kg q6h if temperature >102.5° F	Not well understood; may be related to inhibition of prostaglandin synthesis	***Contraindications:*** Aspirin allergy; hypersensitivity; asthma; last trimester of pregnancy; gastric ulcer; bleeding disorders ***Cost:*** 400-mg tab, 4/day × 5 days: $3 ***Pregnancy category:*** Not recommended	Nausea, heartburn, diarrhea, GI upset and bleeding, dizziness, headache, rash, tinnitus, edema, acute renal failure
Topical decongestants: Oxymetazoline (Afrin, Neo-Synephrine), children 6 years and up, 2 sprays each nostril bid	Sympathomimetic; causes vasoconstriction, which decreases congestion	***Contraindications:*** Hypersensitivity; hypertension; diabetes; heart disease; thyroid disease; difficulty urinating because of enlarged prostate ***Cost:*** OTC: $3-$5 ***Pregnancy category:*** C	Do not use for >3-4 days or exceed dosing—rebound congestion may occur, habituation, stinging of nasal mucosa, dry membranes
Oral decongestants: 130 different products listed in *PDR* for nonprescription drugs; many in combination with an antihistamine; most contain pseudoephedrine, phenylephrine, or phenylpropanolamine; see labels for dosage—do not exceed dosage	Sympathomimetics; cause nasal vasoconstriction, producing decongestion	***Contraindications:*** Hypersensitivity; hypertension (controversial); diabetes; heart or thyroid disease; prostate enlargement ***Cost:*** Varies with product ***Pregnancy category:*** Pseudoephedrine—B; phenylephrine and phenylpropanolamine—C	Drowsiness, dry mouth, insomnia, headache, nervousness, fatigue, irritability, disorientation, rash, palpitations, sore throat, cough

Condyloma Acuminata/Genital Warts

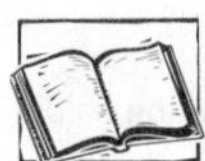

OVERVIEW

Condyloma acuminata are soft, skin-colored warts that appear on the genitalia and occasionally the throat. The condition is considered a sexually transmitted disease (STD). Autoinoculation and mother-child transfer at birth can occur.

Pathogenesis

- Cause—human papillomavirus
- Incubation period—1 to 6 months or longer

Patient Profile

- Males = Females
- Most common in adolescence to young adulthood, but any age group may be affected if sexually active

Signs and Symptoms

- Wartlike growths of varying sizes that may have smooth to very rough surfaces
- Multiple, fingerlike projections
- Warts appear on frenulum, corona, glans, prepuce, meatus, shaft, anus, scrotum, labia, clitoris, periurethral area, perineum, vagina, and cervix
- May have pruritus, dysuria, bleeding (result of trauma)

Differential Diagnosis

- Herpes simplex
- Condyloma lata
- Molluscum contagiosum
- Carcinoma
- Lichen planus

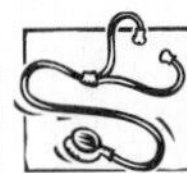

ASSESSMENT

History

Inquire about:

- Onset and duration of symptoms
- Known contact with infected person
- Sexual history and practices
- Past history of condyloma acuminata
- Underlying conditions
- Current medications

Physical Findings

- Wartlike lesions on frenulum, corona, glans, prepuce, meatus, shaft, anus, scrotum, labia, clitoris, periurethral area, perineum, vagina, and cervix
- May be single or multiple; most commonly, multiple

Initial Workup

Laboratory

- Patient should be tested for chlamydial infection, gonorrhea, syphilis
- Consider HIV screen
- No test specific for condyloma acuminata

Radiology: None indicated

Further Workup

Subclinical lesions can be visualized by applying 5% acetic acid—acetowhitening will occur

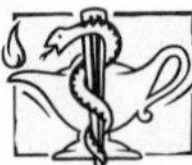

INTERVENTIONS

Office Treatment

For all warts except on cervix or rectal mucosa, cryotherapy with liquid nitrogen, cryoprobe, or podophyllum; repeat weekly until resolution occurs

Lifestyle Modification

Practice safe sex

Patient Education

Teach patient about:

- Condition and treatment options:
  - Cryotherapy or application of medication
  - May take several treatments for resolution
  - May recur; no cure—virus remains in body
- Prevention:
  - Safe sex practices
  - Use of condoms
  - Limit partners
- Importance of yearly Pap smear for females
- How to use medication and side effects (see Pharmacotherapeutics)

Referrals

- To gynecologist for cervical warts
- To surgeon for warts on rectal mucosa

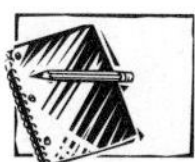

EVALUATION

Outcomes

- Resolve with or without treatment
- Recurrence common

Possible Complications

- Females—cervical dysplasia or carcinoma; rectal carcinoma
- Males—penile or rectal carcinoma; urethral obstruction

Follow-up

Weekly for cryotherapy; every 2 weeks for other treatment

FOR YOUR INFORMATION

Life Span

Pediatric: Consider sexual abuse in child with genital warts
Geriatric: Treatment same as for other age groups
Pregnancy: Treat with cryotherapy

Miscellaneous

The diagnosis of condyloma acuminata can be devastating to the patient. The patient will experience a great deal of anxiety when learning that the condition is not curable and that there is a very high incidence of cervical dysplasia and/or carcinoma. It is important for the NP to provide an atmosphere of support and understanding.

References

Bartlett JG: *Pocket book of infectious disease therapy,* ed 7, Baltimore, 1996, Williams & Wilkins, pp 309-311.

Bennett EC: Vaginitis and sexually transmitted diseases. In Youngkin EQ, Davis MS, editors: *Women's health: a primary care clinical guide,* Norwalk, Conn, 1994, Appleton & Lange, pp 226-231.

NOTES

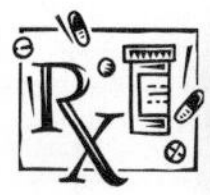

PHARMACOTHERAPEUTICS

Drug of Choice	Mechanism of Action	Prescribing Information	Side Effects
Podofilox 0.5% (Condylox); apply to warts q12h × 3 days; rest 4 days and then repeat; may repeat cycle × 4; may be performed by patient	Necrosis of wart; exact mechanism of action unknown	***Contraindication:*** Hypersensitivity ***Cost:*** 5 mg/ml, 3.5 ml: $50 ***Pregnancy category:*** C	Burning, pain, inflammation, erosion, itching, insomnia, tingling, bleeding, tenderness, malodor, dryness or peeling
Podophyllum (Podocon-25); apply petrolatum to skin around warts to protect; apply solution carefully to wart; wash off in 1-4 hours; repeat in 1 week × 3	Arrests mitosis; interferes with movement of chromosomes	***Contraindications:*** Hypersensitivity; pregnancy; bleeding; poor blood circulation; diabetes ***Cost:*** 30 ml: $50 ***Pregnancy category:*** X	Thrombocytopenia, leukopenia, irritation, peripheral neuropathy, paresthesia, nausea, vomiting, diarrhea, confusion, stupor, convulsions, coma, death

Congestive Heart Failure (CHF)

OVERVIEW

Congestive heart failure (CHF) occurs when the heart no longer pumps efficiently enough to provide sufficient blood flow to peripheral tissue.

Pathogenesis

Causes:
- Ischemic heart disease
- Myocardial infarction
- Dilated cardiomyopathy
- Rheumatic heart disease
- Hypertensive heart disease
- Pericardial disease
- Mitral or tricuspid valve stenosis
- Aortic stenosis or regurgitation

Patient Profile

- Males > Females until age 75
- Males = Females after age 75
- Incidence increases with age

Signs and Symptoms

- Exertional fatigue
- Dyspnea on exertion or at rest
- Ankle edema
- Orthopnea
- Paroxysmal nocturnal dyspnea
- Cough
- Anorexia
- Bloating
- Hemoptysis

Differential Diagnosis

- Nephrotic syndrome
- Cirrhosis
- Chronic lung disease
- Pulmonary emboli

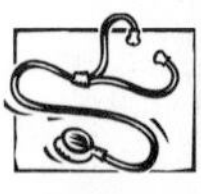

ASSESSMENT

History

Inquire about:
- Onset and duration of symptoms
- History of heart disease or hypertension
- Shortness of breath (how far can patient walk, how many pillows does patient sleep on, waking at night short of breath)
- Risk factors—smoking, elevated cholesterol, diabetes, hypertension
- Family history of heart disease
- Underlying conditions
- Current medications

Physical Findings

- Vital signs—decreased BP, tachycardia, tachypnea
- Pedal edema
- Jugular venous distention
- Hepatojugular reflux
- Lungs—crackles
- Heart—third or fourth heart sound; displaced point of maximum impulse (PMI) to left and down; murmurs
- Abdomen—hepatomegaly, ascites

Initial Workup

Laboratory
- CBC with differential to rule out anemia and infection
- Chemistry panel to include electrolytes, liver function tests, BUN and creatinine, cardiac enzymes
- Thyroid function tests
- Urinalysis

Radiology: Chest film—PA and lateral

Further Workup

- ECG
- Echocardiogram
- Exercise testing

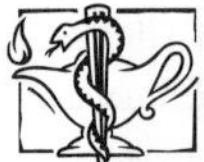

INTERVENTIONS

Office Treatment

In severe cases, immediate transport to local emergency room

Lifestyle Modifications

- Smoking cessation
- Weight reduction
- Stress reduction
- Balance of rest and activity

Patient Education

Teach patient about:
- Condition and treatment
- Treating underlying cause—hypertension, anemia, hyperthyroidism
- Tips for smoking cessation and weight reduction
- Decreasing salt intake
- Balancing activity with rest; not becoming overly fatigued
- Stress reduction—biofeedback, relaxation techniques, yoga, therapeutic massage
- Monitoring weight and reporting weight gain of 2 pounds or more
- Fluid restriction with severe CHF
- Medications used and side effects (see Pharmacotherapeutics)

Referral

Consult with MD or perhaps referral to cardiologist

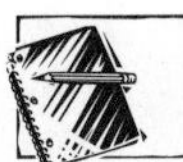

EVALUATION

Outcome

Improved quality of life and prolonged survival

Possible Complications

- Arrhythmias
- Renal failure
- Hepatic dysfunctions
- Electrolyte disturbances
- Death

Follow-up

- If hospitalized to initiate therapy, return to clinic 1 week after discharge
- If managed as outpatient, telephone contact in 24 hours and return to clinic in 1 week; then every 2 weeks until symptom-free and dry weight maintained; then every 3 to 6 weeks

FOR YOUR INFORMATION

Life Span

Pediatric: Usually due to congenital heart disease
Geriatric: Most common in this age group
Pregnancy: Should be treated by specialist

Miscellaneous

N/A

References

Konstam M et al: *Heart failure: management of patients with left-ventricular systolic dysfunction,* Quick Reference Guide for Clinicians No 11, AHCPR Pub No 94-0613, Rockville, Md, 1994, US Department of Health and Human Services, Public Health Service, Agency for Health Care Policy and Research.

Woolliscroft JO: *Current diagnosis and treatment: a quick reference for the general practitioner,* Philadelphia, 1996, Current Medicine, pp 65-67.

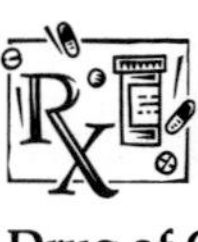

PHARMACOTHERAPEUTICS

Drug of Choice	Mechanism of Action	Prescribing Information	Side Effects
Diuretic therapy for mild or moderate congestive heart failure (CHF):			
Hydrochlorothiazide (HydroDiuril), 25-50 mg PO qd to bid, maximum 200 mg qd; children >6 months, 2.2 mg/kg/day PO in divided doses; children <6 months, 3.3 mg/kg/day in divided doses	Thiazide diuretic; acts on distal tubule and ascending limb of loop of Henle	***Contraindications:*** Hypersensitivity to thiazides or sulfonamides; anuria; renal decompensation; hypomagnesemia ***Cost:*** 25-mg tab, 100 tabs: $2-$12 ***Pregnancy category:*** B	Uremia, glucosuria, drowsiness, dizziness, fatigue, weakness, nausea, vomiting, anorexia, constipation, hepatitis, rash, urticaria, hyperglycemia, aplastic anemia, hemolytic anemia, leukopenia, agranulocytosis, thrombocytopenia, neutropenia, hypokalemia, orthostatic hypotension, hyponatremia, volume depletion
If condition becomes resistant or for more severe edema:			
Furosemide (Lasix), 20 mg PO qd; increase dose by doubling as needed; children, 2 mg/kg/day PO qd; monitor potassium level	Loop diuretic; inhibits reabsorption of sodium and chloride at proximal and distal tubule and at loop of Henle	***Contraindications:*** Hypersensitivity to sulfonamides; anuria; hypovolemia ***Cost:*** 20-mg tab, 100 tabs: $2-$15 ***Pregnancy category:*** C	Headache, fatigue, weakness, orthostatic hypotension, chest pain, circulatory collapse, loss of hearing, hypokalemia, hypomagnesemia, hyperuricemia, hyperglycemia, nausea, diarrhea, renal failure, thrombocytopenia, agranulocytosis, leukopenia, anemia, rash, Stevens-Johnson syndrome, cramps, stiffness
Vasodilator therapy:			
Quinapril (Accupril), 5 mg PO bid; not dosed for children; others: Enalapril, captopril, lisinopril; some authorities believe ACE inhibitors are the preferred drug; may be used in combination with diuretics and digoxin	Prevents conversion of angiotensin I to angiotensin II, producing arterial dilation	***Contraindication:*** Hypersensitivity ***Cost:*** 5-mg tab, 100 tabs: $90 ***Pregnancy category:*** 1st trimester—C; 2nd and 3rd trimesters—D	Cough, hypotension, postural hypotension, syncope, decreased libido, impotence, increased BUN and creatinine, thrombocytopenia, agranulocytosis, angioedema, rash, sweating, photosensitivity, hyperkalemia, nausea, vomiting, gastritis, headache, dizziness, fatigue, somnolence, depression, malaise, back pain, arthralgias, arthritis
To improve cardiac contractility:			
Digoxin (Lanoxin), 0.125-0.5 mg PO qd; monitor therapeutic level q3-6mos once stabilized on maintenance dose	Cardiac glycoside; increases cardiac output	***Contraindications:*** Hypersensitivity; ventricular fibrillation or tachycardia; carotid sinus syndrome; 2nd- or 3rd-degree heart block ***Cost:*** 0.25-mg tab, 100 tabs: $8-$16 ***Pregnancy category:*** C	Headache, drowsiness, apathy, confusion, fatigue, depression, dysrhythmia, hypotension, bradycardia, AV block, blurred vision, yellow-green halos, photophobia, nausea, vomiting, cardiotoxicity, anorexia, abdominal pain, diarrhea
Other vasodilator:			
Isosorbide (Isordil), 10 mg PO tid; may use long-acting nitroglycerin tabs or transdermal patches	Dilates coronary arteries, which improves blood flow	***Contraindications:*** Hypersensitivity; severe anemia; increased intracranial pressure; cerebral hemorrhage ***Cost:*** 10-mg tab, 100 tabs: $2-$30 ***Pregnancy category:*** C	Postural hypotension, tachycardia, syncope, nausea, vomiting, pallor, sweating, rash, headache, flushing, dizziness

Conjunctivitis

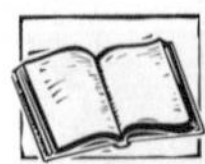

OVERVIEW

Conjunctivitis is inflammation of the conjunctiva. Pink eye refers to bacterial conjunctivitis.

Pathogenesis

Many causes:

- Bacterial—*Staphylococcus aureus, Streptococcus pneumoniae, Haemophilus influenzae, Neisseria gonorrhoeae, Neisseria meningitidis, Pseudomonas, Branhamella catarrhalis,* coliform bacteria, *Klebsiella, Proteus, Corynebacterium diphtheriae, Mycobacterium tuberculosis*
- Chlamydial—*Chlamydia trachomatis, C. oculogenitalis, C. lymphogranulomatis*
- Viral—adenoviruses 3, 4, 7, 8, 11, 19; coxsackie A24; enterovirus 70; herpes simplex; varicella; herpes zoster; measles virus
- Allergic—antigen-antibody reaction to allergen
- Chemical or irritative—topical medications, home/industrial chemicals, wind, smoke, UV light
- Other causes—fungal, parasitic, syphilis, thyroid disease, gout, psoriasis

Patient Profile

- Males = Females
- Any age—depends on cause; most common eye disease in United States

Signs and Symptoms

- Bacterial conjunctivitis:
  - Mucopurulent, profuse discharge
  - Eyelids edematous with matting on awakening
  - Conjunctival hyperemia
  - Burning
  - Tearing
  - Itching
  - Foreign body sensation
  - Photosensitivity
  - Initially one eye—may become bilateral
- Chlamydial conjunctivitis:
  - Thin, mucoid discharge
  - Conjunctival hyperemia
  - Photophobia
  - Moderate to profuse tearing
  - Enlarged, tender preauricular nodes
- Viral conjunctivitis:
  - Profuse tearing
  - Watery discharge
  - Marked conjunctival hyperemia
  - Large preauricular nodes
  - Associated systemic viral symptoms
- Allergic conjunctivitis:
  - Severe itching
  - Tearing
  - No exudate
  - Conjunctival hyperemia
  - Rhinorrhea
- Chemical or industrial conjunctivitis:
  - Burning
  - Tearing
  - Foreign body sensation
  - Conjunctival hyperemia

Differential Diagnosis

- Acute glaucoma
- Iritis
- Corneal abrasion
- Blepharitis
- Lacrimal duct obstruction

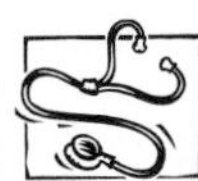

ASSESSMENT

History

Inquire about:

- Onset and duration of symptoms
- Character and quality of discharge
- Ear pain
- Cold symptoms
- Contact with person with "pink eye"
- Use of chemicals
- Visual changes
- Photophobia
- Past history of eye problems
- Family history of allergies
- Underlying conditions
- Current medications

Physical Findings

- Injected conjunctiva
- Absence of foreign body
- Preauricular enlarged nodes
- Visual acuity—within normal limits
- Discharge—may or may not be present
- Rhinorrhea
- Fluorescein staining—no ulcers, keratitis

Initial Workup

Laboratory: None indicated
Radiology: None indicated

Further Workup

- Culture from conjunctiva if management difficult, gonococcus suspected
- Gram and Giemsa stain of discharge

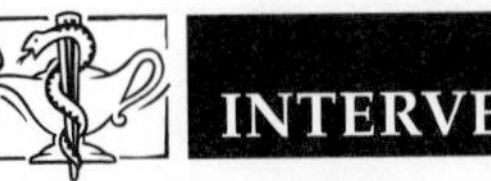

INTERVENTIONS

Office Treatment

If chemical or irritant conjunctivitis, eye irrigation with copious amounts of water or normal saline

Lifestyle Modifications

If bacterial conjunctivitis, patient should avoid contact with others:

- Not share washcloths, towels, etc.
- Stay home from work or school for 24 to 48 hours
- Practice meticulous hand washing to prevent spread

Patient Education

Teach patient about:

- Disease process and treatment options:
  - Bacterial conjunctivitis—antibiotic eye drops
  - Chlamydial conjunctivitis—oral antibiotics and partner needs treatment
  - Viral conjunctivitis—antibiotic eye drops to prevent secondary bacterial infection (if due to herpes refer to ophthalmologist)
  - Allergic conjunctivitis—cromolyn sodium eye drops, antihistamines, cool compresses; warm compresses to remove exudate
- How to prevent spread of disease
- Disposing of contaminated eye makeup
- Not wearing contact lenses; also, lenses may cause reinfection
- About medications—how to apply eye drops (inner aspect lower lid); side effects (see Pharmacotherapeutics)

Referral

To ophthalmologist if suspect herpes simplex or if no improvement in 48 hours

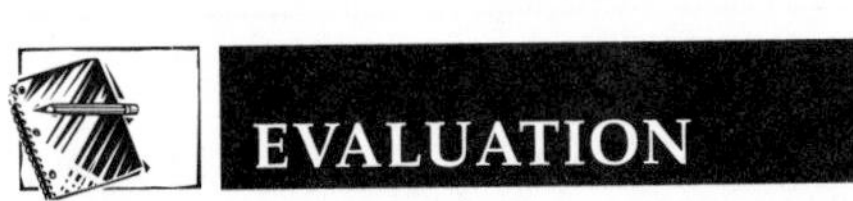

EVALUATION

Outcome

Resolves without sequelae

Possible Complications

- Bacterial conjunctivitis:
  - Chronic marginal blepharitis
  - Conjunctival scar if membrane disrupted
  - Corneal ulcer or perforation
- Viral conjunctivitis:
  - Corneal scars with herpes simplex
  - Corneal scars, lid scars, entropion
  - Misdirected lashes with varicella zoster
  - Bacterial superinfection
- Allergic conjunctivitis—bacterial superinfection

Follow-up

In 48 hours if no improvement; for severe cases, reassess in 10 to 14 days

FOR YOUR INFORMATION

Life Span

Pediatric: May be difficult to instill drops in small children; ensure that parents receive adequate training
Geriatric: May also have difficulty with eye drops or ointment, may need assistance, such as home health nurse
Pregnancy: N/A

Miscellaneous

Conjunctivitis is one of the most common eye disorders.

References

Schachat AP: The red eye. In Barker LR, Burton JR, Zieve PD, editors: *Principles of ambulatory medicine,* ed 4, Baltimore, 1995, Williams & Wilkins, pp 1431-1434.

Uphold CR, Graham MV: *Clinical guidelines in adult health,* Gainesville, Fla, 1994, Barmarrae Books, pp 198-202.

NOTES

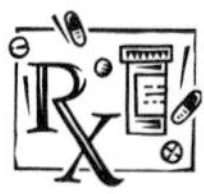

PHARMACOTHERAPEUTICS

Drug of Choice	Mechanism of Action	Prescribing Information	Side Effects
For bacterial or viral conjunctivitis:			
Sodium sulfacetamide (Sulamyd) ophthalmic ointment 10%; adults and children, 0.5-1.0 cm in conjunctival sac qid × 7-14 days or 10% solution 2 qtt q3h × 7-14 days	Bacteriostatic by inhibiting folic acid production; effective against wide range of gram-positive and gram-negative bacteria	***Contraindications:*** Hypersensitivity; hypersensitivity to sulfonamides; incompatible with silver preparations; infants <2 months ***Cost:*** Ointment, 35-g tube: $2; solution, 15-ml bottle: $4 ***Pregnancy category:*** C	Local irritation, stinging, burning
Bacitracin/Polymyxin (Polysporin) ointment; adults and children, 0.5-1 cm in conjunctival sac q4h × 7-14 days	Bactericidal; effective against wide range of gram-positive and gram-negative bacteria	***Contraindication:*** Hypersensitivity to any ingredient ***Cost:*** 3.5-g tube: $4 ***Pregnancy category:*** B	Local irritation, stinging, burning
For chlamydial conjunctivitis:			
Doxycycline (Vibramycin), 100 mg PO bid × 10-21 days—do not use in children <8 years; children >8 years, give 1 mg/lb of body weight in 1 or 2 doses	Bacteriostatic; inhibits protein synthesis; active against gram-positive and gram-negative organisms	***Contraindications:*** Hypersensitivity; pregnancy; nursing mothers; children <8 years ***Cost:*** 100 mg, 2/day × 10 days: $5 ***Pregnancy category:*** D	May increase digoxin level; monitor prothrombin time in patients taking Coumadin; anorexia; nausea, vomiting; enterocolitis; inflammatory lesions; rash; photosensitivity; increased BUN; urticaria; hemolytic anemia, thrombocytopenia; neutropenia
For allergic conjunctivitis:			
Cromolyn sodium (Opticrom); adults and children, 1-2 qtt 4-6 times daily × 4 days—do not wear contact lenses	Inhibits release of histamine	***Contraindication:*** Hypersensitivity ***Cost:*** 10 mg: $35 ***Pregnancy category:*** B	Stinging, burning sensation; eye irritation; watery eyes; puffy eyes
Antihistamines: • Diphenhydramine (Benadryl), 25-50 mg qid PO; children 6-12 years, 12.5-25 mg qid PO • Loratadine (Claritin), 10 mg 1qd PO—do not use in children <12 years • Astemizole (Hismanal), 10 mg 1qd PO—do not use in children <12 years • Fexofenadine (Allegra), 60 mg bid PO—do not use in children <12 years	Compete with histamine for cell receptor sites	***Contraindications:*** Coadministration of erythromycin, ketoconazole, or other drugs metabolized by P450 system with Hismanal; hypersensitivity ***Cost:*** Benadryl, 25 mg, 4/day × 30 days: $4; Claritin, 10-mg tab, 1/day × 30 days: $53; Hismanal, 10-mg tab, 1/day × 30 days: $53; Allegra, 60-mg tab, 2/day × 30 days: $53 ***Pregnancy category:*** Benadryl and Claritin—B; Hismanal and Allegra—C	Sedation—marked with Benadryl and lesser with the others; headache; fatigue; dizziness; nausea, vomiting; dry mouth; cough, rash; nervousness

Constipation

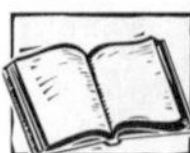

OVERVIEW

Constipation can be described as difficulty in passing stool, diminished frequency of defecation, incomplete evacuation, or infrequent passage of hard stools.

Pathogenesis

Many causes:

- Ignoring urge to defecate
- Abuse of laxatives/cathartics
- Diet low in fiber, or high in fiber but without adequate fluid intake
- Medications (anticholinergic agents, opiates, calcium channel blockers, etc.)
- Congenital abnormalities
- Metabolic and endocrine disorders
- Neurologic disease
- Colonic and/or rectal disorders
- Patient's perception of normal bowel movements

Patient Profile

- Females > Males
- Any age; most common in very young and very old

Signs and Symptoms

- Less frequent defecation than patient perceives as normal
- Lesser volume of stool
- Difficulty expelling feces
- Painful defecation
- Abdominal pain
- Diarrhea (may indicate impacted feces)
- Blood in stool
- Sense of incomplete bowel emptying

Differential Diagnosis

- Partial bowel obstruction
- Irritable bowel syndrome
- Rectal fissures
- Hypothyroidism
- Must differentiate functional from organic cause

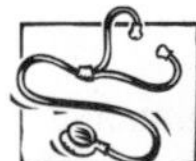

ASSESSMENT

History

Inquire about:

- Onset and duration of symptoms
- What patient's perception of "normal" bowel pattern is
- Dietary and fluid intake (24-hour diet recall)
- Activity level
- Laxative use/abuse
- Consistency of stool
- Underlying conditions
- Current medications

Physical Findings

- Look for bloating, distention, bulges
- Abdominal tenderness
- Firm mass may be palpated
- Bowel sounds—hyperactive (diarrhea or impending obstruction); hypoactive (paralytic ileus, peritonitis)
- Rectal examination—fissures, hemorrhoids, irritation, fecal impaction

Initial Workup

Laboratory

- CBC—should be within normal limits; if anemia, consider neoplasm
- Stool for occult blood; if positive, must rule out neoplasm

Radiology: Flat plate of abdomen

Further Workup

If cancer is suspected:

- Sigmoidoscopy
- Barium enema (air-contrast)

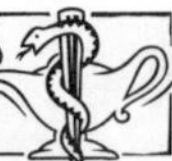

INTERVENTIONS

Office Treatment

None indicated

Lifestyle Modifications

- Increased fluid intake
- High-fiber diet
- Exercise program

Patient Education

Teach patient about:

- Condition and that "normal" patterns vary widely
- High-fiber foods and that bloating may occur as fiber is increased
- Increase in fluid intake—have patient keep record of fluid intake
- Hazards of laxative use/abuse
- Allowing adequate time for bowel evacuation, setting aside a specific time period
- Beginning an exercise program
- Agents that may be tried and side effects (see Pharmacotherapeutics)

Referral

If no improvement in 1 month, to MD

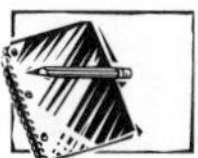

EVALUATION

Outcome
Patient reports resumption of normal bowel activity

Possible Complications
- Acquired megacolon
- Rectal ulceration

Follow-up
Every 2 weeks until normal bowel function resumes

FOR YOUR INFORMATION

Life Span
Pediatric: Consider aganglionic megacolon (Hirschsprung's disease)
Geriatric: Poor diet and inadequate fluid intake major factors; because of advanced age, consider neoplasm
Pregnancy: More trouble in third trimester

Miscellaneous
Constipation is a very common condition that affects the majority of people sometime in their life.

References

Allison OC, Porter ME, Briggs GC: Chronic constipation: assessment and management in the elderly, *J Am Acad Nurse Pract* 6(7):311-317, 1994.

Uphold CR, Graham MV: *Clinical guidelines in adult health,* Gainesville, Fla, 1994, Barmarrae Books, pp 373-375.

NOTES

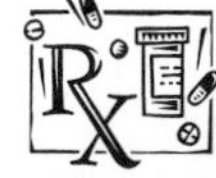

PHARMACOTHERAPEUTICS

Drug of Choice	Mechanism of Action	Prescribing Information	Side Effects
Bulk-forming agents: methylcellulose (Citrucel), psyllium (Effer-Syllium); adults, 1 tsp bid or tid in 8 oz of water or juice, follow with 8 oz water or juice, increase up to 3 tsp; for children, use half the adult dose	Citrucel—attracts water, expands in intestine to increase peristalsis; Effer-Syllium—bulk-forming laxative	***Contraindications:*** Hypersensitivity; GI obstruction; hepatitis ***Cost:*** Varies—OTC ***Pregnancy category:*** Effer-Syllium—C; Citrucel—not categorized	Nausea, vomiting, diarrhea, anorexia, cramps, abdominal distention
Stool softener: docusate sodium (Colace); adults, 50-200 mg/day PO; children 6-12 years, 40-120 mg/day PO; children 3-6 years, 60 mg/day PO; children <3 years, 10-40 mg/day PO	Surface-active agent, helps keep stool soft	***Contraindications:*** None ***Cost:*** Varies—OTC ***Pregnancy category:*** Not categorized	Bitter taste, throat irritation, nausea

Contact Dermatitis

OVERVIEW

Contact dermatitis is a cutaneous reaction that causes inflammation and pruritis.

Pathogenesis

Can be caused by external irritant or allergic reaction to external substance:

- Irritant contact dermatitis:
  - Damage to one of the components of the water-protein-lipid matrix of the outer layer of epidermis caused by irritant
  - Types of irritants—chemicals, dry air, cold air, friction
- Allergic contact dermatitis:
  - Affects individuals previously sensitized
  - First phase—sensitization phase—occurs when allergens penetrate epidermis and produce proliferation of T lymphocytes; can take days or months
  - Second phase—elicitation phase—antigen-specific T lymphocytes combine with subsequent exposures to allergen and produce inflammation
- Causes:
  - Hair care products
  - Makeup
  - Jewelry
  - Chemicals used in hobbies
  - Clothing
  - Detergents
  - Soaps
  - Perfumes
  - Rubber gloves
  - Latex gloves in health care workers
  - Topical medications
  - Can be caused by anything

Patient Profile

- Males = Females
- Any age
- Increased frequency in families with allergies

Signs and Symptoms

- Papules
- Vesicles
- Bullae surrounded by erythema
- Crusting and oozing
- Pruritis
- Scaling
- Fissuring
- Lichenification

Differential Diagnosis

- Herpes simplex
- Atopic dermatitis
- Tinea
- Nummular dermatitis
- Mycosis fungoides

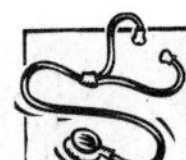

ASSESSMENT

History

Inquire about:

- Onset and duration of symptoms
- Location of eruptions
- Time and rate of onset
- Occupation
- Exposure to chemicals, dyes, detergents, medications, poisonous plants, lubricants, cleansers, rubber gloves
- Family history
- Personal history of allergies, treatments, and results
- Underlying conditions
- Current medications

Physical Findings

- Examine skin thoroughly
- Determine primary lesion
- Determine distribution of lesions—usually where epidermis is thinner (eyelids, genitalia, etc.); palms and soles more resistant
- Linear lesions from leaves brushing skin or from streaking oleoresin when scratching
- Distribution provides clues to offending agent:
  - Scalp and ears—hair care products, jewelry
  - Eyelids—cosmetics, contact lens solution
  - Face/neck—cosmetics, cleaners, medications, jewelry
  - Trunk/axilla—clothing, deodorants
  - Arms/hands—poison oak, ivy, sumac, soaps, detergents, chemicals, jewelry, rubber gloves
  - Legs/feet—clothing, shoes

Initial Workup

Laboratory: Potassium hydroxide (KOH) preparation—rule out tinea
Radiology: None indicated

Further Workup

None indicated

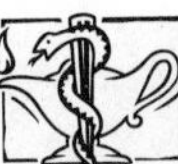

INTERVENTIONS

Office Treatment

None indicated

Lifestyle Modifications

- Depends on severity of reaction and causative agent
- Avoidance of agent if known
- May necessitate change in occupation
- Use of rubber gloves with cotton lining

Patient Education

Teach patient about:

- Condition, cause (if known), and treatment—antihistamines, antipuritic agents, topical steroids, and systemic steroids for severe cases
- Avoiding causative agent (condition usually self-limiting with avoidance of causative agent)
- Stopping any medication that may be causative
- Cleaning of secondary sources of infection—nails (keep trimmed, wash hands frequently), clothing (wash with soap and hot water), etc.
- Skin patch testing, if necessary
- Using cool compresses or cool oatmeal baths to decrease pruritis and erythema
- Worsening symptoms or shortness of breath—patient should report to emergency room
- Medications used and side effects (see Pharmacotherapeutics)

Referrals

None; to allergist for skin patch testing if severe

EVALUATION

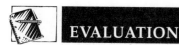

Outcome
Self-limiting; resolves without sequelae

Possible Complication
Secondary bacterial infection

Follow-up
- Mild—none
- Severe—in 48 to 72 hours

FOR YOUR INFORMATION

Life Span
Pediatric: Common problem in this age group
Geriatric: May be more prone to secondary infections or more severe cases because of fragility of skin
Pregnancy: Cautious use of medications

Miscellaneous
Poison ivy, poison oak, and poison sumac produce more cases of allergic contact dermatitis than all other contactants combined.

References

Habif TP: *Clinical dermatology: a color guide to diagnosis and therapy,* ed 3, St Louis, 1996, Mosby, pp 81-99.

Klaus MV, Wieselthier JS: Contact dermatitis, *Am Fam Physician* 48(4):629-632, 1993.

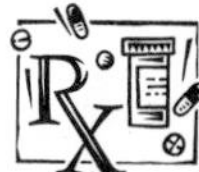

PHARMACOTHERAPEUTICS

Drug of Choice	Mechanism of Action	Prescribing Information	Side Effects
Calamine (Caladryl) lotion; adults and children ≥2 years, apply to affected area after cleaning with soap and water tid to qid	Drying agent; antipruritic	***Contraindication:*** Hypersensitivity ***Cost:*** OTC ***Pregnancy category:*** Unavailable	Usually well-tolerated; if rash worsens, discontinue use
Topical corticosteroid for mild to moderate erythema: hydrocortisone cream, 1% for face (controversial—some feel corticosteroids should not be used on face) and 2.5% elsewhere; apply thin layer 3-4 times daily; for severe erythema, stronger corticosteroid may be needed: mometasone (Elocon), triamcinolone (Kenalog), Betamethasone (Diprolene AF)	Antiinflammatory and antipruritic	***Contraindication:*** Hypersensitivity ***Cost:*** 1%, 30 g: $12; several available OTC; mometasone 0.1%, 45 g: $29; triamcinolone 0.025%, 30 g: $2-$5; betamethasone 0.05%, 15 g: $3-$16 ***Pregnancy category:*** C	Burning, dryness, itching, irritation acne, folliculitis, hypertrichosis, hypopigmentation, atrophy, striae, perioral dermatitis, secondary infection; if used on large area for extended periods of time, can have systemic side effects
Antihistamines: • Diphenhydramine (Benadryl), 25-50 mg PO qid; children 6-12 years, 12.5-25 mg PO qid • Loratadine (Claritin), 10 mg 1 qd PO—do not use in children <12 years • Astemizole (Hismanal), 10 mg 1 qd PO—do not use in children <12 years • Fexofenadine (Allegra), 60 mg PO bid—do not use in children <12 years	Compete with histamine for cell receptor sites	***Contraindications:*** Coadministration of erythromycin, ketoconazole, or other drugs metabolized by P450 system with Hismanal; hypersensitivity ***Cost:*** Benadryl, 25 mg, 4/day × 30 days: $4; Claritin, 10 mg, 1/day × 30 days: $53; Hismanal, 10 mg, 1/day × 30 days: $53; Allegra 60 mg, 2/day × 30 days: $53 ***Pregnancy category:*** Benadryl and Claritin—B; Hismanal and Allegra—C	Sedation—marked with Benadryl and lesser with the others; headache, fatigue, dizziness, nausea and vomiting, dry mouth, cough, rash, nervousness
Systemic steroid for severe cases—prednisone or dexamethasone acetate: • Prednisone, 60-120 mg PO qd, then taper over several days • Dexamethasone acetate, 4-16 mg IM × 1 dose	Corticosteroid; decreases inflammation	***Contraindications:*** Hypersensitivity; psychosis; idiopathic thrombocytopenia; acute glomerulonephritis; amebiasis; nonasthmatic bronchial disease; AIDS; TB; child <2 years old ***Cost:*** Prednisone, 15 mg tab, 100 tabs: $14-$35; dexamethasone acetate, 8 mg/ml, 5 ml: $11-47 ***Pregnancy category:*** C	Hypertension, circulatory collapse, thrombophlebitis, embolism, tachycardia, fungal infections, increased intraocular pressure, diarrhea, nausea, GI hemorrhage, thrombocytopenia, acne, poor wound healing, fractures, osteoporosis, weakness

OVERVIEW

Contraception consists of a wide variety of methods used to prevent pregnancy. These methods are designed to prevent ovulation, prevent implantation, be spermicidal, or prevent the sperm from reaching the egg. There are many different types of contraception. See Table 6 for some of the more common types and the rate of pregnancy.

Pathogenesis
N/A

Patient Profile
- Females > Males
- Female predominant age—menarche to menopause
- Male predominant age—any age after puberty

Signs and Symptoms
N/A

Differential Diagnosis
N/A

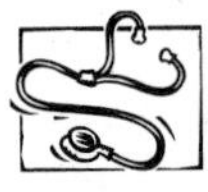

ASSESSMENT

History
There are many individual factors that must be considered when assisting a patient with selection of a birth control method. Some of these factors are:
- Age and maturity
- Desire for future pregnancy
- Marital status
- Cultural and religious beliefs
- Motivation
- Cooperation of partner
- Number of partners
- Cost of method
- Prior experience with birth control methods
- Sexual habits/behaviors
- Frequency of intercourse
- Safety and effectiveness of method
- Confidence in and convenience of method

A comprehensive history must be taken to identify risk factors and other factors that could influence the method selected. Inquire about:
- Smoking history
- Hypertension
- Cardiovascular disease
- Thromboembolic disease
- Diabetes mellitus
- Allergy to latex
- Frequent urinary tract infections
- Migraine headaches
- Other chronic medical conditions
- Current medications
- Age of menarche
- Age of first coitus
- Number of pregnancies and results of pregnancies
- History of sexually transmitted diseases (STDs)
- Number of partners
- Length of menstrual cycle
- Regularity of menstrual cycle
- Prior birth control practices
- Family history of cancer, cardiovascular disease, other significant problems
- Personal and social history, including religious beliefs and practices

Physical Findings
- Females—complete physical examination, including speculum and bimanual examination—should be within normal limits
- Males—complete physical examination before vasectomy

Initial Workup
Laboratory
- Females:
  - Pap smear for cytology
  - Wet mount
  - Cultures for gonorrhea and chlamydial infection
  - Pregnancy test
  - Rapid plasma reagin (RPR)
  - Hemoglobin and hematocrit
  - Urinalysis
  - Lipid profile
  - Blood sugar
  - Preoperative workup for bilateral tubal ligation
- Males:
  - Preoperative workup for vasectomy
  - Postoperative—3 consecutive semen analyses showing no sperm

Radiology: None indicated

Further Workup
None indicated

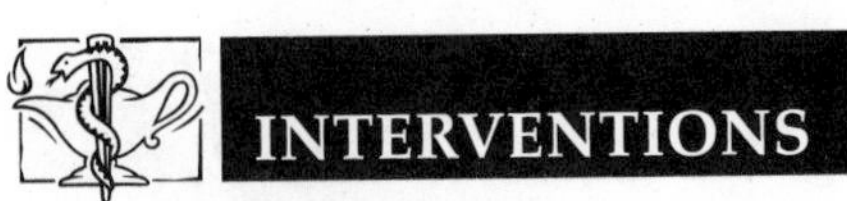

INTERVENTIONS

Office Treatment
None indicated

Lifestyle Modification
Practice safe sex by using barrier method and limiting number of partners

Patient Education
Teach patient about:
- Various methods of birth control:
  - Spermicides—foams, creams, suppositories, tablets; OTC; must be inserted into vagina, close to cervix, before intercourse; protect for 1 hour and 1 encounter; best to use in conjunction with sponge, diaphragm, cervical cap, or condom
  - Coitus interruptus—man withdraws penis from vagina before ejaculation (very unreliable)
  - Condom (male)—sheath that fits over penis; check for holes before application; leave space at tip as reservoir for semen; withdraw penis from vagina before it becomes flaccid; most effective if used with spermicide; OTC; new condom must be used for each encounter; latex helps prevent spread of STDs
  - Condom (female)—sheath that is inserted vaginally; can be inserted up to 2 hours before intercourse; helps prevent spread of STDs; new condom must be used for each encounter
  - Periodic abstinence—need accurate record of menstrual cycles for 12 months; fertile period—shortest cycle minus 18 days and longest cycle minus 11 days; difficult to be accurate for women with irregular cycles; during ovulation basal body temperature will rise 1° for 3 days
  - Diaphragm—inserted vaginally; must use spermicide with it; must be properly fitted by trained professional; helps in preven-

TABLE 6 *Types and Effectiveness of Contraception*

Type of contraception	Description	No. of pregnancies/ 100 women/year
Natural family planning	Avoidance of coitus during ovulation	20
Permanent sterilization	Bilateral tubal ligation or vasectomy	0.15
Oral contraception	Birth control pills	3
Long-acting injectable progestin	Depo-Provera	1
Implantable progestogen	Norplant	1
Intrauterine device	IUD	5
Barrier device	Condom (male or female)	12
	Diaphragm with spermicide	18
	Cervical cap with spermicide	18
Insertion device	Sponge	18-28
Spermicide, alone	Foams, creams, suppositories	21

tion of spread of STDs; leave in for 8 hours after coitus; remove and clean
- Cervical cap—soft, cup-shaped device that fits over cervix; spermicide placed inside cap—not around rim; helps protect against STDs; must be fitted by trained professional
- Sponge—wet with water to activate spermicide, insert into vagina; leave in for 8 hours after coitus; OTC
- Intrauterine device (IUD)—must be placed into uterus by trained professional; string protrudes from vagina; must regularly check for it; not protective against STDs; lasts from 1 to 8 years; not frequently used
- Implantable hormonal contraception—6 Silastic tubes of levonorgestrel implanted in upper arm by trained professional; minor surgical procedure; effective for 5 years; no protection against STDs
- Depo-Provera injections—150 mg of medroxyprogesterone acetate given IM every 3 months; no protection against STDs
- Oral contraception—take pill daily at about same time; no protection against STDs; if pill missed, take 2 the next day and use another method of protection until next period; many types of pills available; should not be used in smoker >35 years of age
- Sterilization—should be considered permanent; preoperative and postoperative teaching
- Postcoital pregnancy prevention ("morning after")—0.5 mg norgestrel and 0.05 mg ethynyl (Ovral)—2 tablets given within 72 hours of unprotected intercourse and 2 more tablets taken 12 hours later; other brands that may be used are Nordette, Levlen, Lo/Ovral (1 dose = 4 white pills), Triphasil, Tri-Levlen (1 dose = 4 yellow pills)

- STDs and prevention
- Females—importance of yearly gynecologic examination; if pregnancy occurs, patient should consult provider immediately
- Medications used and side effects (see Pharmacotherapeutics)

Referrals
Usually none; to surgeon for sterilization

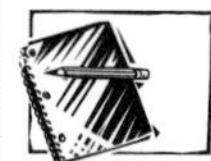

EVALUATION

Outcome
Unwanted pregnancies are prevented

Possible Complications
- Pregnancy
- Oral contraception—thromboembolism, hypertension, myocardial infarction, nausea and vomiting, breakthrough bleeding, amenorrhea, cyclic weight gain, breast tenderness, depression, chloasma, acne, hirsutism, cholestatic jaundice
- IUD—heavy bleeding, salpingitis

Follow-up
- In 1 month to assess effectiveness
- Yearly for annual examination

FOR YOUR INFORMATION

Life Span
Pediatric: Adolescents need careful teaching regarding birth control and sexuality
Geriatric: Postmenopause—contraception is no longer a concern
Pregnancy: Remove IUD and stop all hormonal types of contraception

Miscellaneous
N/A

References
Caufield KA: Controlling fertility. In Youngkin EQ, Davis MS, editors: *Women's health: a primary care clinical guide,* Norwalk, Conn, 1994, Appleton & Lange, pp 101-159.

US Department of Health and Human Services, Public Health Service: *Clinician's handbook of preventive services: put prevention into practice,* Washington DC, 1994, US Government Printing Office, pp 119-121 and 337-342.

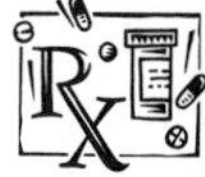

PHARMACOTHERAPEUTICS

Drug of Choice	Mechanism of Action	Prescribing Information	Side Effects
Combination oral contraceptives (many brands available); dosage and instructions vary for different types; see individual package insert for directions	Prevent ovulation by suppressing FSH and LH	***Contraindications:*** Hypersensitivity; breast cancer; thromboembolic disorders; reproductive cancer; undiagnosed vaginal bleeding; pregnancy; hepatic tumor/disease; women 40 years and over; cerebrovascular accident (CVA) ***Cost:*** Varies by brand: $20-$30 ***Pregnancy category:*** X	Dizziness, headache, migraines, depression, hypotension, thrombophlebitis, thromboembolism, pulmonary embolism, myocardial infarction (MI), nausea, vomiting, cholestatic jaundice, weight gain, diplopia, amenorrhea, cervical erosion, breakthrough bleeding, dysmenorrhea, vaginal candidiasis, spontaneous abortion, rash, urticaria, acne, hirsutism, photosensitivity
Medroxyprogesterone acetate, 150 mg IM every 3 months	Inhibits secretion of pituitary gonadotropins; stimulates growth of mammary tissue	***Contraindications:*** Hypersensitivity; breast cancer; thromboembolic disorders; reproductive cancer; undiagnosed vaginal bleeding; pregnancy ***Cost:*** 50 mg/ml, 10 ml: $9-$30; ***Pregnancy category:*** X	Dizziness, headache, migraines, depression, hypotension, thrombophlebitis, thromboembolism, pulmonary embolism, MI, nausea, vomiting, cholestatic jaundice, weight gain, diplopia, amenorrhea, cervical erosion, breakthrough bleeding, dysmenorrhea, vaginal spontaneous abortion, rash, urticaria, acne, hirsutism, photosensitivity

Corneal Ulcer

OVERVIEW

Corneal ulcer occurs as a result of a breakdown in the epithelial barrier due to an abrasive injury, contact lenses, or chronic use of topical steroids. This breakdown allows bacteria, viruses, or fungi to infect the cornea. Ulcers may be central or marginal.

Pathogenesis

Causative organisms:

- Gram-positive organisms—staphylococci, streptococci, bacilli, anaerobes (cocci, bacilli)
- Gram-negative organisms—diplococcus, rods
- *Pseudomonas*
- Viruses

Patient Profile

- Males = Females
- Any age

Signs and Symptoms

- Pain, foreign body sensation
- Blurred vision
- Mucopurulent drainage
- Inflamed eyelid and conjunctiva
- Photophobia

Differential Diagnosis

- Conjunctivitis
- Uveitis
- Keratitis
- Foreign body

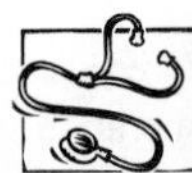

ASSESSMENT

History

Inquire about:

- Onset and duration of symptoms
- Abrasive injury
- Contact lenses
- Chronic topical steroid use
- Past history of corneal ulcer
- Underlying conditions
- Current medications

Physical Findings

- Inflamed eyelid and conjunctiva—circumcorneal infection predominates
- Decreased visual acuity
- Fluorescein stain shows epithelial defect as brilliant green

Initial Workup

Laboratory: None by NP; ophthalmologist may do culture

Radiology: None indicated

Further Workup

None indicated

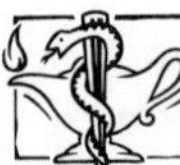

INTERVENTIONS

Office Treatment

If available, stain eye with fluorescein after applying topical anesthetic; observe under ultraviolet lamp—epithelial defect shows brilliant green

Lifestyle Modification

Decreased activity until full vision returns

Patient Education

Teach patient about:

- Disease process and treatment options—prompt referral to ophthalmologist; may treat as inpatient or outpatient, depending on severity
- Preventing corneal ulcers—proper use and handling of contact lenses
- Use of protective eyewear

Referral

Promptly to ophthalmologist

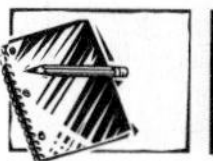

EVALUATION

Outcome
Ulcer heals without any decrease in visual acuity

Possible Complication
Scarring of cornea—loss of vision

Follow-up
Daily with ophthalmologist

FOR YOUR INFORMATION

Life Span
Pediatric: May be easiest to treat if inpatient
Geriatric: Ring ulceration more common
Pregnancy: N/A

Miscellaneous
N/A

Reference
Schachat AP: The red eye. In Barker LR, Burton JR, Zieve PD, editors: *Principles of ambulatory medicine,* ed 4, Baltimore, 1995, Williams & Wilkins, p 1430.

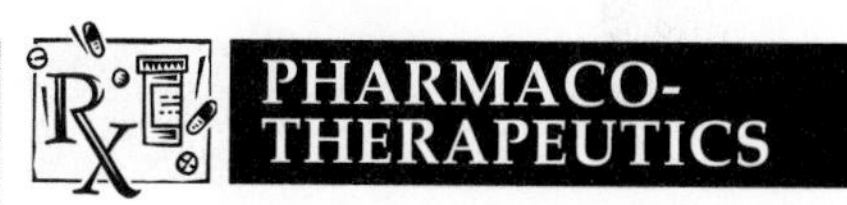

There are a variety of topical eye drops that will be used by the ophthalmologist. The NP's responsibility is diagnosis and prompt referral to the ophthalmologist.

OVERVIEW

Costochondritis is an inflammation that produces anterior chest wall pain in the costochondral and/or costosternal regions. It is also referred to as Tietze's disease or syndrome.

Pathogenesis
Cause—not fully known; may be overuse or trauma

Patient Profile
- Almost exclusively females
- Most common age group—20 to 40 years

Signs and Symptoms
- Insidious onset
- Sharp pain, most commonly in the second through fifth costal cartilage
- Pain worse with movement, coughing, and breathing
- Pain sometimes radiates to arm and shoulder
- Redness and warmth at site of tenderness
- Slight edema and point tenderness

Differential Diagnosis
- Coronary artery disease
- Aortic aneurysm
- Mitral valve prolapse
- Pericarditis
- Gastroesophageal reflux
- Peptic esophagitis
- Gastritis
- Fibromyalgia
- Slipping rib syndrome
- Ankylosing spondylitis
- Anxiety disorder
- Panic attacks
- Asthma
- Pneumonia
- Chronic cough
- Herpes zoster
- Cocaine abuse
- Trauma
- Costoclavicular syndrome

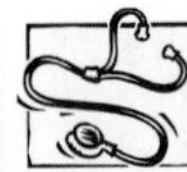

ASSESSMENT

History
Inquire about:
- Onset and duration of symptoms
- Trauma or overuse
- Past history of costochondritis
- Underlying conditions
- Current medications

Physical Findings
- Tenderness on palpation over costochondral junctions
- Redness, warmth, edema at site of tenderness

Initial Workup
Laboratory: Used only to rule out other conditions
Radiology: None indicated

Further Workup
None indicated

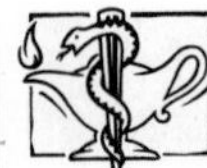

INTERVENTIONS

Office Treatment
None indicated

Lifestyle Modifications
- Smoking cessation
- Avoidance of overuse

Patient Education
Teach patient about:
- Condition and treatment—rest, heat, nonsteroidal antiinflammatory medications
- Course of disease, which is usually self-limiting
- Medications used and side effects (see Pharmacotherapeutics)

Referral
To MD if resistant to treatment

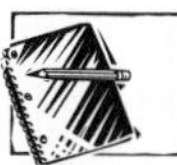

EVALUATION

Outcomes
- Resolves without sequelae; usually takes 3 to 6 weeks for resolution to occur
- Recurrences common

Possible Complications
Usually none

Follow-up
In 1 week to assess response; then in 1 month

FOR YOUR INFORMATION

Life Span
Pediatric: Uncommon; look for other causes of chest pain
Geriatric: Imperative to obtain thorough history and physical; must rule out cardiac origin for pain
Pregnancy: Cautious use of medications

Miscellaneous
N/A

Reference
Smith PL, Britt EJ, Terry PB: Common pulmonary problems: cough, hemoptysis, dyspnea, chest pain, and the abnormal chest x-ray. In Barker LR, Burton JR, Zieve PD, editors: *Principles of ambulatory medicine,* ed 4, Baltimore, 1995, Williams & Wilkins, pp 642-643.

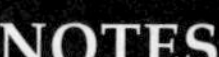

NOTES

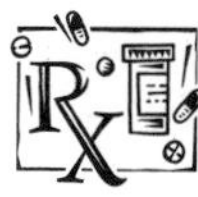

PHARMACOTHERAPEUTICS

Drug of Choice	Mechanism of Action	Prescribing Information	Side Effects
Aspirin, enteric coated, 1 g PO tid or qid; may increase by 300-600 mg/day each week until maximal response seen or toxicity occurs (tinnitus usually 1st symptom); if toxicity occurs, decrease by 600-900 mg/day every 3 days until symptoms resolve	Antiinflammatory action may result from inhibition of synthesis and release of prostaglandins	***Contraindications:*** Hypersensitivity; GI bleeding; bleeding disorders ***Cost:*** OTC ***Pregnancy category:*** Should not be used in 3rd trimester	Dyspepsia, thirst, nausea, vomiting, GI bleeding/ulceration, tinnitus, vertigo, reversible hearing loss, prolongation of bleeding time, leukopenia, thrombocytopenia, purpura, urticaria, angioedema, pruritus, asthma, anaphylaxis, mental confusion, drowsiness, dizziness, headache, fever
Nonsteroidal antiinflammatory drugs (NSAIDs): many different types currently marketed; consult manufacturer's package insert for specific dosing and prescribing information	Exact action unknown; may be caused by inhibition of synthesis of prostaglandins and arachidonic acid	***Contraindications:*** Hypersensitivity to NSAIDs, aspirin; severe hepatic failure; asthma ***Cost:*** Varies with type ***Pregnancy category:*** Depends on product	Stomach distress, flatulence, nausea, abdominal pain, constipation or diarrhea, dizziness, sedation, rash, urticaria, angioedema, anorexia, urinary frequency, increased blood pressure, insomnia, anxiety, visual disturbances, increased thirst, alopecia

Crohn's Disease/Regional Enteritis

OVERVIEW

Crohn's disease is a chronic inflammatory disease, generally of the small intestine and colon, but it may affect any part of the GI tract. It involves all layers of the bowel wall and is most commonly seen in the terminal ileum, jejunum, and colon. The disease may affect several sections of the bowel, with areas of normal bowel in between. It is slowly progressive, with periods of exacerbation and remission. Some patients with mild disease may suffer a couple of acute attacks and go into long periods of remission.

Pathogenesis

- Cause—unknown
- Areas of deep, longitudinal ulceration penetrate between islands of inflamed, edematous mucosa (cobblestone appearance)
- Bowel wall thickens
- Lumen narrows
- Strictures develop, as can abscesses and fistulas

Patient Profile

- Females > Males (slightly)
- Age at onset—15 to 30 years
- More common in Jewish population and in Caucasians in general

Signs and Symptoms

- Depends on location
- Generally—nonbloody diarrhea, fatigue, abdominal pain, weight loss, malnutrition, dehydration, electrolyte imbalance, anemia, pain around umbilicus and in (R) lower abdominal quadrant, arthritis, spondylitis, iritis

Differential Diagnosis

- Ulcerative colitis—very similar (starts distally, spreads in a continuous pattern, and can be cured with surgery)
- Ischemic colitis
- Infection with enteric pathogens
- Malignancy
- Lymphoma
- Drugs

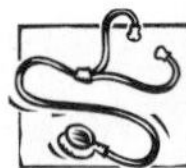

ASSESSMENT

History

Inquire about:

- Onset and duration of symptoms
- Family history
- Underlying conditions
- Current medications

Physical Findings

- Abdominal tenderness
- Weight loss
- May have iritis with tearing
- Photophobia
- Symmetric arthritis
- Pallor of mucous membranes
- Perianal abscess, fistula
- Atrophic glossitis—beefy, red tongue

Initial Workup

Laboratory

- CBC—anemia
- Erythrocyte sedimentation rate (ESR)—increased
- Chemistry profile—electrolyte imbalance; albumin decreased; B_{12} and folate may be decreased

Radiology

- Barium enema
- Flat plate of abdomen

Further Workup

Colonoscopy with ileoscopy and biopsy, by specialist

INTERVENTIONS

Office Treatment

None indicated

Lifestyle Modifications

- Diet—increased fiber, decreased fat
- Stress reduction
- Adequate rest
- Prevention of infections

Patient Education

Teach patient about:

- Disease process and treatment options—medications; nutritional supplement such as total parenteral nutrition; surgery (reserved for severe cases, not curative)
- Diet low in fat and high in fiber
- How to keep record of weight
- Number of stools/day and consistency
- Stress reduction techniques—biofeedback, relaxation, yoga
- Importance of adequate fluid intake
- Living with a chronic illness
- Notifying provider immediately of signs/symptoms of exacerbation (increased stools, fatigue, weight loss)
- Use of medications and side effects (see Pharmacotherapeutics)

Referral

Best handled by specialist in Crohn's disease

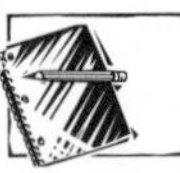

EVALUATION

Outcome

Patient able to resume and maintain normal activities (weight stabilizes; diarrhea stops)

Possible Complications

- Progression with need for surgery; recurrence after surgery (almost certain)
- Fistulas
- Short-bowel syndrome after extensive surgery
- Uveitis
- Arthritis

Follow-up

- Done by specialist
- Close follow-up during exacerbations; every 3 to 6 months when stable

FOR YOUR INFORMATION

Life Span

Pediatric: Rarely occurs

Geriatric: Probably has had disease for a long period of time—close assessment of nutritional and hydration status

Pregnancy: Monitor nutritional status closely

Miscellaneous

If the patient has to have surgery, it is important that he or she understands that it is not curative and that the disease will most likely recur.

References

Heitkemper M, Sawchuck L: Nursing role in management: problems of absorption and elimination. In Lewis SM, Collier IC, Heitkemper MM, editors: *Medical-surgical nursing: assessment and management of clinical problems,* ed 4, St Louis, 1996, Mosby, pp 1231-1235.

Woolliscroft JO: *Current diagnosis and treatment: a quick reference for the general practitioner,* Philadelphia, 1996, Current Medicine, pp 88-89.

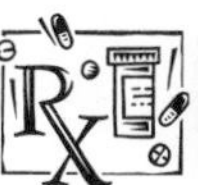

PHARMACOTHERAPEUTICS

The main purpose of medication therapy is to bring acute exacerbations under control.

Drug of Choice	Mechanism of Action	Prescribing Information	Side Effects
Prednisone, 20-60 mg PO qd, taper gradually after 4-6 weeks	Decreases inflammation by suppression of migration of polymorphonuclear leukocytes, fibroblasts; reversal to increase capillary permeability; and lysosomal stabilization	***Contraindications:*** Psychosis; hypersensitivity; idiopathic thrombocytopenia; acute glomerulonephritis; amebiasis; fungal infections; nonasthmatic bronchial disease; child <2 years; AIDS; TB ***Cost:*** 20-mg tab, 100 tabs: \$7-\$18 ***Pregnancy category:*** C	Depression, flushing, sweating, headache, mood change, hypertension, circulatory collapse, thrombophlebitis, embolism, tachycardia, fungal infections, increased intraocular pressure, blurred vision, diarrhea, nausea, abdominal distention, GI hemorrhage, increased appetite, pancreatitis, thrombocytopenia, acne, poor wound healing, fractures, osteoporosis, weakness
Sulfasalazine (Azulfidine), 0.5 g PO bid, increase q4d until reaching 1 g qid; children >2 years, 40-60 mg/kg/day PO in 4-6 divided doses, maximum 2 g/day; maintenance therapy in adults, 2 g/day	Prodrug to deliver sulfapyridine and 5-aminosalicylic acid	***Contraindications:*** Hypersensitivity to sulfonamides or salicylates; pregnancy at term; children <2 years; intestinal/urinary obstruction ***Cost:*** 500-mg tab, 100 tabs: \$10-\$22 ***Pregnancy category:*** C	Anaphylaxis, nausea, vomiting, abdominal pain, stomatitis, hepatitis, glossitis, pancreatitis, headache, confusion, insomnia, hallucinations, convulsions, leukopenia, neutropenia, thrombocytopenia, agranulocytosis, hemolytic anemia, rash, dermatitis, Stevens-Johnson syndrome, renal failure, toxic nephrosis, increased BUN and creatinine, allergic myocarditis
For perirectal disease with fistulas:			
Metronidazole (Flagyl), 250 mg PO tid for maximum of 8 weeks; children, 35-50 mg/kg/day PO in 3 divided doses	Direct-acting amebicide/trichomonacide	***Contraindications:*** Hypersensitivity; renal disease; hepatic disease; contracted visual or color fields; blood dyscrasias; pregnancy 1st trimester; lactation; CNS disorders ***Cost:*** 250-mg tab, 100 tabs: \$5-\$60 ***Pregnancy category:*** B (2nd & 3rd trimesters)	Flat T-waves, headache, dizziness, confusion, irritability, restlessness, depression, fatigue, drowsiness, insomnia, convulsions, blurred vision, sore throat, dry mouth, retinal edema, metallic taste, nausea, vomiting, diarrhea, anorexia, constipation, abdominal cramps, pseudomembranous colitis, darkened urine, albuminuria, neurotoxicity, leukopenia, bone marrow depression, aplasia, rash, pruritus, urticaria
For rectal and left-sided disease:			
Mesalamine (Rowasa); adults, enema 4 g/60 ml PR hs, retain 8 hours, × 3-6 weeks; suppository, 500 mg 1 PR bid × 3-6 weeks; tabs, 800 mg po tid × 6 weeks—not dosed for children	5-Aminosalicylic acid (S-ASA); decreases inflammation by blocking cyclooxygenase; inhibits prostaglandin production in colon	***Contraindication:*** Hypersensitivity to this drug or salicylates ***Cost:*** Enema, 4 g/60 ml × 7: \$62; suppository, 500-mg suppository × 12: \$34; tabs, 400-mg tab, 100 tabs: \$57	Pericarditis, myocarditis, cramps, gas, nausea, diarrhea, headache, fever, dizziness, insomnia, rash, itching, flu, malaise, back pain, peripheral edema, leg and joint pain, sore throat, cough, pharyngitis

Cushing's Disease/Syndrome

OVERVIEW

Cushing's disease/syndrome comprises a group of clinical abnormalities that occur as a result of excess corticosteroids.

Pathogenesis

Causes:

- Most common cause—prolonged use of glucocorticoids and/or adrenocorticotropic hormone (ACTH) (Cushing's syndrome)
- Cushing's disease caused by ACTH-secreting pituitary tumor
- Other causes—adrenal tumors and ACTH-producing tumors outside the hypothalamus-pituitary-adrenal axis (usually lung or pancreas)

Patient Profile

- Females > Males
- Affects all ages

Signs and Symptoms

- Obesity with thin extremities
- Moon face
- Fat deposits on back of neck (buffalo hump)
- Hypertension
- Thin, fragile skin
- Purplish-red striae
- Edema
- Muscle wasting
- Hyperglycemia
- Poor wound healing

Differential Diagnosis

- Obesity associated with diabetes mellitus
- Hypercortisolism secondary to alcoholism

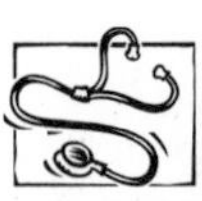

ASSESSMENT

History

Inquire about:

- Onset and duration of symptoms
- Underlying conditions requiring corticosteroid therapy
- Alcohol intake
- Current medications

Physical Findings

- Moon face
- Buffalo hump
- Hypertension
- Purplish-red striae
- Hyperglycemia

Initial Workup

Laboratory

- Chemistry profile—increased glucose, decreased potassium and sodium
- CBC—neutrophilia, polycythemia, lymphopenia
- Urinalysis—glucosuria (possibly)

Radiology

- Chest film
- If pituitary tumor suspected, MRI of pituitary
- If adrenal tumor suspected, CT scan of abdomen

Further Workup

- Dexamethasone suppression test
- Urinary 17-hydroxycorticosteroids and cortisol
- Plasma ACTH concentration
- Corticotropin-releasing hormone test

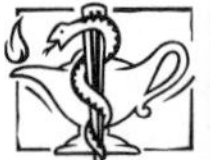

INTERVENTIONS

Office Treatment

None indicated

Lifestyle Modifications

- Stress reduction
- Avoidance of infections
- Smoking cessation
- High-protein and high-potassium diet

Patient Education

Teach patient about:

- Disease process and treatment options—treatment depends on cause:
  - Pituitary adenoma—transsphenoidal removal
  - Adrenal tumor—unilateral adrenalectomy (may need replacement steroids for life)
  - Lung or pancreas tumors—surgical resection with radiation or chemotherapy; may use radiation or chemotherapy alone
  - Prolonged administration of steroids—gradual discontinuance of steroids if possible; gradual reduction in dosage; every-other-day schedule of administration
- May use medications to suppress production of corticosteroids (not very effective)
- Signs and symptoms of infection and need for early treatment
- Monitoring weight daily
- High-protein and high-potassium diet
- Stress reduction techniques, such as biofeedback or relaxation techniques—may help with emotional lability
- Medications used and side effects (see Pharmacotherapeutics)

Referral

To endocrinologist

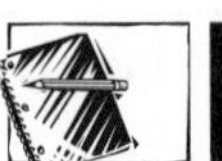

EVALUATION

Outcome

Depends on cause: excess corticosteroids—control of underlying condition with lowest possible dose of steroids may give some relief of symptoms; if surgical intervention performed, prognosis is more favorable

Possible Complications

- Osteoporosis
- Increased susceptibility to infections
- Virilism
- Metastases of malignant tumors
- Diabetes insipidus

Follow-up

- Depends on type of therapy, but frequent monitoring is important
- Will probably be followed by specialist

FOR YOUR INFORMATION

Life Span

Pediatric: Rare—most commonly due to adrenal tumor
Geriatric: Treatment is the same
Pregnancy: May exacerbate condition; needs to be followed by a specialist

Miscellaneous

Cushing's disease/syndrome is usually a chronic condition that has frequent exacerbations with rare remissions.

References

Gregerman RI: Selected endocrine problems: disorders of pituitary, adrenal, and parathyroid glands; pharmacological use of steroids; hypo- and hypercalcemia; osteoporosis; water metabolism; hypoglycemia. In Barker LR, Burton JR, Zieve PD, editors: *Principles of ambulatory medicine,* ed 4, Baltimore, 1995, Williams & Wilkins, pp 1053-1056.

Haas LB: Endocrine problems. In Lewis SM, Collier IC, Heitkemper MM, editors: *Medical-surgical nursing: assessment and management of clinical problems,* ed 4, St Louis, 1996, Mosby, pp 1506-1508.

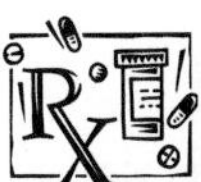

PHARMACOTHERAPEUTICS

Treatment and drug therapy for the patient with Cushing's syndrome should be carried out by an endocrinologist. The following is a list of possible drugs that the endocrinologist may use for treatment. This list is intended only as a guideline for the NP to use to teach the patient about the possible treatment options.

Drug of Choice	Mechanism of Action	Prescribing Information	Side Effects
Ketoconazole (Nizoral), 400-600 mg PO bid (much higher doses than normally recommended)	Acts as a cortisol production inhibitor	***Contraindications:*** Hypersensitivity; coadministration of terfenadine or astemizole ***Cost:*** 200-mg tab, 100 tabs: \$271-\$298 ***Pregnancy category:*** C	Hepatotoxicity, anaphylaxis, hypersensitivity reactions, nausea, vomiting, abdominal pain, pruritus, headache, dizziness, somnolence, fever, chills, photophobia, diarrhea, gynecomastia, impotence, thrombocytopenia, leukopenia, hemolytic anemia, oligospermia, severe depression, ventricular dysrhythmias when used concomitantly with terfenadine
Mitotane (Lysodren); start with 2-6 g daily in divided doses and increase as needed; useful in inoperable carcinoma	Adrenal cytotoxic agent; provides a medical adrenalectomy	***Contraindication:*** Hypersensitivity ***Cost:*** 500-mg tab, 100 tabs: \$204 ***Pregnancy category:*** C	Adrenal insufficiency, sedation, lethargy, vertigo, anorexia, nausea, vomiting, skin rashes
The patient will need corticosteroid replacement therapy if either surgical or medical adrenalectomy is performed. Use the following drugs for replacement:			
Hydrocortisone, 10 mg PO every morning and 5 mg PO every evening as starting dose; may need to adjust according to patient's symptoms; will need higher doses in times of increased stress; patient should not receive immunizations; used with fludrocortisone	Replacement of glucocorticoids lost as a result of hypofunction of adrenal glands	***Contraindications:*** Hypersensitivity; systemic fungal infections; psychosis; idiopathic thrombocytopenia; amebiasis; acute glomerulonephritis ***Cost:*** 10-mg tab, 100 tabs: \$20 ***Pregnancy category:*** C	Sodium retention, hypertension, weight gain, depression, flushing, sweating, circulatory collapse, increased intraocular pressure, diarrhea, nausea, vomiting, GI hemorrhage, pancreatitis, thrombocytopenia, acne, poor wound healing
Fludrocortisone, 0.1-0.2 mg qd; used with hydrocortisone	Replaces mineralocorticoids	***Contraindications:*** Hypersensitivity; systemic fungal infections ***Cost:*** 0.1-mg tab, 100 tabs: \$45 ***Pregnancy category:*** C	Marked effect on sodium retention, hypertension, edema, cardiac enlargement, congestive heart failure, flushing, sweating, headache, circulatory collapse, osteoporosis, weakness

Dementia, Multiinfarct

OVERVIEW

Multiinfarct dementia is a progressive decline in cognitive abilities from a previous level as a result of cerebral infarctions. The decline in cognitive abilities must be generalized and not confined to one function, such as memory or speech, and the patient must not have a decrease in level of consciousness. Deterioration is stepwise with plateaus. Multiinfarct dementia is the second most common form of dementia.

Pathogenesis

Multiple small and large cerebral infarctions secondary to atherosclerosis

Patient Profile

- Males = Females
- Incidence increases with age
- Often associated with hypertension

Signs and Symptoms

- Abrupt onset of symptoms
- Impaired short- and long-term memory
- Distinct episodes of worsening dementia with plateaus
- Impaired abstract thinking
- Impaired judgment
- Aphasia
- Apraxia
- As disease progresses, depression and hemiplegia may develop; may have gait disturbances and pseudobulbar palsy

Differential Diagnosis

- Delirium
- Alzheimer's disease
- Cardiac arrhythmias
- Depression
- Schizophrenia
- Alcoholism
- Drug toxicity

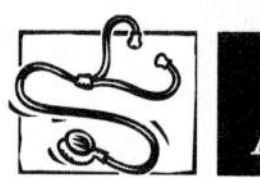

ASSESSMENT

History

- Inquire about:
  - Onset and duration of symptoms
  - Past history of cerebrovascular accident and/or hypertension
  - Depression
  - Alcohol use
  - Past history of mental illness
  - Underlying conditions
  - Current medications
- Include family in history-taking process

Physical Findings

- Results of mini–mental state examination (Table 7)
- May have focal signs such as slight tremors, slightly drooping mouth
- May have gait disturbance
- May have elevated blood pressure

Initial Workup

Laboratory

- No specific laboratory test—must rule out other causes of dementia
- CBC
- Urinalysis, chemistry panel to include electrolytes, creatinine, liver function tests, calcium and phosphate
- Thyroid function panel
- B_{12} and folate level
- Rapid plasma reagin (RPR) or VDRL
- ECG

Radiology: CT scan or MRI of head—small infarcts

Further Workup

Neuropsychologic testing, possibly

TABLE 7 ***Mini–Mental State Examination***

Max score	Score	Questions
Orientation		
5	( )	"What is the (year) (season) (date) (day) (month)?"
5	( )	"Where are we (state) (country) (town) (hospital) (floor)?"
Registration		
3	( )	Name 3 objects: 1 second to say each. Then ask the patient all 3 after you have said them. Give 1 point for each correct answer. Then repeat them until he or she learns all 3. Count trials and record (Trials ________).
Attention and Calculation		
5	( )	Serial 7s (Begin with 100 and count backward by 7). 1 point for each correct answer. Stop after 5 answers. Alternatively, spell "world" backward.
Recall		
3	( )	Ask for 3 objects repeated above. Give 1 point for each correct answer.
Language		
9	( )	Name a pencil and a watch (2 points). Repeat the following: "No ifs, ands, or buts" (1 point). Follow a 3-stage command: "Take a paper in your right hand, fold it in half, and put it on the floor" (3 points). Read and obey the following: "Close your eyes" (1 point). Write a sentence (1 point). Copy design (1 point).
Total Score: ____________		Assess level of consciousness on a continuum:

		Alert Drowsy Stupor Coma
		Persons with dementia usually score <20.

Modified from Folstein MF, Folstein SE, McHugh PR: Mini-mental state: a practical method of grading the cognitive state of patients for the clinician, *J Psychiatr Res 12:*189, 1975, Elsevier Science Ltd., Oxford, England.

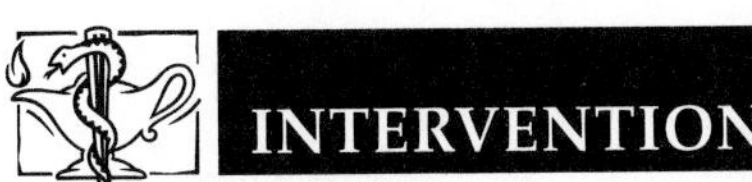

INTERVENTIONS

Office Treatment
Provide supportive environment

Lifestyle Modifications
- Modify home to prevent accidents
- In-home help to care for patient
- Major life crisis that requires drastic lifestyle modifications

Patient Education
Teach patient about:
- Disease process and treatment options—no specific treatment—treat symptoms
- Support groups available for caregiver
- Adult day care programs
- Visiting nurses
- Music therapy—has calming effect on agitated patient
- Nursing home—if necessary
- Exercises to reduce restlessness
- Using short sentences to communicate
- Giving one instruction at a time
- Getting patient's affairs in order
- Legal guardianship
- Importance of taking blood pressure medication
- Medications used and side effects (see Pharmacotherapeutics)

Referrals
- To geriatrician or geriatric NP who specializes in dementia
- To home health agency for nursing
- To physical therapist
- To occupational therapist
- To social worker

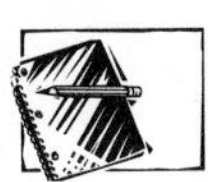

EVALUATION

Outcomes
- Patient maintained in home environment as long as possible
- Caregiver able to adjust and maintain a good quality of life

Possible Complications
- Falls
- Hostile behavior
- Inability to maintain patient in home environment

Follow-up
Every 2 weeks initially to assess medication effects; then as needed

FOR YOUR INFORMATION

Lifespan
Pediatric: N/A
Geriatric: Second most common cause of dementia
Pregnancy: N/A

Miscellaneous
The history given by the patient or the family is the most important element in diagnosing multi-infarct dementia. The sudden onset of symptoms and stairstep progression are key to the diagnosis.

References

Uphold CR, Graham MV: *Clinical guidelines in adult health,* Gainesville, Fla, 1994, Barmarrae Books, pp 560-564.

Wills R: Delirium and dementia. In Carnevali DL, Patrick M, editors: *Nursing management for the elderly,* ed 3, Philadelphia, 1993, JB Lippincott, pp 271-272.

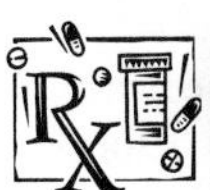

PHARMACOTHERAPEUTICS

Drug of Choice	Mechanism of Action	Prescribing Information	Side Effects
Buspirone (BuSpar), 2.5-5.0 mg PO bid or tid for anxiety	Anxiolytic; inhibits action of serotonin	***Contraindications:*** Hypersensitivity; children <18 years of age ***Cost:*** 5 mg, 3/day × 120 days: $210 ***Pregnancy category:*** B	Dizziness, headache, depression, insomnia, nervousness, numbness, nausea, dry mouth, diarrhea, tachycardia, palpitations, cerebrovascular accident (CVA), congestive heart failure (CHF), myocardial infarction (MI), sore throat, tinnitus, pain, weakness, rash, edema, sweating
Benzodiazepine; for anxiety; use one that is short-acting such as lorazepam (Ativan), 0.25-0.5 mg PO bid or tid	Antianxiety; potentiates actions of gamma-aminobutyric acid (GABA)	***Contraindications:*** Hypersensitivity; narrow-angle glaucoma; psychosis; pregnancy; children <12 years; history of drug abuse; chronic obstructive pulmonary disease (COPD) ***Cost:*** 1 mg, 2/day for 120 days: $6 ***Pregnancy category:*** D	Dizziness, drowsiness, confusion, hallucinations, constipation, dry mouth, rash, orthostatic hypotension, tachycardia, ECG changes, blurred vision
Haloperidol (Haldol); for nighttime irritability and insomnia; 0.25-1 mg PO 1 hour before bedtime	Antipsychotic; depresses cerebral cortex, hypothalamus; limbic system; blocks neurotransmission produced by dopamine; strong alpha-adrenergic	***Contraindications:*** Hypersensitivity; blood dyscrasias; brain damage; bone marrow depression; alcohol and barbiturate withdrawal; Parkinson's disease; angina; epilepsy; urinary retention; narrow-angle glaucoma ***Cost:*** 0.5-mg tab, 100 tabs: $3-$15 ***Pregnancy category:*** C	Laryngospasm, respiratory depression, extrapyramidal symptoms, seizures, neuroleptic malignant syndrome, rash, dry mouth, nausea, vomiting, anorexia, constipation, ileus, hepatitis, orthostatic hypotension, cardiac arrest, tachycardia

OVERVIEW

Depression is an abnormal emotional state or mood disturbance. It is characterized by feelings of sadness, dejection, worthlessness, despair, and discouragement. It is classified as major depression (unipolar disorder), bipolar disorder (episodes of mania with episodes of depression), or dysthymia (less severe than depression)

Pathogenesis

Several theories of causation:

- Biologic theories:
  - Disruption in biogenic amine input to hypothalamus causes neuroendocrine abnormalities
  - Activity of biogenic amines is decreased for an unknown reason
  - Major depression and bipolar disorder—genetically transmitted
- Psychosocial theories:
  - Psychoanalytic—feelings of worthlessness due to rigid superego
  - Cognitive—negative self-view; negative interpretation of experience; negative view of future

Patient Profile

- Females > Males
- Bipolar disorder—mean age, 30 years
- Unipolar disorder—mean age, 40 years
- Lifetime risk of major depression—men: 7% to 12%; women: 20% to 25%

Signs and Symptoms

Major depressive disorder

DSM-III-R criteria—at least 5 of the following symptoms are present during the same period; either the first or the second symptom listed must be present; symptoms must be present most of the day, nearly daily for at least 2 weeks

- Depressed mood (sometimes irritability in children and adolescents) most of the day, nearly every day
- Loss of interest in usual activities most of the day, nearly every day
- Significant weight loss/gain
- Insomnia/hypersomnia
- Psychomotor agitation/retardation
- Fatigue (loss of energy)
- Feelings of worthlessness
- Inability to concentrate
- Recurrent thoughts of death or suicide ideation

Bipolar disorder

Same symptoms as depression, but with periods of mania—elation, expansive mood, increased energy, inflated self-esteem

Dysthymia

Symptoms less severe than major depression; last about 2 years; may have episode of major depression

Differential Diagnosis

- Organic brain disease
- Endocrine disease
- Diabetes mellitus
- Liver failure
- Renal failure
- Chronic fatigue syndrome
- Vitamin deficiency
- Medication side effects
- Medication abuse
- Alcohol or substance abuse or withdrawal
- Dementia

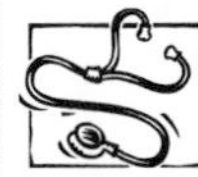

ASSESSMENT

History

Inquire about:

- Onset and duration of symptoms
- Precipitating event
- Loss of libido
- Weight loss/gain
- Low energy level
- Insomnia/hypersomnia
- Constipation/dry mouth
- Usual activities and current activities
- Family history of mental illness
- Alcohol/drug abuse
- Suicidal ideations
- Underlying conditions
- Current medications (steroids, antihypertensives, estrogen, nonsteroidal antiinflammatory drugs, digoxin, anti-Parkinson's drugs—all can cause depression)

Physical Findings

- Note general appearance—may be unkempt
- Personal hygiene may be poor
- Tearful
- Not making eye contact
- Speech slow, soft, and deliberate
- May state, "I feel depressed"
- Physical examination may be normal

Initial Workup

Laboratory: To rule out other causes of symptoms:

- CBC
- Chemistry panel
- Thyroid function
- Urinalysis
- Vitamin B_{12}, folate levels
- Rapid plasma reagin (RPR)

Radiology: If suspect organic brain disease, CT scan or MRI of brain

Further Workup

Based on initial results

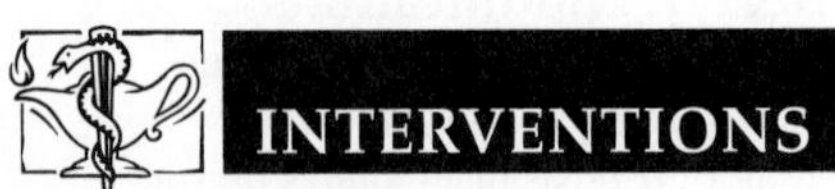

INTERVENTIONS

Office Treatment

Provide support for patient

Lifestyle Modifications

- Nutritionally balanced diet
- Moderate exercise program
- Cessation of alcohol and substance abuse if present

Patient Education

Teach patient about:

- Disease process and treatment options—psychotherapy, medications, or combination of both
- Proper diet and how to establish an exercise program—walking 10 minutes daily is a good place to start
- Enjoying one pleasurable event daily, such as going to a movie or reading a good book
- Alcohol or substance abuse treatment—inpatient or outpatient
- Medications used and side effects—emphasize that antidepressant medications can take from 2 to 4 weeks before improvement will be noticed (see Pharmacotherapeutics)

Referrals

- To psychiatric NP or clinical nurse specialist
- To psychiatrist or psychologist if depression is severe or conservative treatment fails to provide improvement, or as needed

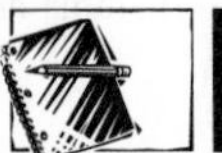

EVALUATION

Outcome

Patient demonstrates improved general appearance, eye contact; states that he or she is not depressed anymore

Possible Complications

- Suicide
- Lack of improvement with deepening despair

Follow-up

- Weekly for first 5 to 6 weeks; then every 2 weeks for 2 months; then monthly
- Depends on severity of depression

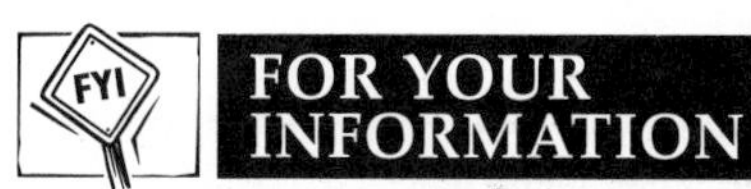

Life Span

Pediatric: Important to differentiate behavioral problems and depression; may coexist, but need to know which is primary

Geriatric: Use lower doses of medications; must differentiate dementia and depression (see Miscellaneous)

Pregnancy: Research currently in progress to assess long-term effects of antidepressant medication taken during pregnancy on children; presently, there do not appear to be any long-term effects

Miscellaneous

It is important for the NP to make an appropriate diagnosis when dealing with the elderly population. Often, elderly patients are diagnosed as being demented when in fact they are depressed. There are 3 major signs that help differentiate depression and dementia: (1) depression develops over days to weeks, whereas dementia is very slow and insidious; (2) the depressed patient can answer questions correctly if given enough time, whereas the demented patient cannot; and (3) a trial of antidepressant medication will yield an improvement in the depressed patient but not in the demented patient.

References

Depaulo JR, Barker LR: Affective disorders. In Barker RL, Burton JR, Zieve PD, editors: *Principles of ambulatory medicine,* ed 4, Baltimore, 1995, Williams & Wilkins, pp 162-168.

Depression Guideline Panel: *Depression in primary care,* vol 1, *Detection and diagnosis,* Clinical Practice Guideline No 5, AHCPR Pub No 93-0550, Rockville, Md, 1993, US Department of Health and Human Services, Public Health Service, Agency for Health Care Policy and Research.

Depression Guideline Panel: *Depression in primary care,* vol 2, *Detection and diagnosis,* Clinical Practice Guideline No 5, AHCPR Pub No 93-0551, Rockville, Md, 1993, US Department of Health and Human Services, Public Health Service, Agency for Health Care Policy and Research.

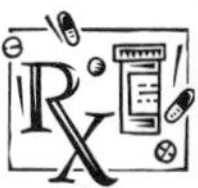

PHARMACOTHERAPEUTICS

There are many antidepressant medications on the market. The following table lists the medications according to their classification, with specific medications also listed. It is important for the NP to teach the patient that it will take some time before the results of the medication are noticed and encourage the patient to take the medication for the prescribed time period. Often, several different medications may need to be tried before the one that produces the best effect is found.

Drug of Choice	Mechanism of Action	Prescribing Information	Side Effects
Selective serotonin reuptake inhibitors (SSRIs): • Fluoxetine (Prozac), 20-80 mg/day • Sertraline (Zoloft), 50-200 mg/day • Paroxetine (Paxil), 10-30 mg/day • None dosed for children; do not use with or within 14 days of monoamine oxidase inhibitors (MAOIs) or drugs metabolized by P450 system	Block reuptake of serotonin	***Contraindication:*** Hypersensitivity ***Cost:*** Fluoxetine, 20-mg tab, 30 tabs: $67; sertraline, 50-mg tab, 100 tabs: $176; paroxetine, 20-mg tab, 30 tabs: $57 ***Pregnancy category:*** Fluoxetine and sertraline—B; paroxetine—C	Dry mouth, constipation, sleepiness, headache, nervousness, anxiety, tremor, abnormal dreams, nausea, diarrhea, dyspepsia, rash, postural hypotension, decreased libido, dysmenorrhea, urinary frequency, impotence, abnormal ejaculation, pain, myalgia, cough
Tricyclic antidepressants: • Amitriptyline (Elavil), 50-150 mg PO hs—not recommended for children <12 years of age • Nortriptyline (Pamelor), 25 mg PO tid—not recommended for children • Trimipramine (Surmontil), 75 mg PO qd in divided doses, maximum 200 mg/day—not recommended for children; do not use with or within 14 days of MAOIs or antiarrhythmics	Unknown	***Contraindications:*** Hypersensitivity; acute recovery phase of MI ***Cost:*** Amitriptyline 50-mg tab, 100 tabs: $2-$66; nortriptyline, 25-mg tab, 100 tabs: $17-$99; trimipramine, 25-mg tab, 100 tabs: $66 ***Pregnancy category:*** C	Dry mouth, dizziness, headache, nausea, weakness, weight gain, unpleasant taste, increased consumption of sweets, drowsiness, extrapyramidal symptoms (elderly patients), constipation, paralytic ileus, hepatitis, acute renal failure, orthostatic hypotension, tachycardia, blurred vision
Nefazodone (Serzone), 50-100 mg PO bid, may be increased weekly—do not use with or within 14 days of MAOIs; do not use with drugs metabolized by P450 system; not dosed for children <18 years	Chemically unrelated to selective serotonin reuptake inhibitors; probably inhibits neuronal uptake of serotonin and epinephrine	***Contraindications:*** Hypersensitivity ***Cost:*** 100-mg tab, 60 tabs: $50 ***Pregnancy category:*** C	Somnolence, dry mouth, nausea, dizziness, constipation, asthenia, lightheadedness, blurred vision, confusion, headache, postural hypotension, tinnitus

Diarrhea, Acute

OVERVIEW

When compared with the patient's normal stools, acute diarrhea is abnormal frequency and liquid consistency of bowel movements.

Pathogenesis

Causes:

- Infections
- Medications (antibiotics, antacids, laxatives)
- Inflammatory bowel disease (Crohn's disease/ulcerative colitis—see sections on specific disease)

Patient Profile

- Males = Females
- Any age

Signs and Symptoms

Depends on cause:

- Infection:
  - Abdominal pain
  - Vomiting
  - Malodorous stools
  - Weight loss (maybe)
- Medications—onset after drug started
- Inflammatory bowel disease:
  - Nocturnal diarrhea
  - Pain
  - Fever

Differential Diagnosis

- Ulcerative colitis
- Crohn's disease
- Drugs
- Irritable colon
- Fecal impaction
- Pseudomembranous colitis
- Diverticulitis
- HIV infection

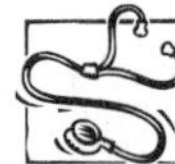

ASSESSMENT

History

Inquire about:

- Onset and duration of symptoms
- Stool volume, frequency, consistency, blood, presence of mucus
- Fever
- Others in household having similar symptoms
- What patient had to eat or drink in last 24 to 48 hours
- Travel to foreign country
- Risk factors for HIV
- Underlying conditions
- Current medications

Physical Findings

- Fever
- Abdominal pain
- Pallor

Initial Workup

Laboratory

- CBC—increased WBC, left shift on differential (infection)
- Chemistry profile—potassium decreased secondary to dehydration
- Stool sample—leukocytes, ova and parasites, culture
- For simple cases of acute diarrhea, no laboratory tests needed

Radiology: Flat plate of abdomen to rule out obstruction, if indicated

Further Workup

Usually none needed unless acute diarrhea becomes chronic

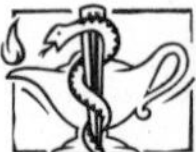

INTERVENTIONS

Office Treatment

None indicated

Lifestyle Modifications

- No solid food—only clear liquids for 24 hours; then bland diet
- Increased fluids (Gatorade to replace electrolytes)
- Avoidance of coffee, dairy products, fruits, and vegetables
- Smoking cessation

Patient Education

Teach patient about:

- Condition and treatment options—if infection, antibiotics
- Increased fluid intake
- Stopping solid food and consuming only clear liquids for 24 hours; then BRAT (Bananas, Rice, Applesauce, Toast) diet; then regular diet
- Recovery time—usually resolves in 72 hours
- Medications used and side effects (see Pharmacotherapeutics)

Referral

Consult with MD when patient's diarrhea is not resolved in 5 days or if patient has bloody diarrhea

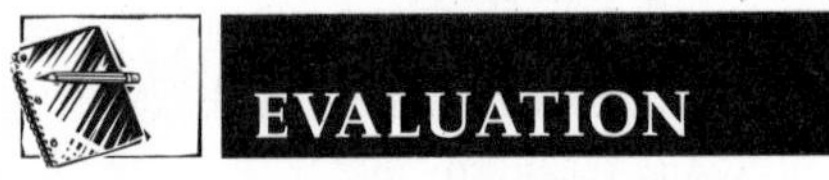

EVALUATION

Outcome

Resolves without sequelae

Possible Complications

- Dehydration
- Sepsis
- Shock
- Anemia

Follow-up

In 5 days if not resolved

FOR YOUR INFORMATION

Life Span

Pediatric: Dehydration can occur much more rapidly in this population
Geriatric: Fecal impaction commonly causes watery diarrhea in the elderly
Pregnancy: Dehydration can cause preterm labor

Miscellaneous

The use of antidiarrheal or antiperistaltic medications is controversial in the patient with infectious diarrhea. Some authorities have reported prolongation of the infection when diarrhea is stopped.

References

Heck JE, Cohen MB: Traveler's diarrhea, *Am Fam Physician* 48(5):793-799, 1993.

Uphold CR, Graham MV: *Clinical guidelines in adult health,* Gainesville, Fla, 1994, Barmarrae Books, pp 375-377.

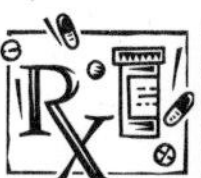

PHARMACOTHERAPEUTICS

Drug of Choice	Mechanism of Action	Prescribing Information	Side Effects
Metronidazole (Flagyl): • For *Giardia,* 250 mg PO tid for 5-10 days; children, 15 mg/kg/day PO in 3 divided doses × 5 days • For *Entamoeba histolytica,* 500-750 mg PO tid × 10 days; children, 35-50 mg/kg/day PO in 3 divided doses × 10 days • For *Clostridium difficile,* 250 mg PO qid × 10-14 days; children, 20 mg/kg/day PO in divided doses q6h × 10-14 days	Direct-acting amebicide/ trichomonacide	***Contraindications:*** Hypersensitivity; renal disease; hepatic disease; contracted visual or color fields; blood dyscrasias; pregnancy 1st trimester; lactation; CNS disorders ***Cost:*** 250-mg tab, 100 tabs: $5-$60 ***Pregnancy category:*** B (2nd & 3rd trimesters)	Flat T-waves, headache, dizziness, confusion, irritability, restlessness, depression, fatigue, drowsiness, insomnia, convulsions, blurred vision, sore throat, dry mouth, retinal edema, metallic taste, nausea, vomiting, diarrhea, anorexia, constipation, abdominal cramps, pseudomembranous colitis, darkened urine, albuminuria, neurotoxicity, leukopenia, bone marrow depression, aplasia, rash, pruritus, urticaria
Ciprofloxacin (Cipro): • For *Shigella,* 500 mg PO bid × 3 days • For traveler's diarrhea, 500 mg PO bid × 3 days—not dosed for children	Fluoroquinolone; interferes with conversion of intermediate DNA fragments in high-molecular-weight-DNA in bacteria	***Contraindication:*** Hypersensitivity ***Cost:*** 250-mg tab, 100 tabs: $262 ***Pregnancy category:*** C	Headache, dizziness, fatigue, insomnia, depression, nausea, diarrhea, increased ALT and AST, flatulence, heartburn, vomiting, rash, pruritus, urticaria, photosensitivity, flushing, fever, blurred vision, tinnitus
Sulfamethoxazole (SMX) and trimethoprim (TMP) (Septra DS): • For *Shigella,* 1 DS tab PO bid × 5 days; children, 8 mg/kg TMP/40 mg/kg/SMZ/day PO in 2 divided doses × 5 days • For traveler's diarrhea, 1 DS tab PO bid × 3 days; children, same as above × 3 days	Sulfamethoxazole interferes with bacterial biosynthesis of proteins; trimethoprim blocks synthesis of tetrahydrofolic acid	***Contraindications:*** Hypersensitivity to either ingredient; pregnancy at term; megaloblastic anemia; infants <2 months; creatinine clearance <15 ml/min; lactation ***Cost:*** DS tab 100 tabs: $8-$70 ***Pregnancy category:*** C	Headache, insomnia, hallucinations, depression, vertigo, fatigue, allergic myocarditis, nausea, vomiting, abdominal pain, stomatitis, hepatitis, glossitis, diarrhea, enterocolitis, renal failure, toxic nephrosis, increased BUN and creatinine, leukopenia, neutropenia, thrombocytopenia, agranulocytosis, hemolytic anemia, hypoprothrombinemia, rash, dermatitis, Stevens-Johnson syndrome, erythema, photosensitivity, anaphylaxis, systemic lupus erythematosus
Kaolin, pectin (Kaopectate), 60-120 ml PO after each loose stool; Children >12 years, 30-60 ml PO after each loose stool; children 3-6 years, 15-30 ml PO after each loose stool	Antidiarrheal	***Contraindication:*** Hypersensitivity ***Cost:*** OTC ***Pregnancy category:*** C	Constipation
Loperamide (Immodium A-D), 4 mg PO then 2 mg after each loose stool; children 8-12 years, 2 mg PO tid day 1, then 0.1 mg/kg PO after each loose stool; children 5-8 years, 2 mg PO bid day 1, then 0.1 mg/kg PO after each loose stool; children 2-5 years, 1 mg PO then 0.1 mg/kg after each loose stool	Antidiarrheal; direct action on intestinal muscles to decrease GI peristalsis; reduces volume, increases bulk, electrolytes not lost	***Contraindications:*** Hypersensitivity; severe ulcerative colitis; pseudomembranous colitis; acute diarrhea associated with *Escherichia coli* ***Cost:*** 2-mg tab, 100 tabs: $35-$70 ***Pregnancy category:*** B	Dizziness, drowsiness, fatigue, fever, nausea, dry mouth, vomiting, constipation, abdominal pain, toxic megacolon, rash, respiratory depression

Diarrhea, Chronic

OVERVIEW

Chronic diarrhea is increased frequency and liquid consistency of stools that lasts for at least 2 weeks or recurs frequently after the initial attack.

Pathogenesis

Causes:
- Malabsorption
- Hyperthyroidism
- Inflammatory bowel diseases
- HIV infection
- Lactose intolerance
- Functional bowel disease
- Irritable bowel syndrome
- Fecal impaction
- Giardiasis
- Laxative abuse

Patient Profile

- Females > Males
- Any age; more frequent in middle-aged and elderly persons

Signs and Symptoms

Depends on cause:
- Malabsorption—large, foul-smelling, light-colored, oily stools
- Hyperthyroidism—frequent, loose stools; weight loss
- Inflammatory bowel disease—nocturnal diarrhea, pain, rectal fistula, fever
- HIV infection—frequent, loose stools; weight loss
- Lactose intolerance—diarrhea that occurs after ingestion of dairy products
- Functional bowel disease—frequent, loose stools; weight loss
- Irritable bowel syndrome—recurrent abdominal pain; diarrhea alternating with constipation
- Fecal impaction—occasional watery stools
- Giardiasis—frequent, foul-smelling stools with weight loss
- Fecal incontinence may occur with all causes

Differential Diagnosis

- Functional disorder versus organic disorder
- Must differentiate from various causes

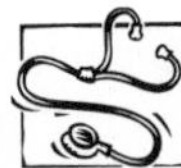

ASSESSMENT

History

Inquire about:
- Onset and duration of symptoms
- Volume, frequency, and consistency of stools
- Use/abuse of laxatives
- Blood and/or mucus in stools
- Fever and/or abdominal pain
- HIV status
- Underlying conditions
- Current medications

Physical Findings

Depends on cause—may find:
- Weight loss
- Abdominal pain
- Perirectal fistula
- Poor skin turgor
- Pallor

Initial Workup

Laboratory
- CBC—anemia
- Chemistry profile—hypokalemia
- Stool for culture and for ova and parasites

Radiology
- Barium enema
- Flat plate of abdomen if indicated

Further Workup

Colonoscopy if indicated

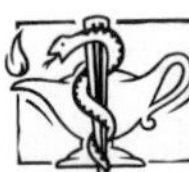

INTERVENTIONS

Office Treatment

Removal of impaction if necessary

Lifestyle Modifications

Depends on cause:
- Avoidance of foods that precipitate or worsen condition
- Increased fluids (Gatorade)
- Cessation of laxative use
- Stress reduction
- Smoking cessation

Patient Education

Teach patient about:
- Condition, cause, and treatment options—avoidance of precipitating factors
- Stress reduction through biofeedback, relaxation techniques
- Normal bowel physiology
- Stopping use of laxatives
- Increased fluid intake to prevent dehydration (Gatorade to replace electrolytes)
- Medications used and side effects (see Pharmacotherapeutics)

Referral

To MD if conservative treatment fails

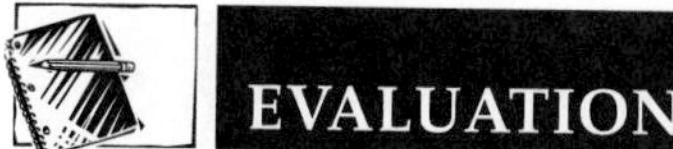

EVALUATION

Outcome
Resolution of diarrhea

Possible Complications
- Dehydration
- Electrolyte imbalance
- Cardiac arrhythmias
- Death

Follow-up
Weekly to every 2 weeks until controlled; depends on severity

FOR YOUR INFORMATION

Lifespan
Pediatric: Dehydration can occur more rapidly
Geriatric: Can be more debilitating
Pregnancy: N/A

Miscellaneous
N/A

References

Heitkemper M, Sawchuck L: Nursing role in management: problems of absorption and elimination. In Lewis SM, Collier IC, Heitkemper MM, editors: *Medical-surgical nursing: assessment and management of clinical problems,* ed 4, St Louis, 1996, Mosby, pp 1207-1213.

Uphold CR, Graham MV: *Clinical guidelines in adult health,* Gainesville, Fla, 1994, Barmarrae Books, pp 375-377.

NOTES

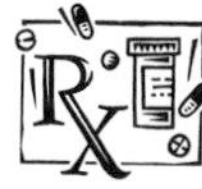

PHARMACOTHERAPEUTICS

Drug of Choice	Mechanism of Action	Prescribing Information	Side Effects
Bulk-forming agent: psyllium (Metamucil), 1-2 tsp in 8 oz water PO bid or tid; children >6 years, 1 tsp in 4 oz water PO; may help reduce incontinence	Bulk-forming laxative	***Contraindications:*** Hypersensitivity; intestinal obstruction; abdominal pain; nausea, vomiting; fecal impaction ***Cost:*** OTC ***Pregnancy category:*** C	Nausea, vomiting, diarrhea, cramps
Metronidazole (Flagyl); for *Giardia,* 250 mg PO tid × 5-10 days; children, 15 mg/kg/day PO in 3 divided doses × 5 days	Direct-acting amebicide/ trichomonacide	***Contraindications:*** Hypersensitivity; renal disease; hepatic disease; contracted visual or color fields; blood dyscrasias; pregnancy 1st trimester; lactation; CNS disorders ***Cost:*** 250-mg tab, 100 tabs: $5-$60 ***Pregnancy category:*** B (2nd & 3rd trimesters)	Flat T-waves, headache, dizziness, confusion, irritability, restlessness, depression, fatigue, drowsiness, insomnia, convulsions, blurred vision, sore throat, dry mouth, retinal edema, metallic taste, nausea, vomiting, diarrhea, anorexia, constipation, abdominal cramps, pseudomembranous colitis, darkened urine, albuminuria, neurotoxicity, leukopenia, bone marrow depression, aplasia, rash, pruritus, urticaria
Kaolin, pectin (Kaopectate), 60-120 ml PO after each loose stool; children >12 years, 30-60 ml PO after each loose stool; children 3-6 years, 15-30 ml PO after each loose stool	Antidiarrheal	***Contraindication:*** Hypersensitivity ***Cost:*** OTC ***Pregnancy category:*** C	Constipation
Loperamide (Immodium A-D), 4 mg PO, then 2 mg after each loose stool; children 8-12 years, 2 mg PO tid day 1, then 0.1 mg/kg PO after each loose stool; children 5-8 years, 2 mg PO bid day 1, then 0.1 mg/kg PO after each loose stool; children 2-5 years, 1 mg PO then 0.1 mg/kg after each loose stool	Antidiarrheal; direct action on intestinal muscles to decrease GI peristalsis; reduces volume, increases bulk, electrolytes not lost	***Contraindications:*** Hypersensitivity; severe ulcerative colitis; pseudomembranous colitis; acute diarrhea associated with *Escherichia coli* ***Cost:*** 2-mg tab, 100 tabs: $35-$70 ***Pregnancy category:*** B	Dizziness, drowsiness, fatigue, fever, nausea, dry mouth, vomiting, constipation, abdominal pain, toxic megacolon, rash, respiratory depression

Digitalis Toxicity

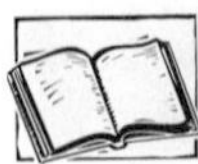

OVERVIEW

Digitalis toxicity is a condition that occurs when there is too much digoxin in the body.

Pathogenesis

Causes:

- May be due to overdosage
- Hypokalemia due to diuretics
- Renal insufficiency
- Medications that interfere with digoxin excretion (quinidine)

Patient Profile

- Males = Females
- Any age if taking digoxin

Signs and Symptoms

- Abdominal pain
- Anorexia
- Nausea
- Vomiting
- Diarrhea
- Confusion
- Delirium
- Psychosis
- Blurred vision
- Bradycardia
- Depression
- Drowsiness
- Fatigue
- Hallucinations
- Headache
- Hypotension
- Weakness
- Restlessness
- Vertigo
- Lethargy
- Irregular pulse
- Nightmares

Differential Diagnosis

- Heart block
- Renal disease

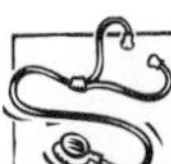

ASSESSMENT

History

Inquire about:

- Onset and duration of symptoms
- Amount and dosage of digoxin being taken
- Contact with plants containing cardiac glycosides, such as oleander or foxglove
- Underlying conditions
- Current medications

Physical Findings

- Impaired sensorium
- Hypotension
- Decreased visual acuity
- Cardiac findings—bradycardia, arrhythmias
- Weight loss
- May have very subtle physical findings

Initial Workup

Laboratory

- Digoxin level >2 ng/ml considered toxic—may be therapeutic level and still be toxic
- Electrolytes—hypokalemia; hyperkalemia with acute ingestion

Radiology: None indicated

Further Workup

- ECG—any number of arrhythmias may be present
- Any change in rhythm suggests digitalis toxicity

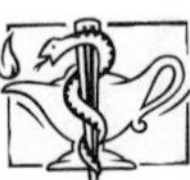

INTERVENTIONS

Office Treatment

If symptoms severe, immediate hospitalization in intensive care unit

Lifestyle Modification

Take medications as directed

Patient Education

Teach patient about:

- Condition and treatment:
  - For mild toxicity—discontinue digoxin temporarily; restart at lower dose
  - For severe toxicity—hospitalization
- High-potassium foods to include in diet (bananas, orange juice)
- Plants that contain cardiac glycosides (oleander, foxglove)
- Medications used and side effects (see Pharmacotherapeutics)

Referral

To primary care physician or cardiologist for severe toxicity

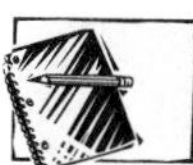

EVALUATION

Outcome

Resolves without sequelae in mild to moderate cases; first 24 hours critical in severe toxicity

Possible Complications

- Life-threatening arrhythmias
- Conduction defects
- Death

Follow-up

- 1 week following hospitalization
- For outpatient, return to clinic in 3 days to redraw digoxin level
- 1 week after restarting digoxin to check level

FOR YOUR INFORMATION

Life Span

Pediatric: Keep out of reach of children
Geriatric: Higher morbidity and mortality rate
Pregnancy: Should be handled by a specialist

Miscellaneous

N/A

References

Gottleib SH: Heart failure. In Barker LR, Burton JR, Zieve PD, editors: *Principles of ambulatory medicine,* ed 4, Baltimore, 1995, Williams & Wilkins, pp 796-797.

House-Fancher MA, Griego L: Nursing role in management: congestive heart failure and cardiac surgery. In Lewis SM, Collier IC, Heitkemper MM, editors: *Medical-surgical nursing: assessment and management of clinical problems,* ed 4, St Louis, 1996, Mosby, p 941.

NOTES

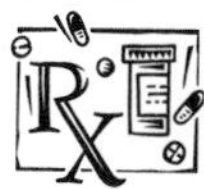

PHARMACOTHERAPEUTICS

Drug of Choice	Mechanism of Action	Prescribing Information	Side Effects
The following drug is used only in the presence of severe, life-threatening arrhythmias:			
Digoxin immune FAB (Digibind); adults and children, dose of digoxin ingested × 0.8 × 66.7 = mg Digibind to give IV; if unknown amount ingested, give 10 vials in 50 ml NS over 30 minutes IV; observe response; if indicated, repeat above dose; draw digoxin level in 4 days	Antibody fragments bind to free digoxin and prevent digoxin from binding to site of action	***Contraindications:*** Hypersensitivity; mild digoxin toxicity ***Cost:*** 40-mg vial, 1 vial: $402 ***Pregnancy category:*** C	Congestive heart failure (CHF), atrial fibrillation, low cardiac output, impaired respiratory function, rapid respiratory rate, hypokalemia, hypersensitivity, facial swelling
For rapid conversion of cardiac arrhythmias, if potassium is low or normal:			
Potassium supplement, 40-80 mEq IV at a rate of 20 mEq/hr	Increases potassium level in body	***Contraindications:*** Severe renal insufficiency; hypersensitivity ***Cost:*** 4 mEq/ml, 50 ml: $137 ***Pregnancy category:*** C	Hyperkalemia, flaccid paralysis, listlessness, confusion, weakness, hypotension, heart block, cardiac arrhythmias, heaviness of legs

Diverticulitis/Diverticulosis

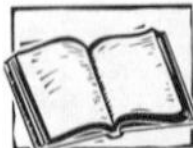

OVERVIEW

Diverticulitis/diverticulosis occurs as a result of the formation of diverticula. Diverticula are outpouchings of the mucosa through the muscular wall of the intestine. They occur most often in the sigmoid colon. When there are multiple, noninflamed diverticula, the disorder is known as diverticulosis. When inflammation occurs in the diverticula, the disorder is known as diverticulitis.

Pathogenesis

- Cause of diverticula formation—unknown; related to low dietary fiber
- Diverticulitis—inflammation occurs as a result of stool and bacteria retention in diverticula

Patient Profile

- Males = Females
- Age >40 years
- More common in Western society because of low-fiber diet

Signs and Symptoms

DIVERTICULOSIS

- Most cases are asymptomatic
- Pain in (L) lower abdominal quadrant
- Diarrhea or constipation
- Firm, tender, mass in (L) lower abdominal quadrant
- Distended abdomen
- Stool positive for occult blood if diverticula bleeding

DIVERTICULITIS

- Pain in (L) lower abdominal quadrant
- Fever
- Chills
- Anorexia
- Nausea
- Vomiting
- Rebound tenderness in (L) lower abdominal quadrant
- Diarrhea or constipation
- Palpable mass
- Distended abdomen
- Tympanic sound on percussion
- Tenderness on rectal examination

Differential Diagnosis

- Irritable bowel syndrome
- Lactose intolerance
- Tumor
- Ulcerative colitis
- Crohn's disease
- Appendicitis

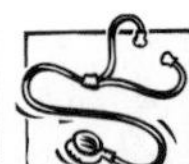

ASSESSMENT

History

Inquire about:

- Onset and duration of symptoms
- Similar episodes in past
- Diet
- Underlying conditions
- Current medications

Physical Findings

DIVERTICULOSIS

- In most cases, normal physical examination
- Slight pain on palpation of (L) lower abdominal quadrant
- Distended abdomen
- Tympany on percussion

DIVERTICULITIS

- Exquisite pain on palpation of (L) lower abdominal quadrant
- Mass in (L) lower abdominal quadrant
- Rebound tenderness
- Muscle rigidity
- Distended abdomen
- Tympany on percussion
- Rectal examination findings—tenderness, induration, mass

Initial Workup

Laboratory

- CBC—increased WBC count in diverticulitis; may also see left shift on differential; anemia possible
- Urinalysis
- Blood culture—positive in diverticulitis with peritonitis
- Stool for occult blood—positive if diverticula bleeding

Radiology

- Barium enema—best means to diagnose diverticulosis
- Flat plate of abdomen—ileus or perforation

Further Workup

Flexible sigmoidoscopy and colonoscopy

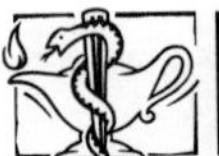

INTERVENTIONS

Office Treatment

None indicated

Lifestyle Modifications

- Increased dietary fiber/low-fat diet
- Smoking cessation
- Regular exercise program

Patient Education

Teach patient about:

- Disease process and treatment options:
  - High fiber diet (may need fiber supplement)
  - Diverticulitis—antibiotics; NPO during acute attack, then progress to fluids and then to high-fiber diet; bed rest, may require hospitalization, surgery for severe cases (2 to 3 recurrences in 1 to 2 years)
- Medications used and side effects (see Pharmacotherapeutics)

Referral

To primary care physician or surgeon in severe cases

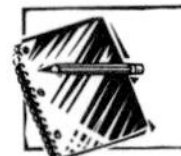

EVALUATION

Outcome

Patient does not develop diverticulitis or will not have a recurrence

Possible Complications

- Hemorrhage
- Perforation
- Peritonitis
- Bowel obstruction
- Abscess
- Fistula

Follow-up

- In 1 week if taking oral antibiotics
- Within 1 week of hospitalization
- Some authorities repeat barium enema in 3 weeks

FOR YOUR INFORMATION

Lifespan

Pediatric: Very rare
Geriatric: Symptoms blunted; may take longer to recuperate
Pregnancy: Increased constipation common—may create problems for patient with diverticulosis

Miscellaneous

Only about 15% of patients with diverticulosis will progress to diverticulitis.

References

Heitkemper M, Sawchuck L: Nursing role in management: problems of absorption and elimination. In Lewis SM, Collier IC, Heitkemper MM, editors: *Medical-surgical nursing: assessment and management of clinical problems,* ed 4, St Louis, 1996, Mosby, pp 1249-1251.

Woolliscroft JO: *Current diagnosis and treatment: a quick reference for the general practitioner,* Philadelphia, 1996, Current Medicine, pp 116-117.

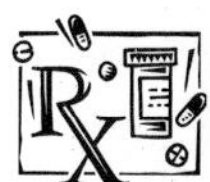

PHARMACOTHERAPEUTICS

Drug of Choice	Mechanism of Action	Prescribing Information	Side Effects
To give stool bulk:			
Psyllium (Metamucil), 1-2 tsp in 8 oz water PO bid or tid; children >6 years, 1 tsp in 4 oz water PO	Bulk-forming laxative	***Contraindications:*** Hypersensitivity; intestinal obstruction; abdominal pain; nausea, vomiting; fecal impaction ***Cost:*** OTC ***Pregnancy category:*** C	Nausea, vomiting, diarrhea, cramps
For relief of bowel spasms:			
Dicyclomine (Bentyl), 10-20 mg PO tid or qid; children >2 years, 10 mg PO tid or qid; children 6 months-2 years, 5 mg PO tid or qid	Inhibits muscarinic actions of acetylcholine at postganglionic parasympathetic neuroeffector sites	***Contraindications:*** Hypersensitivity to anticholinergics; narrow-angle glaucoma; GI obstruction; myasthenia gravis; paralytic ileus; GI atony; toxic megacolon ***Cost:*** 20-mg tab, 100 tabs: $2-$30 ***Pregnancy category:*** B	Confusion, stimulation in elderly, headache, insomnia, dizziness, seizures, coma, dry mouth, constipation, paralytic ileus, heartburn, nausea, vomiting, urinary hesitancy/retention, impotence, palpitations, tachycardia, blurred vision, photophobia, mydriasis, urticaria, rash, fever
For diverticulitis:			
Metronidazole (Flagyl), 250-500 mg PO q8h × 7 days; children, 5 mg/kg PO tid × 5 days	Direct-acting amebicide/ trichomonacide	***Contraindications:*** Hypersensitivity; renal disease; hepatic disease; contracted visual or color fields; blood dyscrasias; pregnancy 1st trimester; lactation; CNS disorders ***Cost:*** 250-mg tab, 100 tabs: $5-$60 ***Pregnancy category:*** B (2nd and 3rd trimesters)	Flat T-waves, headache, dizziness, confusion, irritability, restlessness, depression, fatigue, drowsiness, insomnia, convulsions, blurred vision, sore throat, dry mouth, retinal edema, metallic taste, nausea, vomiting, diarrhea, anorexia, constipation, abdominal cramps, pseudomembranous colitis, darkened urine, albuminuria, neurotoxicity, leukopenia, bone marrow depression, aplasia, rash, pruritus, urticaria
Add one of the following:			
Amoxicillin (Amoxil), 500 mg PO q8h × 7 days; children 20-40 mg/kg/day PO in divided doses q8h	Broad-spectrum antibiotic; interferes with cell wall replication	***Contraindications:*** Hypersensitivity to penicillins; caution if hypersensitive to cephalosporins ***Cost:*** 500-mg tab, 30 tabs: $7-$9 ***Pregnancy category:*** B	Anemia, bone marrow depression, granulocytopenia, nausea, vomiting, diarrhea, increased AST and ALT, abdominal pain, pseudomembranous colitis, headache, fever, anaphylaxis, respiratory distress
Ciprofloxacin 500 mg PO bid—not recommended for children	Fluoroquinolone; interferes with conversion of intermediate DNA fragments in high molecular weight DNA in bacteria	***Contraindication:*** Hypersensitivity ***Cost:*** 250-mg tab, 100 tabs: $262 ***Pregnancy category:*** C	Headache, dizziness, fatigue, insomnia, depression, nausea, diarrhea, increased ALT and AST, flatulence, heartburn, vomiting, rash, pruritus, urticaria, photosensitivity, flushing, fever, blurred vision, tinnitus

Drug Abuse/Substance Abuse

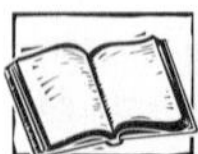

OVERVIEW

Drug and/or substance abuse is an attempt by patients to alter their mood, feelings, thinking, and perception through the use of alcohol, illicit drugs, prescription drugs, or a wide array of synthetic chemicals. It is a maladaptive pattern that leads to significant impairment or distress. DSM-IV criteria for substance abuse is as follows:

A. A maladaptive pattern of substance use leading to clinically significant impairment or distress, as manifested by one or more of the following occurring at any time during the same 12-month period:
   1. Recurrent substance use resulting in a failure to fulfill major role obligations at work, school, or home
   2. Recurrent substance use in situations in which it is physically hazardous, such as driving a car
   3. Recurrent substance-related legal problems
   4. Continued substance use despite having persistent or recurrent social or interpersonal problems caused or exacerbated by the effects of the substance

B. Has never met the criteria for substance dependence for this class of substance

Pathogenesis

Multifactorial and complex:

- Genetic predisposition, learning and behavior problems
- Personality and psychiatric disorders
- Social, environmental, and cultural factors
- Four models to explain drug and/or substance abuse:
  - Moral failure model
  - Legal model
  - Disease model
  - Psychosocial model

Patient Profile

- Males > Females (slightly)
- Any age; usually begins in adolescence

Signs and Symptoms

- Depressants (benzodiazepines, barbiturates, opiates, morphine, heroin, alcohol, sedatives, hypnotics, minor tranquilizers)—nausea/vomiting, myalgia, deep bone or muscle pain, rhinorrhea, sneezing, excessive lacrimation, headache, miosis, euphoria, apathy, dysphoria, depression, drowsiness, psychomotor retardation, slurred speech, impaired attention, impaired memory, impaired social judgment, ataxia, tremors, lack of coordination, mood swings, aggression, combativeness, loss of impulse control, auditory hallucinations, paranoia, fever, perspiration, needle marks
- Stimulants (amphetamines, cocaine, caffeine, tobacco)—restlessness, irritability, anxiety, confusion, aggression, tachycardia, cardiac arrhythmia, chest pain, increased blood pressure, elation, grandiosity, perspiration or chills, hyperthermia or hypothermia, abdominal pain, nausea/vomiting, diarrhea/frequent urination, insomnia, paranoia, hallucinations, dilated pupils, nasal septum ulceration
- Hallucinogens (LSD, nutmeg, phencyclidine, mescaline, peyote, cannabis, hashish)—dilated pupils, vertical and horizontal nystagmus, flushed skin, increased pulse and blood pressure, marked anxiety, panic paranoia, hallucinations, visual and sensory distortions, rapid and severe mood changes, hostility, aggression, violence, depression, suicidal thoughts, grandiosity, euphoria, tremors, flashbacks, insensitivity to pain
- Conditions commonly associated with substance abuse—frequent upper respiratory tract infections, slowly healing skin ulcers, recurrent vaginal infections, hepatitis, sexually transmitted disease, mononucleosis, malnutrition, HIV infection, pancreatitis, tuberculosis

Differential Diagnosis

- Seizure disorder
- Hypothyroidism/hyperthyroidism, thyroid storm
- Hypoglycemia/hyperglycemia
- Schizophrenia
- Mania
- Head injury

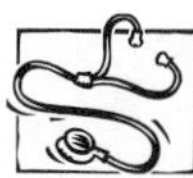

ASSESSMENT

History

Inquire about:

- Onset and duration of symptoms
- Past history of mental illness
- Type of drug abused
- Length of time used
- Age of first use
- Method of using drug (IV, snorting, smoking)
- Amount of drug taken
- Family history of drug abuse
- Work/school history
- Past attempts at sobriety, treatments tried, and results
- Length of time sober
- History of physical, sexual, psychologic abuse
- Perform CAGE questionnaire (see assessment tests in part 3)
- Arrests or incarceration for drug use or distribution
- Underlying conditions
- Current medications

Physical Findings

General findings:

- Unkempt appearance with poor hygiene
- Elevated temperature
- Increased or decreased blood pressure
- Tachycardia
- Tachypnea
- Bruises
- Weight loss
- Peripheral edema
- Tremors
- Peripheral neuropathies
- Hyperactive reflexes
- Burns
- Needle marks
- Infections
- Cellulitis
- Ulcerations
- Pupillary constriction or dilation
- Poor oral hygiene
- Puncture wounds under tongue
- Pharyngitis
- Inflammation and/or erosion of nasal mucosa
- Abdominal tenderness
- Organomegaly
- Dysrhythmia
- Incoordination
- Decreased pain perception
- Alterations in consciousness, attention, sensory perceptions
- In early stages—normal examination

Initial Workup

Laboratory

- CBC—anemia and leukocytosis may be present
- Urinalysis
- Drug screen
- Chemistry profile to include liver function studies, thyroid panel, glucose, creatinine, and BUN

Radiology: Chest film—PA and lateral—evidence of pulmonary disease

Further Workup

Depends on initial workup

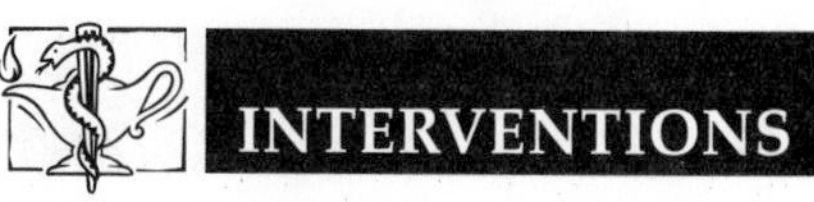

INTERVENTIONS

Office Treatment

If acute intoxication is present, may need life-sustaining measures until transport to emergency room is available

Lifestyle Modifications

- Cessation of use of abused substance
- May necessitate change of environment, including work/school termination for treatment in inpatient program
- Well-balanced diet
- Moderate exercise program if appropriate

Patient Education

Teach patient about:

- Sequelae of substance abuse and treatment options—outpatient and inpatient treatment programs, including Alcoholics Anonymous and Narcotics Anonymous
- Family being included in treatment and give information on Al-Anon, Ala-Teen, and Nar-Anon even if patient refuses treatment
- Medications used and side effects (see Pharmacotherapeutics)

Referral

To drug treatment program—consult Yellow Pages of local phone book for programs

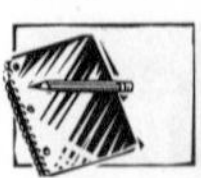

EVALUATION

Outcomes
- Patient is free of substances of abuse
- Patient does not develop end-organ disease from abuse
- Recidivism is high, and constant encouragement is necessary

Possible Complications
- Recidivism
- End-organ disease

Follow-up
- If NP is doing detoxification on an outpatient basis, daily visits are necessary
- If patient is sent to a rehabilitation program, follow-up will be by that program
- NP may see patient for other health problems; it is important to encourage patient to continue with treatment program

FOR YOUR INFORMATION

Life Span
Pediatric: Substance abuse prevention and education are imperative in this age group
Geriatric: More commonly addicted to prescription medication
Pregnancy: Infant can be born addicted; low-birth weight and prematurity common

Miscellaneous
The primary role of the NP in treating drug abuse is one of diagnosis and referral. Detoxification and treatment are best accomplished by professionals specifically trained in this area.

References
Caulker-Burnett I: Primary care screening for substance abuse, *Nurse Pract* 19(6):42-48, 1994.

Sullivan JT, D'Lugoff B: Illicit use and abuse of drugs and substances. In Barker LR, Burton JR, Zieve PD, editors: *Principles of ambulatory medicine,* ed 4, Baltimore, 1995, Williams & Wilkins, pp 251-272.

NOTES

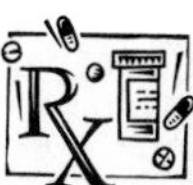

PHARMACOTHERAPEUTICS

Pharmacologic management for drug abuse should be instituted and managed by a professional specially trained in this area. Often the NP may encounter a patient who is currently undergoing treatment and is using a maintenance drug for rehabilitation. It is important for the NP to understand the use of these drugs and to use caution when prescribing other medications for this patient.

Drug of Choice	Mechanism of Action	Prescribing Information	Side Effects
For opioid abuse, use one of the following:			
Methadone, 15-20 mg PO daily; increase if withdrawal symptoms not controlled; must be diluted; should not treat for longer than 21 days and should not repeat treatment for 4 weeks; controlled substance, Schedule II	Synthetic narcotic similar to morphine; interacts with opioid receptors in CNS	***Contraindication:*** Hypersensitivity ***Cost:*** 10 mg/ml, 30 ml: $19 ***Pregnancy category:*** B	Respiratory depression, circulatory depression, cardiac arrest, drowsiness, dizziness, confusion, headache, sedation, nausea, vomiting, anorexia, constipation, cramps, rash, urticaria, bruising, tinnitus, blurred vision, palpitations
Levomethadyl acetate hydrochloride (Orlaam); initially give 20-40 mg PO 3 times weekly, maximum 140 mg; should never be given daily; must be diluted before administration; warn patient that alcohol or other psychoactive drugs used concomitantly can cause fatal overdose	Orlaam: opioid, has longer half-life than methadone; principal action is analgesia and sedation	***Contraindication:*** Hypersensitivity ***Cost:*** 10 mg/ml, 474 ml: $240 ***Pregnancy category:*** C	"Feeling wired," poor concentration, drowsiness, dizziness, withdrawal symptoms if dose too low, addiction, asthenia, back pain, chills, edema, bradycardia, constipation, abdominal pain, dry mouth, arthralgias, abnormal dreams, anxiety, decreased libido, depression, cough, rash, blurred vision, impotence, respiratory depression
Naltrexone hydrochloride (Trexan): patient must be free of opioids for 7-10 days before initiating treatment; initially give 25 mg PO qd; if no symptoms of withdrawal, increase to 50 mg PO qd, then can give 50 mg PO qd, 100 mg PO qd, or 150 mg PO q3d; Narcan challenge test should be performed before administering naltrexone; maintains opioid state in individuals previously opioid dependent; does not lead to physical or psychologic dependence	Pure opioid antagonist; blocks effects of opioids	***Contraindications:*** Patients currently receiving, dependent on, or withdrawing from opioids; patients fail Narcan challenge test or have positive urine for opioids; hypersensitivity; acute hepatitis or liver failure ***Cost:*** 50 mg/tab, 50 tabs: $228 ***Pregnancy category:*** C	Hepatotoxicity; self-administration of heroin or other narcotics may result in coma and death; difficulty sleeping; anxiety; nervousness; abdominal pain/cramps; nausea, vomiting; low energy; joint and muscle pain; headache; loss of appetite; diarrhea; constipation; irritability; dizziness; skin rash; delayed ejaculation; chills; nasal congestion; rhinnorrhea
For alcohol abuse:			
Disulfiram (Antabuse); never administer to a patient with alcohol in his or her system; initially give 500 mg PO daily for 1-2 weeks, then 250 mg PO daily; must abstain from alcohol for at least 12 hours before administration	Produces sensitivity to alcohol, which results in a highly unpleasant reaction to alcohol	***Contraindications:*** Hypersensitivity; severe myocardial disease or coronary occlusion; psychoses; patients who have received metronidazole, paraldehyde, alcohol, or alcohol-containing products ***Cost:*** 500 mg/tab, 50 tablets: $6-$19 ***Pregnancy category:*** Safe usage has not been established	Optic neuritis, peripheral neuritis, polyneuritis, hepatitis, skin eruptions, mild drowsiness, fatigability, impotence, headache, acne, allergic dermatitis, psychotic reactions

Drug Reaction, Cutaneous

OVERVIEW

The most common adverse reaction to drugs is a skin rash. There are many different types of reactions, with the most common being maculopapular, urticarial, and fixed-drug reactions.

Pathogenesis

- Cause—sensitization to a certain drug or components of a drug
- May be immunologically or nonimmunologically mediated
- Sensitization may take weeks or years
- Once sensitization occurs, reaction can occur in minutes to weeks
- Maculopapular reactions—common causes: ampicillin, barbiturates, dolobid, gentamicin, gold salts, isoniazid, phenytoin, sulfonamides, thiazides, many others
- Urticarial reactions—common causes: aspirin (most frequent), penicillin, blood products, almost any drug
- Fixed drug eruptions—common causes: aspirin, barbiturates, methaqualone, sulfonamides, trimethoprin-sulfamethoxazole, tetracycline, many others

Patient Profile

- Females > Males
- Can affect all ages and races

Signs and Symptoms

- Maculopapular reactions—erythematous macules, papules, often confluent and symmetric; pruritis often present
- Urticarial reactions—pruritic, red wheals, hives anywhere on body; may fade in 24 hours, but new urticaria may develop; angioedema can develop and be life-threatening
- Fixed-drug eruptions—red plaques or blisters, which recur at same site each time drug ingested, commonly on penis

Differential Diagnosis

- Viral exanthem can be difficult to distinguish from maculopapular (if rash resolves when drug is stopped, it was a maculopapular drug reaction)
- Primary dermatosis

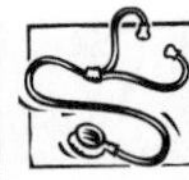

ASSESSMENT

History

Inquire about:

- Onset and duration of symptoms
- Medications used in past month
- Previous history of allergic reactions
- Family history of allergies
- Underlying conditions
- Current medications

Physical Findings

- Complete skin assessment
- Red macules
- Papules
- Pruritis
- Wheals
- Hives
- Morbilliform rash
- Generalized distribution or red plaque or blister in isolated area (commonly found on penis)

Initial Workup

Laboratory

- CBC if secondary infection suspected
- May see eosinophilia in some allergic reactions

Radiology: Usually none

Further Workup

None indicated

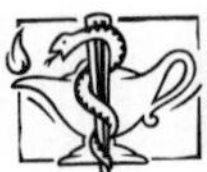

INTERVENTIONS

Office Treatment

None indicated

Lifestyle Modification

Avoidance of the offending agent

Patient Education

Teach patient about:

- Condition and treatment
- Stopping offending agent
- Using antihistamines or topical steroids
- Oatmeal bath or cool compresses to control urticaria
- Need to return to clinic or emergency room if symptoms worsen or breathing problems develop
- Informing all health care providers of allergies
- Obtaining a medical alert tag and wearing it at all times
- Need to avoid reexposure, since subsequent exposures could be very severe or life-threatening
- Medications used and side effects (see Pharmacotherapeutics)

Referral

To MD or emergency room for severe reactions

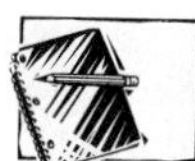

EVALUATION

Outcome

Resolves without sequelae

Possible Complications

- Angioedema
- Bullous reaction
- Stevens-Johnson syndrome
- Anaphylaxis

Follow-up

Telephone contact in 24 hours; return visit in 48 hours; then in 1 week

FOR YOUR INFORMATION

Life Span

Pediatric: Treatment is the same as for other age groups
Geriatric: Higher morbidity and mortality with severe reactions
Pregnancy: Cautious use of medications

Miscellaneous

For patients with urticarial or maculopapular reactions, close follow-up is necessary to ensure that there is no progression of the reaction. It is important for the NP to be aware of cross-sensitivity among classes of drugs. The most common drugs causing reactions are penicillins/cephalosporins and the anticonvulsive drugs hydantoin/barbiturates/carbamazepine.

References

Habif TP: *Clinical dermatology: a color guide to diagnosis and therapy,* ed 3, St Louis, 1996, Mosby, pp 434-441.

Millikan LE: Recognizing drug-related skin eruptions, *Physician Assist* 18(7):44, 49, 53-57, 1994.

NOTES

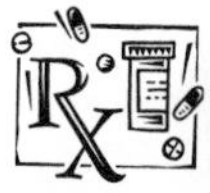

PHARMACOTHERAPEUTICS

Drug of Choice	Mechanism of Action	Prescribing Information	Side Effects
Diphenhydramine (Benadryl); antihistamine to control itching; follow label directions for use	Competes with histamine for cell receptor sites	***Contraindication:*** Hypersensitivity ***Cost:*** Benadryl 25 mg 4/day × 30 days: $4 ***Pregnancy category:*** B	Sedation, headache, fatigue, dizziness, nausea and vomiting, dry mouth, cough, rash
Topical corticosteroid: hydrocortisone cream, 1% for face (controversial) and 2.5% elsewhere; apply thin layer 3-4 times daily; for severe erythema, stronger corticosteroid may be needed: mometasone (Elocon), triamcinolone (Kenalog, Aristocort), betamethasone (Diprolene AF)	Antiinflammatory; antipruritic	***Contraindication:*** Hypersensitivity ***Cost:*** 1%, 30 g: $12; several available OTC; mometasone 0.1%, 45 g: $29; triamcinolone 0.025%, 30 g: $2-$5; betamethasone 0.05%, 15 g: $3-$16 ***Pregnancy category:*** C	Burning, dryness, itching, irritation, acne, folliculitis, hypertrichosis, hypopigmentation, atrophy, striae, perioral dermatitis, secondary infection; if used on large area for extended periods of time, can have systemic side effects

Dysfunctional Uterine Bleeding (DUB)

OVERVIEW

Dysfunctional uterine bleeding (DUB) is abnormal uterine bleeding that is usually associated with anovulation. It is generally not related to lesions of the uterus.

Pathogenesis

Persistent stimulation of endometrium by estrogen—unopposed by progesterone; 90% of cases associated with anovulation

Patient Profile

- Females
- Menarche to menopause
- Highest incidence—puberty and perimenopausal

Signs and Symptoms

- Irregular menses pattern
- Episodes of amenorrhea
- Episodes of heavy, painless, prolonged bleeding

Differential Diagnosis

- Pregnancy
- Ectopic pregnancy
- Anabolic steroids
- Uterine fibroids
- Thyroid disease
- Uterine cancer
- Coagulation defects
- Intrauterine devices
- Medications
- Uterine leiomyomas.

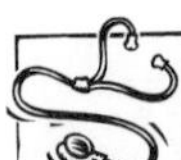

ASSESSMENT

History

Inquire about:

- Onset and duration of symptoms
- Age of menarche; number of days in cycle; number of days menses lasts
- Number of pregnancies, births
- Type of birth control
- Age of first sexual intercourse
- Number of partners
- History of sexually transmitted diseases
- Last menstrual period
- Recent trauma
- Underlying conditions
- Current medications

Physical Findings

Complete physical examination, including pelvic examination and Pap smear, should be within normal limits

Initial Workup

Laboratory: To rule out organic cause:

- CBC
- Thyroid function tests
- PT and PTT
- Urine
- Urine HCG
- Pap smear

Radiology: Pelvic ultrasound or transvaginal ultrasound for suspected organic problems

Further Workup

- Endometrial biopsy
- Hysteroscopy
- Hysterosalpingography if indicated

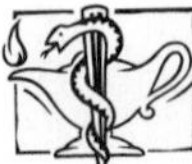

INTERVENTIONS

Office Treatment

None indicated

Lifestyle Modification

Smoking cessation

Patient Education

Teach patient about:

- Condition and treatment options—medications
- Keeping menstrual calendar
- Pad or tampon count
- Usual cause—hormone imbalance
- Medications used and side effects (see Pharmacotherapeutics)

Referral

To MD for severe bleeding or treatment failure

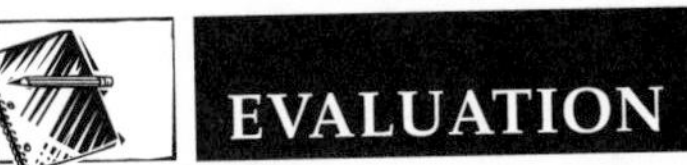

EVALUATION

Outcome

Most patients can successfully be treated with medication

Possible Complications

- Anemia
- Adenocarcinoma
- Side effects of medications

Follow-up

In 2 weeks; then monthly to review menstrual calendar and assess treatment × 2; then annually

FOR YOUR INFORMATION

Life Span

Pediatric: Seen frequently in pubescent girls
Geriatric: In this population, must rule out carcinoma
Pregnancy: Hydatiform mole and ectopic pregnancy can present with similar symptoms

Miscellaneous

N/A

References

Baker S: Menstruation and related problems and concerns. In Youngkin EQ, Davis MS, editors: *Women's health: a primary care clinical guide,* Norwalk, Conn, 1994, Appleton & Lange, pp 83-86.

Uphold CR, Graham MV: *Clinical guidelines in adult health,* Gainesville, Fla, 1994, Barmarrae Books, pp 468-471.

NOTES

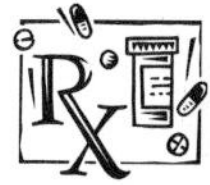

PHARMACOTHERAPEUTICS

Drug of Choice	Mechanism of Action	Prescribing Information	Side Effects
For clients who need contraception:			
Combination oral contraceptives, 35 μg PO qid × 5-7 days, then continue in usual fashion × 3-6 months	Prevent ovulation by suppressing FSH and LH	***Contraindications:*** Hypersensitivity; breast cancer; thromboembolic disorders; reproductive cancer; undiagnosed vaginal bleeding; pregnancy; hepatic tumor/disease; women age 40 years and over; cerebrovascular accident (CVA) ***Cost:*** Varies by brand, \$20-\$30 ***Pregnancy category:*** X	Dizziness, headache, migraines, depression, hypotension, thrombophlebitis, thromboembolism, pulmonary embolism, myocardial infarction (MI), nausea, vomiting, cholestatic jaundice, weight gain, diplopia, amenorrhea, cervical erosion, breakthrough bleeding, dysmenorrhea, vaginal candidiasis, spontaneous abortion, rash, urticaria, acne, hirsutism, photosensitivity
For patients who do not need contraception:			
Medroxyprogesterone acetate, 10 mg PO qd for 10-14 days; continue 10 mg PO qd, days 1-10 to 14 each month or days 16-25 × 3-6 months	Inhibits secretion of pituitary gonadotropins; stimulates growth of mammary tissue	***Contraindications:*** Hypersensitivity; breast cancer; thromboembolic disorders; reproductive cancer; undiagnosed vaginal bleeding; pregnancy ***Cost:*** 50 mg/ml, 10 ml: \$9-\$30; 5-mg tab, 30 tabs: \$16 ***Pregnancy category:*** X	Dizziness, headache, migraines, depression, hypotension, thrombophlebitis, thromboembolism, pulmonary embolism, MI, nausea, vomiting, cholestatic jaundice, weight gain, diplopia, amenorrhea, cervical erosion, breakthrough bleeding, dysmenorrhea, vaginal candidiasis, spontaneous abortion, rash, urticaria, acne, hirsutism, photosensitivity
For heavy bleeding, use one of the following:			
Estrogen (conjugated), 25 mg IV q4h × 3 doses until bleeding lessens; if bleeding not heavy to start and after IV estrogen, 1.25 mg PO qd × 7-10 days, then estrogen, 0.625-1.25 mg PO qd, days 1-25 with medroxyprogesterone, 10 mg PO qd, days 12-25 or estrogen, 1.25 mg PO qd × 7-10 days	Affects release of pituitary gonadotropins; inhibits ovulation	***Contraindications:*** Hypersensitivity; breast cancer; thromboembolic disorders; reproductive cancer; undiagnosed vaginal bleeding; pregnancy ***Cost:*** 1.25-mg tab, 100 tabs: \$50 ***Pregnancy category:*** X	Dizziness, headache, migraines, depression, hypotension, thrombophlebitis, thromboembolism, pulmonary embolism, MI, nausea, vomiting, cholestatic jaundice, weight gain, diplopia, amenorrhea, cervical erosion, breakthrough bleeding, dysmenorrhea, vaginal candidiasis, spontaneous abortion, rash, urticaria, acne, hirsutism, photosensitivity
Mefenamic acid (Ponstel), 500 mg PO tid × 3 days; adults and children > 14 years	Nonsteroidal antiinflammatory; inhibits prostaglandin synthesis	***Contraindications:*** Hypersensitivity; asthma; severe renal disease; severe hepatic disease; ulcer ***Cost:*** 250-mg tab, 100 tabs: \$92 ***Pregnancy category:*** C	Nausea, anorexia, vomiting, diarrhea, cholestatic hepatitis, constipation, flatulence, ulceration, perforation, dizziness, drowsiness, fatigue, tremors, tachycardia, peripheral edema, palpitations, nephrotoxicity, dysuria, hematuria, oliguria, blood dyscrasias, tinnitus, hearing loss

Dyshidrosis (Pompholyx)

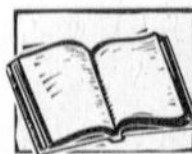

OVERVIEW

Dyshidrosis is a dermatitis that affects the skin of the hands and feet. It is characterized by recurrent vesicular eruptions of the palms of the hands and the soles of the feet.

Pathogenesis

Exact cause unknown:

- Associated with excessive sweating
- Some relationship to stress
- Nickel, chromate, and cobalt ingestion can cause dyshidrosis in some individuals

Patient Profile

- Males = Females
- Usually <40 years of age

Signs and Symptoms

- Red, sweaty palms
- Moderate to severe itching
- Appearance of vesicles; 3 to 4 weeks later, 1- to 3-mm rings of scale
- May lead to erythema, scaling, and lichenification

Differential Diagnosis

- Tinea manuum or pedis
- Contact dermatitis
- Atopic dermatitis
- Drug reaction
- Pustular psoriasis
- Seborrheic dermatitis

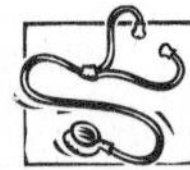

ASSESSMENT

History

Inquire about:

- Onset and duration of symptoms
- Presence of tiny blisters
- Whether palms sweat a lot
- Ingestion of cobalt, nickel, or chromate
- Stress
- Skin allergies
- Treatments tried and results
- Underlying conditions
- Current medications

Physical Findings

- Depends on stage of disease:
  - Initially may consist of intense itching
  - May have vesicles on palms, in finger webs, and on soles of feet
  - Later stage may have erythema, scaling, and lichenification
- Examination of entire skin surface—dyshidrosis occurs only on palms of hands, sides of fingers, and soles of feet

Initial Workup

Laboratory: None indicated
Radiology: None indicated

Further Workup

None indicated

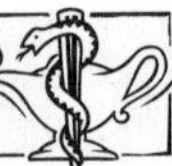

INTERVENTIONS

Office Treatment

None indicated

Lifestyle Modifications

- Stress reduction
- Diet free of metal salts

Patient Education

Teach patient about:

- Condition and treatment—topical steroids; antibiotics
- Keeping hands and feet as dry as possible
- Need for diet free of metal salts—prohibited foods: canned foods, foods cooked in nickel-plated utensils, foods cooked in aluminum or stainless steel utensils, herring, oysters, asparagus, beans, mushrooms, onions, corn, spinach, tomatoes, peas, whole-grain flour, fresh and cooked pears, rhubarb, tea, cocoa and chocolate baking powder
- Stress reduction through biofeedback and relaxation techniques
- Recurrences, which are likely
- Using cold wet compresses to relieve itching
- Medications used and side effects (see Pharmacotherapeutics)

Referral

To dermatologist for resistant cases

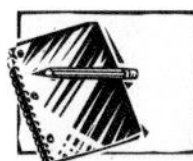

EVALUATION

Outcome
Resolves without sequelae, but recurrences are frequent

Possible Complication
Secondary bacterial infection

Follow-up
In 2 weeks to evaluate treatment

FOR YOUR INFORMATION

Life Span
Pediatric: May start in adolescence
Geriatric: Not usually seen in this age group
Pregnancy: Cautious use of medications

Miscellaneous
N/A

Reference
Habif TP: *Clinical dermatology: a color guide to diagnosis and therapy,* ed 3, St Louis, 1996, Mosby, p 63.

NOTES

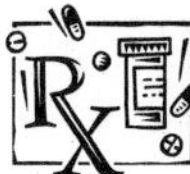

PHARMACOTHERAPEUTICS

Drug of Choice	Mechanism of Action	Prescribing Information	Side Effects
Topical corticosteroid: hydrocortisone cream; apply thin layer 3-4 times daily; for severe erythema, stronger corticosteroid may be needed: mometasone (Elocon), triamcinolone (Kenalog), Betamethasone (Diprolene AF)	Antiinflammatory and antipruritic	***Contraindication:*** Hypersensitivity ***Cost:*** 1%, 30 g: $12; several available OTC; mometasone 0.1%, 45 g: $29; triamcinolone 0.025%, 30 g: $2-$5; betamethasone 0.05%, 15 g: $3-$16 ***Pregnancy category:*** C	Burning, dryness, itching, irritation acne, folliculitis, hypertrichosis, hypopigmentation, atrophy, striae, perioral dermatitis, secondary infection; if used on large area for extended periods of time, can have systemic side effects
Erythromycin (E.E.S.), 500 mg bid or 250 mg qid × 10 days	Inhibits protein synthesis	***Contraindication:*** Hypersensitivity ***Cost:*** 250-mg tabs, 4/day × 10 days: $4 ***Pregnancy category:*** B	Nausea, vomiting, diarrhea, abdominal pain, anorexia, rash, urticaria, pseudomembranous colitis—rarely
For more severe cases:			
Prednisone (Deltasone), 40 mg PO qd × 5 days, 20 mg PO qd × 5 days, 10 mg PO qd × 5 days	Potent antiinflammatory	***Contraindications:*** Systemic fungal infections; psychosis; hypersensitivity; idiopathic thrombocytopenia; acute glomerulonephritis; amebiasis; AIDS; tuberculosis ***Cost:*** 10-mg tab, 100 tabs: $4-$12 ***Pregnancy category:*** C	Depression, flushing, hypertension, circulatory collapse, thrombophlebitis, embolism, diarrhea, nausea, GI hemorrhage, thrombocytopenia, poor wound healing, acne, ecchymosis

Dysmenorrhea

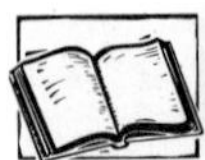

OVERVIEW

Dysmenorrhea is crampy, lower abdominal pain that occurs either immediately before or during menstruation. It is classified as either primary or secondary. Primary dysmenorrhea is dysmenorrhea without pathologic findings; secondary dysmenorrhea has a pathologic cause.

Pathogenesis

- Primary dysmenorrhea—excessive prostaglandin release
- Secondary dysmenorrhea—endometriosis, pelvic infections, intrauterine devices

Patient Profile

- Females
- Primary dysmenorrhea—most commonly occurs in teens to women in their early 20s
- Secondary dysmenorrhea—occurs in women in their 20s to 30s

Signs and Symptoms

PRIMARY DYSMENORRHEA

- "Crampy" lower abdominal pain 12 to 24 hours before start of menses
- Pain intermittent or constant; may extend to back and thighs
- Most severe on first day of menses
- Usually resolves 48 to 72 hours after start
- Fatigue
- Headache
- Bloating
- Nausea, vomiting
- Syncope

SECONDARY DYSMENORRHEA

- Lower abdominal pain a few days to weeks before start of menses
- May extend to back and thighs
- Dyspareunia
- Painful defecation
- Rectal pressure
- Cycle <27 days
- Menstrual bleeding >7 days

Differential Diagnosis

- Cervical stenosis
- Imperforate hymen
- Endometriosis
- Ectopic pregnancy
- Urinary tract infection
- Fibroid
- Carcinoma

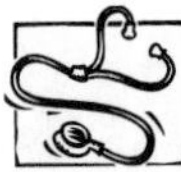

ASSESSMENT

History

Inquire about:

- Onset and duration of symptoms
- Obtain menstrual history, including age of menarche (primary commonly occurs 6 to 12 months after menarche)
- Number of days in cycle
- Duration of bleeding
- Contraceptive history
- Last menstrual period
- Urinary tract symptoms
- Underlying conditions
- Current medications

Physical Findings

Complete physical examination, including pelvic examination:

- Primary dysmenorrhea—within normal limits
- Secondary dysmenorrhea—may have mucopurulent discharge; cervical motion tenderness; small, bluish, endometrial lesions (on labia, cervix, vaginal walls); enlarged uterus; ovarian enlargement and tenderness; or may be within normal limits

Initial Workup

Laboratory: None necessary for primary dysmenorrhea; done to rule out secondary dysmenorrhea:

- CBC—anemia
- Cultures for gonorrhea, chlamydial infection, herpes
- Wet mount
- Pap smear
- Urinalysis

Radiology

- None necessary for primary dysmenorrhea
- Secondary dysmenorrhea—pelvic ultrasound and/or transvaginal ultrasound if indicated

Further Workup

Secondary dysmenorrhea—hysterosalpingogram, hysteroscopy, laparoscopy if indicated

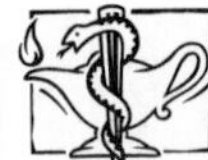

INTERVENTIONS

Office Treatment

None indicated

Lifestyle Modifications

- Regular exercise program
- Decreased salt in diet
- Increased fluids and fiber
- Stress reduction

Patient Education

Teach patient about:

- Primary dysmenorrhea:
  - Treatment—medication
  - Will improve with age and parity
  - Coping strategies
  - Not allowing dysmenorrhea to disrupt life
  - Keeping menstrual record
  - Using a heating pad to decrease discomfort
  - Tips for regular exercise program
  - Decreased salt intake
  - Increased fluids and fiber in diet
  - Stress reduction—relaxation techniques, biofeedback
- Secondary dysmenorrhea—cause and treatment options (will depend on cause)
- Medications used and side effects (see Pharmacotherapeutics)

Referrals

- Primary dysmenorrhea—to MD if treatment failure after 6 months
- Secondary dysmenorrhea—to MD for treatment

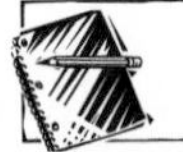

EVALUATION

Outcome

Patient will be able to maintain previous lifestyle

Possible Complications

- Anxiety
- Depression
- Infertility from underlying pathologic condition

Follow-up

Monthly × 3 to assess effectiveness of treatment

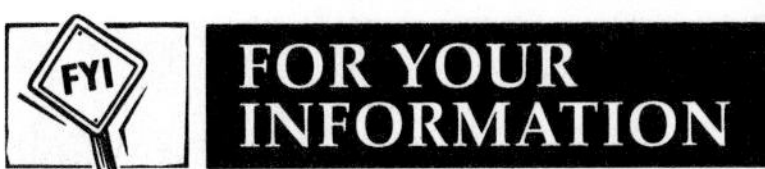

FOR YOUR INFORMATION

Life Span

Pediatric: Primary dysmenorrhea usually begins 6 to 12 months after menarche
Geriatric: N/A
Pregnancy: N/A

Miscellaneous

N/A

Reference

Baker S: Menstruation and related problems and concerns. In Youngkin EQ, Davis MS, editors: *Women's health: a primary care clinical guide,* Norwalk, Conn, 1994, Appleton & Lange, pp 86-89.

NOTES

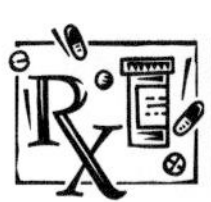

PHARMACOTHERAPEUTICS

Drug of Choice	Mechanism of Action	Prescribing Information	Side Effects
Ibuprofen (Motrin), 400 mg qid PO	Not well understood; may be related to inhibition of prostaglandin synthesis	***Contraindications:*** Aspirin allergy; hypersensitivity; asthma; last trimester of pregnancy; gastric ulcer; bleeding disorders ***Cost:*** 400-mg tab, 4/day × 5 days: $3 ***Pregnancy category:*** Not recommended	Nausea, heartburn, diarrhea, GI upset and bleeding, dizziness, headache, rash, tinnitus, edema, acute renal failure
Naproxen sodium (Anaprox DS), 550 mg PO stat, then 275 mg q6-12h; children, 10 mg/kg/day in 2 divided doses	Nonsteroidal antiinflammatory; inhibits synthesis of prostaglandin to decrease pain	***Contraindications:*** Hypersensitivity; asthma; severe renal disease; severe hepatic disease; ulcer ***Cost:*** 275-mg tab, 100 tabs: $60-$80 ***Pregnancy category:*** B	Nausea, anorexia, vomiting, diarrhea, cholestatic hepatitis, constipation, GI ulceration, GI perforation, dizziness, drowsiness, tachycardia, peripheral edema, nephrotoxicity, dysuria, hematuria, oliguria, azotemia, blood dyscrasias, tinnitus, hearing loss
Mefenamic acid (Ponstel), 500 mg PO tid × 3 days, adults and children >14 years	Nonsteroidal antiinflammatory; inhibits prostaglandin synthesis	***Contraindications:*** Hypersensitivity; asthma; severe renal disease; severe hepatic disease; ulcer ***Cost:*** 250-mg tab, 100 tabs: $92 ***Pregnancy category:*** C	Nausea, anorexia, vomiting, diarrhea, cholestatic hepatitis, constipation, flatulence, ulceration, perforation, dizziness, drowsiness, fatigue, tremors, tachycardia, peripheral edema, palpitations, nephrotoxicity, dysuria, hematuria, oliguria, blood dyscrasias, tinnitus, hearing loss
For clients who need contraception:			
Combination oral contraceptives (many brands available)—dosage and instructions vary for different types; see individual package insert for directions	Prevent ovulation by suppressing FSH and LH	***Contraindications:*** Hypersensitivity; breast cancer; thromboembolic disorders; reproductive cancer; undiagnosed vaginal bleeding; pregnancy; hepatic tumor/disease; women age 40 years and over; cerebrovascular accident (CVA) ***Cost:*** Varies by brand: $20-$30 ***Pregnancy category:*** X	Dizziness, headache, migraines, depression, hypotension, thrombophlebitis, thromboembolism, pulmonary embolism, myocardial infarction (MI), nausea, vomiting, cholestatic jaundice, weight gain, diplopia, amenorrhea, cervical erosion, breakthrough bleeding, dysmenorrhea, vaginal candidiasis, spontaneous abortion, rash, urticaria, acne, hirsutism, photosensitivity

Dyspareunia

OVERVIEW

Dyspareunia is painful sexual intercourse. The pain may occur either when penetration is attempted or on deep penetration by the penis. It may occur in either males or females.

Pathogenesis

Causes:
- Females:
  - Inflammation of genitalia
  - Anatomic abnormalities
  - Pelvic disorder
  - Atrophy
  - Lubrication failure
  - Psychologic disorder
- Males:
  - Muscle spasm of genitals
  - Infection or irritation of genitalia
  - Torsion of spermatic cord
  - Disorder of penile anatomy
  - Prostate infection/enlargement
  - Psychologic disorder

Patient Profile

- Females > Males
- Any age

Signs and Symptoms

- Pain in genitalia or pelvic area
- Degree of pain varies
- Discharge
- Irritation
- Inflammation

Differential Diagnosis

- Vaginismus
- Previous sexual abuse
- Hymenal strands
- Consider any of the causative factors found under Pathogenesis

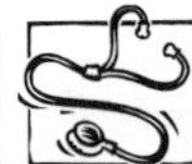

ASSESSMENT

History

Inquire about:
- Onset and duration of symptoms
- Sexual history and practices
- History of trauma or recent surgery
- History of pain on pelvic examination or difficulty with tampon insertion
- Menopausal symptoms
- History of psychologic problems
- History of sexual abuse
- Underlying conditions
- Current medications

Physical Findings

Genital examination:
- Females—may find irritation, inflammation, lesions, atrophy, discharge, involuntary contraction of perianal muscles on speculum or bimanual examination, uterine prolapse, pelvic mass, cervical motion tenderness, cystocele, rectocele
- Males—may find irritation, inflammation, irretractable foreskin, penile discharge, prostate enlargement

Initial Workup

Laboratory
- STD cultures
- Wet mount
- Pap smear
- Urinalysis
- Urine culture
- CBC—WBC increased in infection

Radiology: Pelvic ultrasound if indicated by physical examination

Further Workup

Depends on cause:
- Laparoscopy
- Colposcopy

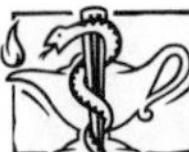

INTERVENTIONS

Office Treatment

Provide supportive environment

Lifestyle Modifications

- Stress reduction
- Smoking cessation
- Alcohol cessation

Patient Education

Teach patient about:
- Condition, cause, and treatment options:
  - Infections—antibiotics
  - Possible surgical interventions—laparoscopy, circumcision (males)
  - Hormonal therapy (females)
  - Water-based lubricants
- Tips for smoking and alcohol cessation, if indicated
- Stress reduction—biofeedback, relaxation technique
- Psychotherapy
- Medications used and side effects (see Pharmacotherapeutics)

Referrals

Dependent on cause:
- To professional sex counselor for psychosexual dysfunction
- To gynecologist (females) or urologist (males or females) for organic cause

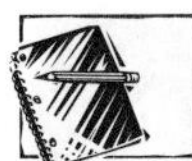

EVALUATION

Outcome

Patient will have normal, healthy, sexual relationship

Possible Complications

- Permanent psychologic damage
- Complications of genital infections

Follow-up

Depends on cause; in 1 month to assess effectiveness of treatment

FOR YOUR INFORMATION

Life Span

Pediatric: May occur at onset of sexual intercourse; careful, thorough counseling is imperative
Geriatric: Vaginal atrophy and lack of lubrication are common after menopause
Pregnancy: Fear of injury to fetus may cause sexual dysfunction; postpartal pain is commonly due to episiotomy

Miscellaneous

For many patients, long-term behavioral therapy, individual therapy, and couple therapy will be necessary to resolve psychologic conflicts

References

Forrest DE: Common gynecologic pelvic disorders. In Youngkin EQ, Davis MS, editors: *Women's health: a primary care clinical guide,* Norwalk, Conn, 1994, Appleton & Lange, pp 256-259.

Schmidt CW: Sexual disorders. In Barker LR, Burton JR, Zieve PD, editors: *Principles of ambulatory medicine,* ed 4, Baltimore, 1995, Williams & Wilkins, p 199.

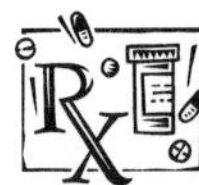

PHARMACOTHERAPEUTICS

For infections, see specific disease for treatment options.

Drug of Choice	Mechanism of Action	Prescribing Information	Side Effects
For females:			
• Estrogen (Premarin), 0.625 mg PO daily • Transdermal estrogen (Estraderm), 0.05 mg—change patch twice a week • Topical estrogen 2-4 g qd × 1-2 weeks; then 1 g 1-3 times weekly	Affects release of pituitary gonadotropins; inhibits ovulation	***Contraindications:*** Hypersensitivity; breast cancer; thromboembolic disorders; reproductive cancer; undiagnosed vaginal bleeding; pregnancy ***Cost:*** 0.625-mg tab, 100 tabs: $28-$37; transdermal and topical estrogen per year: $107 ***Pregnancy category:*** X	Dizziness, headache, migraines, depression, hypotension, thrombophlebitis, thromboembolism, pulmonary embolism, myocardial infarction (MI), nausea, vomiting, cholestatic jaundice, weight gain, diplopia, amenorrhea, cervical erosion, breakthrough bleeding, dysmenorrhea, vaginal candidiasis, spontaneous abortion, rash, urticaria, acne, hirsutism, photosensitivity
For females, if uterus is intact, add the following:			
Medroxyprogesterone acetate, 10 mg PO days 1-12 or days 13-25, or give 2.5 mg PO daily	Inhibits secretion of pituitary gonadotropins; stimulates growth of mammary tissue	***Contraindications:*** Hypersensitivity; breast cancer; thromboembolic disorders; reproductive cancer; undiagnosed vaginal bleeding; pregnancy ***Cost:*** 50 mg/ml, 10 ml: $9-$30; 5-mg tab, 30 tabs: $16 ***Pregnancy category:*** X	Dizziness, headache, migraines, depression, hypotension, thrombophlebitis, thromboembolism, pulmonary embolism, MI, nausea, vomiting, cholestatic jaundice, weight gain, diplopia, amenorrhea, cervical erosion, breakthrough bleeding, dysmenorrhea, vaginal candidiasis, spontaneous abortion, rash, urticaria, acne, hirsutism, photosensitivity
For males or females:			
Water-based lubricant (K-Y Jelly); apply lubricant to vagina or penis as needed	Greaseless water-soluble jelly; safe to use with latex products	***Contraindication:*** Hypersensitivity ***Cost:*** OTC ***Pregnancy category:*** Not categorized	Irritation

Dyspepsia, Nonulcer

OVERVIEW

Nonulcer dyspepsia is a group of upper gastrointestinal symptoms. It occurs in the absence of organic disease.

Pathogenesis

- Cause—generally unknown; may be related to gastric motility disorder or adverse drug effects
- 20% to 30% will go on to develop an ulcer

Patient Profile

- Females > Males
- Any age; more common in adults

Signs and Symptoms

- Belching
- Epigastric pain, gnawing, burning, bloating (food may make it better or worse)
- Anorexia
- Nausea, vomiting
- Borborygmus
- Abdominal tenderness

Differential Diagnosis

- Gastroesophageal reflux disease
- Peptic ulcer disease
- Cholecystitis
- Gastric cancer
- Esophageal spasm
- Malabsorption syndromes
- Irritable bowel syndrome
- Ischemic heart disease
- Thyroid disease
- Diabetes mellitus

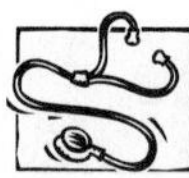

ASSESSMENT

History

Inquire about:

- Onset and duration of symptoms
- Relationship to food intake
- Use of aspirin or nonsteroidal antiinflammatory medications
- Smoking or alcohol use
- Past history of similar symptoms
- Underlying conditions
- Current medications

Physical Findings

- May be none or pain on palpation of mid-epigastric region
- Abdominal tenderness
- Borborygmus

Initial Workup

Laboratory

Done to rule out organic disease:

- CBC—within normal limits
- Chemistry panel—within normal limits
- Stool for occult blood—negative

Radiology

- Upper GI series (usual test done)—within normal limits
- Barium enema—within normal limits
- Gallbladder ultrasound—within normal limits

Further Workup

Endoscopy—within normal limits

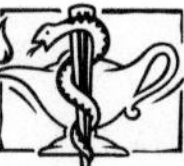

INTERVENTIONS

Office Treatment

None indicated

Lifestyle Modifications

- Smoking cessation
- Alcohol cessation
- Avoidance of aspirin and nonsteroidal antiinflammatory medications
- Avoidance of foods that precipitate attacks
- Stress reduction
- Regular exercise program

Patient Education

Teach patient about:

- Disease process and treatment options—frequent small meals
- Avoidance of foods that exacerbate problem
- Avoidance of foods with caffeine (chocolate, coffee, tea, colas)
- Tips on starting an exercise program
- Tips for smoking and alcohol cessation
- Aspirin and nonsteroidal antiinflammatory drugs and why to avoid
- Stress reduction—relaxation techniques, biofeedback
- Elevating head of bed and not going to bed within 2 hours of eating
- Medications used and side effects (see Pharmacotherapeutics)

Referral

None unless unsure of diagnosis—consult with MD

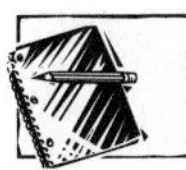

EVALUATION

Outcome
Patient is able to control symptoms

Possible Complications
- Ulcer development
- Tumor
- Other serious pathologic condition

Follow-up
Every 2 weeks until symptoms controlled

FOR YOUR INFORMATION

Life Span
Pediatric: Rare—look for psychologic problems or family dysfunction
Geriatric: More likely to have organic cause
Pregnancy: May cause increase in symptoms

Miscellaneous
Nonulcer dyspepsia is a very common condition. All adults have symptoms at some time in their life.

References
Katz PO: Peptic ulcer disease. In Barker LR, Burton JR, Zieve PD, editors: *Principles of ambulatory medicine,* ed 4, Baltimore, 1995, Williams & Wilkins, pp 467-468.

Talley NJ: Nonulcer dyspepsia: current approaches to diagnosis and treatment, *Am Fam Physician* 47(6):1407-1415, 1993.

NOTES

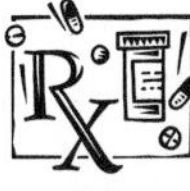

PHARMACOTHERAPEUTICS

There are many OTC preparations available for the treatment of dyspepsia. These should be tried before using the stronger prescription medications. Start with OTC antacids, such as Tums, Rolaids, Maalox, or Mylanta. If no success is achieved with these medications, try the OTC H_2 antagonists, such as Pepcid AC, Tagamet HB, Axid HR, or Zantac. If symptoms are still not relieved, try one of the following prescription medications.

Drug of Choice	Mechanism of Action	Prescribing Information	Side Effects
Famotidine or cimetidine (Pepcid or Tagamet): • Pepcid, 20 mg PO bid—not for children • Tagamet, 300 mg PO with meals and at bedtime—not for children <16 years • Treat for 3-4 weeks, then reduce dosages to OTC strength	Inhibits histamine at H_2 receptor sites	***Contraindication:*** Hypersensitivity ***Cost:*** Pepcid, 20-mg tab, 30 tabs: $45; Tagamet, 300-mg tab, 100 tabs: $45 ***Pregnancy category:*** B	Confusion, headache, depression, dizziness, convulsions, diarrhea, abdominal cramps, paralytic ileus, jaundice, gynecomastia, galactorrhea, increased BUN and creatinine, agranulocytosis, thrombocytopenia, neutropenia, aplastic anemia, urticaria, exfoliative dermatitis
Omeprazole (Prilosec), 20 mg PO qd—not for children	Gastric acid pump inhibitor	***Contraindication:*** Hypersensitivity ***Cost:*** 20-mg tab, 30 tabs: $130 ***Pregnancy category:*** C	Headache, dizziness, asthenia, diarrhea, abdominal pain, vomiting, nausea, constipation, flatulence, acid regurgitation, abdominal swelling, anorexia, cough, epistaxis, rash, dry skin, urticaria, hypoglycemia, increased liver enzymes, weight gain, tinnitus, taste perversion, chest pain, angina, hematuria, bradycardia, tachycardia, urinary tract infection (UTI), pancytopenia, thrombocytopenia, neutropenia, leukocytosis, anemia

Dysphagia

OVERVIEW

Dysphagia is difficulty swallowing. The patient has the sensation that a bolus of food is stuck in the esophagus. Dysphagia is associated with obstruction or motor dysfunction of the oropharyngeal or esophageal portions of the upper gastrointestinal tract. It is a symptom of an underlying disorder.

Pathogenesis

Causes:

- Children:
  - Congenital malformations (esophageal atresia, choanal atresia)
  - Acquired malformations (corrosive esophagitis)
  - Neuromuscular disorders (cerebral palsy, muscular dystrophy)
  - Gastroesophageal reflux disease
- Adults:
  - Tumors (cancer or benign)
  - Strictures (peptic, chemical, trauma)
  - Extrinsic compression
  - (mediastinal tumors, goiter)
  - Gastroesophageal reflux disease
  - Neuromuscular disorder (scleroderma, myasthenia gravis, esophageal spasm)

Patient Profile

- Males = Females
- Any age

Signs and Symptoms

- Patient reports food being "stuck" in esophagus
- Choking
- Pressure in midchest region when swallowing food
- Weight loss
- Heartburn
- Regurgitation
- Burning sensation in throat
- Bad taste in mouth
- Pneumonia

Differential Diagnosis

- Cardiac chest pain
- Must differentiate cause

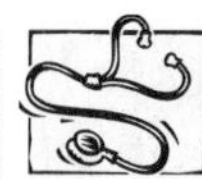

ASSESSMENT

History

Inquire about:

- Onset and duration of symptoms
- What is more difficult to swallow—solids or liquids (motility disorders—both solids and liquids; obstruction—solids)
- Whether dysphagia has occurred before (intermittent dysphagia—motility disorder; chronic/progressive dysphagia—obstruction)
- Pain on swallowing
- Whether temperature extremes make it worse (motility disorders)
- Weight loss
- Underlying conditions
- Current medications

Physical Findings

Look for cause:

- Pallor, sclerodactyly, telangiectasia, calcinosis (scleroderma)
- Hyperkeratotic palms and soles (esophageal carcinoma)
- Pharynx for masses
- Enlarged lymph nodes
- Thyroid enlargement
- Palpate abdomen for pain, masses, organomegaly
- Test tremor, rigidity
- Gag reflex
- Movement of palate, and tongue protrusion

Initial Workup

Laboratory: Tests may provide clue to underlying cause:

- CBC—anemia
- Chemistry profile—electrolyte abnormalities, elevated liver function tests
- Thyroid function tests—increased or decreased

Radiology: Barium swallow, esophageal manometry, neck and chest films, CT scan of chest, as indicated

Further Workup

Endoscopy

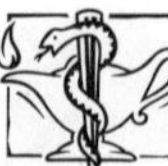

INTERVENTIONS

Office Treatment

None indicated

Lifestyle Modifications

Depends on cause:

- Small, frequent meals
- Avoidance of temperature extremes
- Careful chewing of food
- Smoking cessation

Patient Education

Teach patient about:

- Cause and treatment options:
  - Cancer—radiation, chemotherapy, surgery
  - Neuromuscular disorder—treat spasms and underlying condition
  - Malformations—surgical correction
  - Strictures—esophageal dilation
- Eating small meals
- Chewing food thoroughly
- Avoiding extremes of temperature for foods and liquids
- Tips for smoking cessation
- Medications used and side effects (see Pharmacotherapeutics)

Referral

To gastroenterologist or otolaryngologist

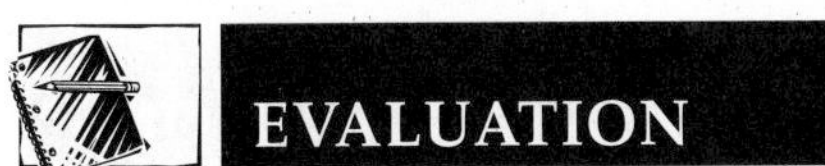

EVALUATION

Outcome
Depends on cause; for all—patient will maintain adequate caloric intake to maintain weight and adequate hydration

Possible Complications
- Aspiration pneumonia
- Esophageal "asthma"
- Death

Follow-up
Usually by specialist

FOR YOUR INFORMATION

Life Span
Pediatric: Congenital malformation most common cause
Geriatric: Look at dental problems for cause
Pregnancy: N/A

Miscellaneous
Dysphagia is a symptom, and a diligent search for the cause of the problem must be made.

References
Katz PO: Peptic ulcer disease. In Barker LR, Burton JR, Zieve PD, editors: *Principles of ambulatory medicine,* ed 4, Baltimore, 1995, Williams & Wilkins, pp 435-443.

Uphold CR, Graham MV: *Clinical guidelines in adult health,* Gainesville, Fla, 1994, Barmarrae Books, pp 377-380.

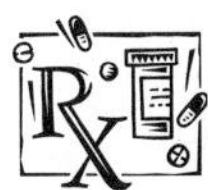

PHARMACOTHERAPEUTICS

The following is a list of the more common medications that may be prescribed by the referring physician.

Drug of Choice	Mechanism of Action	Prescribing Information	Side Effects
Famotidine or cimetidine (Pepcid or Tagamet): • Pepcid, 20 mg PO bid—not for children • Tagamet, 300 mg PO with meals and at bedtime—not for children <16 years • Treat for 3-4 weeks, then reduce dosages to OTC strength	Inhibits histamine at H_2 receptor sites	***Contraindication:*** Hypersensitivity ***Cost:*** Pepcid, 20-mg tab, 30 tabs: $45; Tagamet, 300-mg tab, 100 tabs: $45 ***Pregnancy category:*** B	Confusion, headache, depression, dizziness, convulsions, diarrhea, abdominal cramps, paralytic ileus, jaundice, gynecomastia, galactorrhea, increased BUN and creatinine, agranulocytosis, thrombocytopenia, neutropenia, aplastic anemia, urticaria, exfoliative dermatitis
Omeprazole (Prilosec), 20 mg PO qd—not for children	Gastric acid pump inhibitor	***Contraindication:*** Hypersensitivity ***Cost:*** 20-mg tab, 30 tabs: $130 ***Pregnancy category:*** C	Headache, dizziness, asthenia, diarrhea, abdominal pain, vomiting, nausea, constipation, flatulence, acid regurgitation, abdominal swelling, anorexia, upper respiratory infections, cough, epistaxis, rash, dry skin, urticaria, hypoglycemia, increased liver enzymes, weight gain, tinnitus, taste perversion, chest pain, angina, hematuria, bradycardia, tachycardia, urinary tract infection (UTI), pancytopenia, thrombocytopenia, neutropenia, leukocytosis, anemia, back pain
For spasms, use one of the following:			
Nitroglycerin (Nitrostat), 0.4 mg SL before meals and prn	Nitrate; causes peripheral vasodilation	***Contraindications:*** Hypersensitivity to nitrates or nitrites; severe anemia; increased intraocular pressure; cerebral hemorrhage ***Cost:*** 0.4-mg tab, 60 tabs: $4 ***Pregnancy category:*** C	Postural hypotension, tachycardia, syncope, nausea, vomiting, pallor, sweating, rash, headache, flushing, dizziness
Nifedipine (Procardia), 10-30 mg PO qid	Calcium channel blocker; dilates peripheral arteries	***Contraindication:*** Hypersensitivity ***Cost:*** 10-mg tab, 100 tabs: $30-$50 ***Pregnancy category:*** C	Headache, fatigue, drowsiness, dizziness, anxiety, depression, weakness, light-headedness, dysrhythmias, edema, congestive heart failure (CHF), myocardial infarction (MI), pulmonary edema, nausea, vomiting, diarrhea, gastric upset, constipation, nocturia, polyuria, rash, pruritus, flushing, sexual difficulties, fever, chills

Ectopic Pregnancy

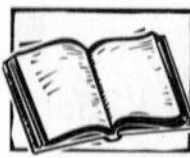

OVERVIEW

An ectopic pregnancy is implantation of a fertilized egg in a fallopian tube (most common), in the cervix, on an ovary, or in the abdominal cavity.

Pathogenesis

Cause—interference in normal ovum transport

Patient Profile

- Females only
- Menarche to menopause
- Risk factors:
  - Intrauterine device (IUD)
  - History of infertility
  - Pelvic inflammatory disease
  - Tubal surgery
  - Prior ectopic pregnancy

Signs and Symptoms

- 1-2 months of amenorrhea
- Morning sickness
- Breast tenderness
- Unilateral abdominal pain
- Mild vaginal bleeding or spotting, possibly
- Pain may be referred to shoulder

Differential Diagnosis

- Pelvic inflammatory disease
- Intrauterine pregnancy
- Recent spontaneous abortion
- Acute appendicitis
- Ovarian cyst
- Ovarian tumor
- Abortion
- Bowel-related disorder

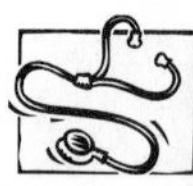

ASSESSMENT

History

Inquire about:

- Onset and duration of symptoms
- Menstrual history and last normal menstrual period
- Sexual history and behaviors
- Past history of ectopic pregnancy
- Risk factors for ectopic pregnancy, particularly use of IUD for birth control
- Underlying conditions
- Current medications

Physical Findings

- Shock symptoms (emergent condition, needs immediate transport to emergency room):
  - Cool, clammy skin
  - Pallor
  - Poor skin turgor
  - Decreased BP
  - Increased pulse
- Other findings more commonly seen in primary care:
  - Unilateral abdominal pain
  - Cervical tenderness
  - Vaginal vault may be bloody
  - Adnexal tenderness
  - Mass
  - Uterus—slightly enlarged

Initial Workup

Laboratory

- Urine pregnancy test—positive
- Serum beta-HCG—low levels suggestive; follow with quantitative
- CBC—to assess blood loss

Radiology: Stat pelvic ultrasound; abdominal CT scan or MRI—may be ordered by NP or MD.

Further Workup

Culdocentesis by MD

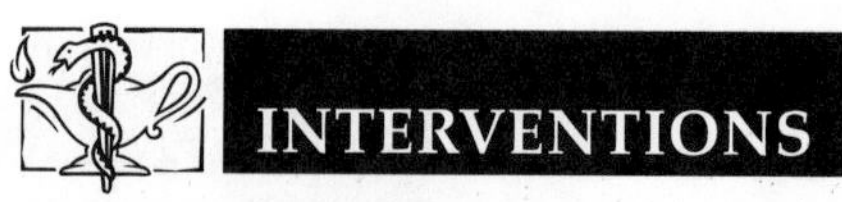

INTERVENTIONS

Office Treatment

Immediate transport to emergency room if shock symptoms present

Lifestyle Modifications

- Preparation for loss of pregnancy
- Possible hospitalization

Patient Education

Teach patient about:

- Condition and need for removal of fetus
- Possible surgical procedures
- Medications used (only used for small, <3.5-cm fetus unruptured) and side effects (see Pharmacotherapeutics)

Referrals

Prompt referral to physician

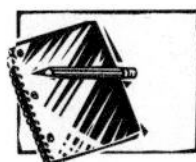

EVALUATION

Outcome
Successful removal of fetus without impairment of fertility

Possible Complications
- Rupture
- Hemorrhage and hypovolemic shock
- Infection
- Loss of reproductive organs
- Disseminated intravascular coagulation
- Any postoperative complications

Follow-up
- Within 1 week of surgery
- If medications used, daily visits for injections and serial beta-HCG levels

FOR YOUR INFORMATION

Life Span
Pediatric: Treatment is same as for adult; may need psychologic counseling
Geriatric: N/A
Pregnancy: Is an abnormal pregnancy

Miscellaneous
On follow-up visits, the patient needs to be assessed for the development of psychologic problems related to the loss of a pregnancy.

References
Corder-Mabe J: Complications of pregnancy. In Youngkin EQ, Davis MS, editors: *Women's health: a primary care clinical guide,* Norwalk, Conn, 1994, Appleton & Lange, pp 447-449.

Patterson KA, Carnago L: Nursing role in management: female reproductive problems. In Lewis SM, Collier IC, Heitkemper MM, editors: *Medical-surgical nursing: assessment and management of clinical problems,* ed 4, St Louis, 1996, Mosby, pp 1598-1601.

NOTES

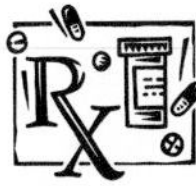

PHARMACOTHERAPEUTICS

The following medications should only be used by individuals familiar with their use, and only in unruptured pregnancies <3.5 cm.

Drug of Choice	Mechanism of Action	Prescribing Information	Side Effects
Methotrexate, 1 mg/kg IM every other day × 4 or 25-30 mg IM × 1	Stops nucleic acid synthesis in cells; clears trophoblastic tissue from site of implantation	***Contraindications:*** Hypersensitivity; leukopenia; thrombocytopenia; anemia; severe hepatic or renal disease ***Cost:*** 25 mg/ml, 2 ml: $15 ***Pregnancy category:*** D	Leukopenia, thrombocytopenia, myelosuppression, anemia, nausea, vomiting, anorexia, diarrhea, stomatitis, hepatotoxicity, cramps, GI hemorrhage, abdominal pain, urinary retention, renal failure, hematuria, azotemia, uric acid nephropathy, rash, alopecia, photosensitivity, dizziness, convulsions
Leucovorin (Wellcovorin), 0.1 mg/kg IM on days not receiving methotrexate—not used with single-dose methotrexate treatment	Protects normal cells	***Contraindications:*** Hypersensitivity; pernicious anemia and other megaloblastic anemias secondary to lack of B_{12} ***Cost:*** 10 mg/ml, 20 ml: $79 ***Pregnancy category:*** C	Wheezing, rash, pruritus, erythema, thrombocytosis, urticaria

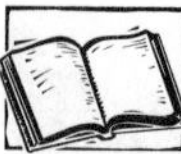

OVERVIEW

Endometriosis is the abnormal growth of endometrial tissue outside the endometrial cavity of the uterus. The most common sites are the ovaries, broad ligaments, fallopian tubes, cul-de-sac, and bowel. Endometrial implants can occur anywhere in the body.

Pathogenesis
Cause—remains unknown; several theories:
- Sampson's theory—retrograde menstruation
- Halban's theory—lymphatic/vascular spread of endometrial tissue
- Meyer's theory—metaplasia of mesothelial cells into endometrial epithelium
- Dioxin theory—linkage between exposure to dioxin and development of endometriosis

Patient Profile
- Females
- Menarche to menopause
- Family history may play a role

Signs and Symptoms
- Most common:
  - Dyspareunia
  - Dysmenorrhea
  - Infertility
  - Perimenstrual back pain
  - Pelvic pain
  - Painful defecation
  - Premenstrual spotting
- Less common:
  - Urinary urgency
  - Hematuria
  - Rectal bleeding

Differential Diagnosis
- Chronic pelvic inflammatory disease
- Acute salpingitis
- Crohn's disease
- Hemorrhagic corpus luteum
- Ectopic pregnancy
- Ruptured ovarian cyst
- Irritable bowel syndrome
- Urinary tract infection

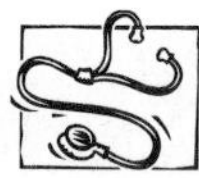

ASSESSMENT

History
Inquire about:
- Onset and duration of symptoms
- Family history of endometriosis
- Menstrual history
- Birth control
- Obstetric history (30% to 40% are infertile)
- Underlying conditions
- Current medications

Physical Findings
- Genitalia and speculum examination may be normal or may see cervical displacement to right or left
- Bimanual examination—tenderness, fixed retroverted uterus, adnexal masses

Initial Workup
Laboratory
- CBC
- Erythrocyte sedimentation rate (ESR)
- CA-125 assay (very expensive; often not covered by insurance)
- If WBC count and ESR are normal and CA-125 is elevated, endometriosis is likely

Radiology: Pelvic ultrasound—identified endometriomas of ovaries

Further Workup
- Biopsy of lesion
- Laparoscopy by MD

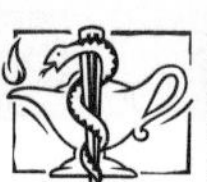

INTERVENTIONS

Office Treatment
None indicated

Lifestyle Modifications
- Major impact on life because of pain, possibility of infertility
- May affect decisions regarding marriage, sexual relationship, career choices

Patient Education
Teach patient about:
- Condition and treatment options—medications, surgery
- Coping mechanisms
- Stress reduction—biofeedback, relaxation techniques, yoga
- Medications used and side effects (see Pharmacotherapeutics)

Referral
To professional experienced in treatment of endometriosis

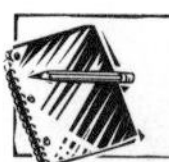

EVALUATION

Outcome
Control of symptoms

Possible Complications
- Infertility
- Chronic pelvic pain
- Major disruption of lifestyle
- Hysterectomy and possible postoperative complications

Follow-up
In 2 weeks after starting medication; then every 3 months to assess effectiveness and side effects; will probably be followed by specialist

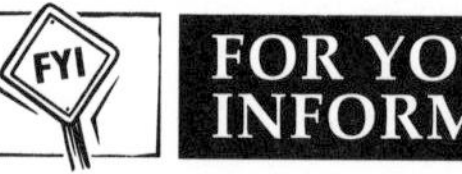

FOR YOUR INFORMATION

Life Span
Pediatric: Tends to occur in patients with early menarche

Geriatric: Signs and symptoms tend to regress with menopause; estrogen therapy may exacerbate symptoms

Pregnancy: To infertility specialist if needed

Miscellaneous
Endometriosis can be a devastating diagnosis. The patient needs a great deal of psychologic support.

References

Forrest DE: Common gynecologic pelvic disorders. In Youngkin EQ, Davis MS, editors: *Women's health: a primary care clinical guide,* Norwalk, Conn, 1994, Appleton & Lange, pp 242-248.

Patterson KA, Carnago L: Nursing role in management: female reproductive problems. In Lewis SM, Collier IC, Heitkemper MM, editors: *Medical-surgical nursing: assessment and management of clinical problems,* ed 4, St Louis, 1996, Mosby, pp 1611-1612.

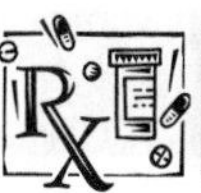

PHARMACOTHERAPEUTICS

The following medications are for use in mild to moderate endometriosis.

Drug of Choice	Mechanism of Action	Prescribing Information	Side Effects
Danazol (Danocrine), 100-800 mg/day PO in 2 divided doses × 6-9 months	Decreases FSH and LH; results in amenorrhea/anovulation	***Contraindications:*** Hypersensitivity; severe renal, cardiac, or hepatic disease; pregnancy; abnormal genital bleeding ***Cost:*** 200-mg tab, 60 tabs: $200 ***Pregnancy category:*** C	Rash, acneiform lesions, oily hair, flushing, sweating, dizziness, headache, fatigue, tremors, paresthesias, anxiety, cramps, muscle spasms, increased blood pressure, hematuria, atrophic vaginitis, decreased libido, decreased breast size, clitoral hypertrophy, nausea, vomiting, weight gain, cholestatic jaundice, nasal congestion
Use one of the following only if danazol is contraindicated or poorly tolerated:			
Medroxyprogesterone acetate (Depo-Provera), 100 mg IM every 2 weeks × 4 doses; then 200 mg IM monthly for 4 more months or 30 mg PO qd × 6 months	Inhibits secretion of pituitary gonadotropins; stimulates growth of mammary tissue	***Contraindications:*** Hypersensitivity; breast cancer; thromboembolic disorders; reproductive cancer; undiagnosed vaginal bleeding; pregnancy ***Cost:*** 50 mg/ml, 10 ml: $9-$30; 5-mg tab, 30 tabs: $16 ***Pregnancy category:*** X	Dizziness, headache, migraines, depression, hypotension, thrombophlebitis, thromboembolism, pulmonary embolism, myocardial infarction (MI), nausea, vomiting, cholestatic jaundice, weight gain, diplopia, amenorrhea, cervical erosion, breakthrough bleeding, dysmenorrhea, vaginal candidiasis, spontaneous abortion, rash, urticaria, acne, hirsutism, photosensitivity
Combination oral contraceptives (many brands available); dosage and instructions vary for different types; see individual package insert for directions	Prevent ovulation by suppressing FSH and LH	***Contraindications:*** Hypersensitivity; breast cancer; thromboembolic disorders; reproductive cancer; undiagnosed vaginal bleeding; pregnancy; hepatic tumor/disease; women age 40 years and over; cerebrovascular accident (CVA) ***Cost:*** Varies by brand: $20-$30 ***Pregnancy category:*** X	Dizziness, headache, migraines, depression, hypotension, thrombophlebitis, thromboembolism, pulmonary embolism, myocardial infarction (MI), nausea, vomiting, cholestatic jaundice, weight gain, diplopia, amenorrhea, cervical erosion, breakthrough bleeding, dysmenorrhea, vaginal candidiasis, spontaneous abortion, rash, urticaria, acne, hirsutism, photosensitivity
Or use one of the following alternatives to danazol or progesterone:			
Leuprolide acetate (Lupron), 0.5-1.0 mg SQ daily × 6 months or 3.75-7.5 mg IM qmo × 6 months	Gonadotropin-releasing hormone; in premenopausal women, decreases estrogen to postmenopausal levels	***Contraindications:*** Hypersensitivity; thromboembolic disorders; undiagnosed vaginal bleeding ***Cost:*** 1 mg/0.2 ml, 2.8 ml: $260 ***Pregnancy category:*** X	Edema, hot flushes, decreased libido, amenorrhea, vaginal dryness
Nafarelin (Synarel) nasal spray, 1 spray (200 μg) into one nostril each morning and 1 spray into other nostril each evening	Analog of gonadotropin-releasing hormone; prevents stimulation of pituitary gland with repeated dosing	***Contraindications:*** Hypersensitivity; pregnancy; lactation; undiagnosed vaginal bleeding ***Cost:*** 10 ml: $323 ***Pregnancy category:*** X	Decreased libido, vaginal dryness, breast tenderness, increased pubic hair, headache, flushing, depression, insomnia, hot flushes, emotional lability, nasal irritation, acne, body odor, rhinitis, chest pain, urticaria

Enuresis

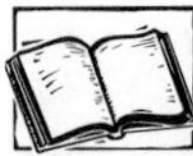

OVERVIEW

Enuresis is defined as involuntary urination. It may be classified as primary enuresis—in a child who has never been completely continent—or as secondary enuresis—return of involuntary urination after an extended period of continence.

Pathogenesis

Causes:

- Primary enuresis:
  - Idiopathic
  - Reduced bladder capacity
- Secondary enuresis:
  - Idiopathic
  - Bacteriuria
  - Glucosuria
  - Insufficient antidiuretic hormone
  - Renal tubular defect
  - Spinal cord malformation (rare)
  - Sickle cell disease
- Either type may be related to maturational lag or deep sleep

Patient Profile

- Males > Females
- Childhood predominant; most commonly, 3- to 6-year-olds; may occur up to age 18 years
- Family history of enuresis increases risk

Signs and Symptoms

- Urinating while asleep at least once a month
- Diurnal may have urinary frequency, dysuria, incontinence with increased intraabdominal pressure

Differential Diagnosis

- Diabetes insipidus
- Diabetes mellitus
- Renal tubular defects
- Spinal cord malformations or tumors
- Sickle cell disease

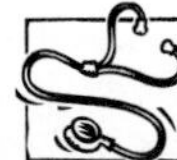

ASSESSMENT

History

Inquire about:

- Onset and duration of symptoms
- Dysuria
- Nocturnal or diurnal
- Family history of enuresis
- Sleep disorders
- Psychologic factors
- Treatments tried and results
- Underlying conditions
- Current medications

Physical Findings

Physical examination may be normal; look for:

- Abdominal masses
- Anomalous genitalia
- Increased BP

Initial Workup

Laboratory: Urinalysis, urine culture, serum glucose, if indicated

Radiology: Intravenous pyelogram, renal ultrasound, voiding cystourethrogram, if indicated

Further Workup

Usually none needed

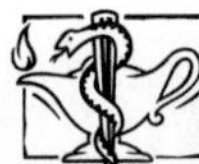

INTERVENTIONS

Office Treatment

Reassurance and support

Lifestyle Modifications

- Parents need to be supportive
- Bed-wetting alarm
- No fluids 2 hours before bed

Patient Education

Teach patient and parents about:

- Condition and treatment—increased fluids during the day and less frequent urination to stretch bladder
- No fluids 2 hours before bed
- Using plastic cover on mattress, extra-thick underwear, towel under child
- Not blaming child (encourage parents *not* to punish child; encourage praise on dry nights)
- Bed-wetting alarms
- Condition usually being self-limiting
- Medications used and side effects (see Pharmacotherapeutics)

Referral

To specialist if indicated

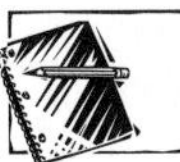

EVALUATION

Outcome
Usually self-limiting problem that resolves by puberty

Possible Complications
- Poor self-esteem
- Urinary tract infection

Follow-up
Initially weekly to provide both parents and child with support and encouragement

FOR YOUR INFORMATION

Life Span
Pediatric: Is primarily a pediatric condition
Geriatric: N/A
Pregnancy: Can be a causative factor

Miscellaneous
Adequate time should be given to trying conservative treatments before starting medications.

References
Driscoll CE: The genitourinary system. In Driscoll CE et al, editors: *The family practice desk reference,* ed 3, St Louis, 1996, Mosby, p 338.

Gilman CM, Mooney KH, Andrews MM: Alterations of renal and urinary tract function in children. In McCance KL, Huether SE, editors: *Pathophysiology: the biologic basis for disease in adults and children,* ed 2, St Louis, 1994, Mosby, pp 1276-1277.

NOTES

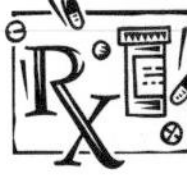

PHARMACOTHERAPEUTICS

Drug of Choice	Mechanism of Action	Prescribing Information	Side Effects
Imipramine (Tofranil), 1-2 mg/kg PO hs, maximum dose 50 mg	Tricyclic antidepressant; increases action of norepinephrine and serotonin by blocking their reuptake	***Contraindications:*** Hypersensitivity; convulsive disorders ***Cost:*** 10-mg tab, 100 tabs: $2-$25 ***Pregnancy category:*** C	Agranulocytosis, thrombocytopenia, eosinophilia, leukopenia, dizziness, drowsiness, confusion, headache, anxiety, tremors, insomnia, nightmares, diarrhea, dry mouth, nausea, vomiting, paralytic ileus, increased appetite, urinary retention, acute renal failure, rash, urticaria, pruritus, orthostatic hypotension, ECG changes, tachycardia, hypertension, tinnitus, blurred vision
Desmopressin (DDAVP), 20-40 μg intranasally hs	Synthetic antidiuretic hormone	***Contraindications:*** Hypersensitivity; nephrogenic diabetes insipidus ***Cost:*** Nasal solution 0.1 mg/ml, 2.5 ml: $54 ***Pregnancy category:*** B	Nasal irritation, nasal congestion, rhinitis, drowsiness, headache, lethargy, flushing, vulvar pain, nausea, heartburn, cramps, increased blood pressure

Epididymitis

OVERVIEW

Epididymitis is inflammation of the epididymis. The epididymis is one of a pair of coiled ducts that carry sperm from the testicles to the vas deferans.

Pathogenesis

- Prepubertal boys:
  - Coliform bacteria
  - Congenital abnormalities
- Postpubertal boys and men up to age 35 years: most common cause—*Neisseria gonorrheae* or *Chlamydia trachomatis*
- Men over age 35 years:
  - Coliform bacteria
  - Pseudomonads
  - Distal urinary tract obstruction
  - Tuberculosis

Patient Profile

- Males
- Most common in postpubertal boys and men up to age 35 years who are sexually active.

Signs and Symptoms

- Acute scrotal pain
- May have gradual onset of pain, dysuria, urethral discharge (possibly)
- Fever
- Scrotal swelling on affected side
- Nausea and vomiting (rarely)

Differential Diagnosis

- Testicular torsion—medical emergency
- Mumps orchitis
- Testicular tumor
- Spermatocele
- Hydrocele
- Varicocele
- Epididymal cyst

ASSESSMENT

History

Inquire about:

- Onset and duration of symptoms (pain begins over several hours)
- Urethral discharge
- Scrotal pain
- Dysuria and urinary frequency and urgency
- Fever
- Symptoms in sexual partner
- New sexual partner
- Underlying conditions
- Current medications

Physical Findings

- Edema and erythema of scrotum
- Tender testis—position, size, consistency normal
- Positive Prehn's sign—passive elevation of testis relieves pain
- Rectal examination—may have prostate tenderness

Initial Workup

Laboratory

- Urinalysis—pyuria, leukocytosis
- Cultures for gonorrhea and chlamydial infection
- Urine culture
- Gram stain of urethral discharge if present

Radiology: Ultrasound of scrotum, radionuclide scan, if uncertain of diagnosis

Further Workup

None indicated

INTERVENTIONS

Office Treatment

None indicated

Lifestyle Modifications

- Safe sex practices
- Increased fluids

Patient Education

Teach patient about:

- Condition and treatment:
  - Antimicrobials
  - Bed rest for 1 to 2 days
  - Scrotal support, elevation
  - Sitz bath
  - Ice packs
- Safe sex practices to prevent future infections (use of condoms and limiting number of partners)
- Importance of finishing all antibiotics
- Alerting sexual partner of need to obtain treatment
- No sexual intercourse until treatment is complete, symptoms resolve, and partner is treated
- Medications used and side effects (see Pharmacotherapeutics).

Referral

To MD for treatment failure

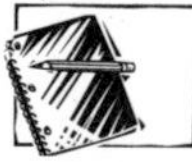

EVALUATION

Outcome

Resolves without sequelae

Possible Complications

- Recurrent epididymitis
- Infertility
- Fournier's gangrene

Follow-up

- For postpubertal boys and men <35 years, none necessary if symptoms resolve
- For older men, repeat urine culture after treatment

FOR YOUR INFORMATION

Life Span

Pediatric: Usually coliform bacteria is causative

Geriatric: Symptoms may not be indicative of severity of disease

Pregnancy: N/A

Miscellaneous

Pain improves within a week or less. Swelling may last weeks or months.

References

Bartlett JG: *Pocket book of infectious disease therapy,* ed 7, Baltimore, 1996, Williams & Wilkins, p 312.

Denman SJ, Murphy PA: Genitourinary infections. In Barker LR, Burton JR, Zieve PD, editors: *Principles of ambulatory medicine,* ed 4, Baltimore, 1995, Williams & Wilkins, p 326.

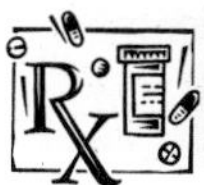

PHARMACOTHERAPEUTICS

For postpubertal boys and men <35 years who are sexually active, treat empirically for STDs.

Drug of Choice	Mechanism of Action	Prescribing Information	Side Effects
For gonorrhea:			
Ceftriaxone (Rocephin), 250 mg IM × 1 dose; children, 125 mg IM × 1 dose	Cephalosporin; inhibits cell wall synthesis	***Contraindication:*** Hypersensitivity ***Cost:*** 250-mg vial, 1 vial: $11 ***Pregnancy category:*** B	Headache; dizziness; weakness; paresthesia; fever; chills; nausea, vomiting; diarrhea; anorexia; pain; glossitis; increased AST, ALT, bilirubin, LDH, and alkaline phosphatase; pseudomembranous colitis; nephrotoxicity; renal failure; leukopenia; thrombocytopenia; agranulocytosis; neutropenia; pancytopenia; rash; urticaria; anaphylaxis
For chlamydial infection, use one of the following:			
Doxycycline (Doryx), 100 mg PO bid × 10-14 days; children >8 years, 4.4 mg/kg/day divided q12h	Tetracycline; inhibits protein synthesis	***Contraindications:*** Hypersensitivity; children <8 years ***Cost:*** 100-mg tab, 20 tabs: $5 ***Pregnancy category:*** D	Eosinophilia, neutropenia, thrombocytopenia, hemolytic anemia, dysphagia, glossitis, nausea, abdominal pain, vomiting, diarrhea, anorexia, hepatotoxicity, flatulence, abdominal cramps, gastritis, pericarditis, rash, urticaria, exfoliative dermatitis, angioedema
Azithromycin (Zithromax), 1 g PO × 1 dose	Macrolide; suppresses protein synthesis	***Contraindication:*** Hypersensitivity ***Cost:*** 250-mg tab, 18 tabs: $147 ***Pregnancy category:*** B	Rash, urticaria, pruritus, dizziness, headache, vertigo, diarrhea, hepatotoxicity, abdominal pain, cholestatic jaundice, flatulence, moniliasis
Erythromycin (E-Base), 500 mg PO qid × 10-14 days; children, 30-50 mg/kg/day in divided doses q12h	Macrolide; suppresses protein synthesis	***Contraindication:*** Hypersensitivity ***Cost:*** 500-mg tab, 100 tabs: $17 ***Pregnancy category:*** B	Rash, urticaria, pruritus, nausea, vomiting, diarrhea, hepatotoxicity, abdominal pain, stomatitis, heartburn, moniliasis
For both gonorrhea and chlamydial infection:			
Ofloxacin, 300 mg PO bid × 10 days (useful for urinary tract infection [UTI] pending culture results)	Fluoroquinolone; interferes with conversion of intermediate DNA fragments into high molecular weight DNA	***Contraindication:*** Hypersensitivity ***Cost:*** 300-mg tab, 50 tabs: $182 ***Pregnancy category:*** C	Headache, dizziness, fatigue, insomnia, depression, nausea, diarrhea, increased ALT and AST, flatulence, rash, pruritus, urticaria, fever, blurred vision, tinnitus
For men >35 years with bacteriuria, use one of the following:			
Trimethoprim/sulfamethoxazole (Septra DS), 1 DS tab PO bid × 10-14 days	Sulfamethoxazole interferes with synthesis of proteins; trimethoprim blocks synthesis of tetrahydrofolic acid	***Contraindications:*** Hypersensitivity; megaloblastic anemia; creatinine clearance <15 ml/min; lactation ***Cost:*** DS tab, 20 tabs: $3-$4 ***Pregnancy category:*** C	Headache, insomnia, hallucinations, vertigo, depression, allergic myocarditis, nausea, vomiting, abdominal pain, stomatitis, hepatitis, enterocolitis, renal failure, toxic nephrosis, leukopenia, neutropenia, agranulocytosis, hemolytic anemia, rash, Stevens-Johnson syndrome, anaphylaxis
Ciprofloxacin (Cipro), 500 mg PO bid × 10 days	Fluoroquinolone; interferes with conversion of intermediate DNA fragments into high molecular weight DNA	***Contraindication:*** Hypersensitivity ***Cost:*** 500-mg tab, 100 tabs: $302 ***Pregnancy category:*** C	Headache, dizziness, fatigue, insomnia, depression, nausea, diarrhea, increased ALT and AST, flatulence, rash, pruritus, urticaria, fever, blurred vision, tinnitus

OVERVIEW

Epiglottitis is an acute inflammation of the epiglottis and its surrounding structures.

Pathogenesis

Cause:

- Children—*Haemophilus influenzae*
- Adults—*H. influenzae* and group A streptococcus

Patient Profile

- Males = Females
- Any age; most common in 3- to 7-year-olds

Signs and Symptoms

- Fever
- Dysphagia
- Drooling
- Sore throat
- Cervical adenopathy
- Respiratory distress
- Muffled voice
- May sit propped up on hands with head forward and tongue out (tripod position)

Differential Diagnosis

- Viral croup
- Aspirated foreign body
- Peritonsillar abscesses
- Sepsis

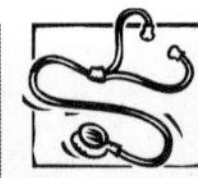

ASSESSMENT

History

Inquire about:

- Onset and duration of symptoms (onset usually sudden)
- Recent upper respiratory tract infection (usually none)
- Underlying conditions
- Current medications

Physical Findings

- Fever
- Drooling
- Assumes tripod position for easier breathing
- Stridor on inspiration
- Cervical adenopathy
- Oropharynx—may be erythematous (important clue to diagnosis, but may be relatively normal-appearing oropharynx)
- *Do not* attempt to visualize epiglottis with tongue blade—total obstruction may occur!

Initial Workup

Laboratory

- Blood culture
- Epiglottis culture—*do not* swab epiglottis outside of an emergency room—have adequate support people and equipment available for possible tracheostomy

Radiology: Chest film—PA and lateral—pneumonia can be a complication

Further Workup

None indicated

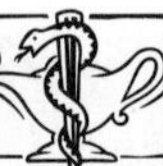

INTERVENTIONS

Office Treatment

Direct hospital admission, possibly to intensive care unit

Lifestyle Modification

Hospitalization

Patient Education

Teach patient about:

- Condition and treatment:
  - Hospitalization
  - Intubation to help with breathing (usually mechanical ventilation not necessary)
  - Intravenous fluids and antibiotics
- Medications used and side effects (see Pharmacotherapeutics)

Referral

To MD for hospitalization if NP does not have privileges

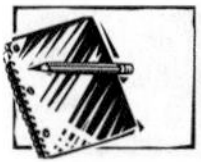

EVALUATION

Outcome
Prognosis good with appropriate treatment

Possible Complications
- Pneumonia
- Meningitis
- Septic arthritis
- Pericarditis
- Death from asphyxia

Follow-up
1 week after hospitalization, by NP or MD

FOR YOUR INFORMATION

Life Span
Pediatric: Most common in this age group
Geriatric: Higher mortality rate
Pregnancy: Cautious use of medications

Miscellaneous
N/A

References
Jackler RK, Kaplan MJ: Ear, nose, and throat. In Tierney LM Jr, McPhee SJ, Papadakis MA, editors: *Current medical diagnosis and treatment,* ed 34, Norwalk, Conn, 1995, Appleton & Lange, p 195.

Koster FT, Barker LR: Respiratory tract infections. In Barker LR, Burton JR, Zieve PD, editors: *Principles of ambulatory medicine,* ed 4, Baltimore, 1995, Williams & Wilkins, p 339.

NOTES

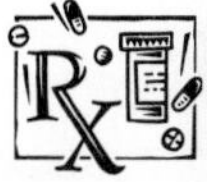

PHARMACOTHERAPEUTICS

Drug of Choice	Mechanism of Action	Prescribing Information	Side Effects
Cefuroxime, (Zinacef), 150 mg/kg/day IV in divided doses q6h	Cephalosporin; inhibits cell wall synthesis	***Contraindication:*** Hypersensitivity ***Cost:*** 1.5-g vial, 10 vials: $140 ***Pregnancy category:*** B	Headache, dizziness, weakness, nausea, vomiting, diarrhea, anorexia, pain, glossitis, pseudomembranous colitis, proteinuria, vaginitis, nephrotoxicity, renal failure, leukopenia, thrombocytopenia, agranulocytosis, neutropenia, lymphocytosis, eosinophilia, hemolytic anemia, rash, urticaria, dyspnea, anaphylaxis

Epistaxis

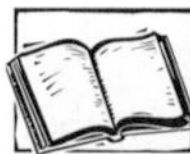

OVERVIEW

Epistaxis is a nosebleed. It may be an anterior bleed, which occurs at Kiesselbach's plexus or at the anterior end of the inferior turbinate; or it may be a posterior bleed, which occurs under the posterior half of the inferior turbinate or at the roof of the nasal cavity.

Pathogenesis

Causes:

- Idiopathic (most common)
- Trauma—nose picking, foreign body, fist
- Infection
- Vascular abnormalities
- Coagulation defects—anticoagulant therapy, hemophilia
- Septal perforation or deviation
- Hypertension
- Neoplasm

Patient Profile

- Males = Females
- Most common—children <10 years and adults >50 years

Signs and Symptoms

- Bleeding from nostril
- Posterior bleed—may present with hemoptysis, nausea, hematemesis, or melena

Differential Diagnosis

Epistaxis may be sign of many other diseases (see Pathogenesis)

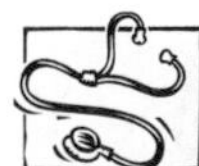

ASSESSMENT

History

Inquire about:

- Onset and duration of symptoms
- Precipitating factors
- Treatments tried and results
- Underlying conditions
- Current medications (especially use of aspirin and NSAIDs)

Physical Findings

Bleeding from one or both nostrils; if not actively bleeding, may see clot; attempt to locate site of bleed—light, suction, nasal speculum needed; clear cavity of blood or remove clot; usually only one bleeding site; if more, suspect systemic disease

Initial Workup

Laboratory: CBC, coagulation studies, if indicated

Radiology: Sinus films, if indicated

Further Workup

None indicated

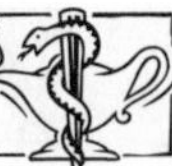

INTERVENTIONS

Office Treatment

- Anterior bleed—insert pledget soaked in vasoconstrictor and local anesthetic; pinch nostril for several minutes; remove pledget; visualize vessel and cauterize with silver nitrate; if unsuccessful, apply second dose of anesthetic and vasoconstrictor and pack with ribbon petrolatum (Vaseline) gauze; insert in folding layers; apply 2 × 2 gauze over nostril
- Posterior bleed or unsuccessful with above treatment—refer to emergency room for further treatment

Lifestyle Modifications

- Application of petrolatum to nostrils to prevent drying
- Smoking cessation and alcohol cessation if appropriate
- Humidification to prevent drying

Patient Education

Teach patient about:

- Cause of nosebleed if known
- How to stop bleed—sit up, lean forward, compress nostrils together, apply ice to bridge of nose
- Medications used and side effects (see Pharmacotherapeutics)

Referral

To emergency room if treatment unsuccessful

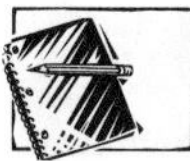

EVALUATION

Outcome
Nosebleed stops—minimal blood loss

Possible Complications
- Shock secondary to large amount of blood loss
- Sinusitis
- Septal hematoma or abscess from packing
- Septal perforation secondary to zealous cauterization
- Vasovagal episode during packing or unpacking

Follow-up
In 24 to 48 hours to remove packing

FOR YOUR INFORMATION

Life Span
Pediatric: Anterior bleed more likely
Geriatric: Posterior bleed more likely; more likely to require hospitalization
Pregnancy: Epistaxis occurs easily because of a high level of circulating estrogen

Miscellaneous
Epistaxis is not a disease, but rather a sign or symptom. The majority of cases are idiopathic, with fewer than 10% being caused by a neoplasm or coagulopathy.

References

Bull TR: *Color atlas of E.N.T. diagnosis,* ed 3, London, 1995, Mosby-Wolfe, pp 140-143.

Uphold CR, Graham MV: Clinical guidelines in adult health, Gainesville, Fla, 1994, Barmarrae Books, pp 239-242.

NOTES

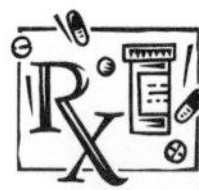

PHARMACOTHERAPEUTICS

Drug of Choice	Mechanism of Action	Prescribing Information	Side Effects
Phenylephrine 0.25%; epinephrine 1:1000; soak pledget in one of these solutions and with one of the anesthetic agents below	Vasoconstrictor; sympathomimetic	***Contraindications:*** Narrow-angle glaucoma; cerebrovascular disease; hypertension ***Cost:*** Minimal ***Pregnancy category:*** C	Anxiety, headache, fear, palpitations, reflex bradycardia, restlessness
Cocaine 4%; lidocaine jelly 2%; lidocaine solution 4%; lidocaine viscous 2%; see instructions above	Local anesthesia; blocks nerve impulse; cocaine also has some vasoconstrictive properties	***Contraindication:*** Hypersensitivity ***Cost:*** Minimal ***Pregnancy category:*** Cocaine—C; lidocaine—B	Resuscitation drugs and equipment should be available when using a local anesthetic, lightheadedness, nervousness, restlessness, drowsiness, blurred vision, bradycardia

Erectile Dysfunction/Impotence

OVERVIEW

Erectile dysfunction can be described as a persistent or recurrent problem with attaining or maintaining penile erection or dissatisfaction with the size or rigidity of the penile erection.

Pathogenesis

Many causes:

- Endocrine disorder—low or high thyroxine level, low testosterone level, high prolactin level, diabetes, high estrogen level, renal failure
- Neurologic disorder—central, spinal, or peripheral nervous system problem
- Vascular disorder—arterial insufficiency, cavernosal insufficiency, venous insufficiency
- Medication—beta-blockers, thiazide diuretics
- Psychologic disorder—schizophrenia, depression, anxiety, personality disorder
- Structural disorder—Peyronie's disease, phimosis, postoperative sequelae
- Idiopathic
- Prostatic infection
- Penile skin infection

Patient Profile

- Males
- Any age after puberty

Signs and Symptoms

- Inability to obtain/maintain erection (may be only symptom)
- Reduced body hair
- Gynecomastia
- Testicular atrophy
- Peripheral vascular disease
- Neuropathy

Differential Diagnosis

Any of the many causes listed under Pathogenesis

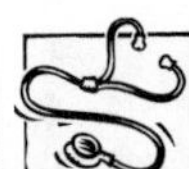

ASSESSMENT

History

Inquire about:

- Onset and duration of symptoms
- Past sexual experiences and behaviors
- Past medical and surgical history (particularly genitourinary history)
- Smoking history
- Underlying conditions
- Current medications

Physical Findings

Physical examination may be within normal limits or may find:

- Decreased body hair
- Diminished peripheral pulses
- Gynecomastia
- Deformed penis
- Abnormal neurologic examination
- Increased BP

Initial Workup

Laboratory

- CBC
- Serum chemistry panel to include electrolytes, BUN, creatinine, albumin, glucose
- TSH
- Prolactin and testosterone levels

Radiology: Doppler studies, angiogram, cavernosogram—depends on possible cause

Further Workup

If indicated:

- Nocturnal penile tumescence testing
- Penile blood pressure
- Sacral evoked response
- Dorsal nerve somatosensory evoked potentials

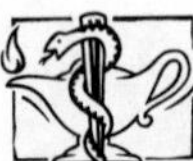

INTERVENTIONS

Office Treatment

None indicated

Lifestyle Modifications

- Smoking and alcohol cessation
- Compliance with treatment plan for any underlying conditions

Patient Education

Teach patient about:

- Condition and treatment options—treat underlying conditions such as diabetes, thyroid dysfunction (may or may not reverse erectile dysfunction)
- Use of vacuum erectile device
- Penile injections (may be used in combination with vacuum device)
- Trial period off of offending medications
- Penile implants
- Importance of including partner in treatment
- Medications used and side effects (see Pharmacotherapeutics)

Referrals

Depends on cause—may need psychiatrist, sex therapist, urologist, plastic surgeon, endocrinologist, neurologist, vascular surgeon

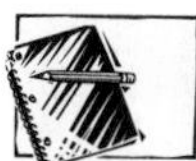

EVALUATION

Outcome
Depends on cause and willingness of patient to follow treatment plan; 15% will have a spontaneous cure

Possible Complications
Side effects of injection therapy:
- Priapism
- Fibrosis
- Hypotension
- Nausea
- Infection

Follow-up
In 2 weeks; then monthly to evaluate treatment; may need more frequent visits for specific underlying condition

FOR YOUR INFORMATION

Life Span
Pediatric: May have congenital anomaly
Geriatric: Impotence is *not* a normal part of aging
Pregnancy: N/A

Miscellaneous
Many patients will not initiate a conversation regarding erectile dysfunction. If the NP is treating the patient for a condition or with medications that can cause erectile dysfunction, it is appropriate to periodically ask the patient if he is experiencing any problems in his sexual experiences. By doing so, it lets the patient know that the NP is willing to discuss this sensitive issue.

Reference
Schmidt CW: Sexual disorders. In Barker LR, Burton JR, Zieve PD, editors: *Principles of ambulatory medicine,* ed 4, Baltimore, 1995, Williams & Wilkins, pp 194-199.

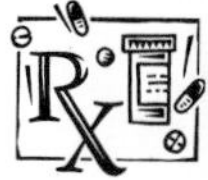

PHARMACOTHERAPEUTICS

Drug of Choice	Mechanism of Action	Prescribing Information	Side Effects
For hypogonadism:			
Testosterone cypionate (Testone LA 200), 200 mg IM q2wk	Replaces testosterone	***Contraindications:*** Hypersensitivity; severe renal, hepatic, or cardiac disease ***Cost:*** 200 mg/ml, 10 ml: $9-$58 ***Pregnancy category:*** X	Rash, acne, oily hair and skin, sweating, dizziness, headache, fatigue, anxiety, insomnia, cramps, muscle spasms, increased blood pressure, hematuria, testicular atrophy, nausea, vomiting, weight gain, cholestatic jaundice, nasal congestion
For hyperprolactinemia:			
Bromocriptine (Parlodel), 2.5-mg ½ tab PO daily; may increase q3-7d; therapeutic range, 2.5-15 mg/day	Inhibits prolactin release	***Contraindications:*** Hypersensitivity to ergot; severe ischemic disease; severe peripheral vascular disease ***Cost:*** 2.5-mg tab, 30 tabs: $44 ***Pregnancy category:*** D	Blurred vision, nasal congestion, headache, depression, restlessness, nervousness, convulsions, hallucinations, anxiety, dizziness, fatigue, urinary frequency and retention, nausea, vomiting, anorexia, cramps, constipation, rash, alopecia, orthostatic hypotension, shock, dysrhythmias
For impotence of vascular, diabetic, or psychogenic origin:			
Yohimbine hydrochloride (Erex), 5.4 mg, 1 tab PO tid; if side effects occur, decrease to ½ tab tid; usually prescribed by a urologist	Alpha-2 adrenergic blocker	***Contraindications:*** Hypersensitivity; renal diseases ***Cost:*** 5.4-mg tab, 100 tabs: $10-$30 ***Pregnancy category:*** Should *not* be used	Antidiuresis, increased BP, increased heart rate, nervousness, irritability, tremor, dizziness, headache, skin flushing

Injection therapy with papaverine and phentolamine should be prescribed by a professional with experience in using this treatment.

Erysipelas

OVERVIEW

Erysipelas is an acute, inflammatory form of cellulitis. It differs from other types of cellulitis in that it involves the lymphatics. It is usually more superficial, with well-defined margins. It is also called St. Anthony's fire.

Pathogenesis
Causes:
- Group A beta-hemolytic streptococcus
- *Streptococcus pyogenes*
- Rarely, *Staphylococcus aureus*
- May be due to trauma to area

Patient Profile
- Males = Females
- Usually infants and adults >40 years
- Highest incidence in elderly >75 years

Signs and Symptoms
- Prodrome of malaise, fever, and chills
- Headache and vomiting
- Arthralgias
- Pruritis
- Skin discomfort
- Vesicles
- Mild, superficial pain
- Erythematous patch with sharply demarcated, raised borders
- Peau d'orange appearance to skin
- Most common areas involved—lower legs, face, and ears; usually unilateral

Differential Diagnosis
- Contact dermatitis
- Angioneurotic edema
- Scarlet fever
- Lupus
- Polychondritis
- Dermatophytid
- Tuberculoid leprosy

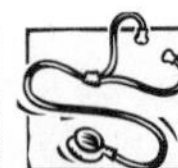

ASSESSMENT

History
Inquire about:
- Onset and duration of symptoms
- Prodromal symptoms
- History of prior erysipelas
- History of wound to area
- Chronic diseases
- Remedies tried and results
- Underlying conditions
- Current medications

Physical Findings
- Previous wound site (will probably not be visible)
- Intense erythema with "streaking" due to involvement of lymphatics
- Peau d'orange appearance to skin
- Mild pain
- Vesicles
- Mild pruritis
- Examination of entire skin area—most common area involved is lower legs, face, and ears, usually unilateral

Initial Workup
Laboratory
- CBC—will have leukocytosis
- Culture of exudate, if any
- Blood culture if concern about systemic infection

Radiology: None indicated

Further Workup
None indicated

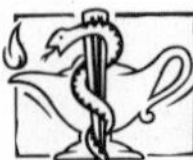

INTERVENTIONS

Office Treatment
None indicated

Lifestyle Modification
Care to avoid injuries

Patient Education
Teach patient about:
- Condition and treatment—antibiotics; warm, moist heat
- Need to seek prompt treatment if symptoms return (chronic form can occur)
- Facial erysipelas—instruct men not to shave during infection and for at least 5 days after resolution
- Medications used and side effects (see Pharmacotherapeutics)

Referral
To MD for resistant cases

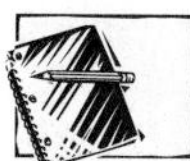

EVALUATION

Outcomes
- Full recovery
- May have chronic edema and scarring

Possible Complications
- Bacteremia
- Scarlet fever
- Pneumonia
- Abscess
- Embolism
- Gangrene
- Meningitis
- Sepsis
- Death

Follow-up
In 48 hours; then in 2 weeks

FOR YOUR INFORMATION

Life Span
Pediatric: In infants, abdomen may be involved

Geriatric: Higher morbidity and mortality

Pregnancy: Cautious use of medication

Miscellaneous
According to Bratton and Neese (1995), erysipelas, a once common disease, had all but disappeared after the advent of antibiotics. However, in the past few years the incidence has been increasing, perhaps because of resistant strains of bacteria.

References

Bratton RL, Nesse RE: St. Anthony's fire: diagnosis and management of erysipelas, *Am Fam Physician* 51(2):401-404, 1995.

Bull TR: *Color atlas of E.N.T. diagnosis,* ed 3, London, 1995, Mosby-Wolfe, p 54.

Habif TP: *Clinical dermatology: a color guide to diagnosis and therapy,* ed 3, St Louis, 1996, Mosby, p 242.

NOTES

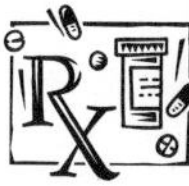

PHARMACOTHERAPEUTICS

Drug of Choice	Mechanism of Action	Prescribing Information	Side Effects
Penicillin VK, 500 mg PO qid for 10 days; children <12 years, 15-50 mg/kg/day PO in divided doses q6h	Bactericidal cell wall inhibitor; effective against gram-positive cocci, most anaerobes, and *Neisseria*	***Contraindications:*** Hypersensitivity; neonates ***Cost:*** 500-mg tab, 40 tabs: $3 ***Pregnancy category:*** B	Hypersensitivity reactions, anaphalaxis or hemolysis, rare neurologic toxicity, neutropenia, nephrotoxicity, bone marrow depression, granulocytopenia, nausea, vomiting, diarrhea, oliguria, proteinuria, vaginitis, anxiety, depression, convulsions
Dicloxacillin (Dynapen), 250-500 mg PO qid; children, 12.5-25 mg/kg/day PO in divided doses q6h	Broad-spectrum penicillin; bactericidal cell wall inhibitor; effective against gram-positive cocci except enterococci; penicillinase resistant	***Contraindication:*** Hypersensitivity ***Cost:*** 500-mg tab, 50 tabs: $19-$88 ***Pregnancy category:*** B	Hypersensitivity reactions, anaphalaxis or hemolysis, rare neurologic toxicity, neutropenia, nephrotoxicity, bone marrow depression, granulocytopenia, nausea, vomiting, diarrhea, oliguria, proteinuria, vaginitis, anxiety, depression, convulsions
Erythromycin (E.E.S.), 500 mg PO bid × 10 days; Children, 30-50 mg/kg/day in 4 divided doses × 10 days; may be used for prophylaxis or established infections	Macrolide; protein synthesis inhibitor; active against bacteria lacking cell walls, most gram-positive aerobes	***Contraindication:*** Hypersensitivity ***Cost:*** 250-mg tabs, 4/day × 10 days: $4 ***Pregnancy category:*** B	Nausea, vomiting, diarrhea, abdominal pain, anorexia, rash, urticaria, pseudomembranous colitis—rarely

Erythema Multiforme

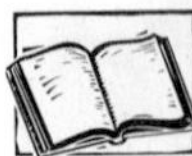

OVERVIEW

Erythema multiforme is a relatively common, acute, self-limiting hypersensitivity reaction. It involves the skin and mucous membranes.

Pathogenesis

- Recent studies—immune complex formation and deposition in cutaneous microvasculature
- Complexes may involve C3, IgM, and fibrin
- 50% of cases—idiopathic
- Other 50% caused by viral infections (herpes simplex), bacterial infections, protozoan infections, collagen vascular disease, medications (penicillins, sulfonamides, barbiturates, salicylates, etc.), vaccines, malignancy, pregnancy, premenstrual hormonal changes, consumption of beer, Reiter's syndrome, sarcoidosis

Patient Profile

- Males > Females
- Peak incidence in 20s and 30s; rare <3 years or >50 years of age

Signs and Symptoms

- May have prodrome of fever, malaise, or itching or burning at site of eruption
- Target lesions and papules—dusky red to purple, round maculopapules or vesicles appear symmetrically on backs of hands, feet, forearms, and lower legs
- Target lesions—papules or vesicles surrounded by normal skin with halo or erythema
- Lesions may ulcerate, encrust, erode, and become infected

Differential Diagnosis

- Urticaria
- Necrotizing vasculitis
- Drug eruptions
- Contact dermatitis
- Pityriasis rosea
- Secondary syphilis
- Ringworm
- Pemphigus vulgaris
- Pemphigoid
- Dermatitis herpetiformis
- Septicemia
- Serum sickness
- Viral exanthems
- Rocky Mountain spotted fever
- Collagen vascular disease
- Mucocutaneous lymph node syndrome
- Meningococcemia
- Lichen planus
- Behçet's syndrome

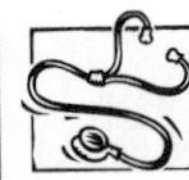

ASSESSMENT

History

Inquire about:

- Onset and duration of symptoms
- Location of lesions
- History of any causative events or agents (see Pathogenesis)
- History of allergies
- Underlying conditions
- Current medications

Physical Findings

- Target lesions and papules—backs of hands, feet, forearms, and lower legs
- Assess entire skin surface
- May have urticarial plaques without target lesions
- May have vesiculobullous formation—red, edematous plaques with vesicles or bullae
- Can progress to Stevens-Johnson syndrome (mucosal erosion and epidermal detachment <10% of involved area) or toxic epidermal necrolysis (more than 30% of involved area shows epidermal detachment)

Initial Workup

Laboratory: None indicated
Radiology: None indicated

Further Workup

None indicated

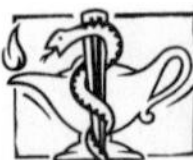

INTERVENTIONS

Lifestyle Modification

Withdrawal of offending agent if identified

Patient Education

Teach patient about:

- Condition and treatment:
  - Mild cases resolve without treatment (few lesions)
  - Many target lesions—oral prednisone over 1 to 3 weeks
- Importance of avoiding offending agent if identified
- Keeping lesions clean—cool compresses for mild cases; Burow's solution or Domeboro solution dressings for more severe cases
- Increasing fluid intake
- Using warm saline rinses or solution of diphenhydramine, lidocaine (Xylocaine), and Kaopectate for oral lesions
- Medications used and side effects (see Pharmacotherapeutics)

Office Treatment

None indicated

Referral

To MD if condition is severe or progressing

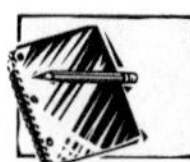

EVALUATION

Outcomes

- Resolves in 4 to 5 weeks, generally without scarring
- May have some hyperpigmentation present
- Risk of recurrence as much as 37%

Possible Complications

- Progression to Stevens-Johnson syndrome or toxic epidermal necrosis
- Secondary infection

Follow-up

Follow closely; return visit 48 hours after initial visit; then weekly until resolution, with telephone contact in between visits

FOR YOUR INFORMATION

Life Span

Pediatric: Rarely seen <3 years of age
Geriatric: Rarely seen >50 years of age
Pregnancy: May be a causative factor; cautious use of medication

Miscellaneous

Stevens-Johnson syndrome and toxic epidermal necrolysis are more severe forms of this disease. These syndromes require prompt hospitalization and aggressive treatment.

Reference

Habif TP: *Clinical dermatology: a color guide to diagnosis and therapy,* ed 3, St Louis, 1996, Mosby, pp 566-571.

NOTES

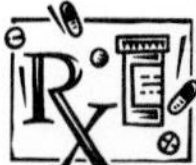

PHARMACOTHERAPEUTICS

Mild cases are not treated systemically.

Drug of Choice	Mechanism of Action	Prescribing Information	Side Effects
Prednisone 40-80 mg/day for 1-3 weeks, then taper quickly over 1 week	Corticosteroid; decreases inflammation	***Contraindications:*** Hypersensitivity; psychosis; idiopathic thrombocytopenia; acute glomerulonephritis; amebiasis; nonasthmatic bronchial disease; AIDS; TB; children <2 years old ***Cost:*** 15-mg tab, 100 tabs: $14-$35 ***Pregnancy category:*** C	Hypertension, circulatory collapse, thrombophlebitis, embolism, tachycardia, fungal infections, increased intraocular pressure, diarrhea, nausea, GI hemorrhage, thrombocytopenia, acne, poor wound healing, fractures, osteoporosis, weakness

Erythema Nodosum

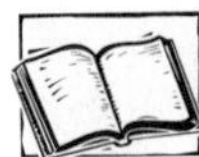

OVERVIEW

Erythema nodosum is characterized by nodular erythematous eruptions. The eruptions occur most commonly on the extensor aspects of the extremities, primarily the shins.

Pathogenesis

- Probably delayed hypersensitivity reaction
- Causes:
  - Idiopathic
  - Bacterial infections—streptococcal infections, tuberculosis, leprosy, *Campylobacter* infections, salmonella, shigella, gonorrhea
  - Sarcoidosis
  - Drugs—sulfonamides, oral contraceptives, bromides
  - Pregnancy
  - Deep fungal infections
  - Viral infections
  - Enteropathies
  - Malignancies
  - Most common causes—streptococcal infection and tuberculosis in children; streptococcal infection and sarcoidosis in adults

Patient Profile

- Females > Males
- Predominant age—20 to 30 years

Signs and Symptoms

- Prodrome of fever, malaise, chills
- Raised, warm, tender, brightly erythematous nodules on anterior shins
- Nodules occur in crops over 2- to 3-week period
- Nodules turn blue in color late in course
- Arthralgias
- Hilar adenopathy

Differential Diagnosis

- Superficial thrombophlebitis
- Cellulitis
- Septic emboli
- Erythema induratum
- Nodular vasculitis
- Cutaneous polyarteritis nodosa
- Sarcoidosis granulomas
- Lymphoma

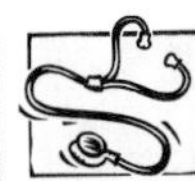

ASSESSMENT

History

Inquire about:

- Onset and duration of symptoms
- Prodrome of fever, malaise, upper respiratory tract infection—precedes eruptions by 1 to 3 weeks
- Previous infections
- History of allergic reactions
- Medications used in previous 2 months
- Underlying conditions
- Current medications

Physical Findings

- Eruptive phase:
  - Flulike symptoms with fever and generalized aching
  - Red nodelike lesions with edema appear on both shins
  - Poorly defined border
  - First week—lesions hard and painful
  - Second week—lesions fluctuant but do not suppurate; color changes from red to bluish; resembles a bruise
  - Individual lesions last about 2 weeks, but further eruptions can occur
- Aching of legs and swelling of ankles may persist for months or years

Initial Workup

Laboratory

- Sedimentation rate—elevated
- CBC—slight leukocytosis
- ASO titer
- Throat culture
- Stool culture and leukocytes if indicated
- Purified protein derivative (PPD) if indicated

Radiology: Chest film for hilar adenopathy or infiltrates

Further Workup

Depends on whether a cause is determined

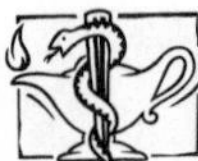

INTERVENTIONS

Office Treatment

Demonstrate use of elastic wraps or support stockings

Lifestyle Modifications

- Discontinuance of any drugs that could be causative agent
- Bed rest with legs elevated—most beneficial
- If other chronic illness identified, may need further lifestyle modifications

Patient Education

Teach patient about:

- Condition, cause if identified, and treatment—nonsteroidal antiinflammatory agents
- Lesions—will resolve in a couple of months
- Bed rest with legs elevated; if not possible, instruct on use of support stockings or elastic wraps
- Scarring does not normally occur
- Arthralgias—may persist for several years
- Recurrence—less than 20%
- Medications used and side effects (see Pharmacotherapeutics)

Referral

To primary care physician or dermatologist for severe cases

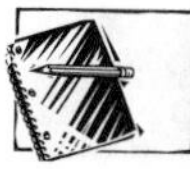

EVALUATION

Outcomes

- Lesions resolve in 3 to 6 weeks without scarring
- Total course—6 to 12 weeks
- Arthralgias may last years

Possible Complications

Complications from underlying condition

Follow-up

In 2 weeks; then monthly depending on causative agent

FOR YOUR INFORMATION

Life Span

Pediatric: Seen rarely in this age group; occurs equally in males and females
Geriatric: Not usually seen in this age group
Pregnancy: May have repeat episodes; pregnancy considered a causative factor

Miscellaneous

Erythema nodosum with hilar adenopathy (Lofgren's syndrome) is seen with multiple causes, not just sarcoidosis.

Reference

Habif TP: *Clinical dermatology: a color guide to diagnosis and therapy,* ed 3, St Louis, 1996, Mosby, pp 575-576.

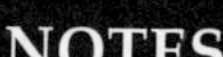

NOTES

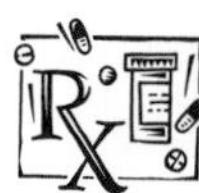

PHARMACOTHERAPEUTICS

Drug of Choice	Mechanism of Action	Prescribing Information	Side Effects
Aspirin, 325-650 mg PO q4-6h for fever and myalgia—do not use in children or adolescents because of risk of Reye's syndrome	Analgesia via peripheral and central nervous systems; may inhibit prostaglandins; antipyretic—acts on hypothalamic system	***Contraindications:*** Hypersensitivity; bleeding disorders or anticoagulant therapy; last trimester of pregnancy; asthma; gastric ulcers ***Cost:*** OTC ***Pregnancy category:*** D	Rash, anaphylactic reaction, GI upset and bleeding, Reye's syndrome in children and adolescents, nausea, vomiting, hepatitis, tinnitus, hearing loss, wheezing, pulmonary edema
Nonsteroidal antiinflammatory agents (NSAIDs): indomethacin, naproxen; dosage varies with agent; check package insert: • Indomethacin 75-150 mg/day in divided doses • Naproxen 500-1000 mg/day divided bid	Exact action unknown; may be caused by inhibition of synthesis of prostaglandins and arachidonic acid	***Contraindications:*** Hypersensitivity to NSAIDs, aspirin; severe hepatic failure; asthma ***Cost:*** Varies with type ***Pregnancy category:*** Depends on product	Stomach distress, flatulence, nausea, abdominal pain, constipation or diarrhea, dizziness, sedation, rash, urticaria, angioedema, anorexia, urinary frequency, increased blood pressure, insomnia, anxiety, visual disturbances, increased thirst, alopecia

Exfoliative Dermatitis

OVERVIEW

Exfoliative dermatitis is a scaling erythematous eruption that is generalized all over the body. It is also known as erythroderma and pityriasis rubra.

Pathogenesis

- 25% are idiopathic; 75% are secondary to cutaneous or systemic disease or medication reaction
- Causes:
  - Atopic dermatitis
  - Colon carcinoma
  - Contact dermatitis
  - Fungal disease with a reaction
  - Leukemia
  - Lichen planus
  - Lung carcinoma
  - Lymphoma
  - Medications such as sulfonamides and sulfones, penicillins, cephalosporins, anticonvulsants, NSAIDS, codeine, heavy metals, INH, quinidine, captopril, iodine, antimalarials
  - Multiple myeloma
  - Mycosis fungoides
  - Pemphigus foliaceus
  - Pityriasis rosea
  - Psoriasis
  - Reiter's syndrome
  - Scabies
  - Seborrheic dermatitis
  - Staphylococcal scaled skin syndrome
  - Stasis dermatitis
  - Toxic epidermal necrolysis

Patient Profile

- Males > Females
- 75% of patients >40 years of age

Signs and Symptoms

- Fine, generalized scales with mild erythema and lichenification of skin
- Initial distribution of rash is dictated by underlying causative condition; with progression, becomes scaly and generalized
- Sensation of skin tightness
- Nail dystrophy
- Hair loss
- Pruritus
- Fever
- Chills
- Malaise/weakness
- Anemia
- Eosinophilia
- Nontender generalized lymphadenopathy
- Steatorrhea
- Hepatomegaly
- Gynecomastia
- Hypoproteinemia
- Dehydration
- High-output cardiac failure
- Tachycardia
- REMEMBER: Signs and symptoms vary with underlying cause

Differential Diagnosis

- Contact dermatitis
- Drug eruptions

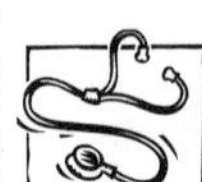

ASSESSMENT

History

Inquire about:

- Onset and duration of symptoms
- Treatments tried and results
- Fever, chills, malaise/weakness
- Past history of exfoliative dermatitis
- Underlying conditions
- Current and past medications

Physical Findings

- Fever, chills, malaise
- Generalized scales with mild erythema and lichenification of skin
- Examination of entire skin surface
- REMEMBER: Findings vary with causative agent

Initial Workup

Laboratory

- None diagnostic
- CBC—leukocytosis and eosinophilia
- Erythrocyte sedimentation rate (ESR)—elevated

Radiology: Chest film or other x-ray studied for underlying diseases

Further Workup

- None unless investigating an underlying disease
- Dermatologist may perform skin biopsy

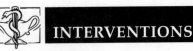

INTERVENTIONS

Office Treatment

None indicated

Lifestyle Modifications

- Avoidance of etiologic agent
- Cool colloid bath, rather than hot baths or showers

Patient Education

Teach patient about:

- Condition, cause, and treatment—topical or systemic steroids; may need to use occlusive dressings with topical steroids
- Stopping any offending agents
- Taking cool Aveeno baths
- Using moisturizing lotions
- Signs and symptoms of infection and to seek care immediately
- Underlying disease treatment and that control of underlying disease will control exfoliative dermatitis
- Idiopathic disease—many cases resolve spontaneously; only symptomatic treatment necessary
- Medications used and side effects (see Pharmacotherapeutics)

Referral

To dermatologist for severe cases or to specialist as determined by underlying cause

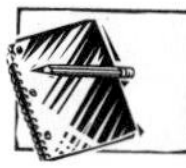

EVALUATION

Outcomes

- Depends on underlying disease or agent
- Idiopathic exfoliative dermatitis—prognosis is poor, with frequent recurrences

Possible Complications

- Secondary infection
- Debility from protein loss
- Dehydration

Follow-up

In 1 week; then every 2 weeks to monitor response to medications and side effects

FOR YOUR INFORMATION

Life Span

Pediatric: Rare in this age group, but may be associated with atopic dermatitis, medications, or inherited dermatoses
Geriatric: Monitor closely for protein depletion and dehydration
Pregnancy: Should be followed by a specialist.

Miscellaneous

N/A

References

Goldstein SM, Odom RB: Skin and appendages. In Tierney LM Jr, McPhee SJ, Papadakis MA, editors: *Current medical diagnosis and treatment,* ed 34, Norwalk Conn, 1995, Appleton & Lange, p 99.

Habif TP: *Clinical dermatology: a color guide to diagnosis and therapy,* ed 3, St Louis, 1996, Mosby, pp 436-438.

NOTES

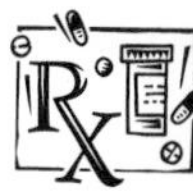

PHARMACOTHERAPEUTICS

Use steroids cautiously in patient with psoriasis. Prolonged use can cause pustular psoriasis.

Drug of Choice	Mechanism of Action	Prescribing Information	Side Effects
Prednisone 40 mg/day with increases of 20 mg/day if no response after 3-4 days; taper to control symptoms; for patients with idiopathic exfoliative dermatitis, may require long-term use to control disease	Corticosteroid; decreases inflammation	***Contraindications:*** Hypersensitivity; psychosis; idiopathic thrombocytopenia; acute glomerulonephritis; amebiasis; nonasthmatic bronchial disease; AIDS; TB; children <2 years old ***Cost:*** 15-mg tab, 100 tabs: $14-$35 ***Pregnancy category:*** C	Hypertension, circulatory collapse, thrombophlebitis, embolism, tachycardia, fungal infections, increased intraocular pressure, diarrhea, nausea, GI hemorrhage, thrombocytopenia, acne, poor wound healing, fractures, osteoporosis, weakness
Hydrocortisone cream, 1% for face (controversial—some feel corticosteroids should not be used on face) and 2.5% elsewhere; apply thin layer 3-4 times daily; for severe erythema, stronger corticosteroid may be needed: mometasone (Elocon), triamcinolone (Kenalog), betamethasone (Diprolene AF)	Antiinflammatory and antipruritic	***Contraindication:*** Hypersensitivity ***Cost:*** 1%, 30 g: $12; several available OTC; mometasone 0.1%, 45 g: $29; triamcinolone 0.025%, 30 g: $2-5; betamethasone 0.05%, 15 g: $3-$16 ***Pregnancy category:*** C	Burning, dryness, itching, irritation, acne, folliculitis, hypertrichosis, hypopigmentation, atrophy, striae, perioral dermatitis, secondary infection; if used on large area for extended periods of time, can have systemic side effects

Fecal Impaction

OVERVIEW

Fecal impaction is a large accumulation of a firm, immovable mass of stool in the rectum, sigmoid flexure, or proximal colon.

Pathogenesis

Causes:

- Diet low in fiber
- Medications
- Neurogenic bowel disorders
- Hypothyroidism
- Hypokalemia
- Hypercalcemia
- Obstructing lesions
- In children, ignoring urge to defecate

Patient Profile

- Males = Females
- Any age; more common >60 years
- Males > Females in children

Signs and Symptoms

- Liquid stool (diarrhea)
- Abdominal pain (particularly after eating)
- Nausea, vomiting
- Tenesmus
- Colic
- Anorexia
- Weight loss
- Headache
- Dehydration
- General malaise
- Fever
- Tachycardia
- Tachypnea
- Urinary frequency
- Incontinence

Differential Diagnosis

- Tumor
- Irritable bowel syndrome
- Gastroenteritis
- Appendicitis
- Diverticulitis

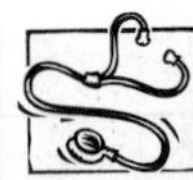

ASSESSMENT

History

Inquire about:

- Onset and duration of symptoms, including date and time of last stool passed
- Amount and consistency of stool being passed
- Associated symptoms
- Underlying conditions
- Current medications

Physical Findings

- Tachycardia
- Tachypnea
- Fever
- Weight loss
- Abdomen—pain on palpation; large mass of stool in (L) lower quadrant
- Rectal examination—large mass of stool

Initial Workup

Laboratory

- CBC—leukocytosis
- Chemistry profile—hyponatremia, hypokalemia

Radiology: Flat plate of abdomen—identifies masses of stool

Further Workup

Usually none needed

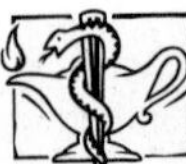

INTERVENTIONS

Office Treatment

- Manual fragmentation and removal of feces
- For complete evacuation after partial removal, insert bisacodyl suppository or use oil-retention enema
- For high impaction beyond digital reach, use polyethylene glycol (Golytely).

Lifestyle Modifications

- Increased dietary fiber and fluid intake
- Bowel program
- Exercise program

Patient Education

Teach patient about:

- Condition and treatment options—manual removal, mineral oil enema, Golytely
- Bowel-training program—set aside time each day for bowel movement
- Importance of taking adequate time to defecate and of heeding defecation urge
- High-fiber diet
- Increased fluid intake
- Tips for starting exercise program
- Avoidance of laxatives
- Use of bulk-forming agents or stool softeners and side effects (see Pharmacotherapeutics)

Referrals

None indicated

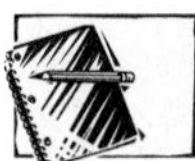

EVALUATION

Outcome
Patient returns to "normal" bowel habits

Possible Complications
- Urinary tract obstruction
- Intestinal obstruction
- Perforation of colon
- Hernia
- Volvulus
- Megacolon
- Rectal prolapse
- Pneumothorax
- Hypoxia
- Shock

Follow-up
In 2 weeks to assess bowel program results

FOR YOUR INFORMATION

Life Span
Pediatric: Children do not want to take time away from play and ignore urge to defecate; this can lead to impaction
Geriatric: Much more common in this population
Pregnancy: Can induce labor

Miscellaneous
Complications can occur as a result of manual disimpaction, such as sepsis, hypotension, and bleeding.

Reference
Cheskin LJ: Constipation and diarrhea. In Barker LR, Burton JR, Zieve PD, editors: *Principles of ambulatory medicine,* ed 4, Baltimore, 1995, Williams & Wilkins, p 487.

NOTES

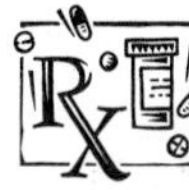

PHARMACOTHERAPEUTICS

Drug of Choice	Mechanism of Action	Prescribing Information	Side Effects
Bisacodyl (Dulcolax), 10-mg suppository PR; same for children >2 years; children <2 years, 5-mg suppository PR	Increases motor activity in intestine	***Contraindications:*** Hypersensitivity; rectal fissures; abdominal pain; nausea, vomiting; appendicitis; acute surgical abdomen; ulcerated hemorrhoids; acute hepatitis; intestinal/biliary tract obstruction ***Cost:*** OTC ***Pregnancy category:*** C	Muscle weakness, nausea, vomiting, anorexia, cramps, diarrhea, rectal burning, hypokalemia, tetany, protein-losing enteropathy
Stool softener: docusate sodium (Colace); adults and children: 50-200 mg/day PO; children 6-12 years, 40-120 mg/day PO; children 3-6 years, 60 mg/day PO; children <3 years, 10-40 mg/day PO	Surface-active agent; helps keep stool soft	***Contraindication:*** None ***Cost:*** Varies—OTC ***Pregnancy category:*** Not categorized	Bitter taste, throat irritation, nausea

Fertility Problems/Infertility

OVERVIEW

Fertility problems can be described as the inability to conceive after 1 year of unprotected sexual intercourse.

Pathogenesis

Multifactorial—30% to 40% of the time due to male dysfunction; 60% to 70% of the time due to female dysfunction

Patient Profile

- Males and Females
- Increases with age; 20% to 25% of couples >40 years of age are infertile

Signs and Symptoms

Signs and symptoms from underlying cause:

- Genital/pelvic infections
- Endocrine dysfunction
- Sexual dysfunction
- Anovulatory cycles
- Endometriosis

Differential Diagnosis

Any of the many causes

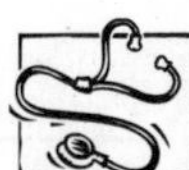

ASSESSMENT

History

Both partners need to be evaluated; inquire about:

- Length of time of unprotected coitus
- Number of sexual encounters per week
- Past sexual history, including history of STDs
- Children with a previous partner
- Women—menstrual history, obstetric history
- Previous use of birth control and type
- Underlying conditions
- Current medications

Physical Findings

Both partners need complete physical examination, which may be within normal limits

Initial Workup

Laboratory

- Male—CBC, chemistry profile, testosterone level, prolactin level, semen analysis, urinalysis, TSH
- Female—CBC, chemistry profile, prolactin level, TSH, urinalysis, Pap smear, FSH, LH

Radiology: Hysterosalpingogram if indicated

Further Workup

Should be done by fertility specialist

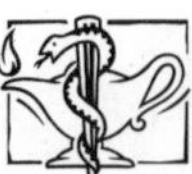

INTERVENTIONS

Office Treatment

Provide supportive environment

Lifestyle Modifications

Depends on underlying cause

Patient Education

Teach patient about:

- Condition and possible causes
- Men with low sperm counts—avoiding hot tubs/saunas; using boxer shorts instead of jockey shorts, having intercourse every 36 hours during woman's fertile period
- Women—keeping basal body temperature chart
- Artificial insemination
- In-vitro fertilization
- Adoption

Referral

To fertility specialist

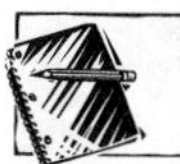

EVALUATION

Outcome
50% of couples will conceive during second year

Possible Complications
- Multiple births with induced ovulation
- Ectopic pregnancy

Follow-up
Done by specialist

FOR YOUR INFORMATION

Life Span
Pediatric: N/A
Geriatric: N/A
Pregnancy: N/A

Miscellaneous
There have been many advances in the field of infertility, and this problem is best handled by a specialist in this area.

Reference
Wood SC: Infertility. In Youngkin EQ, Davis MS, editors: *Women's health: a primary care clinical guide,* Norwalk, Conn, 1994, Appleton & Lange, pp 161-197.

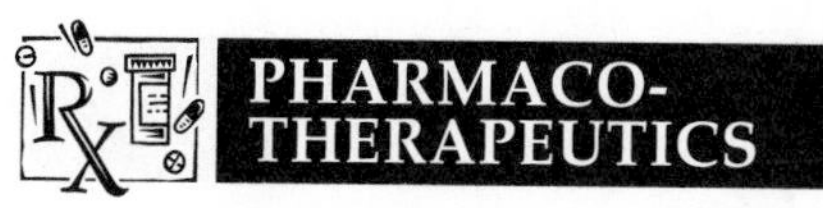

PHARMACOTHERAPEUTICS

There are numerous medications that can be used in the treatment of infertility. The general practitioner's main focus should be in helping the couple to locate the appropriate specialist to meet their needs.

Fever of Unknown Origin (FUO)

OVERVIEW

Current criteria for the diagnosis of fever of unknown origin are a fever greater than 101° F (38.3° C) on at least 4 occasions and illness during a 14-day period, without an obvious cause.

Pathogenesis

Many possible causes:

- Infections—infectious mononucleosis, measles, chickenpox, rubella, viral hepatitis, HIV infection, Rocky Mountain spotted fever, Q fever, Lyme disease, bacterial endocarditis, salmonella, localized bacterial infections of abdominal organs, malaria, Dengue fever, leptospirosis
- Drug hypersensitivity reactions—allopurinol, antihistamines, clofibrate, ibuprofen, isoniazid, nifedipine, phenytoin, propylthiouracil, sulfonamides
- Neoplasms—lymphoma, leukemia, hepatoma, colon cancer
- Collagen vascular diseases—temporal arteritis, polyarteritis nodosa, rheumatic fever, systemic lupus erythematosus, rheumatoid arthritis
- Other—pulmonary emboli, thermoregulatory disorders, factitious/fraudulent fever

Patient Profile

- Males = Females
- Any age

Signs and Symptoms

- Fever
- Headache
- Myalgia
- Malaise

Differential Diagnosis

Any of the many causes listed under pathogenesis

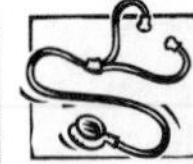

ASSESSMENT

History

Inquire about:

- Onset and duration of fever (usually not helpful in making diagnosis) and associated symptoms
- Amount of fluid intake
- Exposure to infections
- Environmental exposures
- Any new medications
- Recent immunizations
- Other household members being ill
- Treatments tried and results; if medication, when last taken
- Underlying conditions
- Current medications

Physical Findings

Complete physical examination to attempt to uncover cause, with particular attention to:

- General appearance
- Skin—color, rashes, petechiae, purpura, turgor
- Nuchal rigidity
- Lymphadenopathy
- Swollen joints

Initial Workup

Laboratory

- CBC with differential
- C-reactive protein
- Sedimentation rate
- Chemistry profile to include liver function tests
- Blood cultures
- Urinalysis and urine culture
- Start with above tests and add any others indicated from history and physical examination

Radiology: Directed by history and physical examination:

- Chest film, PA and lateral
- Other x-ray studies if indicated—abdominal films, sinus x-ray films, CT scan or MRI of abdomen and pelvis, echocardiogram, ventilation/perfusion scan

Further Workup

- TB skin test
- Sputum cultures
- Serologic tests—Epstein-Barr virus, hepatitis, syphilis, Lyme disease, Q fever
- HIV test
- Rheumatoid factor
- Antinuclear antibody
- Bone marrow biopsy
- Liver biopsy
- Spinal tap
- Exploratory laparotomy

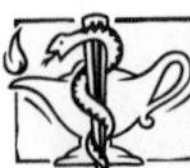

INTERVENTIONS

Office Treatment

None indicated

Lifestyle Modifications

- Adequate fluid intake
- Maintenance of preillness lifestyle as much as possible

Patient Education

Teach patient about:

- Condition
- Diagnostic approach—can be very frustrating for patient to not know what is causing the fever
- Importance of adequate and increased fluid intake
- Importance of finding cause before treatment—therapeutic trials of antibiotics or other medications should not be used until completion of diagnostic workup; they do not solve the problem and may cloud the clinical picture
- Antipyretic medication and side effects (see Pharmacotherapeutics)

Referral

Consult with MD throughout diagnostic process; may need referral to specialist, such as infectious disease specialist

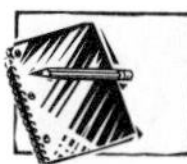

EVALUATION

Outcomes

- In up to 20% of patients, fever resolves without cause being identified
- Prognosis generally good

Possible Complications

Depends on underlying cause

Follow-up

May need daily telephone contact initially, with first follow-up visit 72 hours after initial visit; then weekly until resolution

FOR YOUR INFORMATION

Life Span

Pediatric: Infection and collagen vascular diseases most likely cause

Geriatric: Most common causes—acute leukemia, tuberculosis, temporal arteritis; signs and symptoms may be very subtle

Pregnancy: Must be thoroughly evaluated; perform urinalysis and urine culture first

Miscellaneous

N/A

References

Pierce NF: Undifferentiated acute febrile illness. In Barker LR, Burton JR, Zieve PD, editors: *Principles of ambulatory medicine,* ed 4, Baltimore, 1995, Williams & Wilkins, pp 295-299.

Uphold CR, Graham MV: *Clinical guidelines in adult health,* Gainesville, Fla, 1994, Barmarrae Books, pp 35-39.

NOTES

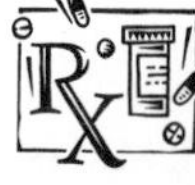

PHARMACOTHERAPEUTICS

The following medications are used for fever and myalgia.

Drug of Choice	Mechanism of Action	Prescribing Information	Side Effects
Acetaminophen (Tylenol), 325-650 mg PO every 4-6 hours; for children, use Children's Tylenol—follow label directions	Decreases fever through action on hypothalamic heat-regulating center of brain	***Contraindications:*** Hypersensitivity; bleeding disorders or anticoagulant therapy; last trimester of pregnancy; asthma; gastric ulcers ***Cost:*** OTC ***Pregnancy category:*** Not categorized	Rash; hepatic toxicity with alcohol ingestion or overdose
Aspirin, 325-650 mg PO q4-6h—do not use in children or adolescents because of risk of Reye's syndrome	Analgesia via peripheral and central nervous systems; may inhibit prostaglandins; antipyretic; acts on hypothalamic system	***Contraindications:*** Hypersensitivity; bleeding disorders or anticoagulant therapy; last trimester of pregnancy; asthma; gastric ulcers ***Cost:*** OTC ***Pregnancy category:*** Not categorized	Rash, anaphylactic reaction, GI upset and bleeding, Reye's syndrome in children and adolescents
Ibuprofen (Motrin), 400 mg qid PO; children 6 months to 12 years, 5 mg/kg PO if temperature <102.5° F (39.1° C); 10 mg/kg PO if temperature >102.5° F every 6 hours	Not well understood; may be related to inhibition of prostaglandin synthesis	***Contraindications:*** Aspirin allergy; hypersensitivity; asthma; last trimester of pregnancy; gastric ulcer; bleeding disorders ***Cost:*** 400-mg tab, 4/day × 5 days: $3 ***Pregnancy category:*** Not categorized but not recommended	Nausea, heartburn, diarrhea, GI upset and bleeding, dizziness, headache, rash, tinnitus, edema, acute renal failure

Fibrocystic Breast Complex

OVERVIEW

Fibrocystic breast complex is a group of benign changes in breast tissue that result in breast masses or nodularity and painful breasts.

Pathogenesis

- Exact cause unknown; appears to be exaggerated response to hormonal changes
- Results in excess fibrous tissue, hyperplasia of epithelial lining of mammary ducts, proliferation of mammary ducts, cyst formation

Patient Profile

- Females almost exclusively
- Menarche and beyond
- Most common in menstruating women
- Appears to run in families

Signs and Symptoms

- Asymptomatic
- Breast pain and tenderness, usually 1 to 2 days before menses and during menses
- Smooth, firm masses
- Bilateral masses
- Movable masses
- Fluctuant masses
- Nipple discharge (milky, watery/milky, yellow, green)
- Breast engorgement

Differential Diagnosis

- Breast cancer
- Pain may have many causes—costochondritis, chest wall muscle spasm, neuralgia, anxiety, depression, angina pectoris, cardiac pain, gastroesophageal reflux disease

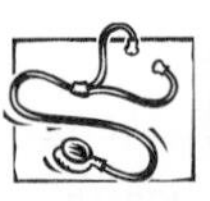

ASSESSMENT

History

Inquire about:

- Onset and duration of symptoms
- Association with menses
- Family history of fibrocystic breasts and breast cancer
- Underlying conditions
- Current medications

Physical Findings

- On thorough breast examination, may find firm, movable mass, fluctuant mass, nipple discharge
- Measure size of abnormality
- Draw picture in progress notes of location and size

Initial Workup

Laboratory: Send nipple discharge for cytology

Radiology: Mammography; in patient <25 years of age, ultrasound more sensitive

Further Workup

Usually performed by MD:

- Fine-needle aspiration
- Core needle biopsy
- Excisional biopsy

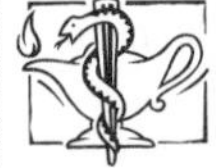

INTERVENTIONS

Office Treatment

None indicated

Lifestyle Modifications

- Monthly self-breast examination
- Stress reduction
- Low-sodium diet
- Exclusion of methylxanthines from diet

Patient Education

Teach patient about:

- Condition and treatment—needle, core, or excisional biopsy
- Self-breast examination and importance of yearly examination by professional
- Diet—low-sodium, especially 10 days before menses; restriction of methylxanthines (chocolate, caffeine)
- Wearing well-fitting supportive bra day and night 1 to 2 days before menses and during menses
- Use of ice packs
- Medications used and side effects (see Pharmacotherapeutics)

Referral

To surgeon for fine-needle aspiration, core biopsy, or excisional biopsy

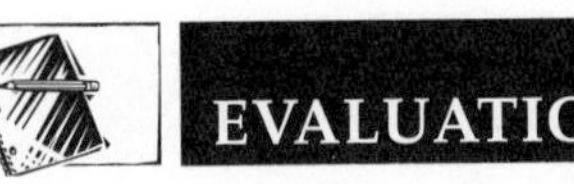

EVALUATION

Outcome

Patient will be able to cope with pain and adequately perform breast self-examination

Possible Complications

- Infection after biopsy
- Atypical hyperplasia could lead to cancer

Follow-up

In 1 month to assess treatment results

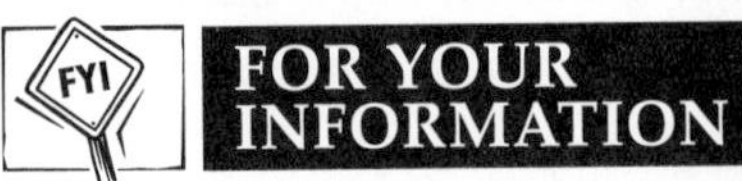

FOR YOUR INFORMATION

Life Span

Pediatric: Biopsy should be avoided

Geriatric: More common for breast masses to be malignant

Pregnancy: Monitor closely; biopsy should be done after delivery, if possible

Miscellaneous

Fibrocystic breasts are a very common condition, with approximately 50% of women being affected. Currently, research is being done to evaluate the usefulness of MRI in the diagnosis of occult breast cancer. MRI is currently being used in several research centers and has been found to have a much higher specificity and sensitivity than mammography or ultrasound.

References

Coons TA: MRI's role in assessing and managing breast disease, *Radiol Technol* 67(4):311-336, 1996.

Vorpahl CL: Nursing role in management: breast disorders. In Lewis SM, Collier IC, Heitkemper MM, editors: *Medical-surgical nursing: assessment and management of clinical problems,* ed 4, St Louis, 1996, Mosby, pp 1546-1547.

PHARMACOTHERAPEUTICS

Drug of Choice	Mechanism of Action	Prescribing Information	Side Effects
Vitamin E, 400 IU/day PO qd	Fat-soluble vitamin	*Contraindication:* Hypersensitivity *Cost:* OTC *Pregnancy category:* A	Weakness, headache, fatigue, nausea, cramps, diarrhea, gonadal dysfunction, blurred vision, contact dermatitis
Pyridoxine (vitamin B_6), 50 mg PO qd	Water-soluble vitamin	*Contraindication:* Hypersensitivity *Cost:* OTC *Pregnancy category:* A	Paresthesia, flushing, warmth, lethargy
To decrease engorgement 2-3 days before menses:			
Hydrochlorothiazide (HCTZ), 25-50 mg PO qd	Thiazide diuretic; acts on distal tubule and ascending limb of loop of Henle	*Contraindications:* Hypersensitivity to thiazides or sulfonamines; anuria; renal decompensation; hypomagnesemia *Cost:* 25-mg tab, 80 tabs: $3 *Pregnancy category:* B	Uremia, glucosuria, drowsiness, paresthesia, dizziness, weakness, nausea, vomiting, anorexia, hepatitis, rash, urticaria, hyperglycemia, hyperuricemia, aplastic anemia, hemolytic anemia, leukopenia, thrombocytopenia, orthostatic hypotension, irregular pulse, hypokalemia, hypercalcemia, hyponatremia, hypochloremia, rash
For more severe condition, use one of the following:			
Danazol (Danocrine), 100-200 mg PO qd × 3 months	Decreases FSH and LH; results in amenorrhea/anovulation	*Contraindications:* Hypersensitivity; severe renal, cardiac, or hepatic disease; pregnancy; abnormal genital bleeding *Cost:* 200-mg tab, 60 tabs: $200 *Pregnancy category:* C	Acneiform lesions, oily hair, flushing, sweating, dizziness, headache, fatigue, tremors, paresthesias, anxiety, cramps, muscle spasms, increased blood pressure, hematuria, atrophic vaginitis, decreased libido, decreased breast size, clitoral hypertrophy, nausea, vomiting, weight gain, cholestatic jaundice, nasal congestion
Bromocriptine (Parlodel), 2.5 mg PO bid × 3 months	Inhibits prolactin release	*Contraindications:* Hypersensitivity to ergot; severe ischemic disease; severe peripheral vascular disease *Cost:* 2.5-mg tab, 30 tabs: $44 *Pregnancy category:* D	Blurred vision, nasal congestion, headache, depression, restlessness, nervousness, convulsions, hallucinations, anxiety, dizziness, fatigue, urinary frequency and retention, nausea, vomiting, anorexia, cramps, constipation, rash, alopecia, orthostatic hypotension, shock, dysrhythmias

Fibromyalgia/Myofascial Pain Syndrome/Fibrositis

OVERVIEW

Fibromyalgia is a common pain syndrome in which there is generalized musculoskeletal pain and stiffness. The pain can be elicited with manual pressure on various "trigger points." Fatigue, sleep disorders, subjective numbness, chronic headaches, and irritable bowel syndrome frequently accompany it.

Pathogenesis

Cause—relatively unknown; sleep disorders, depression, and viral infections have been implicated

Patient Profile

- Females > Males
- Most common age >18 years

Signs and Symptoms

- Generalized pain and stiffness
- Increased pain in the morning, with weather changes, and with stress and anxiety
- Fatigue
- Headache
- Symptoms aggravated with minor exertion
- Depression
- Irritable bowel symptoms

Differential Diagnosis

- Hypothyroidism
- Muscle strain/sprain
- Polymyalgia rheumatica
- Drug-seeking behavior
- Metabolic imbalance
- Depression

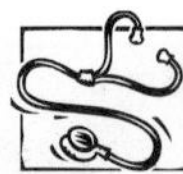

ASSESSMENT

History

Inquire about:

- Onset and duration of symptoms
- What makes pain better or worse
- Amount of activities patient is able to perform
- Sleep problems, particularly early-morning waking
- Recent trauma, stress, viral infection
- Headaches
- Episodes of diarrhea
- Underlying conditions
- Current medications

Physical Findings

- Expression of pain when manual pressure applied to trigger points—most common sites: sternocleidomastoid, low anterior neck, manubriosternal, trapezius ridge, upper and lower rhomboids, iliac crest, medial fat pad of knee, humeral epicondyles
- Usually have 11 or more trigger points
- Rest of physical examination within normal limits

Initial Workup

Laboratory: Done to rule out other diagnoses—all should be within normal limits

- CBC
- Thyroid panel
- Erythrocyte sedimentation rate (ESR)
- Rheumatoid factor

Radiology: None diagnostic

Further Workup

None indicated

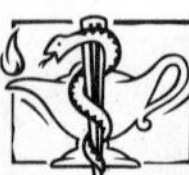

INTERVENTIONS

Office Treatment

None indicated

Lifestyle Modifications

- Smoking cessation
- Stress reduction
- Maintenance of active lifestyle

Patient Education

Teach patient about:

- Condition (assure patient that this is a "real" syndrome) and treatment
  - NSAIDs (usually not very effective), antidepressants, muscle relaxants
  - Physical therapy with ultrasound treatments
  - Hot packs
  - Moderate exercise program
  - Transcutaneous electrical nerve stimulation (TENS)
  - Acupuncture
  - Therapeutic touch and massage
- Stress reduction techniques—relaxation technique, biofeedback, yoga, meditation
- Importance of remaining as active as possible
- Medications used and side effects (see Pharmacotherapeutics)

Referrals

To chiropractor, orthopedist, mental health counselor, as needed

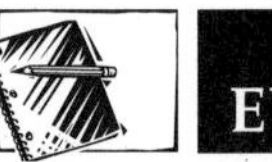

EVALUATION

Outcome

Patient maintains active lifestyle

Possible Complication

Total disability

Follow-up

In 2 weeks × 2; then every 3 months

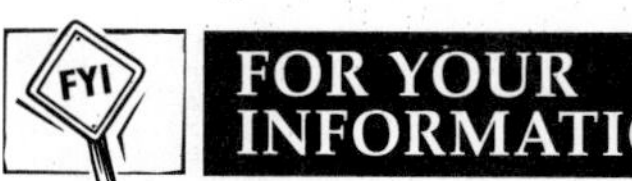

FOR YOUR INFORMATION

Life Span

Pediatric: Rarely seen in patients <18 years of age—explore living situation
Geriatric: Cautious use of medications
Pregnancy: Use nonpharmacologic approach to treatment

Miscellaneous

Fibromyalgia is a very common problem that can be very difficult to treat. There is no one specific treatment to "cure" the problem. The patient needs to understand that it may take a trial of several different types of treatment before results are seen.

References

Hellman DB: Arthritis and musculoskeletal disorders. In Tierney LM Jr, McPhee SJ, Papadakis MA, editors: *Current medical diagnosis and treatment,* ed 34, Norwalk, Conn, 1995, Appleton & Lange, pp 708-709.

Mercier LR: *Practical orthopedics,* ed 4, St Louis, 1995, Mosby, p 289.

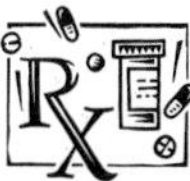

PHARMACOTHERAPEUTICS

Drug of Choice	Mechanism of Action	Prescribing Information	Side Effects
Amitriptyline (Elavil), 10 mg PO hs; may increase up to 50 mg hs	Tricyclic antidepressant; increases action of norepinephrine and serotonin by blocking their reuptake	***Contraindications:*** Hypersensitivity; recovery phase of myocardial infarction (MI) ***Cost:*** 10-mg tab, 100 tabs: $2-$15 ***Pregnancy category:*** C	Agranulocytosis, thrombocytopenia, leukopenia, dizziness, drowsiness, confusion, headache, anxiety, tremor, diarrhea, dry mouth, nausea, paralytic ileus, cramps, epigastric distress, rash, hepatitis, urinary retention, urticaria, orthostatic hypotension, ECG changes, tachycardia, hypertension, blurred vision, tinnitus, mydriasis
Selective serotonin reuptake inhibitors (SSRIs): • Fluoxetine (Prozac), 20-80 mg/day • Sertraline (Zoloft), 50-200 mg/day • Paroxetine (Paxil), 10-30 mg/day • None dosed for children; do not use with or within 14 days of monoamine oxidase inhibitors (MAOIs) or drugs metabolized by the P450 system	Block reuptake of serotonin	***Contraindication:*** Hypersensitivity ***Cost:*** Fluoxetine, 20-mg tab, 30 tabs: $67; sertraline, 50-mg tab, 100 tabs: $176; paroxetine, 20-mg tab, 30 tabs: $57 ***Pregnancy category:*** Fluoxetine and sertraline—B; paroxetine—C	Dry mouth, constipation, sleepiness, headache, nervousness, anxiety, tremor, abnormal dreams, nausea, diarrhea, dyspepsia, rash, postural hypotension, decreased libido, dysmenorrhea, urinary frequency, impotence, abnormal ejaculation, pain, myalgia, cough
Cyclobenzaprine (Flexeril), 10 mg PO hs; maximum dose 60 mg/day; should not be stopped abruptly if used for a long period of time—may produce nausea, headache, and malaise	Tricyclic amine salt; centrally acting skeletal muscle relaxant; action may be related to antidepressant effects	***Contraindications:*** Hypersensitivity; with or within 14 days of MAOIs; acute recovery phase of MI; hyperthyroidism ***Cost:*** 10-mg tab, 100 tabs: $13-$97 ***Pregnancy category:*** B	Dizziness, weakness, drowsiness, diplopia, nausea, vomiting, rash, pruritus, urinary retention, change in libido, anaphylaxis
Nonsteroidal antiinflammatory drugs (NSAIDs): many different types currently marketed; consult manufacturer's package insert for specific dosing and prescribing information; usually do not work well, but trial may be indicated	Exact action unknown; may result from inhibition of synthesis of prostaglandins and arachidonic acid	***Contraindications:*** Hypersensitivity to NSAIDs or aspirin; severe hepatic failure; asthma ***Cost:*** Varies with type ***Pregnancy category:*** Depends on product	Stomach distress, flatulence, nausea, abdominal pain, constipation or diarrhea, dizziness, sedation, rash, urticaria, angioedema, anorexia, urinary frequency, increased blood pressure, insomnia, anxiety, visual disturbances, increased thirst, alopecia

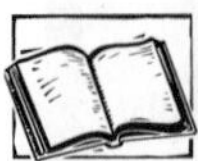

OVERVIEW

Folliculitis is an inflammation of a hair follicle. The inflammation may be superficial or deep. It is a very common condition and is a component of a variety of inflammatory skin diseases.

Pathogenesis

- Can be caused by infection, chemical irritation, or physical injury
- Most commonly, *Staphylococcus aureus* is causative organism of infective folliculitis
- *Pseudomonas aeruginosa* infection occurs in bathing suit areas of hot tub users
- *Candida albicans* infection occurs in patients receiving immunosuppressive therapy or long-term antibiotic therapy
- Immunosuppressed patients and patients with diabetes mellitus are more prone to having folliculitis

Patient Profile

- Males > Females
- Affects all ages

Signs and Symptoms

- Yellow or gray pustules surrounded by erythema with hair in the middle
- Lesions are commonly grouped
- Lesion is nontender or slightly tender
- May be pruritic
- May occur on any body surface area, most commonly on scalp, beard area, and limbs

Differential Diagnosis

- Ingrown hairs
- Keratosis pilaris
- Contact dermatitis
- Tinea
- Acne
- Miliaria
- Flat warts
- Molluscum contagiosum

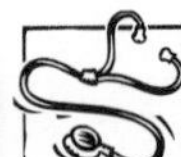

ASSESSMENT

History

Inquire about:

- Onset and duration of symptoms
- Use of hot tub
- History of similar occurrences
- Treatments tried and results
- Recent injury to area
- Nearby surgical wounds or draining abscesses
- Underlying conditions
- Current medications

Physical Findings

- Examination of entire skin surface
- Yellow or gray lesions that are surrounded by erythema and pierced by a hair

Initial Workup

Laboratory

- Gram stain—gram-positive cocci
- Potassium hydroxide preparation—budding yeast or hyphae
- Culture

Radiology: None indicated

Further Workup

None indicated, unless complications arise

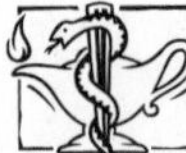

INTERVENTIONS

Office Treatment

None indicated

Lifestyle Modifications

- Avoidance of hot tub use
- Avoidance of tight clothing (jeans folliculitis)
- Good hygiene
- Avoidance of use of topical oils

Patient Education

Teach patient about:

- Condition and treatment—topical antibiotic for small areas; oral antibiotics for more extensive disease
- Not sharing towels or wash cloths
- Shampooing daily with Selsun Blue for scalp lesions
- Applying moist heat to lesions
- Possible causative agents
- Changing razor blade daily; preferable that patient not shave until resolved
- Medications used and side effects (see Pharmacotherapeutics)

Referral

To dermatologist if no resolution within 2 weeks

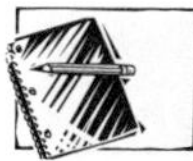

EVALUATION

Outcomes

- Usually resolves with treatment
- May recur in staph carriers; mupirocin (Bactroban) applied to nares may cure carrier state

Possible Complications

- Progression to furuncle/carbuncle
- Scarring

Follow-up

In 2 weeks to assess results of treatment; if unresolved, every 2 weeks until cleared

FOR YOUR INFORMATION

Life Span

Pediatric: Commonly occurs after puberty
Geriatric: Treatment is the same
Pregnancy: Cautious use of medication

Miscellaneous

The entire family may need to be evaluated in an attempt to find a carrier source.

Reference

Habif TP: *Clinical dermatology: a color guide to diagnosis and therapy,* ed 3, St Louis, 1996, Mosby, pp 248-249.

NOTES

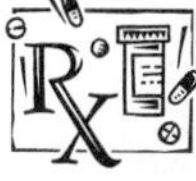

PHARMACOTHERAPEUTICS

Drug of Choice	Mechanism of Action	Prescribing Information	Side Effects
For staphylococcal infection, use one of the following:			
Dicloxacillin 250 mg PO q6h for 10 days; children <40 kg, 12.5-25 mg/kg/d divided q6h	Bactericidal cell wall inhibitor; active against gram-positive cocci except enterococci	***Contraindication:*** Hypersensitivity to penicillins ***Cost:*** 500-mg tab, 50 tabs: $19-$88 ***Pregnancy category:*** B	Bone marrow depression, granulocytopenia, nausea, vomiting, diarrhea, oliguria, proteinuria, hematuria, moniliasis, glomerulonephritis, lethargy, depression, convulsions, anaphylaxis
Erythromycin (E.E.S.), 250 mg PO q6h for 10 days; children, 30-50 mg/kg/d divided q6h × 10 days; for mild cases, use erythromycin 2% solution; apply topically bid × 10 days	Macrolide; protein synthesis inhibitor; active against bacteria lacking cell walls, most gram-positive aerobes	***Contraindication:*** Hypersensitivity ***Cost:*** 250-mg tabs, 4/day × 10 days: $4 ***Pregnancy category:*** B	Nausea, vomiting, diarrhea, abdominal pain, anorexia, rash, urticaria, pseudomembranous colitis—rarely
For Pseudomonas:			
Ciprofloxacin (Cipro), 500 mg PO bid for 10 days—not dosed for children	Fluoroquinilone; interferes with conversion of intermediate DNA fragments into high molecular weight DNA	***Contraindication:*** Hypersensitivity ***Cost:*** 500-mg tab, 100 tabs: $365 ***Pregnancy category:*** C	Headache, dizziness, fatigue, insomnia, depression, seizures, confusion, nausea, diarrhea, increased ALT and AST, flatulence, heartburn, oral candidiasis, rash, pruritus, urticaria, photosensitivity, blurred vision
For mild cases or staphylococcal carriers:			
Mupirocin (Bactroban) ointment; apply to affected area bid or, for carriers, to nares bid	Inhibits bacterial protein synthesis	***Contraindication:*** Hypersensitivity ***Cost:*** 2% ointment, 30 g: $29 ***Pregnancy category:*** B	Burning, stinging, itching, rash, erythema, dry skin, tenderness, swelling, contact dermatitis

Food Allergy

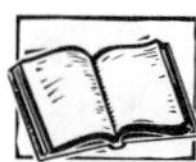

OVERVIEW

Food allergy is a hypersensitivity reaction to a specific food. It results from ingestion of a specific food antigen.

Pathogenesis

- Reaction may be caused by immunologic mechanism or nonimmunologic mechanism
- Any food can elicit reaction
- Most common—cow's milk, egg whites, wheat, soy, peanuts, fish, tree nuts, shellfish, melons, sesame seeds, sunflower seeds, chocolate, food dyes, and additives

Patient Profile

- Males > Females
- More common in children up to age 4
- Positive family history of allergies is risk factor

Signs and Symptoms

- Dermatologic system—urticaria, angioedema, atopic dermatitis, pallor, flushing, contact rashes
- Gastrointestinal system—nausea, vomiting, diarrhea, abdominal pain, occult bleeding, flatulence, bloating, malabsorption, protein-losing enteropathy, eosinophilic gastroenteritis, colitis
- Respiratory system—allergic rhinitis, asthma, bronchospasm, cough, serous otitis media, pulmonary infiltrates
- Neurologic system—hyperkinesis, tension-fatigue syndrome, migraine headaches, syncope
- Other symptoms—systemic anaphylaxis, vasculitis, enuresis, proteinuria, irritability, disinterest, growth retardation

Differential Diagnosis

Essential to obtain a careful history—many diseases can mimic food allergy, such as drug reaction, contact dermatitis, eczema, common cold, or gastrointestinal flu syndrome

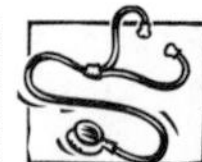

ASSESSMENT

History

Inquire about:

- Onset and duration of symptoms
- Prior history of allergic reaction to specific food
- Family history of food allergy
- If first episode, careful history of all foods ingested in previous 24-hour period, particularly foods not normally eaten (may be difficult to obtain history in a child)
- Underlying conditions
- Current medications

Physical Findings

- Dermatologic system—urticaria, angioedema, atopic dermatitis, pallor or flushing, contact rash
- Gastrointestinal system—nausea, vomiting, diarrhea, abdominal pain, occult bleeding, flatulence, bloating
- Respiratory system—allergic rhinitis, asthma, bronchospasm, cough, serous otitis media
- Neurologic system—hyperkinesis, tension-fatigue syndrome, migraine headache, syncope

Initial Workup

Laboratory

- CBC with differential—eosinophilia
- Stool—mucus and eosinophilia
- None may be needed

Radiology: Usually none

Further Workup

Radioallergosorbent (RAST) test and provocation tests—usually not performed by NP

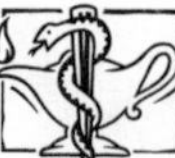

INTERVENTIONS

Office Treatment

None indicated

Lifestyle Modifications

- Elimination of offending food
- If severe reaction is possible, may need to carry epinephrine for self-administration

Patient Education

Teach patient about:

- Condition, cause, and treatment
- Eliminating offending food from diet
- Repeated ingestion of foods resulting in more severe reactions, such as anaphylaxis
- Self-administration of epinephrine
- Fact that sensitivity may be outgrown or endure into adulthood
- Medications used and side effects (see Pharmacotherapeutics)

Referrals

- To nutritionist to help with diet
- To dermatologist for definitive diagnosis of causative agent if uncertain

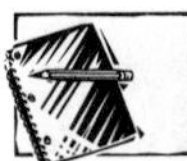

EVALUATION

Outcome
No further episodes or complications

Possible Complications
- Anaphylaxis
- Angioedema
- Bronchial asthma
- Enterocolitis
- Eczematoid lesions

Follow-up
48 hours after first visit; then as needed

FOR YOUR INFORMATION

Life Span
Pediatric: Incidence in children up to 4 years is 8% to 16%; only about 3% to 4% still have allergy after 4 years of age
Geriatric: Rarely develop a new food allergy
Pregnancy: Cautious use of medications

Miscellaneous
N/A

References
Habif TP: *Clinical dermatology: a color guide to diagnosis and therapy,* ed 3, St Louis, 1996, Mosby, pp 120-121.

Valentine MD: Allergy and related conditions. In Barker LR, Burton JR, Zieve PD, editors: *Principles of ambulatory medicine,* ed 4, Baltimore, 1995, Williams & Wilkins, pp 292-293.

NOTES

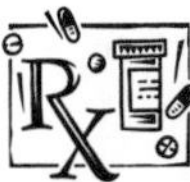

PHARMACOTHERAPEUTICS

Drug of Choice	Mechanism of Action	Prescribing Information	Side Effects
Antihistamines: • Diphenhydramine (Benadryl); adults, 25-50 mg PO qid; children, 6-12 years, 12.5-25 mg PO qid • Hydroxyzine (Atarax), 10-25 mg PO qid • Loratidine (Claritin), 10 mg 1 qd PO—do not use in children <12 years • Astemizole (Hismanal), 10 mg 1 qd PO—do not use in children <12 years • Fexofenadine (Allegra), 60 mg PO bid—do not use in children <12 years	Compete with histamine for cell receptor sites	***Contraindications:*** Coadministration of erythromycin, ketoconazole, or other drugs metabolized by P450 system with Hismanal; hypersensitivity ***Cost:*** Benadryl, 25 mg, 4/day × 30 days: $4.00; Atarax, 10-mg tab, 30 tabs: $2; Claritin, 10-mg tab, 1/day × 30 days: $53; Hismanal, 10-mg tab, 1/day × 30 days: $53; Allegra, 60-mg tab 2/day × 30 days: $53 ***Pregnancy category:*** Benadryl and Claritin—B; Hismanal and Allegra—C	Sedation—marked with Benadryl and lesser with the others; headache, fatigue, dizziness, nausea and vomiting, dry mouth, cough, rash, nervousness

OVERVIEW

Bacterial food poisoning encompasses a variety of illnesses that result from ingesting food contaminated with bacteria. The illness may result from the bacteria itself or from toxins produced by the bacteria.

Pathogenesis

Numerous causes: *Shigella* species, *Salmonella* species, *Bacillus cereus, Clostridium botulinum, Clostridium perfringens, Escherichia coli, Yersinia enterocolitica, Campylobacter jejuni*

Patient Profile

- Males = Females
- All ages

Signs and Symptoms

- Nausea, vomiting
- Cramps
- Diarrhea
- Pseudoappendicitis
- Fever
- Bloody diarrhea
- Sepsis
- Meningitis
- Motor paralysis
- Respiratory paralysis
- Death

Differential Diagnosis

- Inflammatory bowel disease
- Appendicitis
- Infectious gastroenteritis of any kind
- Hepatitis

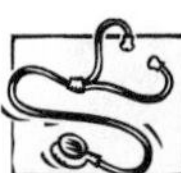

ASSESSMENT

History

Inquire about:

- Onset and duration of symptoms (onset can give clue to causative organisms) (Table 8)
- What was eaten in past 24 hours
- Whether others in group are also ill
- Underlying conditions
- Current medications

Physical Findings

- Abdominal pain
- Fever
- Hyperactive bowel sounds
- Pallor
- Poor skin turgor
- Postural hypotension
- Symmetric motor paralysis

Initial Workup

Laboratory

- CBC with differential—increased WBC count and (L) shift on differential
- Stool culture
- Stool for fecal leukocytes

Radiology: None indicated

Further Workup

None indicated

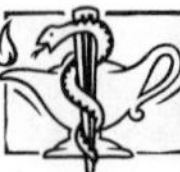

INTERVENTIONS

Office Treatment

For *C. botulinum,* immediate hospitalization in intensive care unit

Lifestyle Modifications

- Bed rest for 1 to 2 days
- Clear liquids for 24 hours; then bland diet

Patient Education

Teach patient about:

- Condition, cause, and treatment options:
  - *Shigella*—antibiotics, increased fluids, rest
  - *Salmonella*—antibiotics only if systemic illness present, increased fluids, rest
  - *B. cereus*—increased fluids, rest
  - *C. botulinum*—immediate hospitalization in intensive care unit
  - *C. perfringens*—increased fluids, rest
  - *E. coli*—antibiotics, increased fluids, rest
  - *Y. enterocolitica*—antibiotics, increased fluids, rest
  - *C. jejuni*—antibiotics, increased fluids, rest
- Diet for all types—liquid or bland
- For diarrhea—kaolin pectin or bismuth subsalicylate *(do not use stronger preparations—may prolong illness)*
- Future preventive measures:
  - No raw seafood, meats, or poultry
  - No unpasteurized dairy products
  - Need to cook food thoroughly
  - Need to keep food refrigerated
  - Need to clean food preparation areas thoroughly
- Medications used and side effects (see Pharmacotherapeutics)

Referral

To MD for *C. botulinum*

TABLE 8 *Symptoms of Food Poisoning and Causative Organisms*

Organism	Onset (hours)	Symptoms
Shigella	12-48	Fever, bloody diarrhea, sepsis, meningitis
Salmonella	12-48	Fever, diarrhea, sepsis, meningitis
Bacillus cereus	2-16	Nausea, vomiting, cramps, diarrhea
Clostridium botulinum	12-36	Vomiting, diarrhea, motor paralysis, respiratory paralysis, death
Clostridium perfringens	12-24	Cramps, diarrhea
Escherichia coli	24-48	Diarrhea, fever (maybe)
Yersinia enterocolitica	3-7 days	Fever, Pseudoappendicitis
Campylobacter jejuni	18-72	Fever, cramps, diarrhea

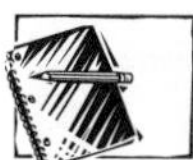

EVALUATION

Outcome
Resolves without sequelae in a few days

Possible Complications
- Electrolyte imbalance
- Cardiac arrhythmias
- Septicemia
- Cardiovascular collapse

Follow-up
In 1 week; sooner if symptoms worsen

FOR YOUR INFORMATION

Life Span
Pediatric: Very young at high risk for severe dehydration and other complications
Geriatric: May dehydrate quickly; require hospitalization more frequently
Pregnancy: *Salmonella* and *Helicobacter* organisms may secondarily infect newborn, resulting in serious consequences

Miscellaneous
The majority of the time, food poisoning is self-limiting and resolved by the time stool cultures are interpreted.

References
Bartlett JG: *Pocket book of infectious disease therapy,* ed 7, Baltimore, 1996, Williams & Wilkins, pp 287-294.

Bennett RG: Acute gastroenteritis and associated conditions. In Barker LR, Burton JR, Zieve PD, editors: *Principles of ambulatory medicine,* ed 4, Baltimore, 1995, Williams & Wilkins, pp 307-318.

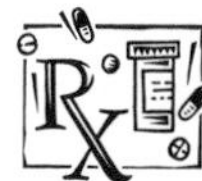

PHARMACOTHERAPEUTICS

Drug of Choice	Mechanism of Action	Prescribing Information	Side Effects
Ciprofloxacin (Cipro): • For *Shigella,* 500 mg PO bid × 3 days • For *Salmonella,* 500 mg PO bid × 14 days • For *Escherichia coli* and *Campylobacter jejuni,* 500 mg PO bid × 3-5 days • Not recommended for children <18 years	Interferes with conversion of intermediate DNA fragments into high molecular weight DNA in bacteria	***Contraindication:*** Hypersensitivity ***Cost:*** 500-mg tab, 100 tabs: $303 ***Pregnancy category:*** C	Headache, dizziness, fatigue, depression, restlessness, nausea, diarrhea, increased ALT and AST, flatulence, heartburn, vomiting, oral candidiasis, rash, pruritus, urticaria, photosensitivity, blurred vision, tinnitus
Sulfamethoxazole (SMZ)/trimethoprim (TMP) (Septra DS): • For *E. coli,* 1 DS PO bid × 7 days • For *Yersinia enterocolitica,* 1 DS PO bid × 3 days • Children, 8 mg/kg (TMP)/40 mg/kg (SMZ) PO bid × 7 days for *E. coli* and 3 days for *Y. en-terocolitica*	Interferes with bacterial biosynthesis of proteins and blocks synthesis of tetrahydrofolic acid	***Contraindications:*** Hypersensitivity; pregnancy at term; megaloblastic anemia; infants *<2 months old; creatinine clearance <15 ml/min; lactation* ***Cost:*** DS tab, 100 tabs: $8-$70 ***Pregnancy category:*** C	Headache, insomnia, hallucinations, depression, vertigo, fatigue, allergic myocarditis, nausea, vomiting, abdominal pain, hepatitis, glossitis, enterocolitis, renal failure, toxic nephrosis, increased BUN and creatinine, leukopenia, neutropenia, thrombocytopenia, agranulocytosis, hemolytic anemia, hypoprothrombinemia, methemoglobinemia, rash, dermatitis, Stevens-Johnson syndrome, anaphylaxis, systemic lupus erythematosus
Ampicillin (Ampicin): • For *Shigella,* 500 mg PO qid × 3-5 days • For *Salmonella,* 500 mg PO qid × 14 days • Children, 50-100 mg/kg/day in divided doses qid × 3-5 days for *Shigella* and 14 days for *Salmonella*	Interferes with cell wall replication	***Contraindication:*** Hypersensitivity to penicillin ***Cost:*** 500-mg tab, 100 tabs: $13-$30 ***Pregnancy category:*** B	Rash, urticaria, anemia, bone marrow depression, granulocytopenia, nausea, vomiting, diarrhea, oliguria, proteinuria, vaginitis, moniliasis, glomerulonephritis, lethargy, hallucinations, anxiety, coma

Frostbite

OVERVIEW

Frostbite is a result of overexposure to the cold. It results in trauma to the skin and subcutaneous tissue. It most commonly affects the fingers, ears, nose, and toes.

Pathogenesis

Overexposure to cold leads to vasoconstriction of peripheral vessels, which leads to decreased blood supply, which leads to tissue damage

Patient Profile

- Males = Females
- Persons more prone to frostbite—the elderly, alcoholics, homeless persons, drug abusers, smokers, and patients with Raynaud's phenomenon

Signs and Symptoms

- First skin appears cold, hard, white, and numb to the touch
- With rewarming, will appear blotchy red, swollen, and painful
- Loss of cutaneous sensation
- Numbness
- Throbbing pain
- Paresthesia
- Excessive sweating
- Joint pain
- Pallor
- Subcutaneous edema
- Blistering
- Blue discoloration
- Skin necrosis
- Gangrene

Differential Diagnosis

Frostnip—superficial cold injury

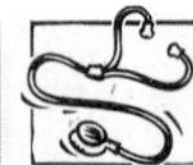

ASSESSMENT

History

Inquire about:

- Onset and duration of symptoms
- Length of time exposed to cold
- Use of alcohol or drugs
- Previous injury to same area
- Tetanus immunization
- Treatments tried
- Underlying conditions (particularly conditions that affect circulation—diabetes, peripheral vascular disease, Raynaud's phenomenon)
- Current medications

Physical Findings

- Skin may appear cold, hard, and white if frostbite is recent, or blotchy red, swollen, and painful if rewarming was attempted
- Blistering
- Swelling and numbness
- May appear blue/black with foul odor if gangrene present

Initial Workup

Laboratory

- CBC
- Electrolytes
- Liver enzymes
- Renal function studies if indicated

Radiology: Depends on severity; if concerned about osteomyelitis, x-ray film of frostbitten area

Further Workup

Depends on severity; usually none

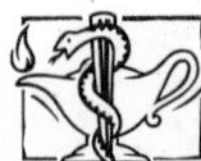

INTERVENTIONS

Office Treatment

- Rewarm injured part in warm water
- Never rub
- Give patient warm fluids to drink
- Protect from injury
- If severe, may need to keep area frozen until transported to acute care facility
- Area may need debridement; can be done with whirlpool therapy

Lifestyle Modifications

- Smoking cessation
- Nutritionally sound diet
- Cessation of drugs and alcohol
- Keeping injured area warm

Patient Education

Teach patient about:

- Condition and treatment
- Rewarming injured area
- Avoiding further trauma to area
- Antibiotics if infection present
- Keeping area clean if open wound present
- Protecting area from cold
- Participating in physical therapy
- Ways to prevent frostbite
- Effects of smoking, drugs, and alcohol
- Tips for smoking, drug, and alcohol cessation
- Dressing in layers
- Need to keep moving and keep dry when out in the cold
- Medications used and side effects (see Pharmacotherapeutics)

Referral

To hospital emergency room if severe

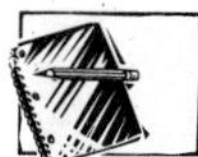

EVALUATION

Outcome

Affected areas heal; may take 6 to 12 months

Possible Complications

- Systemic infection
- Gangrene requiring amputation
- Death

Follow-up

In 48 hours to reassess; then every 2 weeks until healed; assess for signs and symptoms of infection at each visit

FOR YOUR INFORMATION

Life Span

Pediatric: Very young have higher morbidity and mortality
Geriatric: Higher morbidity and mortality; increased risk because of fragility of skin
Pregnancy: Should be handled by specialist

Miscellaneous

Distal parts (fingers and toes) may undergo spontaneous amputation

References

Cohen R, Moelleken B: Disorders due to physical agents. In Tierney LM Jr, McPhee SJ, Papadakis MA, editors: *Current medical diagnosis and treatment,* ed 34, Norwalk, Conn, 1995, Appleton & Lange, pp 1335-1338.

Vaughn K: Emergency care situations. In Lewis SM, Collier IC, Heitkemper MM, editors: *Medical-surgical nursing: assessment and management of clinical problems,* ed 4, St Louis, 1996, Mosby, pp 2009-2010.

NOTES

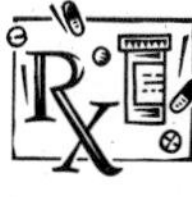

PHARMACOTHERAPEUTICS

The patient needs continual monitoring for the presence of infection. If an infection is suspected, one of the oral antibiotics presented here may be used.

Drug of Choice	Mechanism of Action	Prescribing Information	Side Effects
Dicloxacillin, 250 mg q6h for 10 days; children <40 kg, 12.5-25 mg/kg/d divided q6h	Bactericidal cell wall inhibitor; active against gram-positive cocci except enterococci	***Contraindication:*** Hypersensitivity to penicillins ***Cost:*** 500-mg tab, 50 tabs: $19-$88 ***Pregnancy category:*** B	Bone marrow depression, granulocytopenia, nausea, vomiting, diarrhea, oliguria, proteinuria, hematuria, moniliasis, glomerulonephritis, lethargy, depression, convulsions, anaphylaxis
Erythromycin (E.E.S.), 250 mg q6h for 10 days; children, 30-50 mg/kg/d divided q6h	Macrolide; protein synthesis inhibitor; active against bacteria lacking cell walls, most gram-positive aerobes	***Contraindication:*** Hypersensitivity ***Cost:*** 250-mg tabs, 4/day × 10 days: $4 ***Pregnancy category:*** B	Nausea, vomiting, diarrhea, abdominal pain, anorexia, rash, urticaria, pseudomembranous colitis—rarely
Ciprofloxacin (Cipro), 500 mg bid for 10 days; not dosed for children	Fluoroquinilone; interferes with conversion of intermediate DNA fragments into high molecular weight DNA	***Contraindication:*** Hypersensitivity ***Cost:*** 500-mg tab, 100 tabs: $365 ***Pregnancy category:*** C	Headache, dizziness, fatigue, insomnia, depression, seizures, confusion, nausea, diarrhea, increased ALT and AST, flatulence, heartburn, oral candidiasis, rash, pruritus, urticaria, photosensitivity, blurred vision

Frozen Shoulder/Adhesive Capsulitis

OVERVIEW

Frozen shoulder is a condition in which shoulder motion is restricted in all directions.

Pathogenesis

Cause—unknown; may be bicipital tenosynovitis, rotator cuff tendinitis, or reflex sympathetic dystrophy

Patient Profile

- Females > Males
- Most common age group—middle-aged and elderly persons
- More common in diabetic patients

Signs and Symptoms

- Onset gradual
- Shoulder pain and tenderness
- Decreased range of motion in all directions

Differential Diagnosis

- Posterior shoulder dislocation
- Degenerative arthritis

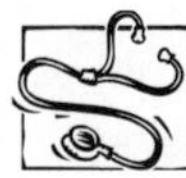

ASSESSMENT

History

Inquire about:

- Onset and duration of symptoms
- Recent or past history of trauma to shoulder
- Difficulty sleeping because of pain in shoulder
- Underlying conditions (diabetes)
- Current medications

Physical Findings

- General appearance—apprehension, holding arm protectively
- Tenderness on palpation
- Decreased range of motion

Initial Workup

Laboratory: None indicated
Radiology: Shoulder—rule out posterior dislocation

Further Workup

None indicated

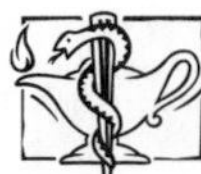

INTERVENTIONS

Office Treatment

None indicated

Lifestyle Modifications

May interfere with occupation and all aspects of lifestyle

Patient Education

Teach patient about:

- Condition and treatment:
  - Overhead pulley exercises, initially every hour
  - Using moist heat
  - Wearing a sling
- Avoiding forceful movement of the shoulder
- Medications used and side effects (see Pharmacotherapeutics)

Referral

To orthopedist for injection of rotator cuff with corticosteroids/lidocaine

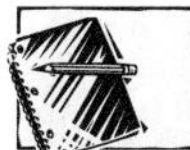

EVALUATION

Outcome
Will eventually resolve, but may take 6 months or longer

Possible Complications
Usually none; may have some mild loss of motion and pain for years

Follow-up
In 2 weeks × 2; then monthly

FOR YOUR INFORMATION

Life Span
Pediatric: Not seen in this age group
Geriatric: More common in this age group; resolution may take longer
Pregnancy: To specialist

Miscellaneous
N/A

References
Hellman DB: Arthritis and musculoskeletal disorders. In Tierney LM Jr, McPhee SJ, Papadakis MA, editors: *Current medical diagnosis and treatment,* ed 34, Norwalk, Conn, 1995, Appleton & Lange, pp 707-708.
Mercier LR: *Practical orthopedics,* ed 4, St Louis, 1995, Mosby, pp 65-66.

NOTES

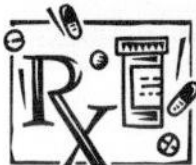

PHARMACOTHERAPEUTICS

Drug of Choice	Mechanism of Action	Prescribing Information	Side Effects
Nonsteroidal antiinflammatory drugs (NSAIDs): many different types currently marketed; consult manufacturer's package insert for specific dosing and prescribing information	Exact action unknown; may be caused by inhibition of synthesis of prostaglandins and arachidonic acid	***Contraindications:*** Hypersensitivity to NSAIDs, aspirin; severe hepatic failure; asthma ***Cost:*** Varies with type ***Pregnancy category:*** Depends on product	Stomach distress, flatulence, nausea, abdominal pain, constipation or diarrhea, dizziness, sedation, rash, urticaria, angioedema, anorexia, urinary frequency, increased blood pressure, insomnia, anxiety, visual disturbances, increased thirst, alopecia

Furuncle/Carbuncle

OVERVIEW

A furuncle is a deep folliculitis that spreads away from the hair follicle into the surrounding dermis. It is a walled-off, pus-filled mass that is painful, and firm or fluctuant. Carbuncles are aggregates of infected follicles and are commonly referred to as boils.

Pathogenesis

Infection usually caused by *Staphylococcus aureus*

Patient Profile

- Males = Females
- Uncommon in children
- Incidence increases after puberty

Signs and Symptoms

FURUNCLE

- Painful, erythematous papule or nodule
- Appears most often in areas of friction—waistline, groin, buttocks, axillae
- May or may not have purulent drainage

CARBUNCLE

- Large, painful, red, swollen mass that drains from several openings
- Occurs in areas of deep dermis (back of neck, lateral aspect of thigh)

Differential Diagnosis

- Folliculitis
- Pseudofolliculitis
- Ruptured epidermal cyst
- Acne pustules
- Keratosis pilaris

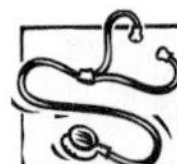

ASSESSMENT

History

Inquire about:

- Onset and duration of symptoms
- Previous history of boils
- Treatments tried and results
- Frequency of occurrence
- Underlying conditions, such as diabetes, alcoholism, malnutrition, immunosuppression
- Current medications

Physical Findings

- Furuncle—painful, hard or fluctuant, erythematous lesion; may have purulent drainage
- Carbuncle—large, painful, red, swollen mass, draining from several openings
- Fever
- Chills
- Malaise—either as prodrome or during active phase

Initial Workup

Laboratory

- Culture and sensitivity of drainage
- If indicated, screen for underlying condition

Radiology: None indicated

Further Workup

- None indicated, unless signs and symptoms of underlying disease present
- If recurrent, culture and sensitivity of nares to determine carrier state

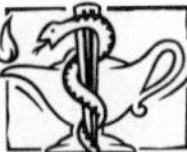

INTERVENTIONS

Office Treatment

- Incision and drainage of fluctuant lesions
- Large wounds may require packing with iodoform; must be removed and repacked twice daily until drainage stops

Lifestyle Modifications

- Good hygiene—daily bathing; frequent hand washing; changing towels, washcloths, and sheets daily
- Avoidance of contact sports such as wrestling
- Avoidance of nose picking (many people carry *Staphylococcus aureus* in their nares)

Patient Education

Teach patient about:

- Condition and treatment:
  - Antibiotics
  - Care of wound if incision and drainage done—need to keep clean, repack with iodoform gauze if necessary, apply dressing
  - Using warm, moist compresses to provide localization and spontaneous drainage
- Causative agent, which may be carried in nares
- Frequent recurrences—have patient shower daily with povidone-iodine (Betadine), chlorhexidine (Hibiclens), or hexachlorophene (Phisohex) soap; after showering apply mupirocin to both nares
- Medications used and side effects (see Pharmacotherapeutics)

Referrals

- To primary care physician for lesions on face, scalp, and neck
- To dermatologist for persistent, recurrent cases

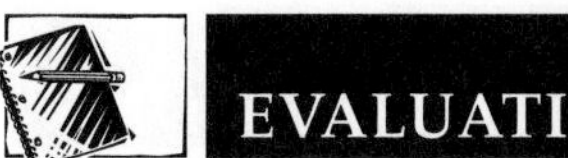

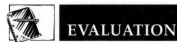

EVALUATION

Outcomes

- Resolves without sequelae
- Recurrences can last for months or years—treat as above to attempt to control

Possible Complications

- Scarring
- Septicemia

Follow-up

In 2 weeks

FOR YOUR INFORMATION

Life Span

Pediatric: Usually occurs after puberty
Geriatric: Treatment is the same; look for underlying condition
Pregnancy: Cautious use of medications

Miscellaneous

Recurrent furuncles/carbuncles could be an indication of an underlying disease process, such as diabetes, primary immunosuppression, or secondary immunosuppression.

References

Habif TP: *Clinical dermatology: a color guide to diagnosis and therapy,* ed 3, St Louis, 1996, Mosby, pp 252-254.

Uphold CR, Graham MV: *Clinical guidelines in adult health,* Gainesville, Fla, 1994, Barmarrae Books, pp 158-159.

PHARMACOTHERAPEUTICS

Drug of Choice	Mechanism of Action	Prescribing Information	Side Effects
For staphylococcal infection, use one of the following:			
Dicloxacillin, 250 mg PO q6h × 10 days; children <40 kg, 12.5-25 mg/kg/d divided q6h	Bactericidal cell wall inhibitor; active against gram-positive cocci except enterococci	***Contraindication:*** Hypersensitivity to penicillins ***Cost:*** 500-mg tab, 50 tabs: $19-$88 ***Pregnancy category:*** B	Bone marrow depression, granulocytopenia, nausea, vomiting, diarrhea, oliguria, proteinuria, hematuria, moniliasis, glomerulonephritis, lethargy, depression, convulsions, anaphylaxis
Erythromycin (E.E.S.), 250 mg PO q6h × 10 days; children, 30-50 mg/kg/d divided q6h	Macrolide; protein synthesis inhibitor; active against bacteria lacking cell walls, most gram-positive aerobes	***Contraindication:*** Hypersensitivity ***Cost:*** 250-mg tabs, 4/day × 10 days-$4 ***Pregnancy category:*** B	Nausea, vomiting, diarrhea, abdominal pain, anorexia, rash, urticaria, pseudomembranous colitis—rarely
For Pseudomonas, *use one of the following:*			
Ciprofloxacin (Cipro), 500 mg PO bid × 10 days—not dosed for children	Fluoroquinilone; interferes with conversion of intermediate DNA fragments into high molecular weight DNA	***Contraindication:*** Hypersensitivity ***Cost:*** 500-mg tab, 100 tabs: $365 ***Pregnancy category:*** C	Headache, dizziness, fatigue, insomnia, depression, seizures, confusion, nausea, diarrhea, increased ALT and AST, flatulence, heartburn, oral candidiasis, rash, pruritus, urticaria, photosensitivity, blurred vision
Cefadroxil (Duricef), 500 mg PO bid × 10 days; children, 30 mg/kg/day PO in divided doses q12h	Cephalosporin; bactericidal; inhibits cell wall synthesis	***Contraindication:*** Hypersensitivity ***Cost:*** 500-mg tab, 50 tabs: $169 ***Pregnancy category:*** B	Diarrhea, pseudomembranous colitis, nausea, vomiting, rash, urticaria, angioedema, vaginitis, neutropenia, Stevens-Johnson syndrome, anaphylaxis, seizures
For mild cases or staphylococcal carriers:			
Mupirocin (Bactroban) ointment; apply to affected area bid or, for carriers, to nares bid	Inhibits bacterial protein synthesis	***Contraindication:*** Hypersensitivity ***Cost:*** 2% ointment, 30 g: $29 ***Pregnancy category:*** B	Burning, stinging, itching, rash, erythema, dry skin, tenderness, swelling, contact dermatitis

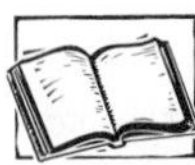

OVERVIEW

Galactorrhea is a milky nipple discharge. It occurs spontaneously and is usually bilateral. It is not related to lactation. Technically, it does not include serous, bloody, or purulent nipple discharge, although some authors may include these under the heading "galactorrhea."

Pathogenesis

Causes:

- Prolactin-producing pituitary adenoma
- Medications (opiates, tricyclics, metoclopramide, verapamil, phenothiazines, alpha-methyldopa, isoniazid, estrogens, reserpine, butyrophenones)
- Birth control pill withdrawal
- Hypothyroidism and other endocrine disorders
- Chest wall conditions (e.g., herpes zoster, postthoracotomy, fibrocystic changes)

Patient Profile

- Females almost exclusively
- Predominant age—reproductive years (15 to 50)

Signs and Symptoms

- Milky discharge from nipples
- Amenorrhea often accompanies galactorrhea
- May have other signs and symptoms, depending on cause

Differential Diagnosis

- Serous discharge—fibrocystic breast disease
- Purulent discharge—mastitis
- Bloody discharge—malignancy

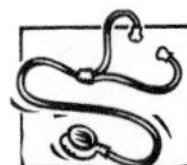

ASSESSMENT

History

Inquire about:

- Onset and duration of symptoms
- Postpartum status and breast-feeding (may have milky discharge up to 5 years after stopping breast-feeding)
- Menstrual history and date of last menstrual period
- Underlying conditions
- Current medications

Physical Findings

- Milky nipple discharge
- Breast examination—no masses should be found
- Depending on history, physical findings of other diseases should be looked for, particularly endocrine diseases:
  - Hypothyroidism—hair loss, weight gain, fatigue
  - Cushing's syndrome—moon face, weight gain
  - Pituitary enlargement/tumor—headache, peripheral visual field loss

Initial Workup

Laboratory

- Sample of discharge placed on slide and stained with Sudan stain—if milk is present, there will be fat globules on microscopic examination
- Tests for prolactin level and thyroid function (TSH, T_3, T_4) in all patients
- Test for FSH/LH level if amenorrheic
- Other laboratory tests according to physical findings

Radiology: CT scan or MRI of pituitary if prolactin level is elevated even minimally

Further Workup

As directed by first set of tests

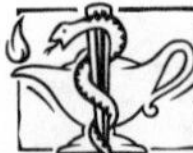

INTERVENTIONS

Office Treatment

None indicated

Lifestyle Modifications

Depends on cause; if idiopathic, patient may wish to wear breast-feeding pads to prevent staining of clothing

Patient Education

Teach patient about:

- Condition and treatment
- Galactorrhea by itself not being harmful
- Underlying causes
- Signs and symptoms of growing pituitary adenoma—central headache, visual field loss
- Stopping any offending medications if possible
- Wearing breast pads to protect clothing
- Treatment options—"watchful waiting" is appropriate in most cases; if large pituitary adenoma is present, may need x-ray therapy or transsphenoidal resection
- Medications used and side effects (see Pharmacotherapeutics)

Referral

Depends on cause—to endocrinologist if endocrine; to gynecologist if amenorrheic

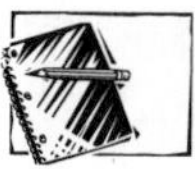

EVALUATION

Outcomes

Depends on cause:

- Physiologic—will resolve with time
- Pituitary adenoma—x-ray therapy has variable success; transsphenoidal resection—90% success rate; symptoms tend to recur with discontinuation of medication

Possible Complications

Depends on cause

Follow-up

Depends on cause

FOR YOUR INFORMATION

Life Span

Pediatric: Usually occurs after puberty
Geriatric: Usually not seen in this population; look for possible cancer
Pregnancy: Pituitary adenomas may grow rapidly

Miscellaneous

The NP needs to assist the patient in coping with this condition, since it causes a great deal of anxiety for many patients. The patient needs to be provided with literature regarding galactorrhea, and the patient needs the support of family and/or friends. Careful evaluation of the patient's anxiety level and coping abilities needs to be performed by the NP, and referral for counseling may be appropriate.

References

Branch LG: Breast health. In Youngkin EQ, Davis MS, editors: *Women's health: a primary care clinical guide,* Norwalk, Conn, 1994, Appleton & Lange, pp 290-292.

Vorpahl CL: Breast disorders. In Lewis SM, Collier IC, Heitkemper MM, editors: *Medical surgical nursing: assessment and management of clinical problems,* ed 4, St Louis, 1996, Mosby, p 1547.

NOTES

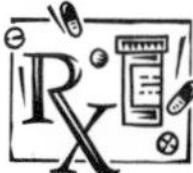

PHARMACOTHERAPEUTICS

Drug of Choice	Mechanism of Action	Prescribing Information	Side Effects
Bromocriptine mesylate (Parlodel); start with ½ to 1 tablet of 2.5 mg/day PO and increase as needed to achieve therapeutic effect; lowest therapeutic dose should be used; may take an average of 6-8 weeks to see results; take with food	Decreases prolactin secretion and, in patients with pituitary adenoma, has been shown to shrink the adenoma	***Contraindications:*** Hypersensitivity; severe ischemia or peripheral vascular disease ***Cost:*** 2.5-mg tab, 30 tabs: $48 ***Pregnancy category:*** B	Nausea, headache, dizziness, fatigue, lightheadedness, vomiting, abdominal cramps, nasal congestion, diarrhea, constipation, drowsiness; incidence of side effects is quite high

Gastritis

OVERVIEW

Gastritis is an inflammation of the lining of the stomach.

Pathogenesis

Several types with different causes:

- Erosive gastritis—mucosal injury due to chemical agent—alcohol, aspirin, NSAID, corticosteroid
- Reflux gastritis—prolonged exposure to bile and pancreatic juice (defective pylorus)
- Hemorrhagic stress ulcer—reaction to hemodynamic disorder (hypovolemia, hypoxia, being in intensive care unit)
- Infectious gastritis—*Helicobacter pylori* (usually component of systemic infection); *Staphylococcus* species
- Atrophic gastritis—gastric mucosal atrophy (seen in the elderly)
- Other causes—shock, sepsis, burns, psychologic stress, renal failure, spicy/irritating foods
- Smoking

Patient Profile

- Males = Females
- Any age

Signs and Symptoms

- Anorexia
- Nausea, vomiting
- Epigastric tenderness—often aggravated by eating
- Feeling of fullness

Differential Diagnosis

- Peptic ulcer disease
- Functional gastrointestinal disorder

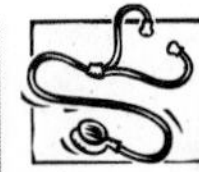

ASSESSMENT

History

Inquire about:

- Onset and duration of symptoms
- Whether food makes it better or worse
- Alcohol intake
- Use of aspirin, nonsteroidal antiinflammatory agents, or steroids
- Smoking history
- Underlying conditions
- Current medications

Physical Findings

- Epigastric pain on palpation
- Weight loss
- Pallor (maybe)
- May have normal physical examination findings

Initial Workup

Laboratory

- CBC—anemia (if bleeding present)
- Serum antigen/antibody test for *H. pylori*

Radiology: Not reliable for gastritis

Further Workup

Endoscopic (gastroscopy) examination with biopsy (precise diagnosis)

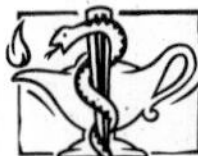

INTERVENTIONS

Office Treatment

None indicated

Lifestyle Modifications

- Smoking cessation
- Avoidance of foods that precipitate symptoms
- Avoidance of aspirin, steroids, and NSAIDs, if possible
- Alcohol cessation

Patient Education

Teach patient about:

- Condition and treatment options:
  - If *H. pylori* found, combination therapy with antibiotics, bismuth subsalicylate, or proton pump inhibitors
  - If non–*H. Pylori,* antacids or H_2 receptor antagonists
- For all—tips on smoking cessation
- Avoidance of alcohol
- Stopping aspirin, steroids, NSAIDs, or, if not possible, treating with misoprostol
- Avoidance of spicy foods that precipitate pain
- Medications used and side effects (see Pharmacotherapeutics)

Referral

To gastroenterologist if treatment fails

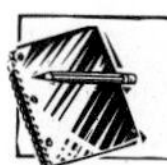

EVALUATION

Outcome
Resolves without sequelae

Possible Complications
- Ulceration
- Bleeding

Follow-up
In 2 weeks × 2; if symptoms unresolved, repeat endoscopy

FOR YOUR INFORMATION

Life Span
Pediatric: Rarely occurs in this age group
Geriatric: Most commonly have chronic atrophic gastritis—may be asymptomatic or have vague symptoms
Pregnancy: Use medications with caution

Miscellaneous
In chronic gastritis, if the acid-secreting cells are lost, intrinsic factor is lost, resulting in vitamin B_{12} deficiency (pernicious anemia). These patients require regular B_{12} injections.

References
Fay M, Jaffe PE: Diagnostic and treatment guidelines for *Helicobacter pylori, Nurse Pract* 21(7):28, 30, 33-34, 1996.

Georges JM, Deters GE. Nursing role in management: problems of digestion. In Lewis SM, Collier IC, Heitkemper MM, editors: *Medical-surgical nursing: assessment and management of clinical problems,* ed 4, St Louis, 1996, Mosby, pp 1174-1176.

NOTES

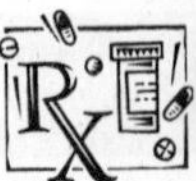

PHARMACOTHERAPEUTICS

There are many OTC preparations available for the treatment of gastritis. These should be tried before using the stronger, prescription medications. Start with OTC antacids, such as Tums, Rolaids, Maalox, or Mylanta. If no success is achieved with these medications, try the OTC H2 antagonists, such as Pepcid AC, Tagamet HB, Axid HR, or Zantac. If symptoms are still not relieved, try one of the prescription medications presented here.

For treatment of *Helicobacter pylori,* use one of the following combination therapies: 3-drug regimens—(1) Pepto-Bismol 2 tabs qid, metronidazole 250 mg tid, and tetracycline 500 mg qid or amoxicillin 500 mg qid × 7 to 14 days; or (2) metronidazole 500 mg bid, omeprazole 20 mg bid, and clarithromycin 250 mg bid × 7 to 14 days; or dual therapy—omeprazole 20 mg bid and clarithromycin 500 mg tid × 2 weeks.

Drug of Choice	Mechanism of Action	Prescribing Information	Side Effects
Famotidine or cimetidine (Pepcid or Tagamet): • Pepcid, 20 mg PO bid—not for children • Tagamet, 300 mg PO with meals and at bedtime—not for children <16 years • Treat for 3-4 weeks, then reduce dosages to OTC strength	Inhibits histamine at H_2 receptor sites	***Contraindication:*** Hypersensitivity ***Cost:*** Pepcid, 20-mg tab, 30 tabs: $45; Tagamet, 300-mg tab, 100 tabs: $45 ***Pregnancy category:*** B	Confusion, headache, depression, dizziness, convulsions, diarrhea, abdominal cramps, paralytic ileus, jaundice, gynecomastia, galactorrhea, increased BUN and creatinine, agranulocytosis, thrombocytopenia, neutropenia, aplastic anemia, urticaria, exfoliative dermatitis
Sucralfate (Carafate), 1 g PO qid on empty stomach—not dosed for children	Protectant; absorbs pepsin	***Contraindication:*** Hypersensitivity ***Cost:*** 1-g tab, 100 tabs: $75 ***Pregnancy category:*** B	Drowsiness, dizziness, dry mouth, constipation, nausea, gastric pain, vomiting, urticaria, rash, pruritus
Misoprostol (Cytotec), 200 μg PO qid with food—not dosed for children	Protectant; inhibits gastric acid secretion	***Contraindications:*** Hypersensitivity; pregnancy ***Cost:*** 200-μg tab, 60 tabs: $41 ***Pregnancy category:*** X	Diarrhea, nausea, vomiting, flatulence, constipation, spotting, cramps, hypermenorrhea, menstrual disorders
For H. pylori:			
Bismuth subsalicylate (Pepto-Bismol), 2 tabs PO qid; children 10-14 years, 15 ml PO qid × 2 weeks	Inhibits prostaglandin synthesis responsible for GI hypermotility; stimulates absorption of fluid and electrolytes	***Contraindication:*** Children <3 years old ***Cost:*** OTC ***Pregnancy category:*** Not categorized	Increased bleeding time, increased fecal impactions, dark stools, confusion, twitching, hearing loss, black gums, black tongue
Omeprazole (Prilosec), 20 mg PO bid × 2 weeks—not for children	Gastric acid pump inhibitor	***Contraindication:*** Hypersensitivity ***Cost:*** 20-mg tab, 30 tabs: $130 ***Pregnancy category:*** C	Headache, dizziness, asthenia, diarrhea, abdominal pain, vomiting, nausea, constipation, flatulence, acid regurgitation, abdominal swelling, anorexia, upper respiratory infections, cough, epistaxis, rash, dry skin, urticaria, hypoglycemia, increased liver enzymes, weight gain, tinnitus, chest pain, angina, hematuria, bradycardia, tachycardia, urinary tract infection (UTI), pancytopenia, thrombocytopenia, neutropenia, leukocytosis, anemia, back pain

Drug of Choice	Mechanism of Action	Prescribing Information	Side Effects
For H. pylori:*—cont'd*			
Metronidazole (Flagyl), 250 mg PO tid × 2 weeks; children, 35-50 mg/kg/day PO in 3 divided doses × 2 weeks	Direct-acting amebicide/trichomonacide	***Contraindications:*** Hypersensitivity; renal disease; hepatic disease; contracted visual or color fields; blood dyscrasias; pregnancy (1st trimester); lactation; CNS disorders ***Cost:*** 500-mg tab, 50 tabs: $5-$40; 250-mg tab, 100 tabs: $5-$110 ***Pregnancy category:*** B (2nd and 3rd trimesters)	Flat T-waves, headache, dizziness, irritability, restlessness, fatigue, convulsions, incoordinations, blurred vision, sore throat, retinal edema, dry mouth, metallic taste, furry tongue, nausea, vomiting, diarrhea, epigastric distress, anorexia, constipation, abdominal cramps, pseudomembranous colitis, darkened urine, vaginal dryness, albuminuria, neurotoxicity, leukopenia, bone marrow depression, rash, urticaria
Tetracycline (Achromycin), 500 mg PO qid 2 weeks; children >8 years, 25-50 mg/kg/day PO in 4 divided doses × 2 weeks	Bacteriostatic; inhibits protein synthesis	***Contraindications:*** Hypersensitivity; children <8 years; pregnancy; lactation ***Cost:*** 250-mg tab, 100 tabs: $6 ***Pregnancy category:*** D	Fever, headache, paresthesia, eosinophilia, neutropenia, thrombocytopenia, leukocytosis, hemolytic anemia, dysphagia, glossitis, discoloration of deciduous teeth, oral candidiasis, nausea, abdominal pain, vomiting, diarrhea, anorexia, hepatotoxicity, pericarditis, increased BUN, rash, photosensitivity, exfoliative dermatitis, pruritus, angioedema
Clarithromycin (Biaxin), 500 mg PO tid × 2 weeks	Binds to 50S ribosomal subunits and suppresses protein synthesis	***Contraindication:*** Hypersensitivity ***Cost:*** 500-mg tab, 60 tabs: $179 ***Pregnancy category:*** C	Rash, urticaria, pruritus, nausea, vomiting, hepatoxicity, diarrhea, heartburn, anorexia, vaginitis, moniliasis, headache
Amoxicillin (Amoxil), 500 mg PO qid; children, 20-40 mg/kg/day PO in 4 divided doses	Interferes with cell wall replication	***Contraindications:*** Hypersensitivity to penicillins; use caution if allergic to cephalosporins ***Cost:*** 500-mg tab, 50 tabs: $9-$20 ***Pregnancy category:*** B	Anemia, increased bleeding time, bone marrow depression, granulocytopenia, nausea, vomiting, diarrhea, increased ALT and AST, abdominal pain, pseudomembranous colitis, headache, fever, anaphylaxis, respiratory distress

Gastroesophageal Reflux Disease (GERD)

OVERVIEW

Gastroesophageal reflux disease (GERD) is a condition in which there is reflux of gastric secretions into the esophagus.

Pathogenesis

Reflux of gastric contents into esophagus secondary to incompetent lower esophageal sphincter, defective esophageal clearance mechanisms, increased gastric secretions, and delayed gastric emptying

Patient Profile

- Males = Females
- Any age
- Risk factors
  - Foods or drugs that decrease lower esophageal sphincter pressure
  - Obesity
  - Cigarette smoking
  - Excessive alcohol
  - Coffee
  - Hiatal hernia
  - Children—Down syndrome, mental retardation, cerebral palsy

Signs and Symptoms

- Heartburn
- Regurgitation—bitter or sour taste in mouth
- Dysphagia
- Laryngitis
- Asthma

Differential Diagnosis

- Cardiac chest pain
- Infectious esophagitis
- Chemical esophagitis
- Peptic ulcer disease
- Esophageal tumor

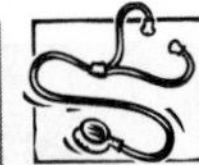

ASSESSMENT

History

Inquire about:

- Onset and duration of symptoms
- Whether symptoms are relieved by sitting up and by taking antacids
- Smoking and alcohol history
- Underlying conditions and current medications

Physical Findings

- Obesity
- Otherwise, physical examination within normal limits

Initial Workup

Laboratory: None indicated
Radiology: Barium swallow

Further Workup

Esophagoscopy with biopsy; diagnosis can usually be made on basis of history

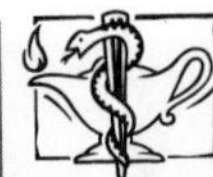

INTERVENTIONS

Office Treatment

None indicated

Lifestyle Modifications

- Smoking and alcohol cessation
- Weight loss—low-fat diet
- Avoidance of foods that precipitate symptoms

Patient Education

Teach patient about:

- Condition and treatment options:
  - Step 1—tips for smoking and alcohol cessation, low-fat diet, and exercise for weight loss; elevating head of bed and not lying down within 2 to 3 hours of eating; eating smaller meals; avoiding foods that precipitate symptoms (chocolate, citrus fruits, dairy products, coffee); antacids
  - Step 2—H_2 receptor blockers (OTC strength, then prescriptive strength)
  - Step 3—higher-dose H_2 receptor blocker, proton pump inhibitor, or prokinetic drug
- Medications used and side effects (see Pharmacotherapeutics)

Referral

To primary care physician or gastroenterologist if step 3 treatment fails

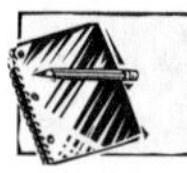

EVALUATION

Outcome

If lifestyle modifications followed, prognosis is good; if not, recurrence is likely on withdrawal of medications

Possible Complications

- Aspiration
- Reflux-induced asthma
- Chronic cough
- Loss of dental enamel
- Halitosis

Follow-up

In 2 weeks; if symptoms relieved, maintain on current therapy for 8 weeks, reevaluating effectiveness periodically

FOR YOUR INFORMATION

Life Span

Pediatric: In infants, reflux generally resolves by 18 months; vomiting, weight loss, and failure to thrive are common symptoms
Geriatric: More prone to aspiration
Pregnancy: Very common; use symptomatic therapy/medications very cautiously and consult obstetrician first

Miscellaneous

Very common condition

References

Heitkemper M, Elrod R: Nursing role in management: problems of digestion. In Lewis SM, Collier IC, Heitkemper MM, editors: *Medical-surgical nursing assessment and management of clinical problems,* ed 4, St Louis, 1996, Mosby, pp 1151-1157.

Sullivan CA, Samuelson WM: Gastroesophageal reflux: a common exacerbating factor in adult asthma, *Nurse Pract* 21(11):82, 1996.

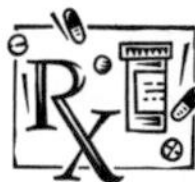

PHARMACOTHERAPEUTICS

There are many OTC preparations available for treatment of GERD. These should be tried before using the stronger, prescription medications. Start with OTC antacids, such as Tums, Gaviscon, Rolaids, Maalox, or Mylanta. If no success is achieved with these medications, try the OTC H_2 antagonists, such as Pepcid AC, Tagamet HB, Axid HR, or Zantac. If symptoms are still not relieved, try one of the prescription medications presented here.

Drug of Choice	Mechanism of Action	Prescribing Information	Side Effects
Famotidine or cimetidine (Pepcid or Tagamet): • Pepcid, 20 mg PO bid—not for children • Tagamet, 300 mg PO with meals and at bedtime—not for children <16 years • Treat for 3-4 weeks, then reduce dosages to OTC strength	Inhibits histamine at H_2 receptor sites	***Contraindication:*** Hypersensitivity ***Cost:*** Pepcid, 20-mg tab, 30 tabs: $45; Tagamet, 300-mg tab, 100 tabs: $45 ***Pregnancy category:*** B	Confusion, headache, depression, dizziness, convulsions, diarrhea, abdominal cramps, paralytic ileus, jaundice, gynecomastia, galactorrhea, increased BUN and creatinine, agranulocytosis, thrombocytopenia, neutropenia, aplastic anemia, urticaria, exfoliative dermatitis
Omeprazole (Prilosec), 20 mg PO qd—not for children	Gastric acid pump inhibitor	***Contraindication:*** Hypersensitivity ***Cost:*** 20-mg tab, 30 tabs: $130 ***Pregnancy category:*** C	Headache, dizziness, asthenia, diarrhea, abdominal pain, vomiting, nausea, constipation, flatulence, acid regurgitation, abdominal swelling, anorexia, upper respiratory infections, cough, epistaxis, rash, dry skin, urticaria, hypoglycemia, increased liver enzymes, weight gain, tinnitus, taste perversion, chest pain, angina, hematuria, bradycardia, tachycardia, urinary tract infection, (UTI), pancytopenia, thrombocytopenia, neutropenia, leukocytosis, anemia, back pain
Cisapride (Propulsid), 10 mg PO qid, maximum 20 mg PO qid; safety in children not established—do not administer with drugs metabolized by cytochrome P450 such as ketoconazole, erythromycin, or clarithromycin	Cholinergic; enhances response to acetylcholine	***Contraindications:*** Hypersensitivity; GI hemorrhage, obstruction, perforation ***Cost:*** 10-mg tab, 100 tabs: $63-$69 ***Pregnancy category:*** C	Dizziness, vomiting, pharyngitis, chest pain, back pain, depression, dehydration, myalgia, diarrhea, abdominal pain, constipation, flatulence, rhinitis, dry mouth, somnolence, palpitation, migraine, tremors, edema

Genital Herpes

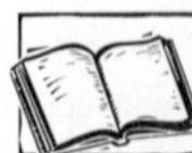

OVERVIEW

Genital herpes is a cutaneous viral infection that produces genital lesions. It is an acute, recurring infection with no known cure.

Pathogenesis

- Cause—herpes simplex virus:
  - HSV-1 usually associated with oral lesions
  - HSV-2 associated with genital lesions (either type may affect either location)
- Incubation 2 to 12 days after contact with lesion or saliva or cervical/penile secretions of infected individual
- After 48 hours, virus finds host ganglia (HSV-1—trigeminal and HSV-2—sacral)
- Stays dormant in ganglia until reactivation; then again causes cutaneous lesions

Patient Profile

- Males = Females
- Any age if sexually active

Signs and Symptoms

- Primary episode:
  - Lesions on genitalia that are painful and tender
  - Itching
  - Burning
  - Dysuria
  - Chills and fever
  - Lymphadenopathy
  - Lesions heal in 21 days
- Recurrent episode:
  - Disease localized to site of lesion
  - Prodrome of burning, itching, or swelling sensation
  - Lesions appear 24 hours later
  - Fewer lesions
  - Heal in 5 to 7 days

Differential Diagnosis

- Syphilis
- Chancroid
- Lymphogranuloma venereum
- Atypical genital warts
- Allergic contact dermatitis
- Scabies

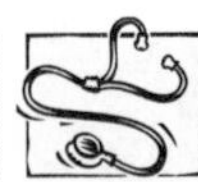

ASSESSMENT

History

Inquire about:

- Onset and duration of symptoms
- Previous occurrence of similar lesions
- Unprotected sexual contact with person known to be infected
- Sexual history and behaviors
- Underlying conditions
- Current medications

Physical Findings

- Multiple, vesicular, painful lesions located on genitalia
- Females may have lesions in vagina and on cervix, as well as on external genitalia; males primarily have lesions on penile glans, shaft, urethra
- Primary episode—fever, tender inguinal lymphadenopathy

Initial Workup

Laboratory

- ELISA testing
- Viral culture (expensive)
- Pap smear—can be used for herpes diagnosis
- Unroof vesicle, use Dacron swab to collect vesicle fluid, place on slide, and fix
- Diagnosis made by finding multinucleated giant cells

Radiology: None indicated

Further Workup

None indicated

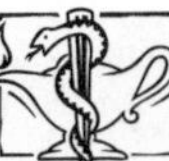

INTERVENTIONS

Office Treatment

None indicated

Lifestyle Modifications

- Practicing safe sex at all times
- Good hand washing to prevent autoinoculation

Patient Education

Teach patient about:

- Disease and treatment options
- No known cure
- Acyclovir—may decrease number of vesicles, decrease healing time, and decrease number of recurrences
- When lesions are present—wearing nonrestricting clothing, taking lukewarm sitz baths, drying lesion with hand-held hair dryer on medium setting
- Abstaining from sexual activity during prodrome and when lesions are present
- Possibility of virus being transmitted even when lesions are not present—use of condoms imperative
- Avoiding use of steroid creams, anesthetic sprays, or any type of lotion or gel on lesions
- Medications used and side effects (see Pharmacotherapeutics)

Referral

May need referral to support group or psychologist for counseling

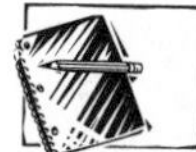

EVALUATION

Outcome
Patient will learn to live and cope with disease

Possible Complications
- Secondary bacterial infection
- Urinary retention
- Aseptic meningitis
- Transmission to neonate

Follow-up
For primary episode—in 2 weeks to evaluate medication tolerance

FOR YOUR INFORMATION

Life Span
Pediatric: With genital lesions in young children, suspect sexual abuse; neonatal infection results in death or significant neurologic impairment
Geriatric: Treatment is the same
Pregnancy: Most risk to fetus occurs if lesions are present at time of delivery; cesarean section should be performed if lesions are present during labor

Miscellaneous
Patients diagnosed with genital herpes need continuous counseling and support. Many educational pamphlets are available and should be given to the newly diagnosed patient.

References
Bartlett JG: *Pocket book of infectious disease therapy,* ed 7, Baltimore, 1996, Williams & Wilkins, pp 307-308.
Bennett EC: Vaginitis and sexually transmitted diseases. In Youngkin EQ, Davis MS, editors: *Women's health: a primary care clinical guide,* Norwalk, Conn, 1994, Appleton & Lange, pp 224-226.

NOTES

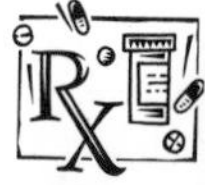

PHARMACOTHERAPEUTICS

Drug of Choice	Mechanism of Action	Prescribing Information	Side Effects
Acyclovir (Zovirax); for first genital episode, 400 mg PO tid × 7-10 days or until resolution occurs; for first rectal episode, 800 mg PO tid × 7-10 days; for recurrent episodes, 400 mg PO tid × 5 days; must start at first sign of lesions; prophylaxis >6 recurrences/year, 400 mg PO bid; dosages are recommendations of CDC	Interferes with DNA synthesis	***Contraindication:*** Hypersensitivity ***Cost:*** 200-mg tab, 100 tabs: $94 ***Pregnancy category:*** C	Tremors, confusion, lethargy, hallucinations, convulsions, dizziness, headache, encephalopathic changes, nausea, vomiting, diarrhea, increased ALT and AST, abdominal pain, oliguria, proteinuria, hematuria, vaginitis, moniliasis, glomerulonephritis, acute renal failure, changes in menses, gingival hyperplasia, rash, urticaria, pruritus, alopecia, joint pain, leg pain, muscle cramps

Giardiasis

OVERVIEW

Giardiasis is an intestinal and/or biliary tract infection.

Pathogenesis

- Cause—*Giardia lamblia,* a flagellated protozoa
- Spread through fecal-oral route
- Incubation period—7 to 14 days

Patient Profile

- Males = Females
- Most common in children, but can affect any age

Signs and Symptoms

- Chronic diarrhea (lasting more than 7 days)
- Abdominal bloating
- Flatulence
- Foul-smelling stools
- Significant weight loss
- Nausea, vomiting
- Often asymptomatic

Differential Diagnosis

- Food allergy
- Irritable bowel syndrome if no weight loss
- Other infectious causes of diarrhea

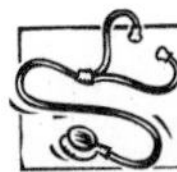

ASSESSMENT

History

Inquire about:

- Onset and duration of symptoms
- Ingestion of unpurified water
- Recent camping trip
- Trips outside United States
- Underlying conditions
- Current medications

Physical Findings

- Weight loss
- Rectal irritation from frequent diarrhea
- Abdominal bloating may be noticeable

Initial Workup

Laboratory

- Stool for ova and parasites repeated 3 times
- String test (Enterotest) to examine duodenal contents for trophozoites

Radiology: None indicated

Further Workup

Esophagogastroduodenoscopy with biopsy

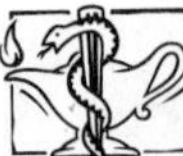

INTERVENTIONS

Office Treatment

None indicated

Lifestyle Modifications

- Good hand washing
- Water purification when camping
- Bottled or potable water when in giardiasis-prone countries

Patient Education

Teach patient about:

- Condition, prevention, and treatment options—medications, well-balanced diet low in lactose and fat
- Good hand-washing technique
- How to purify water when camping
- Medications used and side effects (see Pharmacotherapeutics)

Referral

Usually none; to MD if resistant to treatment

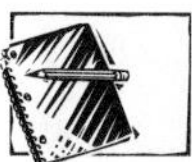

EVALUATION

Outcome
Resolves without sequelae

Possible Complications
- Weight loss (severe)
- Dehydration
- Malnutrition
- Hypokalemia
- Cardiac arrhythmias

Follow-up
In 2 weeks to evaluate treatment results; repeat 3 stools for ova and parasites in 3 to 4 weeks

FOR YOUR INFORMATION

Life Span
Pediatric: More common in early childhood
Geriatric: May dehydrate quickly
Pregnancy: Medications should not be used in pregnancy

Miscellaneous
Patients usually respond to treatment in a few days.

References
Bartlett JG: *Pocket book of infectious disease therapy,* ed 7, Baltimore, 1996, Williams & Wilkins, pp 135, 163, 291.

Goldsmith RS: Infectious diseases: protozoal. In Tierney LM Jr, McPhee SJ, Papadakis MA, editors: *Current medical diagnosis and treatment,* ed 34, Norwalk, Conn, 1995, Appleton & Lange, pp 1227-1229.

NOTES

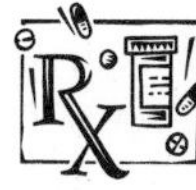

PHARMACOTHERAPEUTICS

Drug of Choice	Mechanism of Action	Prescribing Information	Side Effects
Quinacrine (Atabrine), 100 mg PO tid × 7-10 days; children, 7 mg/kg/day PO in 3 divided doses × 5 days	Causes worm scolex to detach from GI tract; inhibits DNA synthesis	***Contraindications:*** Hypersensitivity; porphyria; psoriasis ***Cost:*** Not available ***Pregnancy category:*** C	Rash, dermatitis, yellow skin, dizziness, headache, insomnia, restlessness, confusion, convulsions, bad taste, oral irritation, corneal deposits, nausea, vomiting, anorexia, diarrhea, cramps, hepatitis, aplastic anemia, agranulocytosis
Metronidazole (Flagyl), 250 mg PO tid × 5 days; children, 15 mg/kg PO tid × 5 days	Direct-acting amebicide/trichomonacide	***Contraindications:*** Hypersensitivity; renal disease; hepatic disease; contracted visual or color fields; blood dyscrasias; pregnancy 1st trimester; lactation; CNS disorders ***Cost:*** 250-mg tab, 100 tabs: $5-$60 ***Pregnancy category:*** B (2nd and 3rd trimesters)	Flat T-waves, headache, dizziness, confusion, irritability, restlessness, depression, fatigue, drowsiness, insomnia, convulsions, blurred vision, sore throat, dry mouth, retinal edema, metallic taste, nausea, vomiting, diarrhea, anorexia, constipation, abdominal cramps, pseudomembranous colitis, darkened urine, albuminuria, neurotoxicity, leukopenia, bone marrow depression, aplasia, rash, pruritus, urticaria

Gingivitis

OVERVIEW

Gingivitis is inflammation and infection of the gingiva.

Pathogenesis

- Poor dental hygiene (most common cause), resulting in plaque buildup
- Plaque composed of bacteria and their by-products
- Causes:
  - Inadequate plaque removal
  - Blood dyscrasia
  - Allergic reactions
  - Chronic debilitating disease
  - Endocrine disturbances
  - Reaction to oral contraceptives

Patient Profile

- Males = Females
- Mostly adults

Signs and Symptoms

- Gum swelling and redness
- Bad mouth odor
- Gum bleeding when brushing or flossing
- If acute, may have significant pain

Differential Diagnosis

- Periodontitis
- Vincent's infection (acute necrotizing ulcerative gingivitis)
- Symptom of chronic illness, such as diabetes, HIV, gingivostomatitis

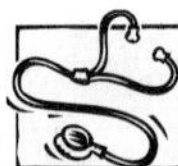

ASSESSMENT

History

Inquire about:

- Onset and duration of symptoms
- Underlying conditions
- Current medications
- Last dental checkup
- Dental hygiene habits

Physical Findings

- Red, swollen gums
- Bad mouth odor

Initial Workup

Laboratory

- CBC—may see leukocytosis
- Culture
- Usually none indicated

Radiology: None indicated

Further Workup

May be done by dentist

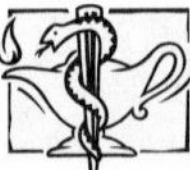

INTERVENTIONS

Office Treatment

None indicated

Lifestyle Modifications

- Smoking cessation
- Daily dental hygiene
- Routine visits to dentist

Patient Education

Teach patient about:

- Cause and prevention of disease
- Importance of good dental hygiene and regular visits to dentist
- Need for about 3 dental visits initially for plaque removal
- Medications used and side effects (see Pharmacotherapeutics)

Referral

To dentist

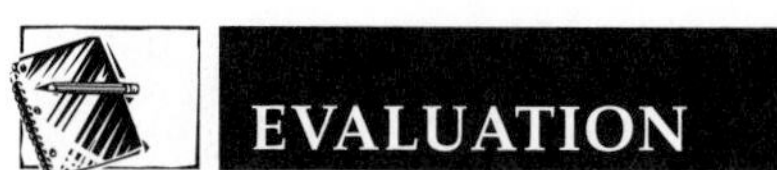

EVALUATION

Outcome
Resolves without sequelae

Possible Complication
Progression to periodontitis

Follow-up
Done by dentist

FOR YOUR INFORMATION

Life Span
Pediatric: Usually milder cases; need to reinforce dental hygiene practices with parents
Geriatric: Seen more frequently because of longevity of plaque buildup
Pregnancy: May have more bleeding because of increased vascularity from hormonal changes

Miscellaneous
Repeated emphasis needs to be placed on daily dental hygiene; recurrences will be frequent if the patient is not followed.

Reference
MacLeod DK: Common problems of the teeth and oral cavity. In Barker LR, Burton JR, Zieve PD, editors: *Principles of ambulatory medicine,* ed 4, Baltimore, 1995, Williams & Wilkins, pp 1484-1485.

NOTES

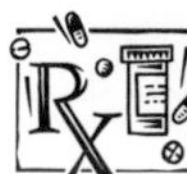

PHARMACOTHERAPEUTICS

Drug of Choice	Mechanism of Action	Prescribing Information	Side Effects
Penicillin (Pen-Vee K), 250-500 mg PO qid × 10 days; children <12 years, 25-50 mg/kg/day PO in divided doses × 10 days	Bactericidal	***Contraindication:*** Hypersensitivity to penicillin or cephalosporins ***Cost:*** 250-mg tab, 40 tabs: $5 ***Pregnancy category:*** B	Nausea and vomiting, epigastric distress, diarrhea, black hairy tongue, anaphylaxis
Erythromycin (E-Mycin), 250 mg PO qid × 10 days; children <12 years, 30-50 mg/kg/day PO qid × 10 days	Inhibits protein synthesis	***Contraindication:*** Hypersensitivity ***Cost:*** 250-mg tab, 40 tabs: $5 ***Pregnancy category:*** B	Pseudomembranous colitis, abdominal cramping, nausea and vomiting, diarrhea, rash, anaphylaxis

Glaucoma

OVERVIEW

Glaucoma is a disease of the eye that is thought to be a result of increased intraocular pressure. It is a group of ocular disorders that can be divided into 2 main types: open-angle glaucoma (most common) and closed-angle glaucoma.

Pathogenesis

- Open-angle glaucoma—decreased outflow of aqueous humor through trabecular meshwork leads to increased aqueous humor, which leads to increased pressure
- Closed-angle glaucoma—decreased outflow of aqueous humor through pupil due to an anatomically narrow anterior chamber angle

Patient Profile

OPEN-ANGLE GLAUCOMA

- Males = Females
- Occurs in patients >40 years of age
- African-Americans have higher frequency

CLOSED-ANGLE GLAUCOMA

- Females > Males
- Occurs in patients 55 to 70 years of age
- Family history

Signs and Symptoms

OPEN-ANGLE GLAUCOMA

- Very slow, progressive disease
- May have peripheral vision loss and later loss of visual acuity
- May be asymptomatic

CLOSED-ANGLE GLAUCOMA

- Ocular pain
- Blurred vision
- Frontal headache
- Lacrimation
- Halos around lights
- Nausea, vomiting
- Lid edema
- Injected conjunctiva
- Increased intraocular pressure

Differential Diagnosis

- Conjunctivitis
- Acute uveitis
- Macular degeneration
- Vascular occlusive disease
- Severe anemia
- Iritis

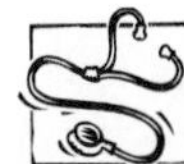

ASSESSMENT

History

Inquire about:

- Onset and duration of symptoms
- Whether one or both eyes affected
- Difficulty with peripheral vision
- Headache, family history, photophobia, or visual blurring (if present, suspect closed-angle glaucoma—a medical emergency)
- Underlying conditions
- Current medications

Physical Findings

- If lid edema, injection of conjunctiva, tearing, and ptosis are present in combination with a positive history, closed-angle glaucoma is suspected and patient is referred immediately to an ophthalmologist
- Normal visual acuity
- Decreased peripheral vision using direct confrontation
- Intraocular pressure may or may not be elevated (measure with hand-held tonometer if available)

Initial Workup

Laboratory: None indicated
Radiology: None indicated

Further Workup

None indicated

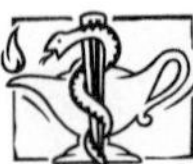

INTERVENTIONS

Office Treatment

None indicated

Lifestyle Modifications

Determined by amount of vision lost, if any

Patient Education

Teach patient about:

- Closed-angle, acute attack:
  - Need for immediate treatment by ophthalmologist (attack can result in blindness in 2 to 3 days)
  - Possible hospitalization
  - Surgery being only treatment option
- Open-angle glaucoma:
  - Disease process
  - Treatment options—eye drops and systemic medications
  - Need for lifelong treatment
  - Need for evaluation and treatment by ophthalmologist
  - Medications that ophthalmologist will likely prescribe (see Pharmacotherapeutics)

Referral

To ophthalmologist

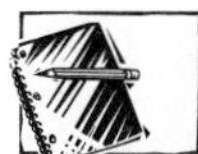

EVALUATION

Outcomes

- Open-angle glaucoma—with continued treatment, prognosis is excellent
- Closed-angle glaucoma—depends on how many acute attacks have occurred

Possible Complication

Both types—blindness

Follow-up

By ophthalmologist

FOR YOUR INFORMATION

Life Span

Pediatric: Very rare
Geriatric: Most common in this population
Pregnancy: N/A

Miscellaneous

Medications that may exacerbate closed-angle glaucoma include systemic or topical anticholinergics, topical sympathomimetics, antihistamines, phenothiazines, and antidepressants.

References

Schachat AP: Glaucoma. In Barker LR, Burton JR, Zieve PD, editors: *Principles of ambulatory medicine,* ed 4, Baltimore, 1995, Williams & Wilkins, pp 1423-1428.

Tucker JB: Practical therapeutics: screening for open-angle glaucoma, *Am Fam Physician* 48(1):75-80, 1993.

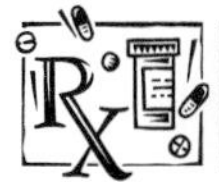

PHARMACOTHERAPEUTICS

The following is an overview of the commonly used medications for open-angle glaucoma. Dosages are not included because this should be managed by the ophthalmologist. However, it is important for the NP to know contraindications and side effects of these medications to be able to treat other conditions the patient may have.

Drug of Choice	Mechanism of Action	Prescribing Information	Side Effects
Tineolol, Betaxolol, levobunolol, carteolol, metipranolol	Beta-adrenergic blocking agents	***Contraindications:*** Asthma; chronic obstructive pulmonary disease, (COPD); sinus bradycardia; 2nd- and 3rd-degree atrioventricular block; overt cardiac failure; cardiogenic shock; hypersensitivity ***Cost:*** 2.5-5.0 ml: $8-$15 ***Pregnancy category:*** C	Headache, fatigue, chest pain, bradycardia, hypertension, syncope, heart block, CVA, palpitations, nausea, diarrhea, dizziness, depression, rash; may mask symptoms of hypoglycemia—use cautiously in diabetics
Epinephrine and dipivefrin	Epinephrine—sympathomimetic; dipivefrin—product of epinephrine	***Contraindications:*** Hypersensitivity; closed-angle glaucoma ***Cost:*** 10 ml: $12-$18 ***Pregnancy category:*** C	Eye pain or ache, headache, injected conjunctiva, allergic lid reactions
Pilocarpine	Direct-acting parasympathomimetic; duplicates muscarinic effects of acetylcholine	***Contraindication:*** Hypersensitivity ***Cost:*** 15 ml: $10 ***Pregnancy category:*** C	Visual blurring resulting from miosis and accommodative spasms, poor dark adaptation, injected conjunctiva
Demecarium bromide	Cholinesterase inhibitor	***Contraindications:*** Hypersensitivity; pregnancy or patients who may get pregnant; active uveal inflammation or iridocyclitis ***Cost:*** 5 ml: $15 ***Pregnancy category:*** X	Stinging, burning, lid muscle twitching, lacrimation, conjunctival and ciliary redness, browache, headache, myopia with visual blurring
Acetazolamide	Carbonic anhydrase inhibitor; controls fluid secretion; nonbacteriostatic sulfonamide	***Contraindications:*** Decreased sodium and/or potassium levels; kidney and liver disease; suprarenal gland failure; hyperchloremic acidosis; cirrhosis ***Cost:*** 125-mg or 250-mg tab, 100 tabs, $6-$12 ***Pregnancy category:*** D	Paresthesias, hearing dysfunction or tinnitus, loss of appetite, taste alteration, nausea, vomiting, diarrhea, polyuria, drowsiness, confusion, urticaria, melena, hematuria, glycosuria, hepatic insufficiency, photosensitivity, convulsions, Stevens-Johnson syndrome

Glomerulonephritis, Acute

OVERVIEW

Acute glomerulonephritis is an inflammatory process that is due to an immunologic response to an infection. It affects the glomeruli of the kidneys.

Pathogenesis

- Cause—most commonly follows a group A beta-hemolytic streptococcal infection
- Other causes of postinfective glomerulonephritis—pneumococcus, staphylococcus, meningococcus, chickenpox, hepatitis
- Infection usually precedes glomerulonephritis by 1 to 3 weeks

Patient Profile

- Males > Females
- Most common age is 2 to 16 years, but can be found in any age group

Signs and Symptoms

- Hematuria
- Oliguria
- Edema
- Hypertension
- Weight gain
- Proteinuria

Differential Diagnosis

- Systemic lupus erythematosus
- IgA nephropathy
- Rapidly progressive glomerulonephritis

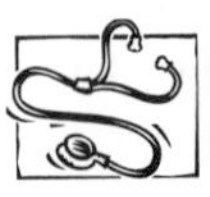

ASSESSMENT

History

Inquire about:

- Onset and duration of symptoms
- Recent known streptococcal infection (pharyngitis, impetigo)
- Recent infection from other cause
- Underlying conditions
- Current medications

Physical Findings

- Increased BP
- Edema
- Abdomen—may have pain on palpation
- Costovertebral angle—may have tenderness

Initial Workup

Laboratory

- CBC with differential—may have anemia
- Streptococcal test—positive if glomerulonephritis due to strep (most common)
- Antistreptolysin O—increased
- Urinalysis—hematuria, proteinuria, microscopic examination—RBC casts
- Serum BUN and creatinine—increased
- 24-hour urine creatinine clearance—decreased

Radiology: None indicated

Further Workup

Renal biopsy if condition appears to be progressive

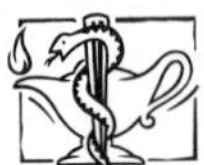

INTERVENTIONS

Office Treatment

None indicated

Lifestyle Modifications

- Sodium-, protein-, and potassium-restricted diet
- Fluid restriction

Patient Education

Teach patient about:

- Condition and treatment:
  - Initial hospitalization to control hypertension and azotemia
  - Limiting fluid intake
  - Low-sodium, low-protein, and low-potassium diet
  - Dialysis—may be required briefly to control excess fluids, hyperkalemia, azotemia
- Medications used and side effects (see Pharmacotherapeutics)

Referral

To primary care physician or nephrologist for hospitalization if NP does not have privileges

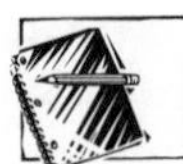

EVALUATION

Outcomes

- Usually resolution occurs in 2 to 3 weeks
- May have hematuria after exercise for up to 2 years
- In some adults hypertension and proteinuria persist; 10 to 20 years later, patient may develop chronic renal failure

Possible Complications

- Hypertensive retinopathy or encephalopathy
- Rapidly progressive glomerulonephritis
- Nephrotic syndrome
- Chronic renal failure

Follow-up

- In 1 week following hospitalization
- If treated as outpatient, telephone contact in 24 hours and return to clinic in 1 week; will probably be followed by primary care physician or nephrologist

FOR YOUR INFORMATION

Life Span

Pediatric: Most common in this age group
Geriatric: Rare in this age group—high morbidity and mortality
Pregnancy: Refer to a specialist

Miscellaneous

N/A

References

Morrison G: Kidney. In Tierney LM Jr, McPhee SJ, Papadakis SA, editors: *Current medical diagnosis and treatment,* ed 34, Norwalk, Conn, 1995, Appleton & Lange, pp 783-784.

Woolliscroft JO: *Current diagnosis and treatment: a quick reference for the general practitioner,* Philadelphia, 1996, Current Medicine, pp 154-155.

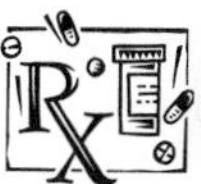

PHARMACOTHERAPEUTICS

Many medications may be used to treat acute glomerulonephritis that are beyond the scope of this book. Only those most commonly used are presented here.

Drug of Choice	Mechanism of Action	Prescribing Information	Side Effects
For hyperkalemia:			
Sodium polystyrene sulfonate (Kayexalate Resin), 1 g/kg PR or PO qd-qid	Removes potassium by exchanging sodium for potassium	***Contraindications:*** Hypersensitivity; hypokalemia ***Cost:*** 60 mg/g of powder, 454 g: $53 ***Pregnancy category:*** C	Constipation, anorexia, nausea, vomiting, diarrhea, gastric irritation, hypocalcemia, hypokalemia, hypomagnesemia, sodium retention
For edema and hypertension:			
Furosemide (Lasix), 1-2 mg/kg PO or IV bid	Loop diuretic; inhibits reabsorption of sodium and chloride at proximal and distal tubule and at loop of Henle	***Contraindications:*** Hypersensitivity to sulfonamides; anuria; hypovolemia ***Cost:*** 20-mg tab, 100 tabs: $2-$15 ***Pregnancy category:*** C	Headache, fatigue, weakness, orthostatic hypotension, chest pain, circulatory collapse, loss of hearing, hypokalemia, hypomagnesemia, hyperuricemia, hyperglycemia, nausea, diarrhea, renal failure, thrombocytopenia, agranulocytosis, leukopenia, anemia, rash, Stevens-Johnson syndrome, cramps, stiffness
For hypertension:			
Quinapril (Accupril), 10-80 mg PO qd; other ACE inhibitors that may be used: captopril, lisinopril, or enalapril; consult manufacturer's insert for prescribing information	Prevents conversion of angiotensin I to angiotensin II, producing arterial dilation	***Contraindication:*** Hypersensitivity ***Cost:*** 10-mg tab, 100 tabs: $90 ***Pregnancy category:*** 1st trimester—C; 2nd and 3rd trimesters—D	Cough, hypotension, postural hypotension, syncope, decreased libido, impotence, increased BUN and creatinine, thrombocytopenia, agranulocytosis, angioedema, rash, sweating, photosensitivity, hyperkalemia, nausea, vomiting, gastritis, headache, dizziness, fatigue, somnolence, depression, malaise, back pain, arthralgias, arthritis
For streptococcal infection:			
Penicillin, (Pen-Vee K), 250-500 mg PO tid or qid × 10 days; children <12 years, 25-50 mg/kg/day PO in divided doses × 10 days	Bactericidal	***Contraindication:*** Hypersensitivity to penicillin or cephalosporins ***Cost:*** 250-mg tab, 40 tabs, $5 ***Pregnancy category:*** B	Nausea, vomiting, epigastric distress, diarrhea, black hairy tongue, anaphylaxis

Gonorrhea

OVERVIEW

Gonorrhea is a sexually transmitted disease (STD) caused by a gram-negative diplococcus.

Pathogenesis

- Cause—*Neisseria gonorrhoeae* (gram-negative diplococcus)
- Transmission—intimate contact, such as sexual acts or parturition
- Incubation period—2 to 7 days

Patient Profile

- Males > Females
- Most common age groups—adolescents and young adults

Signs and Symptoms

- Males:
    - Purulent urethral discharge
    - Dysuria
    - Testicular pain
    - Urethral stricture
- Females:
    - Vaginal discharge
    - Dysuria
    - Asymptomatic
    - Symptoms of pelvic inflammatory disease—dysmenorrhea, metromenorrhagia, lower abdominal pain, fever, cervical motion tenderness, palpable and tender fallopian tubes or ovaries
- Rectal infection—purulent or bloody discharge, tenesmus, rectal burning or itching, asymptomatic
- Pharyngeal infection—Sore throat, exudative pharyngitis, asymptomatic
- Systemic infection—fever, chills, arthralgias, synovial sheath tenderness and swelling, painful skin lesions, endocarditis, meningitis
- Infants and children—same as all of the above
- Neonate—pneumonia, fever, infiltrate on chest x-ray films

Differential Diagnosis

- Chlamydial infection
- Urinary tract infection
- Trichomoniasis

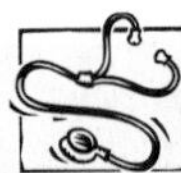

ASSESSMENT

History

Inquire about:

- Onset and duration of symptoms
- Sexual history and number of partners, behaviors, use of condoms
- Past history of STDs
- Known unprotected contact with infected partner
- Underlying conditions
- Current medications

Physical Findings

- Males:
    - Urethral discharge; pain on palpation of testicles
    - If anal sex practiced, rectal examination
- Females:
    - Vaginal/cervical discharge
    - Bartholin's and Skene's glands may be tender
    - Check for cervical motion tenderness
    - Adnexal tenderness/masses
    - If anal sex practiced, rectal examination

Initial Workup

Laboratory:

- Culture for gonorrhea
- Gram stain of exudate—gram-negative diplococci
- Chlamydial culture, rapid plasma reagin (RPR), HIV testing—recommended

Radiology: None indicated

Further Workup

None indicated

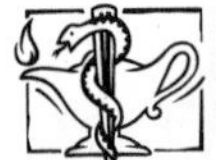

INTERVENTIONS

Office Treatment

None indicated

Lifestyle Modification

Practicing safe sex

Patient Education

Teach patient about:

- Disease and treatment
    - Hospitalization for systemic infection, pneumonia in infants, women with severe pelvic inflammatory disease
    - For others, outpatient treatment with antibiotics
- Abstaining from sexual activity until partner treated, treatment completed, and both are asymptomatic
- Practicing safe sex (use of condoms, limiting number of partners)
- Medications used and side effects (see pharmacotherapeutics)

Referral

To MD for hospitalization unless NP has hospital privileges

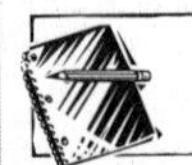

EVALUATION

Outcome

Resolves without sequelae

Possible Complications

- Urethral stricture (males)
- Infertility (females)
- Corneal scarring after eye infections
- Destruction of cardiac valves
- Death

Follow-up

Retest if symptoms recur; some authorities recommend repeat testing in 1 week

FOR YOUR INFORMATION

Life Span

Pediatric: Suspect sexual abuse; can have serious sequelae in young children
Geriatric: Treatment is the same
Pregnancy: Pelvic inflammatory disease can induce labor and delivery

Miscellaneous

Disease must be reported to the local health department

References

Bartlett JG: *Pocket book of infectious disease therapy,* ed 7, Baltimore, 1996, Williams & Wilkins, pp 298-299, 312-314.

Luft J, Carnage LC: Nursing role in management: sexually transmitted diseases. In Lewis SM, Collier IC, Heitkemper MM, editors: *Medical-surgical nursing: assessment and management of clinical problems,* ed 4, St Louis, 1996, Mosby, pp 1565-1567.

PHARMACOTHERAPEUTICS

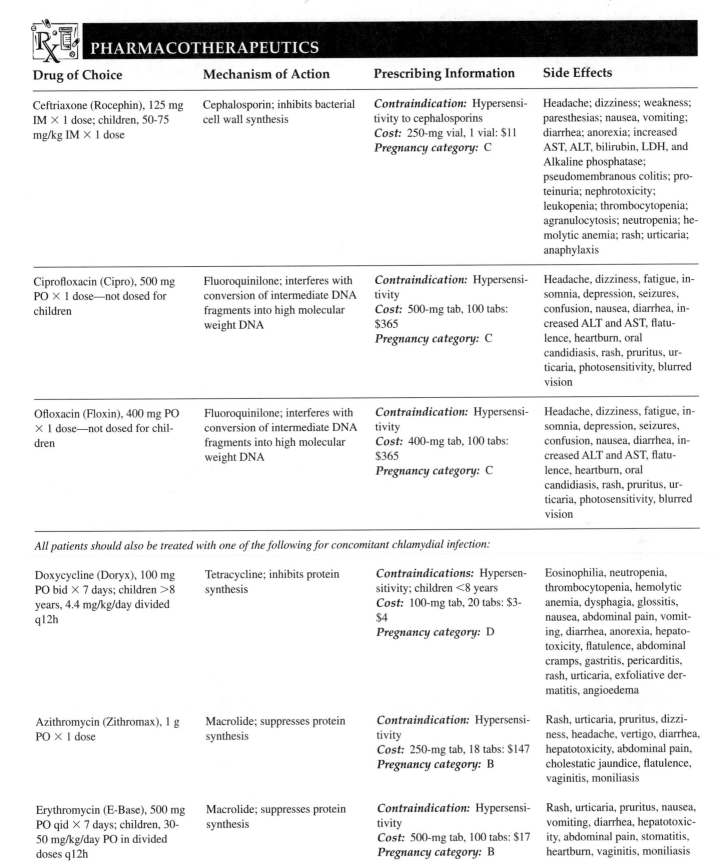

Drug of Choice	Mechanism of Action	Prescribing Information	Side Effects
Ceftriaxone (Rocephin), 125 mg IM × 1 dose; children, 50-75 mg/kg IM × 1 dose	Cephalosporin; inhibits bacterial cell wall synthesis	***Contraindication:*** Hypersensitivity to cephalosporins ***Cost:*** 250-mg vial, 1 vial: $11 ***Pregnancy category:*** C	Headache; dizziness; weakness; paresthesias; nausea, vomiting; diarrhea; anorexia; increased AST, ALT, bilirubin, LDH, and Alkaline phosphatase; pseudomembranous colitis; proteinuria; nephrotoxicity; leukopenia; thrombocytopenia; agranulocytosis; neutropenia; hemolytic anemia; rash; urticaria; anaphylaxis
Ciprofloxacin (Cipro), 500 mg PO × 1 dose—not dosed for children	Fluoroquinilone; interferes with conversion of intermediate DNA fragments into high molecular weight DNA	***Contraindication:*** Hypersensitivity ***Cost:*** 500-mg tab, 100 tabs: $365 ***Pregnancy category:*** C	Headache, dizziness, fatigue, insomnia, depression, seizures, confusion, nausea, diarrhea, increased ALT and AST, flatulence, heartburn, oral candidiasis, rash, pruritus, urticaria, photosensitivity, blurred vision
Ofloxacin (Floxin), 400 mg PO × 1 dose—not dosed for children	Fluoroquinilone; interferes with conversion of intermediate DNA fragments into high molecular weight DNA	***Contraindication:*** Hypersensitivity ***Cost:*** 400-mg tab, 100 tabs: $365 ***Pregnancy category:*** C	Headache, dizziness, fatigue, insomnia, depression, seizures, confusion, nausea, diarrhea, increased ALT and AST, flatulence, heartburn, oral candidiasis, rash, pruritus, urticaria, photosensitivity, blurred vision
All patients should also be treated with one of the following for concomitant chlamydial infection:			
Doxycycline (Doryx), 100 mg PO bid × 7 days; children >8 years, 4.4 mg/kg/day divided q12h	Tetracycline; inhibits protein synthesis	***Contraindications:*** Hypersensitivity; children <8 years ***Cost:*** 100-mg tab, 20 tabs: $3-$4 ***Pregnancy category:*** D	Eosinophilia, neutropenia, thrombocytopenia, hemolytic anemia, dysphagia, glossitis, nausea, abdominal pain, vomiting, diarrhea, anorexia, hepatotoxicity, flatulence, abdominal cramps, gastritis, pericarditis, rash, urticaria, exfoliative dermatitis, angioedema
Azithromycin (Zithromax), 1 g PO × 1 dose	Macrolide; suppresses protein synthesis	***Contraindication:*** Hypersensitivity ***Cost:*** 250-mg tab, 18 tabs: $147 ***Pregnancy category:*** B	Rash, urticaria, pruritus, dizziness, headache, vertigo, diarrhea, hepatotoxicity, abdominal pain, cholestatic jaundice, flatulence, vaginitis, moniliasis
Erythromycin (E-Base), 500 mg PO qid × 7 days; children, 30-50 mg/kg/day PO in divided doses q12h	Macrolide; suppresses protein synthesis	***Contraindication:*** Hypersensitivity ***Cost:*** 500-mg tab, 100 tabs: $17 ***Pregnancy category:*** B	Rash, urticaria, pruritus, nausea, vomiting, diarrhea, hepatotoxicity, abdominal pain, stomatitis, heartburn, vaginitis, moniliasis

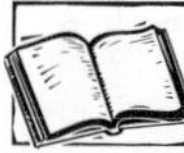

OVERVIEW

Gout is an inflammatory disease caused by urate crystals being deposited in joints, synovia of tendons, and the kidneys. Gout may be classified as primary or secondary.

Pathogenesis

- Primary gout—disturbance in purine metabolism causes underexcretion or overproduction of uric acid, leading to sodium urate crystals; inherited disease
- Secondary gout—increased uric acid from myeloproliferative disease or its treatment—hemolytic anemia, renal disease, psoriasis, use of diuretics, glycogen storage disease, etc.

Patient Profile

- Males > Females
- Most common age—30 to 40 years

Signs and Symptoms

- Acute onset of severe pain—usually in one joint (common sites—metatarsophalangeal joint of great toe [90% of cases], knee, ankle, wrist, and elbow)
- Erythema
- Warmth
- Swelling
- Headache
- Malaise
- Fever
- Chills
- Kidney stones
- Recurrent episodes may be polyarticular
- Deposits of urate crystals in subcutaneous tissue (tophi) may form

Differential Diagnosis

- Cellulitis
- Pseudogout
- Rheumatoid arthritis
- Infectious arthritis
- Amyloidosis
- Lyme disease

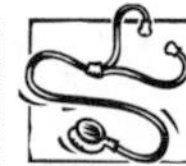

ASSESSMENT

History

Inquire about:

- Onset and duration of symptoms (often starts at night)
- Precipitating causes—aspirin use, alcohol intake, diuretics, ingestion of organ meats
- Family history of gout
- Previous similar attacks
- Underlying conditions
- Current medications

Physical Findings

- Fever
- Tachycardia
- Red, warm, hot, exquisitely tender joint(s)
- Tophi

Initial Workup

Laboratory

- CBC with differential—leukocytosis with left shift
- Erythrocyte sedimentation rate (ESR)-elevated
- Serum uric acid—elevated, but normal uric acid level does *not* rule out gout
- Consider 24-hour urine collection to measure uric acid excretion

Radiology: Plain films of joint—may be normal or have soft tissue swelling, gouty erosions, tophi

Further Workup

Joint aspirate—cloudy, usually with urate crystals

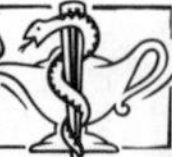

INTERVENTIONS

Office Treatment

None indicated

Lifestyle Modifications

- Low-purine diet
- Cessation of use of causative medications (aspirin, diuretics, nicotinic acid) if possible
- Weight reduction
- Reduction in alcohol intake

Patient Education

Teach patient about:

- Disease and treatment—treating acute attack with NSAID medication first; once controlled, consider preventive agents (used only for frequent recurrences [≥3 per year])
- Immobilizing affected joint
- Low-purine and weight loss diet
- Reducing alcohol intake
- Stopping use of aspirin if possible
- Correcting any diseases or changing any treatments that might be causative
- Medications used and side effects (see Pharmacotherapeutics)

Referral

To orthopedist in cases resistant to treatment

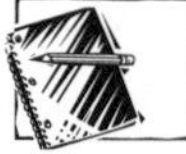

EVALUATION

Outcome

Early treatment produces early resolution

Possible Complications

- Urate nephropathy
- Renal stones
- Large tophi
- Severe joint deterioration

Follow-up

- Telephone contact in 48 hours to assess treatment
- Return to clinic in 1 week; then in 4 weeks
- Start preventive therapy 1 month after resolution of acute attack, if appropriate
- Monitor uric acid level monthly × 2; then every 6 months

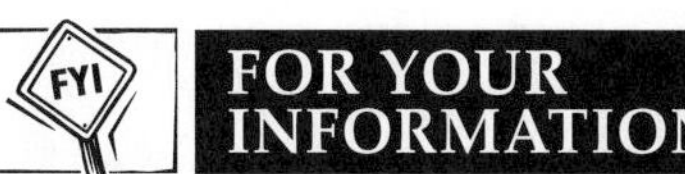

FOR YOUR INFORMATION

Life Span

Pediatric: Rare in this age group
Geriatric: Look for medication as cause
Pregnancy: Cautious use of medication

Miscellaneous

N/A

References

Hellmann DB: Arthritis and musculoskeletal disorders. In Tierney LM Jr, McPhee SJ, Papadakis MA, editors: *Current medical diagnosis and treatment,* ed 34, Norwalk, Conn, 1995, Appleton & Lange, pp 698-702.

Mercier LR: *Practical orthopedics,* ed 4, St Louis, 1995, Mosby, pp 281-283.

NOTES

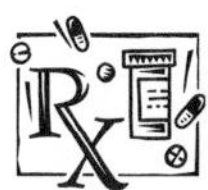

PHARMACOTHERAPEUTICS

Drug of Choice	Mechanism of Action	Prescribing Information	Side Effects
For acute attack, use one of the following:			
Nonsteroidal antiinflammatory drugs (NSAIDs)—any may be used; start with full dosage × 2-3 days, then decrease by 25%-50%; may need to treat with NSAIDs up to 12 months; most commonly used NSAID: Indomethacin (Indocin), 25 mg, 2 tabs PO tid × 3 days, then 1 tab tid until attack resolves	Exact action unknown; may be caused by inhibition of synthesis of prostaglandins and arachidonic acid	***Contraindications:*** Hypersensitivity to NSAIDs, aspirin; severe hepatic failure; asthma ***Cost:*** Varies with type ***Pregnancy category:*** Depends on product	Stomach distress, flatulence, nausea, abdominal pain, constipation or diarrhea, dizziness, sedation, rash, urticaria, angioedema, anorexia, urinary frequency, increased blood pressure, insomnia, anxiety, visual disturbances, increased thirst, alopecia
Colchicine, 0.5-1.2 mg PO every hour until pain decreases or side effects occur (vomiting most common); has high side effect profile—side effects very unpleasant; not used much anymore	Reduces inflammatory response to uric acid crystals	***Contraindications:*** Hypersensitivity; serious GI, renal, hepatic, cardiac disorders ***Cost:*** 0.5-mg tab, 100 tabs: $26 ***Pregnancy category:*** D	Nausea, vomiting, diarrhea (may be severe), abdominal pain, bone marrow depression, agranulocytosis, thrombocytopenia, aplastic anemia
For prevention after acute attack has resolved, use one of the following:			
Probenecid (Benemid), 500 mg PO qd × 1 week; then 500 mg PO bid; increase by 500 mg/day at monthly intervals until uric acid is normal or 2 mg/dl less than during acute attack; interacts with numerous commonly used medications; consult manufacturer's prescribing information before use	Causes increased excretion of uric acid	***Contraindications:*** Hypersensitivity; do not start until acute attack has subsided; do not use in renal disease; severe hepatic disease; history of uric acid calculus ***Cost:*** 500-mg tab, 100 tabs: $12-$35 ***Pregnancy category:*** B	Drowsiness, headache, bradycardia, glycosuria, thirst, nephotic syndrome, gastric irritation, nausea, vomiting, anorexia, hepatic necrosis, rash, dermatitis, acidosis, hypokalemia, apnea
Allopurinol (Zyloprim), 100 mg PO qd; increase by 100 mg/day weekly; maximum dose 800 mg/day	Reduces uric acid synthesis by inhibiting xanthine oxidase	***Contraindications:*** Hypersensitivity to thiazides or sulfonamides; anuria; renal decompensation; hypomagnesemia ***Cost:*** 25-mg tab, 100 tabs: $2-$12 ***Pregnancy category:*** B	Agranulocytosis, thrombocytopenia, aplastic anemia, pancytopenia, bone marrow depression, headache, drowsiness, nausea, vomiting, anorexia, malaise, metallic taste, cramps, myopathy, cholestatic jaundice, renal failure, retinopathy, fever, chills, dermatitis, purpura, alopecia

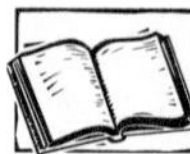

OVERVIEW

Grief is a normal emotional and physical response to a loss or separation. The physical response is due to stimulation of the sympathetic nervous system. The emotional response is thought to occur in stages progressing from alarm to disbelief and denial, to anger and guilt, to finding comfort, and to acceptance of the loss.

Pathogenesis
Loss of something or someone important in the individual's life—family member, friend, pet, home, job, etc.

Patient Profile
- Males = Females
- Any age

Signs and Symptoms
- Physical response—increased heart and respiratory rate, dilated pupils, sweating, bristling of hair, increased blood flow, increased energy, slowed digestion, insomnia
- Emotional response—anger, fear, denial, depression, easy to cry, guilt

Differential Diagnosis
Major depressive episode

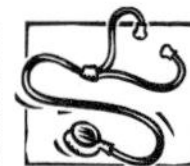

ASSESSMENT

History
Inquire about:
- Onset and duration of symptoms
- When loss occurred
- How patient is coping with loss
- How patient has coped with loss in the past
- Whether patient is carrying out usual daily activities
- Support system
- Suicidal ideation
- Underlying conditions
- Current medications

Physical Findings
Increased heart/respiratory rate, dilated pupils, sweating, bristling of hair

Initial Workup
Laboratory: N/A
Radiology: N/A

Further Workup
N/A

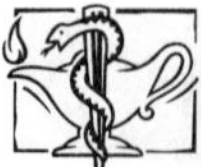

INTERVENTIONS

Office Treatment
Emotional support; allow patient to express feelings

Lifestyle Modifications
- Adjustment to life without deceased
- Return to usual routine within 2 weeks
- Daily exercise program

Patient Education
Teach patient about:
- Grieving process
- Support groups
- Exercise benefits and plan
- Not using psychotropic drugs (they delay normal grieving process)
- Importance of returning to normal activities within 2 weeks

Referral
Only if patient has abnormal response (if patient meets criteria for major depression 2 months after loss)—then to a professional who specializes in this area—psychiatric NP, psychologist, counselor, or psychiatrist

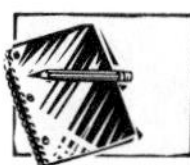

EVALUATION

Outcome
Patient faces pain, expresses emotions, adjusts to altered environment, and lives with memories; is able to resume normal daily activities

Possible Complications
- Major depressive episode
- Development of ineffective coping behaviors, such as alcohol/drug abuse
- Suicide

Follow-up
Weekly × 2; then every 2 weeks × 2; then monthly

FOR YOUR INFORMATION

Life Span
Pediatric: Go through same process as adult
Geriatric: May have more difficulty coping because of more frequent losses that come with aging
Pregnancy: May have more difficulty coping because of emotional lability related to hormonal changes

Miscellaneous
Grief is a complex issue. Cultural variations in coping with losses must be considered.

References
Depression Guidance Panel: *Depression in primary care,* vol 1, *Detection and diagnosis,* Clinical Practice Guideline No 5, AHCPR Pub No 93-0550, Rockville, Md, 1993, US Department of Health and Human Services, Public Health Service, Agency for Health Care Policy and Research, pp 53-54.

Loney M, DuFault K Sr: Loss, grief, and dying. In Phipps WJ et al, editors: *Medical-surgical nursing: concepts and clinical practice,* ed 5, St Louis, 1995, Mosby, pp 239-244.

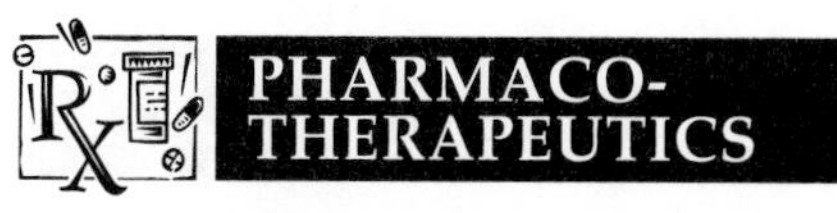

PHARMACOTHERAPEUTICS

The use of drugs during the grieving process should be avoided in order to allow the patient to progress through the process.

Gynecomastia

OVERVIEW

Gynecomastia is usually a benign condition in which there is glandular enlargement of the male breast. Usually the condition is symmetric, but it may be asymmetric.

Pathogenesis

Cause—imbalance between estrogen and androgen levels; excess estrogen results in breast duct proliferation

- Physiologic causes:
    - Puberty
    - Aging
- Pathologic causes:
    - Adrenal, lung, testicular neoplasm
    - Pituitary prolactinoma
    - Hypothyroidism and hyperthyroidism
    - Medications (diazepam, cimetidine, spironolactone, digitalis, and many others)
    - Drug abuse (alcohol, amphetamines, heroin, marijuana)
    - Malnutrition
    - Liver failure
    - Primary gonadal failure
    - Secondary gonadal failure
    - Familial gynecomastia

Patient Profile

- Males
- Most common age—puberty and elderly

Signs and Symptoms

- Puberty—3 types:
    - Type I—1 or more subareolar movable nodules
    - Type II—nodules extend beyond areolar perimeter
    - Type III—resembles female breast development
    - Types I and II may have tenderness; consistency is firm and rubbery
    - Type III—similar to female breast
- Testicles are normal size and consistency; may find mass
- All others—usually asymptomatic
- May have pain and tenderness if it develops rapidly

Differential Diagnosis

- Breast cancer (unilateral)
- Lipoma
- Neurofibroma
- Obesity with increased adipose tissue

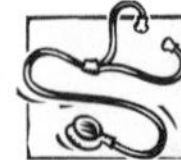

ASSESSMENT

History

Inquire about:

- Onset and duration of breast enlargement
- Pain or discharge
- Breasts increasing or decreasing in size
- Other pubertal events
- Alcohol and illegal drug use
- Diet
- Family history
- Effect on lifestyle and self-esteem
- Underlying conditions
- Current medications

Physical Findings

- Examination of breasts with patient supine—usually will find disklike mound of tissue; should be mobile
- Check for nipple discharge
- Check for axillary lymphadenopathy
- Check for thyroid enlargement
- Abdominal organomegaly
- For pubertal males, do Tanner staging; for others, do testicular examination (masses)

Initial Workup

Laboratory

- Not needed for pubertal gynecomastia
- Serum beta-HCG (increased in carcinomas)
- Plasma testosterone and leutinizing hormone (LH) (increased LH and decreased testosterone indicate testicular failure)
- Serum estradiol
- Serum prolactin
- Thyroid and liver function tests
- BUN and creatinine

Radiology

- Mammogram (atypical gynecomastia)
- Testicular ultrasound (suspected tumor)

Further Workup

Biopsy if suspicious

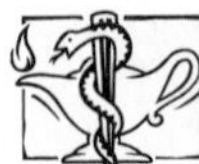

INTERVENTIONS

Office Treatment

None indicated

Lifestyle Modifications

- Weight loss if indicated
- Cessation of alcohol and illegal drug use

Patient Education

Teach patient about:

- Condition and treatment—for pubertal boys, usually resolves without treatment (may take up to 2 years)
- Correcting underlying cause if known
- Diet for weight loss
- Support groups and treatment centers for alcohol and drug abuse
- For severe cases, subcutaneous mastectomy may be performed
- Stopping medication that may be causative factor, if feasible
- Medications that can be used—should be used by individual familiar with their use, and benefit should outweigh risks (see Pharmacotherapeutics)

Referrals

- To surgeon for biopsy or subcutaneous mastectomy, if necessary
- To endocrinologist for medical therapy

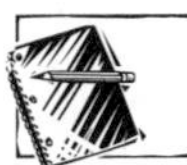

EVALUATION

Outcomes:
- Pubertal—resolves without treatment; withdrawal of causative drugs cures condition
- Others—depends on etiology

Possible Complication
Poor self-esteem

Follow-up
- Pubertal—3- to 6-month intervals
- Others—monitor for side effects of medications if used

FOR YOUR INFORMATION

Life Span
Pediatric: Physiologic gynecomastia seen in neonates and pubertal boys
Geriatric: May be part of normal aging process or, more commonly, drug induced
Pregnancy: N/A

Miscellaneous
Pubertal boys will need a great deal of support and reassurance that this is a transient condition.

Reference
Harman SM, Blackman MR: Common problems in reproductive endocrinology. In Barker LR, Burton JR, Zieve PD, editors: *Principles of ambulatory medicine,* ed 4, Baltimore, 1995, Williams & Wilkins, pp 1125-1126.

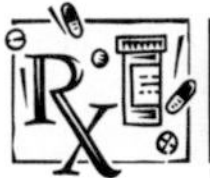

PHARMACOTHERAPEUTICS

The following is a list of medications that may be used by an endocrinologist or primary care physician. Dosages will be determined by the prescribing physician:
- Antiestrogens—clomiphene, tamoxifen
- Testosterone
- Nonaromatizable androgens
- Danazol in pubertal boys
- Diethylstilbestrol in the elderly

Headache, Cluster

OVERVIEW

A cluster headache is a sudden, severe pain in the head that is unilateral. It occurs around the eye and temple, and the attacks typically last 30 minutes to 2 hours. They usually occur 1 to 3 times a day at the same time each day for up to 12 weeks and may remit for up to 5 years. Often the attacks occur at night during the first REM period. They are commonly referred to as Horton's demon.

Pathogenesis

- Cause—unknown
- Vasodilation is extracranial
- Trigeminal nerve may produce pain
- Appears to be a disturbance in circadian rhythm
- Histamine concentration or receptors may dysfunction

Patient Profile

- Males > Females
- Age at onset 30 years or greater
- Women—at menopause or later

Signs and Symptoms

- Sudden, sharp, boring, stabbing pain on one side of upper face, periorbital region, and forehead
- Tearing on side of headache
- Nasal congestion or rhinorrhea on side of headache
- Ptosis and constricted pupil on side of headache
- Patient may pace, cry out, or do bizarre things, such as hitting head against wall

Differential Diagnosis

- Migraine headache
- Facial neuralgias
- Temporal arteritis
- Pheochromocytoma
- Pathologic process in head or neck

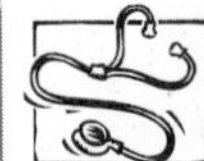

ASSESSMENT

History

Inquire about:

- Onset and duration of symptoms
- Location of symptoms
- Previous treatments tried and results
- Underlying conditions
- Current medications
- May be difficult to obtain history during an acute episode

Physical Findings

- Patient may be pacing, restless, perspiring
- One eye—ptosis, injected conjunctiva, tearing, constricted pupil
- Patient may resist being touched

Initial Workup

Laboratory: None diagnostic for cluster headache

Radiology: If uncertain of diagnosis, CT scan or MRI of head to rule out other disorder

Further Workup

Usually none needed

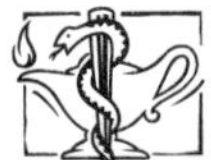

INTERVENTIONS

Office Treatment

- Acute attack—100% O_2, 8 to 10 L/min via tight-fitting mask for 10 to 15 minutes
- Sumatriptan, 6 mg subcutaneously; repeat in 1 hour if necessary, or ergotamine aerosol, 1 to 3 inhalations

Lifestyle Modifications

- During cluster periods may significantly alter lifestyle—may affect employment and social activity
- Smoking cessation
- Avoidance of alcohol during cluster periods; rarely, specific foods may trigger attacks
- Safety during acute attacks

Patient Education

Teach patient about:

- Disease process and self-treatment—O_2 at home, self-administration of sumatriptan or ergotamine during acute attack, or ergotamine to prevent attack
- Possible use of prednisone or methysergide to shorten cluster period and prevent attacks
- Avoiding glare, alcohol, excessive anger
- Avoiding stressful activity or excitement during cluster periods
- Providing education for family
- How to take medications and side effects (see Pharmacotherapeutics)

Referral

Consult with MD on treatment options

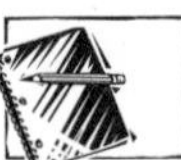

EVALUATION

Outcome

Periods of extended remission; shortened cluster periods with prevention of attacks

Possible Complications

- Self-injury during an attack
- Drug abuse

Follow-up

- During cluster periods, every 2 weeks to assess effectiveness of treatment
- During remission, every 3 to 6 months

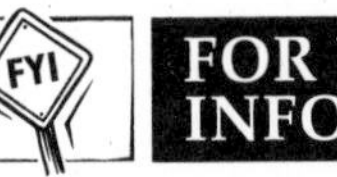

FOR YOUR INFORMATION

Life Span

Pediatric: Very rare

Geriatric: May experience more side effects from medications

Pregnancy: Very rare

Miscellaneous

Other treatments that may be beneficial include:

- Vigorous activity at first sign to abort attack
- Carotid compression on side of attack to reduce pain.
- Temporal artery compression on side of attack may decrease or increase pain

References

Jones JM: The scorn of Horton's demon: understanding cluster headache, *Physician Assist* 18(8):38-50, 1994.

Ozuna JM: Nursing role in management of chronic neurological problems. In Lewis SM, Collier IC, Heitkemper MM, editors: *Medical-surgical nursing: assessment and management of clinical problems,* ed 4, St Louis, 1994, Mosby, pp 1753-1757.

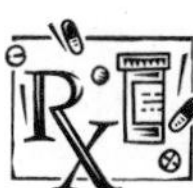

PHARMACOTHERAPEUTICS

Drug of Choice	Mechanism of Action	Prescribing Information	Side Effects
Sumatriptan (Imitrex); used during acute attack; 6 mg SQ via Autoinjector, may repeat in 1 hour, maximum 12 mg/24 hr; 100-mg tab PO, may repeat in 1 hour; safety in children not established	Causes vasoconstriction of cranial arteries	***Contraindications:*** Angina pectoris; myocardial infarction (MI); silent ischemia; Prinzmetal's angina; uncontrolled hypertension; concurrent ergotamine-containing products; hypersensitivity; basilar or hemiplegic migraine ***Cost:*** Two 6-mg syringes: $67 ***Pregnancy category:*** C	Tingling, hot sensation, burning, feeling of pressure, tightness, numbness, dizziness, sedation, flushing, chest tightness, weakness, neck stiffness, sweating, injection site reaction
Ergotamine (Ergostat; Medihaler Ergotamine), 2 mg SL, then 1-2 mg qh—do not exceed 6 mg (3 tabs)/24 hours; inhaler, 1-3 puffs, may repeat in 1 hour, maximum 6 puffs/24 hours—not recommended for children	Constricts smooth muscle in peripheral cranial blood vessels; relaxes uterine muscle; blocks serotonin release	***Contraindications:*** Hypersensitivity; occlusion; coronary artery disease (CAD); hepatic disease; renal disease; peptic ulcer; hypertension ***Cost:*** Ergostat, 2-mg tab, 24 tabs: $18 ***Pregnancy category:*** X	Numbness in fingers and toes, headache, weakness, transient tachycardia, chest pain, edema, bradycardia, claudication, increase or decrease in blood pressure, nausea, vomiting, diarrhea, abdominal cramps, muscle pain
Prednisone; various dosing used: 40 mg/day × 5 days with gradual tapering over 3 weeks; *or* 10-day prednisone burst, 5-mg tabs, days 1-4—4 tabs morning, afternoon, and evening; day 5—4 tabs morning, 3 tabs afternoon and evening; day 6—3 tabs morning and afternoon, 2 tabs evening; day 7—2 tabs morning, afternoon, and evening; day 8—1 tab morning, afternoon, and evening; day 9—1 tab morning and evening; day 10—1 tab morning	Glucocorticoid; antiinflammatory agent	***Contraindications:*** Hypersensitivity; psychosis; idiopathic thrombocytopenia; acute glomerulonephritis; amebiasis; fungal infections; AIDS; TB ***Cost:*** 10-mg tab, 100 tabs: $4-$12 ***Pregnancy category:*** C	Depression, flushing, sweating, headache, mood change, hypertension, circulatory collapse, thrombophlebitis, embolism, fungal infections, increased intraocular pressure, blurred vision, GI hemorrhage, diarrhea, nausea, pancreatitis, thrombocytopenia, acne, poor wound healing, fractures, osteoporosis
For prevention of attacks:			
Methysergide (Sansert), 2 mg PO bid, with meals—no pediatric dosage established	Blocks serotonin HT receptors in peripheral and central nervous systems; potent vasoconstrictor	***Contraindications:*** Hypersensitivity to ergot, tartrazine; occlusion, CAD; hepatic disease; renal disease; peptic ulcer; hypertension; connective tissue disease; fibrotic pulmonary disease ***Cost:*** 2-mg tab, 100 tabs: $155 ***Pregnancy category:*** C	Tremors, anxiety, insomnia, headache, euphoria, confusion, depersonalization, hallucination, drowsiness, retroperitoneal fibrosis, valvular thickening, palpitations, tachycardia, thrombophlebitis, cardiac fibrosis, nausea, vomiting, weight gain, blood dyscrasias

OVERVIEW

Migraine headache is a diffuse, severe, unilateral pain in the head. It is usually described as a throbbing pain and is accompanied by gastrointestinal, visual, or other neurologic signs. There is complete freedom from symptoms between attacks, and attacks vary in frequency from daily to weekly to 1 per year.

Pathogenesis

- Exact cause unknown
- Combination of neurologic, vascular, and chemical factors
- Disturbance of cerebral blood flow, dilation of scalp arteries, and serotonin metabolism abnormality
- May be precipitated by food, alcohol, birth control pills, menses, fatigue, excessive sleep, missing meals, stress, or relief of stress

Patient Profile

- Females > Males
- Any age, but usually <50 years
- Onset most commonly in adolescence to age 30 years
- May be seen in children as young as 5 to 6 years
- Positive family history in 65%

Signs and Symptoms

- Unilateral, severe, throbbing head pain
- Nausea, vomiting
- Photophobia
- Phonophobia
- Sweating
- Scalp tenderness
- Lightheadedness
- Pallor
- Irritability
- 10% to 20% of patients experience aura 10 to 30 minutes before headache
- Sensory dysfunction—tingling or burning sensation, scintillating scotomas, parasthesias
- Motor dysfunction—weakness, paralysis, dizziness, confusion

Differential Diagnosis

- Tension headache
- Cluster headache
- Temporal arteritis
- Head trauma
- Brain tumor
- Cervical radiculopathy
- Drug-seeking behavior
- Epilepsy

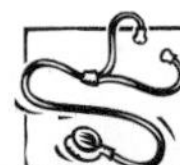

ASSESSMENT

History

Inquire about:

- Onset and duration of symptoms
- Location of symptoms
- Possible precipitating factors
- Treatments tried and results
- Past history of mental illness or head trauma
- Underlying conditions
- Current medications

Physical Findings

- If between attacks, no abnormal findings
- During attack:
    - Increased blood pressure
    - Irritability
    - Photophobia
    - Phonophobia
    - Sweating
    - Scalp tenderness
    - Fever
    - Facial flushing

Initial Workup

Laboratory: None specific for migraine—used to rule out other causes of headache

Radiology: CT scan or MRI of head only to rule out tumor

Further Workup

None indicated

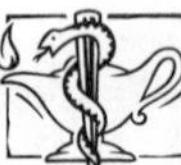

INTERVENTIONS

Office Treatment

For acute, severe attack:

- Sumatriptan, 6 mg subcutaneously, may repeat in 1 hour, or ergotamine inhaler, 1 inhalation, repeat in 5 minutes, maximum 6 inhalations/24 hours
- DHE 45, 1 ml (1 mg/ml) IM or IV, may repeat in 1 hour, maximum 3 ml/day

Lifestyle Modifications

- Smoking cessation
- Diet modification to eliminate precipitating foods
- Avoidance of alcohol
- May need new birth control method if taking oral contraceptives
- Exercise program
- Stress reduction techniques
- Can significantly interfere with lifestyle

Patient Education

Teach patient about:

- Condition and treatment options—during attack, need to lie completely still in dark room, limit noise, use compression of temporal artery on affected side
- Prevention of attack—eliminating precipitating foods
- Keeping headache diary to locate triggers
- Stress reduction through biofeedback or relaxation therapy
- Tips on smoking cessation
- Support groups available
- Alternative birth control methods if taking contraceptives (newer triphasic pills less likely to cause problem)
- How to start aerobic exercise program
- How to avoid alcohol
- Avoiding fatigue and missing meals
- Starting preventive medication—must discontinue acute medication to treat headache before initiating preventive therapy (need to take preventive medication 2 to 3 months to judge effectiveness)
- Medications for acute and preventive use and side effects (see Pharmacotherapeutics)

Referral

Consult with MD if treatment fails

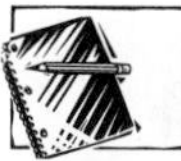

EVALUATION

Outcome
Reduction in severity and frequency of attacks; minimal lifestyle disruption

Possible Complications
- Status migraine
- Cerebral ischemic episode
- If narcotics used for acute attacks, drug addiction

Follow-up
Every 2 weeks until control is gained; then every 3 months to monitor preventive therapy

FOR YOUR INFORMATION

Life Span
Pediatric: May start as early as 5 to 6 years of age; may present with periodic vomiting and abdominal pain, not headache
Geriatric: Onset in this age group is rare—need workup for cranial lesion
Pregnancy: 60% will improve while pregnant; cautious use of medications

Miscellaneous
The NP needs to be alert to the possibility of drug abuse or drug-seeking behavior when seeing a patient for the first time with a complaint of migraine headache.

References
Hoffert MJ: Treatment of migraine: a new era, *Am Fam Physician* 49(3):633-638, 1994.
Smith CW: The nervous system. In Driscoll CE et al, editors: *The family practice desk reference,* ed 3, St Louis, 1996, Mosby, p 454.

NOTES

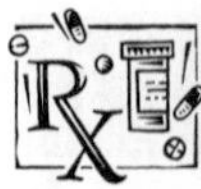

PHARMACOTHERAPEUTICS

There are many drugs used to both treat and prevent migraines. The following table presents only the most commonly used drugs and those approved by the FDA for use in migraines.

Drug of Choice	Mechanism of Action	Prescribing Information	Side Effects
Acetaminophen (Tylenol), 650 mg PO q6h; for children, use Children's Tylenol—follow label directions	Analgesia by increasing pain threshold	***Contraindications:*** Hypersensitivity; bleeding disorders or anticoagulant therapy; last trimester of pregnancy; asthma; gastric ulcers ***Cost:*** OTC ***Pregnancy category:*** Not categorized	Rash, hepatic toxicity with alcohol ingestion or overdose
Aspirin, 650-1000 mg PO q4h—do not use in children or adolescents because of risk of Reye's syndrome	Analgesia via peripheral and central nervous systems; may inhibit prostaglandins	***Contraindications:*** Hypersensitivity; bleeding disorders or anticoagulant therapy; last trimester of pregnancy; asthma; gastric ulcers ***Cost:*** OTC ***Pregnancy category:*** Not categorized	Rash, hepatic toxicity with alcohol ingestion or overdose
Nonsteroidal antiinflammatory drugs (NSAIDs), such as diclofenac (Cataflam), 50 mg, 2 tabs PO at onset; then 1 tab PO q8h—not indicated for children; for children, use naproxen (Naprosyn), 10 mg/kg PO in 2 divided doses	Analgesic; antiinflammatory; inhibits prostaglandin synthesis	***Contraindication:*** Hypersensitivity to aspirin, iodides, other NSAIDs ***Cost:*** Cataflam, 50-mg tab, 30 tabs: $30-$40 ***Pregnancy category:*** B	Nausea, anorexia, dizziness, drowsiness, fatigue, tachycardia, peripheral edema, rash, nephrotoxicity, dysuria, hematuria, oliguria, blood dyscrasias, tinnitus, hearing loss, blurred vision
For more severe attacks, use one of the following:			
Sumatriptan (Imitrex); use during acute attack; 6 mg SQ via Auto-injector, may repeat in 1 hour; maximum dose 12 mg/24 hours, 100-mg tab PO, may repeat in 1 hour—safety in children not established	Causes vasoconstriction of cranial arteries	***Contraindications:*** Angina pectoris; myocardial infarction (MI); silent ischemia; Prinzmetal's angina; uncontrolled hypertension; concurrent ergotomine-containing products; hypersensitivity; basilar or hemiplegic migraine ***Cost:*** Two 6-mg syringes: $67 ***Pregnancy category:*** C	Tingling, hot sensation, burning, feeling of pressure, tightness, numbness, dizziness, sedation, flushing, chest tightness, weakness, neck stiffness, sweating, injection site reaction
Ergotamine (Ergostat; Medihaler Ergotamine), 2 mg SL, then 1-2 mg qh—do not exceed 6 mg (3 tabs)/24 hours; inhaler, 1-3 puffs, may repeat in 1 hour, maximum 6 puffs/24 hours	Constricts smooth muscle in peripheral cranial blood vessels; relaxes uterine muscle; blocks serotonin release	***Contraindications:*** Angina pectoris; MI; silent ischemia; Prinzmetal's angina; uncontrolled hypertension; concurrent ergotomine-containing products; hypersensitivity; basilar or hemiplegic migraine ***Cost:*** Ergostat 2-mg tab, 24 tabs: $18 ***Pregnancy category:*** C	Numbness in fingers and toes, headache, weakness, transient tachycardia, chest pain, edema, bradycardia, claudication, increase or decrease in blood pressure, nausea, vomiting, diarrhea, abdominal cramps, muscle pain
Acetaminophen, dichloralphenazone, isometheptene mucate (Midrin), 2 tabs at onset, then 1 tab qh up to 5 in 12 hours—not recommended for children	Constricts cranial and cerebral arterioles; relaxes patient; pain reducer	***Contraindications:*** Glaucoma, severe renal disease, hypertension, organic heart disease, hepatic disease; patient on monoamine oxidase inhibitor (MAOI) therapy ***Cost:*** 50 tabs: $10-$20 ***Pregnancy category:*** Not classified	Transient dizziness; skin rash

Drug of Choice	Mechanism of Action	Prescribing Information	Side Effects
For rapid control of acute attack:			
Dihydroergotamine mesylate (D.H.E. 45), 1 mg/ml, 1 ml IM or IV, may repeat in 1 hour—do not exceed 3 mg/day or 6 mg/week—not dosed for children	Constricts smooth muscle in periphery, cranial blood vessels; inhibits norepinephrine uptake	***Contraindications:*** Hypersensitivity to ergot; occlusion; coronary artery disease (CAD), hepatic disease; pregnancy; renal disease; peptic ulcer; hypertension; lactation; children; uremia ***Cost:*** 1 mg/ml, 20-ml sol: $195 ***Pregnancy category:*** X	Numbness in fingers and toes, weakness, transient tachycardia, chest pain, bradycardia, increase or decrease in blood pressure, gangrene, nausea, vomiting, muscle pain
The following medications are used for prevention of migraines:			
Aspirin, 325 mg, 1-2 tablets PO hs—do not use in children or adolescents because of risk of Reye's syndrome	Analgesia via peripheral and central nervous systems; may inhibit prostaglandins	***Contraindications:*** Hypersensitivity; bleeding disorders or anticoagulant therapy; last trimester of pregnancy; asthma; gastric ulcers ***Cost:*** OTC ***Pregnancy category:*** Not categorized	Rash, anaphylactic reaction, GI upset and bleeding, Reye's syndrome in children and adolescents
Propranolol (Inderal), 20 mg PO bid, increase gradually, maximum dose 120 mg PO bid; try for 4-6 weeks after reaching maximum dose; if not effective, advisable to withdraw gradually over several weeks; children, 1-2 mg/kg PO bid, maximum dose 16 mg/kg/day; to stop, gradually decrease dosage over 7-14 days	Beta-adrenergic receptor blocking agent	***Contraindications:*** Hypersensitivity; cardiac failure; cardiogenic shock; 2nd- or 3rd-degree heart block; bronchospastic disease; sinus bradycardia; CHF ***Cost:*** 20-mg tabs, 2/day, 100 tabs: $2-$20 ***Pregnancy category:*** C	Bronchospasm, dyspnea, bradycardia, hypotension, congestive heart failure (CHF), palpitations, AV block, agranulocytosis, thrombocytopenia, nausea, vomiting, diarrhea, hepatomegaly, impotence, decreased libido, facial swelling, weight change, depression, hallucinations, dizziness, sore throat, laryngospasm, blurred vision, hyperglycemia; can mask symptoms of hypoglycemia
Amitriptyline (Elavil), 50-100 mg PO hs, maximum dose 200 mg hs; adolescents, 30 mg hs, may increase up to 150 mg hs—do not use in children <12 years	Antidepressant; blocks reuptake of norepinephrine and serotonin	***Contraindications:*** Hypersensitivity to tricyclic antidepressants; recovery phase of MI ***Cost:*** 50-mg tabs, 1/day × 90 days: $3-$10 ***Pregnancy category:*** C	Agranulocytosis, thrombocytopenia, eosinophilia, leukopenia, dizziness, drowsiness, confusion, headache, anxiety, tremors, extrapyramidal symptoms, diarrhea, dry mouth, nausea, vomiting, paralytic ileus, hepatitis, increased appetite, urine retention, rash, urticaria, orthostatic hypotension, ECG changes, tachycardia, hypertension, blurred vision, tinnitus
Methysergide (Sansert), 2 mg PO bid, with meals—no pediatric dosage established	Blocks serotonin HT receptors in CNS and periphery; potent vasoconstrictor	***Contraindications:*** Hypersensitivity to ergot, tartrazine; occlusion; CAD; hepatic disease; renal disease; peptic ulcer; hypertension; connective tissue disease; fibrotic pulmonary disease ***Cost:*** 2-mg tab, 100 tabs: $155 ***Pregnancy category:*** C	Tremors, anxiety, insomnia, headache, euphoria, confusion, depersonalization, hallucination, drowsiness, retroperitoneal fibrosis, valvular thickening, palpitations, tachycardia, thrombophlebitis, cardiac fibrosis, nausea, vomiting, weight gain, blood dyscrasias

Headache, Tension

OVERVIEW

Tension headache is a diffuse, bilateral pain in the head. It usually has a slow onset and is often described as a bandlike sensation around the head. Tension headaches are divided into 2 types: episodic (usually associated with a stressful event) and chronic (daily headaches; must occur 15 days/month for 6 months). Tension headache is the most common type of headache.

Pathogenesis

- Traction on pain-sensitive structures
- Vascular and meningeal inflammation
- Vasodilation
- Contracted muscles of scalp and neck
- Disturbance in serotonin system
- Causative factors—stress, anxiety, depression, cervical osteoarthritis

Patient Profile

- Females > Males
- Onset usually at 20 to 50 years of age
- Positive family history in 40%

Signs and Symptoms

- Bilateral head pain
- Pain is dull, pressing, or bandlike
- Frontooccipital or generalized
- Intensity may vary throughout the day
- May be present on arising or shortly thereafter
- Muscular tightness in neck, occipital, or frontal regions

Differential Diagnosis

- Migrainous headache
- Cluster headache
- Cervical spondylosis
- Caffeine dependency
- Drug-seeking behavior
- Depression
- Head injury
- Dental problems
- Chronic sinusitis
- Eye problems
- Hypertension
- Hypoxia
- Temporal arteritis
- Tumor
- Temporomandibular joint syndrome
- Trigeminal neuralgia

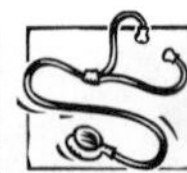

ASSESSMENT

History

Inquire about:

- Onset and duration of symptoms
- Visual difficulties
- Nuchal rigidity
- Fever
- Location of headache
- Severity of pain
- Precipitating factors, such as stress, diet, menses, or depression
- Treatments tried and results
- Mental health problems
- Family history
- Underlying conditions
- Current medications

Physical Findings

- May have normal physical examination if not currently experiencing a headache
- If during attack, patient may have furrowed brow, pallor, increased blood pressure, and muscle tightness or stiffness in neck, occipital, and frontal regions

Initial Workup

Laboratory

- No specific test for tension headache; tests done to rule out other causes of headache:
- CBC
- Chemistry profile to include electrolytes, glucose, BUN, creatinine, liver function studies
- Thyroid panel

Radiology

- CT scan or MRI of head to rule out tumor
- Cervical spine film to rule out cervical spondylosis

Further Workup

Only if headache pattern changes or positive neurologic findings

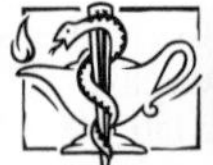

INTERVENTIONS

Office Treatment

None indicated

Lifestyle Modifications

- Smoking cessation
- Stress reduction techniques
- Exercise program—special emphasis on neck range-of-motion and strengthening exercises

Patient Education

Teach patient about:

- Condition and treatment options:
  - Acute episode—resting in quiet, dark room; cool compresses over eyes; hot bath or shower; massage therapy to back of neck and scalp; medications
  - Chronic episodes—antidepressant medications; stress reduction techniques, including relaxation therapy, biofeedback, yoga, exercise program; cervical traction
- Preventive medication
- Tips for smoking cessation
- Keeping a headache diary to help determine any precipitating events
- How to use medications and side effects (see Pharmacotherapeutics)

Referrals

- Consult with MD on patient resistant to treatment
- Possibly to counselor or pain clinic

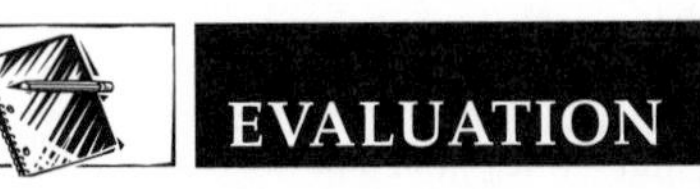

EVALUATION

Outcome

Stressors removed—headaches resolve

Possible Complications

- Drug abuse/dependency
- GI bleeding from NSAIDs

Follow-up

Every 2 weeks until control achieved

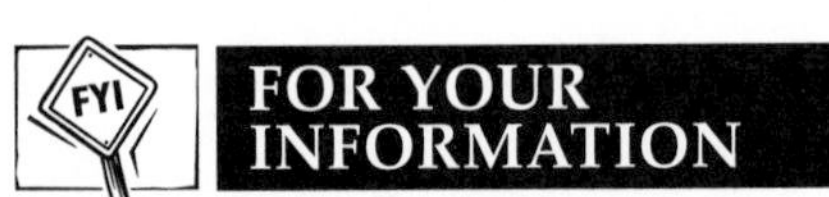

FOR YOUR INFORMATION

Life Span

Pediatric: Not common, but may occur at any age

Geriatric: Onset of new headache should be worked up for possible tumor or temporal arteritis

Pregnancy: Headaches may increase in first trimester because of circulating hormones; usually abate in second and third trimesters

Miscellaneous

The NP must be alert to drug-seeking behavior in the patient complaining of headache.

Reference

Johnner CJ: Headaches and facial pain. In Barker LR, Burton JR, Zieve PD, editors: *Principles of ambulatory medicine,* ed 4, Baltimore, 1995, Williams & Wilkins, pp 1165-1166.

PHARMACOTHERAPEUTICS

Drug of Choice	Mechanism of Action	Prescribing Information	Side Effects
For acute attack, use one of the following:			
Acetaminophen (Tylenol), 650 mg PO q6h; for children, use Children's Tylenol—follow label directions	Analgesia by increasing pain threshold	***Contraindications:*** Hypersensitivity; bleeding disorders or anticoagulant therapy; last trimester of pregnancy; asthma; gastric ulcers ***Cost:*** OTC ***Pregnancy category:*** Not categorized	Rash, hepatic toxicity with alcohol ingestion or overdose
Aspirin, 650-1000 mg PO q4h—do not use in children or adolescents because of risk of Reye's syndrome	Analgesia via peripheral and central nervous systems; may inhibit prostaglandins	***Contraindications:*** Hypersensitivity; bleeding disorders or anticoagulant therapy; last trimester of pregnancy; asthma; gastric ulcers ***Cost:*** OTC ***Pregnancy category:*** Not categorized	Rash, hepatic toxicity with alcohol ingestion or overdose
Nonsteroidal antiinflammatory drugs (NSAIDs), such as diclofenac (Cataflam), 50 mg, 2 tabs PO at onset, then 1 tab PO q8h—not indicated for children; for children, use naproxen (Naprosyn), 10 mg/kg PO in 2 divided doses	Analgesic; antiinflammatory; inhibits prostaglandin synthesis	***Contraindication:*** Hypersensitivity to aspirin, iodides, other NSAIDs ***Cost:*** Cataflam, 50-mg tab, 30 tabs: $30-$40 ***Pregnancy category:*** B	Nausea, anorexia, dizziness, drowsiness, fatigue, tachycardia, peripheral edema, rash, nephrotoxicity, dysuria, hematuria, oliguria, blood dyscrasias, tinnitus, hearing loss, blurred vision
For prevention, use one of the following:			
Propranolol (Inderal), 20 mg PO bid, increase gradually, maximum dose 120 mg bid; try for 4-6 weeks after reaching maximum dose; if not effective, gradually withdraw over several weeks; children, 1-2 mg/kg PO bid, maximum dose 16 mg/kg/day; to stop, gradually decrease dosage over 7-14 days	Beta-adrenergic receptor–blocking agent	***Contraindications:*** Hypersensitivity; cardiac failure; cardiogenic shock; 2nd- or 3rd-degree heart block; bronchospastic disease; sinus bradycardia; congestive heart failure (CHF) ***Cost:*** 20-mg tabs, 2/day, 100 tabs: $2-$20 ***Pregnancy category:*** C	Bronchospasm, dyspnea, bradycardia, hypotension, CHF, palpitations, atrioventricular (AV) block, agranulocytosis, thrombocytopenia, nausea, vomiting, diarrhea, hepatomegaly, impotence, decreased libido, facial swelling, weight change, depression, hallucinations, dizziness, sore throat, laryngospasm, blurred vision, hyperglycemia, can mask symptoms of hypoglycemia
Amitriptyline (Elavil), 50-100 mg PO hs, maximum dose 200 mg hs; adolescents, 30 mg hs, may increase up to 150 mg hs—do not use in children <12 yrs	Antidepressant; blocks reuptake of norepinephrine and serotonin	***Contraindications:*** Hypersensitivity to tricyclic antidepressants; recovery phase of myocardial infarction (MI) ***Cost:*** 50-mg tabs, 1/day × 90 days: $3-$10 ***Pregnancy category:*** C	Agranulocytosis, thrombocytopenia, eosinophilia, leukopenia, dizziness, drowsiness, confusion, headache, anxiety, tremors, extrapyramidal symptoms, diarrhea, dry mouth, nausea, vomiting, paralytic ileus, hepatitis, increased appetite, urine retention, rash, urticaria, orthostatic hypotension, ECG changes, tachycardia, hypertension, blurred vision, tinnitus

Hearing Loss

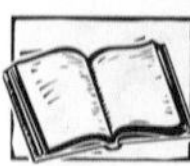

OVERVIEW

Hearing loss is the impairment of an individual's ability to hear. It may be complete or partial and may involve the outer and middle or inner ear. It is classified as either conductive or sensorineural.

Pathogenesis

CONDUCTIVE HEARING LOSS

- Outer and middle ear involved
- Caused by conditions that interfere with air conduction—impacted cerumen, foreign bodies, middle ear disease, otitis externa, otitis media, serous otitis media with effusion, otosclerosis, cholesteatoma, benign or malignant tumors

SENSORINEURAL HEARING LOSS

- Impairment of inner ear and central connections
- Causes—noise exposure, Meniere's disease, presbycusis (degenerative change of inner ear due to aging), trauma, acoustic tumor, maternal rubella, prematurity and/or traumatic delivery (congenital and neonatal loss), syphilis, Paget's disease, diabetes, bacterial meningitis, viral illnesses, multiple sclerosis, ototoxic drugs (antibiotics—streptomycin, gentamycin, vancomycin; diuretics—ethacrynic acid, furosemide; salicylates; antineoplastic agents)

Patient Profile

- Males = Females
- All ages—more common in the elderly

Signs and Symptoms

- Difficulty hearing
- May have tinnitus, dizziness, pain
- Ear may feel "stopped up"

Differential Diagnosis

Must rule out any of the possible causes, particularly cholesteatoma in conductive loss and acoustic tumor in sensorineural loss

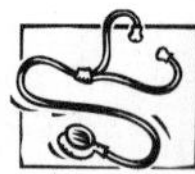

ASSESSMENT

History

Inquire about:

- Onset and duration of symptoms
- Whether loss is unilateral or bilateral
- Fever
- Pain
- Discharge
- Vertigo
- Tinnitus
- Exposure to noise
- Trauma
- Family history
- Underlying conditions
- Past medical history
- Medications used before onset of loss
- Current medications

Physical Findings

- Conductive loss—clarity of sound is normal, but volume must be increased
- Sensorineural loss—sound distorted; increasing volume does *not* improve hearing
- Physical findings depend on cause—thorough physical examination of external canal and tympanic membrane (TM)—check mobility of TM; Rinne test (positive = normal hearing or sensorineural loss; negative = conductive loss; Weber test (conductive loss—sound lateralizes to affected ear; sensorineural loss—sound lateralizes to good ear); audiogram (conductive loss = at least 15-decibel airborne gap; sensorineural loss = loss in decibel levels of 4000-Hz range)

Initial Workup

Laboratory: Rapid plasma reagin (RPR) or VDRL if latent syphilis is possible cause
Radiology: CT scan or MRI if tumor possible

Further Workup

- Pure-tone audiometry
- Vestibular testing
- Electronystagmometry
- Rotational tests
- Posturography (if tinnitus and vertigo present)
- Tympanometry, usually done by specialist

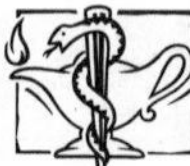

INTERVENTIONS

Office Treatment

Cerumen removal if cerumen impaction present

Lifestyle Modifications

- Noise-induced hearing loss—use of earplugs or ear muffs imperative to prevent further loss
- If loss is progressive and irreversible, learning new ways of communicating—lipreading, sign language

Patient Education

Teach patient about:

- Cause and type of hearing loss patient has
- Treatment options—conductive losses—medications, surgery—usually can be corrected
- Sensorineural loss—may or may not be able to stop progression—need to stop ototoxic drugs; use hearing protection; cannot reverse; hearing aid (may or may not help); ways to communicate—lipreading, sign language; cochlear implants; assisted listening devices
- Medications used and side effects (see Pharmacotherapeutics)

Referral

To audiologist or otolaryngologist

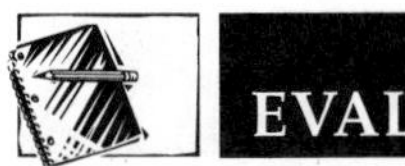

EVALUATION

Outcomes:

- Conductive loss—may be improved, cured, or progression halted
- Sensorineural loss—patient will demonstrate adaptation to hearing loss and learn other means to enhance communications

Possible Complications

- Progresses to chronic problem
- Can lead to increased hearing loss and total deafness
- Chronic tinnitus
- Balance problems

Follow-up

Depends on cause; in 2 weeks for acute otitis media and otitis externa

FOR YOUR INFORMATION

Life Span

Pediatric: Otitis media and eustachian tube problems more common in infants and small children

Geriatric: Most common cause is presbycusis

Pregnancy: Good prenatal care to prevent congenital or neonatal hearing loss

Miscellaneous

For patients with TM perforation or ventilation tubes in place, instruct not to get water in ears

References

Bahadori RS, Bohne BA: Adverse effects of noise on hearing, *Am Fam Physician* 47(5):1219-1226, 1993.

Goldblum K, Collier IC: Vision and hearing problems. In Lewis SM, Collier IC, Heitkemper MM, editors: *Medical-surgical nursing: assessment and management of clinical problems,* ed 4, St Louis, 1996, Mosby, pp 478-480.

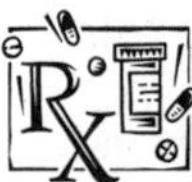

PHARMACOTHERAPEUTICS

Medications are presented only for acute otitis media, serous otitis media, and otitis externa, the most common causes of hearing loss that the NP will treat. Cerumen removal may be accomplished with an ear curette or with Cerumenex, 1:1 hydrogen peroxide and water mixture, or liquid Colace (to soften the cerumen), followed by ear irrigation with a syringe with butterfly tubing or a Water Pik using tepid water.

Drug of Choice	Mechanism of Action	Prescribing Information	Side Effects
For acute otitis media:			
Amoxicillin (Amoxil), PO 250-500 mg q8h × 10 days; children, 20 mg/kg/day PO q8h × 10 days	Bactericidal; broad-spectrum; *not* effective against beta-lactamase–producing pathogens	***Contraindications:*** Hypersensitivity to penicillins; use caution if allergic to cephalosporins ***Cost:*** 500-mg tabs, 3/day × 10 days: $4.00 ***Pregnancy category:*** B	Anaphylactoid reaction, nausea, vomiting, diarrhea, rashes, Stevens-Johnson syndrome, pseudomembranous colitis
For acute otitis media and serous otitis media:			
Erythromycin, 250 mg PO qid × 10 days; children, 30-50 mg/kg/day PO in divided doses × 10 days	Inhibits protein synthesis	***Contraindication:*** Hypersensitivity ***Cost:*** 250-mg tabs, 4/day × 10 days: $4 ***Pregnancy category:*** B	Nausea, vomiting, diarrhea, abdominal pain, anorexia, rash, urticaria, pseudomembranous colitis—rarely
For serous otitis media:			
Oral decongestants; 130 different products listed in *PDR* for nonprescription drugs, many in combination with an antihistamine; most contain pseudoephedrine, phenylephrine, or phenylpropanolamine; see labels for dosage—do not exceed dosage	Sympathomimetics cause nasal vasoconstriction, producing decongestion	***Contraindications:*** Hypersensitivity; hypertension (controversial); diabetes; heart or thyroid disease; prostate enlargement ***Cost:*** Varies with product ***Pregnancy category:*** Pseudoephedrine—B; phenylephrine and phenylpropanolamine—C	Drowsiness, dry mouth, insomnia, headache, nervousness, fatigue, irritability, disorientation, rash, palpitations, sore throat, cough
For otitis externa:			
Hydrocortisone, neomycin sulfate, polymyxin B sulfate (Cortisporin) otic drops, 4 qtt qid; children, 3 qtt qid	Corticoid; suppresses inflammatory response; antiinfective agent	***Contraindications:*** Hypersensitivity; herpes simplex, vaccinia, and varicella infections ***Cost:*** Otic solution, 10 ml: $3-$7 ***Pregnancy category:*** C	Ototoxicity, nephrotoxicity, rash, urticaria, burning, allergic contact dermatitis, secondary infection

Heat Exhaustion

OVERVIEW

Heat exhaustion is a condition that is a result of prolonged exposure to heat. If left untreated, it can progress to heat stroke.

Pathogenesis

Cause—overexposure to heat or failure of the heat-dissipating mechanism of the body, resulting in a rise in core body temperature

Patient Profile

- Males = Females
- Any age, but more likely in children and the elderly
- Risk factors:
  - Poor physical condition
  - Salt or water depletion
  - Obesity
  - Acute febrile or gastrointestinal diseases
  - Chronic condition such as diabetes, hypertension, or cardiac disease; alcohol or other drug abuse; heavy, restrictive clothing

Signs and Symptoms

- Profuse sweating
- Hypotension
- Dehydration
- Tachycardia
- Lack of coordination
- Irritability
- Nausea
- Thirst
- Weakness
- Vomiting
- Fatigue
- Dizziness
- Core temperature elevated, but <103° F (<39.4 degrees C)

Differential Diagnosis

- Febrile illnesses
- Drug-induced fluid loss
- Cardiac arrhythmia or infarction
- Acute cocaine intoxication

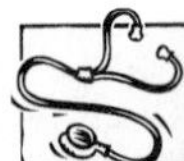

ASSESSMENT

History

Inquire about:

- Onset and duration of symptoms
- Exposure to heat and humidity
- History of previous heat exhaustion
- Alcohol consumption
- Underlying conditions
- Current medications

Physical Findings

- Profuse sweating
- Hypotension
- Tachycardia
- Hyperventilation (can lead to respiratory alkalosis)
- Core temperature elevated, but <103° F (<39.4° C)

Initial Workup

Laboratory: None to diagnose heat exhaustion, but may want to check for end-organ damage:

- Chemistry profile, including electrolytes, creatinine, BUN, liver enzymes
- Urinalysis
- CBC

Radiology: None indicated

Further Workup

None indicated

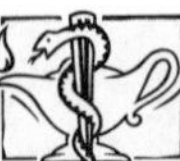

INTERVENTIONS

Office Treatment

- Rapid cooling—undress patient; wet patient down with cool water; apply ice packs
- Fluid and electrolyte replacement with PO fluids (oral saline—4 teaspoons salt in 1 gallon water) or IV fluids such as normal saline
- Have patient rest with legs elevated

Lifestyle Modifications

- If heat exhaustion due to exercise, may need to modify exercise routine until properly conditioned
- Do not wear warm, constrictive clothing
- Drink plenty of fluids without caffeine

Patient Education

Teach patient about:

- Condition and cause
- Proper conditioning before starting vigorous exercise program
- Proper amount of fluids to drink (8 ounces for every 15 minutes of exercise)
- Taking frequent rest breaks in a cool area
- Ways of obtaining an air conditioner or fan (there are many community agencies that will provide these free of charge for the elderly)
- Need to wear cool clothing
- Importance of using fans or air conditioner and assist patient in obtaining help with electric bill (many electric companies have special funds set up for underprivileged people to help pay their electric bill)
- Signs and symptoms of heat exhaustion and to seek help immediately
- Medications—none used to treat heat exhaustion

Referrals

Usually none for heat exhaustion

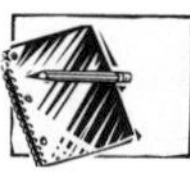

EVALUATION

Outcome
Resolves without sequelae

Possible Complication
Progresses to heat stroke

Follow-up
- Initial event—monitor core body temperature; when it drops to 102° F and stabilizes, patient may be released if no other signs/symptoms present
- Phone call follow-up in 24 hours
- If heat exhaustion is due to living condition, may wish to refer to home health for ongoing evaluation

FOR YOUR INFORMATION

Life Span
Pediatric: Very young more susceptible; teach guardians to monitor fluid intake
Geriatric: Very old more susceptible
Pregnancy: May be more susceptible to volume depletion

Miscellaneous
Very young patients and the elderly may be more appropriately treated in an emergency room, if available.

Reference
Vaughn K: Emergency care situations. In Lewis SM, Collier IC, Heitkemper MM, editors: *Medical surgical nursing: assessment and management of clinical problems,* ed 4, St Louis, 1996, Mosby, p 2010.

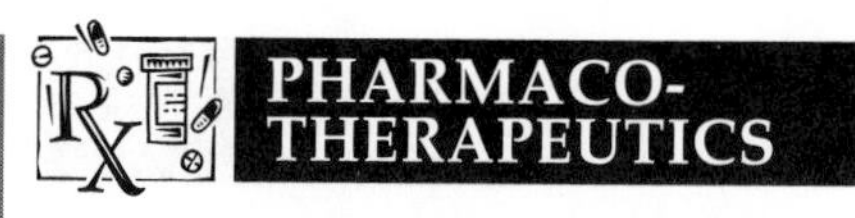

PHARMACOTHERAPEUTICS

There are no specific medications indicated for the treatment of heat exhaustion.

OVERVIEW

Heatstroke is the most serious heat-related illness. It is severe hyperthermia that results when heat exhaustion is left untreated and allowed to progress.

Pathogenesis

Cause—overexposure to heat or failure of heat-dissipating mechanism of body, resulting in rise in core body temperature

Patient Profile

- Males = Females
- Any age, but more common in children and elderly

Signs and Symptoms

- Hot, flushed dry skin
- Exhaustion
- Dehydration
- Confusion
- Disorientation
- Coma
- Core temperature >105° F (>40.5° C)

Differential Diagnosis

- Febrile illnesses
- Drug-induced fluid loss
- Cardiac arrhythmia or infarction
- Acute cocaine intoxication

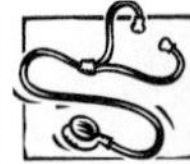

ASSESSMENT

History

Inquire about:

- Onset and duration of symptoms
- Exposure to heat and humidity
- History of previous heat exhaustion
- Underlying conditions
- Current medications (anticholinergics, antihistamines, and phenothiazines can make person more susceptible)

Physical Findings

- Hot, flushed dry skin
- Core temperature >103° F (>40.5° C)
- Confusion
- Dementia
- Disorientation

Initial Workup

Laboratory: Check for end-organ damage:

- Chemistry profile, including electrolytes, creatinine, BUN, liver enzymes
- Urinalysis
- CBC

Radiology: None indicated

Further Workup

If the above tests indicate end-organ damage has occurred, may need additional testing

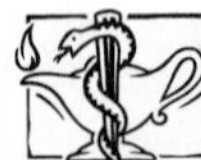

INTERVENTIONS

Office Treatment

- IV fluid and electrolyte replacement with normal saline
- Start cooling process—remove all clothing; may use sheets wet with cool water, icepacks (not placed directly against skin); spray patient with cool water
- Prepare for transport to emergency facility

Lifestyle Modifications

- If heatstroke due to exercise, may need to modify exercise routine until properly conditioned
- Do not wear warm, constrictive clothing
- Drink plenty of fluids without caffeine

Patient Education

Educate patient after initial emergent period; teach patient about:

- Condition and cause
- Proper conditioning to help avoid heat exhaustion
- Proper fluids to drink and amount (8 ounces for every 15 minutes of exercise)
- Taking frequent rest breaks in a cool area
- Having adequate cooling in the home—assist patient in obtaining an air conditioner or fan (there are many community agencies that will provide these free of charge for the elderly)
- Need to wear cool clothing
- Importance of using fans or air conditioner and assist patient in obtaining help with electric bill (many electric companies have special funds set up for underprivileged people to help pay their electric bill)
- Signs and symptoms of heat exhaustion and to seek help immediately
- Medications—no specific ones used to treat heatstroke; treatment is aimed at preventing end-organ damage or healing damage that may have occurred

Referral

To emergency room via emergency transportation

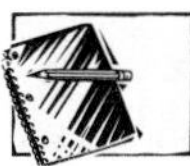

EVALUATION

Outcome
Depends on duration and intensity of hyperthermia and speed and effectiveness of treatment; when mental function is not altered, prognosis is good

Possible Complications
- Cardiac arrhythmias or infarction
- Pulmonary edema and adult respiratory distress syndrome
- Coma
- Seizures
- Acute renal failure
- Rhabdomyolysis
- Disseminated intravascular coagulation
- Hepatocellular necrosis

Follow-up
Within 1 week of hospitalization

FOR YOUR INFORMATION

Life Span
Pediatric: Very young more susceptible
Geriatric: Higher morbidity and mortality
Pregnancy: Needs to be treated by a specialist; close fetal monitoring important

Miscellaneous
Patients with underlying conditions such as diabetes, cardiac disease, hypertension, etc., have a much poorer prognosis.

Reference
Vaughn K: Emergency care situations. In Lewis SM, Collier IC, Heitkemper MM, editors: *Medical-surgical nursing: assessment and management of clinical problems,* ed 4, St Louis, 1996, Mosby, p 2010.

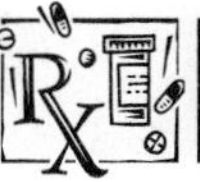

PHARMACOTHERAPEUTICS

There are no specific medications used for the treatment of heatstroke. Treatment is geared to preventing and healing end-organ damage.

Hemorrhoids

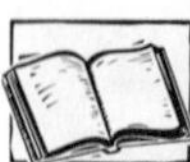

OVERVIEW

Hemorrhoids are varicosities of the hemorrhoidal plexus in the lower rectum or anus. They may be internal (above the internal sphincter) or external (outside the external sphincter).

Pathogenesis

- Cause—dilated veins of the hemorrhoidal plexus due to prolapse of vascular anal cushion and entrapment by internal anal sphincter
- Prolapse occurs as a result of:
  - Passage of large firm stool
  - Increased venous pressure (pregnancy, portal hypertension, straining while lifting)
  - Loss of muscle tone (old age, episiotomy, anal intercourse)

Patient Profile

- Males = Females
- Any age; most common age group—adults

Signs and Symptoms

- Rectal bleeding (bright red)
- Anal pain
- Anal burning
- Anal itching
- Anal protrusion
- Anal fissure
- Anal ulceration

Differential Diagnosis

- Anal tags
- Protruding tumors
- Prolapse of rectal mucosa

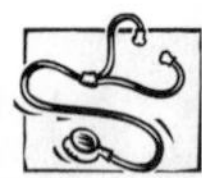

ASSESSMENT

History

Inquire about:

- Onset and duration of symptoms
- Pain
- Itching
- Burning
- Bleeding
- Underlying conditions
- Current medications

Physical Findings

- Large, dilated veins in hemorrhoidal plexus on rectal examination
- External hemorrhoids—mass just outside anus; usually soft and painless
- Thrombosed—painful, firm, bluish discoloration
- Internal hemorrhoids—may or may not be able to visualize; may be able to palpate on internal examination
- If extreme pain on examination, stop and refer to surgeon

Initial Workup

Laboratory: None indicated; may consider hemoglobin and hematocrit if significant bleeding

Radiology: None indicated

Further Workup

None indicated

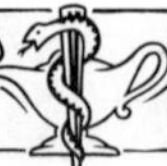

INTERVENTIONS

Office Treatment

None indicated

Lifestyle Modifications

- High-fiber diet
- Increased fluids
- Weight loss
- Avoidance of prolonged sitting
- Proper lifting technique

Patient Education

Teach patient about:

- Condition, causes, and treatment options—ice pack, sitz bath, witch hazel compresses, topical medications
- Avoidance of constipation—high-fiber diet, increased fluids
- Tips for weight loss
- Keeping anal area clean with soap and water
- Avoidance of prolonged sitting on toilet or at work—need to get up and move around periodically
- Proper lifting using legs, not back
- Medications to use and side effects (see Pharmacotherapeutics)

Referral

To surgeon if thrombosed, strangulated, or ulcerated

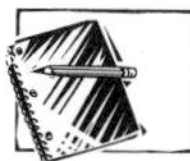

EVALUATION

Outcome
Resolve without sequelae; tend to recur

Possible Complications
- Thrombosis
- Secondary infections
- Ulceration
- Anemia
- Incontinence

Follow-up
In 2 weeks to assess treatment

FOR YOUR INFORMATION

Life Span
Pediatric: Uncommon
Geriatric: Common
Pregnancy: Common

Miscellaneous
If hemorrhoids are severe, surgery may be required. There are several surgical procedures that may be performed, depending on the severity and number of hemorrhoids present.

References
Heitkemper M, Sawchuck L: Nursing role in management: problems of absorption and elimination. In Lewis SM, Collier IC, Heitkemper MM, editors: *Medical-surgical nursing: assessment and management of clinical problems,* ed 4, St Louis, 1996, Mosby, pp 1254-1255.

Smith GW: Benign conditions of the anus and rectum. In Barker LR, Burton JR, Zieve PD, editors: *Principles of ambulatory medicine,* ed 4, Baltimore, 1995, Williams & Wilkins, pp 1351-1356.

NOTES

PHARMACOTHERAPEUTICS

Drug of Choice	Mechanism of Action	Prescribing Information	Side Effects
Stool softener: docusate sodium (Colace); adults, 50-200 mg/day PO; children 6-12 years, 40-120 mg/day PO; children 3-6 years, 60 mg/day PO; children <3 years, 10-40 mg/day PO	Surface-active agent; helps keep stool soft	***Contraindications:*** None ***Cost:*** Varies—OTC ***Pregnancy category:*** Not categorized	Bitter taste, throat irritation, nausea
Hydrocortisone ointment (Anusol HC, Rectasol HC); apply thin film to area tid or qid; children have greater susceptibility to HPA axis suppression and Cushing's syndrome	Steroid preparation; antiinflammatory; antipruritic	***Contraindication:*** Hypersensitivity ***Cost:*** Anusol-HC, 30 g: $16; Rectosol HC, 30 g: $12 ***Pregnancy category:*** C	Burning, itching, irritation, dryness, folliculitis, maceration of skin, secondary infection
Hydrocortisone and pramoxine (Proctocream HC); apply thin film to area tid or qid; children have greater susceptibility to HPA axis suppression and Cushing's syndrome	Steroid—antiinflammatory; antipruritic; pramoxine—surface anesthetic	***Contraindication:*** Hypersensitivity ***Cost:*** Cream 1%, 30 g: $14 ***Pregnancy category:*** C	Burning, itching, irritation, dryness, folliculitis, allergic contact dermatitis, secondary infection

Hepatitis, Viral

OVERVIEW

Viral hepatitis is an inflammatory disease of the liver caused by a distinct group of viruses.

Pathogenesis

5 Viruses identified as causative agents:

- Hepatitis A (HAV):
  - RNA virus of picornavirus group
  - Transmission—fecal-oral route; contaminated food and water
  - Incubation—15 to 50 days
- Hepatitis B (HBV):
  - DNA virus of hepadnaviruses
  - Transmission—sexual contact; blood and blood products; childbirth
  - Incubation: 45 to 160 days
- Hepatitis C (HCV):
  - RNA virus
  - Transmission—blood and blood products; some by sexual contact
  - Incubation: 14-140 days
- Hepatitis D (HDV):
  - RNA virus requiring HBV presence
  - Transmission—only occurs with HBV
  - Incubation—unknown
- Hepatitis E (HEV):
  - RNA virus
  - Transmission—fecal-oral route
  - Incubation—14 to 60 days

Patient Profile

- Males = Females
- Any age

Signs and Symptoms

- HAV:
  - May be asymptomatic
  - Fever, jaundice, anorexia, nausea, malaise, myalgia
  - Infectious 2 weeks before symptoms and 1 week after
  - No carrier state or chronic illness
- HBV:
  - May be asymptomatic
  - Anorexia, nausea, myalgia, malaise, jaundice to fatal hepatitis
  - Infectious 4 to 6 weeks before symptoms and for unpredictable time after symptoms
  - Carrier state and chronic illness
- HCV:
  - Few symptoms
  - Anorexia, nausea, malaise, rarely jaundice, myalgia
  - Infectious 4 to 6 weeks before symptoms and unpredictable after symptoms
  - 50% progress to chronic hepatitis
- HDV:
  - May be asymptomatic
  - Anorexia, nausea, malaise, jaundice, myalgia
  - Infectious 4 to 6 weeks before symptoms and unpredictable after symptoms
  - Only occurs with HBV as coinfection or superinfection in chronic HBV infection
- HEV:
  - May be asymptomatic
  - Fever, jaundice, anorexia, nausea, malaise, myalgia
  - Infectious 2 weeks before symptoms and 1 week after symptoms
  - No carrier or chronic state

Differential Diagnosis

- Infectious mononucleosis
- Drug-induced hepatitis
- Alcoholic hepatitis
- Hepatic malignancy

TABLE 9 ***Laboratory Tests for Viral Hepatitis***

Type	Test	Interpretation
HAV	Anti-HAV IgM Anti-HAV IgG	Acute or recent infection Previous infection
HBV	HBsAg Anti-HB and Anti-HBc HBdAg and HBeAg	Acute or early/carrier state State of recovery More serious or chronic infection
HCV	Anti-HCV	Acute, chronic or recovered
HDV	HDAg and Anti-HDV IgM Anti-HDV IgG	Acute infection Previous infection
HEV	Tests not available	

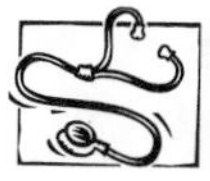

ASSESSMENT

History

Inquire about:

- Onset and duration of symptoms
- Similar illness in other household members
- Dark urine and light-colored stools
- History of blood transfusions or use of blood products
- Sexual behavior
- IV drug use or alcohol use
- Occupation
- Travel to foreign countries (Asia, Africa)
- Underlying conditions (such as chronic renal failure)
- Current medications

Physical Findings

- Jaundice—skin, mucous membranes, sclera
- Tenderness in (R) upper abdominal quadrant
- Splenic enlargement
- Weight loss
- Fever

Initial Workup

Laboratory

- CBC—WBC is low-normal; differential may show few atypical lymphocytes
- Liver function tests—ALT and AST markedly elevated
- Alkaline phosphate—mild to moderate elevation
- Bilirubin—normal to markedly elevated
- Urinalysis—positive for bilirubin
- Prothrombin time—if elevated, suggests severe illness
- Serologic marker for specific type of hepatitis (Table 9)

Radiology: None indicated

Further Workup

Liver biopsy to confirm type and extent of liver damage

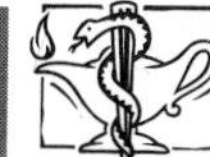

INTERVENTIONS

Office Treatment

- HAV exposure—household and sexual contacts need immune globulin (0.02 ml/kg)
- Known HBV exposure:
    - Unvaccinated—hepatitis B immune globulin (HBIG) (0.06 mg/kg IM); start HB vaccine
    - Vaccinated—test for anti-HBs: adequate—no treatment; inadequate—HB vaccine booster
    - Known nonresponder—HBIG × 2 doses or HBIG × 1 plus HB vaccine × 1
    - Response unknown—test for anti-HBs: adequate—no treatment; inadequate—HBIG × 1 plus HB vaccine booster

Lifestyle Modifications

- Cessation of use of hepatoxic drugs
- Safe sex practices
- Avoidance of alcohol
- Nutritionally sound diet

Patient Education

Teach patient about:

- Condition and treatment options—usually resolves in 4-8 weeks
- Need to rest and increase fluids
- Avoiding hepatoxic drugs such as acetaminophen and aspirin
- How disease is spread and prevention of spread—safe sex, good hand washing, universal precautions for blood and body fluids, sanitary disposal of soiled diapers in day care centers
- Immunization against HAV and HBV for those at risk
- Diet high in protein and carbohydrates and low in fat
- Increased fluids with vomiting and diarrhea
- Medications used and side effects (see Pharmacotherapeutics)

Referral

To MD for severe cases

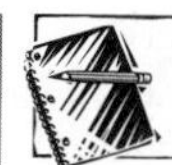

EVALUATION

Outcomes

- HAV—usually resolves without sequelae
- HBV and HDV—may be more severe and result in chronic disease
- HCV—fewer than 50% develop chronic disease; may lead to liver failure
- HEV—resolves without sequelae

Possible Complications

- Acute or subacute necrosis
- Chronic hepatitis
- Cirrhosis
- Liver failure
- Hepatocellular carcinoma
- Death

Follow-up

Depends on severity of disease—liver function tests every 2 weeks; viral biochemical markers in 4 to 6 weeks

FOR YOUR INFORMATION

Life Span

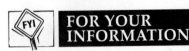

Pediatric: HAV more common in children, especially if they attend day care; HBV more acute, but children usually recover completely

Geriatric: Symptoms may be more severe, and recuperation takes longer

Pregnancy: All should be tested for HBsAg prenatally; if positive, give child hepatitis B immune globulin and HBV vaccine within 12 hours of birth, at 1 month, and at 6 months of age

Miscellaneous

All persons at risk of contracting HAV or HBV should be encouraged to receive the vaccine. CDC recommendations for HAV vaccine recipients include the following: travelers to countries with endemic HAV, gay men, IV drug users, persons with chronic liver disease, and laboratory workers. The following should also be considered: day care workers, food handlers, and staff for institutionally disabled persons. CDC recommendations for HBV vaccine recipients include health care workers, dialysis patients, gay men, and institutionalized persons. Persons at high risk of HBV infection should have postvaccination serologic testing done. If the patient is a nonresponder, up to 3 more vaccinations should be given.

References

Bartlett JG: *Pocket book of infectious disease therapy,* ed 7, Baltimore, 1996, Williams & Wilkins, pp. 113-118, 279-282.

Frymoyer CL: Practical therapeutics: preventing spread of viral hepatitis, *Am Fam Physician* 48(8):1479-1486, 1993.

Woolliscroft JO: *Current diagnosis and treatment: a quick reference for the general practitioner,* Philadelphia, 1996, Current Medicine, pp 178-181.

NOTES

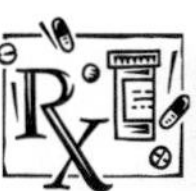

PHARMACOTHERAPEUTICS

Drug of Choice	Mechanism of Action	Prescribing Information	Side Effects
Immune globulin (Gammagard); adults and children, 0.02 ml/kg, not to exceed 2 ml; given IM for passive immunity to HAV	Gamma globulin antibodies	***Contraindication:*** Hypersensitivity ***Cost:*** 2-ml vial: $3 ***Pregnancy category:*** C	Pain at injection site, rash, pruritus, chills, chest pain, arthralgia, lymphadenopathy, anaphylaxis, headache, fatigue, malaise, abdominal pain
Hepatitis B immune globulin (Hep-B, Gammagee); adults and children, 0.06 ml/kg IM plus hepatitis B vaccine	Human immunoglobulin	***Contraindication:*** Hypersensitivity ***Cost:*** 1-ml vial: $50 ***Pregnancy category:*** C	Local pain/tenderness at injection site, urticaria, angioedema, anaphylaxis, arthralgia, headache, fatigue, malaise
Hepatitis A vaccine; adults, 1 ml IM × 1 dose; children, 0.5 ml × 2 doses, 1 month apart; booster dose may be given at 6 months	HAVRX—killed, formalin inactivated	***Contraindication:*** Hypersensitivity ***Cost:*** 0.5-ml vial: $28 ***Pregnancy category:*** C	Induration, redness, and swelling at injection site; fatigue; fever; malaise; anorexia; nausea; rash; urticaria; pharyngitis; arthralgia; lymphadenopathy; insomnia; photophobia
Hepatitis B vaccine (Hep-B); adults and children >10 years: 1 ml IM, then 1 ml IM in 1 month, then 1 ml IM 6 months after initial dose; children 3 months to 10 years, 0.5 ml IM on same schedule as above	Provides active immunity to hepatitis B	***Contraindication:*** Hypersensitivity to immune globulins, thimerosal, glycine ***Cost:*** 3-ml vial: $167 ***Pregnancy category:*** C	Soreness at injection site, urticaria, erythema, swelling, induration, headache, dizziness, fever, nausea, vomiting, anaphylaxis, angioedema
For use in chronic HBV and HCV:			
Interferon alfa-2b, recombinant (Intron-a); HBV—5 mil IU daily or 10 mil IU, 3 times per week IM or SQ × 16 weeks; HCV—3 mil IU, 3 times per week IM or SQ × 24 weeks; should only be done by someone familiar with use; must monitor lab values frequently to assess response	Antiviral action—reprograms virus	***Contraindication:*** Hypersensitivity ***Cost:*** 5 mil IU/ml, 2 ml: $50 ***Pregnancy category:*** C	Dizziness, confusion, numbness, paresthesia, convulsions, coma, edema, hypotension, hypertension, congestive heart failure (CHF), myocardial infarction (MI), cerebrovascular accident (CVA), rash, dry skin, itching, alopecia, weight loss, taste changes, impotence, flulike syndrome, fever, fatigue, myalgia, headache, chills

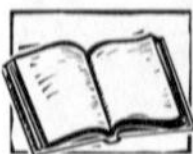

OVERVIEW

A hernia occurs when there is an abnormal opening or weakness in the wall of the abdomen that allows protrusion of an abdominal viscus. There are several types of abdominal hernias—inguinal, femoral, incisional, umbilical, and epigastric. A hernia is classified as either reducible or irreducible/incarcerated. A reducible hernia is one in which the abdominal contents can be put back into the abdominal cavity. An irreducible/incarcerated hernia is one in which the abdominal contents cannot be put back. If intestinal flow and blood supply are cut off, the hernia is said to be strangulated, and the patient needs immediate referral for surgery.

Pathogenesis

Congenital defect or any condition that increases intraabdominal pressure—chronic coughing, obesity, chronic constipation with straining, heavy lifting, hard physical labor

Patient Profile

- Males > Females, especially inguinal hernias
- Any age

Signs and Symptoms

- If reducible or irreducible:
  - May be asymptomatic or have mild pain/discomfort
  - May complain of a soft bulge at the site
- If strangulated:
  - Colicky abdominal pain
  - Nausea, vomiting
  - Abdominal distention

Differential Diagnosis

- For inguinal hernia—adductor muscle strain, hydrocele, varicocele, spermatocele, epididymal cysts, epididymitis, testicular tumor
- For femoral hernia—enlarged lymph node, lipoma, saphenous varix, a direct inguinal hernia
- Incisional, umbilical, and epigastric hernias are usually self-evident

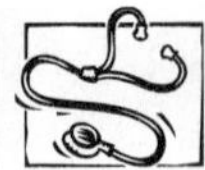

ASSESSMENT

History

Inquire about:

- Onset and duration of symptoms
- What patient was doing at time of onset of symptoms
- Reducibility of hernia
- Nausea, vomiting, abdominal cramping
- Underlying conditions
- Current medications

Physical Findings

- Many hernias are visible on inspection—protruding subcutaneous mass
- If reducible—mass soft and easily pushed back into abdomen
- If not reducible—mass will not push back into abdomen
- If strangulated—discolored and painful—*do not attempt to reduce*
- Inguinal hernias—may be visible soft mass in groin or scrotal sac in males or in labia majora in females; if not visible:
  - Males—invaginate scrotum and advance finger into inguinal canal; patient should cough or strain; will feel bulge on side or tip of finger (Fig. 1)
  - Females—more difficult; locate inguinal ring between inguinal ligament and os pubis; place hand over inguinal ring—will feel bulge when patient coughs
- Femoral hernias—have patient cough, and palpate femoral canal for swelling and impulse
- Umbilical, incisional, and epigastric hernias—with patient lying down, have patient lift head and bear down; will see bulge at site of hernia

Initial Workup

Laboratory: None indicated
Radiology: Abdominal ultrasound if uncertain about abdominal mass

Further Workup

None indicated

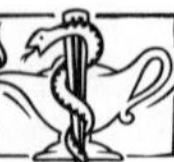

INTERVENTIONS

Office Treatment

Gently reduce hernia if possible

Lifestyle Modifications

- No lifting
- Smoking cessation

Patient Education

Teach patient about:

- Condition and treatment options—surgical repair: if strangulated, need immediate surgery; if irreducible/incarcerated, consult MD for reduction
- Signs and symptoms of strangulation
- Use of support garment
- No heavy lifting before surgery or for 6 weeks postoperatively
- When lifting resumes, using proper technique
- No sex or driving for 2 weeks postoperatively
- May return to light activity in 2 weeks

Referral

To surgeon

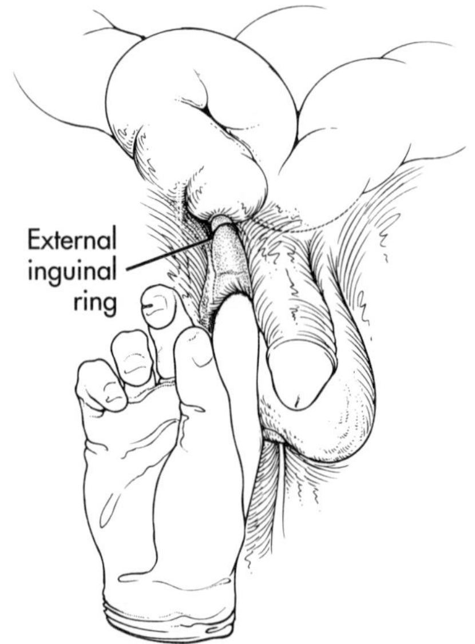

FIG. 1 Inguinal hernia examination.

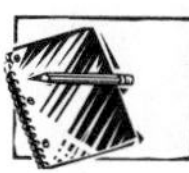

EVALUATION

Outcome
Complete recovery postoperatively

Possible Complications
- Before surgery—strangulation
- Postoperatively—wound infection, bleeding, urine retention

Follow-up
Within 1 week of surgery; if surgery not done immediately, follow-up for problems

FOR YOUR INFORMATION

Life Span
Pediatric: Congenital defect; most common—communicating hydrocele
Geriatric: May have longer recuperation period because of age
Pregnancy: May be causative factor

Miscellaneous
Abdominal hernias are a very common problem. In addition, 75% of all abdominal hernias are inguinal.

Reference
Zenilman ME, Bender JS, Smith GW: Abdominal hernias. In Barker LR, Burton JR, Zieve PD, editors: *Principles of ambulatory medicine,* ed 4, Baltimore, 1995, Williams & Wilkins, pp 1339-1346.

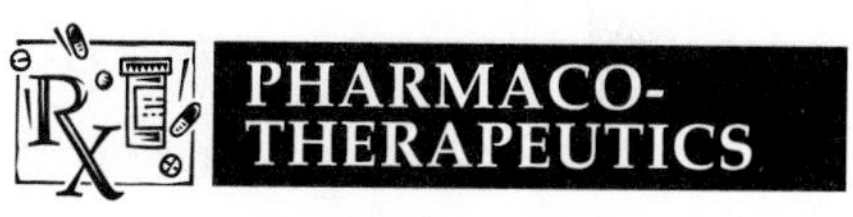

PHARMACOTHERAPEUTICS

There are no medications used specifically for treatment of a hernia.

Herniated Nucleus Pulposus (HNP)

OVERVIEW

Herniated nucleus pulposus occurs when there is rupture of an intervertebral disc with protrusion of the nucleus pulposus into the spinal canal. The protrusion may or may not compress a nerve root.

Pathogenesis
Causes:
- Major or minor trauma
- Improper lifting
- Vibration as results from driving motor vehicles

Patient Profile
- Males = Females
- Most common age—25 to 45 years

Signs and Symptoms
- Sharp, shooting radicular pain
- May have muscle weakness/atrophy
- Paresthesias and numbness in nerve root distribution
- Location of pain and numbness depends on disc involved (Table 10)

Differential Diagnosis
- Spondylolisthesis
- Compression fracture
- Degenerative spondylosis
- Herpes zoster
- Primary tumor
- Vertebral fracture
- Cauda equina syndrome
- Malingering

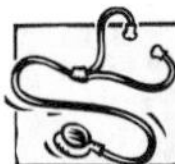

ASSESSMENT

History
Inquire about:
- Onset and duration of symptoms
- Recent injury
- Previous back problems
- Underlying conditions
- Current medications

Physical Findings
- Observe gait and posture (usually cautious and awkward)
- Range of motion (elicits pain)
- Palpate spine (look for muscle spasms)
- Straight and crossed leg raises (usually positive)
- Popliteal compression test (flex leg; apply pressure to popliteal nerve—positive if leg pain reproduced)
- Assess muscle strength in lower extremities
- Assess deep tendon reflexes in lower extremities

Initial Workup
Laboratory: None diagnostic

Radiology
- Plain films of lumbar spine—usually normal
- CT scan or MRI—demonstration of herniation

Further Workup
None indicated

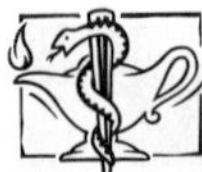

INTERVENTIONS

Office Treatment
None indicated

Lifestyle Modifications
- Smoking cessation
- Weight reduction
- Exercise program
- Proper lifting technique

Patient Education
Teach patient about:
- Condition and treatment:
  - Bed rest for 3 to 7 days (some authors recommend 1 to 2 weeks) with hips moderately flexed
  - Progressive exercise program—pelvic tilt exercises first; then abdominal strengthening exercises
  - Lumbosacral corset
  - Physical therapy
  - Nonsteroidal antiinflammatory drugs
  - Muscle relaxants (use is controversial)
  - Discectomy—many procedures available; absolute indication for surgery—cauda equina
- Medications used and side effects (see Pharmacotherapeutics)

Referral
To orthopedic surgeon or neurosurgeon if conservative treatment fails

TABLE 10 ***Disc Involvement and Location of Symptoms***

Level of herniation	Pain	Numbness
L3-L4	Crosses front of leg from thigh to great toe and crosses buttocks from sacrum to greater trochanter	Anterior thigh and knee
L4-L5	Top of buttocks down side of leg	Outer calf and between great toe and second toe
L5-S1 (most common site)	Top of buttocks down back of leg to ankle	Back of calf and outer aspect of foot
Cauda equina (massive midline protrusion)	Perineum; both legs	Thigh, legs, feet, perineum, often bilateral

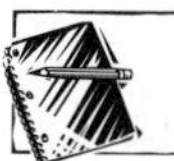

EVALUATION

Outcome
With conservative and surgical treatment and with lifestyle modifications, 80% to 90% have good prognosis

Possible Complications
- Footdrop
- Bladder and sphincter weakness
- Limited movement with restricted activity

Follow-up
Every 2 weeks until full recovery

FOR YOUR INFORMATION

Life Span
Pediatric: Rare before age 20 years
Geriatric: Most commonly suffer from degenerative disc disease
Pregnancy: Commonly causes low-back pain and sciatica; cautious use of medications

Miscellaneous
Narcotic analgesia is rarely indicated and should never be used as first-line treatment except in the most severe cases of HNP.

References
Mercier LR: *Practical orthopedics,* ed 4, St Louis, 1995, Mosby, pp 138-145.
NaKavo KK: Neck and back pain. In Stein JH et al, editors: *Internal medicine,* ed 4, St Louis, 1994, Mosby, pp 1033-1041.

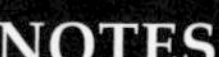

NOTES

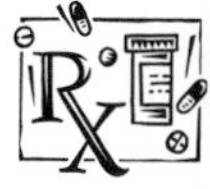

PHARMACOTHERAPEUTICS

Drug of Choice	Mechanism of Action	Prescribing Information	Side Effects
Nonsteroidal antiinflammatory drugs (NSAIDs); many different types currently marketed; consult manufacturer's package insert for specific dosing and prescribing information	Exact action unknown; may result from inhibition of synthesis of prostaglandins and arachidonic acid	***Contraindications:*** Hypersensitivity to NSAIDs, aspirin; severe hepatic failure; asthma ***Cost:*** Varies with type ***Pregnancy category:*** Depends on product	Stomach distress, flatulence, nausea, abdominal pain, constipation or diarrhea, dizziness, sedation, rash, urticaria, angioedema, anorexia, urinary frequency, increased blood pressure, insomnia, anxiety, visual disturbances, increased thirst, alopecia
Muscle relaxants (controversial): orphenadrine (Norflex), 100 mg PO bid; does not normally cause sedation like other muscle relaxants	Not clearly identified; may result from analgesic properties; also has anticholinergic effects	***Contraindications:*** Hypersensitivity; narrow-angle glaucoma; GI obstruction; myasthenia gravis; stenosing peptic ulcer; bladder neck obstruction; cardiospasm ***Cost:*** 100-mg tab, 100 tabs: $127 ***Pregnancy category:*** C	Dry mouth, tachycardia, palpitations, urinary hesitancy/retention, blurred vision, dilation of pupils, increased ocular tension, weakness, nausea, vomiting, headache, dizziness, constipation, drowsiness, hypersensitivity reactions, pruritus, hallucinations, agitation, tremor, gastric irritation

Herpes Simplex

OVERVIEW

Herpes simplex is a recurrent, noncurable, viral disease. It usually manifests itself as painful vesicles that occur in clusters on the skin, eyes, or mucous membranes

Pathogenesis

- Caused by two different virus types—either type 1 or type 2
- HSV1—usually associated with oral herpes
- HSV2—usually associated with genital herpes
- Either type can be found in either location
- Reactivating factors—fever, ultraviolet light, cold wind, systemic illness, menstruation, emotional stress, local trauma, immunosuppression

Patient Profile

- Males = Females
- Widespread
- Affects all ages

Signs and Symptoms

The following are for HSV1 (for HSV2, see section on genital herpes):

- Primary infection—skin:
  - May be asymptomatic
  - May have prodrome of localized pain, tender lymphadenopathy, headache, generalized aching, fever; many have no prodrome
  - Grouped uniform vesicles on an erythematous base appear
  - Lesions erode, crust, last 2 to 6 weeks
  - Virus travels to dorsal root ganglia and remains in latent stage
- Recurrent infection—skin:
  - Some individuals never have recurrent infection
  - Prodrome similar to primary infection—lasts 2 to 24 hours
  - Lesions evolve from an erythematous base
  - In 2 to 4 days, dome-shaped lesions rupture and crust
  - Crust sheds in 8 days
  - Systemic symptoms usually not present

Differential Diagnosis

- Impetigo
- Aphthous stomatitis
- Herpes zoster
- Syphilitic chancre
- Herpangina
- Stevens-Johnson syndrome

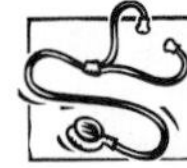

ASSESSMENT

History

Inquire about:

- Onset and duration of symptoms
- Prodromal symptoms
- History of previous herpes infections
- Treatments tried and results
- Contact with infected individual
- Underlying conditions
- Current medications

Physical Findings

Perioral (most common site, but may be anywhere), grouped, uniform vesicles on erythematous base; may be crusted

Initial Workup

Laboratory

- Tzanck smear—multinucleated giant cells
- HSV culture (expensive)
- Herpes antibody titers

Radiology: None indicated

Further Workup

None, unless complications arise

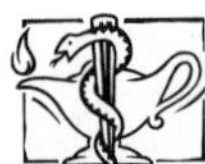

INTERVENTIONS

Office Treatment

Early lesions—unroof and apply Campho-Phenique

Lifestyle Modifications

- Smoking cessation
- Frequent hand washing
- Avoidance of stress (may have implications for recurrence)

Patient Education

Teach patient about:

- Primary infection—length of illness (lesions may last 2 to 6 weeks)
- Disease (noncurable, may have frequent reoccurrences)
- Treatment—antiviral medication—will not cure disease but will shorten length of time lesions are present and decrease recurrences
- Prevention of spread of disease
- Avoiding immunosuppressed individuals
- Seeking treatment at first sign of recurrence
- Support groups available (provide literature)
- Safe sex practices (herpes can be transmitted even when lesions not present)
- Medications used and side effects (see Pharmacotherapeutics)

Referrals

None, unless extensive; then to physician

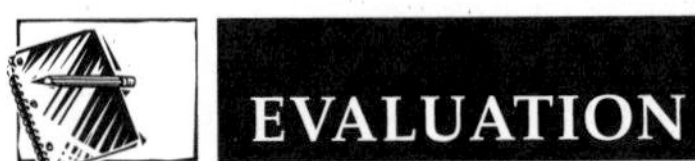

EVALUATION

Outcomes

- Lesions heal without scarring
- Frequent recurrences likely

Possible Complications

- Herpes encephalitis
- Herpes pneumonia
- Aseptic meningitis
- Herpes septicemia

Follow-up

In 1 week; then every 2 weeks until lesions resolve

FOR YOUR INFORMATION

Life Span

Pediatric: Neonate may contract disease during delivery if mother has active lesions
Geriatric: Immune system may not be as competent, putting patient at increased risk
Pregnancy: Acyclovir should only be used in severe or complicated disease

Miscellaneous

Spread of the virus can occur through respiratory droplets, direct contact with lesions, or contact with body fluid containing the virus. It can be spread even when the patient has no active lesions, and education regarding this fact is important in order to try to stop the spread of this disease.

Reference

Habif TP: *Clinical dermatology: a color guide to diagnosis and therapy,* ed 3, St Louis, 1996, Mosby, pp 337-344.

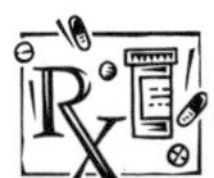

PHARMACOTHERAPEUTICS

Drug of Choice	Mechanism of Action	Prescribing Information	Side Effects
For fever and myalgia, use one of the following:			
Acetaminophen (Tylenol), 325-650 mg q4-6h PO; for children, use Children's Tylenol—follow label directions	Decreases fever through action on hypothalamic heat-regulating center of brain; analgesia by increasing pain threshold	***Contraindication:*** Hypersensitivity ***Cost:*** OTC ***Pregnancy category:*** Not categorized	Anaphylaxis, leukopenia, neutropenia, drowsiness, nausea, vomiting, hepatotoxicity, rash, angioedema, urticaria, toxicity
Aspirin; adults only, 325-650 mg q4-6h PO	Analgesia via peripheral and central nervous systems; may inhibit prostaglandins; antipyretic—acts on hypothalamic system	***Contraindications:*** Hypersensitivity; bleeding disorders or anticoagulant therapy; last trimester of pregnancy; asthma; gastric ulcers ***Cost:*** OTC ***Pregnancy category:*** Not categorized	Rash, anaphylactic reaction, GI upset and bleeding, Reye's syndrome in children and adolescents, nausea, vomiting, hepatitis, tinnitus, hearing loss, wheezing, pulmonary edema
Ibuprofen (Motrin), 400 mg qid PO; children 6 months to 12 years, 5 mg/kg if temperature <102.5° F (39.1° C); 10 mg/kg if temperature >102.5° F q6h	Not well understood; may be related to inhibition of prostaglandin synthesis	***Contraindications:*** Aspirin allergy; hypersensitivity; asthma; last trimester of pregnancy; gastric ulcer; bleeding disorders ***Cost:*** 400-mg tab, 4/day × 5 days: $3 ***Pregnancy category:*** Not recommended	Nausea, heartburn, diarrhea, GI upset and bleeding, dizziness, headache, rash, tinnitus, edema, acute renal failure
Acyclovir (Zovirax); for initial treatment, 200 mg PO 5 times daily × 10 days; for mild symptoms, may use topically every 4 hours for 10 days instead; recurrent treatment, 200 mg PO 5 times daily for 5 days; children, 20 mg/kg PO 4 times daily for 5 days	Interferes with DNA synthesis	***Contraindications:*** Hypersensitivity ***Cost:*** 200-mg tab, 100 tabs: $94 ***Pregnancy category:*** C	Tremors, confusion, lethargy, hallucinations, convulsions, dizziness, headache, encephalopathic changes, nausea, vomiting, diarrhea, increased ALT and AST, abdominal pain, oliguria, proteinuria, hematuria, vaginitis, moniliasis, glomerulonephritis, acute renal failure, changes in menses, gingival hyperplasia, rash, urticaria, pruritus, alopecia, joint pain, leg pain, muscle cramps

Herpes Zoster

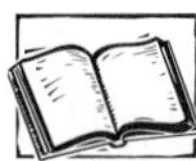

OVERVIEW

Herpes zoster, or shingles, is a cutaneous viral infection, usually involving the skin of a single dermatome.

Pathogenesis

- Caused by reactivation of the varicella zoster virus
- Varicella virus lies dormant in dorsal root ganglia from previous episode of chickenpox
- Immunosuppressive drugs, age, lymphoma, fatigue, emotional upsets, and radiation therapy may initiate reactivation
- Contact with a lesion does not cause a herpes zoster infection in contactant—may cause chickenpox if not immune

Patient Profile

- Males = Females
- Any age, but increases in incidence with age

Signs and Symptoms

- Prodromal symptoms—itching, burning, or knifelike pain—usually along 1 dermatome; more common on trunk, but can appear along any dermatome
- Eruptive phase:
  - Usually only 1 dermatome, but may involve 1 or 2 adjacent dermatomes
  - Red, swollen plaques of various sizes
  - Vesicles arise from erythematous base, usually in clusters; have cloudy or purulent fluid; vary in size; continue to appear for 7 days
  - Crust forms and then falls off in 2 to 3 weeks
  - May have scattered vesicles outside dermatome
  - In the elderly, may have extensive scarring
  - Postherpetic neuralgia increases with age; pain may last for months or years

Differential Diagnosis

- Herpes simplex
- Coxsackievirus
- Contact dermatitis
- Prodromal pain—can mimic may things, including myocardial infarction, cholecystitis, pleuritis

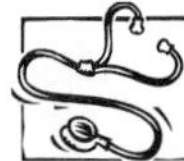

ASSESSMENT

History

Inquire about:

- Onset and duration of symptoms
- Prior history of herpes zoster
- History of chickenpox
- Treatments tried and results
- Underlying conditions
- Current medications

Physical Findings

- Prodromal stage—may complain of pain, burning, itching along dermatome without any objective findings
- Eruptive stage:
  - Erythema, edema, clusters of different-sized vesicles with cloudy or purulent fluid along dermatome
  - Vesicles may umbilicate or rupture, then crust; may have scattered vesicles outside dermatome
  - Lymphadenopathy

Initial Workup

Laboratory

- Generally none
- Viral culture—expensive
- Tzanck smear—does not differentiate from herpes simplex

Radiology: None indicated

Further Workup

None indicated

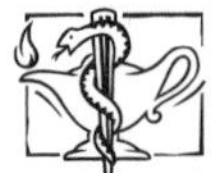

INTERVENTIONS

Office Treatment

Emotional support for patient with postherpetic neuralgia

Lifestyle Modifications

Avoidance of fatigue and emotional upsets—may help prevent recurrences

Patient Education

Teach patient about:

- Disease—self-limiting (usually lasts 2 to 3 weeks) but may recur
- Virus—contagious to susceptible individuals
- Potential for postherpetic neuralgia
- Applying Burow's solution qid for 15 minutes to lesions
- Treatment—symptomatic and not a cure
- Medications used and side effects (See Pharmacotherapeutics)

Referral

To ophthalmologist if eye is involved

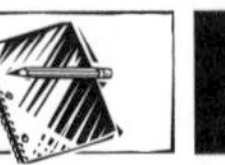

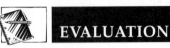

EVALUATION

Outcome

Lesions heal without sequelae

Possible Complications

- Postherpetic neuralgia
- Meningoencephalitis
- Cutaneous dissemination
- Superinfection of skin lesions
- Hepatitis
- Pneumonitis
- Peripheral motor weakness
- Segmental myelitis
- Cranial nerve syndromes
- Corneal ulceration
- Guillain-Barré syndrome

Follow-up

Every 2 weeks

FOR YOUR INFORMATION

Life Span

Pediatric: Rare in this age group
Geriatric: Most commonly seen in this age group
Pregnancy: Pregnant patient should not come in contact with vesicles if patient not immune to chickenpox.

Miscellaneous

In young patients with herpes zoster, always consider the possibility of an underlying chronic illness, such as HIV infection, causing immunosuppression.

Reference

Habif TP: *Clinical dermatology: a color guide to diagnosis and therapy,* ed 3, St Louis, 1996, Mosby, pp 350-359.

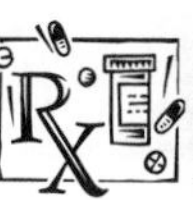

PHARMACOTHERAPEUTICS

Drug of Choice	Mechanism of Action	Prescribing Information	Side Effects
For fever and myalgia, use one of the following:			
Acetaminophen (Tylenol), 325-650 mg q4-6h PO; for children, use Children's Tylenol—follow label directions; caution patient against use of alcohol	Decrease fever through action on hypothalamic heat-regulating center of brain; analgesia by increasing pain threshold	***Contraindication:*** Hypersensitivity ***Cost:*** OTC ***Pregnancy category:*** Not categorized	Anaphylaxis, leukopenia, neutropenia, drowsiness, nausea, vomiting, hepatotoxicity, rash, angioedema, urticaria, toxicity
Aspirin; adults only, 325-650 mg q4-6h PO—do not use in children or adolescents because of risk of Reye's syndrome	Analgesia via peripheral and central nervous systems; may inhibit prostaglandins; antipyretic—acts on hypothalamic system	***Contraindications:*** Hypersensitivity; bleeding disorders or anticoagulant therapy; last trimester of pregnancy; asthma; gastric ulcers ***Cost:*** OTC ***Pregnancy category:*** Not categorized	Rash, anaphylactic reaction, GI upset and bleeding, Reye's syndrome in children and adolescents, nausea, vomiting, hepatitis, tinnitus, hearing loss, wheezing, pulmonary edema
Ibuprofen (Motrin), 400 mg qid PO; children 6 months to 12 years, 5 mg/kg if temperature <102.5° F (39.1° C), 10 mg/kg if temperature >102.5° F	Not well understood; may be related to inhibition of prostaglandin synthesis	***Contraindications:*** Aspirin allergy; hypersensitivity; asthma; last trimester of pregnancy; gastric ulcer; bleeding disorders ***Cost:*** 400-mg tab, 4/day × 5 days: $3 ***Pregnancy category:*** Not recommended	Nausea, heartburn, diarrhea, GI upset and bleeding, dizziness, headache, rash, tinnitus, edema, acute renal failure
The patient may need a narcotic analgesic for relief of pain.			
• Acyclovir (Zovirax), 800 mg 5 times daily for 7 days • Famciclovir (Famvir), 500 mg q8h for 7 days—safety in children <18 years not established • Valacyclovir (Valtrex), 1 g PO tid × 7 days	Interfere with DNA synthesis	***Contraindication:*** Hypersensitivity ***Cost:*** Acyclovir, 200-mg tab, 100 tabs: $94; famciclovir, 500-mg tab, 30 tabs: $184; valacyclovir, 500-mg tab, 42 tabs: $116 ***Pregnancy category:*** acyclovir—C; famciclovir—B; valacyclovir—B	Tremors, confusion, lethargy, hallucinations, convulsions, dizziness, headache, encephalopathic changes, nausea, vomiting, diarrhea, increased ALT and AST, abdominal pain, oliguria, proteinuria, hematuria, vaginitis, moniliasis, glomerulonephritis, acute renal failure, changes in menses, gingival hyperplasia, rash, urticaria, pruritus, alopecia, joint pain, leg pain, muscle cramps
For postherpetic neuralgia, the following may be beneficial. Again, narcotic analgesia may be necessary to control the pain. Use with caution in the elderly.			
Capsaicin cream (Zostrix); adults and children >2 years, apply to area 3-4 times daily; for external use only; do not use over abraded skin; do not use occlusive dressing	Depletes pain impulse transmitter substance P and prevents its resynthesis	***Contraindication:*** Hypersensitivity ***Cost:*** OTC ***Pregnancy category:*** Not available	Irritation, contact dermatitis, excessive burning sensation

Hiccups/Hiccoughs/Singultus

OVERVIEW

A hiccup is a sudden, involuntary sound produced by contraction of the diaphragm, followed by rapid closure of the glottis.

Pathogenesis

Many causes:

- Indigestion
- Rapid eating
- Abdominal surgeries
- Alcoholism
- CNS lesions
- Diaphragmatic irritation
- Mediastinal or other thoracic lesions
- Gastric lesions
- Esophageal lesions
- Hepatic lesions
- Drug induced
- Psychogenic causes
- Idiopathic
- Associated with more than 100 disorders

Patient Profile

- Males > Females
- All ages, even in utero

Signs and Symptoms

- Classic hiccup sound
- Pain in chest wall from intractable hiccups
- Normally last only a few seconds or minutes; if last >48 hours, may indicate underlying disorder

Differential Diagnosis

- Eructation
- Any of over 100 associated disorders

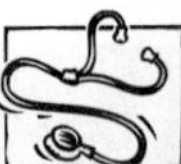

ASSESSMENT

History

Inquire about:

- Onset and duration of hiccups
- Treatments tried and results
- Underlying conditions
- Current medications

Physical Findings

- May appear sleep deprived if hiccups last >48 hours
- Weight loss
- Cardiac arrhythmias

Initial Workup

Laboratory: Usually none, unless looking for underlying cause

Radiology: Usually none

Further Workup

Usually none

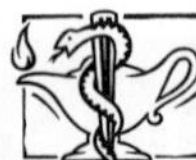

INTERVENTIONS

Office Treatment

May want to try some simple remedies—Valsalva maneuver, tongue traction, smelling salts, rebreathing in paper bag

Lifestyle Modifications

- Smoking cessation
- Alcohol cessation

Patient Education

Teach patient about

- Condition and treatment options:
  - Swallowing a spoonful of sugar
  - Inducing fright
  - Sucking on hard candy
  - Valsalva maneuver
  - Tongue traction
  - Rebreathing into paper bag
  - Smelling salts
  - Sipping ice water
  - Lifting uvula with cold spoon
- Medications used and side effects (see Pharmacotherapeutics)

Referral

Possibly to MD for underlying condition

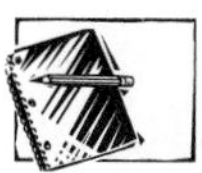

EVALUATION

Outcome
Resolve without sequelae

Possible Complications
- Inability to eat
- Weight loss
- Insomnia
- Exhaustion

Follow-up
In 48 hours; if on maintenance drug therapy, every 3 months to monitor for drug side effects

FOR YOUR INFORMATION

Life Span
Pediatric: May exist in uterus; common; do not harm fetus
Geriatric: Can be very debilitating if intractable hiccups occur
Pregnancy: Common in fetus

Miscellaneous
Intractable hiccups may last for years.

References
Driscoll CE: Blood disorders and cancer. In Driscoll CE et al, editors: *The family practice desk reference,* ed 3, St Louis, 1996, Mosby, p 651.

McQuaid KR: Alimentary tract. In Tierney LM Jr, McPhee SJ, Papadakis MA, editors: *Current medical diagnosis and treatment,* ed 34, Norwalk, Conn, 1995, Appleton & Lange, pp 479-480.

NOTES

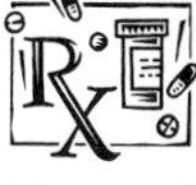

PHARMACOTHERAPEUTICS

Drug of Choice	Mechanism of Action	Prescribing Information	Side Effects
Baclofen (Lioresal), 5-10 mg PO tid; increase at 5-mg intervals, maximum dose 80 mg/day—not recommended for children <18 years	Inhibits synaptic responses in CNS by decreasing GABA, leading to decreased neurotransmitter function, leading to decreased frequency and severity of muscle spasms	***Contraindication:*** Hypersensitivity ***Cost:*** 10-mg tab, 100 tabs: $16-$50 ***Pregnancy category:*** C	Dizziness, weakness, fatigue, headache, insomnia, nasal congestion, blurred vision, mydriasis, hypotension, chest pain, palpitations, edema, nausea, constipation, vomiting, abdominal pain, rash
Metoclopramide (Reglan), 5-10 mg PO qid—not dosed for children <18 years	Enhances response to acetylcholine in upper GI tract; causes contraction of gastric muscle; relaxes pyloric and duodenal segments; increases peristalsis	***Contraindications:*** Hypersensitivity to metoclopramide, procaine, or procainamide; seizure disorder; pheochromocytoma; breast cancer; GI obstruction ***Cost:*** 5-mg tab, 100 tabs: $5-$40 ***Pregnancy category:*** B	Sedation, fatigue, restlessness, headache, sleeplessness, dystonia, dry mouth, constipation, nausea, vomiting, anorexia, decreased libido, prolactin secretion, amenorrhea, hypotension, supraventricular tachycardia, rash
Amitriptyline (Elavil), 50-100 mg PO hs, maximum dose 200 mg PO hs; adolescents, 30 mg PO hs; may increase up to 150 mg q hs—do not use in children <12 years	Antidepressant; blocks reuptake of norepinephrine and serotonin	***Contraindications:*** Hypersensitivity to tricyclic antidepressants; recovery phase of MI ***Cost:*** 50-mg tabs, 1/day × 90 days: $3-$10 ***Pregnancy category:*** C	Agranulocytosis, thrombocytopenia, eosinophilia, leukopenia, dizziness, drowsiness, confusion, headache, anxiety, tremors, extrapyramidal symptoms, diarrhea, dry mouth, nausea, vomiting, paralytic ileus, hepatitis, increased appetite, urine retention, rash, urticaria, orthostatic hypotension, ECG changes, tachycardia, hypertension, blurred vision, tinnitus

Hidradenitis Suppurative

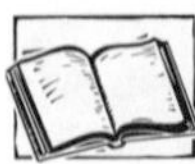

OVERVIEW

Hidradenitis suppurative is a chronic suppurative disease of the sweat glands. Painful abscesses occur most commonly in the axillary region and under the breasts in women and in the anogenital region in men. A hallmark of hidradenitis is a blackhead with multiple surface openings that communicate under the skin, creating sinus tracts.

Pathogenesis

- Disagreement as to actual cause—possibly due to a keratinous follicular plug or to occlusion of a sweat gland
- Plugged structure ruptures and becomes infected, progressing to abscess formation
- Chronic state with secondary bacterial infection is common

Patient Profile

- Females > Males
- Appears after puberty through age 40
- Worse in obese persons

Signs and Symptoms

- Painful, erythematous papules and nodules, one or several, located in sweat glands
- May or may not be fluctuant
- Has multiple surface openings that communicate under the skin

Differential Diagnosis

Furunculosis—single surface opening

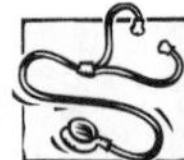

ASSESSMENT

History

Inquire about:

- Onset and duration of symptoms
- Prior history of painful lesions
- Underlying chronic illnesses (diabetes mellitus)
- Treatments tried and results
- Current medications

Physical Findings

- Painful, erythematous papule, nodule, or pustule in axilla, anogenital region, or under the breasts
- May or may not have purulent drainage
- Scarring may be present from previous eruptions
- Lymphadenopathy may be present

Initial Workup

Laboratory

- Culture and sensitivity of wound drainage
- CBC

Radiology: None indicated

Further Workup

None indicated

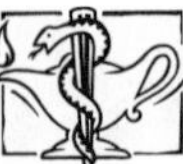

INTERVENTIONS

Office Treatment

- Incision and drainage of fluctuant large lesions
- Injection of smaller lesions with triamcinolone acetomide

Lifestyle Modifications

- Weight reduction diet
- Smoking cessation
- Daily bathing and cleansing of area with antibacterial soap
- Minimized heat exposure
- Avoidance of use of underarm antiperspirants and deodorants (may irritate area)
- Avoidance of tight clothing

Patient Education

Teach patient about:

- Condition and treatment—antibiotics
- Daily bathing and cleansing of area with antibacterial soaps
- Tips for weight reduction and smoking cessation
- Using baking soda as antiperspirant
- Importance of avoiding tight clothing, which may irritate area
- Not shaving affected areas
- Possibility of recurrences
- Possibility of scarring from lesions
- Medications used and side effects—may need long-term antibiotic therapy (see Pharmacotherapeutics)

Referral

To dermatologist for extensive cases

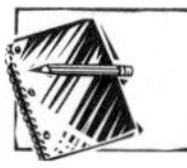

EVALUATION

Outcomes
- Lesions heal with minimal scarring
- Long-term antibiotics may control recurrences
- May require surgical excision for severe cases

Possible Complications
- Scarring
- Lymphedema
- Septicemia
- Rectal fissure formation

Follow-up
- In 2 weeks; then monthly until resolved
- If patient on long-term antibiotic therapy, continue with monthly visits

FOR YOUR INFORMATION

Life Span
Pediatric: Rare before puberty
Geriatric: Rare in this age group
Pregnancy: Cautious use of medications

Miscellaneous
The patient will need a great deal of emotional support to deal with the effects of this disease.

Reference
Habif TP: *Clinical dermatology: a color guide to diagnosis and therapy,* ed 3, St Louis, 1996, Mosby, pp 184-185.

NOTES

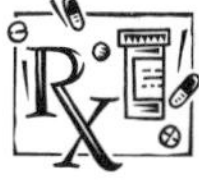

PHARMACOTHERAPEUTICS

Drug of Choice	Mechanism of Action	Prescribing Information	Side Effects
Tetracycline, 500 mg qid × 14 days for active lesion or 500 mg bid for long-term treatment	Inhibits protein synthesis; bacteriostatic	***Contraindications:*** Hypersensitivity; children <8 years ***Cost:*** 500-mg tab, 100 tabs: $6-$20 ***Pregnancy category:*** D	Eosinophilia, neutropenia, thrombocytopenia, leukocytosis, hemolytic anemia, dysphagia, glossitis, oral candidiasis, anorexia, hepatotoxicity, rash, urticaria, photosensitivity, exfoliative dermatitis, angioedema
Erythromycin (E.E.S.), 500 mg qid × 14 days for active disease; 500 mg bid for long-term treatment; children, 30-50 mg/kg/day in 4 divided doses × 10 days; may be used for prophylaxis or for established infections; other antibiotics may be used based on culture and sensitivity results	Macrolide; protein synthesis inhibitor; active against bacteria lacking cell walls, most gram-positive aerobes	***Contraindication:*** Hypersensitivity ***Cost:*** 250-mg tabs, 4/day × 10 days: $4 ***Pregnancy category:*** B	Nausea, vomiting, diarrhea, abdominal pain, anorexia, rash, urticaria, pseudomembranous colitis—rarely

OVERVIEW

Hirsutism is excessive growth of hair on the face and body as a result of excessive production of androgenic hormones. It may be accompanied by acne, obesity, and infertility. Extreme androgenic effects of a deep voice, clitorimegaly, and male-pattern balding are known as virilization.

Pathogenesis

Cause—excessive production of androgenic hormones

Patient Profile

- Females exclusively
- Most commonly occurs in postpubertal age

Signs and Symptoms

- Gradual onset of coarse, dark hair in male-pattern distribution
- Facial hair—beard, moustache, and chest hair
- May have irregular menses, acne, and infertility

Differential Diagnosis

- Excessive ovarian androgen production
- Excessive adrenal androgen production
- Hypothyroidism
- Hyperprolactinemia
- Ovarian tumor
- Adrenal tumor
- Anabolic steroid use in athletes
- Idiopathic
- Rarely, Cushing's disease

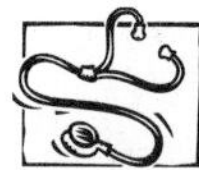

ASSESSMENT

History

Inquire about:

- Onset and duration of symptoms
- Family history of hirsutism
- Menstrual history, including age of menarche, length and regularity of cycle, and length of menses
- Obstetric history
- Underlying conditions
- Current medications

Physical Findings

- Face, chin, and body—fine to coarse dark hair
- Obesity
- Acne

Initial Workup

Laboratory

- Total testosterone level—if >200, need workup to rule out ovarian tumor
- 17-hydroxyprogesterone (17-OHP)—significant elevation suggests adrenal hyperplasia
- Androstenedione >1000—do workup for adrenal tumor
- TSH, FSH, LH, prolactin levels
- If strong suspicion of Cushing's disease, do dexamethasone suppression test—give 1 mg dexamethasone at 11 PM and draw plasma cortisol at 8 AM—if cortisol >10, abnormal
- Corticotropin stimulation test—give 0.25 mg ACTH IV in early morning; draw blood samples for 17-OHP and cortisol 30 to 60 minutes after IV—significant elevation indicates enzyme deficiency or adrenal hyperplasia

Radiology: CT scan of ovaries and/or adrenals to rule out tumors and hyperplasia, cysts

Further Workup

Based on findings from initial workup

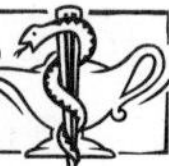

INTERVENTIONS

Office Treatment

Provide counseling and emotional support

Lifestyle Modifications

- Maintenance of ideal body weight or diet for weight reduction
- Smoking cessation

Patient Education

Teach patient about:

- Condition, cause, and treatment—surgical removal if tumor present
- If tumor ruled out—about cosmetic therapy available, such as plucking, bleaching, electrolysis, and cover-up makeup
- Medications to stop further hair growth (but advise patient that they do not always reverse what is present)
- Treatment lasting 6 to 24 months or possibly being lifelong
- Medications used and side effects (see Pharmacotherapeutics)

Referral

Usually none; to endocrinologist if unsure of diagnosis

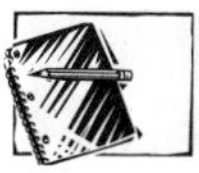

EVALUATION

Outcomes

- Further hair growth halted with long-term therapy
- Unlikely to reverse current hair growth

Possible Complications

- Poor self-esteem
- Increased cardiac risk
- Dysfunctional uterine bleeding
- Infertility

Follow-up

Every 2 weeks × 1 month; then monthly × 3 months

FOR YOUR INFORMATION

Life Span

Pediatric: Can start in adolescence
Geriatric: Can occur after menopause
Pregnancy: If on medication, will need to discontinue

Miscellaneous

Since hirsutism is commonly accompanied by acne and obesity, treatment for these conditions must also be started. Hirsutism can cause the patient to have a poor self-image, and counseling, either by the NP or a specialist, is an important part of the treatment plan.

References

Leach EE, Ruszkowski AM: Integumentary systems. In Lewis SM, Collier IC, Heitkemper MM, editors: *Medical-surgical nursing: assessment and management of clinical problems,* ed 4, St Louis, 1996, Mosby, p 494.

Wood SCW: Infertility. In Youngkin EQ, Davis MS, editors: *Women's health: a primary care clinical guide,* Norwalk, Conn, 1994, Appleton & Lange, pp 176-177.

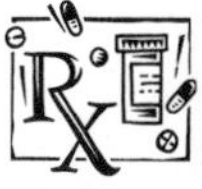

PHARMACOTHERAPEUTICS

Drug of Choice	Mechanism of Action	Prescribing Information	Side Effects
Birth control pills (standard drug used for treatment of hirsutism); usual dosage is 35 μg ethinyl estradiol and 1.0 mg norethindrone or a similar formulation	Prevent ovulation by suppressing FSH and LH	***Contraindications:*** Hypersensitivity; breast cancer; thromboembolic disorders; reproductive cancer; undiagnosed vaginal bleeding; pregnancy; hepatic tumor/disease; women 40 years and over; cerebrovascular accident (CVA) ***Cost:*** Varies by brand: $20-$30 ***Pregnancy category:*** X	Dizziness, headache, migraines, depression, hypotension, thrombophlebitis, thromboembolism, pulmonary embolism, myocardial infarction (MI), nausea, vomiting, cholestatic jaundice, weight gain, diplopia, amenorrhea, cervical erosion, breakthrough bleeding, dysmenorrhea, vaginal candidiasis, spontaneous abortion, rash, urticaria, acne, photosensitivity
Dexamethasone, 0.25-0.5 mg PO hs; or dexamethasone acetate, 4-16 mg IM × 1 dose	Suppression of androgen production; corticosteroid; antiinflammatory	***Contraindications:*** Hypersensitivity; psychosis; idiopathic thrombocytopenia; acute glomerulonephritis; amebiasis; nonasthmatic bronchial disease; AIDS; TB; child <2 years old ***Cost:*** 8 mg/ml, 5 ml: $11-$47 ***Pregnancy category:*** C	Hypertension, circulatory collapse, thrombophlebitis, embolism, tachycardia, fungal infections, increased intraocular pressure, diarrhea, nausea, GI hemorrhage, thrombocytopenia, acne, poor wound healing, fractures, osteoporosis, weakness
Spironolactone (Aldactone), 100-200 mg/day; may be used in combination with birth control pills or dexamethasone; 100-300 mg/day PO in single or divided doses; children, 3.3 mg/kg/day PO in single or divided doses	Antiandrogenic; competes with aldosterone at receptor sites in distal tubule, resulting in excretion of sodium chloride, water, retention of potassium, phosphate	***Contraindications:*** Hypersensitivity; anuria; severe renal disease; hyperkalemia; pregnancy ***Cost:*** 25-mg tab, 100 tabs: $5-$15 ***Pregnancy category:*** D	Headache, confusion, drowsiness, diarrhea, cramps, bleeding, gastritis, vomiting, anorexia, dysrhythmias, rash, pruritus, urticaria, decreased WBC count, platelets, hyperchloremic metabolic acidosis, hyperkalemia, hyponatremia

OVERVIEW

A hordeolum is an infection or inflammation of a hair follicle or gland of the eyelid. The inflammation or infection affects either the follicles of the eyelashes or the meibomian glands. It may be either internal or external. A stye is an external hordeolum.

Pathogenesis
Cause—usually staphylococcal

Patient Profile
- Males = Females
- Any age, but more common in children and adolescents

Signs and Symptoms
- Sudden onset of localized tenderness, redness, and swelling of eyelid
- Discharge
- Itching
- Eye irritation

Differential Diagnosis
- Blepharitis
- Chalazion
- Eyelid neoplasm

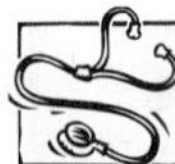

ASSESSMENT

History
Inquire about:
- Onset and duration of symptoms
- Visual disturbances
- Underlying conditions
- Treatment tried and results
- Current medications

Physical Findings
- Redness of eyelid
- Discharge
- Visual acuity—should be within normal limits

Initial Workup
Laboratory: None indicated
Radiology: None indicated

Further Workup
Culture of drainage if resistant to treatment

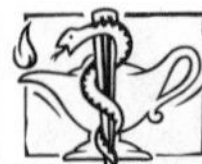

INTERVENTIONS

Office Treatment
None indicated

Lifestyle Modifications
- Refrain from using eye makeup and contact lenses until resolved
- Proper eyelid hygiene

Patient Education
Teach patient about:
- Condition and treatment
- Cleansing eyelid with baby shampoo and tap water
- Using warm compresses to promote drainage
- Never squeezing hordeolum
- Not rubbing eyes
- Not using eye makeup or contact lenses—old eye makeup should be discarded
- How to apply antibiotic ointment and side effects (see Pharmacotherapeutics)

Referrals
None indicated

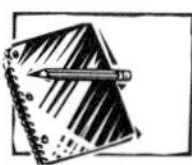

EVALUATION

Outcome
Resolves without sequelae

Possible Complication
Internal hordeolum—generalized cellulitis of eyelid

Follow-up
In 2 weeks to assess effectiveness of treatment

FOR YOUR INFORMATION

Life Span
Pediatric: More common in this age group
Geriatric: May have difficulty applying antibiotic ointment
Pregnancy: N/A

Miscellaneous
If crops of hordeolum occur, do a workup for diabetes mellitus.

Reference
Schachat AP: The red eye. In Barker LR, Burton JR, Zieve PD, editors: *Principles of ambulatory medicine,* ed 4, Baltimore, 1995, Williams & Wilkins, pp 1431-1434.

NOTES

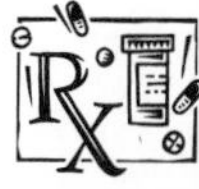

PHARMACOTHERAPEUTICS

Drug of Choice	Mechanism of Action	Prescribing Information	Side Effects
Sodium sulfacetamide (Sulamyd) ophthalmic ointment 10%, 0.5-1.0 cm in conjunctival sac qid × 7-14 days or 10% solution 2 qtt q3h × 7-14 days	Bacteriostatic by inhibiting folic acid production; effective against wide range of gram-positive and gram-negative bacteria	***Contraindications:*** Hypersensitivity; hypersensitivity to sulfonamides; incompatible with silver preparations ***Cost:*** Ointment, 35 g: $2; solution, 15 ml: $4 ***Pregnancy category:*** C	Local irritation, stinging, burning
Bacitracin/polymyxin (Polysporin) ointment, 0.5-1 cm in conjunctival sac q4h × 7-14 days	Bactericidal; effective against wide range of gram-positive and gram-negative bacteria	***Contraindication:*** Hypersensitivity to any ingredient ***Cost:*** 3.5 g: $4 ***Pregnancy category:*** B	Local irritation, stinging, burning

Human Immunodeficiency Virus (HIV) and Acquired Immunodeficiency Syndrome (AIDS)

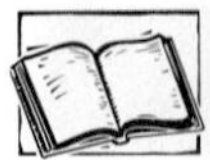

OVERVIEW

Human immunodeficiency virus (HIV) is a type of retrovirus that infects CD4 lymphocytes. The retrovirus kills the CD4 cells, which results in immune dysfunction, leaving the patient prone to opportunistic infections, malignancies, and neurologic lesions. These conditions make up what is known as acquired immunodeficiency syndrome (AIDS). According to the Centers for Disease Control (CDC), to diagnose an individual as having AIDS, one of the following must be present: CD4 <200/mm^3, development of opportunistic infection (candidiasis, cytomegalovirus, coccidioidomycosis, *Pneumocystis carinii, Mycobacterium tuberculosis*), opportunistic cancer (Kaposi's sarcoma, Burkitt's lymphoma, immunoblastic lymphoma), wasting syndrome, or dementia. The time from infection with HIV to the development of AIDS is highly individualized and may take from a few months to many years.

Pathogenesis

- Cause—retrovirus (very fragile virus; can only replicate in living cell)
- Transmitted from human to human through blood, semen, vaginal secretions, and breast milk

Patient Profile

- Males > Females, but is slowly equalizing
- Young adults 25 to 44 years of age
- Persons at risk:
  - All sexually active people with multiple partners
  - IV drug users
  - Recipients of blood products, particularly if received between 1975-1985 (hemophiliacs)
  - Homosexual men
  - Children of HIV-infected women
  - Health care workers because of risk of needle stick (relatively low risk if only risk factor)

Signs and Symptoms

- Acute retroviral syndrome:
  - 2 to 6 weeks after infection with HIV
  - Flulike or mononucleosis-like—fever, myalgias, headache, malaise, rash
  - CD4 count falls but returns to baseline
  - Symptoms mild and self-limiting
- Asymptomatic infection (early HIV infection):
  - Generally healthy
  - May have vague symptoms of headache, fatigue, low-grade fever
- Early symptomatic disease:
  - CD4 count <500/mm^3 but >200/mm^3
  - Generalized lymphadenopathy
  - Persistent fever
  - Chronic diarrhea
  - Headaches
  - Fatigue
  - Myopathies
  - Recurrent night sweats
- CDC classification for diagnosis of AIDS*:
  - CD4 lymphocyte count <200
  - Development of one of the following opportunistic infections: (1) fungal—candidiasis of bronchi, trachea, lungs, or esophagus; disseminated or extrapulmonary histoplasmosis; (2) viral—cytomegalovirus, chronic herpes simplex; (3) protozoal—disseminated or extrapulmonary coccidiomycosis, toxoplasmosis of brain; (4) *Pneumocystis carinii* pneumonia; (5) bacterial—*Mycobacterium tuberculosis, M. avium, M. kansasii*
  - Development of opportunistic cancer: (1) invasive cervical cancer, (2) Kaposi's sarcoma, (3) Burkitt's lymphoma, (4) immunoblastic lymphoma
  - Wasting syndrome
  - Development of dementia

Differential Diagnosis

Depends on stage of HIV infection—many illnesses can mimic HIV infection

*Modified from Centers for Disease Control and Prevention: Recommendations and Reports: 1993 revised classification system for HIV infection and expanded surveillance case definition for AIDS among adolescents and adults, *MMWR* 41(RR-17):1, Dec 18, 1992.

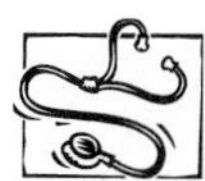

ASSESSMENT

History

Inquire about:

- Onset and duration of symptoms
- Sexual history, including age at first coitus; number of partners; sex with men, women, or both; use of condoms with *every* sexual encounter; sexually transmitted diseases (STDs)
- Drug history, including type of drug and how used
- Use of blood or blood products, particularly between 1975-1985
- Immunizations—flu, pneumonia, tetanus
- Underlying conditions
- Current medications

Physical Findings

- Depends on stage of HIV infection
- Temperature increased
- Weight decreased
- Oral cavity—thrush, ulcers
- Lymphadenopathy
- Pulmonary—crackles indicating pneumonia
- Cardiac—murmur, gallop, heave
- Abdominal examination—hepatomegaly, splenomegaly
- Skin lesions—herpes, psoriasis, seborrhea, Kaposi's sarcoma
- Pelvic and rectal examination—STDs
- Neurologic examination—dementia

Initial Workup

Laboratory

- ELISA—if positive, confirm with Western Blot
- CBC with differential—anemia, leukopenia, thrombocytopenia
- CD4 count
- Chemistry profile
- Urinalysis
- Rapid plasma reagin (RPR)
- Hepatitis screen
- Other tests as determined by history and physical

Radiology: Chest film

Further Workup

As indicated by history and physical

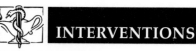

INTERVENTIONS

Office Treatment

None indicated

Lifestyle Modifications

- Cessation of drug use or at least clean needle use
- Safe sex practices
- Learning to live with chronic, terminal illness
- Dealing with societal biases
- Dealing with cost of therapy

Patient Education

Teach patient about:

- Condition and fact that there is no curative treatment at present
- Treatment based on CD4 count:
  - CD4 count $>500/mm^3$ and asymptomatic or minor problems—no treatment, continue to follow
  - CD4 count $200\text{-}499/mm^3$ and asymptomatic or mild immunodeficiency disease—start antiretroviral therapy
  - CD4 count $<200/mm^3$—start antiretroviral therapy and prophylaxis for *Pneumocystis carinii*
- Immunizations—pneumonia vaccine, flu vaccine, TB booster, hepatitis B vaccine
- Method of transmission, safe sex practices
- Importance of notifying sexual partners
- Importance of notifying needle-sharing partners
- Good nutrition and avoidance of raw or potentially contaminated food
- Importance of regular exercise and use of vitamin supplements
- Keeping regular office visits
- Materials and support groups available in local area, including HIV clinics that may be available
- Medications used and side effects (see Pharmacotherapeutics)

Referral

To specialist in HIV/AIDS treatment

Human Immunodeficiency Virus (HIV) and Acquired Immunodeficiency Syndrome (AIDS)—cont'd

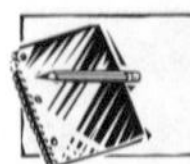

EVALUATION

Outcome
No cure; prolong development of AIDS for as long as possible

Possible Complications
- Opportunistic infections and malignancies
- AIDS meningoencephalitis
- Neuropsychiatric symptoms
- Thrombocytopenia

Follow-up
Based on stage of infection—initially every 3 months for CD4 count and thorough physical examination

FOR YOUR INFORMATION

Life Span
Pediatric: May progress more rapidly in infants; however, some infants who are HIV-positive at birth will revert to negative status; infants born to HIV-positive mothers should have testing done (Table 11)
Geriatric: Progresses rapidly
Pregnancy: Must be handled by specialist in field; patient should be given zidovudine as soon as possible, and the infant should be given zidovudine for 6 weeks after birth

Miscellaneous
It is important for the primary care provider to provide a safe and supportive place for the patient to turn. The diagnosis of HIV infection can be devastating both emotionally and physically for the patient and his or her family. The diagnosis may cause social isolation at a time when family and friends are most needed. It is important for the patient to have access to specialists in the field who can provide the most up-to-date treatment.

References

Bradley-Springer L: Human immunodeficiency virus infection. In Lewis SM, Collier IC, Heitkemper MM, editors: *Medical-surgical nursing: assessment and management of clinical problems,* ed 4, St Louis, 1996, Mosby, pp 235-259.

El-Sadr W et al: *Evaluation and management of early HIV infection,* Clinical Practice Guideline No 7, AHCPR Pub No 94-6572, Rockville, Md, 1994, US Department of Health and Human Services, Public Health Service, Agency for Health Care Policy and Research.

Newmann RE, Nishimoto PW: 1996 human immunodeficiency virus update for primary care provider, *Nurse Pract Forum* 7(1):16-22, 1996.

NOTES

TABLE 11 *Testing for Infants Born to HIV-Positive Mothers*

Age	Test	(+) Result	(−) Result
1 month	HIV culture or polymerase chain reaction test (PCR)	Repeat test to confirm	Repeat test at 3-6 months
3-6 months	HIV culture or PCR	Repeat test to confirm	Test with ELISA at 15 months
15 months	ELISA	Repeat at 18 months	Repeat at 18 months
18 months	ELISA	Child infected	Child not infected

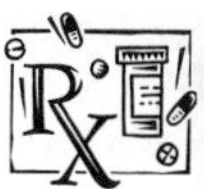

PHARMACOTHERAPEUTICS

There are many drugs used in the treatment of HIV that are beyond the scope of this book. The drugs listed here are the approved antiretroviral medications currently in use and the drug used for prophylaxis against *Pneumocystis carinii.*

Drug of Choice	Mechanism of Action	Prescribing Information	Side Effects
Antiretroviral agents—use one of the following:			
Zidovudine (AZT, Retrovir), 200 mg PO tid or 100 mg PO 5 times/day; if intolerant, decrease dose to 300-400 mg/day in divided doses	Inhibits replication of HIV virus	***Contraindication:*** Hypersensitivity ***Cost:*** 100-mg tab, 100 tabs: $149 ***Pregnancy category:*** C	Fatigue, malaise, headache, rash, nausea, insomnia, paresthesia, myalgia, confusion, agitation, twitching, bone marrow suppression, anemia, granulocytopenia, thrombocytopenia, dyspepsia, flatulence, hepatomegaly, taste change, hearing loss
Didanosine (ddl, Videx), >60 kg, 200 mg PO bid; <60 kg, 125 mg PO bid; must be chewed or dissolved in water; dosage for children based on body surface area (m^2)—1.1-1.4 m^2, PO 100 mg bid; 0.8-1.0 m^2, 75 mg PO bid; 0.5-0.7 m^2, 50 mg PO bid; 0.4 m^2, 25 mg PO bid	Synthetic purine nucleoside of deoxyadenosine that incorporates into cellular DNA and terminates chain	***Contraindication:*** Hypersensitivity ***Cost:*** 150-mg tab, 60 tabs: $130 ***Pregnancy category:*** B	Pancreatitis, peripheral neuropathies, diarrhea, nausea, vomiting, abdominal pain, rash, hyperglycemia, hyperuricemia, hepatic failure, headache, insomnia, seizures, thrombocytopenia, leukopenia, anemia
Zalcitabine (ddc, HIVID), >30 kg, 0.75 mg PO tid; <30 kg, 0.375 mg PO tid; use only in children >13 years old	Inhibits HIV replication by drug's conversion to an active antiviral	***Contraindication:*** Hypersensitivity ***Cost:*** 0.75-mg tab, 100 tabs: $214 ***Pregnancy category:*** C	Painful peripheral neuropathy; rash; oral or esophageal ulcers; pancreatitis; seizures; nausea; diarrhea; fatigue; cardiomyopathy; headache; increased ALT, AST, alkaline phosphatase, amylase, and bilirubin; toxic nephropathy; myalgias; hypertension; leukopenia; thrombocytopenia; anemia
Stavudine (Zerit, d4T), >60 kg, 40 mg PO bid; <60 kg, 20 mg PO bid	Inhibits the enzyme reverse transcriptase, which causes DNA chain termination	***Contraindication:*** Hypersensitivity ***Cost:*** 40-mg tab, 60 tabs: $233 ***Pregnancy category:*** C	Painful peripheral neuropathy, increased AST and ALT, anemia, headache, rash, abdominal pain, diarrhea, nausea, vomiting, myalgia, bone marrow suppression, hepatotoxicity
For prophylaxis of Pneumocystis carinii:			
Trimethoprim (TMP)/sulfamethoxazole (SMZ) (Bactrim DS, Septra DS), 1 DS tab PO per day	SMZ—interferes with synthesis of proteins; TMP—blocks synthesis of tetrahydrofolic acid	***Contraindications:*** Hypersensitivity; pregnancy at term; megaloblastic anemia; creatinine clearance <15 ml/min ***Cost:*** 1 DS/tab, 30 tabs: $2 ***Pregnancy category:*** C	Headache, insomnia, hallucinations, depression, allergic myocarditis, nausea, vomiting, hepatitis, glossitis, enterocolitis, anorexia, renal failure, toxic nephrosis, leukopenia, thrombocytopenia, hemolytic anemia, rash, dermatitis, Stevens-Johnson syndrome, anaphylaxis

Recently the FDA has approved the following new drugs for use in combination with zidovudine: lamivudine (3TC, Epivir), a nucleoside analogue, and saquinavir (Invirase), a protease inhibitor. There are many other new drugs on the horizon, which reemphasizes the importance of being able to refer the patient to a specialist with access to these new medications.

Hydrocele

OVERVIEW

A hydrocele is a collection of fluid within the scrotum. There are several types: communicating hydrocele, which is associated with patent processus vaginalis and indirect inguinal hernia; noncommunicating hydrocele seen frequently in infants, with spontaneous resolution; noncommunicating hydrocele seen in adults, with infrequent resolution; hydrocele of the cord in which the distal portion of the processus vaginalis is closed and fluid filled; hydrocele of the cord in which the proximal end of the cord is open or closed; and acute hydrocele in which the acute process in the tunica vaginalis results in fluid accumulation.

Pathogenesis

- Noncommunicating hydrocele:
  - Processus vaginalis closes, trapping peritoneal fluid (noncommunicating), or distal processus closes, with fluid trapped in middle of processus vaginalis (hydrocele of cord)
  - Causes—infections, tumors, trauma
- Communicating hydrocele—processus vaginalis fails to close

Patient Profile

- Males
- Most common age—childhood, but can occur at any age

Signs and Symptoms

- Scrotal or inguinal canal swelling
- Fluctuation in size of scrotum
- Scrotum may feel heavy
- Occasionally, pain radiating to back

Differential Diagnosis

- Orchitis
- Incarcerated scrotal hernia
- Epididymitis
- Traumatic injury to testicle

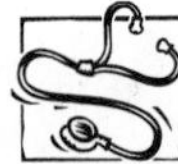

ASSESSMENT

History

Inquire about:

- Onset and duration of symptoms
- Whether condition present since infancy
- History of recent trauma
- Underlying conditions
- Current medications

Physical Findings

- Swelling of scrotum
- Transillumination—hold mass between fingers to make tense, darken room, press flashlight into side of mass (light passes through hydrocele)

Initial Workup

Laboratory: None indicated

Radiology

- Ultrasound of inguinoscrotal area
- Testicular nuclear scan—distinguishes testicular torsion

Further Workup

None needed

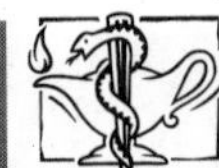

INTERVENTIONS

Office Treatment

None indicated

Lifestyle Modifications

Usually none

Patient Education

Teach patient about condition and treatment:

- Early infancy—observation until communication demonstrated or until 1 to 2 years of age
- Adults—no treatment necessary unless symptomatic, then outpatient surgery
- No medications used for treatment of hydrocele

Referral

To surgeon if necessary

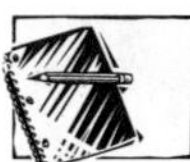

EVALUATION

Outcome
Postoperative recovery is rapid

Possible Complications
- Wound infection
- Hematoma
- Traumatic hydrocele—resolves spontaneously

Follow-up
Every 3 months until decision made for or against surgery

FOR YOUR INFORMATION

Life Span
Pediatric: Common in infancy; frequently resolves spontaneously
Geriatric: N/A
Pregnancy: N/A

Miscellaneous
N/A

Reference
Zenilman ME, Bender JS, Smith GW: Abdominal hernias. In Barker LR, Burton JR, Zieve PD, editors: *Principles of ambulatory medicine,* ed 4, Baltimore, 1995, Williams & Wilkins, pp 1342-1344.

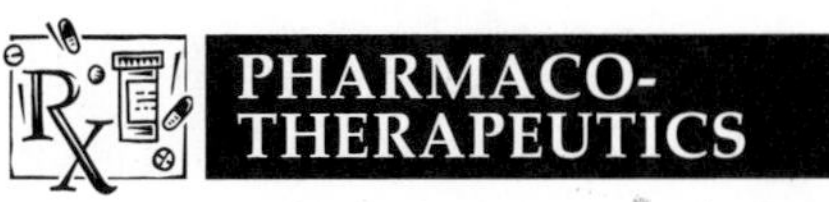

PHARMACOTHERAPEUTICS

There are no medications used for the treatment of hydrocele.

Hypercholesterolemia

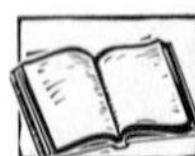

OVERVIEW

Hypercholesterolemia is an increase in the serum cholesterol level to >200 mg/dl. A person is considered at high risk when the cholesterol level is >240 mg/dl. Cholesterol is broken down into two subclasses: high-density lipoproteins (HDLs) and low-density lipoproteins (LDLs). HDLs are protective, or "good cholesterol," and LDLs are arthrogenic, or "bad cholesterol." All patients over the age of 20 years should have their cholesterol checked every 5 years.

Pathogenesis

- Causes of primary hypercholesterolemia—diet, heredity, obesity, sedentary lifestyle, and stress
- Causes of secondary hypercholesterolemia—hypothyroidism, diabetes mellitus, nephrotic syndrome, obstructive liver disease, progestins, anabolic steroids, diuretics (except indapamide), beta-blockers (except those with intrinsic sympathomimetic activity), some immunosuppressants

Patient Profile

- Males > Females
- Prevalence increases with age
- Hereditary

Signs and Symptoms

- May be asymptomatic
- Corneal arcus
- Xanthomas
- Xanthelasma
- Arterial bruits
- Claudication
- Angina pectoris
- Stroke
- Myocardial infarction

Differential Diagnosis

None

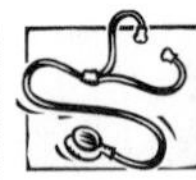

ASSESSMENT

History

Inquire about:

- Onset and duration of symptoms, if any
- Family history of hypercholesterolemia
- Underlying conditions, such as diabetes
- Current medications

Physical Findings

- Patient may not demonstrate any physical findings
- Subcutaneous or cutaneous xanthomas (lipid deposits) found in tendons (tendinous); elbows and knees (tuberous); buttocks, trunk, elbows, and knees (eruptive); skinfolds (planar) (on eyelids, referred to as xanthelasma; in palmar creases, called palmar xanthomas)
- Arterial bruit
- Claudication

Initial Workup

Laboratory

- Serum cholesterol level, including HDL and LDL levels
- Diagnosis of hypercholesterolemia should be based on results of 2 to 3 assays that are averaged (there can be great variability in laboratory results)
- National Cholesterol Education Program and National Institutes of Health have issued the following guidelines for interpreting results: <200 mg/dl, "desirable"; 200 to 239 mg/dl, "borderline high blood cholesterol"; >240 mg/dl "high cholesterol"
- If cholesterol is 200 to 239 mg/dl, HDL level is <35 mg/dl, and patient has 2 or more risk factors—cigarette smoking, family history of premature congestive heart failure, male >45 years or female >55 years or in premature menopause without estrogen replacement, hypertension, or diabetes mellitus, patient is considered to have high cholesterol
- Also check triglyceride level (must be fasting for 12 hours)
- Thyroid function
- Glucose

Radiology: None indicated

Further Workup

None unless evidence of stroke or myocardial infarction (MI)

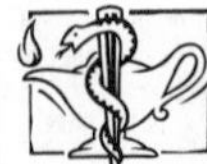

INTERVENTIONS

Office Treatment

None indicated

Lifestyle Modifications

- Diet and exercise
- Smoking cessation

Patient Education

Teach patient about:

- Condition and treatment
- Proper diet:
  - American Heart Association recommendations are step 1 diet first—visible fat restricted to 1 teaspoon per meal; use of unsaturated vegetable oils; only lean meats; skim milk or 1% milk; no more than 3 egg yolks per week; avoidance of food high in fat content; steaming, baking, broiling, grilling, or stir-frying recommended to prepare foods
  - If no decrease in cholesterol after 6 months, place on step 2 diet—only the leanest cuts of meat; no organ meats or shrimp; only 1 egg yolk per week (may use egg white and egg substitutes); use of vegetable oils for cooking (no coconut or palm oil); margarine that contains 2 g or less of saturated fat per tablespoon; skim milk, low-fat yogurt, low-fat cheeses, low-fat ice milk, frozen yogurt, or sherbet may be used
  - If no reduction in cholesterol in 6 months, consider pharmacologic intervention
- The fact that this is a lifelong commitment
- Importance of exercise to increase HDL level and decrease weight; exercise should be at least 3 times per week
- Medications used and side effects (see Pharmacotherapeutics)

Referrals

None if no symptoms of more life-threatening conditions, such as stroke or MI

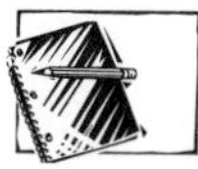

EVALUATION

Outcome

Decrease in total cholesterol and LDL levels and increase in HDL level

Possible Complications

- Coronary artery disease
- Stroke
- MI

Follow-up

Every 3 months for cholesterol level

FOR YOUR INFORMATION

Life Span

Pediatric: Children over 2 years of age should be screened if a parent has a cholesterol level >240 mg/dl or if there is a family history of premature cardiac disease
Geriatric: Most authorities recommend screening up to 65 to 70 years of age
Pregnancy: N/A

Miscellaneous

Diet, exercise, and smoking cessation are major lifestyle changes for most patients. It will take a great deal of encouragement and support from the NP to help the patient make these changes.

References

Blackman MR, Busby-Whitehead MJ: Clinical implications of abnormal lipoprotein metabolism. In Barker LR, Burton JR, Zieve PD, editors: *Principles of ambulatory medicine,* ed 4, Baltimore, 1995, Williams & Wilkins, pp 1075-1100.

Griego L, House-Fancher MA: Coronary artery disease. In Lewis SM, Collier IC, Heitkemper MM, editors: *Medical surgical nursing: assessment and management of clinical problems,* ed 4, St Louis, 1996, Mosby, pp 890-893.

US Department of Health and Human Services, Public Health Service, Office of Disease Prevention and Health Promotion: *Clinician's handbook of preventive services: put prevention into practice,* Washington, DC, 1994, US Government Printing Office, pp 13-16, 163-169, 303.

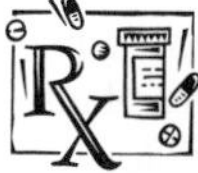

PHARMACOTHERAPEUTICS

Drug of Choice	Mechanism of Action	Prescribing Information	Side Effects
Bile acid–sequestering agents: • Cholestyramine (Questran); adults, 4 g PO ac and hs, maximum dose 32 g/day; children, 240 mg/kg/day PO in 3 divided doses • Colestipol (Colestid); adults, 15-30 g/day PO in 2-4 divided doses • Drugs must be mixed with either liquid or applesauce; give other medications 1 hour before or 4 hours after	Bind with bile acids in intestine and complex is excreted in feces	***Contraindications:*** Hypersensitivity; biliary obstruction ***Cost:*** Cholestyramine—4-g to 5-g packet, 60 packets: $83; Colestipol—5-g packet, 90 packets: $110 ***Pregnancy category:*** Safe use has not been established	Constipation, abdominal discomfort, flatulence, nausea, vomiting, dyspepsia, eructation, anorexia, decreased vitamins A, D, and K
Niacin or nicotinic acid (Nicolar), 250 mg PO qd following evening meal; may increase q4-7d until reach 1.5-2 g daily; after 2 months, check cholesterol level; if not adequately controlled, increase at 2- to 4-week intervals up to 3 g/day; maximum dose 6 g/day—rarely necessary	Interferes with synthesis of cholesterol and lipoproteins	***Contraindications:*** Hypersensitivity; hepatic dysfunction; active peptic ulcer disease; arterial bleeding ***Cost:*** 500-mg tab, 100 tabs: $2-$64 ***Pregnancy category:*** C	Severe hepatic toxicity; generalized flushing—can block with an aspirin taken with niacin; atrial fibrillation and other cardiac arrhythmias can occur; dyspepsia; vomiting; diarrhea; peptic ulceration; decreased glucose tolerance; hyperuricemia
• Lovastatin (Mevacor); patient should be on low-cholesterol, low-fat diet; starting dose, 20 mg PO qd with evening meal • Pravastatin (Pravachol), 10-20 mg PO qd at bedtime • Neither drug recommended for children	HMG-CoA reductase inhibitors	***Contraindications:*** Pregnancy and lactation; hypersensitivity; active liver disease ***Cost:*** Lovastatin—20-mg tab, 100 tabs: $212; Pravastatin—20-g tab, 90 tabs: $170 ***Pregnancy category:*** X	Marked increase in serum transaminases and acid regurgitation; dry mouth; vomiting; leg pain; shoulder pain; insomnia; eye irritation; alopecia; pruritus

Hyperparathyroidism

OVERVIEW

Hyperparathyroidism is the overproduction of parathyroid hormone (PTH). The normal regulatory feedback loop is out of control, resulting in an inability to maintain a normal serum calcium level.

Pathogenesis

- Primary hyperparathyroidism—increased secretion of PTH due to benign tumor or adenoma
- Secondary hyperparathyroidism—caused by hypocalcemia induced by vitamin D deficiency, chronic renal failure, malabsorption, or hyperphosphatemia
- Tertiary hyperparathyroidism—caused by hyperplasia of parathyroid gland; seen in patients who underwent dialysis for an extended period of time and then received a transplant

Patient Profile

- Females > Males
- Age >50 years or any age and sex if patient has chronic renal failure

Signs and Symptoms

Many signs and symptoms:

- Renal—nephrolithiasis, nephrocalcinosis, pancreatitis, pancreatic calcification, constipation, vomiting, anorexia, weight loss
- Gastrointestinal—abdominal distress, gastroduodenal ulcer, pancreatitis, pancreatic calcification, constipation, vomiting, anorexia, weight loss
- Orthopedic—bone pain and tenderness, cystic bone lesions, skeletal demineralization, spontaneous fracture, vertebral collapse, osteoporosis, arthralgia, gout, pseudogout, periarticular calcification
- Mental—fatigue, apathy, anxiety, depression, psychosis
- Neurologic—somnolence, coma, diffuse EEG abnormalities
- Neuromuscular—muscle fatigue, weakness, hypotonia
- Ocular—band keratopathy, conjunctivitis, conjunctival calcium deposits
- Cardiovascular—hypertension, short QT interval

Differential Diagnosis

Other causes of increased serum calcium level must be ruled out (i.e., bronchogenic carcinoma; carcinoma of kidney; breast carcinoma; multiple myeloma; lymphoma; leukemia; prostate cancer; Paget's disease; granulomatous diseases, such as sarcoidosis, tuberculosis, berylliosis, histoplasmosis, and coccidioidomycosis; drugs—thiazide diuretics, furosemide, vitamin D intoxication, vitamin A excess, lithium, milk alkali syndrome, exogenous calcium intake; hyperthyroidism; hypothyroidism; acute adrenal insufficiency; vipoma; pheochromocytoma; immobilization)

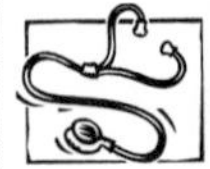

ASSESSMENT

History

Inquire about:

- Onset and duration of symptoms
- Family history
- Underlying conditions, such as chronic renal failure, vitamin D deficiency, malabsorption
- Current medications

Physical Findings

- General appearance of ill health
- Hypertension
- Weight loss
- Abdominal pain
- Joint pain, tenderness, swelling, redness
- May have bone pain, muscle wasting

Initial Workup

Laboratory

- Serum calcium levels >10.2 mg/dl on 3 successive occasions
- Serum phosphate level <2.5 mg/dl
- Serum chloride level—elevated
- Serum immunoreactive parathyroid hormone level—elevated

Radiology

- Ultrasound of neck
- Thallium technetium scan
- MRI
- CT scan with and without contrast, as indicated

Further Workup

- None by NP
- Needle biopsy or open surgical removal with frozen section by surgeon

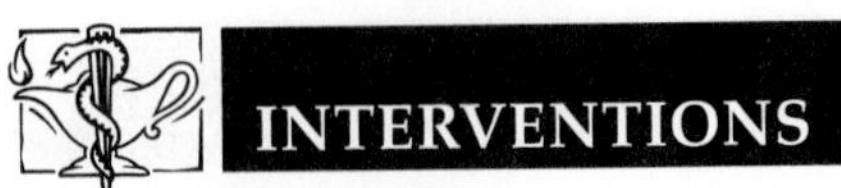

INTERVENTIONS

Office Treatment

None indicated

Lifestyle Modifications

- If cause is chronic renal failure, then numerous changes will need to occur (see section on renal failure)
- If primary hyperparathyroidism, need to ensure that patient maintains adequate levels of hydration before surgery—avoids damage to other organs

Patient Education

Teach patient about:

- Condition and treatment options:
  - Only curative treatment is surgical resection of diseased gland
  - If patient is not surgical candidate or symptoms are mild, maintain high fluid intake, moderate dietary calcium intake, phosphorus supplementation, and stress importance of continued ambulation—must avoid immobilization
  - Use of diuretics to enhance urinary excretion of calcium and estrogen therapy to decrease serum calcium and urinary calcium levels in postmenopausal women (not all patients respond to this therapy)
- Medications used and side effects (see Pharmacotherapeutics)

Referral

To endocrinologist or surgeon who specializes in neck surgery

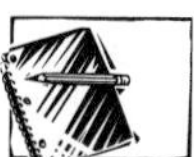

EVALUATION

Outcomes

- Primary hyperparathyroidism—postoperative prognosis is excellent
- Secondary hyperparathyroidism—postoperative prognosis is poor because of primary disease state of chronic renal failure

Possible Complications

- Pathologic fractures
- Renal damage
- Urinary tract infections

Follow-up

Depends on treatment; if conservative treatment and NP continues to follow patient, need to perform laboratory tests every 3 months

FOR YOUR INFORMATION

Life Span

Pediatric: Usually have secondary hyperparathyroidism as a result of renal failure
Geriatric: Primary hyperparathyroidism more common in this age group; may cause confusion
Pregnancy: Needs specialist to follow

Miscellaneous

The NP's primary responsibility for the patient with primary hyperparathyroidism is initial diagnosis and coordination of care with specialists in the field.

References

Gregerman RI: Selected endocrine problems: disorders of pituitary, adrenal, and parathyroid glands; pharmacological use of steroids; hypo and hypercalcemia; osteoporosis; water metabolism; hypoglycemia. In Barker LR, Burton JR, Zieve PD, editors: *Principles of ambulatory medicine,* ed 4, Baltimore, 1995, Williams & Wilkins, pp 1063-1064.

Haas LB: Endocrine problems. In Lewis SM, Collier IC, Heitkemper MM, editors: *Medical-surgical nursing: assessment and management of clinical problems,* ed 4, St Louis, 1996, Mosby, pp 1498-1504.

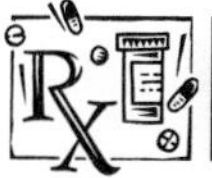

PHARMACOTHERAPEUTICS

Drug of Choice	Mechanism of Action	Prescribing Information	Side Effects
Furosemide (Lasix), 20-40 mg/day; use cautiously; patient must be well hydrated; children, 2 mg/kg/day PO, increase to maximum of 6 mg/kg/day	Inhibits reabsorption of sodium and chloride at proximal and distal tubule and in loop of Henle	***Contraindications:*** Hypersensitivity to sulfonamides; anuria; hypovolemia; infants; lactation; electrolyte depletion ***Cost:*** 20-mg tab, 30 tabs: $2 ***Pregnancy category:*** C	Headache, fatigue, weakness, orthostatic hypotension, chest pain, ECG changes, circulatory collapse, loss of hearing, ear pain, tinnitus, hypokalemia, hypochloremic alkalosis, hypomagnesemia, hyperuricemia, hypocalcemia, hyperglycemia, nausea, diarrhea, dry mouth, vomiting, polyuria, renal failure, thrombocytopenia, agranulocytosis, leukopenia, neutropenia, rash, pruritus, Stevens-Johnson syndrome, cramps
Estrogen therapy, 0.625 mg PO 1 tab daily; estrogen is available in pills, as a transdermal patch, or as a vaginal cream; method of administration should be decided on by NP and patient together by determining which method best meets patient's needs	Affects release of pituitary gonadotropins; inhibits ovulation	***Contraindications:*** Hypersensitivity; breast cancer; thromboembolic disorders; reproductive cancer; undiagnosed vaginal bleeding; pregnancy ***Cost:*** 0.625-mg tab, 100 tabs: $50 ***Pregnancy category:*** X	Dizziness, headache, migraines, depression, hypotension, thrombophlebitis, thromboembolism, pulmonary embolism, myocardial infarction (MI), nausea, vomiting, cholestatic jaundice, weight gain, diplopia, amenorrhea, cervical erosion, breakthrough bleeding, dysmenorrhea, vaginal candidiasis, spontaneous abortion, rash, urticaria, acne, hirsutism, photosensitivity
If patient has intact uterus, add:			
Medroxyprogesterone acetate (Provera), 10 mg PO on days 1-12 or days 13-25; or can give 2.5 mg PO daily; estrogen and medroxyprogesterone acetate are now available in 1 tab sold under trade name Prempro	Inhibits secretion of pituitary gonadotropins; stimulates growth of mammary tissue	***Contraindications:*** Hypersensitivity; breast cancer; thromboembolic disorders; reproductive cancer; undiagnosed vaginal bleeding; pregnancy ***Cost:*** 5-mg tab, 30 tabs: $16 ***Pregnancy category:*** X	Dizziness, headache, migraines, depression, hypotension, thrombophlebitis, thromboembolism, pulmonary embolism, MI, nausea, vomiting, cholestatic jaundice, weight gain, diplopia, amenorrhea, cervical erosion, breakthrough bleeding, dysmenorrhea, vaginal candidiasis, spontaneous abortion, rash, urticaria, acne, hirsutism, photosensitivity

Hypertension, Essential

OVERVIEW

Essential hypertension is high blood pressure (BP) for which there is no identifiable cause.

Pathogenesis
Cause—unknown; increased prevalence with aging, in African-Americans, and in lower socioeconomic groups

Patient Profile
- Males > Females
- Most common age—30 to 50 years

Signs and Symptoms
- Most are asymptomatic
- May have some signs or symptoms of target organ disease:
  - Cardiovascular system—coronary artery disease, left ventricular hypertrophy, left ventricular dysfunction, cardiac failure
  - Peripheral vascular disease—absence or diminished peripheral pulse, intermittent claudication
  - Renal system—proteinuria, increased creatinine level
  - Eyes—hemorrhage, exudates, papilledema
- See Table 12 for diagnostic criteria of the Joint National Committee on Detection, Evaluation, and Treatment of High Blood Pressure (average of 2 or more readings on 2 or more visits)

Differential Diagnosis
For secondary hypertension—polycystic kidney disease, renovascular disease, coarctation of aorta, Cushing's syndrome, pheochromocytoma

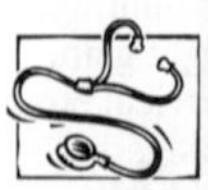

ASSESSMENT

History
Inquire about:
- Past history of elevated BP and readings
- Symptoms of secondary hypertension
- Physical activity
- Smoking and alcohol use
- Diet
- Family history of hypertension
- Coronary heart disease, diabetes, elevated cholesterol level
- Underlying conditions
- Current medications

Physical Findings
Complete physical examination:
- Fundoscopic examination—arteriolar narrowing, arteriovenous nicking, hemorrhages
- Assessment for distended neck veins, carotid bruit, thyromegaly
- Cardiovascular examination—tachycardia, murmurs, clicks, gallops, third and fourth heart sounds
- Abdominal examination—bruit, enlarged kidneys
- Palpation of peripheral pulses

Initial Workup
Laboratory
- CBC
- Urinalysis
- Chemistry profile to include electrolytes, BUN, creatinine, glucose, uric acid, cholesterol profile

Radiology: Based on history and physical examination—possible chest film; ultrasound (abdominal) if indicated

Further Workup
Baseline ECG

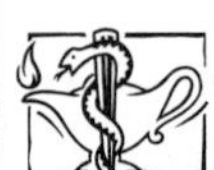

INTERVENTIONS

Office Treatment
None indicated

Lifestyle Modifications
- Smoking and alcohol cessation
- Weight loss
- Stress reduction
- Exercise program
- Possibly low-salt diet

Patient Education
Teach patient about:
- Condition
- First line of treatment:
  - Lifestyle modifications
  - Tips for smoking and alcohol cessation
  - Weight-loss diet
  - Starting a moderate exercise program (exercise found to be most important modification)
  - Stress reduction—biofeedback, relaxation therapy, yoga
  - Chronicity of hypertension and need for lifelong commitment to lifestyle changes and treatment
  - How to check own blood pressure and keep a record
  - Target organ disease
- Next line of treatment—medication—preferably using step approach: diuretics, beta-blockers, calcium channel blockers, angiotensin-converting enzyme inhibitors, alpha-adrenergic agents, and side effects (see Pharmacotherapeutics)

Referrals
Usually none indicated

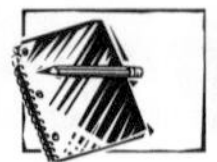

EVALUATION

Outcome
BP returns to normal

Possible Complications
- Stroke
- Myocardial infarction
- Renal failure
- Hypertensive heart disease

Follow-up
- Every 2 weeks until BP stabilized; then every 3 to 6 months
- Have patient bring BP record to visit if applicable

TABLE 12 *Diagnostic Criteria for High Blood Pressure*

Category	Systolic	Diastolic
Normal	<130 mm Hg	<85 mm Hg
High normal	130-139 mm Hg	85-89 mm Hg
Hypertension stage I (mild)	140-159 mm Hg	90-99 mm Hg
Stage II (moderate)	160-179 mm Hg	100-109 mm Hg
Stage III (severe)	180-209 mm Hg	110-119 mm Hg
Stage IV (very severe)	≥210 mm Hg	≥120 mm Hg

From *The Fifth Report of the Joint National Committee on Detection, Evaluation, and Treatment of High Blood Pressure,* NIH Pub No 93-1088, Washington, DC, 1993, National Institutes of Health, National Heart, Lung, and Blood Institute.

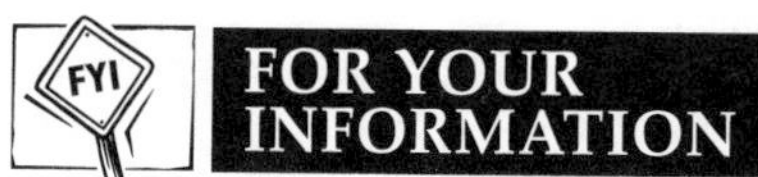

FOR YOUR INFORMATION

Life Span

Pediatric: Less common in this age group
Geriatric: Isolated systolic hypertension seen in this age group; treatment is recommended—use lowest dose of medications possible
Pregnancy: Cautious use of medications

Miscellaneous

N/A

References

Blake GH: Primary hypertension: the role of individualized therapy, *Am Fam Physician* 50(1):138-146, 1994.

Frolich ED: The JNC-V: consensus recommendations for the treatment of hypertension, *Physician Assist* 10:45-46, 50-61, 1993.

Massie BM: Systemic hypertension. In Tierney LM Jr, McPhee SJ, Papadakis MA, editors: *Current medical diagnosis and treatment,* ed 34, Norwalk, Conn, 1995, Appleton & Lange, pp 373-390.

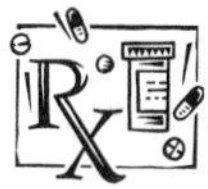

PHARMACOTHERAPEUTICS

There are many antihypertensive medications on the market. A representative of each category of drug is presented here. Consult the manufacturer's insert for prescribing information on other medications.

Drug of Choice	Mechanism of Action	Prescribing Information	Side Effects
Diuretics: • Hydrochlorothiazide (HydroDiuril), 12.5-50 mg PO qd; children >6 months, 2.2 mg/kg/day in divided doses • Others: chlorothiazide, chlorthalidone, indapamide	Thiazide diuretic; acts on distal tubule and ascending limb of loop of Henle	***Contraindications:*** Hypersensitivity to thiazides or sulfonamides; anuria; renal decompensation; hypomagnesemia ***Cost:*** 25-mg tab, 100 tabs: $2-$12 ***Pregnancy category:*** B	Uremia, glucosuria, drowsiness, dizziness, fatigue, weakness, nausea, vomiting, anorexia, constipation, hepatitis, rash, urticaria, hyperglycemia, aplastic anemia, hemolytic anemia, leukopenia, agranulocytosis, thrombocytopenia, neutropenia, hypokalemia, orthostatic hypotension, hyponatremia, volume depletion
Beta-blockers: • Propranolol (Inderal), 40-240 mg/day PO in divided doses; children, 1 mg/kg/day PO • Others: atenolol, betaxolol, metoprolol, nadolol, timolol	Reduce myocardial O_2 requirement by decreasing heart rate, myocardial contractility and blood pressure	***Contraindications:*** Hypersensitivity; cardiac failure; cardiogenic shock; 2nd- or 3rd-degree heart block; bronchospastic disease; sinus bradycardia; congestive heart failure (CHF) ***Cost:*** 40-mg tab, 100 tabs: $2-$40 ***Pregnancy category:*** C	Headache, fatigue, drowsiness, dizziness, anxiety, depression, weakness, insomnia, tinnitus, dysrhythmias, edema, CHF, hypotension, pulmonary edema, nausea, vomiting, diarrhea, constipation, nocturia, polyuria, rash, pruritus, photosensitivity, flushing, sexual difficulties, fever, chills, impotence
Calcium channel blockers: • Nifedepine (Procardia XL), 30-120 mg PO qd—not dosed for children • Others: diltiazem, verapamil, amlodipine, felodipine, isradipine, nicardipine	Induce coronary artery vasodilation, which reduces myocardial O_2 requirements	***Contraindication:*** Hypersensitivity ***Cost:*** 30-mg tab, 100 tabs: $95 ***Pregnancy category:*** C	Headache, fatigue, drowsiness, dizziness, anxiety, depression, weakness, insomnia, tinnitus, dysrhythmias, edema, CHF, hypotension, pulmonary edema, nausea, vomiting, diarrhea, constipation, nocturia, polyuria, rash, pruritus, photosensitivity, flushing, sexual difficulties, fever, chills
Angiotensin-converting enzyme inhibitors: • Quinapril (Accupril), 10-80 mg PO qd—not dosed for children • Others: benazepril, captopril, enalapril, fosinopril, lisinopril	Prevent conversion of angiotensin I to angiotensin II, producing arterial dilation	***Contraindication:*** Hypersensitivity ***Cost:*** 10-mg tab, 100 tabs: $90 ***Pregnancy category:*** 1st trimester—C; 2nd and 3rd trimesters—D	Cough, hypotension, postural hypotension, syncope, decreased libido, increased BUN and creatinine, thrombocytopenia, agranulocytosis, angioedema, rash, sweating, photosensitivity, hyperkalemia, nausea, vomiting, gastritis, headache, dizziness, fatigue, somnolence, depression, malaise, back pain, arthralgias, arthritis
Alpha-adrenergic agents: • Terazosin (Hytrin), 1-20 mg PO qd—not dosed for children • Others: prazosin, doxazosin	Relaxation of smooth muscle resulting from blockade of alpha-1 adrenoceptors in bladder neck and prostate	***Contraindication:*** Hypersensitivity ***Cost:*** 5-mg tab, 100 tabs: $123 ***Pregnancy category:*** C	Palpitations, orthostatic hypotension, tachycardia, edema, dizziness, headache, drowsiness, anxiety, depression, vertigo, nausea, vomiting, diarrhea, urinary frequency, incontinence, impotence, blurred vision, epistaxis, dry mouth, dyspnea

Hypertensive Urgencies and Emergencies

OVERVIEW

Hypertensive urgencies are situations in which the blood pressure (BP) needs to be reduced in 24 hours. Such situations include heart failure, renal ischemia, and angina. Hypertensive emergencies are defined as those situations in which the BP must be reduced within 1 hour to prevent or limit target organ damage. Such situations include intracranial hemorrhage, acute myocardial infarction, encephalopathy, and dissecting aortic aneurysm.

Pathogenesis

Causes:

- Many possible causes; exact cause unknown
- More common in secondary hypertension
- Noncompliance with antihypertensive therapy (abrupt withdrawal of medication)
- Failure of autoregulatory mechanisms
- Stress
- Genetic predisposition (more common in African-Americans)
- Obesity
- Tobacco use

Patient Profile

- Males > Females
- Most common age—40 years

Signs and Symptoms

- Urgent situations—asymptomatic but BP markedly elevated >240/>130
- Emergent:
  - Headache, heart failure, angina with BP >240/>130
  - Blurred vision
  - Chest pain
  - Dyspnea
  - Nausea, vomiting
  - Retinopathy, commonly with papilledema
  - Pulmonary edema
  - Stupor
  - Coma
  - Seizures
  - Restlessness
  - Nephropathy that may rapidly progress to renal failure

Differential Diagnosis

- Pheochromocytoma
- Tyramine ingestion
- Illicit drug use (crack cocaine, methamphetamine)

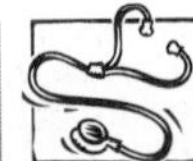

ASSESSMENT

History

Inquire about:

- Onset and duration of symptoms
- History of hypertension
- Family history
- Use of tobacco or illicit street drugs
- Underlying conditions
- Current medications

Physical Findings

- Markedly elevated BP (BP is not always indicative of end organ damage)
- Urgent situations—mental status intact, pedal edema, bounding pulse
- Emergent situations—irritability, confusion, stupor, bounding pulse, arrhythmias, pulmonary edema, pedal edema
- Fundoscopic examination—papilledema

Initial Workup

Laboratory

- Urinalysis—hematuria, proteinuria, RBC casts
- Electrolytes—hypokalemia
- BUN and creatinine—both increased
- CBC—anemia, thrombocytopenia
- Fibrin degradation products—elevated

Radiology: Renal ultrasound and/or scan

Further Workup

None indicated

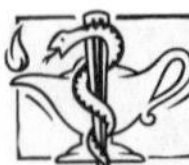

INTERVENTIONS

Office Treatment

- Emergent situations—severe encephalopathy, nephropathy, and papilledema present—immediate transport to emergency department
- Urgent situations—prompt administration of nifedipine (immediate release), 10 mg PO, or captopril, 25 mg PO; may repeat in 30 minutes

NOTE: Recently many organizations have adopted the policy of *not* attempting to rapidly lower a patient's blood pressure in outpatient clinic settings. Check with your organization regarding their policies and procedures.

Lifestyle Modifications

- Compliance with medication regimen
- Low-salt diet—may be helpful for some
- Weight loss
- Regular exercise
- Stress reduction
- Alcohol and tobacco cessation

Patient Education

Teach patient about:

- Condition and importance of taking medication as directed
- Tips for weight loss
- Tips for alcohol and smoking cessation
- Stress reduction—relaxation therapy, biofeedback, yoga
- How to check own BP and keep record
- Starting a moderate, regular exercise program
- Medications used and side effects (see Pharmacotherapeutics)

Referral

To MD for hospitalization if NP does not have privileges, or to MD if resistant to treatment

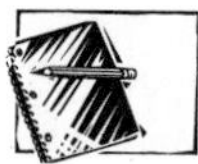

EVALUATION

Outcome
BP returns to normal, and patient follows treatment regimen

Possible Complications
- Renal failure
- Stroke
- Congestive heart failure
- Retinopathy

Follow-up
Every 2 weeks until BP stable; if possible, have patient check BP 3 times per week and keep record to bring to visit

FOR YOUR INFORMATION

Life Span
Pediatric: Look for secondary cause
Geriatric: Higher morbidity and mortality rate
Pregnancy: Needs to be managed by a specialist

Miscellaneous
N/A

References

Barker LR: Hypertension. In Barker LR, Burton JR, Zieve PD, editors: *Principles of ambulatory medicine,* ed 4, Baltimore, 1995, Williams & Wilkins, pp 812-817.

Massie BM: Systemic hypertension. In Tierney LM Jr, McPhee SJ, Papadakis MA, editors: *Current medical diagnosis and treatment,* ed 34, Norwalk, Conn, 1995, Appleton & Lange, pp 388-390.

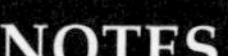

NOTES

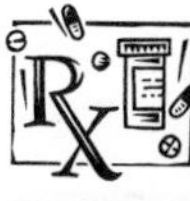

PHARMACOTHERAPEUTICS

There are many medications used in the treatment of hypertensive emergencies that are beyond the scope of this book. Only the oral medications for hypertensive urgencies are presented here. For others, consult an acute care text. NOTE: Recently many organizations have adopted the policy of *not* attempting to lower a patient's blood pressure in outpatient clinic settings. Check with your organization regarding their policies and procedures.

Drug of Choice	Mechanism of Action	Prescribing Information	Side Effects
Nifedipine (Procardia), 10 mg PO, may repeat after 30 minutes; onset of action, 10 minutes; in the past, many clinicians used Procardia sublingually; this practice has gone out of favor because sublingual administration may result in very rapid hypotension, causing inadequate cerebral or cardiac blood flow	Induces coronary artery vasodilation, which reduces myocardial O_2 requirements	***Contraindication:*** Hypersensitivity ***Cost:*** 30-mg tab, 100 tabs: $95 ***Pregnancy category:*** C	Headache, fatigue, drowsiness, dizziness, anxiety, depression, weakness, insomnia, tinnitus, dysrhythmias, edema, congestive heart failure (CHF), hypotension, pulmonary edema, nausea, vomiting, diarrhea, constipation, nocturia, polyuria, rash, pruritus, photosensitivity, flushing, sexual difficulties, fever, chills
Captopril (Capoten), 25 mg PO, may repeat in 30 minutes; monitor closely because may cause excessive BP reduction	Angiotensin-converting enzyme inhibitor; causes vasodilation by blocking conversion of angiotensin I to angiotensin II	***Contraindication:*** Hypersensitivity ***Cost:*** 25-mg tab, 100 tabs: $65-$75 ***Pregnancy category:*** C	Headache, fatigue, drowsiness, dizziness, anxiety, depression, weakness, insomnia, tinnitus, dysrhythmias, edema, CHF, hypotension, pulmonary edema, nausea, vomiting, diarrhea, constipation, nocturia, polyuria, rash, pruritus, photosensitivity, flushing, sexual difficulties, fever, chills

Hyperthyroidism

OVERVIEW

Hyperthyroidism is a condition that occurs as a result of excess production of thyroid hormones. The most common conditions producing hyperthyroidism are Graves' disease and toxic multinodular goiter.

Pathogenesis

- Graves' disease—autoimmune disorder; thyroid-stimulating immunoglobulins bind to thyrotropin (TSH) receptors, mimic the action of TSH, and cause excess excretion of thyroxine (T_4) and triiodothyronine (T_3)
- Toxic multinodular goiter—multiple, small nodules, function independently and secrete thyroid hormones
- Other causes may be found but are extremely rare and are not included here

Patient Profile

- Females > Males
- Any age, peaks in third and fourth decades
- Toxic multinodular goiter—more common later in life (fifth and sixth decades)

Signs and Symptoms

- Palpitations
- Tachycardia
- Nervousness
- Increased sweating
- Heat intolerance
- Weight loss
- Fatigue and weakness
- Increased appetite
- Ophthalmopathy (exophthalmos)
- Goiter
- Tremor
- Warm and moist skin
- Emotional lability

Differential Diagnosis

- Malignancy
- Diabetes
- Pregnancy
- Menopause
- Pheochromocytoma
- Anxiety

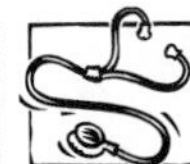

ASSESSMENT

History

Inquire about:

- Onset and duration of symptoms (may be insidious in onset)
- Family history of thyroid disease
- Past history of thyroid disease
- Underlying conditions
- Current medications

Physical Findings

- Warm and moist skin
- Exophthalmos (protrusion of eyeball from orbit)
- Tachycardic heart rate
- Palpable thyroid enlargement

Initial Workup

Laboratory

- Thyroid panel: T_3—elevated; T_4—elevated; TSH—below normal; free thyroxine index (FTI)—elevated
- Numerous drugs can interfere with laboratory test results; these include anabolic steroids, estrogens, heparin, iodine-containing compounds, phenytoin, rifampin, salicylates, thyroxine

Radiology: Thyroid scan

Further Workup

- Radioiodine uptake (RIU)—elevated in Graves' disease; elevated or normal in toxic multinodular goiter
- Immunoradioactive assays

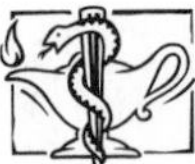

INTERVENTIONS

Office Treatment

None indicated

Lifestyle Modifications

Sufficient calories to prevent weight loss

Patient Education

Teach patient about:

- Disease process and treatment options—most commonly treated with medications; occasionally subtotal thyroidectomy done
- Graves' disease—self-limiting; usually resolves in 1 to 2 years; medications needed until euthyroid state obtained and maintained
- Adequate diet to prevent weight loss
- Weight gain expected after thyroid hormones revert to normal
- Using artificial tears for moisture
- Needing to tape eyes shut for sleep; wearing dark glasses to prevent irritation, if exopthalmos present
- Medications used and side effects (see Pharmacotherapeutics)

Referral

To endocrinologist if possible

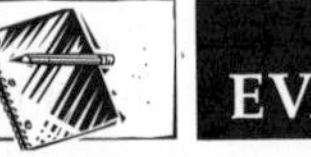

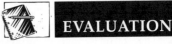

EVALUATION

Outcome

Thyroid function returns to normal range

Possible Complications

- Thyroid storm—a life-threatening condition—can cause heart failure, mania, or coma—requires inpatient treatment
- Hypothyroidism—overtreatment with medications
- Visual loss—due to severe ophthalmopathy
- Muscle wasting
- Nephrocalcinosis

Follow-up

Repeat thyroid tests at 6-week intervals until euthyroid state achieved; then every 3 months × 2; then every 6 months

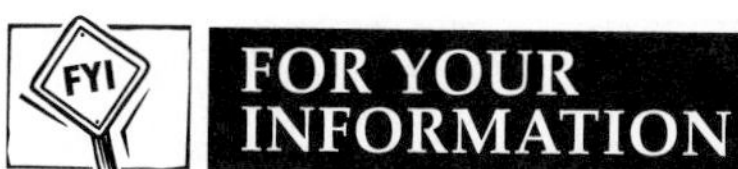

FOR YOUR INFORMATION

Life Span

Pediatric: Should be treated by a specialist
Geriatric: May be harder to diagnose, since classic signs and symptoms may be absent
Pregnancy: Treat with small doses of propylthiouracil (PTU); should be handled by specialist

Miscellaneous

Often, female patients are hesitant to comply with treatment because they are enjoying the weight loss that goes with hyperthyroidism. It is important for the NP to adequately explain the condition and the harm that it will do if left untreated. It is also important to assist the patient in dealing with this changing body image.

References

Gregerman RI: Thyroid disorders. In Barker LR, Burton JR, Zieve PD, editors: *Principles of ambulatory medicine,* ed 4, Baltimore, 1995, Williams & Wilkins, pp 1027-1035.
Haas LB: Endocrine problems. In Lewis SM, Collier IC, Heitkemper MM, editors: *Medical-surgical nursing: assessment and management of clinical problems,* ed 4, St Louis, 1996, Mosby, pp 1486-1490.
Zaldel LB: Guidelines on thyroid disease to improve diagnosis, *Nurse Pract* 21(8):8, 1996.

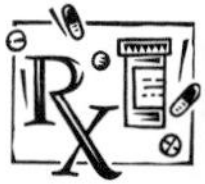

PHARMACOTHERAPEUTICS

Drug of Choice	Mechanism of Action	Prescribing Information	Side Effects
Beta-adrenergic blocker: Propranolol (Inderal), 40-240 mg PO qd in single or divided doses; children, 1 mg/kg/day PO in single or divided doses; does not correct problem of increased thyroid hormones; only controls symptoms	Reduces myocardial O_2 requirement by decreasing heart rate, myocardial contractility, and blood pressure	***Contraindications:*** Hypersensitivity; cardiac failure; cardiogenic shock; 2nd- or 3rd-degree heart block; bronchospastic disease; sinus bradycardia; congestive heart failure (CHF) ***Cost:*** 40-mg tab, 100 tabs: $2-$40 ***Pregnancy category:*** C	Headache, fatigue, drowsiness, dizziness, anxiety, depression, weakness, insomnia, tinnitus, dysrhythmias, edema, CHF, hypotension, pulmonary edema, nausea, vomiting, diarrhea, constipation, nocturia, polyuria, rash, pruritus, photosensitivity, flushing, sexual difficulties, fever, chills
Propylthiouracil (PTU), initially 100 mg PO tid; increase as needed to obtain euthyroid state; check laboratory values every 6 weeks; maintenance dose usually 100-150 mg PO qd; children >10 years, start with 150-300 mg PO in 3 divided doses; preferred drug in pregnancy, elderly, and patients with cardiac disease	Inhibits synthesis of thyroid hormones	***Contraindications:*** Hypersensitivity; lactating mothers ***Cost:*** 50-mg tab, 100 tabs: $5-$10 ***Pregnancy category:*** D	Agranulocytosis (most serious side effect), leukopenia, thrombocytopenia, aplastic anemia, drug fever, lupuslike syndrome, hepatitis, periarteritis, nephritis, interstitial pneumonitis, erythema nodosum, skin rash, urticaria, nausea, vomiting, hair loss, pruritus, drowsiness, edema
Methimazole (Tapazole), 15-60 mg PO qd in 3 doses separated by 8 hours; maintenance dose 5-15 mg PO qd; children, 0.4 mg/kg/day PO in 3 divided doses at 8-hour intervals; maintenance dose about half the initial dose	Inhibits synthesis of thyroid hormone	***Contraindications:*** Hypersensitivity; lactating mothers ***Cost:*** 5-mg tab, 100 tabs: $13 ***Pregnancy category:*** D	Agranulocytosis (most serious side effect), leukopenia, thrombocytopenia, aplastic anemia, drug fever, lupuslike syndrome, hepatitis, periarteritis, nephritis, interstitial pneumonitis, erythema nodosum, skin rash, urticaria, nausea, vomiting, hair loss, pruritus, drowsiness, edema

For radioiodide therapy (sodium iodide ^{131}I), the dosage calculation is the estimated thyroid weight multiplied by 80 μCi/g, divided by the 24-hour radioiodide uptake. Radioiodide accumulates in thyroid tissue and damages or destroys it. Although it is uniformly effective, relatively inexpensive, and simple to administer, radioiodide can only be administered by an endocrinologist or nuclear medicine physician. Antithyroid drugs must be given with it until a response is felt—usually in 3 months. Full radiation precautions should be taken for 24 hours after administration. The patient must be instructed on precautions to take after discharge. Patients are usually given the initial dose in the hospital.

OVERVIEW

Hypertriglyceridemia is an increase in the synthesis and/or a decrease in the degradation of triglycerides. Triglycerides are a part of the total lipoprotein makeup of plasma, along with the various types of cholesterol. Hypertriglyceridemia can be either primary or secondary in nature. The major lipoproteins containing triglycerides are chylomicrons, very low density lipoproteins (VLDLs), and intermediate-density lipoproteins (IDLs).

Pathogenesis
Causes:
- Primary—usually genetic
- Secondary—certain diseases such as diabetes mellitus, chronic renal failure, hypothyroidism, or dysglobulinemia, or drugs such as corticosteroids, estrogens, thiazide diuretics, alcohol, beta-blockers, or isotretinoin

Patient Profile
- Males > Females
- Any age
- Genetic types:
  - Familial combined hyperlipidemia—autosomal dominant
  - Polygenic hyperlipidemia—autosomal dominant
  - Familial hypertriglyceridemia—autosomal dominant
  - Familial dyslipoproteinemia—autosomal recessive

Signs and Symptoms
- Usually asymptomatic
- If triglycerides very high (>1000), may have abdominal pain, acute pancreatitis, eruptive xanthoma, lipemia retinalis, hepatosplenomegaly, memory loss/dementia, peripheral neuropathy
- Atherosclerosis

Differential Diagnosis
None

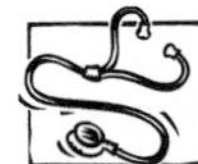

ASSESSMENT

History
Inquire about:
- Onset and duration of symptoms
- Family history of hypertriglyceridemia
- Underlying conditions such as diabetes, chronic renal failure, hypothyroidism
- Current medications, particularly estrogen, thiazide diuretics, steroids

Physical Findings
May be negative; if triglycerides very high, may find abdominal tenderness, eruptive xanthoma, lipemia retinalis, hepatosplenomegaly, peripheral neuropathy

Initial Workup
Laboratory: Serum triglyceride level obtained after 12-hour fast—normal: <150 mg/dl in adults, <100 mg/dl in children; borderline hypertriglyceridemia: 250-500 mg/dl hypertriglyceridemia: >500 mg/dl
Radiology: None indicated

Further Workup
- Serum cholesterol level if high triglycerides found
- Search for underlying cause—either disease process or drugs

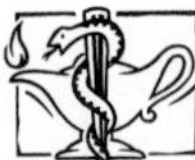

INTERVENTIONS

Office Treatment
None indicated

Lifestyle Modifications
- Diet and exercise to reduce weight to ideal
- Smoking cessation
- Elimination of alcohol

Patient Education
Teach patient about:
- Proper diet:
  - American Heart Association recommendations are step 1 diet first—visible fat restricted to 1 teaspoon per meal; use of unsaturated vegetable oils; only lean meats; skim milk or 1% milk; no more than 3 egg yolks per week; avoidance of food high in fat content; steaming, baking, broiling, grilling, or stir-frying recommended to prepare foods
  - If no decrease in triglycerides after 6 months, place on step 2 diet—only the leanest cuts of meat; no organ meats or shrimp; only 1 egg yolk per week (may use egg white and egg substitutes); use of vegetable oils for cooking (no coconut or palm oil); margarine that contains 2 g or less of saturated fat per tablespoon; skim milk, low-fat yogurt, low-fat cheeses, low-fat ice milk, frozen yogurt, or sherbet may be used
  - If no reduction in triglycerides in 6 months consider pharmacologic intervention
- The fact that this is a lifelong commitment
- Importance of exercise to decrease weight; exercise should be at least 3 times per week
- Tips for smoking cessation and alcohol cessation
- Medications used and side effects (see Pharmacotherapeutics)

Referral
To nutritionist for diet instruction

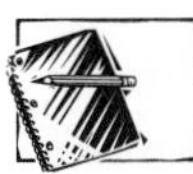

EVALUATION

Outcome
Reduction in triglyceride level

Possible Complications
- Acute pancreatitis
- Atherosclerosis leading to myocardial infarction or cerebrovascular accident

Follow-up
Every 3 months for fasting lipid profile, liver function tests

FOR YOUR INFORMATION

Life Span
Pediatric: Usually due to heredity
Geriatric: More common in this group; decision to use pharmacologic agents must be individualized
Pregnancy: Drugs are contraindicated

Miscellaneous
The NP needs to search thoroughly for any underlying causes of hypertriglyceridemia. If one is found, treating or eliminating it can greatly reduce the triglycerides. If the patient is found to have primary hypertriglyceridemia, lifelong therapy will be needed.

References
Blackman MR, Busby-Whitehead MJ: Clinical implications of abnormal lipoprotein metabolism. In Barker LR, Burton JR, Zieve PD, editors: *Principles of ambulatory medicine,* ed 4, Baltimore, 1995, Williams & Wilkins, pp 1075-1100.

Griego L, House-Fancher MA: Coronary artery disease. In Lewis SM, Collier IC, Heitkemper MM, editors: *Medical-surgical nursing: assessment and management of clinical problems,* ed 4, St Louis, 1996, Mosby, pp 888-894.

NOTES

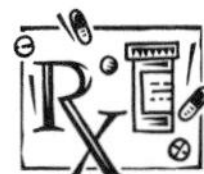

PHARMACOTHERAPEUTICS

Drug of Choice	Mechanism of Action	Prescribing Information	Side Effects
Niacin or nicotinic acid (Nicolar), 500 mg to 3 g qd, bid, or tid; start with low dose and increase as needed—not recommended for children	Interferes with synthesis of cholesterol and lipoproteins	***Contraindications:*** Hypersensitivity; hepatic dysfunction; active peptic ulcer disease; arterial bleeding ***Cost:*** 500-mg tab, 100 tabs: $2-$64 ***Pregnancy category:*** C	Severe hepatic toxicity; generalized flushing—can block with an aspirin taken with niacin; atrial fibrillation and other cardiac arrhythmias can occur; dyspepsia; vomiting; diarrhea; peptic ulceration; decreased glucose tolerance; hyperuricemia
Gemfibrozil (Lopid), 600 mg, 1 tab 30 minutes before breakfast and 1 tab 30 minutes before supper—not dosed for children; do not use in combination with HMG-CoA reductase inhibitors such as lovastatin; rhabdomyolysis can occur	Lipid-regulating agent that decreases triglycerides and VLDLs	***Contraindications:*** Hypersensitivity; hepatic or severe renal dysfunction; preexisting gallbladder disease ***Cost:*** 600-mg tab, 60 tabs: $14-$72 ***Pregnancy category:*** C	Dyspepsia, abdominal pain, acute appendicitis, atrial fibrillation, diarrhea, nausea, vomiting, eczema, fatigue, rash, vertigo, constipation, headache

Hypertrophic Cardiomyopathy

OVERVIEW

Hypertrophic cardiomyopathy is a disease of the cardiac muscle in which there is inappropriate hypertrophy of the left ventricular septum. The hypertrophy is considered inappropriate because it is not related to any pressure or volume overload. There may or may not be obstruction of the ventricular outflow tract. Obstruction occurs as a result of the thickened septum impinging on the anterior leaflet of the mitral valve.

Pathogenesis

Cause—60% of cases familial; others occur sporadically

Patient Profile

- Males = Females
- Most commonly present in young adulthood, but may be seen throughout life span

Signs and Symptoms

- Angina, relieved by recumbent position
- Syncope
- Palpitations
- Fatigue
- Congestive heart failure
- Sudden death

Differential Diagnosis

- Aortic stenosis
- Mitral regurgitation
- Pulmonic stenosis
- Ventricular septal defect

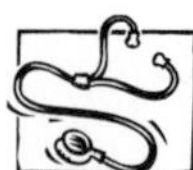

ASSESSMENT

History

Inquire about:

- Onset and duration of symptoms
- Family history of hypertrophic cardiomyopathy
- Underlying conditions
- Current medications

Physical Findings

Heart examination:

- Double apical impulse
- S_4 and possible S_3; split S_2
- Crescendo-decrescendo systolic murmur—apex and (L) sternal border
- Murmur—increases and lengthens with Valsalva maneuver, standing
- Decreases with squatting, lying down, passive leg raising, and isometric handgrip

Initial Workup

Laboratory: None indicated
Radiology: Chest film—normal cardiac size to cardiomegaly

Further Workup

- ECG—nonspecific ST abnormalities; (L) ventricular hypertrophy
- Echocardiogram
- Thallium stress test
- Cardiac catheterization
- Angiography, as indicated

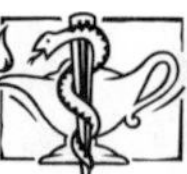

INTERVENTIONS

Office Treatment

None indicated

Lifestyle Modifications

- No strenuous activity or competitive sports (high risk of sudden death)
- Smoking cessation

Patient Education

Teach patient about:

- Condition and treatment
- Restricting strenuous activity and not participating in competitive sports
- Limiting caloric intake because of restricted activity
- Coping with a chronic condition and learning to live with restricted activity
- Medications used and side effects (see Pharmacotherapeutics)

Referrals

- To counselor
- To cardiologist
- Refer family to learn cardiopulmonary resuscitation (CPR)

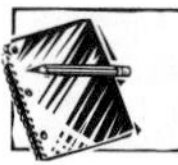

EVALUATION

Outcome
Patient learns to live with chronic illness and restricted activity

Possible Complications
- Sudden death
- Congestive heart failure
- Arrhythmias

Follow-up
Every 2 weeks until stable; then every 6 to 12 months

FOR YOUR INFORMATION

Life Span
Pediatric: Sudden death while participating in sports may be presenting feature
Geriatric: More prevalent in this age group
Pregnancy: Should be handled by a specialist

Miscellaneous
N/A

References
DeSantis RW, Dee GW: Cardiomyopathies. In Dale DC, Federman DD, editors: *Scientific American:* Medicine, vol 1, New York, 1995, Scientific American, pp 11-12.

Massie BM: Systemic hypertension. In Tierney LM Jr, McPhee SJ, Papadakis MA, editors: *Current medical diagnosis and treatment,* ed 34, Norwalk, Conn, 1995, Appleton & Lange, pp 360-361.

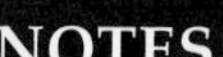

NOTES

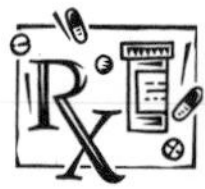

PHARMACOTHERAPEUTICS

Drug of Choice	Mechanism of Action	Prescribing Information	Side Effects
Propranolol (Inderal), 30-120 mg PO bid or tid or 160 mg PO qd extended-release form; may increase dose up to 320 mg/day; children, 1 mg/kg/day PO—do not use doses above 16 mg/kg/day	Reduce myocardial O_2 requirement by decreasing heart rate, myocardial contractility, and blood pressure	***Contraindications:*** Hypersensitivity; cardiac failure; cardiogenic shock; 2nd- or 3rd-degree heart block; bronchospastic disease; sinus bradycardia; congestive heart failure (CHF) ***Cost:*** 40-mg tab, 100 tabs: $2-$40 ***Pregnancy category:*** C	Bronchospasm, dyspnea, bradycardia, hypotension, CHF, palpitations, atrioventricular (AV) block, agranulocytosis, thrombocytopenia, nausea, vomiting, diarrhea, constipation, impotence, decreased libido, joint pain, arthralgia, facial swelling, rash, pruritus, depression, hallucinations, dizziness, fatigue, lethargy, sore throat, laryngospasm, blurred vision
Verapamil (Calan), 80 mg PO tid or qid, or 240 mg PO qd sustained-release form; maximum dose 480 mg/day—not dosed for children <18 years	Calcium channel blocker; dilates coronary arteries; decreases SA/AV node conduction; dilates peripheral arteries	***Contraindications:*** Sick sinus syndrome; 2nd- and 3rd-degree AV block; hypotension; cardiogenic shock; severe CHF; hypersensitivity ***Cost:*** 240-mg tab, 100 tabs: $54-$126 ***Pregnancy category:*** C	Edema, CHF, bradycardia, hypotension, nausea, diarrhea, gastric upset, constipation, nocturia, polyuria, headache, drowsiness, dizziness, anxiety, depression, weakness, insomnia, confusion

OVERVIEW

Hypothyroidism is a condition that results from a decrease in thyroid hormones.

Pathogenesis

Many causes:

- Cretinism—occurs in infancy; due to thyroid deficiencies during fetal or early neonatal life
- Secondary hypothyroidism—follows radioactive iodine therapy or thyroid surgery (most common adult cause)
- Primary hypothyroidism—autoimmune thyroiditis or idiopathic
- With goiter—most commonly due to autoimmune disease, such as Hashimoto's thyroiditis

Patient Profile

- Females > Males
- Age >40, but can occur at any age

Signs and Symptoms

- Insidious onset
- Weakness, fatigue, lethargy
- Cold intolerance
- Decreased memory
- Modest weight gain
- Muscle cramps
- Arthralgias
- Paresthesias
- Decreased sweating
- Menorrhagia
- Hoarseness
- Dry, coarse skin
- Periorbital puffiness
- Swelling of hands and feet
- Husky voice
- Bradycardia
- Hypothermia
- Delayed relaxation of deep tendon reflexes
- Reduced body and scalp hair

Differential Diagnosis

- Nephrotic syndrome
- Chronic nephritis
- Depression
- Congestive heart failure
- Primary amyloidosis
- Dementia from other causes
- Euthyroid sick syndrome

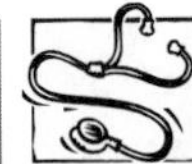

ASSESSMENT

History

Inquire about:

- Onset and duration of symptoms
- History of treatment for hyperthyroidism
- Family history of thyroid problems
- Underlying conditions
- Current medications

Physical Findings

- Dry, coarse skin
- Reduced systolic blood pressure
- Increased diastolic blood pressure
- Periorbital puffiness
- Dull facial expression
- Swelling of hands and feet
- Bradycardia
- Huskiness of voice
- Reduced body and scalp hair
- Delayed relaxation of deep tendon reflexes

Initial Workup

Laboratory

- Serum triiodothyronine (T_4) and thyroxine (T_3) levels—low
- Serum TSH level—high if thyroid diseased; low if pituitary diseased
- CBC—anemia may be present
- Serum chemistry panel—may find increased cholesterol, CPK, LDH, and AST levels and decreased sodium level

Radiology: Chest film—PA and lateral—may show enlarged heart

Further Workup

None indicated

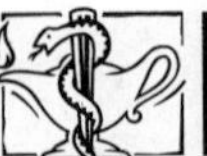

INTERVENTIONS

Office Treatment

None indicated

Lifestyle Modifications

- Adjustment to chronic illness and need for lifelong medication therapy
- Diet to decrease weight and constipation
- Smoking cessation

Patient Education

Teach patient about:

- Disease process and need for lifelong medication therapy
- Reporting any signs/symptoms of infection or heart problems (palpitations, chest pain)
- Medications used and side effects (see Pharmacotherapeutics)

Referral

Consider referral to endocrinologist if available

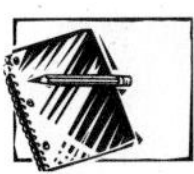

EVALUATION

Outcome
Patient returns to euthyroid state with marked improvement in physical appearance and mental function

Possible Complications
- Myxedema coma—life-threatening, severe hypothermia, coma
- Increased susceptibility to infection
- Megacolon
- Treatment-induced congestive heart failure in patient with coronary heart disease
- Organic psychoses
- Adrenal crisis
- Infertility
- Hypersensitivity to opiates

Follow-up
- Every 6 weeks to monitor TSH until stable; then every 3 to 6 months
- May need to follow older patient more closely—monthly

FOR YOUR INFORMATION

Life Span
Pediatric: Usually congenital hypothroidism
Geriatric: Thyroxine may exacerbate angina pectoris and cardiac arrhythmias; may also decrease bone mineral density
Pregnancy: Monitoring should be done on a monthly basis (TSH level) during first trimester; adjustment of medication usually necessary during this time; should be followed by specialist

Miscellaneous
N/A

References
Gregerman RI: Thyroid disorders. In Barker LR, Burton JR, Zieve PD, editors: *Principles of ambulatory medicine,* ed 4, Baltimore, 1995, Williams & Wilkins, pp 1035-1039.

Haas LB: Endocrine problems. In Lewis SM, Collier IC, Heitkemper MM, editors: *Medical-surgical nursing: assessment and management of clinical problems,* ed 4, St Louis, 1996, Mosby, pp 1496-1498.

NOTES

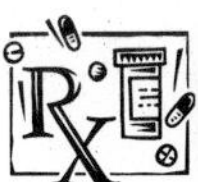

PHARMACOTHERAPEUTICS

Drug of Choice	Mechanism of Action	Prescribing Information	Side Effects
Levothyroxine (Synthroid, Levothroid, etc.), 50-100 μg/day PO; increase by 25-μg increments until TSH level is normal; children, 10-15 μg/kg/day PO; adjust as needed until TSH level is normal	Replacement of decreased thyroid hormone; thyroid hormone increases metabolic rate of tissue	***Contraindications:*** Untreated thyrotoxicosis; hypersensitivity; uncorrected adrenal insufficiency ***Cost:*** 50-μg tab, 100 tabs: $4-$21 ***Pregnancy category:*** A	Thyrotoxicosis caused by overdose; rash; urticaria; hair loss; pseudotumor cerebri—can occur in pediatric patients

Impetigo

OVERVIEW

Impetigo is a superficial, common, contagious skin infection. It presents as either bullous or nonbullous impetigo.

Pathogenesis

Causes:

- *Staphylococcus aureus*
- Group A beta-hemolytic streptococci
- Occasionally *Streptococcus pyogenes*
- Bullous impetigo caused by staphylococci
- Nonbullous impetigo usually caused by streptococci

Patient Profile

- Males = Females
- Bullous impetigo more common in children; nonbullous impetigo—any age
- Risk factors:
  - Warm, humid environment
  - Tropical or subtropical climate
  - Summer or fall season
  - Minor trauma, such as insect bites
  - Poor hygiene, epidemics, during war
  - Familial spread
  - Poor health with anemia and malnutrition
  - Complication of pediculosis, scabies, chickenpox, eczema
  - Contact dermatitis

Signs and Symptoms

BULLOUS IMPETIGO

- Usually on face
- One or more vesicles that enlarge to form bullae
- Contents clear to cloudy
- After vesicle ruptures, a thin, flat, honey-colored crust appears; if removed, reveals bright-red, inflamed, moist base that oozes serum
- May dry without crust, leaving red base with rim of scale

NONBULLOUS IMPETIGO

- Small vesicles or pustules, rupture—expose red, moist base
- Honey-yellow to white-brown crust forms
- Little erythema

Differential Diagnosis

BULLOUS IMPETIGO

- Burns
- Pemphigus vulgaris
- Bullous pemphigoid
- Stevens-Johnson syndrome

NONBULLOUS IMPETIGO

- Chickenpox
- Herpes
- Folliculitis
- Erysipelas
- Insect bites
- Severe eczematous dermatitis
- Scabies
- Tinea corporis

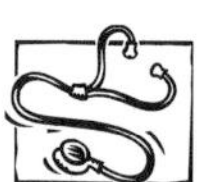

ASSESSMENT

History

Inquire about:

- Onset and duration of symptoms
- Infection in other family members
- History of previous infections
- History of injury to skin, such as insect bite
- Treatment tried and results
- Underlying conditions
- Current medications

Physical Findings

- Vesicles, erythematous base
- Yellow crust in bullous impetigo
- Yellow to white-brown crust, usually on face, in nonbullous impetigo

Initial Workup

Laboratory: Culture taken from base of lesion after crust removed

Radiology: None indicated

Further Workup

None indicated

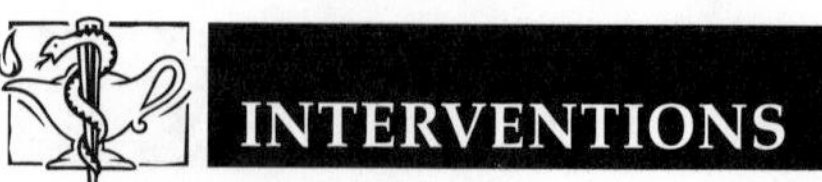

INTERVENTIONS

Office Treatment

None indicated

Lifestyle Modifications

- Good hygiene to prevent spread
- Smoking cessation

Patient Education

Teach patient about:

- Condition and treatment—antibiotics
- Nonbullous—prevention by avoiding skin trauma
- Importance of good hygiene
- Spreading within family
- Signs and symptoms of poststreptococcal acute glomerulonephritis—weight gain, gross hematuria, headache may indicate elevated BP
- Medications used and side effects (see Pharmacotherapeutics)

Referral

To dermatologist for resistant cases

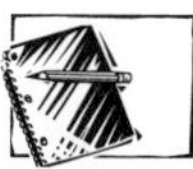

EVALUATION

Outcome
Resolution of lesion within 7 to 10 days

Possible Complications
- Ecthyma
- Erysipelas
- Poststreptococcal acute glomerulonephritis
- Bacteremia

Follow-up
- Usually none needed; return to clinic if no resolution
- Poststreptococcal acute glomerulonephritis most commonly occurs 1 to 5 weeks after onset—average 10 days; most common in children 2 to 4 years of age

FOR YOUR INFORMATION

Life Span
Pediatric: Most commonly seen in this age group
Geriatric: Higher morbidity and mortality
Pregnancy: Cautious use of medications

Miscellaneous
Treatment with antibiotics will not prevent the development of acute glomerulonephritis, so careful observation and education of the patient are important.

References

Habif TP: *Clinical dermatology: a color guide to diagnosis and therapy,* ed 3, St Louis, 1996, Mosby, pp 236-241.

Woolliscroft JO: *Current diagnosis and treatment: a quick reference for the general practitioner,* Philadelphia, 1996, Current Medicine, pp 364-365.

NOTES

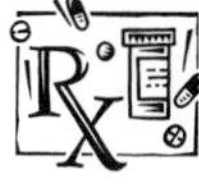

PHARMACOTHERAPEUTICS

Drug of Choice	Mechanism of Action	Prescribing Information	Side Effects
Dicloxacillin, 250 mg PO q6h × 10 days; children, 12.5-25 mg/kg/day divided q6h	Bactericidal cell wall inhibitor; active against gram-positive cocci except enterococci	***Contraindication:*** Hypersensitivity to penicillins ***Cost:*** 500-mg tab, 50 tabs: $19-$88 ***Pregnancy category:*** B	Bone marrow depression, granulocytopenia, nausea, vomiting, diarrhea, oliguria, proteinuria, hematuria, moniliasis, glomerulonephritis, lethargy, depression, convulsions, anaphylaxis
Erythromycin (E.E.S.), 250 mg PO q6h × 10 days; children, 30-50 mg/kg/day divided q6h	Macrolide; protein synthesis inhibitor; active against bacteria lacking cell walls, most gram-positive aerobes	***Contraindication:*** Hypersensitivity ***Cost:*** 250-mg tabs, 4/day × 10 days: $4 ***Pregnancy category:*** B	Nausea, vomiting, diarrhea, abdominal pain, anorexia, rash, urticaria, pseudomembranous colitis—rarely
Cefadroxil (Duricef), 500 mg PO bid × 10 days; children, 30 mg/kg/day PO in divided doses q12h	Cephalosporin; bactericidal; inhibits cell wall synthesis	***Contraindication:*** Hypersensitivity ***Cost:*** 500-mg tab, 50 tabs: $169 ***Pregnancy category:*** B	Diarrhea, pseudomembranous colitis, nausea, vomiting, rash, urticaria, angioedema, vaginitis, neutropenia, Stevens-Johnson syndrome, anaphylaxis, seizures

Influenza (Flu)

OVERVIEW

Influenza (flu) is an acute viral infection that affects the nasopharynx, conjunctiva, and respiratory tract. It is usually a self-limiting disease, with outbreaks occurring during the winter months.

Pathogenesis
- Cause—influenza virus types A, B, and C
- Transmission is from person to person through direct or indirect contact
- Incubation period—1 to 5 days

Patient Profile
- Males = Females
- Any age

Signs and Symptoms
- Abrupt onset
- High fever
- Malaise
- Myalgia
- Headache
- Sore throat
- Nonproductive cough
- Rhinorrhea
- Conjunctivitis
- Symptoms usually last 3 to 4 days; cough and malaise may linger 1 to 2 weeks

Differential Diagnosis
- Common cold
- Bronchitis
- Pneumonia
- Infectious mononucleosis
- Other viral infections

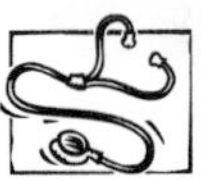

ASSESSMENT

History
Inquire about:
- Onset and duration of symptoms
- Other affected household members
- Status of influenza vaccine
- Underlying conditions
- Current medications

Physical Findings
- General—fever, ill appearance, dry mucous membranes or poor skin turgor if dehydrated, injected conjunctiva
- Enlarged cervical lymph nodes
- Nose—mucosa red; clear drainage; turbinates may be swollen
- Lungs—may be clear or have adventitious sounds

Initial Workup
Laboratory
- Consider CBC—leukopenia (leukocytosis may indicate secondary bacterial infection)
- Culture of nasopharyngeal secretions
- No laboratory tests are diagnostic; diagnosis based on history, physical findings, and epidemiologic data

Radiology: Consider chest film—PA and lateral—usually normal; may show basilar streaking or patchy infiltrate

Further Workup
Usually none needed

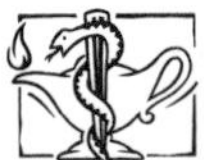

INTERVENTIONS

Office Treatment
None indicated

Lifestyle Modifications
- Smoking cessation
- Rest
- Increased fluids
- Good hand-washing technique

Patient Education
Teach patient about:
- Condition and treatment:
  - Fever control
  - Using saline nasal spray for congestion
- Proper hand washing and disposal of tissues to prevent spread
- Using a cool mist vaporizer to humidify air
- Tips for smoking cessation
- Prevention of disease through yearly vaccination
- Medications used and side effects (see Pharmacotherapeutics)

Referrals
Usually none needed

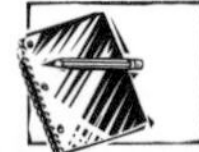

EVALUATION

Outcome
Usually resolves without sequelae

Possible Complications
- Secondary bacterial infections, such as otitis media, pneumonia, sinusitis, bronchitis, rhabdomyolysis
- Death

Follow-up
- Mild—none required
- More severe cases—weekly until symptoms resolve

FOR YOUR INFORMATION

Life Span
Pediatric: Do *not* give aspirin to children with influenza because of risk of Reye's syndrome

Geriatric: Higher morbidity and mortality—may require hospitalization

Pregnancy: Influenza vaccine should only be given to those women with medical problems that would place them at high risk for complications from influenza; if possible, vaccination should be delayed until after first trimester; benefits must outweigh risks

Miscellaneous
U.S. Department of Health and Human Services influenza vaccine guidelines:
- Groups at increased risk of complications from influenza:
  - ≥65 years of age
  - Residents of nursing homes or chronic care facilities
  - Chronic pulmonary or cardiovascular disorders—adults and children, including children with asthma
  - Chronic metabolic diseases, renal impairment, hemoglobinopathies or immunosuppression—adults and children
- Groups that can transmit influenza to high-risk individuals:
  - Health care providers—all settings
  - Nursing home and chronic care facility employees
  - Home care providers
  - Household members of high-risk individuals

References

Koster FT, Barker LR: Respiratory tract infections. In Barker LR, Burton JR, Zieve PD, editors: *Principles of ambulatory medicine,* ed 4, Baltimore, 1995, Williams & Wilkins, pp 331-333.

US Department of Health and Human Services: Public Health Service: *Clinician's handbook of preventive services: put prevention into practice,* Washington, DC, 1994, US Government Printing Office, pp 257-260.

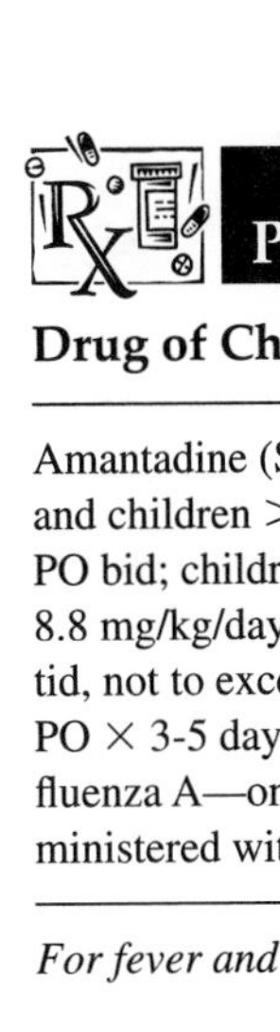

PHARMACOTHERAPEUTICS

Drug of Choice	Mechanism of Action	Prescribing Information	Side Effects
Amantadine (Symmetrel); adults and children >9 years, 100 mg PO bid; children 1-9 years, 4.4-8.8 mg/kg/day PO divided bid to tid, not to exceed 200 mg/day PO × 3-5 days; only for influenza A—only effective if administered within first 48 hours	Prevents penetration of virus into host by preventing uncoating of nucleic acid in viral cell	***Contraindications:*** Hypersensitivity; children <1 year; lactation ***Cost:*** 100-mg tab, 100 tabs: $19-$62 ***Pregnancy category:*** C	Headache, dizziness, fatigue, anxiety, hallucinations, convulsions, orthostatic hypotension, congestive heart failure (CHF), photosensitivity, blurred vision, leukopenia, nausea, vomiting, constipation, urinary frequency, urinary retention
For fever and myalgia, use one of the following:			
Acetaminophen (Tylenol), 325-650 mg PO q4-6h; for children, use Children's Tylenol—follow label directions	Decreases fever through action on hypothalamic heat-regulating center of brain; analgesia by increasing pain threshold	***Contraindications:*** Hypersensitivity; bleeding disorders or anticoagulant therapy; last trimester of pregnancy; asthma; gastric ulcers ***Cost:*** OTC ***Pregnancy category:*** Not categorized	Rash, hepatic toxicity with alcohol ingestion or overdose
Aspirin, 325-650 mg PO q4-6h—do not use in children or adolescents because of risk of Reye's syndrome	Analgesia via peripheral and central nervous systems; may inhibit prostaglandins; antipyretic—acts on hypothalamic system	***Contraindications:*** Hypersensitivity; bleeding disorders or anticoagulant therapy; last trimester of pregnancy; asthma; gastric ulcers ***Cost:*** OTC ***Pregnancy category:*** Not categorized	Rash, anaphylactic reaction, GI upset and bleeding, Reye's syndrome in children and adolescents
Influenza vaccine, whole- or split-virus types: adult and child >9 years, 0.5 ml IM × 1 dose—may give whole or split; children 3-9 years, 0.5 ml IM; children 6-35 months, 0.25 ml IM; if child not previously vaccinated, give 2nd dose 1 month after 1st dose	Produces antibodies to influenza vaccine; split vaccine causes fewer adverse reactions	***Contraindications:*** Hypersensitivity to eggs, chicken; active infection; Guillain-Barré syndrome ***Cost:*** 5-ml vial: $34-$48 ***Pregnancy category:*** C	Fever, Guillain-Barré syndrome, urticaria, erythema, anaphylaxis, malaise, myalgia

Insect Bites and Stings

OVERVIEW

Insect bites and stings affect people by inoculating poisons, invading tissue, and transmitting disease. This section discusses only the effects of irritative, poisonous, and allergic reactions of insect bites and stings.

Pathogenesis

Caused by arthropods, either allergic reaction (local tissue inflammation from poison) or toxic reaction from large inoculation of poison vectors—wasps, bees, ants, brown recluse spiders, black widow spiders, scorpions, mosquitoes, flies, lice, fleas, mites, ticks, caterpillars, centipedes

Patient Profile

- Males = Females
- All ages
- Seasonal

Signs and Symptoms

- Local reactions:
  - Erythema
  - Pain
  - Heat
  - Swelling
  - Itching
  - Blisters
  - Necrosis
  - Ulceration
  - Drainage
  - Secondary infection
- Toxic reactions:
  - Nausea, vomiting
  - Headache
  - Fever
  - Diarrhea
  - Lightheadedness
  - Syncope
  - Drowsiness
  - Muscles spasms
  - Edema
  - Convulsions
- Allergic systemic reactions:
  - Itching eyes
  - Facial flushing
  - Generalized urticaria
  - Dry cough
  - Chest/throat constriction
  - Wheezing
  - Dyspnea
  - Cyanosis
  - Abdominal cramps
  - Diarrhea
  - Nausea, vomiting
  - Vertigo
  - Chills/fever
  - Stridor
  - Shock
  - Loss of consciousness
  - Involuntary bowel/bladder activity
  - Frothy sputum
  - Respiratory failure
  - Cardiovascular collapse
  - Death
- Delayed reactions
  - Serum-sickness–like reactions
  - Fever, malaise
  - Headache
  - Urticaria
  - Lymphadenopathy
  - Polyarthritis

Differential Diagnosis

- Local reactions:
  - Cellulitis
  - Infection
  - Dermatoses
  - Punctures
  - Foreign bodies
- Toxic reactions:
  - Chemical exposure/ingestion
  - Medications
  - IV drug abuse
  - Environmental
- Allergic reactions:
  - Medications
  - Illicit drugs
  - Food
  - Topical products
  - Environmental
  - Plants
  - Chemicals

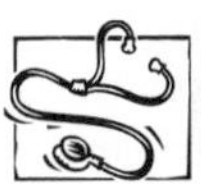

ASSESSMENT

History

Inquire about:

- Onset and duration of symptoms
- Exposure to arthropods
- History of stinging or biting sensation
- Prior history of reaction
- Treatments tried and results
- Last tetanus booster
- Underlying diseases
- Current medications

Physical Findings

Inflammation, ulceration, vesiculation, pustulation, rupture, eschar, swelling, usually very localized at site of bite or sting

Initial Workup

Laboratory

- CBC—leukocytosis, thrombocytopenia
- Urinalysis—proteinuria, hemoglobinuria, myoglobinuria

Radiology: None indicated

Further Workup

None indicated

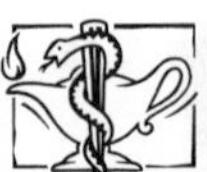

INTERVENTIONS

Office Treatment

- If severe reaction, activate 911 system and provide life support as needed
- For mild reactions:
  - Remove stinger and cleanse wound
  - Apply ice pack to bite or sting site (10 minutes on/10 minutes off)
  - Elevate affected part
  - Rest affected part
  - Give tetanus booster if indicated

Lifestyle Modification

Avoidance of areas with causative agents

Patient Education

Teach patient about:

- Condition and treatment—epinephrine, antihistamines, steroids
- Need to wear medical alert tag
- Using epinephrine for severe anaphylactic reactions
- Keeping epinephrine kit available at all times
- Using insect repellents
- Checking clothing, skin, and hair for insects when returning from outdoors
- Medications used and side effects (see Pharmacotherapeutics)

Referral

Immediately to emergency room for severe reactions

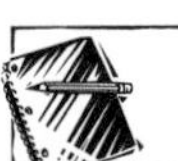

EVALUATION

Outcome

Resolves without complications

Possible Complications

- Infection
- Scarring
- Drug reactions
- Multisystem failure
- Death

Follow-up

In 72 hours; then in 1 week

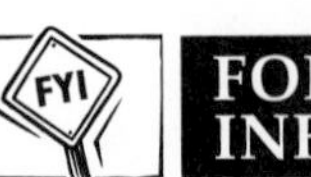

FOR YOUR INFORMATION

Life Span

Pediatric: Treatment is the same
Geriatric: Treatment is the same; higher morbidity and mortality
Pregnancy: Treatment is the same; monitor fetus closely

Miscellaneous

Patients who have very severe reactions to commonly encountered insects may need a referral to an allergist for desensitization with immunotherapy.

Reference

Habif TP: *Clinical dermatology: a color guide to diagnosis and therapy,* ed 3, St Louis, 1996, Mosby, pp 478-482.

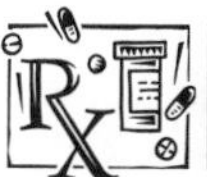

PHARMACOTHERAPEUTICS

Drug of Choice	Mechanism of Action	Prescribing Information	Side Effects
Epinephrine 1:1000; children, 0.01 ml/kg SQ; adults, 0.3-0.5 ml SQ; may need to carry epinephrine kit at all times	B_1 and B_2 agonist; produces bronchodilation and cardiac and CNS stimulation; large doses—vasoconstriction; small doses—vasodilation	***Contraindications:*** Hypersensitivity to sympathomimetics; narrow-angle glaucoma ***Cost:*** 0.1 mg/ml of 1:1000 sol, 10 ml: $12-$14 ***Pregnancy category:*** C	Urinary retention, tremors, anxiety, insomnia, headache, dizziness, cerebral hemorrhage, palpitations, tachycardia, hypertension, dysrhythmias, anorexia, nausea, vomiting, dyspnea
For pain, use one of the following:			
Acetaminophen (Tylenol), 325-650 mg q4-6h PO; for children, use Children's Tylenol—follow label directions	Decreases fever through action on hypothalamic heat-regulating center of brain; analgesia by increasing pain threshold	***Contraindication:*** Hypersensitivity ***Cost:*** OTC ***Pregnancy category:*** Not categorized	Anaphylaxis, leukopenia, neutropenia, drowsiness, nausea, vomiting, hepatotoxicity, rash, angioedema, urticaria, toxicity
Aspirin; adults only, 325-650 mg q4-6h PO	Analgesia via peripheral and central nervous systems; may inhibit prostaglandins; antipyretic—acts on hypothalamic system	***Contraindications:*** Hypersensitivity; bleeding disorders or anticoagulant therapy; last trimester of pregnancy; asthma; gastric ulcers ***Cost:*** OTC ***Pregnancy category:*** D	Rash, anaphylactic reaction, GI upset and bleeding, Reye's syndrome in children and adolescents, nausea, vomiting, hepatitis, tinnitus, hearing loss, wheezing, pulmonary edema
Ibuprofen (Motrin, Advil); dose varies with type of drug	Not well understood; may be related to inhibition of prostaglandin synthesis	***Contraindications:*** Aspirin allergy; hypersensitivity; asthma; last trimester of pregnancy; gastric ulcer; bleeding disorders ***Cost:*** 400-mg tab, 4/day × 5 days: $3 ***Pregnancy category:*** Not recommended	Nausea, heartburn, diarrhea, GI upset and bleeding, dizziness, headache, rash, tinnitus, edema, acute renal failure
Diphenhydramine (H_1) (Benadryl), 25-50 mg IV, IM, or PO q6h × 24 hours; children 2-6 years, 6.25 mg q4-6h; children 6-12 years, 12.5-25 mg q4-6h	Blocks histamine at H_1 receptor sites	***Contraindications:*** Hypersensitivity; acute asthma attack ***Cost:*** 25-mg tab, 100 tabs: $2-$20; 50-mg/ml, 10 ml: $4-$17 ***Pregnancy category:*** C	Dizziness, drowsiness, fatigue, anxiety, euphoria, increased thick secretions, wheezing, chest tightness, thrombocytopenia, agranulocytosis, hemolytic anemia, dry mouth, nausea, anorexia, photosensitivity, urinary retention, dysuria, blurred vision, dilated pupils, tinnitus, nasal stuffiness, dry nose, throat
For anaphylactoid reaction, may need both H_1 and H_2 receptor antagonists.			
Cimetidine (H_2) (Tagamet), 300 mg IV over 3-5 minutes—not recommended for children <16 years	Blocks histamine at H_2 receptor sites	***Contraindication:*** Hypersensitivity ***Cost:*** 300 mg/2 ml, 50 ml: $45-$100 ***Pregnancy category:*** B	Confusion, headache, depression, dizziness, anxiety, weakness, convulsions, bradycardia, tachycardia, diarrhea, paralytic ileus, jaundice, gynecomastia, agranulocytosis, thrombocytopenia, neutropenia, aplastic anemia, increased prothrombin time, urticaria, exfoliative dermatitis
Prednisone, 20-40 mg/day × 1 week	Corticosteroid; decreases inflammation	***Contraindications:*** Hypersensitivity; psychosis; idiopathic thrombocytopenia; acute glomerulonephritis; amebiasis; nonasthmatic bronchial disease; AIDS; TB; children <2 years old ***Cost:*** 15-mg tab, 100 tabs: $14-$35 ***Pregnancy category:*** C	Hypertension, circulatory collapse, thrombophlebitis, embolism, tachycardia, fungal infections, increased intraocular pressure, diarrhea, nausea, GI hemorrhage, thrombocytopenia, acne, poor wound healing, fractures, osteoporosis, weakness

Insomnia

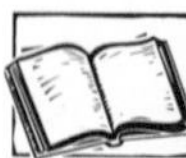

OVERVIEW

Insomnia is persistent difficulty in either falling asleep, staying asleep, or early-morning awakening, or it may be a combination of all three problems. Insomnia may be transient or chronic.

Pathogenesis

- 50% of cases from underlying psychiatric disorder
- 10% of cases from drug and/or alcohol abuse
- 10% of cases from underlying medical condition
- 10% of cases primary sleep disorder, such as sleep apnea or nocturnal myoclonus
- 20% of cases idiopathic

Patient Profile

- Males = Females
- More common in elderly, obese individuals and heavy smokers

Signs and Symptoms

- Fatigue, tiredness
- Daytime sleepiness
- Napping
- May have difficulty falling asleep
- Waking in middle of night
- "Tossing and turning"
- Waking early in morning

Differential Diagnosis

Look for possible cause

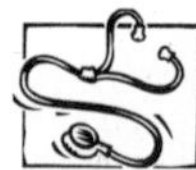

ASSESSMENT

History

Inquire about:

- Onset and duration of symptoms
- Recent stressful events
- Alcohol and drug use
- Pattern of insomnia (difficulty falling asleep, staying asleep, or waking early)
- Daytime napping
- Shift work
- History of psychiatric illness
- Frequent travel
- Number of hours in bed
- Treatments tried and results
- Interviewing a family member
- Underlying conditions
- Current medications

Physical Findings

Physical examination—within normal limits unless there is some underlying medical condition, such as arthritis, hyperthyroidism, gastroesophageal reflux disease, duodenal ulcer, or respiratory distress

Initial Workup

Laboratory: None for primary insomnia
Radiology: Chest film if indicated

Further Workup

Sleep studies

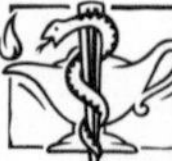

INTERVENTIONS

Office Treatment

None indicated

Lifestyle Modifications

- Smoking cessation
- Caffeine withdrawal
- Avoidance of heavy, late-night snacks
- No alcohol after 5 PM
- Exercise program

Patient Education

Teach patient about:

- Condition and treatment options:
  - If specific cause found, treat underlying condition
  - If no underlying cause, patient to keep sleep diary for 2 weeks; include bedtime, hours in bed, time when sleep initiated, hours slept, number of awakenings, time of arising, quality of sleep
- Establishing a bedtime routine
- No daytime napping
- Starting a regular exercise program (not close to bedtime)
- Unwinding before going to bed
- No reading or watching TV in bed
- Avoidance of caffeine, alcohol, nicotine, and stimulating medications just before bedtime
- Medications used and side effects (see Pharmacotherapeutics)

Referral

For counseling if underlying psychologic problem

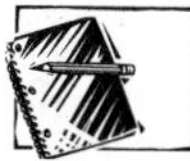

EVALUATION

Outcome
Resolves without sequelae in 3 to 4 weeks

Possible Complications
- Becomes chronic
- Increased daytime sleepiness

Follow-up
In 2 weeks × 2; if no improvement, consider counseling

FOR YOUR INFORMATION

Life Span
Pediatric: Very rare; look for underlying cause, such as enuresis
Geriatric: Educate regarding age-related changes in sleep
Pregnancy: May experience insomnia in later stages of pregnancy because of difficulty in finding a comfortable position

Miscellaneous
The use of medication should be reserved for only the most severe cases of insomnia that may or may not have an underlying cause.

References
Goldberg RJ: *Practical guide to the care of the psychiatric patient,* St Louis, 1995, Mosby, pp 119-131.

Neubauer DN, Smith PL, Early CJ: Sleep disorders. In Barker LR, Burton JR, Zieve PD, editors: *Principles of ambulatory medicine,* ed 4, Baltimore, 1995, Williams & Wilkins, pp 1257-1271.

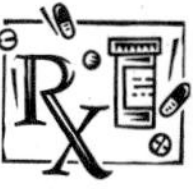

PHARMACOTHERAPEUTICS

Drug of Choice	Mechanism of Action	Prescribing Information	Side Effects
Diphenhydramine (Benadryl), 25-50 mg PO hs; children 6-12 years, 12.5-25 mg PO hs	Competes with histamine for H_1-receptor sites	***Contraindications:*** Hypersensitivity; acute asthma attack; lower respiratory tract disease ***Cost:*** 25-mg tab, 100 tabs, $4 ***Pregnancy category:*** C	Dizziness, drowsiness, anxiety, euphoria, confusion, wheezing, thrombocytopenia, agranulocytosis, hemolytic anemia, dry mouth, nausea, anorexia, urinary retention, dysuria, blurred vision, dilated pupils, tinnitus, nasal stuffiness
Zolpidem (Ambien), 5 mg PO hs, maximum dose 10 mg; for short-term treatment, 7-10 days—safety in children <18 years not established	Sedative-hypnotic; produces CNS depression at limbic, thalamic, and hypothalamic levels	***Contraindication:*** Hypersensitivity to benzodiazepines ***Cost:*** 10-mg tab, 1/day × 7 days: $11 ***Pregnancy category:*** B	Leukopenia, headache, lethargy, daytime sedation, dizziness, confusion, anxiety, irritability, amnesia, nausea, vomiting, diarrhea, chest pain, palpitations
Triazolam (Halcion), 0.125 mg PO hs, maximum dose 0.25 mg; has shortest half-life—safety in children <18 years not established	Benzodiazepine; CNS depression at limbic, thalamic, and hypothalamic levels	***Contraindications:*** Hypersensitivity to benzodiazepines; pregnancy; lactation; intermittent porphyria ***Cost:*** 0.125-mg tab, 50 tabs: $30-$60 ***Pregnancy category:*** X	Leukopenia, headache, lethargy, drowsiness, daytime sedation, dizziness, confusion, lightheadedness, amnesia, poor coordination, nausea, vomiting, diarrhea, heartburn, abdominal pain, chest pain, pulse changes
Amitriptyline (Elavil), 50-100 mg PO hs, maximum dose 200 mg hs; adolescents, 30 mg PO hs; may increase up to 150 mg hs—do not use in children <12 years	Antidepressant; blocks reuptake of norepinephrine and serotonin	***Contraindications:*** Hypersensitivity to tricyclic antidepressants; recovery phase of myocardial infarction (MI) ***Cost:*** 50-mg tabs, 1/day × 90 days: $3-$10 ***Pregnancy category:*** C	Agranulocytosis, thrombocytopenia, eosinophilia, leukopenia, dizziness, drowsiness, confusion, headache, anxiety, tremors, extrapyramidal symptoms, diarrhea, dry mouth, nausea, vomiting, paralytic ileus, hepatitis, increased appetite, urine retention, rash, urticaria, orthostatic hypotension, ECG changes, tachycardia, hypertension, blurred vision, tinnitus

Insulin-Dependent Diabetes Mellitus (IDDM)

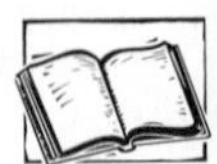

OVERVIEW

Insulin-dependent diabetes mellitus (IDDM), also referred to as type I diabetes, is a chronic condition characterized by the body's inability to produce enough insulin to maintain the blood glucose level within normal range. This lack of insulin leads to hyperglycemia and end-organ damage, such as nephropathy, neuropathy, retinopathy, and accelerated atherosclerosis. IDDM is characterized by insulinopenia, which, if left untreated, results in ketoacidosis.

Pathogenesis

Cause—autoimmune process—results in progressive destruction of beta cells; islet cell antibodies and insulin autoantibodies cause destruction

Patient Profile

- Males = Females
- Age—normally begins in childhood around adolescence; can occur at any age
- Hereditary factors not as important in IDDM as in non–insulin-dependent diabetes mellitus

Signs and Symptoms

Signs and symptoms develop abruptly and include polyuria, polydypsia, polyphagia, anorexia, weight loss (patients with IDDM are usually very thin), increased fatigue, muscle cramps, irritability, emotional lability, headaches, anxiety attacks, chest pain, vision changes, abdominal discomfort/pain, nausea, diarrhea

Differential Diagnosis

- Non–insulin-dependent diabetes mellitus
- Glucose intolerance
- Benign renal glycosuria
- Secondary diabetes—pancreatic diseases, hormonal disorders, inborn errors of metabolism, genetic disorders, obesity, cytogenetic syndromes, drug or chemical-induced glucose intolerance, acute poisonings such as salicylate poisoning

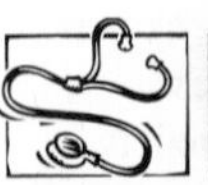

ASSESSMENT

History

Inquire about:

- Onset and duration of symptoms
- Family history of diabetes
- Underlying conditions
- Current medications, including OTC medications
- Dietary intake of caffeine, sugar-containing syrups, fish oils
- Use of the following drugs, which may cause hyperglycemia (particularly in patients prone to diabetes): glucagon, glucocorticoids, growth hormone, epinephrine, estrogen and progesterone, thyroid preparations, thiazide diuretics, furosemide, acetazolamide, diazoxide, beta-blockers, alpha-agonists, calcium channel blockers, phenytoin, phenobarbital sodium, nicotinic acid, cyclophosphamide, I-asparaginase, decongestant and diet pills, nonsteroidal antiinflammatory agents, nicotine

Physical Findings

- Findings may be subjective
- Patients usually thin with little body fat
- May find retinal changes on fundoscopic examination

Initial Workup

Laboratory

- Blood glucose level—elevated
- Urinanalysis—glucose and ketones present
- CBC—WBC count may be elevated
- Hemoglobin A1C
- C-peptide insulin level
- Islet-cell antibodies

Radiology: None indicated

Further Workup

Oral glucose tolerance test if diagnosis questionable; many clinicians use 2-hour postprandial test after a high-sugar meal for diagnosis

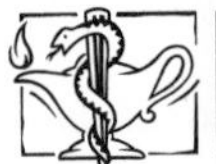

INTERVENTIONS

Office Treatment

None indicated

Lifestyle Modifications

- Diabetic diet
- Smoking cessation
- Regular aerobic exercise
- Adjustment to administering injections and monitoring blood glucose
- Adjustment to living with a chronic illness

Patient Education

- Teach patient about:
  - Disease process and possible complications of diabetes—nephropathy, retinopathy, accelerated atherosclerosis, neuropathy, etc.
  - Diabetic diet
  - Administering insulin injections and, if necessary, how to mix insulins
  - Performing blood glucose monitoring
  - Signs and symptoms of hyperglycemic/hypoglycemic reactions
  - Proper foot care and why necessary
  - Proper diet for child—needs to be adjusted to meet age requirements
  - Ongoing process of education and that each visit will have a question-and-answer period to help with problems
  - Treatment options—2, 3, or 4 insulin injections per day using an intermediate-, long-, or short-acting insulin or, for selected individuals, an insulin pump
  - Condition being lifelong and that, at the present time, there is no cure
  - Medications used and side effects (see Pharmacotherapeutics)
- For children, parents need to be included in the teaching
- Teach child and parents that a "normal" life is possible—school attendance, goals, and career plans should be encouraged
- Instruct parents to allow child to participate in his or her care as much as possible

Referrals

- To dietitian
- To social worker
- To diabetes educator
- If resistant to treatment, may need referral to endocrinologist

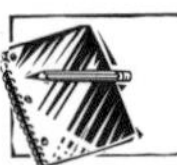

EVALUATION

Outcomes

- Normoglycemia
- Monitor hemoglobin A1C—ideal is for level to be within normal limits
- Current research has demonstrated that tight control can slow progression of end-organ damage
- Tight control can also lead to more episodes of hypoglycemia, long-term effects of which are unknown
- Patient will continue to lead a normal, productive life

Possible Complications

- Hyperlipidemia
- Microvascular diseases
- Macrovascular diseases
- Foot problems
- Hypoglycemia
- Diabetic ketoacidosis
- Psychologic problems related to chronic disease

Follow-up

- Weekly until control is achieved; then every 2 weeks × 1 month; then monthly × 2 months; then every 3 months
- Teaching needs to be incorporated into every clinic visit
- Monitor hemoglobin A1C and do foot examination every 3 months
- Yearly chemistry panel to measure lipids, renal function, thyroid function
- Yearly eye examination

FOR YOUR INFORMATION

Life Span

Pediatric: Onset of type I common
Geriatric: May have difficulty performing glucose monitoring and administering insulin because of various aspects of aging, such as decreased visual acuity or arthritis
Pregnancy: Needs close monitoring and to be followed by specialist.

Miscellaneous

The diagnosis of diabetes can have a major impact on the patient and family. The NP needs to treat the psychosocial aspects of the disease, as well as the physical aspects.

References

The Diabetes Control and Complications Trial Research Group: The effect of intensive treatment of diabetes on the development and progression of long-term complications in insulin-dependent diabetes mellitus, *N Engl J Med* 329(14):977-986, 1993.

Gregerman RI: Diabetes mellitus. In Barker LR, Burton JR, Zieve PD, editors: *Principles of ambulatory medicine,* ed 4, Baltimore, 1995, Williams & Wilkins, pp 977-1018.

Valentine V: Patient with diabetes. In Lewis SM, Collier IC, Heitkemper MM, editors: *Medical-surgical nursing: assessment and management of clinical problems,* ed 4, St Louis, 1996, Mosby, pp 1438-1474.

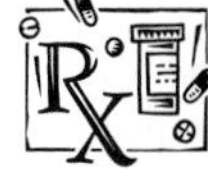

PHARMACOTHERAPEUTICS

The patient with insulin-dependent diabetes has an absolute deficiency in insulin and requires insulin replacement for treatment. There are many treatment regimens used for diabetes and also a wide variety of insulin preparations available. To provide information on all of the available preparations is beyond the scope of this book; only the three main types of insulin are presented: short-acting (regular), intermediate-acting (NPH or Lente), and long-acting (Ultralente). For more detailed information, consult another reference. The most common treatment used is 2 insulin injections per day, with two thirds of the daily requirement given in the morning and the remaining one third given in the evening. For intensive therapy, 3 or more injections are used. The 2-injection regimen consist of two thirds intermediate-acting insulin (NPH or Lente) and one third short-acting insulin (regular). To calculate the amount of insulin needed, find the patient's weight in kilograms and multiply that by 0.4 to 0.6 units of insulin, basing the number used on the patient's body size. For instance, if the patient is 5 foot 1 inch tall and weighs 50 kg, use 0.4 units/kg; in this example, the patient would require a total of 20 units of insulin per day. Two thirds of this would be 13 units in the morning, and one third would be 7 units in the evening. These numbers are then broken down to determine the amount of NPH and regular insulin to use. Using the above formula, the morning dose of 13 units would be administered as 9 units of NPH and 4 units of regular insulin, and the evening dose of 7 units total would be 5 units of NPH and 2 units of regular insulin.

Drug of Choice	Mechanism of Action	Prescribing Information	Side Effects
Regular insulin (human, pork, or pork/beef); see above for dosages; administer SQ or IV	Replaces body's natural insulin; onset of action 30 minutes-1 hour; peak effect 2-4 hours; duration of action 5-7 hours	***Contraindication:*** Hypersensitivity to beef or pork ***Cost:*** 100 U/ml, 10 ml: $16-$18 ***Pregnancy category:*** B	Hypoglycemia; hyperglycemia if dosage is inadequate; lipodystrophy; increased exercise can decrease insulin requirements
NPH insulin (intermediate-acting; available in human and purified pork); administered SQ only; see above for dosages	Replaces body's natural insulin; onset of action 3-4 hours; peak action 6-12 hours; duration of action 18-28 hours	***Contraindication:*** Hypersensitivity to pork ***Cost:*** 100 U/ml, 10 ml: $16-$17 ***Pregnancy category:*** B	Hypoglycemia, particularly if regular meals not eaten; hyperglycemia if dosage too low; lipodystrophy
Lente insulin (intermediate-acting; available in human and purified pork); administered SQ only; see above for dosages	Replaces body's natural insulin; onset of action 1-3 hours; peak action 8-12 hours; duration of action 18-28 hours	***Contraindication:*** Hypersensitivity to pork ***Cost:*** 100 U/ml, 10 ml: $16-$17 ***Pregnancy category:*** B	Hypoglycemic reaction, especially if meals not eaten regularly; hyperglycemia if dosage too low; lipodystrophy
Ultralente insulin (long-acting; available in human and purified pork); administered SQ only; see above for dosages	Replaces body's natural insulin; onset of action 4-6 hours; peak action 18-24 hours; duration of action 36 hours	***Contraindication:*** Hypersensitivity to pork ***Cost:*** 100 U/ml, 10 ml: $16-$17 ***Pregnancy category:*** B	Hypoglycemia if patient not eating regular meals; hyperglycemia if dosage too low; lipodystrophy

There are also combination preparations available: 70/30 and 50/50. The 70/30 preparation is 70% NPH and 30% regular, and the 50/50 preparation is 50% NPH and 50% regular. With these preparations, the patient does not have to mix the two different types of insulin.

Irritable Bowel Syndrome (IBS)

OVERVIEW

Irritable bowel syndrome (IBS) is a chronic disorder of the gastrointestinal (GI) system characterized by altered bowel habits (diarrhea and/or constipation), abdominal pain, and gaseousness in the absence of a detectable pathologic condition.

Pathogenesis

- Exact cause unknown
- Patient has abnormal gut motility with increased response to stress and stimulants

Patient Profile

- Females > Males
- Predominant age—late teens and 20s
- Rare for onset after age 50 years

Signs and Symptoms

- Abdominal pain—lower part of abdomen associated with change in consistency or frequency of stools and relieved by defecation (hallmark of IBS)
- Mucus in stools
- Constipation
- Diarrhea
- Increased symptoms after eating
- Abdominal distention
- Gas
- Urgency of defecation
- Nausea, vomiting

Differential Diagnosis

- Ulcerative colitis
- Crohn's disease
- Lactose intolerance
- Infections
- Diverticula
- Celiac sprue
- Adenocarcinoma of colon
- Hypothyroidism/hyperthyroidism
- Diabetes mellitus

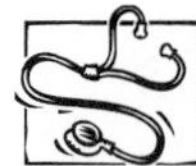

ASSESSMENT

History

Inquire about:

- Onset and duration of symptoms
- Predominant symptom—abdominal pain, constipation, diarrhea
- Blood in diarrheal stool or waking at night with diarrhea (if yes to either question, consider inflammatory bowel disease)
- Weight loss (should not occur)
- Stressors in life
- Diet history
- Bloating or gaseousness with eating
- Family history
- Underlying conditions
- Current medications

Physical Findings

- May be no abnormal findings or tenderness in (L) lower abdominal quadrant
- May have excessive tenderness on rectal examination

Initial Workup

Laboratory

- CBC
- Erythrocyte sedimentation rate
- Stool for occult blood
- Stool for ova and parasites
- Tests used to rule out other conditions
- All normal in irritable bowel syndrome

Radiology: Severe symptoms—barium enema

Further Workup

Severe symptoms—sigmoidoscopy

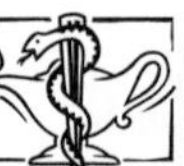

INTERVENTIONS

Office Treatment

None indicated

Lifestyle Modifications

- Smoking cessation
- Increased dietary fiber
- Stress management

Patient Education

Teach patient about:

- Condition and treatment—balanced diet with increased fiber, avoiding aggravating foods, bulking agents
- Tips for smoking cessation
- Stress reduction techniques—biofeedback, relaxation techniques
- Medications (antispasmodic agents) used and side effects (see Pharmacotherapeutics)

Referral

To MD if above therapy fails

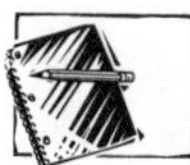

EVALUATION

Outcome
Patient able to manage symptoms, which will recur throughout life, especially in times of stress

Possible Complications
Usually none

Follow-up
Every 2 weeks until symptoms improve; then every 6 months

FOR YOUR INFORMATION

Life Span
Pediatric: Possibility exists that recurrent abdominal pain in childhood is a form of IBS or leads to IBS
Geriatric: Onset rare after age 50; consider another diagnosis
Pregnancy: Symptoms may worsen during pregnancy

Miscellaneous
IBS is thought to be the most common GI disorder seen in primary care.

References

Dalton C, Drossman DA: Calming the irritable bowel: close-up on new diagnostic criteria, *Adv Nurse Pract* 4(12):30-34, 1996.

Schuster MM: Irritable bowel syndrome. In Barker LR, Burton JR, Zieve PD, editors: *Principles of ambulatory medicine,* ed 4, Baltimore, 1995, Williams & Wilkins, pp 492-499.

NOTES

PHARMACOTHERAPEUTICS

Drug of Choice	Mechanism of Action	Prescribing Information	Side Effects
To give stool bulk:			
Psyllium (Metamucil), 1-2 tsp in 8 oz water PO bid or tid; children >6 years, 1 tsp in 4 oz water PO; may help reduce incontinence	Bulk-forming laxative	***Contraindications:*** Hypersensitivity; intestinal obstruction; abdominal pain; nausea, vomiting; fecal impaction ***Cost:*** OTC ***Pregnancy category:*** C	Nausea, vomiting, diarrhea, cramps
For gas control:			
Mylanta Gas Relief, 1 tablet PO qid pc and hs; tablets should be thoroughly chewed—not for use in children	High-capacity antiflatulent	***Contraindication:*** Hypersensitivity ***Cost:*** OTC ***Pregnancy category:*** Not categorized	None known
Dicyclomine (Bentyl); adult, 10-20 mg PO tid-qid; children >2 years, 10 mg PO tid-qid; children 6 months-2 years, 5 mg PO tid-qid	Antispasmodic, anticholinergic	***Contraindications:*** Hypersensitivity to anticholinergics; narrow-angle glaucoma; GI obstruction; myasthenia gravis; paralytic ileus; GI atony; toxic megacolon ***Cost:*** 20-mg tab, 100 tabs: $2-$30 ***Pregnancy category:*** B	Confusion, stimulation in the elderly, headache, insomnia, dizziness, seizures, coma, dry mouth, constipation, paralytic ileus, heartburn, nausea, vomiting, dysphagia, urinary hesitancy or retention, palpitations, blurred vision, photophobia, cycloplegia, urticaria, rash, pruritus, anhidrosis, fever

Juvenile Rheumatoid Arthritis/Still's Disease

OVERVIEW

Juvenile rheumatoid arthritis is a form of rheumatoid arthritis that occurs in children. The different types are systemic (20%), pauciarticular (30%), and polyarticular (50%).

Pathogenesis

Causes: multifactorial—abnormal immune response, genetic predisposition, environmental triggers, infections

Patient Profile

- Females > Males
- Most common ages—1 to 4 years and 9 to 14 years

Signs and Symptoms

SYSTEMIC TYPE

- Spiking fevers
- Rash
- Arthralgias
- Chest pain
- Fatigue
- Pericarditis
- Myocarditis
- Generalized lymphadenopathy
- Splenomegaly

PAUCIARTICULAR TYPE

- Arthralgias of larger joints; ≤4 joints involved
- Eye pain, redness (uveitis)
- Leg length difference
- Morning stiffness
- Abnormal gait

POLYARTICULAR TYPE

- Arthralgias, symmetric involvement of small joints of hands and feet
- Cervical spine involvement common
- Cold intolerance
- Fatigue
- Growth retardation
- Rheumatoid nodules
- Synovial cysts and thickening
- Limited range of motion

Differential Diagnosis

- Systemic lupus erythematosus
- Hemoglobinopathies
- Malignancy
- Rheumatic fever
- Lyme disease
- Sympathetic dystrophy

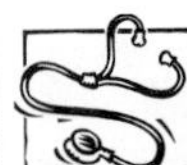

ASSESSMENT

History

Inquire about:

- Onset and duration of symptoms
- Fever and rash
- Family history
- Underlying conditions
- Current medications

Physical Findings

SYSTEMIC TYPE

- Joint pain with range of motion
- Fever
- Weight loss
- Rash
- Enlarged inguinal and cervical lymph nodes
- Pericardial friction rub
- Abdominal examination—splenomegaly

PAUCIARTICULAR TYPE

- Abnormal gait
- Leg length difference
- Large joint pain with range of motion (≤4 joints)
- Joint swelling
- Eye pain, redness (uveitis—needs prompt referral to opthalmologist)

POLYARTICULAR TYPE

- Symmetric joint pain on range of motion
- Delayed growth
- Weak hand grips
- Weight loss

Initial Workup

Laboratory

- CBC with differential:
  - Leukocytes—normal or elevated (systemic)
  - Hemoglobin—normal or low (systemic)
  - Platelet count—normal or elevated
- Antinuclear antibody (ANA)—positive in 40% (polyarticular or pauciarticular)
- Erythrocyte sedimentation rate (ESR)—elevated
- Rheumatoid factor—positive in only 10% of cases

Radiology: Plain films of involved joints—osteoporosis; joint destruction minimal, with erosions and cysts

Further Workup

Joint aspiration if indicated

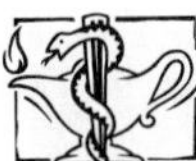

INTERVENTIONS

Office Treatment

None indicated

Lifestyle Modifications

- Home exercise program
- Keeping warm when sleeping to prevent morning stiffness

Patient Education

Teach patient about:

- Disease and treatment
- Importance of home exercise program
- Keeping joints warm to prevent morning stiffness
- Maintaining previous lifestyle as much as possible
- Well-balanced diet with adequate calcium, iron, and protein
- Importance of regular ophthalmic examinations for patients with pauciarticular type
- Medications used and side effects (see Pharmacotherapeutics)

Referrals

- To rheumatologist if resistant to treatment with NSAIDs
- To social worker
- To physical therapist
- To counselor

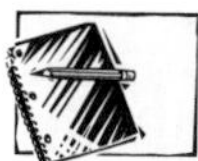

EVALUATION

Outcomes

- 70% to 80% of patients will go into remission
- Functional ability dependent on severity

Possible Complications

- Debilitating joint disease
- Blindness
- Glaucoma
- Side effects of treatment

Follow-up

Every 2 weeks × 2; then every 3 to 4 months if stable

FOR YOUR INFORMATION

Life Span

Pediatric: Disease can have major impact on child's psychosocial development
Geriatric: N/A
Pregnancy: Should be seen by a specialist

Miscellaneous

The goal of treatment is to maintain musculoskeletal function at as near normal as possible.

References

Hellman DB: Arthritis and musculoskeletal disorders. In Tierney LM Jr, McPhee SJ, Papadakis MA, editors: *Current medical diagnosis and treatment,* ed 34, Norwalk, Conn, 1995, Appleton & Lange, pp 716-717.

Mercier LR: *Practical orthopedics,* ed 4, St Louis, 1995, Mosby, pp 285-286.

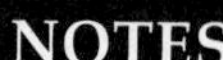

NOTES

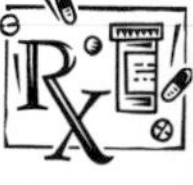

PHARMACOTHERAPEUTICS

Drug of Choice	Mechanism of Action	Prescribing Information	Side Effects
Aspirin, 75-90 mg/kg/day PO in divided doses—do not use if viral infection present	Antiinflammatory action may be caused by inhibition of synthesis and release of prostaglandins	***Contraindications:*** Hypersensitivity; GI bleeding; bleeding disorders ***Cost:*** OTC ***Pregnancy category:*** Should not be used in 3rd trimester	Dyspepsia, thirst, nausea, vomiting, GI bleeding/ulceration, tinnitus, vertigo, reversible hearing loss, prolongation of bleeding time, leukopenia, thrombocytopenia, purpura, urticaria, angioedema, pruritus, asthma, anaphylaxis, mental confusion, drowsiness, dizziness, headache, fever
Other nonsteroidal antiinflammatory drugs (NSAIDs): usually ibuprofen, 40 mg/kg/day PO in divided doses, or naproxen, 10-20 mg/kg/day PO in divided doses	Exact action unknown; may result from inhibition of synthesis of prostaglandins and arachidonic acid	***Contraindications:*** Hypersensitivity to NSAIDs, aspirin; severe hepatic failure; asthma ***Cost:*** Varies with type ***Pregnancy category:*** Depends on product	Stomach distress, flatulence, nausea, abdominal pain, constipation or diarrhea, dizziness, sedation, rash, urticaria, angioedema, anorexia, urinary frequency, increased blood pressure, insomnia, anxiety, visual disturbances, increased thirst, alopecia

Kaposi's Sarcoma

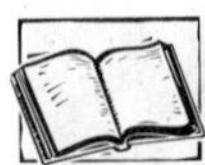

OVERVIEW

Kaposi's sarcoma is a malignant skin lesion. The different types of Kaposi's sarcoma are classic, African cutaneous, African lymphadenopathic, AIDS, and immunosuppressive.

Pathogenesis

- Classic and AIDS-associated type—may be caused by a new herpesvirus
- Other types—cause is unknown

Patient Profile

CLASSIC TYPE

- Males > Females (3:1)
- Age 50 to 70 years
- Jewish, Greek, or Italian descent

AFRICAN CUTANEOUS TYPE

- Females > Males
- Age <10 years or >20 years

AFRICAN LYMPHADENOPATHIC TYPE

- Females > Males
- Age <10 years

AIDS–ASSOCIATED TYPE

- Males > Females
- Age 25 to 42 years

IMMUNOSUPPRESSIVE TYPE

- Males > Females (10:1)
- Age 20 to 80 years

Signs and Symptoms

CLASSIC TYPE

- Site—feet and lower legs
- Violet-colored macules and papules progress to plaques with red-purple nodules

AFRICAN CUTANEOUS TYPE

- Site—extremities, lower legs
- Purple nodules

AFRICAN LYMPHADENOPATHIC TYPE

- Site—nodes
- Lymphadenopathy

AIDS-ASSOCIATED TYPE

- Site—head, neck, upper aspect of trunk
- Initially—raised, oval or elongated, rust-colored infiltrates; rapidly progress to red-purple nodules with plaques to follow
- Node involvement common

IMMUNOSUPPRESSIVE TYPE

- Site—variable
- Red-purple nodules

Differential Diagnosis

Bacillary angiomatosis

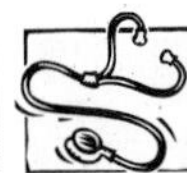

ASSESSMENT

History

Inquire about:

- Onset and duration of symptoms
- Living in Zaire or Uganda
- HIV status
- History of immunosuppressive drug treatment, such as for transplant patient
- Underlying diseases
- Current medications

Physical Findings

- Depends on type, but all will have a red-purple macule or papule with or without nodules
- May find lymphadenopathy
- Need to examine entire skin surface thoroughly

Initial Workup

Laboratory: Usually none, unless looking for underlying condition—HIV

Radiology: CT scan of chest and abdomen for visceral involvement

Further Workup

Usually none

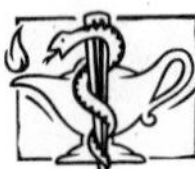

INTERVENTIONS

Office Treatment

- Cryotherapy—3 treatments 3 weeks apart—may have blister formation (avoid fluid in blisters—may contain HIV virus; probably won't be done by NP)
- Counseling and support important

Lifestyle Modifications

- Smoking cessation
- Good hygiene if immunosuppressed
- Need to remain active as long as possible
- Need help getting affairs in order
- May need assistance in preparing for death

Patient Education

Teach patient about:

- Disease, prognosis, and treatment:
  - Classic type—10 year survival
  - Other types—poor prognosis
  - Reducing or stopping immunosuppressive medication (risk acute rejection in transplant patient)
  - Cryotherapy
  - Intralesional chemotherapy
  - Surgical excision
  - Radiotherapy
  - Systemic chemotherapy
- Medications used and side effects (see Pharmacotherapeutics)

Referral

To oncologist or dermatologist

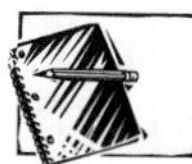

EVALUATION

Outcomes
- Good cosmetic effect
- Improved quality of life
- Patient accepts prognosis and is able to put affairs in order

Possible Complications
Debility and death

Follow-up
- By specialist for treatment
- By NP for counseling, possibly weekly

FOR YOUR INFORMATION

Life Span
Pediatric: Uncommon in this age group
Geriatric: Classic type most commonly seen in this age group
Pregnancy: Specialist must handle; may need to make decision regarding fetus

Miscellaneous
Homosexual men have a greater than 30% incidence of developing AIDS-related Kaposi's sarcoma. Also, it has been found that homosexual men who live in or travel to San Francisco, Los Angeles, or New York City are far more likely to develop AIDs-related Kaposi's sarcoma.

References

Habif TP: *Clinical dermatology: a color guide to diagnosis and therapy,* ed 3, St Louis, 1996, Mosby, pp 733-734.

Huether SE, Kravitz M: Structure, function, and disorders of the integument. In McCance KL, Huether SE, editors: *Pathophysiology: the biological basis for disease in adults and children,* ed 2, St Louis, 1994, Mosby, pp 1542-1544.

NOTES

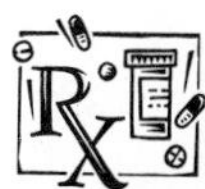

PHARMACOTHERAPEUTICS

Drug of Choice	Mechanism of Action	Prescribing Information	Side Effects
Doxorubicin (Adriamycin), bleomycin (Blenoxane), vinblastine (Velban), vincristine (Oncovin); dosage individualized for each patient; given intralesionally or IV	Doxorubicin—probably binds to DNA and inhibits nucleic acid synthesis; bleomycin—exact mechanism unknown, but main mode is inhibition of DNA; vinblastine—interferes with metabolic pathways of amino acids; vincristine—arrests dividing cells	***Contraindications:*** Doxorubicin—marked myelosuppression; bleomycin— hypersensitivity; vinblastine—significant granulocytopenia, bacterial infections; vincristine—demyelinating form of Charcot-Marie-Tooth disease ***Cost:*** Doxorubicin—20-mg vial: $92-$96; bleomycin—15-U ampule: $280; vinblastine—1 mg/ml, 10 ml: $21-$35; vincristine—1 mg/ml, 5 ml: $57-$73 ***Pregnancy category:*** D	Myelosuppression, impairment of fertility, mutagenic, cardiotoxicity, reversible alopecia, acute severe nausea and vomiting, stomatitis, anorexia, diarrhea, hypersensitivity

Keloids

OVERVIEW

A keloid is an unusually large, hypertrophic scar that does not subside on its own.

Pathogenesis

- Overgrowth of fibrous tissue
- Caused by injury or surgery

Patient Profile

- Males = Females
- African-Americans, Hispanics, Asians > Caucasians
- All ages

Signs and Symptoms

May be asymptomatic or may have pain, tenderness, hyperesthesia, pruritis

Differential Diagnosis

- Hypertrophic scar (usually regresses spontaneously)
- Dermatofibroma
- Infiltrating basal cell carcinoma

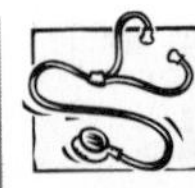

ASSESSMENT

History

Inquire about:

- Onset and duration of symptoms
- Previous injury or surgery at site
- Previous keloids
- Family history of keloids
- Ethnic background
- Treatments tried and results
- Underlying conditions
- Current medications

Physical Findings

- Firm, smooth, elevated scar with sharply demarcated borders
- Most common sites—chest, back, earlobe, face from acne

Initial Workup

Laboratory: None indicated
Radiology: None indicated

Further Workup

None indicated

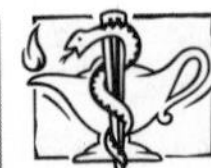

INTERVENTIONS

Office Treatment

Fresh, small, narrow lesions—intralesional steroid injections with triamcinolone acetate; use 25- to 27-gauge needle with TB syringe; disperse steroid by injecting while advancing needle; pressure of injection should be firm until lesion blanches (most commonly *not* performed by NP)

Lifestyle Modifications

- Cessation of body piercing
- Safety measures to avoid injuries

Patient Education

Teach patient about:

- Condition and treatment
  - Intralesional steroid injections
  - Surgery in combination with intralesional steroid injections
  - Cryotherapy
  - Silicone gel sheeting (used for fresh surgical incisions)
- Results of therapy—does not always result in resolution and recurrence is common
- Medications used and side effects (see Pharmacotherapeutics)

Referral

To surgeon, dermatologist, or plastic surgeon for more extensive keloids

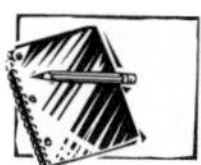

EVALUATION

Outcome
Resolution of keloid

Possible Complication
Recurrence of keloid

Follow-up
Reinject with steroid every 4 weeks until resolution

FOR YOUR INFORMATION

Life Span
Pediatric: More common in adolescents
Geriatric: Treatment is the same
Pregnancy: May be best to withhold treatment until after delivery

Miscellaneous
Compressive pressure dressings immediately after injury, as well as local steroid injection postoperatively, may be beneficial in the high-risk patient.

References
Habif TP: *Clinical dermatology: a color guide to diagnosis and therapy,* ed 3, St Louis, 1996, Mosby, p 637.

Lewis SL: Nursing role in management: cell injury and inflammation. In Lewis SM, Collier IC, Heitkemper MM, editors: *Medical-surgical nursing: assessment and management of clinical problems,* ed 4, St Louis, 1996, Mosby, p 196.

NOTES

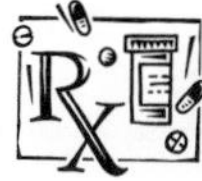

PHARMACOTHERAPEUTICS

Drug of Choice	Mechanism of Action	Prescribing Information	Side Effects
Triamcinolone acetonide (Kenalog), 10 mg/ml solution; inject 1 ml in each lesion; treat up to 3 lesions; if no response, may need higher dose	Antiinflammatory	***Contraindications:*** Hypersensitivity; systemic fungal infection ***Cost:*** 10 mg/ml, 5 ml: $7 ***Pregnancy category:*** C	Skin atrophy; ulceration; depigmentation; telangiectasias; systemic absorption with adrenal suppression—rare with 10 mg/ml dosage; burning; itching; irritation; sodium and fluid retention; osteoporosis; muscle weakness; congestive heart failure (CHF); hypertension; peptic ulcer; impaired wound healing; convulsions; cushingoid state

Labyrinthitis

OVERVIEW

Labyrinthitis is an infection or inflammation of the vestibular labyrinth of the inner ear.

Pathogenesis:

- Many causes:
  - Infections, especially viruses
  - Tumors
  - Vasculitis
  - Ototoxic drugs
  - Head injury neuronitis
- Physiologic mismatch of visual, somatosensory, and vestibular systems—external stimulus triggers it

Patient Profile

- Males = Females
- Any age—more common in the elderly

Signs and Symptoms

- Vertigo
- Nausea and vomiting
- Tinnitus
- Perspiration
- Malaise
- Nystagmus
- Hearing loss

Differential Diagnosis

- Meniere's disease
- Postconcussion syndrome
- Chronic bacterial otomastoiditis
- Drug-induced damage
- Benign positional vertigo
- Multiple sclerosis
- Temporal lobe epilepsy

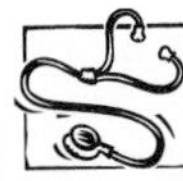

ASSESSMENT

History

Inquire about:

- Onset and duration of symptoms
- Underlying conditions
- Current medications including medications used just before onset of symptoms

Physical Finding

Spontaneous nystagmus using Bárány's maneuver

Initial Workup

Laboratory: CBC—will probably be within normal limits (low WBC count if viral infection present; high WBC count if bacterial infection present)

Radiology: CT scan or MRI if tumor suspected

Further Workup

- Electronystagmography
- Caloric test (Bárány's maneuver)

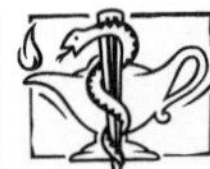

INTERVENTIONS

Office Treatment

None indicated

Lifestyle Modifications

Depends on severity of symptoms—may be a major disability resulting in lost income and strain on family relationships

Patient Education

Teach patient about:

- Disease process and treatment options—depends on cause; treat symptoms with medications
- How to take medications and side effects (see Pharmacotherapeutics)

Referral

To otolaryngologist if no improvement in 2 weeks

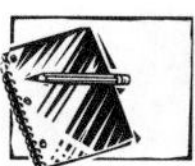

EVALUATION

Outcome
Resolves without sequelae

Possible Complication
Permanent hearing loss

Follow-up
In 1 week × 2; then consider referral if no improvement

FOR YOUR INFORMATION

Life Span
Pediatric: Unusual in this age group
Geriatric: Benign positional vertigo most common cause in this population
Pregnancy: Avoid medications

Miscellaneous
N/A

References

Bass EB, Lewis RF: Dizziness, vertigo, motion sickness, near syncope, syncope, and disequilibrium. In Barker LR, Burton JR, Zieve PD, editors: *Principles of ambulatory medicine,* ed 4, Baltimore, 1995, Williams & Wilkins, pp 1203-1204.

Goldblum K, Collier IC: Vision and hearing problems. In Lewis SM, Collier IC, Heitkemper MM, editors: *Medical-surgical nursing assessment and management of clinical problems,* ed 4, St Louis, 1996, Mosby, pp 478-480.

NOTES

PHARMACOTHERAPEUTICS

Drug of Choice	Mechanism of Action	Prescribing Information	Side Effects
Promethazine (Phenergan), 25 mg PO q6h; children, 12.5-25 mg bid	Histamine receptor antagonist; phenothiazine derivative	***Contraindications:*** Hypersensitivity; asthma ***Cost:*** 25-mg tab, 30 tabs: $2 ***Pregnancy category:*** C	Sedation, sleepiness, blurred vision, dry mouth, dizziness, increased or decreased blood pressure, rash, nausea, vomiting
Diazepam (Valium), 5 mg PO qid; elderly, 2 mg PO bid initially; increase as needed to control symptoms; children, 1 mg PO bid	Benzodiazipine; acts on limbic system, thalamus, and hypothalamus	***Contraindications:*** Hypersensitivity; closed-angle glaucoma; psychoses; pregnancy ***Cost:*** 5-mg tab, 30 tabs: $2 ***Pregnancy category:*** D	Dizziness, drowsiness, confusion, headache, anxiety, tremors, orthostatic hypotension, ECG changes, tachycardia, blurred vision, tinnitus, constipation, dry mouth, nausea, vomiting, rash, dermatitis
Prochlorperazine suppositories (Compazine), 25 mg PR bid; children, 2.5 mg bid-tid PR for vomiting—do not use in children <2 years	Phenothiazine; centrally blocks chemoreceptor trigger zone, which acts on vomiting center	***Contraindications:*** Hypersensitivity; coma; seizures; encephalopathy; bone marrow depression ***Cost:*** 25-mg suppository, 12 suppositories: $22 ***Pregnancy category:*** C	Euphoria, depression, extrapyramidal symptoms, restlessness, dizziness, nausea, vomiting, anorexia, dry mouth, diarrhea, constipation, weight loss, circulatory failure, tachycardia, respiratory depression
For vertigo:			
Meclizine (Antivert), 25 mg PO tid-qid—not recommended for children <12 years	Antihistamine	***Contraindications:*** Hypersensitivity; shock; lactation ***Cost:*** 25-mg tab, 30 tabs: $6 ***Pregnancy category:*** B	Drowsiness, fatigue, restlessness, headache, insomnia, nausea, anorexia, dry mouth, blurred vision

OVERVIEW

Lacrimal disorders comprise a group of disorders in which tear production is either increased or decreased. The most common disorder is decreased tear production, resulting in "dry eyes," which is the topic covered here.

Pathogenesis
Decreased tear production—may be due to blocked lacrimal gland, diuretics, atropine-like agents, rheumatoid arthritis, allergies, Bell's palsy, thyroid disease, or eyelid abnormalities, or may be idiopathic

Patient Profile
- Males = Females
- Arid climates—Southwest
- Most common in the elderly

Signs and Symptoms
- Gritty sensation in eyes
- Redness
- Visual blurring
- Inadequate tear production on ocular surface

Differential Diagnosis
- Allergies
- Eye infection

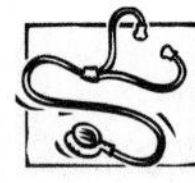

ASSESSMENT

History
Inquire about:
- Onset and duration of symptoms
- Underlying conditions
- Current medications

Physical Findings
- Conjunctival redness, possibly mucus production
- May appear dry

Initial Workup
Laboratory: Can measure tear production using Schirmer's filter strip—adequate wetting of strip 15 mm or greater in 5 minutes indicates sufficient tear production
Radiology: None indicated

Further Workup
None indicated

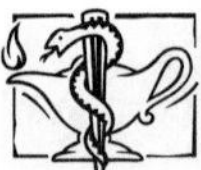

INTERVENTIONS

Office Treatment
May need to milk lacrimal gland

Lifestyle Modifications
- May need to stop wearing contact lenses
- Use of artificial tears on regular basis
- Cool-mist vaporizer in home to provide humidification
- Smoking cessation

Patient Education
Teach patient about:
- Condition and treatment—artificial tears
- Not wearing contacts
- Using cool mist vaporizer in home for humidification
- Medications used and side effects (see Pharmacotherapeutics)

Referrals
None indicated

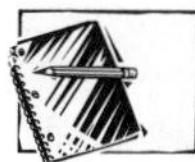

EVALUATION

Outcome

Adequate management with artificial tears

Possible Complications

- Severe dryness leading to corneal breakdown
- Invasion by bacteria

Follow-up

In 2 weeks to assess treatment; then every 3 months or as needed

FOR YOUR INFORMATION

Life Span

Pediatric: Lacrimal duct blockage in infants
Geriatric: Common in this age group
Pregnancy: Dry eyes are frequently part of pregnant state

Miscellaneous

Prevention of exposure to eye irritants, such as pollution, cigarette/cigar/pipe smoke, or sun exposure will help to prevent further drying.

Reference

Riordan-Eva P, Vaughn DG: Eye. In Tierney LM Jr, McPhee SJ, Papadakis MA, editors: *Current medical diagnosis and treatment,* ed 34, Norwalk, Conn, 1995, Appleton & Lange, pp 144-150.

NOTES

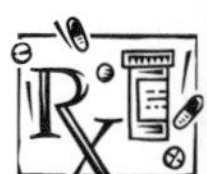

PHARMACOTHERAPEUTICS

Drug of Choice	Mechanism of Action	Prescribing Information	Side Effects
Artificial tears (Murine), 1-2 qtt each eye prn—do not touch tip of container to anything	Hypotonic solution to match natural eye fluid	***Contraindication:*** Hypersensitivity ***Cost:*** 15 ml: $4 ***Pregnancy category:*** Not categorized	Eye pain; changes in vision; worsening redness or irritation—discontinue use

Lactose Intolerance

OVERVIEW

Lactose intolerance is the inability of the body to break down lactose into glucose and galactose because of a deficiency in lactase enzyme

Pathogenesis

- Primary lactose intolerance—decline in lactase activity
- Secondary lactose intolerance—acquired lactase deficiency due to ulcerative colitis, Crohn's disease, gastroenteritis, sprue, immunoglobulin deficiencies

Patient Profile

- Males = Females
- Primary lactose intolerance—teens and early adulthood predominant age
- Secondary lactose intolerance—depends on cause
- Highest incidence in Native-Americans, African-Americans, Mexican-Americans, Jewish-Americans

Signs and Symptoms

- Bloating
- Cramping
- Abdominal pain
- Diarrhea
- Flatulence
- Borborygmi
- Symptoms usually occur 30 minutes to several hours after ingesting milk or milk products

Differential Diagnosis

- Gastroenteritis
- Sprue
- Ulcerative colitis
- Crohn's disease

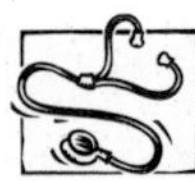

ASSESSMENT

History

Inquire about:

- Onset and duration of symptoms
- Relationship of symptoms to consumption of milk or milk products
- Family history
- Ethnic background
- Underlying conditions
- Current medications

Physical Findings

- Physical examination usually within normal limits
- If patient recently ingested milk or milk products, may find hyperactive bowel sounds or mild tenderness on abdominal palpation

Initial Workup

Laboratory

- Usually diagnosed by history and 3-week trial of lactose-free diet
- Hydrogen breath test after ingestion of lactose—abnormal
- Lactose intolerance test—failure of blood glucose to rise >20 mg/dl after ingestion of lactose suggests lactase deficiency

Radiology: None indicated

Further Workup

None indicated

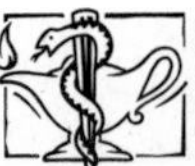

INTERVENTIONS

Office Treatment

None indicated

Lifestyle Modification

Reduction or restriction of lactose in diet

Patient Education

Teach patient about:

- Condition and treatment—reduced or restricted lactose diet
- Reading labels on products
- Better tolerance of lactose when consumed with other foods
- Use of commercially available lactase preparations and calcium carbonate (see Pharmacotherapeutics)

Referrals

Usually none needed

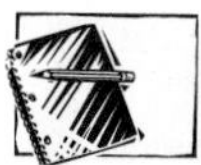

EVALUATION

Outcome
Patient is able to control symptoms

Possible Complication
Calcium deficiency

Follow-up
In 2 weeks to evaluate therapy and symptom control

FOR YOUR INFORMATION

Life Span
Pediatric: Use lactose-free formulas for infants; malnutrition can occur in children
Geriatric: If recent onset, look for cause of secondary lactose intolerance
Pregnancy: Many lactose-intolerant women can tolerate lactose during pregnancy

Miscellaneous
N/A

Reference
Heitkemper M, Sawchuck L: Nursing role in management: problems of absorption and elimination. In Lewis SM, Collier IC, Heitkemper MM, editors: *Medical-surgical nursing: assessment and management of clinical problems,* ed 4, St Louis, 1996, Mosby, pp 1253-1254.

NOTES

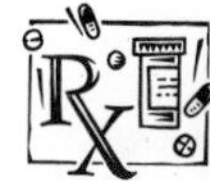

PHARMACOTHERAPEUTICS

Drug of Choice	Mechanism of Action	Prescribing Information	Side Effects
Lactase enzyme (Lactaid); swallow or chew 3 capsules with first bite of dairy product	Replenishes lactase enzyme	***Contraindication:*** Hypersensitivity ***Cost:*** OTC ***Pregnancy category:*** Not categorized	Warning label: "If you experience any symptoms that are unusual or seem unrelated to condition, contact your provider before taking more"
Calcium carbonate (Tums), 2 tabs after each meal and at bedtime for calcium supplement	Each tablet provides 200 mg calcium	***Contraindications:*** Hypersensitivity; hypercalcemia; hyperparathyroidism; bone tumors ***Cost:*** OTC ***Pregnancy category:*** C	Constipation, anorexia, obstruction, nausea, vomiting, flatulence, diarrhea, hemorrhage, rebound hypertension, hypercalcemia, renal dysfunction, renal failure, renal stones

Laryngitis

OVERVIEW

Laryngitis is an inflammation of the mucosa of the larynx with edema of the vocal cords. It may be acute or chronic.

Pathogenesis

ACUTE LARYNGITIS

- Viral or bacterial infection
- Inhalation of irritating fumes
- Aspiration of caustic chemical
- Damage during surgery

CHRONIC LARYNGITIS

- Excessive use of voice (singers, public speakers)
- Continuous inhalation of irritating fumes
- Aging changes—muscle atrophy, loss of moisture in larynx, bowing of vocal cords
- Heavy smoking
- Esophageal reflux
- Alcohol abuse

Patient Profile

- Males = Females
- All ages; chronic form—more common in adults

Signs and Symptoms

- Voice huskiness
- Hoarseness
- Total loss of voice
- Throat tickles
- Throat pain
- Rawness of throat
- Need to clear throat frequently
- Fever
- Malaise
- Cough
- Difficulty swallowing
- Regional lymphadenopathy

Differential Diagnosis

- Vocal nodules
- Malignancy
- Diphtheria
- Croup

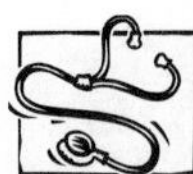

ASSESSMENT

History

Inquire about:

- Onset and duration of symptoms
- Smoking history
- Occupation and exposure to irritants
- Contact with individual with laryngitis
- History of esophageal reflux
- Underlying conditions
- Current medications

Physical Findings

Depends on cause—may not have any physical findings or may have any combination of the following: pharyngeal erythema, tonsillar enlargement, tonsillar exudate, fever, cough, lymphadenopathy

Initial Workup

Laboratory

- CBC—WBC count increased in bacterial infection
- Throat culture and sensitivity if indicated

Radiology: None indicated

Further Workup

Laryngoscopy with biopsy if chronic and history of smoking or alcohol abuse

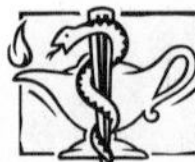

INTERVENTIONS

Office Treatment

None indicated

Lifestyle Modifications

- Smoking cessation
- Occupational change or modification
- Cessation of alcohol abuse
- Humidification of home or workplace

Patient Education

Teach patient about:

- Disorder and treatment:
  - Resting voice, increasing fluid intake, smoking cessation, alcohol cessation, avoidance of irritants
  - Antipyretics, antibiotics if indicated and analgesics
  - Warm saltwater gargles
  - Vocal cord stripping
- Medications used and side effects (see Pharmacotherapeutics)

Referral

Usually none; to otolaryngologist if symptoms continue beyond 2 months

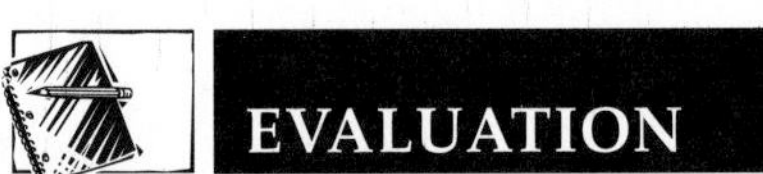

Outcome

Usually self-limited and resolves without sequelae

Possible Complication

Chronic hoarseness

Follow-up

In 2 weeks for reevaluation; further follow-up as needed

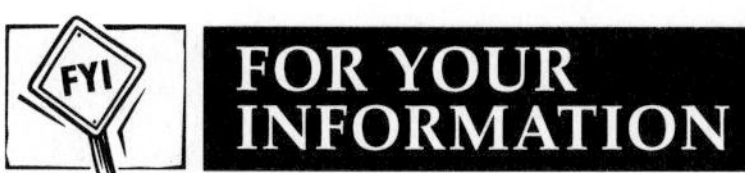

FOR YOUR INFORMATION

Life Span

Pediatric: Fairly common
Geriatric: More likely to develop chronic laryngitis
Pregnancy: N/A

Miscellaneous

For patients who make their living with their voice, chronic laryngitis can have a devastating effect.

Reference

Phipps WJ: Management of persons with problems of the upper airway. In Phipps WJ et al: *Medical-surgical nursing: concepts and clinical practice,* ed 5, St Louis, 1995, Mosby, p 1015.

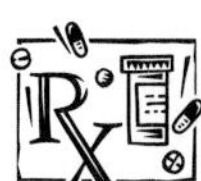

PHARMACOTHERAPEUTICS

Drug of Choice	Mechanism of Action	Prescribing Information	Side Effects
For fever and myalgia, use one of the following:			
Acetaminophen (Tylenol), 325-650 mg PO q4-6h; for children, use Children's Tylenol—follow label directions	Decreases fever through action on hypothalamic heat-regulating center of brain; analgesia by increasing pain threshold	***Contraindications:*** Hypersensitivity; bleeding disorders or anticoagulant therapy; last trimester of pregnancy; asthma; gastric ulcers ***Cost:*** OTC ***Pregnancy category:*** Not categorized	Rash; hepatic toxicity with alcohol ingestion or overdose
Aspirin, 325-650 mg PO q4-6h—do not use in children or adolescents because of risk of Reye's syndrome	Analgesia via peripheral and central nervous systems; may inhibit prostaglandins; antipyretic—acts on hypothalamic system	***Contraindications:*** Hypersensitivity; bleeding disorders or anticoagulant therapy; last trimester of pregnancy; asthma; gastric ulcers ***Cost:*** OTC ***Pregnancy category:*** Not categorized	Rash, anaphylactic reaction, GI upset and bleeding, Reye's syndrome in children and adolescents
Ibuprofen (Motrin), 400 mg qid PO; children 6 months-12 years, 5 mg/kg PO if temperature <102.5° F (39.1° C); 10 mg/kg PO q6h if temperature >102.5° F	Not well understood; may be related to inhibition of prostaglandin synthesis	***Contraindications:*** Aspirin allergy; hypersensitivity; asthma; last trimester of pregnancy; gastric ulcer; bleeding disorders ***Cost:*** 400-mg tab, 4/day × 5 days: $3 ***Pregnancy category:*** Not categorized but not recommended	Nausea, heartburn, diarrhea, GI upset and bleeding, dizziness, headache, rash, tinnitus, edema, acute renal failure
For suspected bacterial infection, use one of the following:			
Amoxicillin (Amoxil), 250-500 mg PO q8h × 10 days; children, 20 mg/kg/day PO q8h × 10 days	Bactericidal, broad-spectrum; not effective against beta-lactamase–producing pathogens	***Contraindications:*** Hypersensitivity to penicillins; use caution if allergic to cephalosporins ***Cost:*** 500-mg tabs, 3/day × 10 days: $4 ***Pregnancy category:*** B	Anaphylactoid reaction, nausea, vomiting, diarrhea, rashes, Stevens-Johnson syndrome, pseudomembranous colitis
Erythromycin, 250 mg PO qid × 10 days; children, 30-50 mg/kg/day PO in 4 divided doses × 10 days	Inhibits protein synthesis	***Contraindication:*** Hypersensitivity ***Cost:*** 250-mg tab, 4/day × 10 days: $4 ***Pregnancy category:*** B	Nausea, vomiting, diarrhea, abdominal pain, anorexia, rash, urticaria, pseudomembranous colitis—rarely

Laxative Abuse

OVERVIEW

Laxative abuse is the continual use of laxatives to either promote diarrhea or promote the patient's perception of "normal" bowel habits.

Pathogenesis

- Psychologic causes:
  - Bulimia nervosa
  - Hysterical behavior
  - Secondary gain of attention
  - Inappropriate perception of "normal" bowel habits
- Physical cause—chronic constipation (may also be caused by laxative abuse)

Patient Profile

- Females > Males
- Adolescence to early adulthood—bulimia nervosa
- Elderly—misperception of "normal" bowel habits

Signs and Symptoms

- Diarrhea
- Abdominal pain
- Rectal pain
- Nausea and vomiting
- Weight loss
- Muscle weakness
- Incontinence
- Hypokalemia
- Finger clubbing
- Edema

Differential Diagnosis

- Crohn's disease
- Ulcerative colitis
- Gastroenteritis
- Amebiasis
- Pseudomembranous colitis
- Whipple's disease
- Amyloidosis

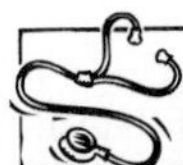

ASSESSMENT

History

Inquire about:

- Onset and duration of diarrhea
- Number of stools per day
- Consistency and color of stool
- Amount of laxative used
- Length of time used
- Why laxatives are being used (weight control)
- Underlying conditions
- Current medications

Physical Findings

- Weight loss
- May or may not have abdominal pain on palpation
- Arrhythmias (if hypokalemic)
- Finger clubbing
- Edema
- Rectal sphincter tone decreased

Initial Workup

Laboratory

- Chemistry profile—electrolyte abnormalities
- Urinalysis
- Stool pH (alkaline = phenolphthalein)
- CBC with differential

Radiology: Barium enema if indicated

Further Workup

Proctoscopy—melanosis coli

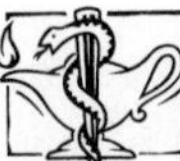

INTERVENTIONS

Office Treatment

None

Lifestyle Modifications

- Cessation of laxative use
- Nutritionally sound diet with increased fiber and fluids
- Moderate exercise program

Patient Education

Teach patient about:

- Harmful effects of laxative use
- "Normal" bowel habits
- Proper nutrition—use of fiber and increased fluids
- Starting an exercise program
- Need for psychologic support
- Using stool softeners or bulk-forming agents (see Pharmacotherapeutics)

Referrals

May need psychologic counseling—to psychiatric NP, therapist, psychiatrist, psychologist, as indicated

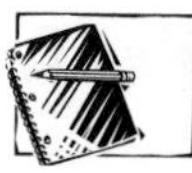

EVALUATION

Outcomes

- Patient stops using laxatives
- Bowels function properly

Possible Complications

- Malnutrition
- Electrolyte imbalance
- Renal failure
- Cardiac arrhythmias
- Death

Follow-up

Monthly × 3, if being seen by mental health professional

FOR YOUR INFORMATION

Life Span

Pediatric: Lifelong laxative dependence; death with lesser amounts
Geriatric: Rectal incontinence; death with lesser amounts
Pregnancy: May be harmful to fetus

Miscellaneous

Laxative abuse may be difficult to diagnose. Many patients will not readily admit to laxative use. Suspect it in a patient with chronic diarrhea and question the patient during several visits.

References

Cheskin LJ: Constipation and diarrhea. In Barker LR, Burton JR, Zieve PD, editors: *Principles of ambulatory medicine,* ed 4, Baltimore, 1995, Williams & Wilkins, pp 484-485.

Kresevic DM, Lincoln RA: Nursing practice with elders. In Phipps WJ et al, editors: *Medical-surgical nursing: concepts and clinical practice,* ed 5, St Louis, 1995, Mosby, p 78.

NOTES

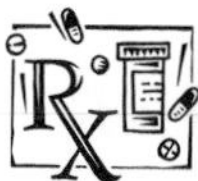

PHARMACOTHERAPEUTICS

Drug of Choice	Mechanism of Action	Prescribing Information	Side Effects
Stool softener: dicusate sodium (Colace); adults and children >12 years, 50-200 mg/day PO; children 6-12 years, 40-120 mg/day PO; children 3-6 years, 20-60 mg/day PO; children <3 years, 10-40 mg/day PO	Acts like a detergent; permits water and fatty substances to mix with fecal material	***Contraindications:*** None known ***Cost:*** 100 tabs: $2-$4 ***Pregnancy category:*** C	Incidence of side effects very small; bitter taste, throat irritation, nausea, rash
Bulk-forming agent: psyllium hydrophilic mucilloid (Metamucil, Citrucel); adult dose, 1 tsp or 1 Tbsp mixed with 8 oz liquid—dose depends on formulation; follow label directions; children 6-12 years, ½ adult dose; must be taken with at least 8 oz fluid—may cause choking; teach patients to seek immediate medical attention if they experience chest pain, vomiting, or difficulty swallowing or breathing	Natural fiber that promotes elimination by its bulking effect	***Contraindications:*** Intestinal obstruction; fecal impaction; known allergy; abdominal pain; nausea and vomiting; difficulty swallowing ***Cost:*** $3-$10, depending on size ***Pregnancy category:*** B	Choking, allergic reaction, abdominal pain, nausea, chest pain

Lead Poisoning

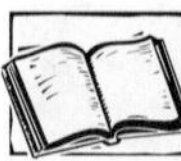

OVERVIEW

Lead poisoning occurs when there are high levels of lead found in the blood.

Pathogenesis

Cause—ingestion of lead or inhalation of lead dust

Patient Profile

- Males = Females
- Any age; more common in young children

Signs and Symptoms

May be asymptomatic:

- Acute lead poisoning:
  - Abdominal pain
  - Hemolytic anemia
  - Hepatitis
  - Fatigue
  - Irritability
  - Lethargy
  - Difficulty concentrating
  - Headache
  - Vomiting
  - Myalgia
- Chronic lead poisoning:
  - Anorexia
  - Metallic taste
  - Weight loss
  - Severe abdominal cramps
  - Peripheral neuritis
  - Seizures
  - Coma
  - Irritability
  - Impaired mental development
  - Decreased intelligence

Differential Diagnosis

- Iron deficiency anemia
- Hemolytic anemia
- Acute abdomen
- Other polyneuropathies
- Mental retardation
- Attention deficit disorder
- Autism
- Dementia
- Epilepsy

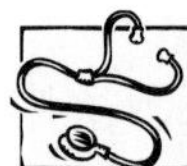

ASSESSMENT

History

Inquire about:

- Onset and duration of symptoms
- Living in or regularly visiting a home with peeling or chipped paint built before 1978
- Anyone else in the household being diagnosed with lead poisoning
- Living with someone whose job or hobby involves exposure to lead
- Living near an active lead smelter, battery-recycling plant, or other industry likely to release lead
- Patient's occupation—plumber, pipe fitter, auto repair person, printer, etc.
- Underlying conditions
- Current medications

Physical Findings

- Abdominal examination—may have abdominal rigidity, pain on palpation
- Irritability
- Poor performance on development tests
- Weight loss
- Tremor
- Hyperactivity

Initial Workup

Laboratory

- Blood lead level *(CDC classification):*

Class	Lead
I	<0.48 μmol/L, <10 μg/dl
II	0.48-0.92 μmol/L, 10-19 μg/dl
III	0.97-2.12 μmol/L, 20-44 μg/dl
IV	2.17-3.33 μmol/L, 45-69 μg/dl
V	>3.38 μmol/L, >70 μg/dl

- CBC—hemoglobin and hematocrit slightly decreased, eosinophilia or basophilic stippling on differential

Radiology

- Abdominal x-ray film—lead particles
- X-ray film of long bones—lines of increased density in metaphyseal plate

Further Workup

Usually none

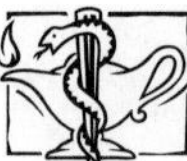

INTERVENTIONS

Office Treatment

None indicated

Lifestyle Modifications

- Removal of lead paint
- Proper protective wear for work or hobbies
- If asymptomatic, avoidance of excess fluid intake
- Low-fat diet to reduce absorption and retention of lead

Patient Education

Teach patient about:

- Disease process and treatment:
  - For class I or II, diet teaching—low-fat diet to reduce retention; adequate calcium and iron
  - Oral chelation for class III or IV if asymptomatic
  - Parenteral chelation for class III, IV, or V if symptomatic
- Sources of lead and ways to avoid lead poisoning:
  - Monitoring children to ensure that they do not eat lead paint
  - If working around lead, remove clothing before entering home
  - Shower immediately on returning home
  - Wet mopping and dusting with high-phosphate solution to control lead-bearing dust
- Long-term effects on children
- Medications used and side effects (see Pharmacotherapeutics)

Referral

Consult with MD regarding parenteral chelation for patients with class V lead poisoning and for patients with class III or IV lead poisoning who are symptomatic

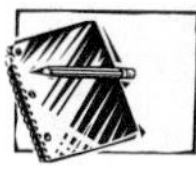

EVALUATION

Outcomes
- Without encephalopathy, improves with chelation
- If encephalopathy occurs, permanent sequelae, such as mental retardation, seizure disorder, blindness
- Hemiparesis may occur in up to 50% of cases

Possible Complications
- CNS toxicity with long-term effects
- Chronic renal failure
- Mental retardation
- Seizure disorder
- Blindness
- Hemiparesis

Follow-up
In 7 to 10 days for repeat lead level—may see rebound from stored lead in bones; then monitor lead level every 2 weeks × 2; then monthly × 1

FOR YOUR INFORMATION

Life Span
Pediatric: Most commonly seen in this age group; CDC recommends screening all children between 6 and 72 months of age; child 6 to 16 years of age should be screened if developmentally disabled or positive past history of exposure
Geriatric: Not commonly seen in this age group
Pregnancy: Low birth weight and premature birth

Miscellaneous
Many hobbies and occupations put people at risk of lead poisoning. Some more common ones include lead-glazed ceramics, target shooting at firing ranges, preparing lead shot or fishing sinkers, stained-glass making, car or boat repair, plumbing, pipe-fitting, shipbuilding, printing, plastic manufacturing, lead smelting, gas station attending. Lead poisoning is a reportable disease. Report results to local health department.

References

Carter BL: Poisoning and overdose. In Driscoll CE et al: *The family practice desk reference,* ed 3, St Louis, 1996, Mosby, pp 584-587.

Olsen KR: Poisoning. In Tierney LM Jr, McPhee SJ, Papadakis MA, editors: *Current medical diagnosis and treatment,* ed 34, Norwalk, Conn, 1995, Appleton & Lange, p 1513.

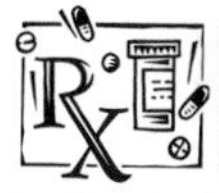

PHARMACOTHERAPEUTICS

Drug of Choice	Mechanism of Action	Prescribing Information	Side Effects
Succimer (Chemet), 10 mg/kg PO q8h × 5 days, then 10 mg/kg PO q12h × 2 weeks; may need a second course—allow 2 weeks between courses; for young children, contents of capsule may be sprinkled on food—not recommended for children <1 year	Binds with lead ions to form water-soluble complex excreted by kidneys	***Contraindication:*** Hypersensitivity ***Cost:*** 100-mg tab, 100 tabs: $318 ***Pregnancy category:*** C	Back, stomach, rib, flank pain; abdominal cramps; chills; fever; flu-like syndrome; increased platelets; intermittent eosinophilia; proteinuria; decreased urination; increased ALT, AST, alkaline phosphatase, and cholesterol; nausea, vomiting; diarrhea; metallic taste; anorexia; drowsiness; dizziness; sore throat; rhinorrhea; nasal congestion; otitis media; watery eyes; plugged ears
Dimercaprol (British Anti-Lewisite, BAL), 4 mg/kg IM, q4h × 5 days with IV infusion of edetate calcium disodium (CaEDTA)—see below	Chelating agent; binds with mercury, gold, arsenic, lead, copper—forms water-soluble complex excreted by kidneys	***Contraindications:*** Hypersensitivity; anuria, hepatic insufficiency; poisoning of other metals; severe renal disease; <3 years of age; pregnancy ***Cost:*** 100 mg/ml: $10 ***Pregnancy category:*** D	Headache, paresthesia, anxiety, tremors, convulsions, shock, rash, pain at injection site, fever, burning lips, hypertension, tachycardia, nausea, vomiting, rhinorrhea, throat pain or constriction, lacrimation, burning sensation in penis
Edetate calcium sodium (CaEDTA), 1500 mg/m^2/day continuous IV infusion over 5 days with BAL	Binds lead ions to form water-soluble complex excreted by kidneys	***Contraindications:*** Hypersensitivity; anuria; poisoning with other metals; children <3 years ***Cost:*** Variable; 150 mg/ml, 20 ml: $5 ***Pregnancy category:*** C	Headache, paresthesias, urticaria, fever, cheilosis, hypertension, dysrhythmias, thrombophlebitis, vomiting, diarrhea, abdominal cramps, anorexia, nasal congestion, sneezing, leg cramps, hematuria, renal tubular necrosis, proteinuria

Lumbar Strain

OVERVIEW

Lumbar strain occurs when there is injury to the muscles, tendons, ligaments, or fascia of the back.

Pathogenesis

Cause—often unknown

Patient Profile

- Males = Females
- Most common age group—20- to 40-year-olds
- Risk factors:
  - Obesity
  - Chronic poor posture
  - Chronic, repetitive, improper lifting
  - Exaggerated lumbar lordosis
  - Leg length discrepancy

Signs and Symptoms

- Pain in lower back, buttocks, hips
- Pain increases with movement
- Muscle spasms

Differential Diagnosis

- Herniated nucleus pulposus
- Osteomyelitis
- Metabolic bone disease
- Neoplasm
- Abdominal aneurysm
- Pyelonephritis
- Osteoarthritis
- Osteoporosis
- Malingering

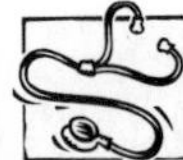

ASSESSMENT

History

Inquire about:

- Onset and duration of symptoms
- Recent trauma
- Whether pain worsens with bending, lifting
- Previous history of back injury
- Occupational history
- Systemic symptoms, such as weight loss, fever (malignant disease)
- Bowel or bladder incontinence
- Loss of sensation
- Underlying conditions
- Current medications

Physical Findings

- Pain on palpation of lumbar spine and paraspinal musculature
- Decreased lumbar range of motion
- Motor, sensory, reflex examination—normal
- Straight leg raises—cause low-back pain but not leg pain; if positive in lying position, perform distracted leg raises with patient sitting (if negative, consider malingering)
- Apply pressure to top of head (if causes pain, consider malingering)

Initial Workup

Laboratory: Only necessary if concerned about neoplasm; inflammatory, diffuse bone disease; or renal disease

Radiology: Plain films of lumbar spine if recurrent or unresponsive to treatment

Further Workup

CT scan or MRI if concerned about disc herniation

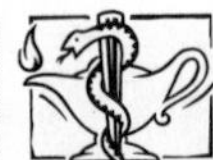

INTERVENTIONS

Office Treatment

None indicated

Lifestyle Modifications

- Smoking cessation
- Weight loss
- Exercise program
- Proper lifting technique

Patient Education

Teach patient about:

- Condition and treatment:
  - Bed rest for 1 day, light activity for 1 to 2 days, then full activity
  - Using ice pack for 20 to 30 minutes 4 times daily for 24 hours
  - Using heat 20 to 30 minutes 4 times daily after first 24 hours
  - Using nonsteroidal antiinflammatory drugs
- Exercises to strengthen back and stomach
- Proper lifting technique
- Medications used and side effects (see Pharmacotherapeutics)

Referral

To orthopedist if conservative treatment fails

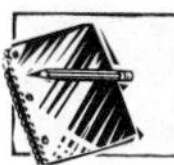

EVALUATION

Outcomes

- Resolves without sequelae
- Resolution may be hindered by litigation

Possible Complication

Chronic low-back pain

Follow-up

In 1 week; then in 4 weeks

FOR YOUR INFORMATION

Life Span

Pediatric: Uncommon in this age group; thorough workup necessary
Geriatric: Most common cause of low-back pain—degenerative disc disease
Pregnancy: Commonly associated with low-back pain

Miscellaneous

Avoid use of narcotic analgesia.

Reference

Mercier LR: *Practical orthopedics,* ed 4, St Louis, 1995, Mosby, pp 146-147.

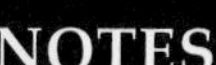

NOTES

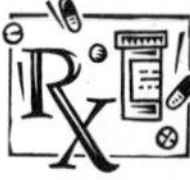

PHARMACOTHERAPEUTICS

Drug of Choice	Mechanism of Action	Prescribing Information	Side Effects
Nonsteroidal antiinflammatory drugs (NSAIDs): many different types currently marketed; consult manufacturer's package insert for specific dosing and prescribing information	Exact action unknown; may result from inhibition of synthesis of prostaglandins and arachidonic acid	***Contraindications:*** Hypersensitivity to NSAIDs, aspirin; severe hepatic failure; asthma ***Cost:*** Varies with type ***Pregnancy category:*** Depends on product	Stomach distress, flatulence, nausea, abdominal pain, constipation or diarrhea, dizziness, sedation, rash, urticaria, angioedema, anorexia, urinary frequency, increased blood pressure, insomnia, anxiety, visual disturbances, increased thirst, alopecia
Muscle relaxant (controversial): Orphenadrine (Norflex), 100 mg PO bid	Not clearly identified; relief may result from analgesic properties; also has anticholinergic effects	***Contraindications:*** Hypersensitivity; narrow-angle glaucoma; GI obstruction; myasthenia gravis; stenosing peptic ulcer; bladder neck obstruction; cardiospasm ***Cost:*** 100-mg tab, 100 tabs: $127 ***Pregnancy category:*** C	Dry mouth, tachycardia, palpitations, urinary hesitancy/retention, blurred vision, dilation of pupils, increased ocular tension, weakness, nausea, vomiting, headache, dizziness, constipation, drowsiness, hypersensitivity reactions, pruritus, hallucinations, agitation, tremor, gastric irritation

Lung Abscess

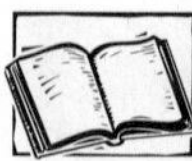

OVERVIEW

Lung abscess is a pus-filled cavity within the lung. It occurs as a result of a lung infection with either aerobic or anaerobic bacteria.

Pathogenesis

Cause—aerobic or anaerobic bacteria:

- *Prevotella, Bacteroides,* streptococci, *Fusobacterium*—anaerobes found in gingival crevice and aspirated
- *Staphylococcus aureus* and *Klebsiella pneumoniae*—most common aerobic pathogens

Patient Profile

- Males > Females
- Any age

Signs and Symptoms

- Cough
- Purulent, foul-smelling sputum
- Fever and chills
- Chest pain
- Dyspnea
- Fatigue
- Malaise
- Weight loss
- Anorexia
- Night sweats

Differential Diagnosis

- Lung cancer
- Bronchiectasis
- Tuberculosis
- Wegener's granulomatous
- Mycotic lung infection

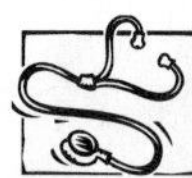

ASSESSMENT

History

Inquire about:

- Onset and duration of symptoms
- Purulent, foul-smelling sputum
- Underlying conditions
- Current medications

Physical Findings

- General—weight loss, fever, diaphoresis
- Lungs—decreased breath sounds, rales, wheezing, tachypnea, dullness to percussion, cavernous breath sounds
- Heart—tachycardia

Initial Workup

Laboratory

- CBC with differential—leukocytosis with left shift
- Anemia
- Sputum culture and Gram stain

Radiology: Chest film—PA and lateral—consolidation with radiolucency, air-fluid level, pleural effusion

Further Workup

Transtracheal aspirate for culture

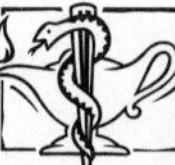

INTERVENTIONS

Office Treatment

None indicated

Lifestyle Modification

Smoking cessation

Patient Education

Teach patient about:

- Condition and treatment:
  - Hospitalization if severely ill
  - Treatment with antimicrobials—lengthy
  - Chest percussion and postural drainage (teach significant other to perform if treated as outpatient)
- Importance of taking medication as directed and for proper time
- Increasing fluid intake
- Medications used and side effects (see Pharmacotherapeutics)

Referral

To MD if hospitalization is required and NP does not have privileges

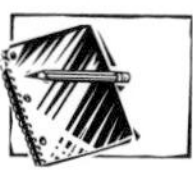

EVALUATION

Outcomes:
- Prognosis is guardedly favorable
- Recurrence can occur with inadequate treatment

Possible Complications
- Brain abscess
- Meningitis
- Empyema
- Pneumothorax
- Recurrent lung abscess
- Treatment failure requiring surgical resection of lung

Follow-up
- Weekly × 2; then every 2 weeks until resolution
- Chest x-ray film should be done every 2 weeks

FOR YOUR INFORMATION

Life Span
Pediatric: *Staphylococcus* is most common causative organism in children
Geriatric: Higher morbidity and mortality; always consider hospitalization
Pregnancy: Hospitalization for close monitoring

Miscellaneous
This condition is most commonly seen in patients who are prone to aspiration, such as alcoholics, drug abusers, epileptics, comatose patients, and patients with gastroesophageal reflux disease.

References
Bartlett JG: Ambulatory care for selected infections including osteomyelitis, lung abscess, and endocarditis. In Barker LR, Burton JR, Zieve PD, editors: *Principles of ambulatory medicine,* ed 4, Baltimore, 1995, Williams & Wilkins, pp 376-379.

Stauffer JL: Lung. In Tierney LM Jr, McPhee SJ, Papadakis MA, editors: *Current medical diagnosis and treatment,* ed 34, Norwalk, Conn, 1995, Appleton & Lange, pp 231-232.

NOTES

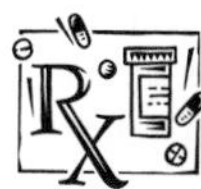

PHARMACOTHERAPEUTICS

Drug of Choice	Mechanism of Action	Prescribing Information	Side Effects
Penicillin G, 6-12 mil U/day IV in divided doses q6h until improved, then 750 mg (1.2 mil U) PO qid × several weeks or may start with PO medications in mild illness; children, 25,000-300,000 U/day IV in divided doses q6h, then 25,000-90,000 U/kg/day PO in divided doses q6h	Penicillin; interferes with cell wall replication; makes cell wall osmotically unstable	***Contraindication:*** Hypersensitivity ***Cost:*** 10,000,000 U/vial, 10 vials: \$66; 400,000-U tab, 100 tabs: \$8-\$12 ***Pregnancy category:*** B	Bone marrow depression, granulocytopenia, nausea, vomiting, diarrhea, oliguria, proteinuria, hematuria, vaginitis, moniliasis, glomerulonephritis, lethargy, hallucinations, anxiety, coma, convulsions, hyperkalemia, hypokalemia
Clindamycin, 600 mg IV q8h until improvement, then 300 mg PO q6h; children, 15-40 mg/kg/day IV in divided doses q8h, then 9-25 mg/kg/day PO in divided doses q6h	Lincomycin derivative; suppresses protein synthesis by binding to 50 S subunit of bacterial ribosome	***Contraindications:*** Hypersensitivity; ulcerative colitis/enteritis ***Cost:*** 150 mg/ml, 2 ml: \$11; 150-mg tab, 100 tabs: \$70-\$112 ***Pregnancy category:*** B	Leukopenia; eosinophilia; agranulocytosis; thrombocytopenia; nausea, vomiting; abdominal pain; diarrhea; pseudomembranous colitis; anorexia; weight loss; increased AST, ALT, bilirubin, and alkaline phosphatase; vaginitis; rash; pruritus

Lung Cancer

OVERVIEW

Lung cancer is a malignant neoplasm of the lung. It is broadly classified as non–small cell carcinoma or small cell carcinoma. Non–small cell cancer is the most common type and includes squamous cell, large cell, adenocarcinoma, and bronchioloalveolar carcinoma. All types except bronchioloalveolar carcinoma are related to cigarette smoking. In bronchioloalveolar carcinoma, 50% of those affected have never smoked.

Pathogenesis

Causes:

- Smoking
- Secondhand smoke
- Asbestos exposure
- Arsenic
- Halogen ethers
- Nickel and nickel compounds
- Radon
- Radioisotopes
- Atmospheric pollution

Patient Profile

- Males > Females
- Most common age—50 to 70 years

Signs and Symptoms

- May be asymptomatic
- Chronic cough
- Shortness of breath
- Hemoptysis
- Chest pain
- Hoarseness
- Wheezing
- Extreme fatigue
- Shoulder/arm pain
- Weight loss
- Anemia
- Edema and rubor of upper trunk and face, occasionally with syncope (superior vena cava syndrome)

Differential Diagnosis

- Metastatic cancer
- Granuloma

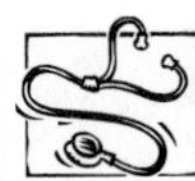

ASSESSMENT

History

Inquire about:

- Onset and duration of symptoms
- Smoking history
- Occupational history
- Underlying conditions
- Current medications

Physical Findings

- May be normal
- Weight loss
- Lungs—wheezing, crackles, absent breath sounds at site of tumor; dullness to percussion

Initial Workup

Laboratory

- CBC with differential—may have decreased Hgb and Hct
- Chemistry profile to include sodium, potassium, calcium, and liver enzymes
- Sputum cytology—cancer cells

Radiology

- Chest—PA and lateral—reveals a mass
- CT scan of chest—defines the cancer better

Further Workup

Bronchoscopy

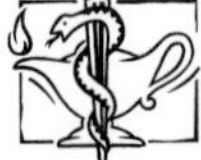

INTERVENTIONS

Office Treatment

None indicated

Lifestyle Modifications

- Smoking cessation
- Living with a chronic, possibly terminal, illness

Patient Education

Teach patient about:

- Condition and treatment
  - Hospitalization for surgical resection for non–small cell carcinoma
  - Outpatient chemotherapy or radiation therapy
- Tips for smoking cessation
- Using oxygen at home and safety measures
- Pain control—medication, biofeedback, relaxation therapy
- Medications used and side effects (see Pharmacotherapeutics)

Referrals

- To surgeon and/or oncologist
- To social worker
- To home health agency

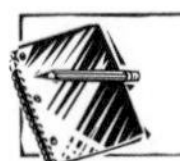

EVALUATION

Outcomes

Depends on type and stage:

- Stage I non–small cell carcinoma—50% 5-year survival
- Small cell carcinoma—very poor prognosis

Possible Complications

- Metastatic disease
- Death

Follow-up

- If surgically resected, 1 week after hospitalization; then every 3 months
- If no surgical resection, every 2 weeks to assess pain management

FOR YOUR INFORMATION

Life Span

Pediatric: Not seen in this age group
Geriatric: Most common in this age group
Pregnancy: N/A

Miscellaneous

The NP can assist in the battle against this deadly disease by educating patients on the dangers of smoking and encouraging smoking cessation.

References

Barr L, Smith PL: Lung cancer. In Barker LR, Burton JR, Zieve PD, editors: *Principles of ambulatory medicine,* ed 4, Baltimore, 1995, Williams & Wilkins, pp 678-689.

Stauffer JL: Lung. In Tierney LM Jr, McPhee SJ, Papadakis MA, editors: *Current medical diagnosis and treatment,* ed 34, Norwalk, Conn, 1995, Appleton & Lange, pp 240-244.

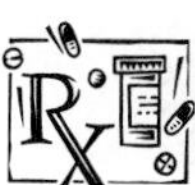

PHARMACOTHERAPEUTICS

Pain control can be a challenge when caring for the patient with lung cancer. Always start with nonnarcotic medication and change medication as needed. Never withhold narcotic pain medication for fear of patient addiction.

Drug of Choice	Mechanism of Action	Prescribing Information	Side Effects
For mild to moderate pain, use one of the following:			
Aspirin, 325-650 mg PO q4-6h for fever and myalgia—do not use in children or adolescents because of risk of Reye's syndrome	Analgesia via peripheral and central nervous systems; may inhibit prostaglandins; antipyretic—acts on hypothalamic system	***Contraindications:*** Hypersensitivity; bleeding disorders or anticoagulant therapy; last trimester of pregnancy; asthma; gastric ulcers ***Cost:*** OTC ***Pregnancy category:*** Not categorized	Rash, anaphylactic reaction, GI upset and bleeding, Reye's syndrome in children and adolescents
Acetaminophen (Tylenol), 325-650 mg PO q4-6h for fever or myalgia; for children, use Children's Tylenol—follow label directions	Decreases fever through action on hypothalamic heat-regulating center of brain; analgesia by increasing pain threshold	***Contraindications:*** Hypersensitivity; bleeding disorders or anticoagulant therapy; last trimester of pregnancy; asthma; gastric ulcers ***Cost:*** OTC ***Pregnancy category:*** Not categorized	Rash; hepatic toxicity with alcohol ingestion or overdose
Nonsteroidal antiinflammatory drugs (NSAIDs): many different types currently marketed; consult manufacturer's package insert for specific dosing and prescribing information	Exact action unknown; may result from inhibition of synthesis of prostaglandins and arachidonic acid	***Contraindications:*** Hypersensitivity to NSAIDs, aspirin; severe hepatic failure; asthma ***Cost:*** Varies with type ***Pregnancy category:*** Depends on product	Stomach distress, flatulence, nausea, abdominal pain, constipation or diarrhea, dizziness, sedation, rash, urticaria, angioedema, anorexia, urinary frequency, increased blood pressure; insomnia, anxiety, visual disturbances, increased thirst, alopecia
For moderate pain, use one of the following:			
Tramadol hydrochloride (Ultram), 50-100 mg PO q4-6h, not to exceed 400 mg/day	Centrally acting analgesic—exact mechanism of action unknown	***Contraindications:*** Hypersensitivity; acute intoxication with alcohol, hypnotics, centrally acting analgesics, opioids, or psychotropic drugs ***Cost:*** 50-mg tab, 100 tabs: $60 ***Pregnancy category:*** C	Dependence, dizziness, vertigo, nausea, vomiting, constipation, headache, somnolence, pruritus, CNS stimulation, sweating, dyspepsia, dry mouth, hypotension, tachycardia, anxiety, confusion, coordination disturbance, nervousness, sleep disorder, flatulence, abdominal pain, rash
Acetaminophen/hydrocodone (Vicodin), 5 mg hydrocodone/500 mg acetaminophen, 1-2 tabs PO q4-6h, not to exceed 8 tabs daily; avoid alcohol and other CNS depressants; Schedule III narcotic	Hydrocodone—similar to codeine, acts on central nervous system; specific mechanism unknown; acetaminophen—inhibits prostaglandin synthesis, specific mechanism unknown	***Contraindications:*** Hypersensitivity to either component ***Cost:*** 5/500-tab, 100 tabs: $20-$98 ***Pregnancy category:*** C	Physical/psychologic dependence, drowsiness, mental clouding, lethargy, anxiety, fear, nausea, vomiting, urinary retention, respiratory depression, rash, pruritus
For moderate to severe pain:			
Morphine (M.S. Contin, sustained release), 15 mg PO q12h—do not break, chew, or crush; Schedule II narcotic	Centrally acting analgesic	***Contraindications:*** Hypersensitivity; respiratory depression; acute or severe bronchial asthma; paralytic ileus ***Cost:*** 15-mg tab, 100 tabs: $64-$77 ***Pregnancy category:*** C	Respiratory depression, apnea, circulatory depression, respiratory arrest, shock, cardiac arrest, constipation, lightheadedness, dizziness, sedation, nausea, vomiting, sweating, dysphoria, euphoria, weakness, headache, agitation, tremor, seizures, uncoordinated muscle movement, dry mouth, anorexia, diarrhea, cramps, tachycardia, facial flushing, palpitations, syncope, urinary retention, pruritus, rash, edema, blurred vision

Lyme Disease

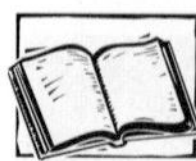

OVERVIEW

Lyme disease is a multisystem disease that is spread by the bite of the ixodid tick. The infection occurs in 3 stages.

Pathogenesis

- Caused by spirochete *Borrelia burgdorferi*
- Certain mice and deer are sources of infection for tick

Patient Profile

- Males = Females
- Any age; usually more common in children
- Most cases in United States occur in Northeast coastal region, Minnesota and Wisconsin, and parts of California

Signs and Symptoms

- Stage I (begins 3 to 32 days after bite)—expanding skin rash and flulike symptoms (fever, chills, malaise, headache)
- Stage II (begins months after bite):
  - Cardiac—fluctuating degrees of atrioventricular (AV) block, myopericarditis, left ventricular dysfunction
  - Arthritis
  - Brief attacks of swelling and pain
  - Multiple annular secondary lesions
  - Neurologic abnormalities
  - Fluctuating symptoms of meningitis
- Stage III (begins months to years after bite):
  - Chronic arthritis
  - Acrodermatitis chronica atrophicans (rare in United States)
  - Chronic neurologic symptoms—subtle encephalopathy affecting mood, memory, or sleep

Differential Diagnosis

- Juvenile rheumatoid arthritis
- Viral syndromes
- Later stages may mimic many other diseases

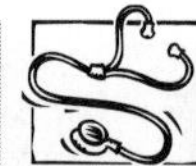

ASSESSMENT

History

Inquire about:

- Onset and duration of symptoms
- Being outdoors in the woods
- Finding a tick on skin surface
- Any skin lesions—course, characteristics
- Travel to endemic areas
- Treatment tried and results
- Underlying chronic illness
- Current medications

Physical Findings

- Stage I:
  - Red papule at site of tick bite; lesion expands with central clearing or may have scaly center (erythema migrans–type rash)
  - Stiff neck
  - Fever
  - Regional lymphadenopathy
- Stage II:
  - Multiple smaller, annular lesions
  - Facial palsies
  - Headaches
  - Neck pain and stiffness
  - Heart block
  - Joint pain and stiffness
- Stage III:
  - Joint inflammation, pain, stiffness
  - Joint erosion, erythematous atrophic plaque (acrodermatitis chronica atrophicans—rare in United States)
  - Neurologic symptoms—mood, memory, or sleep changes; distal paresthesias; spinal or radicular pain

Initial Workup

Laboratory

- IgG and IgM for *B. burgdorferi* antibodies (ELISA and Western Blot)—may be negative in early stages; look for high titers
- Depending on stage, culture of cerebrospinal fluid

Radiology: None indicated, except for later in disease to look for arthritic changes

Further Workup

ECG—heart block

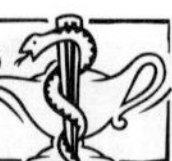

INTERVENTIONS

Office Treatment

Tick removal if still present

Lifestyle Modification

Use of tick repellents and avoidance of areas with high concentration of ticks, if possible

Patient Education

Teach patient about:

- Condition and treatment—antibiotics
- Prevention of tick bites—wear lightly colored clothes; tuck pant legs into socks; tuck shirt into pants; wear hat and long-sleeved shirt; avoid overhanging grass and brush; spray clothes with DEET; remove clothing and wash and dry in high temperature
- Tick removal—use tweezers; pull straight back with slow, steady force; disinfect skin before and after
- Medications used and side effects (see Pharmacotherapeutics)

Referral

To MD if in stage II or III

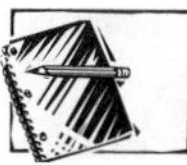

EVALUATION

Outcome
Resolves without development of stage II symptoms

Possible Complications
- Recurrent synovitis, tendinitis, bursitis
- Chronic neurologic symptoms

Follow-up
- Mild disease—at end of antimicrobial treatment or in 2 weeks
- Moderate disease—weekly until condition stabilizes

FOR YOUR INFORMATION

Life Span
Pediatric: Treat with amoxicillin
Geriatric: Higher morbidity and mortality
Pregnancy: Spirochete can cross placenta; IV antibiotics preferred treatment

Miscellaneous
In areas where anxiety about Lyme disease is high, overdiagnosis of Lyme disease leads to the overuse of antibiotics. Attention needs to be paid to patient anxieties, and there needs to be an increased awareness of musculoskeletal problems in order to avoid this overuse of antibiotics.

References

Habif TP: *Clinical dermatology: a color guide to diagnosis and therapy,* ed 3, St Louis, 1996, Mosby, pp 464-471.

Peters S: Hitting the bull's eye: practical diagnosis and treatment of lyme disease, *Adv Nurse Pract* 4(11):14-17, 49, 57, 1996.

NOTES

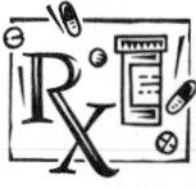

PHARMACOTHERAPEUTICS

Drug of Choice	Mechanism of Action	Prescribing Information	Side Effects
Doxycycline (Vibramycin) 100 mg PO bid × 10-30 days; children >8 years, 4.4 mg/kg/day PO divided q12h × 7 days	Tetracycline; inhibits protein synthesis	***Contraindications:*** Hypersensitivity; children <8 years ***Cost:*** 100-mg tab, 20 tabs: $5 ***Pregnancy category:*** D	Eosinophilia, neutropenia, thrombocytopenia, hemolytic anemia, dysphagia, glossitis, nausea, abdominal pain, vomiting, diarrhea, anorexia, hepatotoxicity, flatulence, abdominal cramps, gastritis, pericarditis, rash, urticaria, exfoliative dermatitis, angioedema
Amoxicillin (Amoxil), PO 250-500 mg q8h × 10-30 days; children, 20 mg/kg/day PO q8h × 10-30 days	Bactericidal; broad-spectrum; *not* effective against beta-lactamase–producing pathogens	***Contraindications:*** Hypersensitivity to penicillins; use caution if allergic to cephalosporins ***Cost:*** 500-mg tabs, 3/day × 10 days: $4 ***Pregnancy category:*** B	Anaphylactoid reaction, nausea, vomiting, diarrhea, rash, Stevens-Johnson syndrome, pseudomembranous colitis
Erthromycin (E.E.S.), 500 mg PO q6h × 10 days; children, 30-50 mg/kg/day in 4 divided doses × 10 days	Macrolide; protein synthesis inhibitor; active against bacteria lacking cell walls, most gram-positive aerobes	***Contraindication:*** Hypersensitivity ***Cost:*** 250-mg tabs, 4/day × 10 days: $4 ***Pregnancy category:*** B	Nausea, vomiting, diarrhea, abdominal pain, anorexia, rash, urticaria, pseudomembranous colitis—rarely

Lymphogranuloma Venereum

OVERVIEW

Lymphogranuloma venereum is a systemic, sexually transmitted disease that affects the inguinal lymph nodes.

Pathogenesis

- Cause—virulent serovar of *Chlamydia trachomatis:* L_1, L_2, or L_3
- Infects lymphoid tissue instead of columnar epithelial cells

Patient Profile

- Males > Females
- Rare in United States, but increasing incidence of anorectal infection in male homosexuals
- Common in Africa, Asia, South America, Haiti, and Jamaica

Signs and Symptoms

- Primary stage:
  - Superficial papules, vesicles, ulcers, or erosions on external genitalia
  - Painless
  - Heal without scarring
- Secondary stage:
  - Fever
  - Chills
  - Inguinal lymphadenopathy (may be unilateral)—begins a week to months after primary stage
  - Nodes (buboes) are firm and tender
  - Eventually involve overlying skin—severe pain
  - In 1 to 2 weeks buboes become fluctuant and rupture—drain, heal, and scar
- Tertiary stage:
  - Anogenital stage—inflammation of genitalia or anorectal canal
  - Rectum inoculated through direct contact or through posterior lymphatic spread
  - Predominantly seen in women and homosexual men
  - Proctitis
  - Fever
  - Tenesmus
  - Anal pruritus
  - Lymphatic obstruction
  - Perirectal abscess
  - Anal fistulas
  - Rectal stricture/stenosis

Differential Diagnosis

- Chancroid
- Genital herpes
- Syphilis
- Gonorrhea
- Irritable bowel syndrome

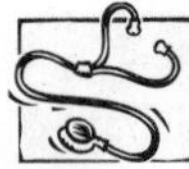

ASSESSMENT

History

Inquire about:

- Onset and duration of symptoms
- Primary lesions and when they occurred
- Travel to Africa, South America, Haiti, Jamaica, East Asia, Indonesia
- Sexual history and behaviors
- Known unprotected contact with an infected partner
- Past history of sexually transmitted diseases
- Underlying conditions
- Current medications

Physical Findings

Depends on stage:

- Primary stage—papules, vesicles, ulcers, or erosions on external genitalia
- Secondary stage—fever, chills, enlarged inguinal lymph nodes (unilateral, may be firm or fluctuant, painful)
- Tertiary stage—genital or anorectal inflammation, proctitis, fever, tenesmus, rectal discharge, perianal growths, perirectal abscesses, fistulas, rectal strictures or stenosis

Initial Workup

Laboratory

- CBC with differential—slightly increased WBC count
- Lymphocytosis or monocytosis
- Serologic testing using fixation, neutralizing antibody, or immunofluorescence (check with laboratory on availability—not widely done)
- Rapid plasma reagin (RPR)
- HIV screening

Radiology: Barium enema—elongated strictures

Further Workup

Incision and drainage of fluctuant buboes for culture and sensitivity

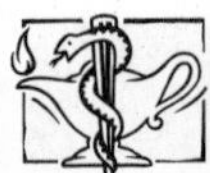

INTERVENTIONS

Office Treatment

Incision and drainage of fluctuant buboes

Lifestyle Modification

Practice safe sex

Patient Education

Teach patient about:

- Disease and treatment—antibiotics
- Safe sex practices—proper use of condom; avoidance of multiple partners; partners need to be treated
- No sexual intercourse until treatment completed
- Medications used and side effects (see Pharmacotherapeutics)

Referrals

Usually none; to infectious disease specialist if treatment fails

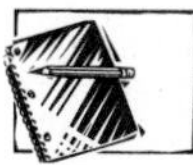

EVALUATION

Outcomes

- Early treatment resolves without sequelae
- Relapse with inadequate treatment

Possible Complications

- Scarring results in renal or bowel obstructions
- Fistulas
- Destruction of anal canal, anal sphincter, perineum

Follow-up

Weekly during treatment

FOR YOUR INFORMATION

Life Span

Pediatric: Consider sexual abuse
Geriatric: Recovery may take longer and may be more complications
Pregnancy: May be acquired by neonate during passage through infected birth canal

Miscellaneous

N/A

References

Bennett EC: Vaginitis and sexually transmitted diseases. In Youngkin EQ, Davis MS, editors: *Women's health: a primary care clinical guide,* Norwalk, Conn, 1994, Appleton & Lange, pp 231-232.

Goens JL, Schwartz RA, DeWolf K: Mucocutaneous manifestations of chancroid, lymphogranuloma venereum, and granuloma inguinale, *Am Fam Physician* 49(2):415-418, 423-425, 1994.

NOTES

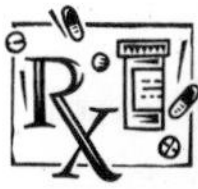

PHARMACOTHERAPEUTICS

Drug of Choice	Mechanism of Action	Prescribing Information	Side Effects
Doxycycline (Doryx), 100 mg PO bid × 21 days; children >8 years, 4.4 mg/kg/day divided q12h × 21 days	Tetracycline; inhibits protein synthesis	***Contraindications:*** Hypersensitivity; children <8 years ***Cost:*** 100-mg tab, 20 tabs: $5 ***Pregnancy category:*** D	Eosinophilia, neutropenia, thrombocytopenia, hemolytic anemia, dysphagia, glossitis, nausea, abdominal pain, vomiting, diarrhea, anorexia, hepatotoxicity, flatulence, abdominal cramps, gastritis, pericarditis, rash, urticaria, exfoliative dermatitis, angioedema
Erythromycin (E-Base), 500 mg PO qid × 21 days; children, 30-50 mg/kg/day PO in divided doses q12h × 21 days	Macrolide; suppresses protein synthesis	***Contraindication:*** Hypersensitivity ***Cost:*** 500-mg tab, 100 tabs: $17 ***Pregnancy category:*** B	Rash, urticaria, pruritus, nausea, vomiting, diarrhea, hepatotoxicity, abdominal pain, stomatitis, heartburn, vaginitis, moniliasis

Mastalgia

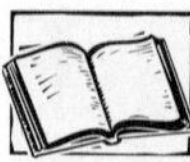

OVERVIEW

Mastalgia is defined as pain in the breasts. It is usually due to congestion in the breasts from any number of causes. There are 3 distinct patterns of breast pain: cyclical, noncyclical, and chest wall pain.

Pathogenesis

- Cyclical pain
  - Waxes and wanes with menstrual cycle
  - Most common type
  - Exact cause unknown
- Noncyclical pain
  - No relationship to menstrual cycle
  - Pain is usually localized to a single spot
  - Exact cause unknown
- Chest wall pain—usually costochondritis
- Mastalgia may be associated with:
  - Fibrocystic breast disease
  - Premenstrual syndrome
  - Pregnancy
  - Hormone replacement therapy or oral contraceptives
  - Infection
  - Advanced breast cancer
  - Trauma, such as abuse

Patient Profile

- Females
- Menarche to menopause
- Mild pain—very common; severe pain—uncommon

Signs and Symptoms

- Cyclical pain:
  - Breasts aching, heavy, tender, bilateral; pain is diffuse
  - Patient may report inability to sleep on stomach because of pain
  - Breasts may enlarge
- Noncyclical pain—pain may be diffuse or localized to a single spot
- Chest wall pain—pain begins in midchest and radiates to breast

Differential Diagnosis

Must differentiate various associated conditions

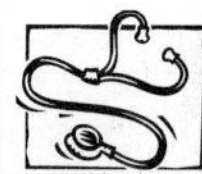

ASSESSMENT

History

Inquire about:

- Onset and duration of symptoms
- Relationship to menstrual cycle
- Severity of pain
- Lumps or masses in breasts
- Amount of coffee, tea, cola, chocolate consumed
- Menstrual and obstetric history
- Treatments tried and results
- Underlying conditions
- Current medications

Physical Findings

- Breast examination—may be normal or may find lump or mass
- Nipple discharge
- Skin dimpling
- Abscess
- Compare size of breasts

Initial Workup

Laboratory

- Possible TSH and prolactin
- Usually none necessary

Radiology: Mammogram if indicated by age or presence of suspicious lump

Further Workup

- Fine-needle aspiration for cysts
- Breast biopsy if indicated

INTERVENTIONS

Office Treatment

None indicated

Lifestyle Modifications

- Weight reduction if indicated
- Smoking cessation
- Low-fat, low-salt diet and decreased methylxanthines

Patient Education

Teach patient about:

- Condition and cause if found
- Treatment—many treatments can be tried (hormone therapy, gammalinolenic acid, vitamins B_6 and E, danazol, bromocriptine), no one treatment proven effective
- Decreased methylxanthine intake
- Decreased salt intake, especially 1 to 2 days before menses
- Decreased fat intake
- Wearing good support bra day and night during worst pain
- Ice packs
- Fact that breast pain does not mean cancer
- Medications used and side effects (see Pharmacotherapeutics)

Referral

Usually none needed; to surgeon if biopsy necessary

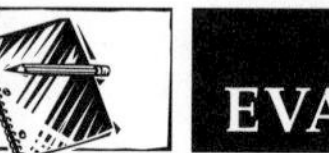

EVALUATION

Outcome

Patient will have reduced pain

Possible Complications

Side effects of medications used

Follow-up

In 1 month to assess effectiveness of treatment and for repeat breast examination

FOR YOUR INFORMATION

Life Span

Pediatric: May begin at menarche
Geriatric: Look for an advanced cancer
Pregnancy: May have breast pain due to hormonal changes

Miscellaneous

N/A

References

Baker S: Menstruation and related problems and concerns. In Youngkin EQ, Davis MS, editors: *Women's health: a primary care clinical guide,* Norwalk, Conn, 1994, Appleton & Lange, pp 92-98.

Perna WC: Pearls for practice: mastalgia: diagnosis and treatment, *J Am Acad Nurse Pract* 8(12):579-584, 1996.

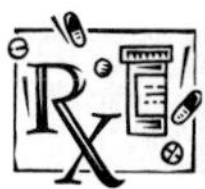

PHARMACOTHERAPEUTICS

Drug of Choice	Mechanism of Action	Prescribing Information	Side Effects
Combination oral contraceptives: many brands available; dosage and instructions vary for different types; see individual package insert for directions	Prevent ovulation by suppressing FSH and LH	***Contraindications:*** Hypersensitivity; breast cancer; thromboembolic disorders; reproductive cancer; undiagnosed vaginal bleeding; pregnancy; hepatic tumor/disease; women 40 years and over; cerebrovascular accident (CVA) ***Cost:*** Varies by brand: $20-$30 ***Pregnancy category:*** X	Dizziness, headache, migraines, depression, hypotension, thrombophlebitis, thromboembolism, pulmonary embolism, myocardial infarction (MI), nausea, vomiting, cholestatic jaundice, weight gain, diplopia, amenorrhea, cervical erosion, breakthrough bleeding, dysmenorrhea, vaginal candidiasis, spontaneous abortion, rash, urticaria, acne, hirsutism, photosensitivity
Gamma-linolenic acid (Evening Primrose), 3 g PO qd	Contains essential fatty acids that help control prolactin secretion	***Contraindication:*** Hypersensitivity ***Cost:*** OTC; at health food stores ***Pregnancy category:*** Not categorized	Mild GI disturbances
Danazol (Danocrine), 100-800 mg/day PO in 2 divided doses × 6-9 months	Decreases FSH and LH; results in amenorrhea/anovulation	***Contraindications:*** Hypersensitivity; severe renal, cardiac, or hepatic disease; pregnancy; abnormal genital bleeding ***Cost:*** 200-mg tab, 60 tabs: $200 ***Pregnancy category:*** C	Rash, acneiform lesions, oily hair, flushing, sweating, dizziness, headache, fatigue, tremors, paresthesias, anxiety, cramps, muscle spasms, increased blood pressure, hematuria, atrophic vaginitis, decreased libido, decreased breast size, clitoral hypertrophy, nausea, vomiting, weight gain, cholestatic jaundice, nasal congestion
Bromocriptine mesylate (Parlodel); start with ½ to 1 tablet of 2.5 mg/day PO and increase as needed to achieve therapeutic affect; lowest therapeutic dose should be used; may take an average of 6-8 weeks to see results; take with food	Decreases prolactin secretion and, in patients with pituitary adenoma, has been shown to shrink the adenoma	***Contraindications:*** Hypersensitivity; severe ischemia or peripheral vascular disease ***Cost:*** 2.5-mg tab, 30 tabs: $48 ***Pregnancy category:*** B	Nausea, headache, dizziness, fatigue, lightheadedness, vomiting, abdominal cramps, nasal congestion, diarrhea, constipation, drowsiness; incidence of side effects is quite high
Ibuprofen (Motrin), 400 mg PO qid	Not well understood; may be related to inhibition of prostaglandin synthesis	***Contraindications:*** Aspirin allergy; hypersensitivity; asthma; last trimester of pregnancy; gastric ulcer; bleeding disorders ***Cost:*** 400-mg tab, 4/day × 5 days: $3 ***Pregnancy category:*** Not categorized but not recommended	Nausea, heartburn, diarrhea, GI upset and bleeding, dizziness, headache, rash, tinnitus, edema, acute renal failure
Pyridoxine (vitamin B_6), 50 mg PO qd	Water-soluble vitamin	***Contraindication:*** Hypersensitivity ***Cost:*** OTC ***Pregnancy category:*** A	Paresthesia, flushing, warmth, lethargy
Vitamin E, 150-600 IU PO qd	Fat-soluble vitamin	***Contraindication:*** Hypersensitivity ***Cost:*** OTC ***Pregnancy category:*** A	Altered metabolism of hormones, altered immunity, weakness, headache, fatigue, nausea, cramps, diarrhea, gonadal dysfunction, blurred vision, contact dermatitis
Spironolactone (Aldactone), 25 mg PO qd, maximum 200 mg PO qd; use lowest effective dose; children, 3.3 mg/kg/day PO	Competes with aldosterone at receptor sites in distal tubules; results in excretion of sodium, chloride, and water, retention of potassium	***Contraindications:*** Hypersensitivity; anuria; severe renal disease; hyperkalemia ***Cost:*** 25-mg tab, 100 tabs: $4-$37 ***Pregnancy category:*** D	Headache, confusion, drowsiness, diarrhea, cramps, bleeding, gastritis, vomiting, anorexia, dysrhythmias, rash, pruritus, urticaria, amenorrhea, decreased WBC count, hyperkalemia

Mastoiditis

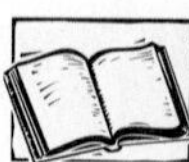

OVERVIEW

Mastoiditis is an inflammatory and infective process of the mastoid air cells. Mastoid air cells are air-filled sinuses in the mastoid process.

Pathogenesis

Causes:

- Acute otitis media
- Inadequately treated suppurative otitis media
- Cholesteatoma

Patient Profile

- Males = Females
- Most common age groups—children and middle-aged adults

Signs and Symptoms

- Ear pain
- Protrusion of auricle
- Bulging tympanic membrane
- Erythematous tympanic membrane
- Postauricular edema
- Tenderness
- Fever

Differential Diagnosis

- Severe otitis externa
- Postauricular cellulitis
- Benign or malignant neoplasm

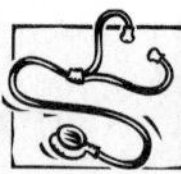

ASSESSMENT

History

Inquire about:

- Onset and duration of symptoms
- History of ear infection, how treated, and whether all medication was taken
- Underlying conditions
- Current medications

Physical Findings

- Auricle and mastoid process may be extremely painful to palpation
- Tympanic membrane bulging and erythematous
- Fever

Initial Workup

Laboratory: CBC with differential—elevated WBC count and left shift on differential

Radiology: Mastoid films—clouding of mastoid air cells

Further Workup

Audiogram—to assess hearing

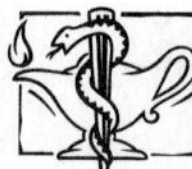

INTERVENTIONS

Office Treatment

None indicated

Lifestyle Modifications

- No swimming
- Earplugs when showering

Patient Education

Teach patient about:

- Disease process and cause
- Treatment:
  - Hospitalization during acute phase for IV antibiotics
  - Myringotomy
  - PO antibiotics after discharge
- Importance of taking all medications
- Avoidance of water in ear
- How to take medication and side effects (see Pharmacotherapeutics)

Referral

To physician for hospitalization if NP does not have hospital privileges

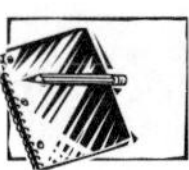

EVALUATION

Outcome

Depends on severity—if treated early, resolves without sequelae

Possible Complications

- Hearing loss
- Subperiosteal abscess, sigmoid sinus thrombosis
- Meningitis
- Intracranial abscess

Follow-up

Within 48 hours of hospital discharge; then in 2 weeks

FOR YOUR INFORMATION

Life Span

Pediatric: Common in this age group—parents need thorough teaching to ensure compliance

Geriatric: May require longer hospitalization

Pregnancy: Cautious use of medications

Miscellaneous

Patients who are immunocompromised are at increased risk of developing mastoiditis.

References

Bull TR: *Color atlas of E.N.T. diagnosis,* ed 3, London, 1995, Mosby-Wolfe, pp 73-75, 85.

Jackler RK, Kaplan MJ: Ear, nose, and throat. In Tierney LM Jr, McPhee SJ, Papadakis MA, editors: *Current medical diagnosis and treatment,* ed 34, Norwalk, Conn, 1995, Appleton & Lange, p 175.

NOTES

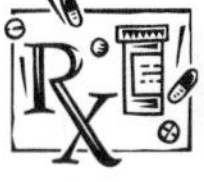

PHARMACOTHERAPEUTICS

Drug of Choice	Mechanism of Action	Prescribing Information	Side Effects
Ampicillin/sulbactam (Unasyn), 750 mg q8h IV—do not use in children <12 years	Bactericidal; effective against beta-lactamase–producing organisms; interferes with cell wall replication	***Contraindications:*** Hypersensitivity to any penicillin; may have cross-sensitivity if allergic to cephalosporins ***Cost:*** 1.5-g vial, 10 vials: $64 ***Pregnancy category:*** B	Anaphylaxis, pseudomembranous colitis, bone marrow depression, nausea, vomiting, diarrhea, vaginitis, glomerulonephritis, convulsions, coma
Cefuroxime (Zinacef), 750 mg PO q8h IV; children >3 months, 50-100 mg/kg/day in divided doses q8h IV	Cephalosporin; bactericidal; inhibits cell wall synthesis; effective against beta-lactamase–producing organisms	***Contraindications:*** Hypersensitivity to cephalosporins; may have cross-sensitivity if allergic to penicillins ***Cost:*** 1.5-g vial, 10 vials: $140 ***Pregnancy category:*** B	May have cross-sensitivity if allergic to penicillins; anaphylaxis, pseudomembranous colitis, nausea, vomiting, diarrhea, nephrotoxicity, leukopenia, agranulocytosis, rash, urticaria
Amoxicillin/clavulanate potassium (Augmentin), 875 mg 1 PO bid × 14 days; children, 25-45 mg/kg/day PO in 2 divided doses × 14 days	Penicillin; broad-spectrum; bactericidal; effective against beta-lactamase–producing organisms	***Contraindication:*** Hypersensitivity to penicillins ***Cost:*** 875-mg tab, 2/day: $78 ***Pregnancy category:*** B	May have cross-sensitivity if allergic to cephalosporins; anaphylaxis, bone marrow depression, leukopenia, nausea, vomiting, diarrhea, pseudomembranous colitis, vaginitis, glomerulonephritis
For patients who are hypersensitive to penicillin/cephalosporins:			
Erythromycin (E-mycin); adults and children, 15-20 mg/kg/day IV in divided doses q6h; adults, 250-500 mg PO q6h; children, 30-50 mg/kg/day PO in divided doses q6h	Macrolide; suppresses protein synthesis	***Contraindication:*** Hypersensitivity ***Cost:*** 1-g vial: $18; 250-mg tabs, 4/day × 14 days: $12-$15 ***Pregnancy category:*** B	Rash, urticaria, nausea, vomiting, diarrhea, hepatotoxicity, stomatitis, anorexia, vaginitis

Measles (Rubella)

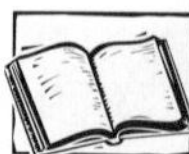

OVERVIEW

Rubella is a benign, contagious viral disease. The disease can cause fetal infection with resultant birth defects. The disease is also known as German measles or 3-day measles.

Pathogenesis

- Cause—single-stranded RNA virus
- Spread by airborne droplets; replicates in nasopharynx and regional lymph nodes
- Incubation period—14 to 21 days
- Invades bloodstream; either spreads to skin or to fetus of pregnant woman
- Can produce disseminated fetal infection—most hazardous in first trimester
- Three phases—incubation phase, prodromal phase, eruptive phase

Patient Profile

- Males = Females
- Predominantly children ages 5 to 9 years
- Incidence decreased because of vaccine, but still have outbreaks in hospitals, colleges, prisons, religious communities, etc.

Signs and Symptoms

- Incubation phase—asymptomatic
- Prodromal phase—malaise, headache, fever, lymphadenopathy, petechiae of soft palate (late prodromal or early eruptive; only 2% of cases)
- Eruptive phase—rash of 1-cm, round or oval, pinkish to rosy red macules or maculopapules; begins on face and neck and rapidly spreads to trunk and extremities
- Fades in 24 to 48 hours in same order
- Congenital rubella—cataracts, microphthalmia, chorioretinitis, patent ductus arteriosus, pulmonic stenosis, atrial and ventricular septal defects, sensorineural deafness, microcephaly, meningoencephalitis, mental retardation, low birth weight, purpuric skin lesions, radiolucent bone disease, hepatosplenomegaly, large anterior fontanel, language and behavior disorders, cryptorchidism, inguinal hernia

Differential Diagnosis

- Measles, scarlet fever, infectious mononucleosis, toxoplasmosis, roseola infantum, erythema infectiosum, drug eruptions
- Congenital rubella—cytomegalovirus, varicella-zoster, picornavirus, poliovirus, herpes simplex, Western equine encephalitis, measles, hepatitis B, mumps, influenza, toxoplasmosis, congenital syphilis, malaria

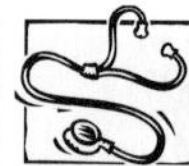

ASSESSMENT

History

Inquire about:

- Onset and duration of symptoms, including prodromal symptoms
- Contact with other infected individuals
- Status of immunizations
- Living conditions
- Treatments tried
- Underlying diseases
- Current medications

Physical Findings

- Lymphadenopathy—usually postauricular, suboccipital, and cervical
- Pinpoint to 1-cm pinkish to rosy red macular or maculopapular rash

Initial Workup

Laboratory

- CBC—mild leukopenia with lymphocytosis
- Rubella antibody titer—fourfold rise
- Rubella virus culture from pharynx, nose, or blood—positive for rubella virus

Radiology: None indicated

Further Workup

None indicated

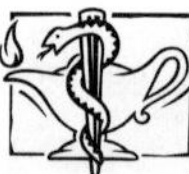

INTERVENTIONS

Office Treatment

Rubella vaccine for those not immunized

Lifestyle Modifications

- Contact isolation for 7 days after rash erupts
- Avoid exposure to pregnant women

Patient Education

Teach patient and parents about:

- Condition and treatment
- Fever control
- Importance of vaccination at appropriate times
- Avoiding contact with pregnant women and why
- Vaccine—educate female patients not to become pregnant for 3 months after receiving vaccine
- Medications used and side effects—avoid use of aspirin (see Pharmacotherapeutics)

Referrals

None indicated; to MD for congenital rubella

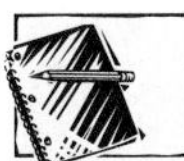

EVALUATION

Outcome
Complete and full recovery without sequelae

Possible Complications
- Postinfectious encephalitis
- Thrombocytopenic purpura
- Testicular pain
- Mild hepatitis
- Congenital rubella:
  - Spontaneous abortion
  - Stillbirth
  - Premature delivery
- Progressive rubella panencephalitis
- Endocrine disturbances

Follow-up
Telephone follow-up in 72 hours

FOR YOUR INFORMATION

Life Span
Pediatric: Most common in this age group
Geriatric: N/A
Pregnancy: Rubella in first trimester can cause congenital rubella syndrome

Miscellaneous
Rubella vaccine should be given to the following individuals if they have not been immunized as children: prepubertal boys and girls, postpartum women, college students, day care personnel, health care workers, and military personnel

References
Fries LF, Halsey NA: Immunization to prevent infectious disease. In Barker LR, Burton JR, Zieve PD, editors: *Principles of ambulatory medicine,* ed 4, Baltimore, 1995, Williams & Wilkins, pp 388-389.

Habif TP: *Clinical dermatology: a color guide to diagnosis and therapy,* ed 3, St Louis, 1996, Mosby, p 417.

NOTES

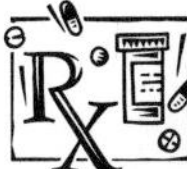

PHARMACOTHERAPEUTICS

Drug of Choice	Mechanism of Action	Prescribing Information	Side Effects
For fever and myalgia:			
Acetaminophen (Tylenol), 10-15 mg/kg/dose in children; adults, 325-650 mg q4-6h PO	Decreases fever through action on hypothalamic heat-regulating center of brain; analgesia by increasing pain threshold	***Contraindication:*** Hypersensitivity ***Cost:*** OTC ***Pregnancy category:*** Not categorized	Anaphylaxis, leukopenia, neutropenia, drowsiness, nausea, vomiting, hepatotoxicity, rash, angioedema, urticaria, toxicity
Rubella vaccine; unless contraindicated, all nonimmunized individuals should receive combination measles, mumps, and rubella vaccine; for adults and children, 0.5 ml SQ; adults receive 1 dose; children, 1 dose at 12-15 months of age, another at either 4-6 years or 11-12 years of age	Live virus that causes body to build antibodies against the disease	***Contraindications:*** Anaphylactoid reaction to neomycin; pregnancy; anaphylactoid reaction to eggs ***Cost:*** 0.5-ml vial: $36 ***Pregnancy category:*** C	Burning/stinging at site of injection, malaise, sore throat, cough, rhinitis, headache, dizziness, fever, rash, nausea, vomiting, diarrhea, regional lymphadenopathy, nerve deafness, allergic reaction, anaphylaxis, optic neuritis

Measles (Rubeola)

OVERVIEW

Measles is a highly contagious viral infection. It is spread by respiratory droplets from infected individuals who cough.

Pathogenesis

- Cause—RNA virus
- Spread by airborne droplets
- Incubation period—7 to 14 days
- Contagious from right before prodromal phase to 4 days after rash appears

Patient Profile

- Males = Females
- Unvaccinated preschool children
- Previously vaccinated adolescents and young adults in secondary schools and colleges

Signs and Symptoms

- Prodromal period—brassy cough, coryza and conjunctivitis, fever, malaise, photophobia, Koplik's spots (minute whitish spots over buccal mucosa, rapidly increase; underlying mucosa bright red and granular)
- Eruptive period—maculopapular, slightly elevated dark red to purple rash (starts on face and behind ears; rapidly spreads to trunk and extremities; early stage blanches easily; fading rash yellowish brown and does not blanch)

Differential Diagnosis

- Drug eruptions
- Infectious mononucleosis
- *Mycoplasma pneumoniae*
- Rubella
- Erythema infectiosum
- Roseola
- Enterovirus
- Rocky Mountain spotted fever

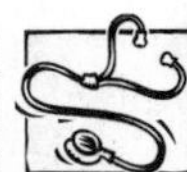

ASSESSMENT

History

Inquire about:

- Onset and duration of symptoms
- Spread of rash (face to trunk and extremities)
- History of vaccination (until 1989, most only vaccinated once; from 1963 to 1968, vaccination was with killed vaccine instead of live)
- Treatments tried and results
- Underlying diseases
- Current medications

Physical Findings

- Prodromal period—Koplik spots (minute whitish spots on buccal mucosa; underlying mucosa bright red and granular)
- Eruptive period—dark red to purple maculopapule rash starting on face and spreading to trunk and extremities; lymphadenopathy

Initial Workup

Laboratory

- Usually none needed
- Measles-specific IgM or substantial rise in IgG titers
- Viral isolation in tissue culture

Radiology: None indicated

Further Workup

None indicated

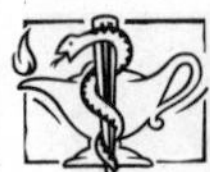

INTERVENTIONS

Office Treatment

- Vaccine administration—effective after exposure if within 72 hours
- Administration of 150,000U of vitamin A palmitate IM

Lifestyle Modifications

- Respiratory isolation until 4 days after onset of rash
- Activity restricted during febrile stage; if immunocompromised, restrict activity during entire disease process

Patient Education

Teach patient and family about:

- Condition and treatment:
  - Immunoglobulin for those exposed and not immunized
  - Vitamin A supplement—found to decrease morbidity and mortality from disease—levels are greatly reduced early in disease
  - Fever control with acetaminophen
- Proper vaccination of children
- Disposing of tissues, covering mouth when coughing, washing hands frequently
- Medications used and side effects (see Pharmacotherapeutics)

Referrals

Usually none

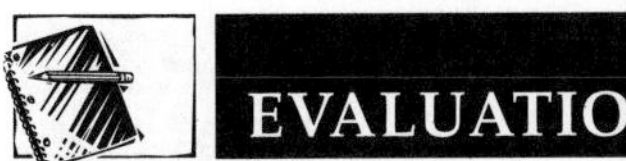

EVALUATION

Outcome
Resolves without sequelae

Possible Complications
- Otitis media
- Laryngotracheitis
- Bronchopneumonia
- Encephalitis
- Hemorrhagic lesions
- Thrombocytopenic purpura
- Myocarditis and pericarditis
- Panencephalitis

Follow-up
None needed unless complications occur

FOR YOUR INFORMATION

Life Span
Pediatric: Most common in this age group
Geriatric: N/A
Pregnancy: Increased fetal morbidity and mortality

Miscellaneous
Recipients of killed measles vaccine (those vaccinated between 1963 and 1968) can develop an atypical measles. Atypical measles has the same prodromal period, and then 3 to 5 days later a maculopapular rash develops on the wrists and ankles. It spreads to the soles of the feet and palms and then to the extremities and trunk. The face is usually spared.

References

Fries, LF, Halsey NA: Immunization to prevent infectious disease. In Barker LR, Burton JR, Zieve PD, editors: *Principles of ambulatory medicine,* ed 4, Baltimore, 1995, Williams & Wilkins, pp 388-389.

Habif TP: *Clinical dermatology: a color guide to diagnosis and therapy,* ed 3, St Louis, 1996, Mosby, pp 409-412.

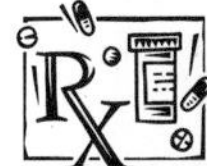

PHARMACOTHERAPEUTICS

Drug of Choice	Mechanism of Action	Prescribing Information	Side Effects
Vitamin A palmitate, 150,000 U IM initially, then 15,000 U PO × 7 days	Increases level of vitamin A, which is reduced early in disease process	***Contraindications:*** Hypersensitivity; hypervitaminosis A ***Cost:*** 50,000 μ/ml, 20-ml vial: $197 ***Pregnancy category:*** X	Allergic reactions, anaphylaxis
For fever and myalgia:			
Acetaminophen (Tylenol), 325-650 mg PO q4-6h; for children, use Children's Tylenol—follow label directions	Decreases fever through action on hypothalamic heat-regulating center of brain; analgesia by increasing pain threshold	***Contraindication:*** Hypersensitivity ***Cost:*** OTC ***Pregnancy category:*** Not categorized	Anaphylaxis, leukopenia, neutropenia, drowsiness, nausea, vomiting, hepatotoxicity, rash, angioedema, urticaria, toxicity
Postexposure prophylaxis:			
Immune globulin; immunocompetent individual, 0.25 ml/kg IM, maximum dose 15 ml; immunocompromised individual, 0.5 ml/kg IM, maximum dose 15 ml	Prevents or modifies disease in person exposed to measles less than 6 days before administration	***Contraindications:*** Anaphylactoid or severe allergic response in past; severe thrombocytopenia; severe vitamin A deficiency ***Cost:*** 10 ml: $9-$18 ***Pregnancy category:*** C	Local pain and tenderness, urticaria, angioedema, anaphylaxis
Rubella vaccine; unless contraindicated, all nonimmunized individuals should receive combination measles, mumps, and rubella vaccine; for adults and children, 0.5 ml SQ; adults receive 1 dose; children, 1 dose at 12-15 months of age, another at either 4-6 years or 11-12 years of age	Live virus, which causes body to build antibodies against the disease	***Contraindications:*** Anaphylactoid reaction to neomycin; pregnancy; anaphylactoid reaction to eggs ***Cost:*** 0.5-ml vial: $36 ***Pregnancy category:*** C	Burning/stinging at site of injection, malaise, sore throat, cough, rhinitis, headache, dizziness, fever, rash, nausea, vomiting, diarrhea, regional lymphadenopathy, nerve deafness, allergic reaction, anaphylaxis, optic neuritis

Melanoma

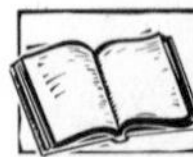

OVERVIEW

Melanoma is a malignancy that arises from the melanocyte system. It is a dangerous tumor that has the ability to metastasize to any organ system.

Pathogenesis

Cause—malignant degeneration of cells in melanocyte system

Patient Profile

- Males = Females
- Median age = 53, but high incidence in 25- to 29-year-old age group
- Risk factors:
  - Fair-skinned, blond hair, freckles, and blue eyes, but does occur in African-Americans
  - Previous pigmented lesions
  - History of blistering sunburn during childhood or adolescence (acute sun exposure with burning more harmful than frequent mild sun exposure)

Signs and Symptoms

- Pigmented lesion—bleeds, scales, changes in size, changes in texture, and changes in color
- Common sites:
  - Whites—back and lower legs
  - African-Americans—hands, feet, and nails

Differential Diagnosis

- Dysplastic nevi
- Vascular skin tumors
- Squamous cell carcinoma
- Basal cell carcinoma
- Seborrheic keratosis

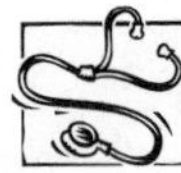

ASSESSMENT

History

Inquire about:

- Onset and duration of lesion
- Change in color, texture, size; bleeding, crusting
- History of previous pigmented lesion in same site
- History of sun exposure with sunburn (blistering) in childhood or adolescence
- History of malignant melanoma
- Treatments tried and results
- Underlying conditions
- Current medications

Physical Findings

Careful examination of entire skin surface, using the ABCDEs of melanoma diagnosis: A = Asymmetry, B = Border irregularity, C = Color variegations, D = Diameter >6 mm, E = Elevation above skin surface

Initial Workup

Laboratory: None indicated
Radiology: Only if concerned about metastasis to brain, lung, lymph system

Further Workup

None indicated by NP

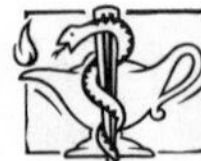

INTERVENTIONS

Office Treatment

None by NP

Lifestyle Modifications

- Avoidance of excessive sun exposure
- Smoking cessation
- Use of sunscreens—needs to protect against UVA, but most protect against UVB (use of hats and proper clothing more effective)

Patient Education

Teach patient about:

- Condition and treatment—surgical excision, chemotherapy
- Performing a skin self-examination (see section on basal cell carcinoma)
- Posttreatment regimen—thorough skin examination every 3 to 6 months by professional, with self-examination weekly
- Protecting children from sunburn
- Medications used and side effects (see Pharmacotherapeutics)

Referral

Prompt referral to dermatologist or surgeon

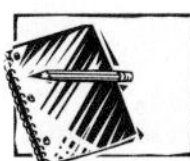

EVALUATION

Outcomes

- Lesion removed with good cosmetic results
- No metastasis
- Best prognosis—lesions <0.85 mm in depth: 95% to 100% 5-year survival
- Worst prognosis—spread to lymphatics: <5% 5-year survival

Possible Complications

- Metastasis
- Death

Follow-up

With dermatologist or surgeon on regular basis

FOR YOUR INFORMATION

Life Span

Pediatric: Need early education of children and parents regarding use of sunscreen and avoidance of sunburn

Geriatric: Higher morbidity and mortality

Pregnancy: If occurs during pregnancy, there is risk to fetus, and consideration should be given to termination of pregnancy

Miscellaneous

The incidence of melanoma, with its resultant mortality, has risen rapidly over the past 2 decades. The most rapidly increasing form of cancer, melanoma may be due in part to alterations in the upper atmosphere by pollutants increasing the amount of radiation that people exposed to the sun are receiving.

References

Habif TP: *Clinical dermatology: a color guide to diagnosis and therapy,* ed 3, St Louis, 1996, Mosby, pp 699-718.

Runkle GP, Zaloznik AJ: Malignant melanoma, *Am Fam Physician* 49(1):91-98, 1994.

NOTES

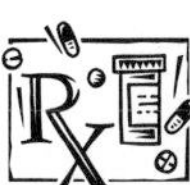

PHARMACOTHERAPEUTICS

There is no clear drug of choice for the treatment of melanoma. Each oncologist will have his or her own treatment recommendations. The following are just two of the options that might be used.

Drug of Choice	Mechanism of Action	Prescribing Information	Side Effects
Dacarbazine (DTIC-Dome), 2-4.5 mg/kg/day IV × 10 days; may be repeated in 4 weeks	Exact mechanism unknown; 3 hypotheses—inhibition of DNA synthesis, action as an alkylating agent, or interaction with SH groups	***Contraindication:*** Hypersensitivity ***Cost:*** 10 mg/ml, 10 ml: $86 ***Pregnancy category:*** C	Hematopoietic depression, hepatic necrosis, anorexia, nausea, vomiting, alopecia, facial flushing
Cisplatin (Platinol), 100 mg/m^2 IV once every 4 weeks; must be administered by individual experienced in use of chemotherapeutic agents	Alkylates DNA, RNA; inhibits enzymes that allow synthesis of amino acids in proteins	***Contraindications:*** Renal impairment; myelosuppression; hearing impairment; hypersensitivity ***Cost:*** 1 mg/ml, 50 mg: $156-$163 ***Pregnancy category:*** D	Severe nausea and vomiting, renal tubular damage, ototoxicity, peripheral neuropathies, hypokalemia and hypomagnesemia, myelosuppression, anemia, anaphylaxis

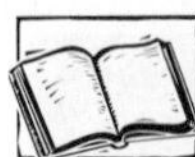

OVERVIEW

Meniere's disease is a disease of the inner ear in which there is increased endolymph, which creates increased pressure in the inner ear.

Pathogenesis

Cause—unknown; several possibilities:

- Excess endolymph in membranous labyrinth—pressure increases; membranous labyrinth ruptures
- High-potassium endolymph mixes with low-potassium perilymph
- Degeneration of vestibular and cochlear hair cells occurs
- Recent theory—intracranial compression of balance nerve by blood vessel

Patient Profile

- Males = Females
- 20 to 60 years of age, most commonly around 40 years of age
- 85% have only one ear affected

Signs and Symptoms

- Sudden, severe attacks of vertigo; may be preceded by an aura—sense of fullness in ear
- Tinnitus
- Decrease in hearing
- Sweating
- Nausea, vomiting
- Falling
- Prostration
- Hearing loss

Differential Diagnosis

- Viral labyrinthitis
- Acoustic tumor
- Syphilis
- Perilymph fistula
- Benign positional vertigo

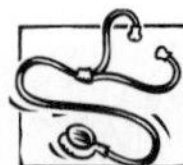

ASSESSMENT

History

Inquire about:

- Onset and duration of symptoms
- Prior injuries to inner ear
- Underlying conditions
- Current medications

Physical Findings

- Between attacks:
  - Low-frequency sensorineural hearing loss
  - Spontaneous nystagmus may be present
- During severe attack:
  - Pallor, sweating, increased heart and respiratory rate
  - Vomiting
  - Falling
  - Decreased hearing
  - Spontaneous nystagmus
  - Patient will not want to move, since this increases symptoms

Initial Workup

Laboratory: Done to rule out other conditions—rapid plasma reagin (RPR) or fluorescent treponemal antibody, thyroid studies

Radiology: MRI to rule out acoustic tumor

Further Workup

To be done by otolaryngologist

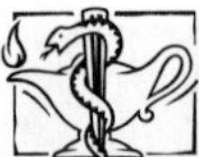

INTERVENTIONS

Office Treatment

If during acute attack, lay patient down, turn off lights, provide emesis basin, have patient close eyes, protect from falling

Lifestyle Modifications

- Must learn to live with unpredictability of attacks—may necessitate change in occupation and change in social life
- Can be very debilitating condition

Patient Education

Teach patient about:

- Need for prompt treatment by otolaryngologist
- Disease process and treatment options—several surgical procedures that are used for incapacitating vertigo
- Medications used (primarily for symptom relief) and side effects (see Pharmacotherapeutics)

Referral

Promptly to otolaryngologist for definitive diagnosis and treatment

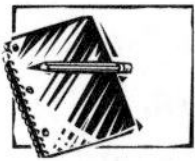

EVALUATION

Outcomes

- Balance problem may improve
- Hearing usually worsens

Possible Complications

- Loss of hearing, injury during attack
- Total disability

Follow-up

By otolaryngologist

FOR YOUR INFORMATION

Life Span

Pediatric: Rarely seen in this population
Geriatric: Higher risk of severe injury due to falls
Pregnancy: Difficult to treat—most drugs used for treatment should not be used in pregnancy

Miscellaneous

An acoustic tumor produces a clinical picture identical to that of Meniere's disease. *Do not overlook that possibility!*

References

Bull TR: *Color atlas of E.N.T. diagnosis,* ed 3, London, 1995, Mosby-Wolfe, pp. 23-25.

Niparko JK: Hearing loss and associated problems. In Barker LR, Burton JR, Zieve PD, editors: *Principles of ambulatory medicine,* ed 4, Baltimore, 1995, Williams & Wilkins, pp 1412-1413.

NOTES

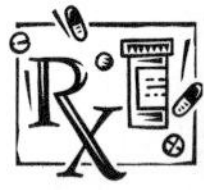

PHARMACOTHERAPEUTICS

Drug of Choice	Mechanism of Action	Prescribing Information	Side Effects
Promethazine (Phenergan), 25 mg PO q6h; children, 12.5-25 mg PO bid	Histamine receptor antagonist; phenothiazine derivative	***Contraindications:*** Hypersensitivity; asthma ***Cost:*** 25-mg tab, 30 tabs: $2 ***Pregnancy category:*** C	Sedation, sleepiness, blurred vision, dry mouth, dizziness, increased or decreased blood pressure, rash, nausea, vomiting
Diazepam (Valium), 5 mg PO qid; elderly, 2 mg PO bid initially; increase as needed to control symptoms; children, 1 mg PO bid	Benzodiazepine; acts on limbic system, thalamus, and hypothalamus	***Contraindications:*** Hypersensitivity; closed-angle glaucoma; psychoses; pregnancy ***Cost:*** 5-mg tab, 30 tabs: $2 ***Pregnancy category:*** D	Dizziness, drowsiness, confusion, headache, anxiety, tremors, orthostatic hypotension, ECG changes, tachycardia, blurred vision, tinnitus, constipation, dry mouth, nausea, vomiting, rash, dermatitis
For vomiting:			
Prochlorperazine suppositories (Compazine), 25 mg PR bid; children, 2.5 mg PR bid-tid—do not use in children <2 years	Phenothiazine; centrally blocks chemoreceptor trigger zone, which acts on vomiting center	***Contraindications:*** Hypersensitivity; coma; seizures, encephalopathy; bone marrow depression ***Cost:*** 25-mg suppository, 12 suppositories: $22 ***Pregnancy category:*** C	Euphoria, depression, extrapyramidal symptoms, restlessness, dizziness, nausea, vomiting, anorexia, dry mouth, diarrhea, constipation, weight loss, circulatory failure, tachycardia, respiratory depression
For vertigo:			
Meclizine (Antivert), 25 mg PO tid-qid—not recommended for children <12 years	Antihistamine	***Contraindications:*** Hypersensitivity; shock; lactation ***Cost:*** 25-mg tab, 30 tabs: $6 ***Pregnancy category:*** B	Drowsiness, fatigue, restlessness, headache, insomnia, nausea, anorexia, dry mouth, blurred vision

Meningitis, Bacterial

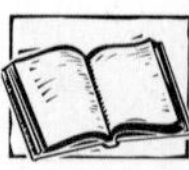

OVERVIEW

Bacterial meningitis is an inflammation of the membranes covering the brain and spinal cord in response to a bacterial infection. It also involves the fluid in the subarachnoid space and the ventricles.

Pathogenesis

- 70% to 90% caused by *Neisseria meningitidis, Haemophilus influenzae,* or *Streptococcus pneumoniae*
- Other organisms—Enterobacteriaceae, group B streptococci, and *Listeria monocytogenes* (neonates, immunocompromised); *Mycobacterium tuberculosis* (from developing countries or immunocompromised); staphylococci (head trauma or neurosurgical shunts)

Patient Profile

- Males = Females
- Any age
- Most common in neonates, infants, and the elderly

Signs and Symptoms

- Headache
- Neck pain and stiffness
- Back pain and stiffness
- Vomiting
- Nausea
- Photophobia
- Fever
- Seizures
- Altered level of consciousness
- Confusion
- Rash—macular and erythematous at onset; then petechial or purpuric

Differential Diagnosis

- Viral meningitis
- Sepsis
- Brain abscess
- Sinusitis
- Subarachnoid hemorrhage
- Vasculitis
- Autoimmune diseases

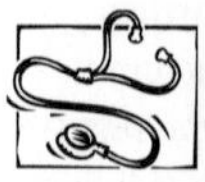

ASSESSMENT

History

Inquire about:

- Onset and duration of symptoms
- Recent upper respiratory tract infection
- Neurosurgical procedures or head injuries
- Alcoholism
- Underlying conditions
- Current medications

Physical Findings

- Fever
- Tachycardia
- Shock
- Confusion or altered level of consciousness
- Nuchal rigidity on flexion only
- Positive Kernig's and Brudzinski's signs
- Meningeal (high-pitched) cry in infants
- Papilledema
- Bulging fontanel in infant
- Rash

Initial Workup

Laboratory

- Lumbar puncture—turbid CSF
- Neonates:
  - WBCs increased in CSF
  - Blood glucose ratio <0.6
  - Protein >150 mg/dl
- Infants/children:
  - WBCs increased in CSF
  - Blood glucose ratio <0.6
  - Protein >50 mg/dl
- Adults:
  - WBCs increased in CSF
  - Blood glucose ratio <0.4
  - Protein >45 mg/dl
- All ages:
  - Gram stain positive in 75%
  - Cultures positive in 70% to 80%
  - CBC—↑ WBC count—may see left shift on differential
  - Blood culture

Radiology

- Chest film—pneumonitis or abscess
- CT scan of head if concerned about increased intracranial pressure
- Sinus/skull films—cranial osteomyelitis, paranasal sinusitis, skull fracture

Further Workup

None indicated

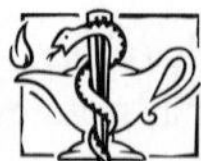

INTERVENTIONS

Office Treatment

Prompt referral to emergency room

Lifestyle Modification

Depends on outcome; if residual neurologic deficits present, may need to make significant modifications

Patient Education

- Teaching will need to be done during recovery phase of illness—patient needs prompt referral to emergency room
- Family members need teaching regarding:
  - Chemoprophylaxis, treatment of patient—possibly intensive care unit, IV antibiotics, steroids
  - Seriousness of condition
  - Medications used and side effects (see Pharmacotherapeutics)

Referral

To emergency room immediately

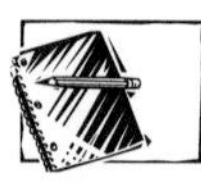

EVALUATION

Outcomes

- Mortality:
  - *H. influenzae*—5% to 10%
  - *N. meningitidis*—5% to 10%
  - *S. pneumoniae*—10% to 30%
- Long-term sequelae—5% to 40%

Possible Complications

- Death
- Neurologic complications
- Sensorineural hearing loss
- Learning deficits
- Subdural effusions

Follow-up

1 week after hospitalization; then every 3 months

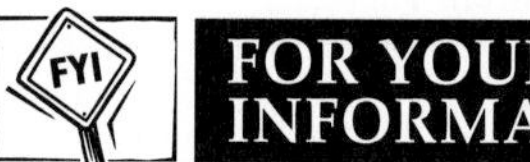

FOR YOUR INFORMATION

Life Span

Pediatric: Most common in neonates and infants

Geriatric: Signs and symptoms may be more subtle

Pregnancy: Cautious use of medications; protection of fetus

Miscellaneous

The NP needs to ensure that household contacts receive the proper chemoprophylaxis. Hearing loss may be permanent.

References

Bartlett JG: *Pocket book of infectious disease therapy,* ed 7, Baltimore, 1996, Williams & Wilkins, pp 252-259.

Woolliscroft JO: *Current diagnosis and treatment: a quick reference guide for the general practitioner,* Philadelphia, 1996, Current Medicine, pp 248-249.

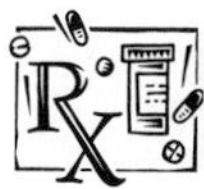

PHARMACOTHERAPEUTICS

Drug of Choice	Mechanism of Action	Prescribing Information	Side Effects
Use one of the following for chemoprophylaxis of household contacts:			
Rifampin (Rifampicin), 600 mg PO bid × 2 days; children >1 month, 10 mg/kg PO bid × 2 days; children <1 month, 5 mg/kg PO bid × 2 days	Inhibits DNA-dependent polymerase; decreases tubercle bacilli replication	***Contraindication:*** Hypersensitivity ***Cost:*** 300-mg tab, 30 tabs: $50 ***Pregnancy category:*** C	Rash, pruritis, visual disturbances, weakness, flulike syndrome, edema, shortness of breath, nausea, vomiting, anorexia, diarrhea, pseudomembranous colitis, pancreatitis, hematuria, acute renal failure, hemoglobinuria, hemolytic anemia, thrombocytopenia, leukopenia
Ciprofloxacin (Cipro), 500 mg PO × 1 dose—not recommended for children <18 years	Interferes with conversion of intermediate DNA fragments into high molecular weight DNA	***Contraindication:*** Hypersensitivity to quinolones ***Cost:*** 500-mg tab, 1 tab: $3 ***Pregnancy category:*** C	Headache, dizziness, fatigue, insomnia, depression, restlessness, nausea, diarrhea, increased AST and ALT, flatulence, heartburn, vomiting, dysphagia, oral candidiasis, rash, pruritis, photosensitivity, fever, chills, pruritus, urticaria, blurred vision, tinnitus
There are many IV antibiotics that may be used for treatment. Treatment should be based on culture results, but should start immediately. For empiric treatment until culture results are known, give both of the following:			
Ceftriaxone (Rocephin), 2 g IV q12h; children, 100 mg/kg/day IV divided q12h	Cephalosporin; inhibits bacterial cell wall synthesis	***Contraindication:*** Hypersensitivity to cephalosporins ***Cost:*** 250-mg vial: $11 ***Pregnancy category:*** C	Headache; dizziness; weakness; paresthesias; nausea; vomiting; diarrhea; anorexia; increased AST, ALT, bilirubin, LDH, and alkaline phosphatase; pseudomembranous colitis; proteinuria; nephrotoxicity; leukopenia; thrombocytopenia; agranulocytosis; neutropenia; hemolytic anemia; rash; urticaria; anaphylaxis
Vancomycin (Vancocin), 1 g IV q12h; children, 60 mg/kg/day IV divided q12h	Inhibits bacterial cell wall synthesis	***Contraindication:*** Hypersensitivity ***Cost:*** 1-gm vial: $23-$63 ***Pregnancy category:*** C	Renal failure, nausea, pseudomembranous colitis, hearing loss, vertigo, dizziness, tinnitus, rashes, reversible agranulocytosis, chills, anaphylaxis
Consider adding:			
Rifampin (Rifampicin), 300 mg PO or IV; children, 20 mg/kg/day IV	Antitubercular; decreases replication of bacilli	***Contraindication:*** Hypersensitivity ***Cost:*** 300-mg tab, 60 tabs: $89-$126 ***Pregnancy category:*** C	Rash, pruritus, visual disturbances, flulike syndrome, nausea, vomiting, anorexia, diarrhea, pseudomembranous colitis, heartburn, pancreatitis, hematuria, acute renal failure, hemoglobinuria, headache, fatigue, hemolytic anemia, eosinophilia, thrombocytopenia, leukopenia; discoloration of urine, stool, saliva, sputum, sweat, tears to red-orange color
To reduce neurologic sequelae in children and high-risk adults (with impaired mental status, cerebral edema, and/or very high intracranial pressure), consider giving the following:			
Dexamethasone 0.15 mg/kg IV q6h × 4 days	Corticosteroid; antiinflammatory	***Contraindications:*** Hypersensitivity; psychosis; idiopathic thrombocytopenia; acute glomerulonephritis; amebiasis; nonasthmatic bronchial disease; AIDS; TB; children <2 years old ***Cost:*** 8 mg/ml, 5 ml: $11-$47 ***Pregnancy category:*** C	Hypertension, circulatory collapse, thrombophlebitis, embolism, tachycardia, fungal infections, increased intraocular pressure, diarrhea, nausea, GI hemorrhage, thrombocytopenia, acne, poor wound healing, fractures, osteoporosis, weakness

OVERVIEW

Viral meningitis is inflammation of the membranes covering the brain and spinal cord in response to a viral infection. It also involves the fluid in the subarachnoid space and in the ventricles.

Pathogenesis
Caused by:
- Coxsackievirus A, B
- Enteroviruses
- Poliovirus
- Mumps
- Herpes simplex and zoster
- Epstein-Barr virus
- Cytomegalovirus
- Adenovirus

Patient Profile
- Males = Females
- Any age; most commonly young adults
- Peaks in summertime

Signs and Symptoms
- Severe headache
- Fever
- Nausea
- Vomiting
- Stiff neck
- Photophobia
- Myalgias
- Occasionally rash

Differential Diagnosis
- Bacterial meningitis
- Encephalitis
- Migraine headache
- Brain abscess
- Postinfectious encephalomyelitis

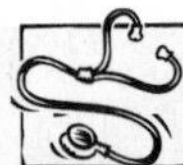

ASSESSMENT

History
Inquire about:
- Onset and duration of symptoms
- Fever
- Underlying conditions
- Current medications

Physical Findings
- Fever
- Tachycardia
- Shock
- Nuchal rigidity on flexion
- Positive Kernig's and Brudzinski's signs
- Papilledema

Initial Workup
Laboratory
- Lumbar puncture:
  - CSF cell count up to 3000 to 4000 (usually 50-200)
  - CSF increased pressure
  - CSF protein increased, but usually <150
  - CSF glucose normal
  - Negative CSF Gram stain and culture
- CBC—WBC normal or slightly elevated

Radiology: CT scan or MRI of brain

Further Workup
EEG if encephalitis is a concern

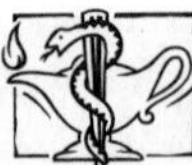

INTERVENTIONS

Office Treatment
None indicated; consult with MD regarding hospital admission

Lifestyle Modification
Hospitalization for 1 week

Patient Education
Teach patient about:
- Disease process and treatment options—inpatient, symptomatic treatment; antibiotics not indicated but may be started if unsure if bacterial or viral
- Low probability of transmission to contacts
- May need IV fluids if oral intake poor or vomiting present
- Medications used and side effects (see Pharmacotherapeutics)

Referral
To MD for hospital admission

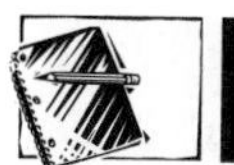

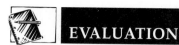

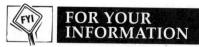

EVALUATION

Outcome
Complete recovery in 2 to 7 days

Possible Complications
- Fatigue
- Irritability
- Muscle weakness
- Rarely, seizures

Follow-up
In 7 days after hospitalization

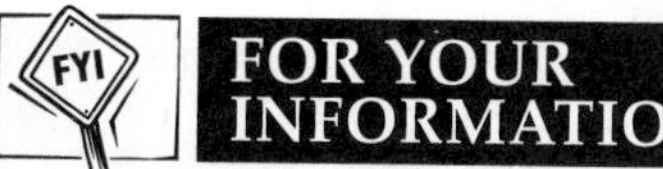

FOR YOUR INFORMATION

Life Span
Pediatric: Uncommon
Geriatric: Rarely seen in this population—look for alternative diagnosis
Pregnancy: Cautious use of medications

Miscellaneous
Although it may be permanent after bacterial meningitis, hearing loss is not a complication of viral meningitis.

References

Jacobs RA: General problems in infectious diseases. In Tierney LM Jr, McPhee SJ, Papadakis MA, editors: *Current medical diagnosis and treatment,* ed 35, Norwalk, Conn, 1995, Appleton & Lange, pp 1086-1089.

Kerr ME, Walleck CA: Nursing role in management: intracranial problems. In Lewis SM, Collier IC, Heitkemper MM, editors: *Medical-surgical nursing assessment and management of clinical problems,* ed 4, St Louis, 1996, Mosby, pp 1715-1718.

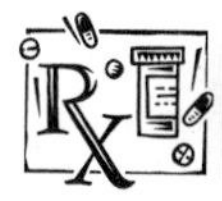

PHARMACOTHERAPEUTICS

Drug of Choice	Mechanism of Action	Prescribing Information	Side Effects
May need parenteral narcotic analgesia, such as one of the following:			
Meperidine (Demerol), 25-50 mg IM q4h; children, 1 mg/kg IM q4h	Depresses pain impulse transmission at spinal cord	***Contraindications:*** Hypersensitivity; narcotic addiction ***Cost:*** 25 mg/ml, 1 ml: $5 ***Pregnancy category:*** C	Drowsiness, dizziness, confusion, headache, sedation, euphoria, increased intracranial pressure, palpitations, bradycardia, tachycardia, tinnitus, blurred vision, miosis, diplopia, nausea, vomiting, anorexia, cramps, constipation, urinary retention, rash, urticaria, respiratory depression
Morphine, 2-5 mg IM or IV q3-4h; children, 0.1-0.2 mg/kg SQ q4h	Depresses pain impulse transmission at spinal cord by interacting with opioid receptors	***Contraindications:*** Hypersensitivity; narcotic addiction; hemorrhage; bronchial asthma; increased intracranial pressure ***Cost:*** 10 mg/ml, 10 ml: $7-$13 ***Pregnancy category:*** B	Drowsiness, dizziness, confusion, headache, sedation, euphoria, palpitations, change in blood pressure, bradycardia, tinnitus, blurred vision, miosis, nausea, vomiting, anorexia, constipation, cramps, urinary retention, rash, urticaria, respiratory depression
For nausea and vomiting:			
Prochlorperazine suppositories (Compazine), 25 mg PR bid; children 2.5 mg PR bid-tid—do not use in children <2 years	Phenothiazine; centrally blocks chemoreceptor trigger zone, which acts on vomiting center	***Contraindications:*** Hypersensitivity; coma; seizures, encephalopathy; bone marrow depression ***Cost:*** 25-mg suppository, 12 suppositories: $22 ***Pregnancy category:*** C	Euphoria, depression, extrapyramidal symptoms, restlessness, dizziness, nausea, vomiting, anorexia, dry mouth, diarrhea, constipation, weight loss, circulatory failure, tachycardia, respiratory depression
For fever and myalgia:			
Acetaminophen (Tylenol), 650 mg PO q4h; children, 10-15 mg/kg/dose PO q4h	Decreases fever through action on hypothalamic heat-regulating center of brain; analgesia by increasing pain threshold	***Contraindications:*** Hypersensitivity; bleeding disorders or anticoagulant therapy; last trimester of pregnancy; asthma; gastric ulcers ***Cost:*** OTC ***Pregnancy category:*** Not categorized	Rash; hepatic toxicity with alcohol ingestion or overdose

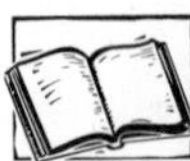

OVERVIEW

Menopause is defined as cessation of menses for 6 months or a serum follicle-stimulating hormone (FSH) level >40 mIU/ml on 2 occasions 1 week apart. There is a 7- to 10-year period before cessation of menses in which physiologic changes of the reproductive system occur that is known as the climacteric period.

Pathogenesis

Cause:
- Physiologic changes in ovarian follicles occur with aging
- After age 35, few follicles responsive to FSH
- As follicles decrease, production of estrogen and progesterone decreases

Patient Profile

- Females
- Before age 30—premature menopause
- Age 31 to 40 years—early menopause
- Age >40 years—normal menopause

Signs and Symptoms

- Cessation of menses
- Hot flushes
- Sweating, especially at night
- Depression
- Nervousness
- Insomnia
- Dyspareunia
- Vulvar atrophy
- Vaginal atrophy
- Stress incontinence
- Urge incontinence
- Nocturia
- Skin—wrinkles, dryness

Differential Diagnosis

- Pregnancy
- Hypothalamic dysfunction
- Polycystic ovarian disease
- Obstruction of uterine outflow tract
- Thyroid disease

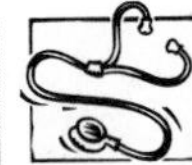

ASSESSMENT

History

Inquire about:
- Onset and duration of symptoms
- Severity of symptoms
- Menstrual and obstetric history
- Birth control
- Underlying conditions
- Current medications

Physical Findings

- Skin—dry and wrinkled
- Speculum examination—vaginal atrophy and dryness, small uterus; check for uterine prolapse, rectocele, cystocele
- Thyroid may be irregular or nodular
- May find fractures as a result of osteoporosis (late finding)

Initial Workup

Laboratory
- FSH level >40 mIU (diagnostic of menopause)
- E_2 level <50 pq/ml
- For patient considering hormone replacement therapy (HRT)—chemistry profile, including lipid panel and liver function tests
- Pap smear
- Mammogram
- Thyroid studies

Radiology: Bone mineral density if concerned about osteoporosis

Further Workup

Endometrial biopsy (controversial)

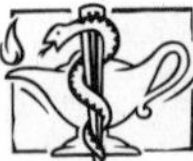

INTERVENTIONS

Office Treatment

None needed

Lifestyle Modifications

- Smoking cessation
- Regular exercise program

Patient Education

Teach patient about:
- Condition and treatment options for various symptoms—HRT alleviates most symptoms
- Benefits of HRT—prevention of osteoporosis, protection against coronary heart disease, alleviation of symptoms
- Risks of HRT—breast cancer (remains controversial), endometrial cancer (only if on unopposed estrogen)
- Hypercoagulability and thrombosis (estrogen dosage usually low enough not to cause this problem)
- For urinary incontinence—pelvic floor exercises
- For skin and vaginal dryness—lubrication
- Sexuality and birth control
- Weight-bearing exercise to prevent osteoporosis
- Medications used and side effects (see Pharmacotherapeutics)

Referral

Usually none needed

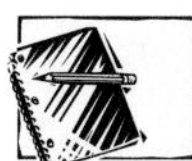

EVALUATION

Outcome
Relief of menopausal symptoms

Possible Complications
- Coronary heart disease
- Osteoporosis with resultant fractures

Follow-up
In 1 month to assess effectiveness of therapy; then every 3 to 6 months

FOR YOUR INFORMATION

Life Span
Pediatric: N/A
Geriatric: Menopausal symptoms may exist for 15 to 20 years after cessation of menses
Pregnancy: Until menses have ceased for 6 months and FSH >40 mIU, there is still a possibility that pregnancy could occur

Miscellaneous
The NP should support and encourage the patient who is going through menopause. Assure the patient that this is a normal part of the aging process.

References

Garner CH: The climacteric, menopause, and the process of aging. In Youngkin EQ, Davis MS, editors: *Women's health: a primary care clinical guide,* Norwalk, Conn, 1994, Appleton & Lange, pp 309-338.

Jones JM, Jones KD: What's happening: pearls and perils of the perimenopause, *J Am Acad Nurse Pract* 8(11):531-535, 1996.

Scharbo-Dehaan M: Hormone replacement therapy, part 2, *Nurse Pract* 21(12):1-13, 1996.

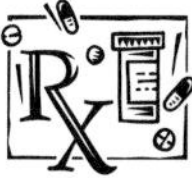

PHARMACOTHERAPEUTICS

Absolute contraindications to estrogen and progestin use include the following: known or suspected estrogen-dependent malignancies; unexplained abnormal uterine bleeding; active thrombophlebitis; pregnancy; otosclerosis; malignant melanoma; acute liver disease; and breast cancer. Relative contraindications to estrogen use include the following: a history of breast cancer; uterine leiomyoma; endometriosis; hypertriglyceridemia; gallbladder disease; migraine headache; and a history of thrombosis or thrombophlebitis.

Drug of Choice	Mechanism of Action	Prescribing Information	Side Effects
Estrogen (Premarin), 0.625 mg PO 1 tab daily; estrogen is available in pills, as transdermal patch, or as vaginal cream; method of administration should be decided on by NP and patient together	Affects release of pituitary gonadotropins; inhibits ovulation	***Contraindications:*** Hypersensitivity; breast cancer; thromboembolic disorders; reproductive cancer; undiagnosed vaginal bleeding; pregnancy ***Cost:*** 0.625-mg tab, 100 tabs: $50; transdermal or topical estrogen per year: $107 ***Pregnancy category:*** X	Dizziness, headache, migraines, depression, hypotension, thrombophlebitis, thromboembolism, pulmonary embolism, myocardial infarction (MI), nausea, vomiting, cholestatic jaundice, weight gain, diplopia, amenorrhea, cervical erosion, breakthrough bleeding, dysmenorrhea, vaginal candidiasis, spontaneous abortion, rash, urticaria, acne, hirsutism, photosensitivity
If patient has intact uterus, add the following:			
Medroxyprogesterone acetate (Provera), 10 mg PO on days 1-12 or days 13-25, or can give 2.5 mg PO daily; estrogen and medroxyprogesterone acetate are now available in 1 tablet sold under trade name Prempro	Inhibits secretion of pituitary gonadotropins; stimulates growth of mammary tissue	***Contraindications:*** Hypersensitivity; breast cancer; thromboembolic disorders; reproductive cancer; undiagnosed vaginal bleeding; pregnancy ***Cost:*** 5-mg tab, 30 tabs: $16 ***Pregnancy category:*** X	Dizziness, headache, migraines, depression, hypotension, thrombophlebitis, thromboembolism, pulmonary embolism, MI, nausea, vomiting, cholestatic jaundice, weight gain, diplopia, amenorrhea, cervical erosion, breakthrough bleeding, dysmenorrhea, vaginal candidiasis, spontaneous abortion, rash, urticaria, acne, hirsutism, photosensitivity

Mitral Stenosis

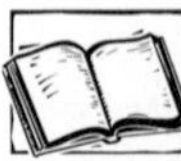

OVERVIEW

Mitral stenosis is a narrowing of the mitral valve between the left atrium and ventricle of the heart. Because of this narrowing, the left atrium becomes hypertrophied, which leads to pulmonary congestion and right-sided heart failure.

Pathogenesis

Cause—rheumatic heart disease due to rheumatic fever

Patient Profile

- Females > Males
- Symptoms usually develop between 30 and 70 years of age

Signs and Symptoms

- Dyspnea
- Orthopnea
- Paroxysmal nocturnal dyspnea
- Palpitations
- Fatigue with exertion
- Recumbent cough
- Hoarseness
- Chest pain
- Peripheral edema
- Jugular venous distention
- Hepatomegaly
- Development of emboli

Differential Diagnosis

- Atrial myxoma
- Endocarditis

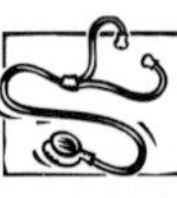

ASSESSMENT

History

Inquire about:

- Onset and duration of symptoms
- History of heart murmur
- History of rheumatic fever
- History of arrhythmia or pulmonary edema
- Underlying conditions
- Current medications

Physical Findings

- Early in disease:
  - Increased middiastolic rumbling murmur with presystolic accentuation (heard at apex with bell of stethoscope—may need to turn patient to left lateral position)
  - Loud S_1 and opening snap
- Late disease:
  - P_2 increased
  - High-pitched decrescendo diastolic murmur
  - Jugular venous distention
  - Hepatomegaly
  - Peripheral edema

Initial Workup

Laboratory: None diagnostic
Radiology: Chest film—left atrial enlargement

Further Workup

- 2-D echocardiogram
- Cardiac catherization

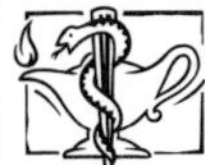

INTERVENTIONS

Office Treatment

None indicated

Lifestyle Modifications

- Adequate rest
- Low-salt diet
- Moderate exercise program

Patient Education

Teach patient about:

- Condition and treatment:
  - Mild disease—treat with medication (mildly symptomatic—diuretics; atrial fibrillation—warfarin; rapid atrial fibrillation—digoxin); prophylaxis before dental procedures; sodium-restricted diet
  - Severe disease—surgical intervention, commissurotomy, balloon valvuloplasty, prosthetic valve
- Adequate rest and moderate physical activity
- Medications used and side effects (see Pharmacotherapeutics)

Referral

To cardiologist for evaluation and recommendations

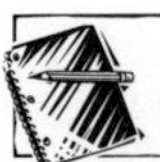

EVALUATION

Outcome

Prognosis good if treatment plan followed

Possible Complications

- Thromboembolism
- Recurrent rheumatic fever
- Bacterial endocarditis
- Pulmonary hypertension
- Pulmonary edema

Follow-up

Every 4 weeks for prophylaxis if taking IM prophylaxis; otherwise every 3 to 6 months

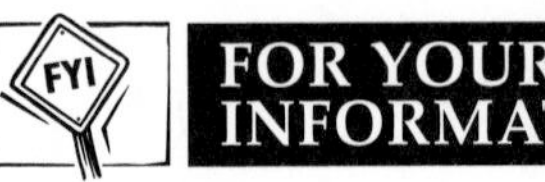

FOR YOUR INFORMATION

Life Span

Pediatric: Most common time for rheumatic fever to occur
Geriatric: High morbidity and mortality; atrial fibrillation more common
Pregnancy: Needs to be followed by a specialist

Miscellaneous

Even though rheumatic heart disease is the most common cause of mitral stenosis, 50% of patients will not report having rheumatic fever.

References

Massie BM: Systemic hypertension. In Tierney LM Jr, McPhee SJ, Papadakis MA, editors: *Current medical diagnosis and treatment,* ed 34, Norwalk, Conn, 1995, Appleton & Lange, pp 292-298.

Shapiro EP: Common cardiac disorders revealed by auscultation of the heart. In Barker LR, Burton JR, Zieve PD, editors: *Principles of ambulatory medicine,* ed 4, Baltimore, 1995, Williams & Wilkins, pp 775-776.

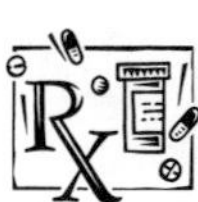

PHARMACOTHERAPEUTICS

Drug of Choice	Mechanism of Action	Prescribing Information	Side Effects
Rheumatic fever prophylaxis:			
Penicillin G benzathine, 1.2 mil units IM monthly for at least 5 years; consult with MD if patient allergic to penicillin; adults normally do not need prophylaxis unless they have had rheumatic fever in the past 5-10 years	Interferes with cell wall replication	***Contraindication:*** Hypersensitivity ***Cost:*** 600,000 U/ml, 10 ml: $68 ***Pregnancy category:*** B	Anemia, bone marrow depression, granulocytopenia, nausea, vomiting, diarrhea, increased AST and ALT, oliguria, proteinuria, hematuria, vaginitis, moniliasis, glomerulonephritis, lethargy, coma, convulsions, local pain and tenderness at injection site, rash, anaphylaxis
For mild symptoms of heart failure, use one of the following:			
Hydrochlorothiazide (Hydrodiuril), 25-50 mg PO qd-bid, maximum 200 mg qd; children >6 months, 2.2 mg/kg/day PO in divided doses; children <6 months, 3.3 mg/kg/day in divided doses	Thiazide diuretic; acts on distal tubule and ascending limb of loop of Henle	***Contraindications:*** Hypersensitivity to thiazides or sulfonamides; anuria; renal decompensation; hypomagnesemia ***Cost:*** 25-mg tab, 100 tabs: $2-$12 ***Pregnancy category:*** B	Uremia, glucosuria, drowsiness, dizziness, fatigue, weakness, nausea, vomiting, anorexia, constipation, hepatitis, rash, urticaria, hyperglycemia, aplastic anemia, hemolytic anemia, leukopenia, agranulocytosis, thrombocytopenia, neutropenia, hypokalemia, orthostatic hypotension, hyponatremia, volume depletion
Furosemide (Lasix), 20 mg PO qd, increase dose by doubling as needed; children, 2 mg/kg/day PO qd; monitor potassium level	Loop diuretic; inhibits reabsorption of sodium and chloride at proximal and distal tubule and at loop of Henle	***Contraindications:*** Hypersensitivity; anuria; hypovolemia ***Cost:*** 20-mg tab, 100 tabs: $2-$15 ***Pregnancy category:*** C	Headache, fatigue, weakness, orthostatic hypotension, chest pain, circulatory collapse, loss of hearing, hypokalemia, hypomagnesemia, hyperuricemia, hyperglycemia, nausea, diarrhea, renal failure, thrombocytopenia, agranulocytosis, leukopenia, anemia, rash, Stevens-Johnson syndrome, cramps, stiffness
For atrial fibrillation:			
Warfarin (Coumadin); usually start with 10-15 mg PO qd, then titrate to maintain prothrombin time INR between 2.0-3.0	Depresses synthesis of coagulation factors that are dependent on vitamin K (II, VII, IX, X)	***Contraindications:*** Hypersensitivity; hemophilia; peptic ulcer disease; thrombocytopenic purpura; severe hepatic disease; severe hypertension; subacute bacterial endocarditis; acute nephritis; blood dyscrasias; pregnancy ***Cost:*** 5-mg tab, 100 tabs: $30-$50 ***Pregnancy category:*** D	Diarrhea, nausea, vomiting, anorexia, stomatitis, cramps, hepatitis, hematuria, rash, dermatitis, fever, hemorrhage, agranulocytosis, leukopenia, eosinophilia
Use the following only for rapid atrial fibrillation or flutter:			
Digoxin (Lanoxin), 0.125-0.5 mg PO qd; monitor therapeutic level every 3-6 months once stabilized on maintenance dose	Cardiac glycoside; increases cardiac output	***Contraindications:*** Hypersensitivity; ventricular fibrillation or tachycardia; carotid sinus syndrome; 2nd- or 3rd-degree heart block ***Cost:*** 0.25-mg tab, 100 tabs: $8-$16 ***Pregnancy category:*** C	Headache, drowsiness, apathy, confusion, fatigue, depression, dysrhythmia, hypotension, bradycardia, arteriovenous (AV) block, blurred vision, yellow-green halos, photophobia, nausea, vomiting, anorexia, abdominal pain, diarrhea
Bacterial endocarditis prophylaxis for dental procedures:			
Amoxicillin (Amoxil), 3 g PO 1 hour before procedure and 1.5 g PO 6 hours later	Broad-spectrum antibiotic; interferes with cell wall replication	***Contraindication:*** Hypersensitivity to penicillin ***Cost:*** 500-mg tab, 30 tabs: $6-$13 ***Pregnancy category:*** B	Anemia, bone marrow depression, granulocytopenia, nausea, vomiting, diarrhea, pseudomembranous colitis, headache, anaphylaxis, respiratory distress

Mitral Valve Prolapse

OVERVIEW

Mitral valve prolapse is bulging of the leaflets of the mitral valve into the left atrium during systole.

Pathogenesis

Cause:
- Myxomatous degeneration of mitral valve
- May have familial tendency

Patient Profile

- Females > Males
- Early adulthood

Signs and Symptoms

- Most are asymptomatic
- Chest pain
- Palpitations
- Orthostatic hypotension
- Fatigue
- Shortness of breath

Differential Diagnosis

Hypertrophic cardiomyopathy

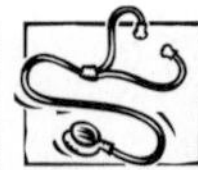

ASSESSMENT

History

Inquire about:
- Onset and duration of symptoms
- Family history of mitral valve prolapse
- Underlying conditions
- Current medications

Physical Findings

- Heart examination:
  - Midsystolic click at lower left sternal border
  - Midsystolic or late-systolic murmur
- Thin body habitus
- Commonly associated with scoliosis and pectus excavatum

Initial Workup

Laboratory: None indicated
Radiology: Chest film—narrow AP diameter; elongated cardiac silhouette

Further Workup

- 2-D echocardiography—diagnostic test of choice
- Color Doppler—Shows amount of regurgitation
- Exercise testing (possibly)

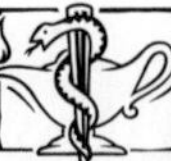

INTERVENTIONS

Office Treatment

None indicated

Lifestyle Modification

Avoidance of smoking or smoking cessation

Patient Education

Teach patient about:
- Condition and treatment:
  - If asymptomatic—no treatment or limitations
  - If symptomatic—medication
  - Rarely, mitral valve replacement
- Benign nature of condition
- Medication used and side effects (see Pharmacotherapeutics)

Referral

To cardiologist if severe symptoms present

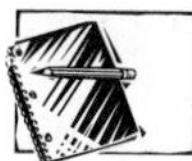

EVALUATION

Outcome
Prognosis good; condition usually benign

Possible Complications
Rare:
- Bacterial endocarditis
- Stroke
- Congestive heart failure
- Arrhythmias
- Mitral regurgitation
- Sudden death

Follow-up
Every 3 to 6 months if taking medications; otherwise, reevaluate every 2 to 3 years

FOR YOUR INFORMATION

Life Span
Pediatric: Usually not seen in this age group
Geriatric: Usually diagnosed before age 50
Pregnancy: Usually no problems; murmur may become more prominent

Miscellaneous
It is important for the NP to encourage the patient to discuss any fears he or she may have regarding mitral valve prolapse. Many patients suffer undue anxiety related to the diagnosis of a "heart problem."

References
Kupper NS, Duke ES: Nursing role in management: inflammatory and valvular heart disease. In Lewis SM, Collier IC, Heitkemper MM, editors: *Medical-surgical nursing: assessment and management of clinical problems,* ed 4, St Louis, 1996, Mosby, pp 1025-1026.

Shapiro EP: Common cardiac disorders revealed by auscultation of the heart. In Barker LR, Burton JR, Zieve PD, editors: *Principles of ambulatory medicine,* ed 4, Baltimore, 1995, Williams & Wilkins, pp 774-775.

NOTES

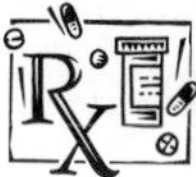

PHARMACOTHERAPEUTICS

Drug of Choice	Mechanism of Action	Prescribing Information	Side Effects
Propranolol (Inderal), 10-40 mg/day PO tid-qid; other beta-blockers may also be used, such as atenolol, metoprolol, nadolol, penbutolol, timolol	Reduces myocardial O_2 requirement by decreasing heart rate, myocardial contractility, and blood pressure	***Contraindications:*** Hypersensitivity; cardiac failure; cardiogenic shock; 2nd- or 3rd-degree heart block; bronchospastic disease; sinus bradycardia; congestive heart failure (CHF) ***Cost:*** 40-mg tab, 100 tabs: $2-$40 ***Pregnancy category:*** C	Headache, fatigue, drowsiness, dizziness, anxiety, depression, weakness, insomnia, tinnitus, dysrhythmias, edema, CHF, hypotension, pulmonary edema, nausea, vomiting, diarrhea, constipation, nocturia, polyuria, rash, pruritus, photosensitivity, flushing, sexual difficulties, fever, chills

Molluscum Contagiosum

OVERVIEW

Molluscum contagiosum is a contagious viral disease. In children lesions occur on the face, trunk, and extremities. In adults lesions occur on the groin and genitalia. In adults transmission is primarily sexual, but in children transmission is usually by fomites.

Pathogenesis

- Cause—DNA virus of poxvirus group; spread by autoinoculation through scratching
- Lesions frequently grouped; may be few or many
- Face, trunk, and extremities affected in children, and groin and genitalia affected in adults
- Lesions differ from warts—do not affect palms of hands or soles of feet
- Incubation period 2 weeks to 2 months

Patient Profile

- Males = Females
- Children and young adults
- All ethnic backgrounds

Signs and Symptoms

- Pearly white to flesh-colored firm papules
- Usually grouped in one or two areas
- Centrally umbilicated
- Found anywhere on body, but more common on face, trunk, and extremities in children, and on groin and genitalia in adults

Differential Diagnosis

- Furunculosis
- Keratoacanthomas
- Warts
- Pyodermas
- Vesicular skin disorders

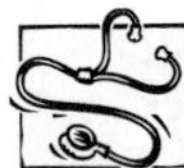

ASSESSMENT

History

Inquire about:

- Onset and duration of symptoms
- Contact with another individual with similar lesions
- Treatments tried and results
- Underlying conditions
- Current medications

Physical Findings

- Dome-shaped, white to flesh-colored, small lesions on face, trunk, and extremities in children; on groin and genitalia in adults
- May be grouped
- If present for a time, center is soft and umbilicated

Initial Workup

Laboratory

- Remove small lesion with curette; place on slide; mix with potassium hydroxide; place another slide on top; heat; crush with firm, twisting pressure; place under microscope; look for large intracytoplasmic inclusion bodies
- Or punch biopsy may be performed

Radiology: None indicated

Further Workup

None indicated

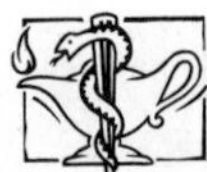

INTERVENTIONS

Office Treatment

Cryotherapy with nitrogen, curettage, cantharidin application

Lifestyle Modification

Avoidance of contact with infected individual

Patient Education

Teach patient about:

- Disease and treatment:
  - Is self-limiting in most cases and resolves in 6 to 12 months
  - Treatment options if so desired—curettage, cryosurgery, cantharidin, laser therapy—remember, scarring is an important consideration
- Safe sex and use of condoms to prevent spread
- Not scratching to prevent autoinoculation
- Treatment/medication used and side effects (see Pharmacotherapeutics)

Referral

To dermatologist for extensive number of lesions

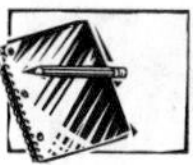

EVALUATION

Outcome
Lesions resolve without scarring

Possible Complication
Extensive infection if immunocompromised

Follow-up
In 2 weeks; may need to retreat

FOR YOUR INFORMATION

Life Span
Pediatric: Generally obtained through fomite; however, if lesions present in genital area, consider sexual abuse, particularly if no lesions present elsewhere
Geriatric: Uncommon in this age group
Pregnancy: Allow to resolve on its own or treat after delivery

Miscellaneous
N/A

References
Bennett EC: Vaginitis and sexually transmitted diseases. In Youngkin EQ, Davis MS, editors: *Women's health: a primary care clinical guide,* Norwalk, Conn, 1994, Appleton & Lange, pp 232-233.

Habif TP: *Clinical dermatology: a color guide to diagnosis and therapy,* ed 3, St Louis, 1996, Mosby, pp 304-305, 335-336.

NOTES

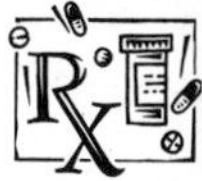

PHARMACOTHERAPEUTICS

Drug of Choice	Mechanism of Action	Prescribing Information	Side Effects
Cantharidin 0.7%; apply small amount to lesions, avoiding surrounding skin—will blister and heal; usually only requires 1 application	Keratolytic	***Contraindication:*** Hypersensitivity ***Cost:*** 7.5 ml: $19 ***Pregnancy category:*** C	Scar formation; painful—may be too painful for genital lesions

Mononucleosis, Infectious

OVERVIEW

Infectious mononucleosis is an acute viral infection.

Pathogenesis

- Cause—Epstein-Barr virus (EBV)
- Spread—person to person by oropharyngeal route
- Incubation period—4 to 6 weeks

Patient Profile

- Males = Females
- Most common age group—adolescents to young adults, but can occur at any age

Signs and Symptoms

- Malaise
- Fatigue
- Headache
- Fever
- Adenopathy
- Sore throat
- Splenomegaly
- Hepatomegaly
- Eyelid edema
- Palatal petechiae
- Generalized maculopapular rash

Differential Diagnosis

- Streptococcal pharyngitis
- Viral tonsillitis
- Hepatitis
- Rubella
- Cytomegalovirus
- Adenovirus
- Toxoplasmosis
- Vincent's angina
- Lymphocytic leukemia

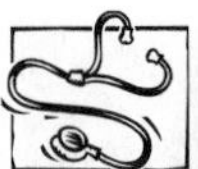

ASSESSMENT

History

Inquire about:

- Onset and duration of symptoms
- Exposure to person with mononucleosis
- Difficulty breathing or swallowing
- Severe headache, confusion
- Underlying conditions
- Current medications

Physical Findings

- May appear generally ill
- Fever
- Mouth and throat—enlarged tonsils, palatal petechiae, white membrane covering one or both tonsils
- Posterior cervical adenopathy
- Abdominal examination—hepatomegaly and/or splenomegaly
- Skin—possibly maculopapular confluent rash

Initial Workup

Laboratory

- CBC with differential—increased WBC count; lymphocytosis with atypical lymphocytes
- Monospot or test for heterophil antibody—positive (if negative and patient symptomatic, repeat in 7 to 10 days)
- EBV titer—positive
- Liver function tests—elevated
- Throat culture—30% also have streptococcal infection

Radiology: Usually none needed

Further Workup

Usually none

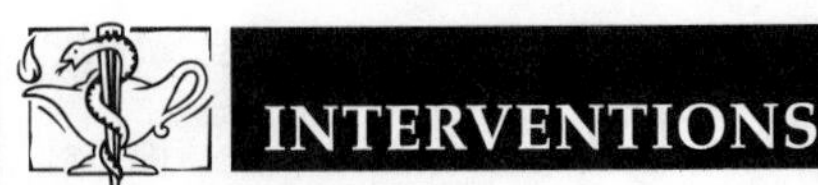

INTERVENTIONS

Office Treatment

None indicated

Lifestyle Modifications

- Adequate rest (may need bed rest during acute phase)
- Nutritious diet
- Avoidance of strenuous physical activity and contact sports

Patient Education

Teach patient about:

- Condition and treatment—symptomatic: antibiotics for strep infection
- Length of illness—may take several weeks to fully recover; may miss school for extended time
- Importance of adequate rest
- Avoiding contact sports and strenuous activity due to splenomegaly
- Healthy diet—may use milk shakes, juices, and soft foods if throat sore
- Using warm saltwater gargles for sore throat
- Good hand-washing technique to prevent spread
- Medications used and side effects (see Pharmacotherapeutics)

Referral

Refer to MD if patient has marked tonsillar swelling and difficulty swallowing or has CNS complications

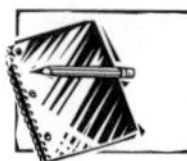

EVALUATION

Outcome
Usually resolves without sequelae—fever resolves in about 10 days, and adenopathy and splenomegaly resolve in 4 weeks

Possible Complications
Many can occur—chronic EBV infection, splenic rupture, hemolytic anemia, thrombocytopenic purpura, coagulopathy, aplastic anemia, seizures, nerve palsies, pericarditis, myocarditis, pneumonitis, pleural effusion, erythema multiforma, orchitis, parotitis, etc.

Follow-up
Every 1 to 2 weeks until symptoms resolve

FOR YOUR INFORMATION

Life Span
Pediatric: Commonly seen in adolescents
Geriatric: Rare in this population
Pregnancy: Symptomatic treatment same as with others

Miscellaneous
N/A

References
Bull TR: *Color atlas of E.N.T. diagnosis,* ed 3, London, 1995, Mosby-Wolfe, pp 188-189.

Waterbury L, Zieve PD: Selected illnesses affecting lymphocytes: mononucleosis, chronic lymphocytic leukemia and the undiagnosed patient with lymphadenopathy. In Barker LR, Burton JR, Zieve PD, editors: *Principles of ambulatory medicine,* ed 4, Baltimore, 1995, Williams & Wilkins, pp 624-628.

NOTES

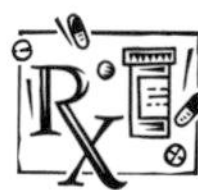

PHARMACOTHERAPEUTICS

Drug of Choice	Mechanism of Action	Prescribing Information	Side Effects
For fever and myalgia:			
Acetaminophen (Tylenol), 325-650 mg PO q4-6h; for children, use Children's Tylenol—follow label directions	Decreases fever through action on hypothalamic heat-regulating center of brain; analgesia by increasing pain threshold	***Contraindications:*** Hypersensitivity; bleeding disorders or anticoagulant therapy; last trimester of pregnancy; asthma; gastric ulcers ***Cost:*** OTC ***Pregnancy category:*** Not categorized	Rash; hepatic toxicity with alcohol ingestion or overdose
For streptococcal pharyngitis:			
Erythromycin (E-mycin), 250 mg PO qid × 10 days—do not use amoxicillin or ampicillin because there seems to be an increased incidence of hypersensitivity reactions causing a rash, which can also be caused by mononucleosis; if patient hypersensitive to erythromycin, consult with MD on treatment	Macrolide; binds to 50 S ribosomal subunit and suppresses protein synthesis	***Contraindication:*** Hypersensitivity ***Cost:*** 250-mg tab, 40 tabs: $5-$10 ***Pregnancy category:*** B	Rash, urticaria, pruritus, nausea, vomiting, diarrhea, hepatotoxicity, abdominal pain, heartburn, anorexia, vaginitis, moniliasis, tinnitus

Motion Sickness

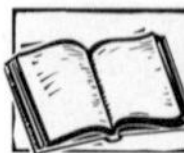

OVERVIEW

Motion sickness occurs when there are erratic or rhythmic motions in any combination of directions. It is a normal response to an abnormal situation.

Pathogenesis

Cause—sensory conflict between visual receptors, vestibular receptors, and body proprioceptors about body motion; induced by planes, trains, boats, cars, amusement park rides, 3-D movies

Patient Profile

- Males = Females
- All ages, although may become more prone to motion sickness with age

Signs and Symptoms

- Nausea
- Vomiting
- Malaise
- Drowsiness
- Yawning
- Salivation
- Hyperventilation
- Headache
- Flushing
- Anxiety
- Panic
- Confusion
- Diaphoresis

Differential Diagnosis

- Vestibular disease
- Gastroenteritis
- Metabolic disorders

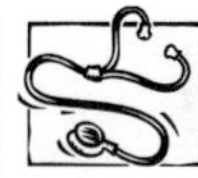

ASSESSMENT

History

Inquire about:

- Onset and duration of symptoms
- Trigger for sickness, such as reading or staring
- Underlying conditions
- Current medications

Physical Findings

Physical examination—within normal limits

Initial Workup

Laboratory: None indicated
Radiology: None indicated

Further Workup

None indicated

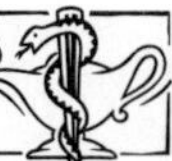

INTERVENTIONS

Office Treatment

None indicated

Lifestyle Modifications

- Depends on severity and whether treatment works
- May need to change mode of transportation if possible

Patient Education

Teach patient about:

- Condition and preventive measures:
  - Sitting in middle of plane or boat
  - Not staring at moving objects
  - Ensuring adequate ventilation
  - Avoiding reading
  - Semirecumbent seating
  - Having a small meal before trip
  - Avoiding alcohol
- Medications to use and side effects (see Pharmacotherapeutics)

Referrals

None indicated

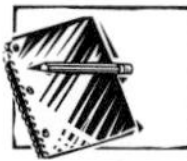

EVALUATION

Outcome
Patient will be able to travel without having motion sickness

Possible Complications
- Hypotension
- Dehydration
- Panic

Follow-up
After next exposure to assess treatment success or failure

FOR YOUR INFORMATION

Life Span
Pediatric: Not as common
Geriatric: Use caution with medications—sedation may be more pronounced in this age group
Pregnancy: May be more prone to motion sickness

Miscellaneous
N/A

Reference
Bass EB, Lewis RF: Dizziness, vertigo, motion sickness, near syncope, syncope, and disequilibrium. In Barker LR, Burton JR, Zieve PD, editors: *Principles of ambulatory medicine,* ed 4, Baltimore, 1995, Williams & Wilkins, p 1207.

NOTES

PHARMACOTHERAPEUTICS

Drug of Choice	Mechanism of Action	Prescribing Information	Side Effects
For vertigo:			
Meclizine (Antivert), 25 mg PO tid-qid; not recommended for children <12 years	Antihistamine	*Contraindications:* Hypersensitivity; shock; lactation *Cost:* 25-mg tab, 30 tabs, $6 *Pregnancy category:* B	Drowsiness, fatigue, restlessness, headache, insomnia, nausea, anorexia, dry mouth, blurred vision
Dimenhydrinate (Dramamine), 50 mg PO q4h; rectal, 100 mg qd or bid; children, 5 mg/kg in 4 equal divided doses	Decreases vestibular stimulation	*Contraindications:* Hypersensitivity; shock *Cost:* 50-mg tab, 100 tabs: $7 *Pregnancy category:* B	Drowsiness, restlessness, confusion, convulsions in young children, nausea, anorexia, diarrhea, dry mouth, blurred vision, rash, urticaria
Scopolamine transdermal disc (Transderm-Scop), 1 disc behind ear; leave for 3 days—not for children; use with great caution in elderly	Inhibition of vestibular input to CNS; antagonizes acetylcholine at receptor sites in eyes, smooth muscle, cardiac muscle	*Contraindications:* Hypersensitivity; glaucoma *Cost:* 12 discs: $45 *Pregnancy category:* C	Dizziness, drowsiness, confusion, disorientation, blurred vision, dilated pupils, dry mouth, acute narrow-angle glaucoma, rash, erythema

Multiple Sclerosis (MS)

OVERVIEW

Multiple sclerosis (MS) is a chronic, progressive, demyelinization of the white matter of the brain and spinal cord. This demyelinization process causes multiple neurologic signs and symptoms.

Pathogenesis

- Cause—Unknown; several theories: autoimmune theory, viral theory, combined theory (autoimmune response triggered by environmental toxin or virus)
- Process—loss of myelin, disappearance of oligodendrocytes, proliferation of astrocytes—plaque formation throughout CNS

Patient Profile

- Females > Males
- Onset at age 15 to 50 years
- Most commonly, Caucasians of European descent

Signs and Symptoms

- Onset usually insidious
- May have chronic progressive deterioration or periods of remission and exacerbation
- Ataxia
- Blurred, double, or loss of vision (optic neuritis) in one eye
- Clumsiness
- Emotional lability
- Clonus
- Genital anesthesia in women
- Hand paralysis
- Sexual dysfunction
- Hemiparesis
- Hyperactive deep tendon reflexes
- Incoordination
- Loss of position sense
- Loss of vibration sense
- Urinary frequency, hesitancy, incontinence

Differential Diagnosis

- Amyotrophic lateral sclerosis
- Behçet's disease
- Brainstem tumors
- CNS infections
- Leukodystrophies
- Ruptured intervertebral disc
- Small cerebral infarcts
- Syphilis
- Systemic lupus erythematosus
- Spinal cord tumors

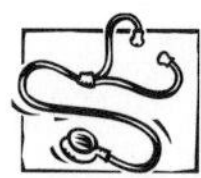

ASSESSMENT

History

Inquire about:

- Onset and duration of symptoms
- Ethnic background
- Family history of MS
- Underlying conditions
- Current medications

Physical Findings

- Weakness or paralysis of limbs
- Spasticity of muscles
- Incoordination
- Nystagmus
- Decreased or loss of vision in one eye
- Decreased sensation—position and vibration

Initial Workup

Laboratory

- No definitive diagnostic test for MS—diagnosis based on history and physical examination
- Cerebrospinal fluid—may show lymphocytes or monocytes; abnormal colloidal gold curve; normal or slightly elevated protein level

Radiology: MRI or CT scan of head and spinal cord—may show plaques or be normal

Further Workup

Visual-evoked response testing—delayed because of decreased nerve conduction

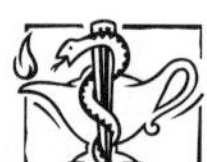

INTERVENTIONS

Office Treatment

Careful observation of patient over time helps in diagnosis

Lifestyle Modifications

Major lifestyle modifications will need to be made:

- Making home wheelchair/walker accessible
- Safety bars around toilet and shower
- Wheelchair lift or ramps
- May require a change in occupation or adaptation to condition
- Family support and assistance needed

Patient Education

Teach patient about:

- Disease process and treatment options—no specific treatment for progressive MS; treatment aimed at symptom relief; prednisone useful for treating acute exacerbations; immunosuppressive drugs of some benefit; Interferon β (Betaseron) used for patients with exacerbating and remitting MS
- Support groups available
- Making plans for the future, such as equipping home, caring for children, maintaining activity as long as possible
- Importance of avoiding fatigue, extremes of hot and cold, and exposure to infection—can trigger exacerbation
- Importance of well-balanced diet, high in fiber
- Exercise plan
- Including family in treatment and care
- How to avoid contractures and pressure sores during periods of immobility
- Medications used and side effects (see Pharmacotherapeutics)

Referrals

To specialist in MS

- To home health nurse
- To local chapter of MS Society

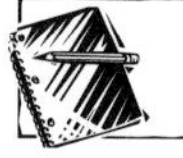

EVALUATION

Outcomes

- Highly variable
- Average duration >25 years
- Patient will adjust to disease process and be able to live active, productive life

Possible Complications

- Coma
- Delirium
- Contractures and pressure sores
- Paraplegia
- Optic nerve atrophy

Follow-up

Usually done by specialist or may be done by NP monthly to monitor for side effects of medications

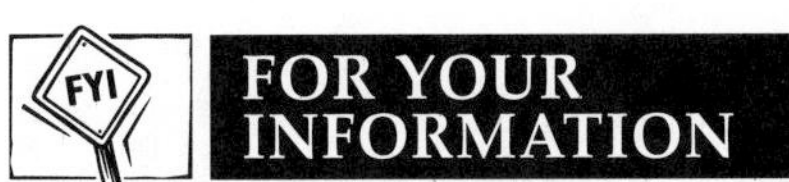

FOR YOUR INFORMATION

Life Span

Pediatric: Rarely seen before puberty
Geriatric: Less likely to have remissions
Pregnancy: Some studies show no effect on MS, and others show exacerbation of condition

Miscellaneous

This can be a devastating disease for both the patient and the family. There is a need for a great deal of support, particularly during times of exacerbation.

Reference

Ozuna JM: Nursing role in management: chronic neurologic problems. In Lewis SM, Collier IC, Heitkemper MM, editors: *Medical-surgical nursing: assessment and management of clinical problems,* ed 4, St Louis, Mosby, 1995, pp 1766-1770.

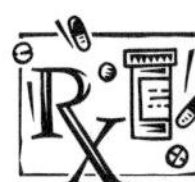

PHARMACOTHERAPEUTICS

There are many drugs currently in use to manage the patient with MS. The following is a partial list of some of the commonly used medications to attempt to control the acute exacerbations. There are many other medications used to help control symptoms of the disease.

Immunosuppressive drugs such as azathioprine (Inuran), cyclosporine, and cyclophosphamide (Cytoxan) are currently under investigation and have produced some beneficial effects. These drugs are currently not approved by the FDA for treatment of MS.

Drug of Choice	Mechanism of Action	Prescribing Information	Side Effects
To control acute exacerbations:			
Methylprednisolone, 1000 mg IV × 5 days, followed by tapered oral dose	Glucocorticoid; decreases inflammation	***Contraindications:*** Hypersensitivity; psychosis; idiopathic thrombocytopenia; acute glomerulonephritis; amebiasis; fungal infections; nonasthmatic bronchial disease; AIDS; TB ***Cost:*** 125-mg vial: $7-$12 ***Pregnancy category:*** C	Depression, flushing, sweating, headache, mood changes, hypertension, circulatory collapse, thrombophlebitis, embolism, tachycardia, fungal infections, increased intraocular pressure, diarrhea, nausea, abdominal distention, GI hemorrhage, thrombocytopenia, acne, poor wound healing, fractures, osteoporosis
For ambulatory patients with relapsing or remitting MS:			
Interferon β (Betaseron), 0.25 mg SQ qod	Antiviral; immunoregulatory; action not understood	***Contraindication:*** Hypersensitivity to natural or recombinant interferon β or human albumin ***Cost:*** 0.3-mg vial: $72 ***Pregnancy category:*** C	Headache, fever, pain, chills, mental changes, hypertonia, suicide attempts, migraine, palpitations, hypertension, tachycardia, conjunctivitis, blurred vision, diarrhea, constipation, irregular menses, metrorrhagia, cystitis, breast pain, decreased WBC and lymphocytes, lymphadenopathy, sweating, myalgia, myasthenia, sinusitis
For spasticity:			
Baclofen (Lioresal), 5 mg PO 1-3 × 1 day	Skeletal muscle relaxant; inhibits synaptic response in CNS by decreasing gamma-aminobutyric acid (GABA)	***Contraindication:*** Hypersensitivity ***Cost:*** 10-mg tab, 100 tabs: $20 ***Pregnancy category:*** C	Dizziness; weakness; fatigue; drowsiness; headache; insomnia; disorientation; nasal congestion; blurred vision; hypotension; chest pain; palpitations; nausea, vomiting; constipation; increased AST, ALK, and phosphates; abdominal pain; urinary frequency; rash; pruritis

Mumps

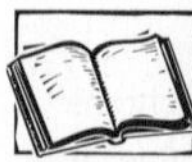

OVERVIEW

Mumps is an acute viral disease characterized by swelling of one or both parotid glands.

Pathogenesis

Cause—paramyxovirus; communicable from 2 days before onset of swelling to 6 to 10 days after parotitis onset; incubation 14 to 21 days

Patient Profile

- Males = Females
- Most common age—5 to 15 years, but can affect any age
- Once common, but incidence decreasing because of immunizations

Signs and Symptoms

- May have prodrome of fever, malaise, headache, anorexia
- Parotid gland pain and swelling (either or both)
- Fever up to 104° F (40° C)
- Pain when chewing sour foods
- 15% have meningeal signs
- Rarely, maculopapular erythematous rash
- Rarely, develop arthritis, orchitis, thyroiditis, mastitis, pancreatitis
- May be asymptomatic

Differential Diagnosis

- Parainfluenza parotitis
- Allergic parotitis
- Lymphadenitis
- Salivary gland tumors

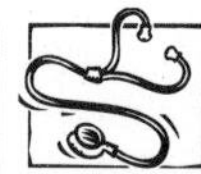

ASSESSMENT

History

Inquire about:

- Onset and duration of symptoms
- Immunizations
- Contact with individual known to have mumps
- Underlying conditions
- Current medications

Physical Findings

- Fever
- Parotid gland swelling, which obscures angle of mandible and elevates earlobe
- Orchitis, maybe

Initial Workup

Laboratory

- CBC—leukopenia
- Can isolate virus from blood, urine, spinal fluid, throat washings—rarely necessary

Radiology: Usually none needed; testicular scan may be useful to differentiate mumps orchitis from testicular torsion

Further Workup

None indicated

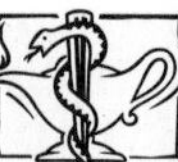

INTERVENTIONS

Office Treatment

None indicated

Lifestyle Modification

Bed rest during acute phase

Patient Education

Teach patient about:

- Condition and treatment—symptomatic (antipyretics and analgesics)
- Mumps orchitis—scrotal support or athletic supporter; rarely causes sterility
- Staying out of school until no longer contagious (about 9 days)
- Immunization—will protect against later exposure but not current one
- Medication used and side effects (see Pharmacotherapeutics)

Referrals

None indicated

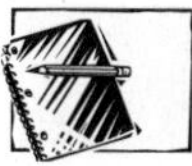

EVALUATION

Outcome
Resolves without sequelae

Possible Complications
- Meningoencephalitis
- Orchitis
- Oophoritis
- Pancreatitis
- Nephritis
- Arthritis
- Myocarditis,
- Deafness

Follow-up
Usually none needed

FOR YOUR INFORMATION

Life Span
Pediatric: Orchitis more commonly occurs in adolescents; most commonly seen in this population, but decreasing because of immunizations
Geriatric: Most are immune; more complications if occurs in this age group
Pregnancy: Vaccinate after delivery

Miscellaneous
It is important for the NP to ensure that children receive the appropriate vaccinations.

References
Bope ET: Care of children. In Driscoll CE et al, editors: *The family practice desk reference,* ed 3, St Louis, 1996, Mosby.
Bull TR: *Color atlas of E.N.T. diagnosis,* ed 3, London, 1995, Mosby-Wolfe, pp 227, 230.

NOTES

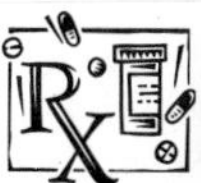

PHARMACOTHERAPEUTICS

Drug of Choice	Mechanism of Action	Prescribing Information	Side Effects
For fever and myalgia:			
Acetaminophen (Tylenol), 325-650 mg PO q4-6h; for children, use Children's Tylenol—follow label directions	Decreases fever through action on hypothalamic heat-regulating center of brain; analgesia by increasing pain threshold	***Contraindications:*** Hypersensitivity; bleeding disorders or anticoagulant therapy; last trimester of pregnancy; asthma; gastric ulcers ***Cost:*** OTC ***Pregnancy category:*** Not categorized	Rash; hepatic toxicity with alcohol ingestion or overdose
Measles, mumps, rubella vaccine; adults and children: 0.5 ml SQ; adults receive 1 dose; children, 1 dose at 12-15 months of age, another at either 4-6 years or 11-12 years of age	Live virus, which causes body to build antibodies against the disease	***Contraindications:*** Anaphylactoid reaction to neomycin; pregnancy; anaphylactoid reaction to eggs ***Cost:*** 0.5-ml vial: $36 ***Pregnancy category:*** C	Burning/stinging at site of injection, malaise, sore throat, cough, rhinitis, headache, dizziness, fever, rash, nausea, vomiting, diarrhea, regional lymphadenopathy, nerve deafness, allergic reaction, anaphylaxis, optic neuritis

Myocardial Infarction (MI)

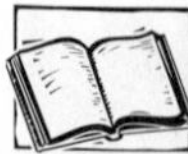

OVERVIEW

Myocardial infarction (MI) is said to have occurred when there is necrosis of a portion of the heart muscle due to obstruction of a coronary artery.

Pathogenesis
Obstruction of coronary artery from atherosclerosis, coronary artery spasm, embolism, congenital coronary abnormalities

Patient Profile
- Males > Females until age 70, then Males = Females
- Most common over age 40, but may occur at any age

Signs and Symptoms
- Pain—chest, jaw, arm, back, neck, abdomen
- Anxiety
- Diaphoresis
- Dyspnea
- Lightheadedness
- Pallor
- Weakness
- Nausea
- Vomiting
- Hypertension or hypotension

Differential Diagnosis
- Angina pectoris
- Aortic dissection
- Pulmonary embolism
- Acute pericarditis
- Spontaneous pneumothorax

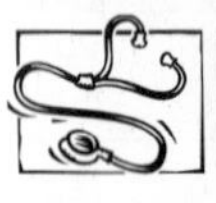

ASSESSMENT

History
Inquire about:
- Onset and duration of symptoms:
  - Pain—quality, intensity, duration, location; what, if anything, provides relief
  - Associated symptoms of nausea, vomiting, diaphoresis, dyspnea
- History of heart disease
- Family history of heart disease
- Risk factors—smoking, increased cholesterol
- Underlying conditions
- Current medications

Physical Findings
- Pallor
- Dyspnea
- Weakness
- Confusion
- Hypertension or hypotension
- Heart examination—gallop rhythm, murmur, tachycardia or bradycardia, pulsus alternans
- Lungs—rales, wheezes

Initial Workup
Laboratory
- Creatinine kinase (CK) and its isoenzymes—elevated CK (within 4 to 8 hours of MI) and CK-MB indicative of MI
- LDH—elevated within 24 hours
- CBC—leukocytosis

Radiology
- Chest—PA and lateral
- Thallium scan

Further Workup
- ECG
- 2-D echocardiogram
- Cardiac catherization

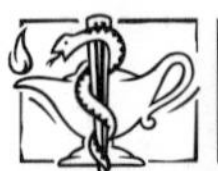

INTERVENTIONS

Office Treatment
- Immediate transport to emergency room
- Administer oxygen if available
- Keep quiet

Lifestyle Modifications
- Smoking cessation
- Low-salt and low-fat diet
- Stress reduction

Patient Education
Teach patient about:
- Condition and treatment:
  - Coronary reperfusion if possible
  - Medications for pain control, arrhythmia control, vasodilation
  - Cholesterol—lowering
  - After acute episode—balloon angioplasty, coronary artery bypass graft
  - Tips for smoking cessation
  - Low-salt, low-fat diet
  - Stress reduction—biofeedback, relaxation techniques, yoga
  - Participating in cardiac rehabilitation and continuing exercise program
- Medications used and side effects (see Pharmacotherapeutics)

Referral
To cardiologist

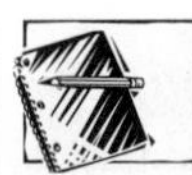

EVALUATION

Outcome
Prognosis good with early intervention

Possible Complications
- Congestive heart failure
- Cardiogenic shock
- Myocardial rupture
- Dysrrythmias
- Cardiac arrest
- Death

Follow-up
- 1 week after hospitalization; then in 3 to 6 weeks for exercise stress test
- ECG in 3 months
- Cardiac rehabilitation center

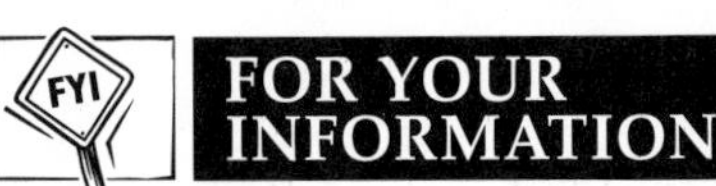

Life Span
Pediatric: Very rare; usually due to congenital anomaly
Geriatric: Higher rate of morbidity and mortality
Pregnancy: N/A

Miscellaneous
N/A

References
Braunwald E et al: *Diagnosing and managing unstable angina,* Quick Reference Guide for Clinicians No 10, AHCPR Pub No 94-0603, Rockville, Md, 1994, US Department of Health and Human Services, Public Health Service, Agency for Health Care Policy and Research and Nation Heart, Lung, and Blood Institute.

Thamer MA, Stewart KJ: Post-myocardial infarction care, cardiac rehabilitation, and physical conditioning. In Barker LR, Burton JR, Zieve PD, editors; *Principles of ambulatory medicine,* ed 4, Baltimore, 1995, Williams & Wilkins, pp 712-730.

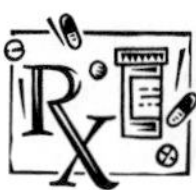

PHARMACOTHERAPEUTICS

Many medications are used during the acute phase of an MI. It is beyond the scope of this book to present them here; The most commonly used post-MI medications are presented here., For others, consult an acute care text.

Drug of Choice	Mechanism of Action	Prescribing Information	Side Effects
Aspirin, 80-325 mg PO qd	Decreases platelet aggregation	***Contraindications:*** Hypersensitivity; bleeding disorders or anticoagulant therapy; last trimester of pregnancy; asthma; gastric ulcers ***Cost:*** OTC ***Pregnancy category:*** Not categorized	Rash, anaphylactic reaction, GI upset and bleeding; Reye's syndrome in children and adolescents
Propranolol (Inderal), 30-120 mg PO bid or tid or 160 mg PO qd extended-release form; others: atenolol, metoprolol, nadolol, penbutolol, timolol; consult package insert for prescribing information	Reduces myocardial O_2 requirement by decreasing heart rate, myocardial contractility, and blood pressure	***Contraindications:*** Hypersensitivity; cardiac failure; cardiogenic shock; 2nd- or 3rd-degree heart block; bronchospastic disease; sinus bradycardia; congestive heart failure (CHF) ***Cost:*** 40-mg tab, 100 tabs: $2-$40 ***Pregnancy category:*** C	Bronchospasm, dyspnea, bradycardia, hypotension, CHF, palpitations, arteriovenous (AV) block, agranulocytosis, thrombocytopenia, nausea, vomiting, diarrhea, constipation, impotence, decreased libido, joint pain, arthralgia, facial swelling, rash, pruritus, depression, hallucinations, dizziness, fatigue, lethargy, sore throat, laryngospasm, blurred vision
Cholesterol-lowering agents:			
Bile acid–sequestering agents: • Cholestyramine (Questran); adult 4 g PO ac and hs, maximum dose 32 g/day; children, 240 mg/kg/day PO in 3 divided doses • Colestipol (Colestid); adults, 15-30 g/day PO in 2-4 divided doses • Drugs must be mixed with either liquid or applesauce; give other medications 1 hour before or 4 hours after	Bind with bile acids in intestine, and complex is excreted in feces	***Contraindications:*** Hypersensitivity; biliary obstruction ***Cost:*** Cholestyramine: 4 g in 5-g packet, 60 packets: $83; colestipol: 5-g packet, 90 packets: $110 ***Pregnancy category:*** Safe use has not been established	Constipation, abdominal discomfort, flatulence, nausea, vomiting, dyspepsia, eructation, anorexia, decreased levels of vitamin A, D, and K
Niacin or nicotinic acid (Nicolar), 250 mg PO qd following evening meal; may increase every 4-7 days until 1.5-2 g daily is reached; after 2 months, check cholesterol level; if not adequately controlled, increase at 2- to 4-week intervals up to 3 g/day; maximum dose 6 g/day, rarely necessary	Interferes with synthesis of cholesterol and lipoproteins	***Contraindications:*** Hypersensitivity; hepatic dysfunction; active peptic ulcer disease; arterial bleeding ***Cost:*** 500-mg tab, 100 tabs: $2-$64 ***Pregnancy category:*** C	Severe hepatic toxicity; generalized flushing—can block with an aspirin taken with niacin; atrial fibrillation and other cardiac arrhythmias can occur; dyspepsia, vomiting, diarrhea, peptic ulceration, decreased glucose tolerance, hyperuricemia
HMG-CoA reductase inhibitors: • Lovastatin (Mevacor); patient should be on low-cholesterol, low-fat diet; starting dose is 20 mg PO qd with evening meal • Pravastatin (Pravachol), 10-20 mg PO qd at bedtime • Neither drug recommended for children	HMG-CoA reductase inhibitors	***Contraindications:*** Pregnancy and lactation; hypersensitivity; active liver disease ***Cost:*** Lovastatin: 20-mg tab, 100 tabs: $212; pravastatin: 20-g tab; 90 tabs: $170 ***Pregnancy category:*** X	Marked increase in serum transaminase, acid regurgitation, dry mouth, vomiting, leg pain, shoulder pain, insomnia, eye irritation, alopecia, pruritus

Nephrotic Syndrome

OVERVIEW

Nephrotic syndrome is a condition that occurs as a result of damage to the glomerular apparatus of the kidney. It is characterized by increased (>3.5 g/24 hours) protein excretion. It is classified as either primary (idiopathic) or secondary.

Pathogenesis

Causes:

- Primary syndrome:
  - Minimal-change disease
  - Focal glomerulosclerosis
  - Membranous glomerulonephritis
  - IgA nephropathy
  - Fibrillary glomerulopathy
- Secondary syndrome:
  - Allergens
  - Carcinoma
  - Diabetes
  - Erythema multiforme
  - HIV infection
  - Lymphomas
  - Leukemias
  - Malignant hypertension
  - NSAIDs
  - Sarcoidosis
  - Toxemia of pregnancy

Patient Profile

- Males = Females
- Any age

Signs and Symptoms

- Peripheral edema
- Ascites
- Anorexia
- Abdominal distention
- Hypertension
- Oliguria
- Puffy eyelids
- Scrotal swelling
- Shortness of breath
- Weight gain

Differential Diagnosis

- Consider all possible secondary causes
- Congestive heart failure

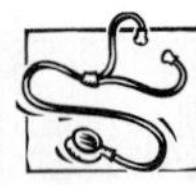

ASSESSMENT

History

Inquire about:

- Onset and duration of symptoms
- Decreased urine output
- Weight gain
- Underlying conditions
- Current medications

Physical Findings

- Weight gain
- Peripheral edema
- Increased BP
- Puffy eyes
- Heart—tachycardia
- Lungs—crackles, tachypnea, shortness of breath

Initial Workup

Laboratory

- Urinalysis—proteinuria, hematuria, microscopic examination—RBC count, granular, hyaline casts
- 24-hour urine protein >3.5 g/24 hours
- Chemistry panel—to include electrolytes, cholesterol, triglycerides, BUN, and creatinine—increased cholesterol and triglycerides; may have increased potassium, decreased sodium, and increased BUN and creatinine
- Serum albumin—decreased

Radiology

- Renal ultrasound
- CT scan

Further Workup

Renal biopsy—gold standard

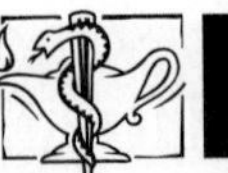

INTERVENTIONS

Office Treatment

None indicated

Lifestyle Modifications

- Diet—low sodium, slightly decreased protein
- May require fluid restriction

Patient Education

Teach patient about:

- Condition and treatment—if secondary nephrotic syndrome exists, vigorous treatment of cause
- Fluid restriction
- Proper diet
- Avoiding nephrotoxic drugs
- Importance of regular health maintenance, such as flu vaccine and pneumonia vaccine
- Signs and symptoms of infection and to report promptly
- Medications used and side effects (see Pharmacotherapeutics)

Referral

To nephrology NP or nephrologist for management

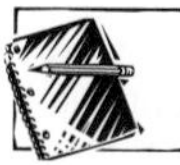

EVALUATION

Outcome
If underlying cause is treatable, may have complete reversal; otherwise may progress to end-stage renal disease

Possible Complications
- Acute renal failure
- Chronic renal failure
- Pulmonary emboli
- Renal vein thrombosis
- Infection
- Pleural effusion

Follow-up
By nephrologist

FOR YOUR INFORMATION

Life Span
Pediatric: Minimal-change disease commonly seen in young children
Geriatric: High morbidity and mortality
Pregnancy: May be due to toxemia—should be handled by specialist

Miscellaneous
N/A

References

Kraus ES: Proteinuria. In Barker LR, Burton JR, Zieve PD, editors: *Principles of ambulatory medicine,* ed 4, Baltimore, 1995, Williams & Wilkins, pp 525-526.

Morrison G: Kidney. In Tierney LM Jr, McPhee SJ, Papadakis SA, editors: *Current medical diagnosis and treatment,* ed 34, Norwalk, Conn, 1995, Appleton & Lange, pp 786-789.

NOTES

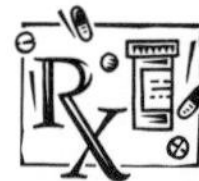

PHARMACOTHERAPEUTICS

There are many medications that may be used in the treatment of nephrotic syndrome. These are beyond the scope of this book.

Drug of Choice	Mechanism of Action	Prescribing Information	Side Effects
Mainstay of therapy:			
Furosemide, 40 mg PO qd, increase as needed to control edema	Loop diuretic; inhibits reabsorption of sodium and chloride at proximal and distal tubule and at loop of Henle	***Contraindications:*** Hypersensitivity; anuria; hypovolemia ***Cost:*** 20-mg tab, 100 tabs: $2-$15 ***Pregnancy category:*** C	Headache, fatigue, orthostatic hypotension, chest pain, circulatory collapse, hypokalemia, hypomagnesemia, hyperuricemia, hyperglycemia, nausea, diarrhea, renal failure, thrombocytopenia, agranulocytosis, anemia, rash, Stevens-Johnson syndrome

Non–Insulin-Dependent Diabetes Mellitus (NIDDM)

OVERVIEW

Non–insulin-dependent diabetes mellitus (NIDDM), or type II diabetes, is a chronic condition in which the body is unable to maintain a normal blood glucose level. It is characterized by the fact that the patient is *not* ketosis prone, as in insulin-dependent diabetes mellitus (IDDM). It accounts for 80% to 90% of all cases of diabetes.

Pathogenesis

- Caused by defects in insulin secretion and peripheral insulin action
- Strong genetic influence
- Insulin present, but ineffective; may actually have increased amounts of insulin

Patient Profile

- Females > Males
- Higher prevalence rate in African-Americans and Native Americans
- Predominant age >35 years, but may occur at any age

Signs and Symptoms

- Polyuria
- Polydipsia
- Polyphagia
- Weight loss
- Weakness
- Fatigue
- Frequent infections (furuncles, yeast infections)

Differential Diagnosis

- IDDM
- Pancreatic insufficiency
- Pheochromocytoma
- Cushing's syndrome
- Corticosteroid use
- Stress hyperglycemia

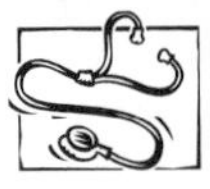

ASSESSMENT

History

Inquire about:

- Onset and duration of symptoms
- Family history of diabetes
- Ethnic background
- Underlying conditions
- Current medications
- Drugs that may cause hyperglycemia in patients prone to diabetes—glucagon, glucocorticoids, growth hormone, epinephrine, estrogen and progesterone, thyroid preparations, thiazide diuretics, furosemide, acetazolamide, diazoxide, beta-blockers, alpha-agonists, calcium channel blockers, phenytoin, phenobarbital sodium, nicotinic acid, cyclophosphamide, I-asparaginase, decongestants and diet pills, nonsteroidal antiinflammatory agents, nicotine

Physical Findings

- BP—increased or normal
- Eyes—may have decreased visual acuity
- Fundoscopic—may find evidence of retinopathy, such as microaneurysms and hard exudates
- May have candidiasis, furuncles, carbuncles, or other infection

Initial Workup

Laboratory

- Fasting blood glucose level >126 mg/dl on 2 occasions is diagnostic
- Random glucose >200 mg/dl with classic symptoms is diagnostic
- Lipid panel—may have elevated cholesterol level
- Urinalysis—glucose present

Radiology: None indicated

Further Workup

- Hemoglobin A1C
- 2-hour glucose challenge after 75-g glucose load—over 200 mg/dl after 2 hours is diagnostic

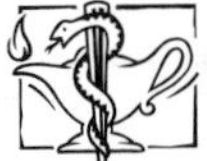

INTERVENTIONS

Office Treatment

Usually none indicated; if furuncle present, may need incision and drainage

Lifestyle Modifications

- Diabetic diet
- Smoking cessation
- Regular aerobic exercise
- Adjustment to living with a chronic illness
- Adjustment to taking daily medication

Patient Education

Education should be ongoing process; ideally should include dietitian, social worker, and specially trained diabetic educator—teach patient about:

- Condition and treatment:
  - Diabetic diet and exercise—first-line treatment
  - If normoglycemia not reached, medications with diet and exercise—oral agents first, insulin last
- Disease process and possible complications of diabetes—nephropathy, retinopathy, accelerated atherosclerosis, neuropathy
- Performing blood glucose monitoring
- Signs and symptoms of hyperglycemic and hypoglycemic reactions
- Proper foot care and why necessary
- This being a lifelong condition, for which, at the present time, there is no cure
- Medications used and side effects (see Pharmacotherapeutics)

Referrals

To dietitian, social worker, and diabetic educator if possible; if resistant to treatment may need to refer to endocrinologist

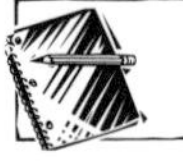

EVALUATION

Outcomes

- Normoglycemia
- May see "honeymoon phase" when insulin requirement is diminished—usually lasts from 3 to 12 months
- Monitor hemoglobin A1C—ideal is for level to be within normal limits
- Current research concerning tight glucose control was done with patients with IDDM; unknown whether same benefits can be seen with NIDDM patients

Possible Complications

- Hyperlipidemia
- Microvascular diseases
- Macrovascular diseases
- Foot problems
- Skin ulcerations
- Hypoglycemia
- Hyperosmolar coma
- Psychologic problems related to chronic disease

Follow-up

- Weekly until control is achieved; then every 2 weeks × 1 month; then monthly × 2 months; then every 3 months
- Teaching incorporated into every clinic visit
- Monitoring of hemoglobin A1C and foot examination every 3 months
- Yearly chemistry panel to measure lipids, renal function, thyroid function
- Yearly eye examination

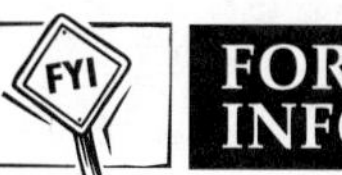

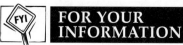

FOR YOUR INFORMATION

Life Span

Pediatric: Generally is an adult disease; best handled by specialist
Geriatric: Very common cause of blindness in this age group
Pregnancy: Needs to be placed on insulin regimen and will need intense management by specialist

Miscellaneous

The diagnosis of diabetes can have a major impact on the patient and his or her family. It is important for the NP to remember to treat the psychosocial aspect of the disease, as well as the physical aspect.

References

Cunningham MA: Non–insulin-dependent diabetes: getting the attention it deserves, *Clin Excel Nurse Pract* 1(2):95-104, 1997.

Valentine V: Patient with diabetes. In Lewis SM, Collier IC, Heitkemper MM, editors: *Medical-surgical nursing: assessment and management of clinical problems,* ed 4, St Louis, 1996, Mosby, pp 1438-1474.

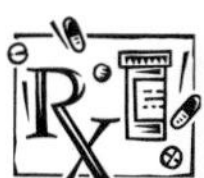

PHARMACOTHERAPEUTICS

Drug of Choice	Mechanism of Action	Prescribing Information	Side Effects
First-generation sulfonylureas: • Tolbutamide (Orinase), 500-3000 mg/day PO in 2-3 divided doses • Tolazamide (Tolinase), 100-1000 mg/day PO in 1-2 divided doses • Chlorpropamide (Diabinese), 100-500 mg/day PO in 1 dose • These drugs should not be used in the elderly or renally impaired; chlorpropamide has a very long half-life; use extreme caution when changing to another drug or to insulin therapy	Stimulate release of insulin from pancreas	***Contraindications:*** Hypersensitivity; known ketoacidosis; hypersensitivity to sulfonamides ***Cost:*** Tolbutamide: 500-mg tab, 100 tabs: $3-$27; tolazamide: 100-mg tab, 100 tabs: $5-$28; chlorpropamide: 100-mg tab, 100 tabs: $3-$35 ***Pregnancy category:*** C	Hypoglycemia, increased risk of cardiovascular mortality, epigastric discomfort, hypersensitivity reactions, nausea, heartburn, pruritus, leukopenia, agranulocytosis, thrombocytopenia, hemolytic anemia, headache
Second-generation sulfonylureas: • Glyburide (Micronase), 1.5-20 mg/day PO in 1-2 doses • Glipizide (Glucotrol), 2.5-40 mg/day PO in 1-2 doses • Glimepiride (Amaryl), 1-8 mg/day PO in 1 dose	Stimulate release of insulin from functioning beta cells	***Contraindications:*** Hypersensitivity; ketoacidosis; hypersensitivity to sulfonamides ***Cost:*** Glyburide: 5-mg tab, 100 tabs: $51-$61; glipizide: 5-mg tab, 100 tabs: $18-$35; glimepiride: 1-mg tab, 100 tabs: $22 ***Pregnancy category:*** C	Increased risk of cardiovascular mortality, severe hypoglycemia, allergic skin reactions, dizziness, drowsiness, headache
Metformin (Glucophage); usual starting dose 500 mg with morning and evening meals; maximum dose 2500 mg; if 2500 mg is given, may be better tolerated given tid; may also start with 850 mg given once daily with morning meal, increase by 1 tab every other week; may be used as monotherapy or with sulfonylureas	Decreases hepatic glucose production and intestinal absorption and improves insulin sensitivity	***Contraindications:*** Renal disease or renal dysfunction; withhold drug if patient is to have radiologic studies using iodinated contrast material; hypersensitivity; diabetic ketoacidosis ***Cost:*** 500-mg tab, 100 tabs: $46 ***Pregnancy category:*** B	Can cause lactic acidosis—rare but serious; increased risk of cardiovascular mortality, diarrhea, nausea, vomiting, abdominal bloating, flatulence, anorexia, unpleasant taste, rash, dermatitis
Acarbose (Precose); starting dose 25 mg (half of 50-mg tab) given tid with first bite of each meal; increase at 4- to 8-week intervals based on 1-hour postprandial blood sugar; maximum dose 100 mg tid	Alpha-glucosidase; delays digestion of ingested carbohydrates, thereby delaying absorption of glucose	***Contraindications:*** Hypersensitivity; ketoacidosis; inflammatory bowel disease; colonic ulceration; partial intestinal obstruction; digestive problems ***Cost:*** 50-mg tab, 100 tabs: $46 ***Pregnancy category:*** B	Abdominal pain, diarrhea, flatulence, decreased hematocrit
If the above treatments fail to control the blood glucose level, try insulin. For information on insulin, see section on insulin-dependent diabetes mellitus			
Troglitazone (Rezulin), 200 mg PO 1 time/day with food; maximum dose 600 mg/day; currently for use with patients receiving >30 units/day of insulin; may soon have indication as monotherapy.	Insulin-resistance reducer	***Contraindications:*** Type I diabetes; hepatic impairment; nursing mothers; use caution when using with drugs metabolized by CYP450 enzyme system ***Cost:*** Unavailable ***Pregnancy category:*** B	Hypoglycemia—monitor glucose closely, may need to lower insulin dose; asthenia; dizziness; GI disturbance

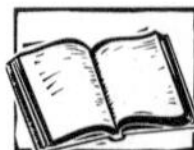

OVERVIEW

Obesity is a condition of increased body weight or excessive accumulation of body fat. It can also be defined as weight 20% greater than an individual's desirable body weight for the person's age, height, and sex.

Pathogenesis
- Caloric intake exceeds caloric output
- Multi-factorial—genetic, social, developmental, metabolic, psychologic

Patient Profile
- Females > Males
- 30%-40% of all adults; increasing at rapid rate

Signs and Symptoms
Increased weight and adipose tissue

Differential Diagnosis
- Hypothyroidism
- Cushing's syndrome

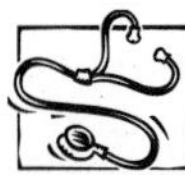

ASSESSMENT

History
Inquire about:
- Onset and duration of symptoms
- Lowest and highest weight
- Dietary habits, including number of meals per day and snacks
- Emotional stresses at home and work
- Amount of physical activity each week
- Motivation for weight loss
- Past diets tried and results
- Occupation
- Family history
- Underlying conditions
- Current medications

Physical Findings
- Increased weight and adipose tissue
- Gynecoid pattern (pear-shaped)—heaviest in hips, thighs, buttocks (lower risk of cardiovascular diseases)
- Android pattern (apple shape)—heaviest in abdominal area (high risk of cardiovascular disease)
- Skin may have striae, irritation in fat folds
- Boils
- Fungal infections

Initial Workup
Laboratory
- None for diagnosis
- Thyroid panel—rule out hypothyroidism
- Cardiac risk factors—cholesterol, triglycerides, glucose

Radiology: None indicated

Further Workup
Figure patient's body mass index (BMI):
- Weight in kilograms ÷ height in meters^2
- Men—desirable, 22-24; >28.5, obese
- Women—desirable, 21-23; >27.5, obese

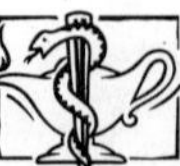

INTERVENTIONS

Office Treatment
None indicated

Lifestyle Modifications
Nutritionally sound, low-fat diet with reduced calories—long-term commitment

Patient Education
Teach patient about:
- Condition and health risks
- Setting realistic goals for weight loss and exercise plan
- Dieting and cutting calories—switch from whole milk to 2% milk and then to skim milk; use artificial sweetener instead of sugar; eat fruit for snacks instead of high-fat/high-calorie snacks; increase amount of vegetables in diet; avoid frying foods—bake, broil, or grill
- Support group and diet programs in community, such as TOPS, Overeaters Anonymous, Weight Watchers
- Avoiding programs or medications that promise "lose all the weight you want, while eating all the food you want"
- Obesity being a chronic disease that requires a lifelong commitment to change

Referrals
- To nutritionist
- For morbid obesity (BMI >40), to specialist

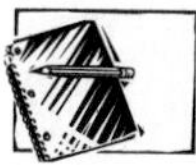

EVALUATION

Outcome
Patient loses weight, approximately 2 pounds per week, and develops healthy lifestyle

Possible Complications
- Cardiovascular disease
- Diabetes mellitus
- Hypertension
- Hyperlipidemia
- Gallbladder disease
- Osteoarthritis
- Gout
- Sleep apnea
- Poor self-esteem

Follow-up
Every 2 weeks × 2; then monthly for several months

FOR YOUR INFORMATION

Life Span
Pediatric: Prevalence increasing, possibly because of decreased physical activity
Geriatric: Metabolic rate decreases 2% every 10 years
Pregnancy: Common time for onset of obesity

Miscellaneous
N/A

References
Horton ES: Obesity. In Stein JH et al, editors: *Internal medicine,* ed 4, St Louis, 1994, Mosby, pp 1263-1266.

Long BC: Healthy lifestyles: nutrition, exercise, rest, and sleep. In Phipps WJ et al, editors: *Medical-surgical nursing: concepts and clinical practice,* ed 5, St Louis, 1995, Mosby, pp 145-146.

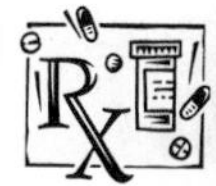

PHARMACOTHERAPEUTICS

As a general rule, drug therapy is not recommended for the treatment of obesity. At the present time, there is no "magic bullet" that will allow the patient to eat as he or she pleases and still lose weight. Current medications must be used in conjunction with diet and exercise. Current prescription medications available are either Schedule III or Schedule IV drugs, which, in many parts of the country, NPs are unable to prescribe. These medications should only be used by someone experienced in their use because many have serious addictive potential and side effects. A great deal of research is currently being done in the area of obesity, and perhaps in the very near future we will be able to cure and prevent obesity.

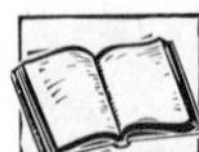

OVERVIEW

Onychomycosis is an infection of the toenails and fingernails caused by a fungus. It is also called tinea unguium.

Pathogenesis

- Cause—*Trichophyton rubrum, Trichophyton mentagrophytes;* also caused by *Candida* organisms
- Trauma predisposes to infection
- Four distinct patterns of infection—distal subungual onychomycosis, white superficial onychomycosis, proximal subungual onychomycosis, candidal onychomycosis

Patient Profile

Depends on type:

- Tinea:
  - Males = Females
  - Adults
- Candidal infection:
  - Females > Males
  - Adults

Signs and Symptoms

Depends on pattern:

- Distal subungual onychomycosis—most common; invades distal area of nail bed; distal nail plate turns yellow or white and rises and separates from nail bed
- White superficial onychomycosis—invasion of nail plate; nail is soft, dry, and powdery
- Proximal subungual onychomycosis—posterior nail fold–cuticle area invaded; migrate to matrix and invade nail plate; debris accumulates, and nail separates; white bands begin at proximal nail plate and grow outward
- Candida onychomycosis—involves all fingernails; nail plate thickens, turns yellow-brown

Differential Diagnosis

- Black nail paronychia
- Herpetic whitlow
- Eczema
- Pustular psoriasis
- Tumor
- Darier's disease
- Pityriasis rubra pilaris
- Trophic changes
- Peripheral vascular disease
- Endocrine disease
- Drugs
- Trauma
- Alopecia areata
- Lichen planus
- Yellow nail syndrome

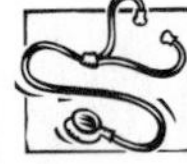

ASSESSMENT

History

Inquire about:

- Onset and duration of symptoms
- History of constant contact with warmth and moisture
- Trauma to nails
- Contact with other infected areas
- Treatments tried and results
- Underlying conditions (psoriasis, diabetes)
- Current medications

Physical Findings

Examination of nails of toes and hands—depending on type, may see thickened yellow or white nails; nails may be powdery, soft, and dry; separation of nail from nail bed, yellowish-brown nails

Initial Workup

Laboratory

- Potassium hydroxide preparation
- Fungal culture
- CBC and initial liver function studies (done before starting medications)

Radiology: None indicated

Further Workup

None indicated

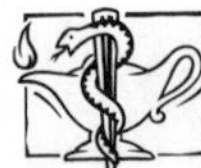

INTERVENTIONS

Office Treatment

Obtain specimens for potassium hydroxide preparation and culture

Lifestyle Modifications

- Avoidance of prolonged immersion in warm water
- Changing socks frequently; wearing loose-fitting shoes
- Control of underlying chronic illnesses

Patient Education

Teach patient about:

- Condition and treatment:
  - Oral antifungals
  - Difficult and frustrating to treat
  - Lengthy treatment—6 to 9 months for fingernails, 9 to 12 months for toenails, 12 to 24 months for great toe
- Medications used and side effects (see Pharmacotherapeutics)

Referral

To dermatologist if extensive

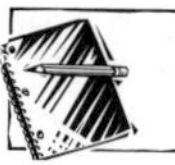

EVALUATION

Outcome
Resolves without sequelae; treatment must be for long period of time, and recurrence after stopping medication very common

Possible Complications
- Cellulitis
- Osteomyelitis

Follow-up
Every 3 months for liver function studies if taking antifungal agent

FOR YOUR INFORMATION

Life Span
Pediatric: Rarely occurs before puberty
Geriatric: Look for underlying condition
Pregnancy: Should attempt to wait to treat until after pregnancy

Miscellaneous
Treatment with topical agents is of little value. The only value of using topical agents is to control inflammation at the nail folds.

Reference
Habif TP: *Clinical dermatology: a color guide to diagnosis and therapy,* ed 3, St Louis, 1996, Mosby, pp 765-770.

NOTES

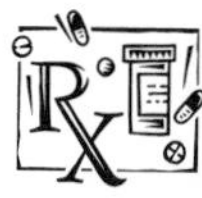

PHARMACOTHERAPEUTICS

Drug of Choice	Mechanism of Action	Prescribing Information	Side Effects
Griseofulvin (Fulvicin), 250-500 mg PO bid with food for 6-9 months—fingernails; 9-12 months—toenails; 12-24 months—great toenail; children, 5 mg/lb/day PO; take with food to increase absorption; baseline liver function tests should be performed and evaluated on regular basis (every 3 months)	Fungistatic	***Contraindications:*** Porphyria; hepatocellular failure; hypersensitivity ***Cost:*** 250-mg tab, 100 tabs: $33-$69 ***Pregnancy category:*** C	Porphyria, hepatocellular failure, leukopenia, persistent anemia, skin rash, urticaria, oral thrush, nausea, vomiting, diarrhea, headache, fatigue, dizziness, insomnia, mental confusion, proteinuria, leukopenia
Fluconazole (Diflucan), 150-mg tab PO weekly for 6-9 months—fingernails; 9-12 months—toenails; 12-24 months—great toenail; significant drug interactions can occur; consult manufacturer's prescribing information; take with food to increase absorption	Fungistatic; inhibits fungal cytochrome P-450	***Contraindication:*** Hypersensitivity ***Cost:*** 150-mg tab, 12 tabs: $107 ***Pregnancy category:*** C	Hepatotoxicity—monitor liver function tests on initiation and every 3 months; hypersensitivity reactions, nausea, vomiting, diarrhea, anaphylaxis, seizures, leukopenia, thrombocytopenia, Stevens-Johnson syndrome
Itraconazole (Sporanox); pulse dosing—400 mg/day PO for first week of each month; 6-9 months—fingernails; 9-12 months—toenails; 12-24 months—great toenail; many drug interactions; consult manufacturer's prescribing information	Inhibits cytochrome P-450-dependent synthesis of ergosterol—vital component of cell membrane	***Contraindications:*** Coadministration of terfenadine, astemizole, cisapride; coadministration with triazolam, midazolam; pregnancy or those contemplating pregnancy; hypersensitivity ***Cost:*** 100-mg tab, 30 tabs: $162 ***Pregnancy category:*** C	Take with food to increase absorption; hepatotoxicity can occur—monitor liver function tests initially and every 3 months; hypersensitivity reactions, nausea, vomiting, rash, hypertension, headache, malaise, myalgia, vasculitis, vertigo, abdominal pain, anorexia, fatigue, fever
Terbinafine (Lamisil), 250 mg/day PO for 12 weeks—toenail, 6 weeks—fingernails; safety in children not established	Fungistatic	***Contraindication:*** Hypersensitivity ***Cost:*** 250-mg tab, 12 tabs: $170 ***Pregnancy category:*** B	Rare hepatobiliary dysfunction, headache, diarrhea, dyspepsia, abdominal pain, nausea, flatulence, rash, pruritus, urticaria, taste disturbance, visual disturbance

Osteoarthritis (OA)/Degenerative Arthritis/ Degenerative Joint Disease

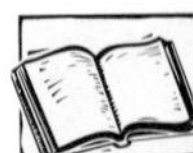

OVERVIEW

Osteoarthritis is a noninflammatory arthritis in which there is deterioration of the articular cartilage and bony overgrowth of the joint surface.

Pathogenesis

Cause—unknown

Patient Profile

- Males = Females
- Most common age >40 years
- Risk factors:
  - Past joint trauma
  - Obesity
  - Normal aging process
  - Occupational overuse

Signs and Symptoms

- Dull, aching joint pain, tenderness
- Decreased range of motion in joint
- Joint enlargement (Heberden's nodes—distal interphalangeal joints; Bouchard's nodes—proximal interphalangeal joints)
- Joint crepitus
- Joint stiffness—occurs with rest; improves with activity

Differential Diagnosis

- Osteoporosis
- Malignancy
- Tendinitis
- Bursitis
- Vasculitis
- Rheumatoid arthritis
- Gout
- Pseudogout

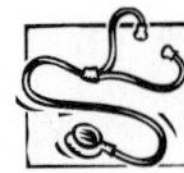

ASSESSMENT

History

Inquire about:

- Onset and duration of symptoms (slow, gradual onset, asymmetric)
- Past history of joint trauma
- Amount of disability or limitations from joint pain and stiffness
- Treatments tried and results
- Underlying conditions
- Current medications

Physical Findings

Joint enlargement, swelling, crepitus, and decreased range of motion

Initial Workup

Laboratory: Only needed to rule out other causes

Radiology: Plain films of affected joint(s)—narrowed joint space, bone cysts, osteophytes

Further Workup

None indicated

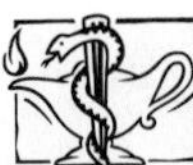

INTERVENTIONS

Office Treatment

None indicated

Lifestyle Modifications

- Weight loss
- Exercise program

Patient Education

Teach patient about:

- Condition and treatment
- Warm, moist heat may be beneficial
- Starting a moderate exercise program to strengthen surrounding muscles
- Tips for weight loss
- Pain control—biofeedback, relaxation therapy, meditation
- Medications used and side effects (see Pharmacotherapeutics)

Referrals

- Consider physical and/or occupational therapy
- To orthopedic surgeon for intraarticular steroid injections or joint replacement surgery if necessary

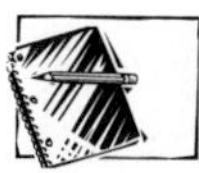

EVALUATION

Outcome

Maintenance of function for as long as possible

Possible Complications

- Side effects of medications
- Total loss of joint function

Follow-up

- Every 2 weeks × 2
- If stable, every 3 to 6 months—monitor for medication side effects, such as peptic ulcer

FOR YOUR INFORMATION

Life Span

Pediatric: Very rare in this age group—look for another cause of joint pain
Geriatric: Most common in this age group—use lowest effective dose of medications
Pregnancy: Cautious use of medications

Miscellaneous

N/A

Reference

Mercier LR: *Practical orthopedics,* ed 4, St Louis, 1995, Mosby, pp 279-280.

Peters S: Osteoarthritis options: new guidelines for primary care, *Adv Nurse Pract* 4(12):41-42, 50, 1996.

PHARMACOTHERAPEUTICS

Drug of Choice	Mechanism of Action	Prescribing Information	Side Effects
Acetaminophen (Tylenol), 325 mg, 2 tabs PO q4-6h; may increase up to 4000 mg/day	Analgesia by increasing pain threshold	***Contraindications:*** Hypersensitivity; bleeding disorders or anticoagulant therapy; last trimester of pregnancy; asthma; gastric ulcers ***Cost:*** OTC ***Pregnancy category:*** Not categorized	Rash; hepatic toxicity with alcohol ingestion or overdose
Aspirin, 325 mg, 2 tabs PO q4h	Antiinflammatory action may result from inhibition of synthesis and release of prostaglandins	***Contraindications:*** Hypersensitivity; GI bleeding; bleeding disorders ***Cost:*** OTC ***Pregnancy category:*** Should not be used in 3rd trimester	Dyspepsia, thirst, nausea, vomiting, GI bleeding/ulceration, tinnitus, vertigo, reversible hearing loss, prolongation of bleeding time, leukopenia, thrombocytopenia, purpura, urticaria, angioedema, pruritus, asthma, anaphylaxis, mental confusion, drowsiness, dizziness, headache, fever
Nonsteroidal antiinflammatory drugs (NSAIDs): many different types currently marketed; consult manufacturer's package insert for specific dosing and prescribing information	Exact action unknown; may result from inhibition of synthesis of prostaglandins and arachidonic acid	***Contraindications:*** Hypersensitivity to NSAIDs, aspirin; severe hepatic failure; asthma ***Cost:*** Varies with type ***Pregnancy category:*** Depends on product	Stomach distress, flatulence, nausea, abdominal pain, constipation or diarrhea, dizziness, sedation, rash, urticaria, angioedema, anorexia, urinary frequency, increased blood pressure, insomnia, anxiety, visual disturbances, increased thirst, alopecia, peptic ulcer
Capsaicin 0.025% (Capsaicin-P); apply lotion to affected joints 3-4 times daily; avoid contact with eyes and mucous membranes	Analgesic rub; exact mechanism of action unknown	***Contraindications:*** Hypersensitivity; open wounds or irritated skin ***Cost:*** OTC ***Pregnancy category:*** Not categorized	Transient burning or stinging; rash, irritation

Osteomyelitis

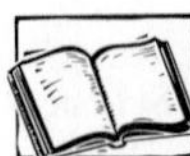

OVERVIEW

Osteomyelitis is an infection of the bone or bone marrow. It may be acute or chronic. Acute osteomyelitis is generally a disease of childhood, and chronic osteomyelitis is a disease of adulthood. The most common site of acute osteomyelitis in children is the metaphyseal end of a single long bone; in adults over age 50 years, the spine is the most common site. Chronic osteomyelitis in adults can occur in any bone that has been subjected to an open fracture or wound.

Pathogenesis

Causes:

- Acute osteomyelitis:
  - Hematogenous route—*Staphylococcus aureus, Haemophilus influenzae,* streptococci, less common—gram-negative organisms
  - Vertebral osteomyelitis—*S. aureus,* gram-negative enteric organisms, *Mycobacterium tuberculosis,* fungi
- Chronic osteomyelitis—polymicrobial

Patient Profile

- Males > Females
- Most common age groups:
  - Acute osteomyelitis—infants and children, adults >50 years
  - Chronic osteomyelitis—adults, most commonly older adults

Signs and Symptoms

- Acute osteomyelitis in children:
  - Abrupt onset of high fever, irritability, malaise, anorexia, inflammation over bone, bone pain and tenderness, swelling, restriction of movement
  - Vertebral osteomyelitis—insidious onset, history of genitourinary disease and/or manipulation, limitation of joint motion, bone pain
- Chronic osteomyelitis—nonhealing ulcer or sinus, fever, bone pain, inflammation, soft tissue swelling, limitation of joint motion, erythema

Differential Diagnosis

- Acute suppurative arthritis
- Rheumatic fever
- Cellulitis
- Tumor
- Gout

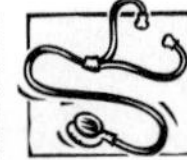

ASSESSMENT

History

Inquire about:

- Onset and duration of symptoms
- Recent history of infection (in those >50 years of age, ask about genitourinary infection)
- Recent history of trauma to area
- Recent history of surgical procedure involving bone
- Underlying conditions
- Current medications

Physical Findings

- Fever (may or may not be present)
- Pain, swelling, erythema, tenderness over bone
- May find draining ulcer/sinus

Initial Workup

Laboratory

- Blood cultures—may or may not be positive
- Needle aspiration over involved bone or bone biopsy—culture or histology
- CBC—leukocytosis in acute cases
- Erythrocyte sedimentation rate (ESR)—elevated

Radiology: Plain films of bone—acute infection—initially, x-ray film may be normal; sclerotic bone may be seen later, as in chronic osteomyelitis

Further Workup

None indicated

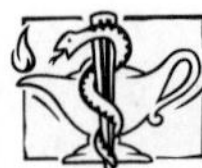

INTERVENTIONS

Office Treatment

None indicated

Lifestyle Modification

Hospitalization with bed rest

Patient Education

Teach patient about:

- Condition and treatment:
  - Hospitalization and IV antibiotic therapy initially
  - Length of antimicrobial therapy—4 to 6 weeks for acute osteomyelitis; longer for chronic osteomyelitis
  - Immobilizing affected extremity
  - Importance of regular follow-up
- Medications used and side effects (see Pharmacotherapeutics)

Referral

To physician for hospitalization if NP does not have privileges

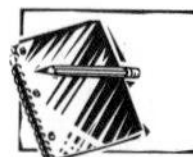

EVALUATION

Outcomes

- Acute osteomyelitis—prognosis good, but 6 weeks of treatment required
- Chronic osteomyelitis—unpredictable course

Possible Complications

- Amputation
- Abscess formation
- Bacteremia
- Fracture

Follow-up

Within 1 week of hospitalization; then every 2 weeks until resolved

FOR YOUR INFORMATION

Life Span

Pediatric: Acute, hematogenous osteomyelitis of long bones most common
Geriatric: Vertebral osteomyelitis most common form of acute osteomyelitis; onset very insidious; higher morbidity and mortality
Pregnancy: Cautious use of medications

Miscellaneous

N/A

References

Bartlett JG: *Pocket book of infectious disease therapy,* ed 7, Baltimore, 1996, Williams & Wilkins, pp 244-245.

Mercier LR: *Practical orthopedics,* ed 4, St Louis, 1995, Mosby, pp 262-267.

NOTES

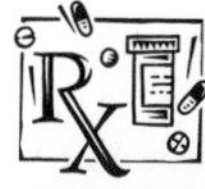

PHARMACOTHERAPEUTICS

Antibiotic therapy should be based on the results of culture and sensitivity tests. However, treatment should not wait for culture results, and it is fairly safe to begin treatment with a penicillinase-resistant penicillin (see below). It is beyond the scope of this book to cover all of the intravenous medications that may be used. Consult an acute care or infectious disease text.

Drug of Choice	Mechanism of Action	Prescribing Information	Side Effects
Nafcillin (Unipen), 1 g IV q4-6h; children <40 kg, 25 mg/kg IM bid × 4-6 weeks	Interferes with cell wall replication	***Contraindication:*** Hypersensitivity to penicillins ***Cost:*** 1-g vial, 10 vials: $45 ***Pregnancy category:*** B	Anemia, bone marrow depression, granulocytopenia, nausea, vomiting, diarrhea, increased ALT and AST, pseudomembranous colitis, oliguria, proteinuria, hematuria, vaginitis, moniliasis, glomerulonephritis, coma, convulsions

Osteoporosis

OVERVIEW

Osteoporosis is an abnormality of bone metabolism that results in loss of bone mass. It is a generalized and progressive disorder that increases susceptibility to fractures. It may be classified as either primary or secondary.

Pathogenesis

Causes:

- Primary osteoporosis:
  - Type I—postmenopausal endocrine changes: imbalance between bone formation and resorption
  - Type II—age-related reduction in vitamin D
- Secondary osteoporosis:
  - Hyperthyroidism
  - Hyperparathyroidism
  - Hypogonadism
  - Hyperprolactinism
  - Diabetes mellitus
  - Corticosteroids
  - Ethanol
  - Tobacco
  - Barbiturates
  - Chronic renal failure
  - Liver disease
  - Chronic obstructive pulmonary disease (COPD)
  - Rheumatoid arthritis
  - Malignancy
  - Cushing's syndrome

Patient Profile

- Females > Males
- Any age

Signs and Symptoms

- Asymptomatic initially
- Back pain
- Traumatic fractures of vertebrae, hip, forearm
- Loss of height

Differential Diagnosis

- See various causes of secondary osteoporosis under Pathogenesis
- Multiple myeloma
- Other neoplasia
- Osteomalacia
- Paget's disease

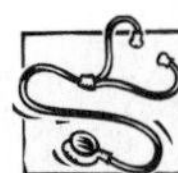

ASSESSMENT

History

Inquire about:

- Onset and duration of symptoms
- Previous fractures/back pain
- Noticeable loss of height
- Physical activity (amount and frequency)
- Smoking history
- Diet history, particularly caffeine consumption, alcohol intake, low-calcium/vitamin D intake
- Age at menopause
- Underlying conditions, such as diabetes
- Current medications

Physical Findings

- Back—dorsal kyphosis (Dowager's hump), cervical lordosis
- Painful area—look for deformity from fracture

Initial Workup

Laboratory

- Tests performed to rule out secondary osteoporosis:
  - CBC
  - Erythrocyte sedimentation rate (ESR)
  - Serum protein electrophoresis (to rule out multiple myeloma)
  - Thyroid-stimulating hormone (TSH)
  - Glucose level
  - Estrogen level (to rule out endocrine disease)
- Calcium level
- Vitamin D level—normal
- Alkaline phosphatase—normal or increased if healing fracture

Radiology: Only if fracture suspected; may wish to do bone mineral density studies

Further Workup

None indicated

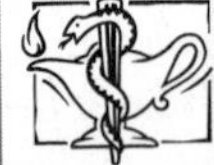

INTERVENTIONS

Office Treatment

None indicated

Lifestyle Modifications

- Smoking cessation
- Weight-bearing exercise program
- Reduction of alcohol intake

Patient Education

Teach patient about:

- Condition and treatment—consider hormone replacement therapy
- Weight-bearing exercises (walking)
- Tips for smoking cessation
- High-calcium diet (sardines, cheese, green vegetables, skim milk)
- Reducing alcohol intake
- Medications used and side effects (see Pharmacotherapeutics)

Referrals

Usually none needed; to orthopedist for resistant cases with repeated fractures

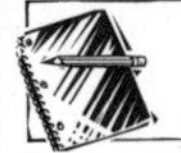

EVALUATION

Outcome

Stabilization of osteoporotic process

Possible Complications

- Severe, disabling pain
- Neurologic deficits secondary to vertebral fractures
- Inability to perform self-care activities

Follow-up

In 1 month × 2; then every 3 to 6 months

FOR YOUR INFORMATION

Life Span

Pediatric: Juvenile osteoporosis—rare and beyond the scope of this book

Geriatric: Most commonly affected age-group

Pregnancy: Rare type of acute osteoporosis may occur during pregnancy

Miscellaneous

Primary prevention of osteoporosis should begin with adequate calcium and vitamin D intake in childhood.

References

Kessenich CR: Update on pharmacologic therapies for osteoporosis, *Nurse Pract* 21(8):19-24, 1996.

Mercier LR: *Practical orthopedics,* St Louis, 1995, Mosby, pp 164-167.

Miller JL: Clinical evaluation and treatment of osteoporosis, *Physician Assist* 18(3):23-33, 1994.

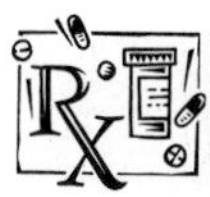

PHARMACOTHERAPEUTICS

Drug of Choice	Mechanism of Action	Prescribing Information	Side Effects
Calcium carbonate (Os-Cal), 1 tab qd to tid, or Tums, 1 tab bid or tid; men, 1.0-1.5 g/day—number of tabs depends on dosage/tab	Calcium supplement; neutralizes gastric acidity	***Contraindications:*** Hypersensitivity; hypercalcemia; hyperparathyroidism; bone tumors ***Cost:*** OTC ***Pregnancy category:*** C	Constipation, anorexia, obstruction, nausea, vomiting, flatulence, diarrhea, hemorrhage, rebound hypertension, hypercalcemia, metabolic alkalosis, renal dysfunction
Hormone replacement therapy (for progressive disease, patient may need both calcium supplement and hormone replacement therapy):			
Estrogen (Premarin), 0.625 mg PO 1 tab daily; estrogen is available in pills, as transdermal patch, or as vaginal cream; method of administration should be decided on by NP and patient together by determining which method best meets patient's needs	Affects release of pituitary gonadotropins; inhibits ovulation	***Contraindications:*** Hypersensitivity; breast cancer; thromboembolic disorders; reproductive cancer; undiagnosed vaginal bleeding; pregnancy ***Cost:*** 0.625-mg tab, 100 tabs: $50; transdermal or topical estrogen per year: $107 ***Pregnancy category:*** X	Dizziness, headache, migraines, depression, hypotension, thromboembolism, pulmonary embolism, myocardial infarction (MI), nausea, vomiting, cholestatic jaundice, weight gain, diplopia, amenorrhea, cervical erosion, breakthrough bleeding, dysmenorrhea, vaginal candidiasis, spontaneous abortion, rash, urticaria, acne, hirsutism, photosensitivity
If patient has intact uterus, add:			
Medroxyprogesterone acetate (Provera), 10 mg PO on days 1-12 or days 13-25; or can give 2.5 mg PO daily; estrogen and medroxyprogesterone acetate are now available in 1 tab sold under trade name Prempro	Inhibits secretion of pituitary gonadotropins; stimulates growth of mammary tissue	***Contraindications:*** Hypersensitivity; breast cancer; thromboembolic disorders; reproductive cancer; undiagnosed vaginal bleeding; pregnancy ***Cost:*** 5-mg tab, 30 tabs: $16 ***Pregnancy category:*** X	Dizziness, headache, migraines, depression, hypotension, thromboembolism, pulmonary embolism, MI, nausea, vomiting, cholestatic jaundice, weight gain, diplopia, amenorrhea, cervical erosion, breakthrough bleeding, dysmenorrhea, vaginal candidiasis, spontaneous abortion, rash, urticaria, acne, hirsutism, photosensitivity
For patients with bone mineral density ≥2 standard deviations below the mean for young, normal persons and/or history of osteoporotic fractures:			
Alendronate (Fosamax), 10 mg PO qd 30 minutes before breakfast with full glass of water; patient should wait at least 30 minutes in upright position before eating or drinking anything else	Biophosphonate; acts to decrease bone resorption and prevent bone loss	***Contraindications:*** Abnormalities of esophagus that delay emptying; inability to stand or sit upright for 30 minutes; hypersensitivity; hypocalcemia ***Cost:*** 10-mg tab, 100 tab: $167 ***Pregnancy category:*** C	Abdominal pain, nausea, dyspepsia, constipation, diarrhea, flatulence, acid regurgitation, vomiting, dysphagia, gastritis, muscle cramp, headache, dizziness
For women unable to take hormone replacement therapy:			
Calcitonin (salmon) (Calcimar), 100 IU/day SQ or IM daily or every other day; may also be given by nasal spray—1 spray in one nostril daily or every other day; each spray 200 IU	Decreases bone resorption, blood calcium levels; increases deposits of calcium in bone	***Contraindication:*** Hypersensitivity ***Cost:*** 200 units/ml, 2 ml: $28 ***Pregnancy category:*** C	Rash, pruritus of earlobes, edema of feet, headache, flushing, tetany, chills, weakness, dizziness, nausea, diarrhea, vomiting, anorexia, abdominal pain, salty taste, swelling, tingling of hands
For those institutionalized or house bound:			
Multiple vitamins with 800 units of vitamin D, 1 tab daily	Vitamin supplement	***Contraindication:*** Hypersensitivity ***Cost:*** OTC ***Pregnancy category:*** A	Usually well tolerated
For hypogonadal men:			
Testosterone, 100-200 mg IM every 2 weeks	Increases bone development	***Contraindications:*** Hypersensitivity; severe renal, hepatic, and cardiac disease; genital bleeding ***Cost:*** 100 mg/ml, 10 ml: $6-$32 ***Pregnancy category:*** X	Rash, acneiform lesions, oily hair and skin, flushing, sweating, acne, dizziness, headache, fatigue, tremors, paresthesias, anxiety, lability, cramps, spasms, increased blood pressure, hematuria, cholestatic jaundice, nasal congestion

Otitis Media, Acute

OVERVIEW

Acute otitis media is an inflammation and infection of the middle ear.

Pathogenesis

- Usually preceded by viral upper respiratory tract infection; causes eustachian tube dysfunction; congestion in eustachian tube increases, impeding flow of middle ear secretions; as fluid increases, bacteria flourish
- Most common pathogens—pneumococci, *Hemophilus influenzae, Moraxella catarrhalis,* group A streptococci, *Staphylococcus aureus,* viruses

Patient Profile

- Males = Females
- Any age, but peak age is 6 to 12 months

Signs and Symptoms

- Earache—infant may pull on ear
- Nasal discharge
- Cough
- Otorrhea
- Fever
- Hearing loss
- Vertigo

Differential Diagnosis

- Otitis externa
- Mastoiditis
- Temporomandibular joint dysfunction
- Dental abscess
- Foreign body
- Trauma

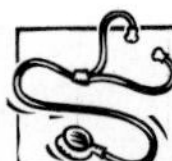

ASSESSMENT

History

Inquire about:

- Onset and duration of symptoms
- Ear pain
- Dizziness
- Recent upper respiratory tract infection
- Current cough
- Sore throat
- Drainage from ear
- Nasal congestion
- Fever
- Underlying conditions
- Current medications

Physical Findings

- Tympanic membrane—full or bulging; decreased or absent mobility; absent or obscured bony landmarks; opaque, yellow, or red (redness alone not a reliable sign)
- Discharge if tympanic membrane perforated
- Fever (maybe)

Initial Workup

Laboratory

- Usually none
- Tympanocentesis for culture and sensitivity if treatment fails or for recurrent infections

Radiology: Sinus films in recurrent cases

Further Workup

Audiometry after treatment, possibly

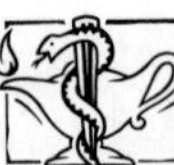

INTERVENTIONS

Office Treatment

None indicated

Lifestyle Modifications

- Smoking cessation
- Avoidance of secondhand smoke

Patient Education

Teach patient about:

- Disease process and treatment—antibiotics
- Tips for smoking cessation (if patient is a child, parents need to understand importance of not smoking around child)
- How to take medications, importance of taking all medication, and side effects (see Pharmacotherapeutics)

Referral

To ear, nose, and throat specialist for recurrent cases

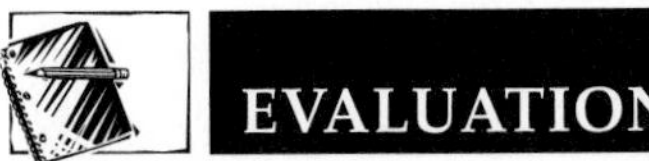

EVALUATION

Outcome

Resolves without sequelae; symptoms usually improve in 48 to 72 hours

Possible Complications

- Perforation of tympanic membrane
- Mastoiditis
- Facial nerve paralysis
- Recurrent acute otitis media—atrophy and scarring of tympanic membrane, cholesteatoma, permanent hearing loss, chronic mastoiditis, brain abscess

Follow-up

In 3 days if symptoms not improved; otherwise, in 2 weeks

FOR YOUR INFORMATION

Life Span

Pediatric: More common in this population

Geriatric: More likely to develop serous otitis media

Pregnancy: N/A

Miscellaneous

In an otherwise healthy adult who has recurrent otitis media, rule out nasopharyngeal cancer.

References

Bull TR: *Color atlas of E.N.T. diagnosis,* ed 3, London, 1995, Mosby-Wolfe, pp 16, 69, 71, 84-85.

Niparko JK: Hearing loss and associated problems. In Barker LR, Burton JR, Zieve PD, editors: *Principles of ambulatory medicine,* ed 4, Baltimore, 1995, Williams & Wilkins, pp 1409-1410.

NOTES

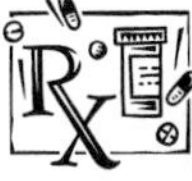

PHARMACOTHERAPEUTICS

NOTE: Otitis media will usually resolve on its own. Many authors recommend using antibiotics for only the most severe cases.

Drug of Choice	Mechanism of Action	Prescribing Information	Side Effects
Use one of the following:			
Amoxicillin (Amoxil), 250-500 mg PO q8h × 10 days; children, 20 mg/kg/day PO q8h × 10 days	Bactericidal; broad spectrum; *not* effective against beta-lactamase–producing pathogens	***Contraindications:*** Hypersensitivity to penicillins; use caution if allergic to cephalosporins ***Cost:*** 500-mg tab, 3/day × 10 days: $4 ***Pregnancy category:*** B	Anaphylactoid reaction, nausea, vomiting, diarrhea, rash, Stevens-Johnson syndrome, pseudomembranous colitis
Erythromycin, 250 mg PO qid × 10 days; children, 30-50 mg/kg/day in divided doses × 10 days	Inhibits protein synthesis	***Contraindication:*** Hypersensitivity ***Cost:*** 250-mg tabs, 4/day × 10 days: $4 ***Pregnancy category:*** B	Nausea, vomiting, diarrhea, abdominal pain, anorexia, rash, urticaria, pseudomembranous colitis—rarely
If no response to above medication in 3 days, switch to:			
Trimethoprim-sulfamethoxazole (Bactrim DS), 1 tab PO q12h × 10 days; children, 8 mg/kg trimethoprim and 40 mg/kg sulfamethoxazole in 24 hours given in 2 doses q12h × 10 days	Blocks 2 steps in biosynthesis of nucleic acids and proteins	***Contraindications:*** Hypersensitivity to trimethoprim or sulfonamides; megaloblastic anemia caused by folic acid deficiency; pregnancy at term or lactation ***Cost:*** 800 mg/160 mg, 20 tabs: $3; 400 mg/80 mg, 20 tabs: $2 ***Pregnancy category:*** C	Headache, insomnia, hallucinations, depression, vertigo, anxiety, allergic myocarditis, nausea, vomiting, abdominal pain, hepatitis, enterocolitis, renal failure, toxic nephrosis, leukopenia, neutropenia, thrombocytopenia, hemolytic anemia, Stevens-Johnson syndrome, anaphylaxis

Otitis Media with Effusion/Serous Otitis Media

OVERVIEW

Otitis media with effusion is an accumulation of serous fluid in the middle ear that persists for 3 months or longer. It may follow acute otitis media.

Pathogenesis

- Loss of patency of eustachian tube
- Causes:
  - Adenoidal hypertrophy
  - Recent upper respiratory tract infection
  - Allergies
  - Deviated nasal septum
  - Recent acute otitis media
  - Nasopharyngeal carcinoma (new onset of serous otitis that does not resolve—must rule out)

Patient Profile

- Males = Females
- Any age, but more common in children

Signs and Symptoms

- May be asymptomatic
- Sensation of stuffiness or fullness
- Popping or crackling sounds when chewing
- Hearing loss

Differential Diagnosis

- Nasopharyngeal carcinoma
- Anatomic abnormalities

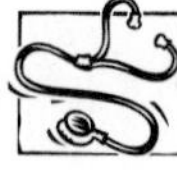

ASSESSMENT

History

Inquire about:

- Onset and duration of symptoms
- Recent upper respiratory tract infection
- Rhinitis
- Cough
- Fever
- Pain and hearing loss
- History of allergies/allergic rhinitis
- Underlying conditions
- Current medications

Physical Findings

- Tympanic membrane—bubbles or fluid level; may have yellow color
- Decreased movement on insufflation
- Decreased hearing acuity

Initial Workup

Laboratory: Usually none indicated
Radiology: None indicated

Further Workup

- Tympanometry
- Audiometry before and after treatment, if indicated

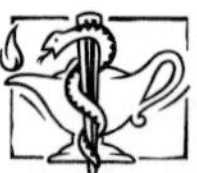

INTERVENTIONS

Office Treatment

None indicated

Lifestyle Modifications

- Smoking cessation
- Adjusting to possibility of hearing loss

Patient Education

Teach patient about:

- Disease process and treatment options:
  - If asymptomatic, observation for 6 weeks may be indicated
  - Antibiotics, nasal spray, surgery
- Importance of follow-up care
- Tips for smoking cessation (if patient is a child, parents need to understand importance of not smoking around child)
- How to take medications and side effects (see Pharmacotherapeutics)

Referral

To ear, nose, and throat specialist after second failure with antibiotics

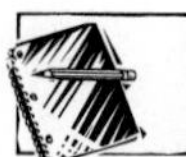

EVALUATION

Outcome

Resolves without sequelae

Possible Complications

- Hearing loss
- Atrophy and scarring of tympanic membrane
- Cholesteatoma
- Chronic mastoiditis
- Brain abscess

Follow-up

Monthly until condition resolves

FOR YOUR INFORMATION

Life Span

Pediatric: More common in this age group
Geriatric: Hearing loss may be more pronounced, since elderly patient may also have presbycusis
Pregnancy: N/A

Miscellaneous

In adults with new-onset serous otitis media, consider the possibility of nasopharyngeal carcinoma.

References

Niparko JK: Hearing loss and associated problems. In Barker LR, Burton JR, Zieve PD, editors: *Principles of ambulatory medicine,* ed 4, Baltimore, 1995, Williams & Wilkins, p 1409.

Otitis Media Guideline Panel, US Department of Health and Human Services, Public Health Service, Agency for Health Care Policy and Research: *Quick reference guide for clinicians:* managing otitis media with effusion in young children, *J Am Acad Nurse Pract* 6(10):493-500, 1995.

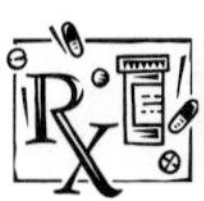

PHARMACOTHERAPEUTICS

Drug of Choice	Mechanism of Action	Prescribing Information	Side Effects
Use one of the following:			
Amoxicillin (Amoxil), PO 250-500 mg q8h × 14 days; children, 20 mg/kg/day PO q8h × 14 days	Bactericidal; broad spectrum; *not* effective against beta-lactamase–producing pathogens	***Contraindications:*** Hypersensitivity to penicillins; use caution if allergic to cephalosporins ***Cost:*** 500-mg tabs, 3/day × 14 days: $4 ***Pregnancy category:*** B	Anaphylactoid reaction, nausea, vomiting, diarrhea, rash, Stevens-Johnson syndrome, pseudomembranous colitis
Erythromycin, 250 mg PO qid × 14 days; children, 30-50 mg/kg/day PO in divided doses × 14 days	Inhibits protein synthesis	***Contraindication:*** Hypersensitivity ***Cost:*** 250-mg tabs, 4/day × 14 days: $4 ***Pregnancy category:*** B	Nausea, vomiting, diarrhea, abdominal pain, anorexia, rash, urticaria, pseudomembranous colitis—rarely
Trimethoprim-sulfamethoxazole (Bactrim DS), 1 tab PO q12h × 14 days; children, 8 mg/kg trimethoprim and 40 mg/kg sulfamethoxazole in 24 hours given in 2 doses q12h × 14 days	Blocks 2 steps in biosynthesis of nucleic acids and proteins	***Contraindications:*** Hypersensitivity to trimethoprim or sulfonamides; megaloblastic anemia caused by folic acid deficiency; pregnancy at term or lactation ***Cost:*** 800 mg/160 mg, 20 tabs: $3; 400 mg/80 mg, 20 tabs: $2 ***Pregnancy category:*** C	Headache, insomnia, hallucinations, depression, vertigo, anxiety, allergic myocarditis, nausea, vomiting, abdominal pain, hepatitis, enterocolitis, renal failure, toxic nephrosis, leukopenia, neutropenia, thrombocytopenia, hemolytic anemia, Stevens-Johnson syndrome, anaphylaxis
Add one of the following or use alone:			
Intranasal cromolyn (Nasalcrom); adults and children >6 years, 1 spray each nostril, 3-4 times daily	Inhibits release of antihistamine; inhibits sensitized mast cell degranulation	***Contraindication:*** Hypersensitivity ***Cost:*** 13 ml: $22 ***Pregnancy category:*** B	Sneezing; nasal stinging, burning, and irritation; headaches; bad taste
Topical decongestant: oxymetazoline (Afrin, NeoSynephrine); children 6 years and up, 2 sprays each nostril bid	Sympathomimetic; causes vasoconstriction that decreases congestion	***Contraindications:*** Hypersensitivity; hypertension; diabetes; heart disease; thyroid disease; difficulty urinating because of enlarged prostate ***Cost:*** OTC; $3-$5 ***Pregnancy category:*** C	Do not use for >3-4 days or exceed dosing—rebound congestion may occur; habituation, stinging of nasal mucosa, dry membranes
Oral decongestants: 130 different products listed in *PDR* for nonprescription drugs; many in combination with an antihistamine; most contain pseudoephedrine, phenylephrine, or phenylpropanolamine; see labels for dosage—do not exceed dosage	Sympathomimetics; cause nasal vasoconstriction, producing decongestion	***Contraindications:*** Hypersensitivity; hypertension (controversial); diabetes; heart or thyroid disease; prostate enlargement ***Cost:*** Varies with product ***Pregnancy category:*** Pseudoephedrine—B; phenylephrine and phenylpropanolamine—C	Drowsiness, dry mouth, insomnia, headache, nervousness, fatigue, irritability, disorientation, rash, palpitations, sore throat, cough

Pain Management (Acute and Chronic Pain)

OVERVIEW

Pain is defined as an unpleasant sensation. Acute pain is short-lived and slowly resolves as the area of injury heals. Chronic pain is pain that lasts longer than 6 months.

Pathogenesis

- Acute pain—caused by hyperactivity of the sympathetic nervous system as a result of injury, trauma, spasm, or disease
- Chronic pain:
  - Rarely caused by hyperactivity of the sympathetic nervous system
  - Characterized by location—visceral pain (abdominal or thoracic), somatic pain (muscles and connective tissue), neurologic pain (diabetic neuropathy)

Patient Profile

- Males = Females
- Any age

Signs and Symptoms

- Subjective complaint of pain
- Acute pain—may be accompanied by tachycardia, tachypnea, diaphoresis, increased BP, dilated pupils
- Chronic pain—may have depressive symptoms

Differential Diagnosis

- Drug-seeking behavior
- Malingering
- Anxiety
- Depression

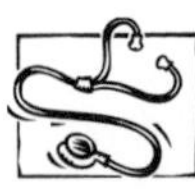

ASSESSMENT

History

Inquire about:

- Onset and duration of symptoms
- Information based on the following Mnemonic:
  - **P**recipitating factors
  - **Q**uality of pain
  - **R**adiation of pain
  - **S**ubjective description of severity of pain
  - **T**iming of pain
- Intensity of pain (have patient rate pain on scale of 1 to 10)
- Treatment tried and results
- Associated symptoms
- Underlying conditions
- Current medications

Physical Findings

- Acute pain:
  - Increased BP, heart rate, respirations
  - Diaphoresis
  - General appearance—pallor, anxious
- Chronic pain—physical examination may reveal only subjective complaints of pain on palpation or movement

Initial Workup

Laboratory: Depends on cause of pain
Radiology: Depends on cause of pain

Further Workup

Depends on cause of pain

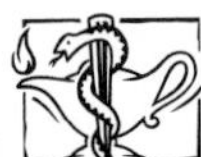

INTERVENTIONS

Office Treatment

None indicated

Lifestyle Modification

Chronic pain—learning to live with chronic condition

Patient Education

Teach patient about:

- Condition and treatment options:
  - Using biofeedback, relaxation techniques, yoga, distraction, therapeutic touch, massage therapy
  - Importance of using analgesics as directed and not prn
  - Using analgesics for specified period of time before trying others
  - Possible surgical procedures
  - Using dorsal column stimulators (DCS) or transcutaneous electrical nerve stimulators (TENS)
- Maintaining as active a lifestyle as possible
- Medications used and side effects (see Pharmacotherapeutics)

Referral

To pain control clinic

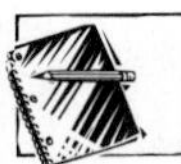

EVALUATION

Outcome

Pain is controlled with minimal to no disruption in lifestyle

Possible Complication

Total disability

Follow-up

Every 2 weeks until pain is controlled

FOR YOUR INFORMATION

Life Span

Pediatric: Treatment is the same as for adults, with medication dosages adjusted accordingly
Geriatric: May be unwilling to take pain medication because of fear of falls, altered mental state, and fear of loss of independence; medication must be started at lowest dose possible
Pregnancy: Cautious use of medications

Miscellaneous

Pain management can be very challenging for the NP. There are many emotional and cultural factors that influence the patient's perception of pain, and these, along with the subjective and objective data, must be considered when deciding on a plan of care.

References

Acute Pain Management Guideline Panel, *Acute pain management: operative or medical procedures and trauma,* Clinical Practice Guideline 1, AHCPR Pub No 92-0032, Rockville, Md, 1992, US Department of Health and Human Services, Public Health Service, Agency for Health Care Policy and Research.

Jacox A et al: *Management of cancer pain,* Clinical Practice Guideline No 9, AHCPR Pub No 94-0592, Rockville, Md, 1994, US Department of Health and Human Services, Public Health Service, Agency for Health Care Policy and Research.

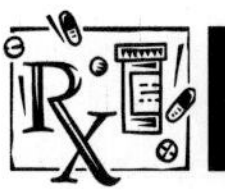

PHARMACOTHERAPEUTICS

Drug of Choice	Mechanism of Action	Prescribing Information	Side Effects
For mild to moderate pain:			
Aspirin, 325-650 mg PO q4-6h for fever and myalgia—do not use in children or adolescents because of risk of Reye's syndrome	Analgesia via peripheral and central nervous systems; may inhibit prostaglandins; antipyretic—acts on hypothalamic system	***Contraindications:*** Hypersensitivity; bleeding disorders or anticoagulant therapy; last trimester of pregnancy; asthma; gastric ulcers ***Cost:*** OTC ***Pregnancy category:*** Not categorized	Rash, anaphylactic reaction, GI upset and bleeding, Reye's syndrome in children and adolescents
Acetaminophen (Tylenol), 325-650 mg PO q4-6h for fever and myalgia; for children, use Children's Tylenol—follow label directions	Decreases fever through action on hypothalamic heat-regulating center of brain; analgesia by increasing pain threshold	***Contraindications:*** Hypersensitivity; bleeding disorders or anticoagulant therapy; last trimester of pregnancy; asthma; gastric ulcers ***Cost:*** OTC ***Pregnancy category:*** Not categorized	Rash; hepatic toxicity with alcohol ingestion or overdose
Nonsteroidal antiinflammatory drugs (NSAIDs): many different types currently marketed; consult manufacturer's package insert for specific dosing and prescribing information	Exact action unknown; may result from inhibition of synthesis of prostaglandins and arachidonic acid	***Contraindications:*** Hypersensitivity to NSAIDs, aspirin; severe hepatic failure; asthma ***Cost:*** Varies with type ***Pregnancy category:*** Depends on product	Stomach distress, flatulence, nausea, abdominal pain, constipation or diarrhea, dizziness, sedation, rash, urticaria, angioedema, anorexia, urinary frequency, increased blood pressure, insomnia, anxiety, visual disturbances, increased thirst, alopecia
For moderate pain:			
Tramadol hydrochloride (Ultram), 50-100 mg PO q4-6h, not to exceed 400 mg/day; no dosage established for children <16 years	Centrally acting analgesic; exact mechanism of action unknown	***Contraindications:*** Hypersensitivity; acute intoxication with alcohol, hypnotics, centrally acting analgesics, opioids, psychotropic drugs ***Cost:*** 50-mg tab, 100 tabs: $60 ***Pregnancy category:*** C	Dependence, dizziness, vertigo, nausea, vomiting, constipation, headache, somnolence, pruritus, CNS stimulation, sweating, dyspepsia, dry mouth, hypotension, tachycardia, anxiety, confusion, coordination disturbance, nervousness, sleep disorder, flatulence, abdominal pain, rash
Acetaminophen/hydrocodone (Vicodin), 5 mg hydrocodone/ 500 mg acetaminophen; 1-2 tabs PO q4-6h, not to exceed 8 tabs daily; avoid alcohol and other CNS depressants; Schedule III narcotic	Hydrocodone—similar to codeine; acts on central nervous system; specific mechanism unknown; acetaminophen—inhibits prostaglandin synthesis; specific mechanism unknown	***Contraindication:*** Hypersensitivity to either component ***Cost:*** 5 mg/500 mg tab, 100 tabs: $20-$98 ***Pregnancy category:*** C	Physical/psychologic dependence, drowsiness, mental clouding, lethargy, anxiety, fear, nausea, vomiting, urinary retention, respiratory depression, rash, pruritus
For moderate to severe pain:			
Morphine (MS Contin, sustained-release), 15 mg PO q12h—do not break, chew, or crush; Schedule II narcotic	Centrally acting analgesic	***Contraindications:*** Hypersensitivity; respiratory depression; acute or severe bronchial asthma; paralytic ileus ***Cost:*** 15-mg tab, 100 tabs: $64-$77 ***Pregnancy category:*** C	Respiratory depression, apnea, circulatory depression, respiratory arrest, shock, cardiac arrest, constipation, lightheadedness, dizziness, sedation, nausea, vomiting, sweating, dysphoria, euphoria, weakness, headache, agitation, tremor, seizures, uncoordinated muscle movement, dry mouth, anorexia, diarrhea, cramps, tachycardia, facial flushing, palpitations, syncope, urinary retention, pruritus, rash, edema, blurred vision

Pancreatitis

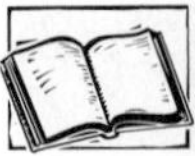

OVERVIEW

Pancreatitis is an inflammatory process of the pancreas. It may be acute or chronic. Chronic pancreatitis may follow acute pancreatitis or may occur in the absence of any acute episode.

Pathogenesis

- Injury to pancreas
- Many causes—trauma, viral infections (mumps), duodenal ulcer, cysts, abscesses, cystic fibrosis, drugs (steroids, NSAIDs, sulfonamides), biliary tract disease, alcoholism
- Acute pancreatitis—autodigestion of pancreas occurs as a result of injury to pancreatic cells or activation of enzymes in pancreas rather than in intestine
- Chronic pancreatitis—either obstructive or calcifying:
  - Obstructive type—usually associated with biliary disease
  - Calcifying type—inflammation and sclerosis in head of pancreas and around ducts

Patient Profile

- Males = Females
- Acute pancreatitis—any age
- Chronic pancreatitis—35 to 45 years (usually alcohol related)

Signs and Symptoms

ACUTE PANCREATITIS

- Abdominal pain—epigastric; may radiate to back
- Nausea, vomiting
- Abdominal distention
- Fever
- Hypotension
- Shock
- Jaundice
- Flank discoloration
- Periumbilical discoloration (Cullen's sign)
- Pleural effusion

CHRONIC PANCREATITIS

- All of the above to a lesser degree with weight loss
- Constipation
- Steatorrhea
- Diabetes

Differential Diagnosis

- Penetrating or perforating ulcer
- Cholecystitis
- Aortic aneurysm
- Intestinal obstruction
- Choledocholithiasis
- Pancreatic cancer
- Cholelithiasis

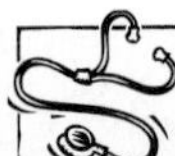

ASSESSMENT

History

Inquire about:

- Onset and duration of symptoms
- Whether patient is able to keep food and fluids down
- Alcohol intake
- History of prior illness
- Underlying conditions
- Current medications

Physical Findings

- Epigastric pain that may radiate to back
- Diminished or absent bowel sounds
- Hypotension
- Bluish flank discoloration (Grey Turner's sign)
- Bluish periumbilical discoloration (Cullen's sign)
- Mild jaundice
- Crackles in lungs
- Weight loss
- Dark urine
- Frothy urine/stool

Initial Workup

Laboratory

ACUTE PANCREATITIS

- Serum amylase, serum lipase—elevated
- Bilirubin, ALT, AST, alkaline phosphate—elevated when associated with alcoholic hepatitis or choledocholithiasis
- Glucose—increased
- Calcium—decreased
- CBC—WBC count elevated

CHRONIC PANCREATITIS

- Laboratory values may be normal or as above
- Fecal fat determination—steatorrhea

Radiology

ACUTE PANCREATITIS

- Flat plate of abdomen—signs of ileus
- Chest film—pleural effusion
- Ultrasound or CT scan of abdomen

CHRONIC PANCREATITIS

- Flat plate of abdomen—pancreatic calcification
- Ultrasound or CT scan of abdomen—pseudocyst/calcification

Further Workup

Secretin stimulation test—most useful in diagnosing chronic pancreatitis

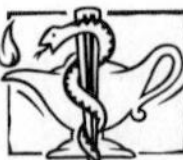

INTERVENTIONS

Office Treatment

None indicated

Lifestyle Modifications

- Cessation of alcohol ingestion or drugs that may have been causative
- Hospitalization if acute pancreatitis

Patient Education

Teach patient about:

- Disease process and treatment options:
  - Acute pancreatitis—refer to MD; most require hospitalization
  - Chronic pancreatitis—pain control (avoid narcotics); pancreatic enzyme supplements; alcohol abstinence—support groups, inpatient treatment programs; diabetes mellitus—how to administer insulin, monitoring blood sugar, signs and symptoms of hypoglycemia, proper diabetic diet
- Medications used and side effects (see Pharmacotherapeutics)

Referral

Most should be referred to MD; NP may follow stable patient with chronic pancreatitis

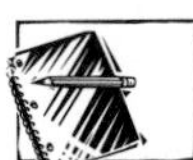

EVALUATION

Outcomes

- Acute pancreatitis—85% to 90% resolve without sequelae
- Chronic pancreatitis—recurrent episodes of acute or slowly progressive pancreatitis—no cure; a patient learns to live with disease

Possible Complications

- Acute pancreatitis—pseudocyst
- Chronic pancreatitis—pseudocyst, abscess, biliary/duodenal obstruction

Follow-up

- Acute pancreatitis—within 1 week of hospital discharge, then every 2 weeks × 3 for serum amylase evaluation
- Chronic pancreatitis—every 2 weeks × 4 to assess alcohol abstinence; then monthly × 3; if stable, every 3 months

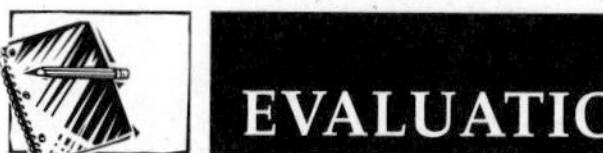

EVALUATION

Life Span

Pediatric: Mumps can cause pancreatic injury and pancreatitis
Geriatric: May have more lengthy recuperation after acute pancreatitis
Pregnancy: N/A

Miscellaneous

When treating the patient with chronic pancreatitis, an attempt should be made to control the pain initially with nonnarcotics. As the disease progresses, narcotic pain relievers will need to be used, particularly during acute attacks.

References

Elrod R: Nursing role in management: problems of the liver, biliary tract, and pancreas. In Lewis SM, Collier IC, Heitkemper MM, editors: *Medical-surgical nursing: assessment and management of clinical problems,* ed 4, St Louis, 1996, Mosby, pp 1287-1296.

Woolliscroft JO: *Current diagnosis and treatment: a quick reference for the general practitioner,* Philadelphia, 1996, Current Medicine, pp 294-297.

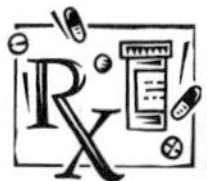

PHARMACOTHERAPEUTICS

Drug of Choice	Mechanism of Action	Prescribing Information	Side Effects
For fever and myalgia:			
Acetaminophen (Tylenol), 325-650 mg PO q4-6h; for children, use Children's Tylenol—follow label directions	Decreases fever through action on hypothalamic heat-regulating center of brain; analgesia by increasing pain threshold	***Contraindications:*** Hypersensitivity; bleeding disorders or anticoagulant therapy; last trimester of pregnancy; asthma; gastric ulcers ***Cost:*** OTC ***Pregnancy category:*** Not categorized	Rash; hepatic toxicity with alcohol ingestion or overdose
For myalgia:			
Ibuprofen (Motrin), 400 mg PO qid; children 6 months to 12 years, 5 mg/kg	Not well understood; may be related to inhibition of prostaglandin synthesis	***Contraindications:*** Aspirin allergy; hypersensitivity; asthma; last trimester of pregnancy; gastric ulcer; bleeding disorders ***Cost:*** 400-mg tab, 4/day × 5 days: $3 ***Pregnancy category:*** Not categorized but not recommended	Nausea, heartburn, diarrhea, GI upset and bleeding, dizziness, headache, rash, tinnitus, edema, acute renal failure
Pancrelipase (Pancrease MT); adults and children, 1-3 caps ac or with meals or 1 cap with snack	Pancreatic enzyme needed for proper pancreatic functioning	***Contraindications:*** Allergy to pork; acute pancreatitis; acute exacerbations of chronic pancreatitis ***Cost:*** $25 ***Pregnancy category:*** C	Anorexia, nausea, vomiting, diarrhea, hyperuricuria, hyperuricemia
Famotidine or cimetidine (Pepcid or Tagamet): • Pepcid, 20 mg PO bid—not for children • Tagamet, 300 mg PO with meals and at bedtime—not for children <16 years; • Treat for 3-4 weeks, then reduce dosages to OTC strength	Inhibits histamine at H_2 receptor sites; reducing gastric acid increases availability of pancreatic enzymes	***Contraindication:*** Hypersensitivity ***Cost:*** Pepcid, 20-mg tab, 30 tabs: $45; Tagamet, 300-mg tab, 100 tabs: $45 ***Pregnancy category:*** B	Confusion, headache, depression, dizziness, convulsions, diarrhea, abdominal cramps, paralytic ileus, jaundice, gynecomastia, galactorrhea, increased BUN and creatinine, agranulocytosis, thrombocytopenia, neutropenia, aplastic anemia, urticaria, exfoliative dermatitis

For management of pain caused by chronic pancreatitis, see section on pain management.

Parkinson's Disease

OVERVIEW

Parkinson's disease is a chronic neurodegenerative disorder of the central nervous system.

Pathogenesis

- Cause—unknown
- Loss of dopamine-producing neurons in substantia nigra
- Decrease in dopamine-synthesizing enzymes and metabolites, also in gamma aminobutyric acid (GABA), serotonin, and norepinephrine
- Four theories—accelerated aging, intrinsic or extrinsic toxin, genetic predisposition, oxidation of dopamine

Patient Profile

- Males = Females
- Age >50 years; can occur at younger age
- Rare in African-Americans

Signs and Symptoms

- Gradual onset
- Initial clues—recent onset of clumsiness, changes in handwriting, frequent falls
- Tremor—may be unilateral initially; more prominent at rest; thumb and forefinger move in rotary ("pill-rolling") motion
- "Cogwheel rigidity"—jerky movement of limbs when moved through range of motion (ROM)
- Bradykinesia—problem initiating movement; postural abnormalities
- Patient lacks spontaneous movement—mask facies; drooling; shuffling gait; decreased blinking; low-volume, poorly enunciated, clipped speech
- Dementia
- Depression
- Dysphagia

Differential Diagnosis

- Parkinsonism from other causes; will not respond to levodopa
- Side effects of neuroleptic medications, toxins, infections
- Multisystem atrophy
- Benign essential tremor

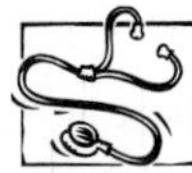

ASSESSMENT

History

Inquire about:

- Onset and duration of symptoms
- Ability to perform activities of daily living
- Occupational and environmental history to uncover exposure to toxins
- History of neuroleptic drug use
- Underlying conditions
- Current medications

Physical Findings

- "Pill-rolling" tremor (particularly at rest)
- Limb rigidity when moved through ROM
- Stooped posture
- Shuffling gait
- Deadpan expression
- Slightly hyperactive reflexes
- Extraocular movements—difficulty with upward gaze
- Blink reflex decreased
- Sense of smell may be lost
- Mini–mental state examination—should be >20; if <20, consider Alzheimer's disease or other dementing disorder

Initial Workup

Laboratory: None indicated; diagnosis based on history, physical examination, and response to antiparkinsonian drugs; may wish to get baseline CBC, chemistry profile, urinalysis

Radiology: None indicated

Further Workup

None indicated

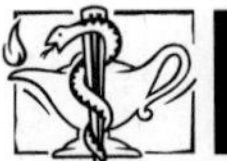

INTERVENTIONS

Office Treatment

None indicated

Lifestyle Modifications

Chronic, progressive illness—lifestyle modifications depend on severity of disability

- Safety major concern
- Smoking cessation
- Exercise plan
- Special chairs
- Elevated toilet seat
- Special eating utensils

Patient Education

Teach patient and family about:

- Disease process and treatment options—medications must be individualized, based on severity
- Life span—usually not shortened; patient should remain functional for as long as possible
- Exercise plan
- Depression—common; need to report symptoms
- Importance of high fluid intake
- Small, frequent meals if difficulty eating
- High-bulk foods
- Medications used and side effects (see Pharmacotherapeutics)

Referrals

- To MD or consult with MD regarding treatment approach
- To physical, occupational, speech therapists

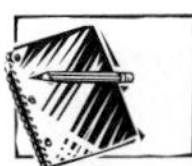

EVALUATION

Outcome

Patient will remain functional and in own home

Possible Complications

- Dementia
- Depression
- Fractures from falls
- Aspiration pneumonia

Follow-up

Every 2 weeks when initiating drug therapy; during stable periods, monthly; must be individualized

FOR YOUR INFORMATION

Life Span

Pediatric: Very rare
Geriatric: Most commonly seen in this age group
Pregnancy: Cautious use of medications

Miscellaneous

N/A

References

Reich SG: Common disorders of movement: tremor and Parkinson's disease. In Barker LR, Burton JR, Zieve PD, editors: *Principles of ambulatory medicine,* ed 4, Baltimore, 1995, Williams & Wilkins, pp 1217-1228.

Sandroni P, Young RR: *Tremor: classification, diagnosis, and management, Am Fam Physician* 50(7):1505-1512, 1994.

NOTES

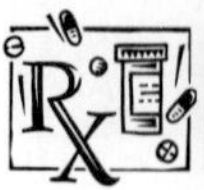

PHARMACOTHERAPEUTICS

There are many medications used for Parkinson's disease, and treatment must be individualized. The following is a brief overview of commonly used medications. The NP should consult with a physician regarding the treatment plan.

Drug of Choice	Mechanism of Action	Prescribing Information	Side Effects
As symptoms progress, use one of the following:			
Anticholinergic such as trihexyphenidyl (Artane), 1 mg PO qd, increase by 2 mg every 3-5 days until reach dose of 6-10 mg PO qd	Blocks central muscarinic receptors	***Contraindications:*** Hypersensitivity; narrow-angle glaucoma; myasthenia gravis; GI/GU obstruction; tachycardia; myocardial ischemia; unstable cardiovascular disease; prostatic hypertrophy ***Cost:*** 2-mg tab, 100 tabs: $5-$20 ***Pregnancy category:*** C	Confusion, anxiety, restlessness, irritability, hallucinations, headache, sedation, depression, incoherence, dizziness, flushing, blurred vision, difficulty swallowing, dry eyes, angle-closure glaucoma, palpitations, tachycardia, postural hypotension, urticaria, rash, nasal congestion, decreased sweating, increased temperature, numbness of fingers, paralytic ileus, dryness of mouth, urinary hesitancy or retention
Amantadine (Symmetrel), 200 mg PO qd	Causes release of dopamine from neurons	***Contraindications:*** Hypersensitivity; lactation; eczematic rash ***Cost:*** 100-mg tab, 100 tabs: $20-$80 ***Pregnancy category:*** C	Headache, dizziness, drowsiness, anxiety, psychosis, depression, hallucinations, tremors, convulsions, orthostatic hypotension, congestive heart failure (CHF), photosensitivity, leukopenia, nausea, vomiting, urinary frequency or retention
As disability progresses, add:			
Carbidopa-levodopa (Sinemet); start with half of 25 mg/100 mg tab PO tid; maximum 8 tabs/day in divided doses	Carbidopa inhibits decarboxylation of levodopa; more levodopa available	***Contraindications:*** Hypersensitivity; narrow-angle glaucoma; undiagnosed skin lesions ***Cost:*** 25 mg/100 mg tab, 100 tabs: $50-$70 ***Pregnancy category:*** C	Hemolytic anemia, leukopenia, agranulocytosis, hand tremors, fatigue, headache, anxiety, twitching, numbness, weakness, insomnia, agitation, nightmares, psychosis, hypomania, hallucinations, nausea, vomiting, anorexia, abdominal distress, dry mouth, flatulence, dysphagia, rash, sweating, orthostatic hypotension, tachycardia, palpitations, blurred vision, dilated pupils, urinary retention or incontinence

Drug of Choice	Mechanism of Action	Prescribing Information	Side Effects
As adjunct for levodopa:			
Selegiline (Eldepryl), 5 mg PO breakfast and lunch; after 2-3 days, begin to reduce dose of carbidopa-levodopa	Increases dopaminergic activity by inhibition of MAO type B activity	***Contraindication:*** Hypersensitivity ***Cost:*** 5-mg tab, 60 tabs: $130 ***Pregnancy category:*** C	Increased tremors, chorea, restlessness, blepharospasm, increased bradykinesia, grimacing, tardive dyskinesia, dystonic symptoms, involuntary movements, hallucinations, dizziness, mood changes, delusions, lethargy, apathy, sleep disturbances, migraine, numbness, muscle cramps, orthostatic hypotension, dysrhythmia, palpitations, tachycardia, edema, nausea, vomiting, weight loss, anorexia, slow urination, nocturia, prostatic hypertrophy, increased sweating, alopecia, hematoma, rash, photosensitivity, asthma
May be used with carbidopa-levodopa:			
Bromocriptine (Parlodel), 1.25 mg PO bid with meals; maximum dose 100 mg qd	Activation of striatal dopamine receptors	***Contraindications:*** Hypersensitivity to ergot; severe ischemic disease; pregnancy; severe peripheral vascular disease ***Cost:*** 2.5-mg tab, 30 tabs: $44 ***Pregnancy category:*** D	Blurred vision, diplopia, nasal congestion, headache, depression, restlessness, anxiety, nervousness, convulsions, hallucinations, dizziness, fatigue, drowsiness, urinary frequency, urinary retention, nausea, vomiting, anorexia, cramps, dry mouth, rash, alopecia, orthostatic hypotension, decreased blood pressure, shock, palpitations, bradycardia
For depression:			
Amitriptyline (Elavil), 50-100 mg hs; maximum dose 200 mg hs	Antidepressant; blocks reuptake of norepinephrine and serotonin	***Contraindications:*** Hypersensitivity to tricyclic antidepressants; recovery phase of myocardial infarction (MI) ***Cost:*** 50-mg tab, 90 tabs: $3-$10 ***Pregnancy category:*** C	Agranulocytosis, thrombocytopenia, eosinophilia, leukopenia, dizziness, drowsiness, confusion, headache, anxiety, tremors, extrapyramidal symptoms, diarrhea, dry mouth, nausea, vomiting, paralytic ileus, hepatitis, increased appetite, urine retention, rash, urticaria, orthostatic hypotension, ECG changes, tachycardia, hypertension, blurred vision, tinnitus

Paronychia

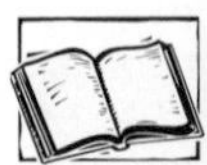

OVERVIEW

Paronychia is an acute or chronic inflammation of the folds around the fingernails or toenails. It is an infectious process.

Pathogenesis

Causes:

- Acute paronychia—*Staphylococcal aureus* most common cause; also caused by streptococci and *Pseudomonas*
- Chronic paronychia—*Candida albicans* or gram-positive or gram-negative organisms

Patient Profile

- Females > Males
- All ages
- Common

Signs and Symptoms

- Swelling of skin around nail—red, painful, may be purulent
- Separation of nail fold from nail plate

Differential Diagnosis

Herpetic whitlow, felon

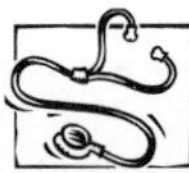

ASSESSMENT

History

Inquire about:

- Onset and duration of symptoms
- Treatments tried and results
- Type of occupation (hands need to be kept dry)
- Underlying conditions
- Current medications

Physical Findings

- Red, painful swelling at nail fold; may have purulent drainage
- Separation of nail fold from nail bed

Initial Workup

Laboratory

- CBC
- Gram stain
- Potassium hydroxide preparation (pseudohyphae and spores if *Candida* present)
- Culture and sensitivity of drainage as indicated

Radiology: None indicated

Further Workup

None indicated

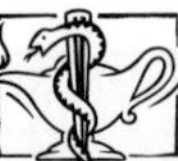

INTERVENTIONS

Office Treatment

- Obtain samples of drainage if present
- Incision and drainage of abscess
- Subungual abscess—may need partial or complete nail removal

Lifestyle Modifications

- Patient may need a change of employment—need to keep hands dry for healing to occur
- If toes involved—encourage loose-fitting shoes and cotton socks, changing socks frequently to keep feet dry

Patient Education

Teach patient about:

- Condition and treatment—antibiotics, topical antifungal creams
- If underlying chronic condition present (e.g., diabetes mellitus), need to control
- Keeping fingers and toes dry
- Medications used and side effects (see Pharmacotherapeutics)

Referral

To dermatologist, surgeon, or podiatrist

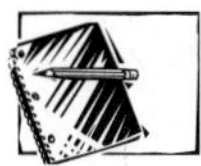

EVALUATION

Outcome
Resolves without sequelae

Possible Complications
- Subungual abscess
- Thickening and discoloration of nail
- Nail loss

Follow-up
In 1 week, then every 2 weeks until healed

FOR YOUR INFORMATION

Life Span
Pediatric: May occur as a result of thumb or finger sucking
Geriatric: Treatment is the same
Pregnancy: Cautious use of medications

Miscellaneous
For patients involved in occupations requiring them to immerse their hands in water frequently, this may be considered a work-related illness.

Reference
Habif TP: *Clinical dermatology: a color guide to diagnosis and therapy,* ed 3, St Louis, 1996, Mosby, pp 763-764.

NOTES

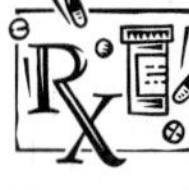

PHARMACOTHERAPEUTICS

Drug of Choice	Mechanism of Action	Prescribing Information	Side Effects
For suppurative lesions with conditions such as diabetes mellitus:			
Dicloxacillin (Dynapen): adults and children >40 kg; 250 mg PO q6h × 10 days; children <40 kg, 12.5-25 mg/kg/day PO in equally divided doses q6h	Bactericidal cell wall inhibitor; active against gram-positive cocci except enterococci	***Contraindication:*** Hypersensitivity to penicillins ***Cost:*** 500-mg tab, 50 tabs: $19-$88 ***Pregnancy category:*** B	Bone marrow depression, granulocytopenia, nausea, vomiting, diarrhea, oliguria, proteinuria, hematuria, moniliasis, glomerulonephritis, lethargy, depression, convulsions, anaphylaxis
For prophylaxis or established infections:			
Erythromycin (E.E.S.), 500 mg PO bid × 10 days; children, 30-50 mg/kg/day in 4 divided doses × 10 days	Macrolide; protein synthesis inhibitor; active against bacteria lacking cell walls, most gram-positive aerobes	***Contraindication:*** Hypersensitivity ***Cost:*** 250-mg tab, 4/day × 10 days: $4 ***Pregnancy category:*** B	Nausea, vomiting, diarrhea, abdominal pain, anorexia, rash, urticaria, pseudomembranous colitis—rarely
For chronic paronychia:			
Topical antifungals may be beneficial; many available: ketoconazole cream (Nizoral), terbinafine cream (Lamisil), clotrimazole cream (Lotrimin); apply to affected area bid; clotrimazole may be used for children; may require long-term therapy (at least 2-3 months and often longer); patient must keep hands dry	All are fungistatic	***Contraindication:*** Hypersensitivity ***Cost:*** Ketoconazole, 15-g tube: $13; terbinafine, 15-g tube: $25; clotrimazole 1%, 15-g tube: $8-$9 ***Pregnancy category:*** Ketoconazole—C; terbinafine—B; clotrimazole—B	Burning, stinging, erythema, itching

Pediculosis (Lice)

OVERVIEW

Pediculosis is an infestation of the skin of the scalp, trunk, or body by a parasite.

Pathogenesis

- Three species of lice:
  - *Pediculus capitis*—head louse
  - *Pediculus corporis*—body louse
  - *Phthirus pubis*—crab or pubic louse
- Parasite survives by sucking blood
- Transmission—by direct contact for head and body lice; through sexual contact for pubic lice

Patient Profile

- Females > Males
- Adults—most common form, pubic lice
- Children—most common form, head lice

Signs and Symptoms

- Intense itching
- Excoriation from scratching
- Presence of louse or nit
- *P. capitis*—lice and nits usually found on back of head and nape of neck; nits appear cemented to hair shaft
- *P. corporis*—lice and nits found in seams of clothing
- *P. pubis:*
  - Lice and nits found in pubic hair and hair of chest, abdomen, and thighs; may also be found on eyelashes of children
  - Gray-blue macules may be found in adjacent groin area

Differential Diagnosis

- Scabies
- Neurodermatosis
- Seborrheic dermatitis

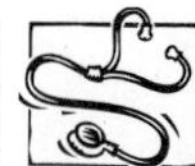

ASSESSMENT

History

Inquire about:

- Onset and duration of symptoms
- Visualization of lice or nits and itching—especially at night
- Nits or lice observed in close contacts
- Underlying conditions
- Current medications

Physical Findings

- Excoriated areas from scratching
- Use of magnifying glass may help in finding lice or nits
- Lice or nits may be found in seams of clothing

Initial Workup

Laboratory: None indicated (with pubic lice, look for other sexually transmitted diseases)

Radiology: None indicated

Further Workup

None indicated

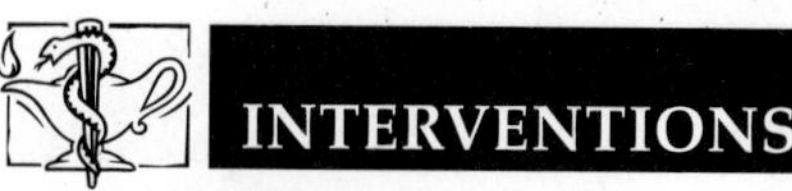

INTERVENTIONS

Office Treatment

None indicated

Lifestyle Modification

Good personal hygiene imperative

Patient Education

Teach patient about:

- Condition and treatment—pediculicides
- Transmission of disease
- Importance of good personal hygiene
- Laundering all bed linen and clothes (especially hats and jackets with hoods) in very hot water; if garments cannot be laundered, dry clean and seal in plastic bag for 2 weeks
- Soaking combs and brushes in hot water for 10 minutes
- Removing nits from hair after treatment—soak hair with solution of half water and half white vinegar; let sit for 15 minutes; use fine-toothed comb to comb hair and remove nits
- Medications—cannot be used on eyelashes—for eyelashes, manually remove lice and nits or apply petroleum jelly 3 to 4 times a day for 8 to 10 days
- Medications used and side effects (see Pharmacotherapeutics)

Referrals

None needed

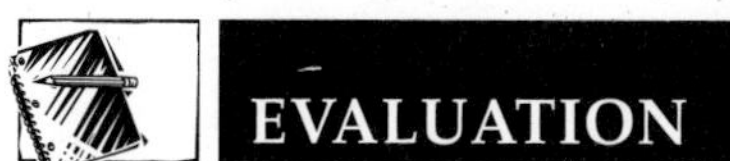

EVALUATION

Outcome
Resolves without sequelae

Possible Complication
Secondary bacterial infection from scratching

Follow-up
Return to clinic if treatment fails

FOR YOUR INFORMATION

Life Span
Pediatric: More common in children attending day care or school
Geriatric: Treatment is the same
Pregnancy: Do not exceed recommended dosage of lindane, and do not treat more than twice during pregnancy

Miscellaneous
N/A

References
Habif TP: *Clinical dermatology: a color guide to diagnosis and therapy,* ed 3, St Louis, 1996, Mosby, pp 454-456.
Sokoloff F: Identification and management of pediculosis, *Nurse Pract* 19(8):62-64, 1994.

NOTES

PHARMACOTHERAPEUTICS

Drug of Choice	Mechanism of Action	Prescribing Information	Side Effects
Permethrin (Nix); shampoo and rinse hair, towel dry—apply permethrin and leave on 10 minutes, rinse with hot water	Pediculicidal and ovacidal	***Contraindication:*** Hypersensitivity ***Cost:*** OTC ***Pregnancy category:*** Not categorized	Itching, swelling, and redness of scalp; hypersensitivity; difficulty breathing; asthma attack
Synergized pyrethrins 0.3% (RID, A-200); apply to affected area until all hair is wet; leave on for 10 minutes; add water to work up lather; and rinse thoroughly with hot water; a second treatment must be done in 7-10 days; do not use near eyes or allow contact with mucous membranes	Pediculicidal	***Contraindications:*** Hypersensitivity; use with caution in persons allergic to ragweed ***Cost:*** OTC ***Pregnancy category:*** Not categorized	Itching, swelling, and redness of scalp; difficulty breathing
Lindane 1% (Kwell); shampoo or lotion; shampoo for scalp—apply to dry hair and work in thoroughly; leave on for 10 minutes; add water to work up lather; rinse thoroughly; lotion for body and pubic area—apply cream from neck down; leave on for 8-12 hours; wash off thoroughly	Parasiticidal and ovacidal	***Contraindications:*** Hypersensitivity; premature neonates; seizure disorder ***Cost:*** Lotion, 60 ml: $2-$6; shampoo, 2 oz: $3-$6 ***Pregnancy category:*** B	CNS stimulation ranging from dizziness to convulsions; skin irritation; hypersensitivity reaction; nausea, vomiting; diarrhea; liver damage

Pelvic Inflammatory Disease (PID)

OVERVIEW

Pelvic inflammatory disease (PID) is an infection of the uterus, fallopian tubes, and ovaries. It begins with cervicitis and can progress to endometritis and salpingitis.

Pathogenesis

- Cause—Polymicrobial infection:
  - Usually starts with *Neisseria gonorrhoeae, Chlamydia trachomatis,* or both.
  - Other organisms—*Gardnerella vaginalis, Escherichia coli,* diphtheroids
  - Mix of aerobic and anaerobic organisms
- Transmission—sexual intercourse

Patient Profile

- Females
- Most common age group—adolescents and young adults, but can occur at any age
- Risk factors:
  - Multiple sex partners
  - Sexually transmitted diseases
  - Recent IUD insertion
  - Attempted abortion
  - Nulliparity

Signs and Symptoms

- More likely to occur during or within 1 week of menses
- Lower abdominal pain
- Abnormal vaginal discharge
- Fever
- Chills
- Nausea, vomiting
- Postcoital bleeding
- Spotting between menstrual periods
- Adnexal tenderness
- Cervical motion tenderness

Differential Diagnosis

- Ectopic pregnancy
- Appendicitis
- Ruptured ovarian cyst
- Endometriosis
- Endometritis
- Ovarian torsion
- Pyelonephritis
- Ulcerative colitis
- Irritable bowel syndrome

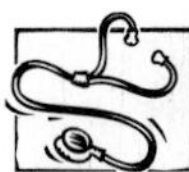

ASSESSMENT

History

Inquire about:

- Onset and duration of symptoms
- Fever
- Vaginal discharge and abnormal vaginal bleeding
- Recent attempted abortion
- Sexual history and behaviors; number of partners
- Use of IUD
- Menstrual history and last menstrual period
- Known sexual intercourse with a partner with untreated urethritis
- Underlying conditions
- Current medications

Physical Findings

- Fever
- Lower abdominal tenderness; may have rebound tenderness
- Hypoactive bowel sounds
- Speculum examination—cervical inflammation, yellow discharge
- Bimanual examination—adnexal tenderness, uterine tenderness, cervical motion tenderness
- Minimum CDC criteria for PID diagnosis (all 4 required):
  - Lower abdominal tenderness
  - Adnexal tenderness
  - Cervical motion tenderness
  - Absence of a competing diagnosis
- Additional CDC criteria
  - Oral temperature >38.3° C
  - Abnormal cervical or vaginal discharge
  - Elevated erythrocyte sedimentation rate (ESR)
  - C-reactive protein
  - Cervical infection with *N. gonorrhoeae* or *C. trachomatis*
  - Histopathologic evidence in endometrial biopsy specimen
  - Tubo-ovarian abscess by sonography or other radiologic test
  - Laparoscopy

Initial Workup

Laboratory

- Pregnancy test
- C-reactive protein
- CBC with differential—increased WBC count, left shift
- Rapid plasma reagin (RPR)
- Cultures for gonorrhea and chlamydial infection
- Wet mount—if number of WBCs > number of epithelial cells, *may* indicate PID; if number of epithelial cells > number of WBCs, diagnosis *not* PID
- ESR—elevated

Radiology: Pelvic ultrasound—fluid in cul-de-sac, distended tubes, masses, pelvic abscess

Further Workup

Laparoscopy—best for diagnosis but impractical for routine use

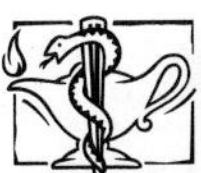

INTERVENTIONS

Office Treatment

Must make decision to treat as inpatient or outpatient; CDC guidelines for inpatient treatment:

- Diagnosis uncertain
- Pelvic abscess suspected
- Pregnancy
- Patient is child or adolescent
- Severe illness
- Patient is unable to follow or tolerate outpatient therapy
- Failure of outpatient treatment
- Unable to do follow-up in 72 hours
- Patients with HIV infection

Lifestyle Modifications

Safe sex practices

Patient Education

Teach patient about:

- Disease and treatment—if requires hospitalization, explain reason to patient
- Safe sex—use of condoms with every sexual encounter; single partner
- Importance of following treatment regimen and finishing all medication
- Importance of having partners treated
- Medications used and side effects (see Pharmacotherapeutics)

Referral

To MD if hospitalization required and NP does not have hospital privileges

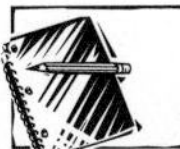

EVALUATION

Outcome

Resolves without sequelae, and patient practices safe sex

Possible Complications

- Pelvic abscess
- Recurrent infection
- Increased risk of ectopic pregnancy
- Infertility
- Chronic pelvic pain

Follow-up

In 72 hours and again in 2 weeks

FOR YOUR INFORMATION

Life Span

Pediatric: Adolescents very vulnerable; requires hospitalization
Geriatric: Rare after menopause
Pregnancy: Rare in pregnancy

Miscellaneous

Contraception with an IUD is contraindicated in patients with a history of PID.

References

Bartlett JG: *Pocket book of infectious disease therapy,* ed 7, Baltimore, 1996, Williams & Wilkins, pp 313-314.

Forrest DE: Common gynecologic pelvic disorders. In Youngkin EQ, Davis MS, editors: *Women's health: a primary care clinical guide,* Norwalk, Conn, 1994, Appleton & Lange, pp 249-253.

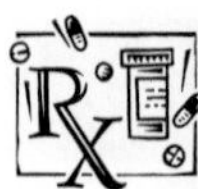

PHARMACOTHERAPEUTICS

Only outpatient therapy is discussed here.

Drug of Choice	Mechanism of Action	Prescribing Information	Side Effects
Regimen A—use one of the following:			
Ceftriaxone (Rocephin), 250 mg IM × 1 dose; children 50-75 mg/kg IM × 1 dose	Cephalosporin; inhibits bacterial cell wall synthesis	***Contraindication:*** Hypersensitivity to cephalosporins ***Cost:*** 250-mg vial: $11 ***Pregnancy category:*** C	Headache; dizziness; weakness; paresthesias; nausea, vomiting; diarrhea; anorexia; increased AST, ALT, bilirubin, LDH, and alkaline phosphatase; pseudomembranous colitis; proteinuria; nephrotoxicity; leukopenia; thrombocytopenia; agranulocytosis; neutropenia; hemolytic anemia; rash; urticaria; anaphylaxis
Cefoxitin (Mefoxin), 2 g IM × 1 dose	Inhibits bacterial wall synthesis	***Contraindications:*** Hypersensitivity to cephalosporins; infants <1 month ***Cost:*** 2-mg vial, 10 vials: $170 ***Pregnancy category:*** B	Headache; dizziness; weakness; paresthesias; nausea; vomiting; diarrhea; anorexia; glossitis; increased AST, ALT, bilirubin, LDH, and alkaline phosphatase; abdominal pain; nephrotoxicity; renal failure; leukopenia; thrombocytope- nia; agranulocytosis; pancytopenia; rash; urticaria; anaphylaxis
With cefoxitin, concurrently administer:			
Probenecid (Benemid) 1 g PO × 1 dose	Inhibits tubular reabsorption of urates; increases excretion of uric acids; inhibits tubular secretion of penicillin and cephalosporin	***Contraindications:*** Hypersensitivity; severe hepatic disease; blood dyscrasias; severe renal disease; history of uric acid calculus ***Cost:*** 500-mg tab, 100 tabs: $9-$30 ***Pregnancy category:*** B	Drowsiness, headache, bradycardia, glycosuria, nephrotic syndrome, gastric irritation, nausea, vomiting, anorexia, hepatic necrosis, rash, acidosis, hypokalemia, hyperchloremia, apnea, irregular respirations
Plus (with either ceftriaxone or cefoxitin):			
Doxycycline (Doryx), 100 mg PO bid × 14 days; children >8 years, 4.4 mg/kg/day divided q12h	Tetracycline; inhibits protein synthesis	***Contraindications:*** Hypersensitivity; children <*8 years* ***Cost:*** 100-mg tab, 20 tabs: $5 ***Pregnancy category:*** D	Eosinophilia, neutropenia, thrombocytopenia, hemolytic anemia, dysphagia, glossitis, nausea, vomiting, nephrotoxicity, abdominal pain, diarrhea, anorexia, flatulence, abdominal cramps, gastritis, pericarditis, rash, urticaria, exfoliative dermatitis, angioedema

Drug of Choice	Mechanism of Action	Prescribing Information	Side Effects
Regimen B:			
Ofloxacin, 400 mg PO bid × 14 days—not dosed for children	Fluoroquinilone; interferes with conversion of intermediate DNA fragments into high molecular weight DNA	***Contraindication:*** Hypersensitivity ***Cost:*** 400-mg tab, 100 tabs: $365 ***Pregnancy category:*** C	Headache, dizziness, fatigue, insomnia, depression, seizures, confusion, nausea, diarrhea, increased ALT and AST, flatulence, heartburn, oral candidiasis, rash, pruritus, urticaria, photosensitivity, blurred vision
Plus one of the following:			
Clindamycin (Cleocin), 450 mg PO qid × 14 days; children >1 month, 8-25 mg/kg/day PO in 4 divided doses	Suppresses protein synthesis	***Contraindications:*** Hypersensitivity to clindamycin or lincomycin; ulcerative colitis/ enteritis ***Cost:*** 300-mg tab, 16 tabs: $38; 150-mg tab, 16 tabs: $19 ***Pregnancy category:*** B	Nausea, vomiting; abdominal pain; diarrhea; pseudomembranous colitis; anorexia; weight loss; increased AST, ALT, and bilirubin; jaundice; vaginitis; rash; urticaria; pruritus
Metronidazole (Flagyl), 500 mg PO bid × 14 days	Direct-acting amebicide/trichomonacide	***Contraindications:*** Hypersensitivity; 1st-trimester pregnancy; CNS disorders ***Cost:*** 500-mg tab, 50 tabs: $5-$90 ***Pregnancy category:*** B after 1st trimester	Flat T-waves, headache, dizziness, confusion, irritability, restlessness, convulsions, blurred vision, sore throat, retinal edema, dry mouth, nausea, vomiting, diarrhea, an-orexia, abdominal cramps, pseudomembranous colitis, albuminuria, neurotoxicity, leukopenia, bone marrow depression, aplasia, rash, pruritus

Peptic Ulcer Disease

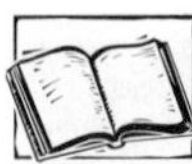

OVERVIEW

Peptic ulcer disease results from loss of the mucosal membrane of the gastrointestinal (GI) tract. It may be acute or chronic and is described by its location within the GI tract. Duodenal ulcers are by far the most common, followed by gastric and esophageal ulcers.

Pathogenesis

Cause—multifactorial:
- Impaired mucosal barrier leads to hydrochloric acid and pepsin acting on impaired mucosa, resulting in ulcer
- *Helicobacter pylori* present in >90% of duodenal and >75% of gastric ulcers
- Drugs may be ulcerogenic

Patient Profile

DUODENAL ULCER
- Males > Females
- Peak age—35 to 45 years

GASTRIC ULCER
- Females > Males
- Peak age—45 to 55 years

Signs and Symptoms

DUODENAL ULCER
- Burning, cramping, pressurelike pain in midepigastrium and upper abdomen 2 to 4 hours after meals
- Nocturnal pain
- Nausea, vomiting
- Heartburn
- Melena
- Pain relieved by antacids and/or food
- Symptoms last a few weeks, then patient symptom-free for several weeks

GASTRIC ULCER
- Burning or pressure high in (L) epigastrium, upper abdomen, back
- Pain may or may not be associated with food
- Occasional nausea, vomiting, weight loss

Differential Diagnosis

- Gastroesophageal reflux
- Nonulcer dyspepsia
- Gastric carcinoma
- Pancreatitis
- Diverticulitis
- Cholelithiasis

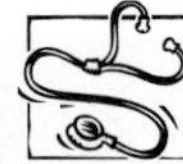

ASSESSMENT

History

Inquire about:
- Onset and duration of symptoms
- Effect of food on symptoms
- Nausea, vomiting, weight loss
- Smoking and alcohol history
- Family history
- Use of nonsteroidal antiinflammatory medication or steroids
- Underlying conditions
- Current medications

Physical Findings

- Physical exam may be within normal limits
- Possibly, pain on palpation of epigastric area
- Rectal examination—stool for occult blood negative or positive

Initial Workup

Laboratory
- CBC—look for anemia
- Serum *H. pylori* test

Radiology: Upper GI series

Further Workup

Endoscopy

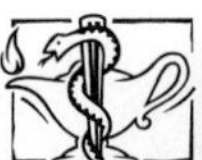

INTERVENTIONS

Office Treatment

None indicated

Lifestyle Modifications

- Smoking cessation
- Discontinuance of use of nonsteroidal antiinflammatory agents
- Stress reduction techniques
- Alcohol—moderate amounts and with food

Patient Education

Teach patient about:
- Disease process and treatment options:
  - For *H. pylori*—combination therapy with antibiotics, bismuth subsalicylate, or proton pump inhibitors
  - If non–*H. pylori*—antacids or H_2 receptor antagonists
- Tips on smoking cessation
- Avoidance of alcohol
- Stopping aspirin, steroids, NSAIDs; if not possible, treat with sucralfate or misoprostol
- Avoidance of spicy foods that precipitate pain
- Medications used and side effects (see Pharmacotherapeutics)

Referral

To gastroenterologist for patients resistant to treatment or if bleeding

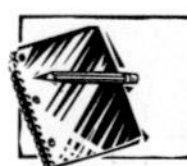

EVALUATION

Outcome

If *H. pylori* eradicated, <10% recur in first year

Possible Complications

- Hemorrhage
- Perforation
- Gastric outlet obstruction

Follow-up

- Every 2 weeks × 2
- Repeat endoscopy to assess healing

FOR YOUR INFORMATION

Life Span

Pediatric: Uncommon before puberty
Geriatric: May not have symptoms, especially if related to use of NSAIDs; may present with hemorrhage
Pregnancy: Use medication with caution

Miscellaneous

The patient with bleeding ulcers will require long-term therapy, as will the patient who remains positive for *H. pylori.*

References

Fay M, Jaffe PE: Diagnostic and treatment guidelines for *Helicobacter pylori, Nurse Pract* 21(7):28-34, 1996.

Woolliscroft JO: *Current diagnosis and treatment: a quick reference for the general practitioner,* Philadelphia, 1996, Current Medicine, pp 118-119, 150-151.

NOTES

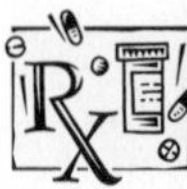

PHARMACOTHERAPEUTICS

Drug of Choice	Mechanism of Action	Prescribing Information	Side Effects
Famotidine or cimetidine (Pepcid or Tagamet): • Pepcid, 20 mg PO bid—not for children • Tagamet, 300 mg PO with meals and at bedtime—not for children <16 years • Treat for 3-4 weeks, then reduce dosages to OTC strength	Inhibits histamine at H_2 receptor sites	***Contraindication:*** Hypersensitivity ***Cost:*** Pepcid, 20-mg tab, 30 tabs: $45; Tagamet, 300-mg tab, 100 tabs: $45 ***Pregnancy category:*** B	Confusion, headache, depression, dizziness, convulsions, diarrhea, abdominal cramps, paralytic ileus, jaundice, gynecomastia, galactorrhea, increased BUN and creatinine, agranulocytosis, thrombocytopenia, neutropenia, aplastic anemia, urticaria, exfoliative dermatitis
For patients needing to continue use of aspirin, NSAIDs, or steroids:			
Sucralfate (Carafate), 1 g PO qid on empty stomach—not dosed for children	Protectant; absorbs pepsin	***Contraindication:*** Hypersensitivity ***Cost:*** 1-g tab, 100 tabs: $75 ***Pregnancy category:*** B	Drowsiness, dizziness, dry mouth, constipation, nausea, gastric pain, vomiting, urticaria, rash, pruritus
Misoprostol (Cytotec), 200 μg PO qid with food—not dosed for children	Protectant; inhibits gastric acid secretion	***Contraindications:*** Hypersensitivity; pregnancy ***Cost:*** 200-μg tab, 60 tabs: $41 ***Pregnancy category:*** X	Diarrhea, nausea, vomiting, flatulence, constipation, spotting, cramps, hypermenorrhea, menstrual disorders
For H. pylori:			
Bismuth subsalicylate (Pepto-Bismol), 2 tabs PO qid; children 10-14 years, 15 ml PO qid × 2 weeks	Inhibits prostaglandin synthesis responsible for GI hypermotility; stimulates absorption of fluid and electrolytes	***Contraindication:*** Children <3 years old ***Cost:*** OTC ***Pregnancy category:*** Not categorized	Increased bleeding time, increased fecal impactions, dark stools, confusion, twitching, hearing loss, tinnitus, metallic taste, black gums, black tongue
Omeprazole (Prilosec), 20 mg PO bid × 2 weeks—not for children	Gastric acid pump inhibitor	***Contraindication:*** Hypersensitivity ***Cost:*** 20-mg tab, 30 tabs: $130 ***Pregnancy category:*** C	Headache, dizziness, asthenia, diarrhea, abdominal pain, vomiting, nausea, constipation, flatulence, acid regurgitation, abdominal swelling, anorexia, upper respiratory infections, cough, epistaxis, rash, dry skin, urticaria, hypoglycemia, increased liver enzymes, weight gain, tinnitus, taste perversion, chest pain, angina, hematuria, bradycardia, tachycardia, urinary tract infection (UTI), pancytopenia, thrombocytopenia, neutropenia, leukocytosis, anemia, back pain

Drug of Choice	Mechanism of Action	Prescribing Information	Side Effects
Metronidazole (Flagyl), 250 mg PO tid or qid × 2 weeks; children, 35-50 mg/kg/day in 3 divided doses × 2 weeks	Direct-acting amebicide/trichomonacide	***Contraindications:*** Hypersensitivity; renal disease; hepatic disease; contracted visual or color fields; blood dyscrasias; pregnancy (1st trimester); lactation; CNS disorders ***Cost:*** 500-mg tab, 50 tabs: $5-$40; 250-mg tab, 100 tabs: $5-$110 ***Pregnancy category:*** B (2nd and 3rd trimesters)	Flat T-waves, headache, dizziness, irritability, restlessness, fatigue, drowsiness, convulsions, incoordination, blurred vision, sore throat, retinal edema, dry mouth, metallic taste, furry tongue, nausea, vomiting, diarrhea, epigastric distress, anorexia, constipation, abdominal cramps, pseudomembranous colitis, darkened urine, vaginal dryness, albuminuria, neurotoxicity, leukopenia, bone marrow depression, aplasia, rash, pruritus, urticaria, flushing
Tetracycline (Achromycin), 500 mg PO qid × 2 weeks; children >8 years, 25-50 mg/kg/day in 4 divided doses × 2 weeks	Bacteriostatic; inhibits protein synthesis	***Contraindications:*** Hypersensitivity; children <8 years; pregnancy or lactation ***Cost:*** 250-mg tab, 100 tabs: $6 ***Pregnancy category:*** D	Fever, headache, paresthesia, eosinophilia, neutropenia, thrombocytopenia, leukocytosis, hemolytic anemia, dysphagia, glossitis, discoloration of deciduous teeth, oral candidiasis, nausea, abdominal pain, vomiting, diarrhea, anorexia, hepatotoxicity, pericarditis, increased BUN, rash, urticaria, photosensitivity, increased pigmentation, exfoliative dermatitis, pruritus, angioedema
Amoxicillin (Amoxil), 500-750 mg PO qid × 2 weeks; children, 20-40 mg/kg/day in 4 divided doses × 2 weeks	Interferes with cell wall replication	***Contraindications:*** Hypersensitivity to penicillins; use caution if allergic to cephalosporins ***Cost:*** 500-mg tab, 50 tabs: $9-$20 ***Pregnancy category:*** B	Anemia, increased bleeding time, bone marrow depression, granulocytopenia, nausea, vomiting, diarrhea, increased ALT and AST, abdominal pain, pseudomembranous colitis, headache, fever, anaphylaxis, respiratory distress
Clarithromycin (Biaxin), 500 mg PO tid × 2 weeks—not dosed for children	Binds to 50 S ribosomal subunits and suppresses protein synthesis	***Contraindication:*** Hypersensitivity ***Cost:*** 500-mg tab, 60 tabs: $179 ***Pregnancy category:*** C	Rash, urticaria, pruritus, nausea, vomiting, hepatoxicity, diarrhea, heartburn, anorexia, vaginitis, moniliasis, headache

- For treatment of *H. pylori,* use one of the following combination therapies:
  - Triple therapy: (1) bismuth subsalicylate, 2 tabs qid, plus metronidazole, 250 mg tid or qid, plus tetracycline, 500 mg qid, *or* amoxicillin, 500 mg qid, × 7-14 days; or (2) metronidazole, 500 mg bid, plus omeprazole, 20 mg bid, plus clarithromycin, 250 mg bid
  - Dual therapy: clarithromycin, 500 mg tid, plus omeprazole, 20 mg bid, × 14 days
- For acute ulcer:
  - Triple therapy plus ranitidine: bismuth subsalicylate, 2 tabs qid, plus metronidazole, 250 mg tid or qid, plus tetracycline, 500 mg qid, *or* amoxicillin, 500 mg qid, plus ranitidine, 300 mg hs, × 2 weeks
  - Dual therapy with acid pump inhibitor: omeprazole, 20 mg bid, plus clarithromycin, 500 mg tid, × 2 weeks; then omeprazole, 20 mg qd, × 2 weeks or 4-6 weeks with full-dose H_2 receptor

Pericarditis, Acute

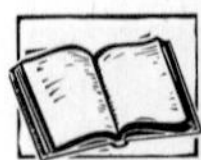

OVERVIEW

Acute pericarditis is defined as an acute inflammation of the pericardium.

Pathogenesis
Causes:
- Idiopathic
- Several viral causes suspected
- Uremia
- Bacterial infection
- Acute myocardial infarction
- Tuberculosis
- Neoplasm
- Trauma

Patient Profile
- Males > Females
- Most common age group—adolescents and young adults

Signs and Symptoms
- Chest pain—sudden onset; over precordium or retrosternally; may radiate to trapezius, neck, abdomen, or epigastrium; relieved by leaning forward and sitting up
- Dyspnea
- Fever
- Anxiety
- Myalgia
- Pericardial friction rub

Differential Diagnosis
- Myocardial infarction
- Unstable angina
- Ulcer
- Acute aortic dissection
- Spontaneous pneumothorax
- Pulmonary embolism

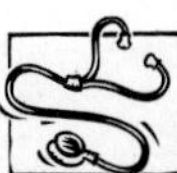

ASSESSMENT

History
Inquire about:
- Onset and duration of symptoms
- Recent history of viral or bacterial infection
- Exposure to tuberculosis
- Recent chest trauma
- Past history of heart problems
- Underlying conditions
- Current medications

Physical Findings
- General appearance—anxious
- Dyspnea
- Lungs—localized rales
- Heart—pericardial friction rub, arrhythmias
- Fever

Initial Workup
Laboratory
- CBC—leukocytosis
- Erythrocyte sedimentation rate (ESR)—increased

Radiology: Chest film—PA and lateral

Further Workup
- ECG
- Echocardiogram
- Pericardiocentesis

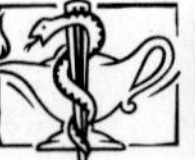

INTERVENTIONS

Office Treatment
None indicated

Lifestyle Modifications
- Smoking cessation
- Weight loss if overweight

Patient Education
Teach patient about:
- Condition and treatment
- Tips for weight loss
- Tips for smoking cessation
- Activity—only restricted by symptoms
- Medications used and side effects (see Pharmacotherapeutics)

Referral
To cardiologist if treatment fails

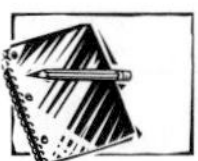

EVALUATION

Outcomes
- Most resolve without sequelae
- 15% will have recurrence
- Very small number develop right-sided heart failure

Possible Complications
- Recurrence
- Pericardial tamponade
- Chronic, constrictive pericarditis

Follow-up
In 2 weeks

FOR YOUR INFORMATION

Life Span
Pediatric: Commonly seen in adolescents
Geriatric: Rare in this age group
Pregnancy: Cautious use of medications; should see a specialist

Miscellaneous
Pericardiectomy may be necessary for the rare patient who does not respond to medication.

References
Massie BM: Systemic hypertension. In Tierney LM Jr, McPhee SJ, Papadakis MA, editors: *Current medical diagnosis and treatment,* ed 34, Norwalk, Conn, 1995, Appleton & Lange, p 364.

Woolliscroft JO: *Current diagnosis and treatment: a quick reference guide for the general practitioner,* Philadelphia, 1996, Current Medicine, pp 304-305.

NOTES

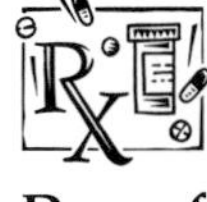

PHARMACOTHERAPEUTICS

Drug of Choice	Mechanism of Action	Prescribing Information	Side Effects
Aspirin, 80-650 mg PO q4h × 2 weeks	Decreases platelet aggregation	***Contraindications:*** Hypersensitivity; bleeding disorders or anticoagulant therapy; last trimester of pregnancy; asthma; gastric ulcers ***Cost:*** OTC ***Pregnancy category:*** Not categorized	Rash, anaphylactic reaction, GI upset and bleeding, Reye's syndrome in children and adolescents
Ibuprofen (Motrin), 400-600 mg PO q6h × 2 weeks; children, 20-30 mg/kg/day PO in 4 divided doses; other NSAIDs may work equally as well; take with food	Not well understood; may be related to inhibition of prostaglandin synthesis	***Contraindications:*** Aspirin allergy; hypersensitivity; asthma; last trimester of pregnancy; gastric ulcer; bleeding disorders ***Cost:*** 400-mg tab, 30 tabs: $4 ***Pregnancy category:*** Not categorized but not recommended	Nausea, heartburn, diarrhea, GI upset and bleeding, dizziness, headache, rash, tinnitus, edema, acute renal failure

Peyronie's Disease

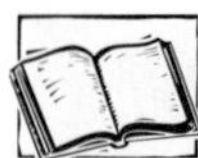

OVERVIEW

Peyronie's disease is a disease of the penis that is characterized by a painful, curved, erection.

Pathogenesis

- Cause—unknown
- Vasculitis-like inflammatory reaction leads to decreased tissue oxygenation = fibrosis and calcification of corpora cavernosa (plaque formation), associated with Dupuytren contracture, diabetes, and tendency to develop keloids

Patient Profile

- Males
- Middle age

Signs and Symptoms

- Painful, curved, erection
- Painful intercourse for both partners or inability to have intercourse
- Absence of pain when flaccid

Differential Diagnosis

Priapism

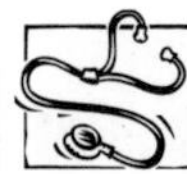

ASSESSMENT

History

Inquire about:

- Onset and duration of symptoms
- Ability to have intercourse
- Underlying conditions
- Current medications

Physical Findings

- Dense, fibrous plaque palpable on dorsum of penis
- May find Dupuytren's contracture (flexion deformity of fingers or toes) or keloids

Initial Workup

Laboratory

- None diagnostic for Peyronie's disease
- Serum glucose—to assess for diabetes

Radiology: Penile ultrasound—assess amount of plaque formation

Further Workup

Nocturnal penile tumescence testing

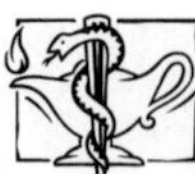

INTERVENTIONS

Office Treatment

None indicated

Lifestyle Modification

Psychologic and physical adjustment to inability to have sexual intercourse

Patient Education

Teach patient about:

- Condition and treatment:
  - 50% will have spontaneous remission
  - Trial of medication (vitamin E, aminobenzoate potassium [Potaba])—may help speed remission
  - If severe, may need surgical intervention—several different procedures may be used
- Medications used and side effects (see Pharmacotherapeutics)

Referral

To urologic surgeon

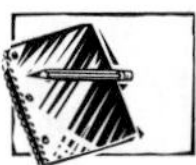

EVALUATION

Outcome
Patient has decreased pain and is able to have intercourse

Possible Complications
- Debilitating pain
- Impotency
- Usual postoperative complications

Follow-up
Monthly if using medications to assess results

FOR YOUR INFORMATION

Life Span
Pediatric: Extremely rare
Geriatric: Rare
Pregnancy: N/A

Miscellaneous
N/A

References
Driscoll CE: The genitourinary system. In Driscoll CE et al, editors: *The family practice desk reference,* ed 3, St Louis, 1996, Mosby, p 423.

Robinson KM, McCance KL, Gray DP: Alterations of the reproductive system. In McCance KL, Huether SE, editors: *Pathophysiology: the biological basis for disease in adults and children,* ed 2, St Louis, 1994, Mosby, pp 770-771.

NOTES

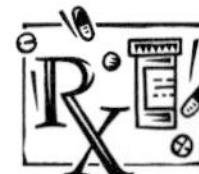

PHARMACOTHERAPEUTICS

Drug of Choice	Mechanism of Action	Prescribing Information	Side Effects
Vitamin E, 100-200 IU PO qid, may need to take for extended period of time	Fat-soluble vitamin; increases oxygenation	***Contraindication:*** Hypersensitivity ***Cost:*** OTC ***Pregnancy category:*** A	Weakness, headache, fatigue, altered metabolism of hormones, nausea, cramps, diarrhea, increased risk of thrombophlebitis, blurred vision, sterile abscess, contact dermatitis
Aminobenzoate potassium (Potaba), 2 g PO 6 times daily	Member of vitamin B complex; increases oxygenation	***Contraindications:*** Do not administer to patients taking sulfonamides; hypersensitivity ***Cost:*** 2-g envule, 50 envules: $41 ***Pregnancy category:*** Not categorized	Anorexia, nausea, fever, rash

Pharyngitis

OVERVIEW

Pharyngitis is an inflammation of the pharynx.

Pathogenesis

Cause—acute infection, usually either bacterial or viral:

- Bacterial infection—group A beta-hemolytic streptococci, *Neisseria gonorrhoeae, Corynebacterium diphtheriae, Haemophilus influenzae, Moraxella catarrhalis*
- Viral infection—rhinovirus, adenovirus, parainfluenza virus, coxsackievirus, Epstein-Barr virus
- Chronic infection—irritation from postnasal discharge, chemical irritation, neoplasms

Patient Profile

- Males = Females
- All ages, but greatest incidence in 5- to 18-year-olds

Signs and Symptoms

- Sore throat
- Enlarged tonsils with exudate
- Fever
- Anorexia
- Chills
- Malaise
- Headache
- Cervical adenopathy
- Rash

Differential Diagnosis

- Stomatitis
- Rhinitis or sinusitis
- Epiglottitis
- Must differentiate causative factor

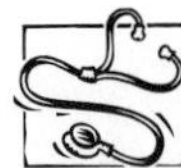

ASSESSMENT

History

Inquire about:

- Onset and duration of symptoms
- Upper respiratory tract symptoms
- Excessive drooling and/or dysphagia (may indicate peritonsillar abscess)
- Rash
- Headache
- Abdominal pain
- Fatigue
- Past history of sore throat
- Smoking
- Sexual practices
- Underlying conditions
- Current medications

Physical Findings

- Erythematous pharynx
- Enlarged tonsils with yellow, white, or gray exudate (may not be any)
- Fever
- Anterior cervical node enlargement
- May have enlarged nodes elsewhere, depending on cause

Initial Workup

Laboratory

- Rapid strep test (low sensitivity)
- Throat culture and sensitivity
- CBC—increased WBC count in bacterial infections and decreased WBC count in viral infections
- Monospot if indicated
- Gonorrhea culture if indicated
- Viral cultures if indicated; usually not necessary

Radiology: None indicated

Further Workup

Usually none

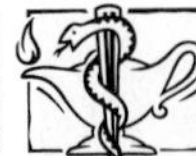

INTERVENTIONS

Office Treatment

None indicated

Lifestyle Modifications

- Smoking cessation
- Increased fluid intake
- Cool mist vaporizer for humidification of home

Patient Education

Teach patient about:

- Disease process and treatment options:
  - Viral infection—symptomatic treatment: acetaminophen or ibuprofen for fever; warm saltwater gargles; rest
  - Bacterial infection—addition of antibiotics to treatment; importance of completing all antibiotics
- Need to call office immediately if symptoms worsen
- Increasing fluid intake
- Tips to quit smoking
- Discarding old toothbrush
- Not sharing drinking glasses or utensils
- How to take medication and side effects (see Pharmacotherapeutics)

Referral

To MD if unresponsive to treatment or if complications arise

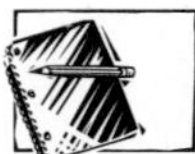

EVALUATION

Outcome
Resolves without sequelae

Possible Complications
- Rheumatic fever
- Poststreptococcal glomerulonephritis
- Peritonsillar abscess
- Systemic infection
- Otitis media
- Sinusitis
- Pneumonia

Follow-up
If no significant improvement in 3 to 4 days, recheck; otherwise recheck in 2 weeks

FOR YOUR INFORMATION

Life Span
Pediatric: Most common in this age group
Geriatric: Much less common; may be sicker
Pregnancy: Cautious use of medication

Miscellaneous
Patients with streptococcal infection should not return to school or work until they have been treated with antibiotics for 24 hours

References
Kiselica D: Group A beta-hemolytic streptococcal pharyngitis: current clinical concepts, *Am Fam Physician* 49(5):1147-1153, 1994.

Koster FT, Barker LR: Respiratory tract infections. In Barker LR, Burton JR, Zieve PD, editors: *Principles of ambulatory medicine,* ed 4, Baltimore, 1995, Williams & Wilkins, pp 333-335.

NOTES

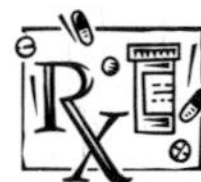

PHARMACOTHERAPEUTICS

Drug of Choice	Mechanism of Action	Prescribing Information	Side Effects
• Penicillin (Pen-Vee K), 250-500 mg PO tid or qid × 10 days; children <12 years, 25-50 mg/kg/day PO in divided doses × 10 days • Benzathine penicillin, 1.2 mil units IM	Bactericidal	***Contraindication:*** Hypersensitivity to penicillin or cephalosporins ***Cost:*** 250-mg tab, 40 tabs: $5 ***Pregnancy category:*** B	Nausea, vomiting; epigastric distress; diarrhea; black, hairy tongue; anaphylaxis
Erythromycin (E-Mycin), 250 mg PO qid × 10 days; children <12 years, 30-40 mg/kg/day PO qid × 10 days	Inhibits protein synthesis	***Contraindication:*** Hypersensitivity ***Cost:*** 250-mg tab, 40 tabs: $5 ***Pregnancy category:*** B	Pseudomembranous colitis, abdominal cramping, nausea, vomiting, diarrhea, rash, anaphylaxis
For pharyngeal gonorrhea:			
Ceftriaxone (Rocephin), 250 mg IM; children, 50-75 mg/kg/day × 1 dose	Cephalosporin; bactericidal; inhibits cell wall synthesis	***Contraindications:*** Hypersensitivity to cephalosporins; caution in patients allergic to penicillin—may have cross-sensitivity ***Cost:*** 250-mg vial, 1-vial: $12 ***Pregnancy category:*** B	Anaphylaxis; diarrhea; headache; dizziness; pain, induration, or tenderness at injection site; rash; leukopenia; pseudomembranous colitis

Pheochromocytoma

OVERVIEW

Pheochromocytoma is a condition in which there is a neoplasm that produces excessive amounts of catecholamines. The neoplasm is most commonly found on the adrenal medulla.

Pathogenesis

Cause—catecholamine-producing neoplasm:

- 10% are extraadrenal
- 10% are multiple or bilateral
- 10% are malignant
- 10% recur after surgical removal
- 10% occur in children
- 10% are familial

Patient Profile

- Males = Females
- Any age, but more common in 40- to 60-year-olds
- Risk factors:
  - Familial pheochromocytoma
  - Multiple endocrine neoplasia types II A and B
  - Neurofibromatosis
  - Von Hippel-Lindau syndrome

Signs and Symptoms

- Constipation
- Weight loss
- Tremor
- Anxiety
- Paroxysmal spells (the "5 Ps"):
  - **P**ressure—sudden increase in blood pressure
  - **P**ain—headache, chest, and abdominal pain
  - **P**erspiration
  - **P**alpitations
  - **P**allor
- Orthostatic hypotension
- Grade II to IV retinopathy
- Fever
- Hyperglycemia
- Hypercalcemia
- Erythrocytosis

Differential Diagnosis

- Labile essential hypertension
- Anxiety and panic attacks
- Paroxysmal cardiac arrhythmia
- Thyrotoxicosis
- Menopausal syndrome
- Hypoglycemia
- Withdrawal of adrenergic-inhibiting medications
- Angina
- Hyperventilation
- Migraine headache
- Amphetamine or cocaine use
- Sympathomimetic ingestion

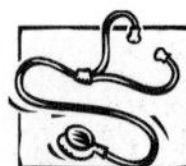

ASSESSMENT

History

Inquire about:

- Onset and duration of symptoms
- Family history of pheochromocytoma
- Episodes of severe pounding headache and sweating
- Underlying conditions
- Current medications

Physical Findings

- May not have any
- If during a paroxysmal attack, may find severe hypertension, perspiration, bounding pulse, and pallor
- May appear anxious
- Grade II to IV retinopathy

Initial Workup

Laboratory

- Chemistry panel—elevated glucose and calcium levels
- CBC—elevated RBC count
- 24-hour urine metanephrine (catecholamine metabolites)—elevated
- 24-hour urine catecholamines—elevated

Radiology: CT scan or MRI of abdomen—to locate tumor

Further Workup

None indicated

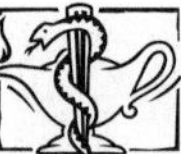

INTERVENTIONS

Office Treatment

None indicated

Lifestyle Modifications

- Lifestyle interrupted by hospitalization for tumor removal
- Postoperative recuperation may be lengthy

Patient Education

Teach patient about:

- Disease process and treatment options:
  - Initially, use of medications to control symptoms (alpha-adrenergic blockers and beta-adrenergic blockers; start alpha-blocker first)
  - Surgical removal of tumor—for 75% of patients, having surgery controls hypertension; in other 25%, medication will be needed for rest of life
- Medications used and side effects (see Pharmacotherapeutics)

Referral

To surgeon experienced in this type of surgery

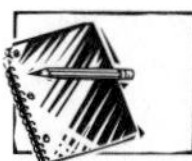

EVALUATION

Outcomes

- 75% will have hypertension cured
- 25% will continue with hypertension, or it will recur; usually, easily controlled with conventional treatment
- If tumor is malignant, less than 50% survival after 5 years

Possible Complications

- Postural hypotension with alpha-adrenergic blockade
- Pulmonary edema with beta-adrenergic blockade

Follow-up

- Daily blood pressure monitoring before surgery
- Postoperatively, weekly 24-hour urinalysis for catecholamine and metanephrine for 2 weeks
- If normal, monitor laboratory values yearly for 5 years

FOR YOUR INFORMATION

Life Span

Pediatric: Very rare in this age group
Geriatric: Treatment is the same
Pregnancy: First and second trimester, surgical resection; third trimester, cesarean section together with surgical resection

Miscellaneous

Several conditions are associated with pheochromocytoma, including multiple endocrine neoplasia types IIA and IIB, neurofibromatosis, Von Hippel-Lindau syndrome, ataxia-telangiectasia, tuberous sclerosis, Sturge-Weber syndrome, cholelithiasis, and renal artery stenosis.

References

Barker LR: Hypertension. In Barker LR, Burton JR, Zieve PD, editors: *Principles of ambulatory medicine,* ed 4, Baltimore, 1995, Williams & Wilkins, p 816.

Haas L: Endocrine problems. In Lewis SM, Collier IC, Heitkemper MM, editors: *Medical-surgical nursing: assessment and management of clinical problems,* ed 4, St Louis, 1996, Mosby, p 1515.

NOTES

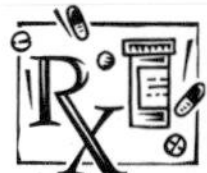

PHARMACOTHERAPEUTICS

Drug of Choice	Mechanism of Action	Prescribing Information	Side Effects
Phenoxybenzamine (Dibenzyline), 10 mg/day; increase q2d until blood pressure controlled; start this drug first—safety and effectiveness in children not established	Alpha-adrenergic blocker; blocks sympathetic nervous system; controls hypertension and sweating	***Contraindications:*** Conditions in which fall in blood pressure is undesirable ***Cost:*** 10-mg tab, 100 tabs: $62 ***Pregnancy category:*** C	Postural hypotension, tachycardia, inhibition of ejaculation, nasal congestion, miosis, GI irritation, drowsiness, fatigue
Propranolol (Inderal); adults and children, 10 mg q6h; increase as necessary to control tachycardia	Nonselective beta-adrenergic blocker	***Contraindications:*** Hypersensitivity; cardiac failure; cardiogenic shock; 2nd- or 3rd-degree heart block; bronchospastic disease; sinus bradycardia; congestive heart failure (CHF) ***Cost:*** 40-mg tab, 100 tabs: $2-$40 ***Pregnancy category:*** C	Bronchospasm, dyspnea, bradycardia, hypotension, CHF, palpitations, atrioventricular block, agranulocytosis, thrombocytopenia, nausea, vomiting, diarrhea, constipation, impotence, decreased libido, joint pain, arthralgia, facial swelling, rash, pruritus, depression, hallucinations, dizziness, fatigue, lethargy, sore throat, laryngospasm, blurred vision

Phimosis and Paraphimosis

OVERVIEW

Phimosis is a condition in which the foreskin of the penis cannot be retracted back over the glans. Paraphimosis is a condition in which the foreskin is retracted behind the glans and cannot be moved forward over the glans. This causes a constrictive band behind the glans. Both conditions can cause penile pathology.

Pathogenesis

Causes:

- Phimosis:
  - Physiologic—present at birth and normally resolves by 2 to 3 years of age
  - Congenital—unresolved physiologic phimosis
  - Acquired—result of repeated infections and irritation
- Paraphimosis—foreskin not placed back over glans after cleaning, catheter insertion, cystoscopy

Patient Profile

- Males
- Any age
- Risk factors—phimosis: poor hygiene, diabetes

Signs and Symptoms

- Phimosis—inability to retract foreskin, painful erection, inflammation of glans (balanitis)
- Paraphimosis—edema of glans, pain, drainage

Differential Diagnosis

- Insect bite
- Trauma
- Allergic reaction

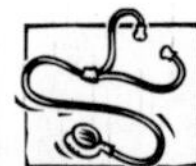

ASSESSMENT

History

Inquire about:

- Onset and duration of symptoms
- History of infection
- Pain
- Underlying conditions
- Current medications

Physical Findings

- Phimosis—inability to retract foreskin
- Paraphimosis:
  - Inability to replace foreskin over glans
  - Swelling of glans
  - Drainage

Initial Workup

Laboratory: Culture of any drainage
Radiology: None needed

Further Workup

None needed

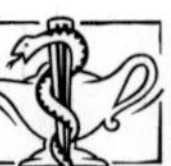

INTERVENTIONS

Office Treatment

Paraphimosis:

- Attempt to reduce
- May require sedation

Lifestyle Modification

Appropriate hygiene

Patient Education

Teach patient about:

- Condition and treatment:
  - Phimosis—circumcision
  - Paraphimosis—if reduction unsuccessful, will need dorsal slit with eventual circumcision
- After circumcision, no sexual intercourse until completely healed
- No medications for this condition

Referral

To urologic surgeon

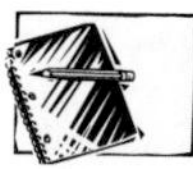

EVALUATION

Outcome
Uneventful recovery after circumcision

Possible Complications
- Gangrene from paraphimosis
- Posthitis from phimosis

Follow-up
1 to 2 weeks after circumcision

FOR YOUR INFORMATION

Life Span
Pediatric: Recurrent balanitis can lead to an acquired phimosis, as can forced reduction of a physiologic phimosis
Geriatric: Recurrent infection and irritation most common causes
Pregnancy: N/A

Miscellaneous
N/A

References
Meredith C: Nursing role in management: male genitourinary problems. In Lewis SM, Collier IC, Heitkemper MM, editors: *Medical-surgical nursing: assessment and management of clinical problems,* ed 4, St Louis, 1996, Mosby, pp 1639-1640.

Robinson KM, McCance KL, Gray DP: Alterations of the reproductive system. In McCance KL, Huether SE, editors: *Pathophysiology: the biological basis for disease in adults and children,* ed 2, St Louis, 1994, Mosby, pp 770-771.

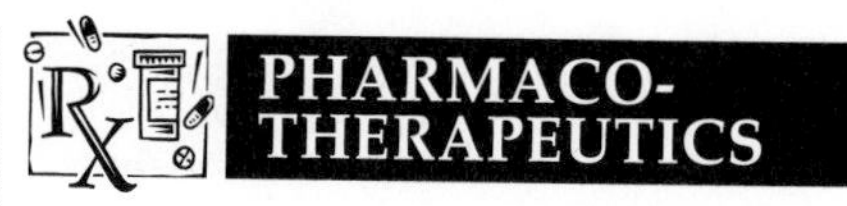

PHARMACOTHERAPEUTICS

No medications are used for this condition.

Pinworms (Enterobiasis)

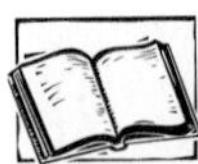

OVERVIEW

Enterobiasis is an intestinal infestation with *Enterobius vermicularis,* commonly known as the pinworm. Pinworms are white, thread-like worms.

Pathogenesis

Cause—*E. vermicularis:*

- Gravid female deposits eggs in perianal area
- Autoinoculation through perianal scratching, poor hand-washing technique, and ingestion of eggs

Patient Profile

- Males = Females
- Preschool and school-age children most commonly
- Also, mothers of infected children and institutionalized persons

Signs and Symptoms

- Perianal pruritus and excoriation
- Restlessness
- Insomnia
- Poor appetite
- Weight loss
- Diarrhea
- Mild abdominal pain
- Pruritus vulvae
- Vaginitis

Differential Diagnosis

- Other intestinal parasites
- Poor hygiene
- Contact dermatitis

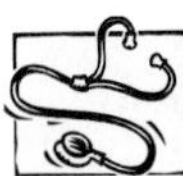

ASSESSMENT

History

Inquire about:

- Onset and duration of symptoms
- Others in household having similar symptoms
- Underlying conditions
- Current medications

Physical Findings

Excoriated perianal area from scratching

Initial Workup

Laboratory: Cellophane tape examination:

- Patient will need to obtain first thing in morning
- Put cellophane tape on tongue blade, sticky side out
- Place against anal opening and then place on slide
- Examine with microscope under low power

Radiology: None indicated

Further Workup

None indicated

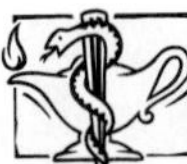

INTERVENTIONS

Office Treatment

None indicated

Lifestyle Modification

Good hand-washing technique

Patient Education

Teach patient about:

- Condition and treatment—antihelminthic medication
- Good hand-washing technique
- Proper sanitation
- Medications used and side effects (see Pharmacotherapeutics)

Referral

None needed

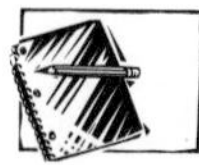

EVALUATION

Outcome
Resolves without sequelae

Possible Complications
Worms may migrate to other parts of the body, causing:
- Cholangitis
- Pancreatitis
- Diverticulitis
- Liver abscess
- Intestinal obstruction
- Intussusception

Follow-up
Usually none

FOR YOUR INFORMATION

Life Span
Pediatric: Most common in this age group
Geriatric: May be seen in nursing home patients
Pregnancy: Cautious use of medications

Miscellaneous
N/A

References

Bope ET: Care of children. In Driscoll CE et al, editors: *The family practice desk reference,* ed 3, St Louis, 1996, Mosby, p 526.

Goldsmith RS: Infectious diseases: helminthic. In Tierney LM Jr, McPhee SJ, Papadakis MA, editors: *Current medical diagnosis and treatment,* ed 34, Norwalk, Conn, 1995, Appleton & Lange, pp 1262-1263.

NOTES

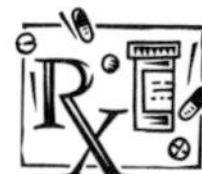

PHARMACOTHERAPEUTICS

Drug of Choice	Mechanism of Action	Prescribing Information	Side Effects
Mebendazole (Vermox); adults and children >2 years: 100 mg PO × 1 dose	Anthelmintic; inhibits formation of worm's microtubules and depletes its glucose	***Contraindication:*** Hypersensitivity ***Cost:*** 100-mg tab, 12 tabs: $55 ***Pregnancy category:*** C	Dizziness, fever, transient diarrhea, abdominal pain, rash, urticaria, angioedema
Pyrantel pamoate (Antiminth); adults and children >2 years, 11 mg/kg PO as a single dose; not to exceed 1 g; repeat in 2 weeks	Paralyzes worm; worm is then expelled by normal peristalsis	***Contraindication:*** Hypersensitivity ***Cost:*** 250 mg/5 ml: $5-$15 ***Pregnancy category:*** C	Rash, dizziness, headache, drowsiness, insomnia, fever, nausea, vomiting, anorexia, diarrhea, distention

Pityriasis Alba

OVERVIEW

Pityriasis alba is a common skin condition that appears usually before puberty. The lesions are small, white or hypopigmented patches or plaques. The condition affects the face, neck and arms.

Pathogenesis

Cause—unknown, but individual is usually atopic

Patient Profile

- Males = Females
- Most common age—3 to 10 years; rare after 25 years of age

Signs and Symptoms

- Begins with slightly erythematous patch, which turns scaly and hypopigmented or white
- Most common areas—face, neck, and arms
- Lesions will not tan when exposed to sun (instead, redden)

Differential Diagnosis

- Pityriasis versicolor
- Vitiligo
- Milia
- Keratosis pilaris

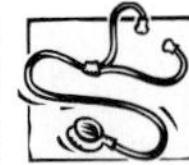

ASSESSMENT

History

Inquire about:

- Onset and duration of symptoms
- History of atopy
- Treatments tried and results
- Underlying conditions
- Current medications

Physical Findings

- Early—slightly erythematous patch or plaque
- Later—small amount of scale on hypopigmented or white patch or plaque
- Usually on face, neck, or arms

Initial Workup

Laboratory: None indicated
Radiology: None indicated

Further Workup

None indicated

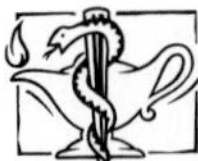

INTERVENTIONS

Office Treatment

None indicated

Lifestyle Modification

Keep affected areas covered from direct sunlight, either with clothing or sunscreen with at least 25 SPF rating

Patient Education

Teach patient about:

- Condition and treatment:
  - Topical steroids for inflammation (will not shorten disease or improve pigmentation)
  - Chronicity of condition—usually will resolve in second or third decade of life
  - No definitive treatment available
- Keeping areas lubricated with emollient such as Lubriderm cream
- Protecting from sunlight with clothing or sunscreen (25 SPF rating)
- Using makeup to help conceal areas
- Medications used and side effects (see Pharmacotherapeutics)

Referrals

None

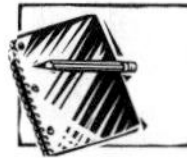

EVALUATION

Outcome
Resolution of lesions in second or third decade of life

Possible Complications
None expected

Follow-up
As needed

FOR YOUR INFORMATION

Life Span
Pediatric: Most common in this age group
Geriatric: Rare in this age group
Pregnancy: Use emollients only

Miscellaneous
Adolescents may need a great deal of support and encouragement because of the cosmetic effects of the condition. Counseling done either by the NP or by a social worker may be extremely beneficial and allow the adolescent to voice his or her concerns about the condition.

References
Habif TP: *Clinical dermatology: a color guide to diagnosis and therapy,* ed 3, St Louis, 1996, Mosby, pp 620-621.

Whitmore E: Common problems of the skin. In Barker LR, Burton JR, Zieve PD, editors: *Principles of ambulatory medicine,* ed 4, Baltimore, 1995, Williams & Wilkins, p 1446.

NOTES

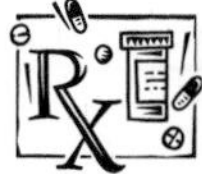

PHARMACOTHERAPEUTICS

Drug of Choice	Mechanism of Action	Prescribing Information	Side Effects
Topical corticosteroid: hydrocortisone cream, 1% for face (controversial—some feel corticosteroids should not be used on face) and 2.5% elsewhere; apply thin layer 3-4 times daily; for severe erythema, stronger corticosteroid may be needed: mometasone (Elocon), triamcinolone (Kenalog), betamethasone (Diprolene AF)	Antiinflammatory and antipruritic	***Contraindication:*** Hypersensitivity ***Cost:*** 1%, 30 g: $12; several available OTC; mometasone 0.1%, 45 g: $29; triamcinolone 0.025%, 30 g: $2-$5; betamethasone 0.05%, 15 g: $3-$16 ***Pregnancy category:*** C	Burning, dryness, itching, irritation acne, folliculitis, hypertrichosis, hypopigmentation, atrophy, striae, perioral dermatitis, secondary infection; if used on large area for extended periods of time, can have systemic side effects

Pityriasis Rosea

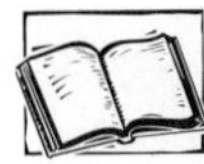

OVERVIEW

Pityriasis rosea is a common, usually mild, skin disorder. It is usually characterized by salmon pink to light brown oval lesions in light-skinned individuals; dark-skinned individuals will have hyperpigmentation, primarily on the trunk and proximal extremities. The condition is self-limiting; it lasts for several weeks to several months.

Pathogenesis

Cause—unknown; there is some (unproven) evidence that condition is viral in nature

Patient Profile

- Female > Males
- Most common age—10 to 35 years, but can occur at any age
- Incidence higher during colder months

Signs and Symptoms

- Starts with "herald patch"—2- to 10-mm pink to light brown oval patch in light-skinned individuals; in dark-skinned individuals hyperpigmentation appears suddenly on trunk or proximal extremities; 7 to 14 days later, smaller, similar lesions erupt, usually on trunk, particularly on lower abdominal region, and proximal extremities
- Lesions have fine white scale attached
- Frequently lesions are along skin cleavage lines in "Christmas tree" pattern
- Mild pruritis

Differential Diagnosis

- Secondary syphilis
- Tinea corporis
- Viral rash
- Drug rash
- Psoriasis
- Eczema
- Lichen planus

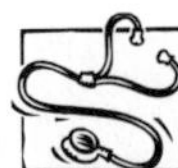

ASSESSMENT

History

Inquire about:

- Onset and duration of symptoms, particularly appearance of "herald patch"
- Presence of itching
- Treatments tried and results
- Underlying conditions
- Current medications

Physical Findings

- Early—2- to 10-cm oval, pink to light brown or hyperpigmented lesion with fine-scale "herald patch"
- Later—smaller, 1- to 2-cm lesions of same color present on trunk and proximal extremities; in extensive cases may develop on arms, legs, and face

Initial Workup

Laboratory

- Rapid plasma reagin (RPR) to rule out syphilis
- Potassium hydroxide preparation to rule out tinea

Radiology: None indicated

Further Workup

None indicated

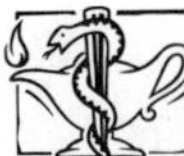

INTERVENTIONS

Office Treatment

None indicated

Lifestyle Modifications

- Lukewarm showers or baths (hot water may intensify itching)
- Exposing lesions to sun hastens resolution; caution against overexposure

Patient Education

Teach patient about:

- Condition and treatment:
  - Antihistamines for itching
  - Topical or oral steroids
  - Usually self-limiting, resolving in several weeks to months
- Good hygiene to prevent secondary infection; need to take lukewarm baths or showers (hot water may exacerbate condition)
- Avoiding strenuous activity, which may increase body temperature, aggravating rash
- Medications used and side effects (see Pharmacotherapeutics)

Referrals

Usually none; to dermatologist for extensive cases

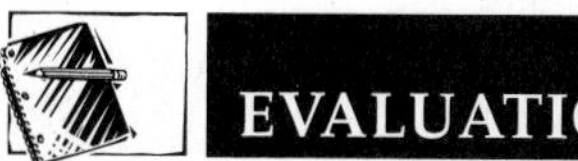

EVALUATION

Outcome
Resolves without sequelae

Possible Complication
Secondary bacterial infection

Follow-up
Monthly until lesions resolve

FOR YOUR INFORMATION

Life Span
Pediatric: Most commonly seen in this age group
Geriatric: Rare in this age group
Pregnancy: Cautious use of medications

Miscellaneous
The cosmetic effects of this condition can be devastating for the patient. Counseling and reassurance can help to ease the patient's anxieties about the condition.

References
American Academy of Dermatology: *Pityriasis rosea,* Schaumburg, Ill, 1993, American Academy of Dermatology.

Habif TP: *Clinical dermatology: a color guide to diagnosis and therapy,* ed 3, St Louis, 1996, Mosby, pp 218-220.

NOTES

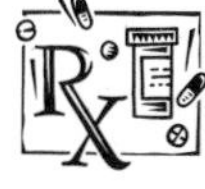

PHARMACOTHERAPEUTICS

Drug of Choice	Mechanism of Action	Prescribing Information	Side Effects
Topical corticosteroid: hydrocortisone cream, 1% for face (controversial—some feel corticosteroids should not be used on face) and 2.5% elsewhere; apply thin layer 3-4 times daily; for severe erythema, stronger corticosteroid may be needed: mometasone (Elocon), triamcinolone (Kenalog), betamethasone (Diprolene AF)	Antiinflammatory and antipruritic	***Contraindication:*** Hypersensitivity ***Cost:*** 1%, 30 g: $12; several available OTC; mometasone 0.1%, 45 g: $29; triamcinolone 0.025%, 30 g: $2-$5; betamethasone 0.05%, 15 g: $3-$16 ***Pregnancy category:*** C	Burning, dryness, itching, irritation acne, folliculitis, hypertrichosis, hypopigmentation, atrophy, striae, perioral dermatitis, secondary infection; if used on large area for extended periods of time, can have systemic side effects
Diphenhydramine (Benadryl), 25-50 mg PO qid; children 6-12 years, 12.5-25 mg PO qid	Competes with histamine for cell receptor sites	***Contraindication:*** Hypersensitivity ***Cost:*** Benadryl, 25 mg, 4/day × 30 days: $4 ***Pregnancy category:*** B	Sedation, headache, fatigue, dizziness, nausea, vomiting, dry mouth, cough, rash, nervousness
Prednisone, 60-120 mg PO qd, then taper over several days	Corticosteroid; decreases inflammation	***Contraindications:*** Hypersensitivity; psychosis; idiopathic thrombocytopenia; acute glomerulonephritis; amebiasis; nonasthmatic bronchial disease; AIDS; TB; children <2 years old ***Cost:*** 15-mg tab, 100 tabs: $14-$35 ***Pregnancy category:*** C	Hypertension, circulatory collapse, thrombophlebitis, embolism, tachycardia, fungal infections, increased intraocular pressure, diarrhea, nausea, GI hemorrhage, thrombocytopenia, acne, poor wound healing, fractures, osteoporosis, weakness

Plague

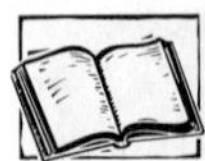

OVERVIEW

Plague is an infectious disease transmitted to humans by the bite of a flea from an infected wild rodent. Untreated bubonic plague may progress to pneumonic plague, which can be spread by respiratory droplets to other humans.

Pathogenesis

Cause—*Yersinia pestis,* a bacillus

Patient Profile

- Males = Females
- Any age
- Seen in Southwestern United States

Signs and Symptoms

- Sudden onset—high fever, malaise, muscular pain and prostration
- Pustule or ulcer at site of flea bite
- Lymph nodes—painful and enlarged with edema (bubo); eventually may drain
- Delirium
- Seizures
- Shock
- Primary or secondary pneumonic plague:
  - Fever
  - Chills
  - Cough
  - Chest pain
  - Hemoptysis
  - Dyspnea
  - Lethargy
  - Hypotension
  - Shock

Differential Diagnosis

- Lymphadenitis mistaken for streptococcal or staphylococcal infection
- Lymphogranuloma venereum
- Syphilis
- Tularemia
- Other manifestations resembling malaria
- Rickettsial fever
- Influenza
- Other bacterial pneumonias

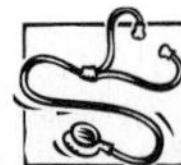

ASSESSMENT

History

Inquire about:

- Onset and duration of symptoms (can be quickly fatal if not treated promptly)
- Contact with wild rodents/fleas
- Recent travel to Southwestern United States
- Underlying conditions
- Current medications

Physical Findings

- Appearance—severely ill
- Fever
- Ulcer/lesion at site of flea bite
- Lymphadenopathy—painful to palpation with erythema and edema (bubo)
- Tachycardia
- Hypotension
- Lungs—crackles, dyspnea
- Abdominal examination—hepatomegaly/splenomegaly

Initial Workup

Laboratory

- CBC with differential—increased WBC count, left shift
- Gram stain of aspirate from bubo—gram-negative coccobacilli
- Cultures of aspirate, blood, and sputum—contact public health department for help with cultures

Radiology: Chest film—PA and lateral—pulmonary consolidation if pneumonia present

Further Workup

None indicated

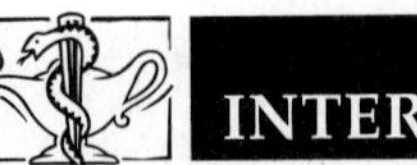

INTERVENTIONS

Office Treatment

None indicated

Lifestyle Modification

Avoidance of wild rodents and flea control

Patient Education

Teach patient about:

- Disease, how contracted, treatment:
  - Hospitalization—if pneumonic plague suspected, respiratory isolation
  - Antimicrobials
  - Bed rest
  - Hot, moist compresses for buboes
  - IV fluids
- Avoiding contact with wild rodents
- Controlling rat and flea population
- Antimicrobial prophylaxis for other people at risk
- Medications used and side effects (see Pharmacotherapeutics)

Referral

To MD for hospitalization if NP does not have privileges

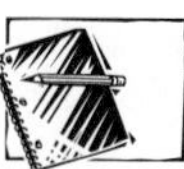

EVALUATION

Outcomes

- With prompt treatment, full resolution
- With primary pneumonic plague, delay in treatment >24 hours usually results in death

Possible Complications

- Pericarditis
- Adult respiratory distress syndrome
- Meningitis
- Death

Follow-up

1 week after hospitalization

FOR YOUR INFORMATION

Life Span

Pediatric: Seizures common in children
Geriatric: Higher mortality rate
Pregnancy: Consult with specialist

Miscellaneous

Plague vaccine is available for people at high risk of exposure. However, efficacy is not clearly established.

Reference

Chambers HF: Infectious diseases: bacterial & chlamydial. In Tierney LM Jr, McPhee SJ, Papadakis MA, editors: *Current medical diagnosis and treatment,* ed 34, Norwalk, Conn, 1995, Appleton & Lange, pp 1183-1184.

NOTES

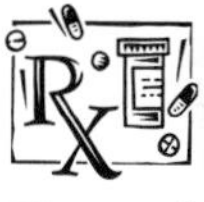

PHARMACOTHERAPEUTICS

Drug of Choice	Mechanism of Action	Prescribing Information	Side Effects
Streptomycin, 15 mg/kg IM bid × 10 days	Aminoglycoside; interferes with protein synthesis	***Contraindications:*** Hypersensitivity; severe renal disease ***Cost:*** 1-g vial: $4 ***Pregnancy category:*** B	Oliguria, hematuria, renal damage, renal failure, nephrotoxicity, confusion, depression, numbness, neurotoxicity, ototoxicity, agranulocytosis, thrombocytopenia, anemia, nausea, vomiting, anorexia, hepatic necrosis, hypotension, myocarditis, rash, dermatitis, alopecia
Tetracycline (Achromycin): for severe infection—give 2 g/day PO in divided doses with streptomycin; for mild infection—give 25-50 mg/kg/day in 4 divided doses × 10 days; for prophylaxis—give 500 mg PO bid × 5 days	Inhibits protein synthesis	***Contraindications:*** Hypersensitivity; children <8 years old; lactation ***Cost:*** 500-mg tab, 100 tabs: $6-$15 ***Pregnancy category:*** D	Fever, headache, paresthesia, eosinophilia, neutropenia, thrombocytopenia, leukocytosis, hemolytic anemia, dysphagia, glossitis, oral candidiasis, nausea, diarrhea, hepatotoxicity, flatulence, abdominal cramps, stomatitis, pericarditis, rash, urticaria, photosensitivity, exfoliative dermatitis, angioedema
For meningitis:			
Chloramphenicol, 60 mg/kg/day PO in 4 divided doses × 10 days	Interference or inhibition of protein synthesis	***Contraindications:*** Hypersensitivity; severe renal or hepatic disease; minor infections ***Cost:*** 250-mg tab, 100 tabs: $25-$125 ***Pregnancy category:*** C	Anemia, thrombocytopenia, aplastic anemia, granulocytopenia, optic neuritis, nausea, vomiting, diarrhea, abdominal pain, glossitis, colitis, itching, rash, gray syndrome in newborns, headache, depression, confusion

Pneumonia, Bacterial

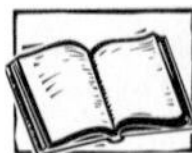

OVERVIEW

Bacterial pneumonia is an acute bacterial infection of the lung. The disease is usually said to be community acquired or hospital acquired.

Pathogenesis

- Spread by hematogenous means, inhalation, or aspiration from oropharynx
- Causes—*Streptococcus pneumoniae* (pneumococcal), *Haemophilus influenzae, Staphylococcus aureus, Moraxella catarrhalis, Klebsiella pneumoniae, Pseudomonas aeruginosa, Escherichia coli*

Patient Profile

- Males > Females
- All ages; bacterial pneumonia more common in adults

Signs and Symptoms

- Fever
- Chills
- Cough
- Chest pain
- Dark, thick, rusty sputum
- Anxiety
- Anorexia
- Confusion
- Dehydration
- Headache
- Facial flush
- Malaise
- Myalgia
- Prostration
- Restlessness
- Shoulder pain
- Weakness

Differential Diagnosis

- Other causes of pneumonia
- Tuberculosis
- Pulmonary embolism
- Pneumothorax

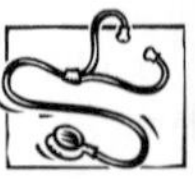

ASSESSMENT

History

Inquire about:

- Onset and duration of symptoms
- Cough and sputum
- Underlying conditions
- Current medications

Physical Findings

- General—fever, ill-appearing, facial flush
- Lungs—crackles, wheezing, pleural friction rub, rhonchi, bronchial breath sounds, decreased breath sounds, whispered pectoriloquy
- Heart—tachycardia

Initial Workup

Laboratory

- CBC with differential—leukocytosis with left shift
- Increased Hgb and Hct resulting from dehydration
- Chemistry panel to include electrolytes, liver function studies, renal function tests
- Sputum culture and Gram stain

Radiology: Chest film—PA and lateral—lobar or segmental consolidation

Further Workup

- With pleural effusion, thoracentesis should be done
- Blood cultures

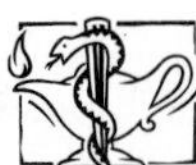

INTERVENTIONS

Office Treatment

None indicated

Lifestyle Modifications

- Smoking cessation
- Increased fluid intake
- Adequate rest

Patient Education

Teach patient about:

- Condition and treatment:
  - If over 65 years with coexisting illnesses or if severely ill with the pneumonia, hospitalization may be appropriate
  - Outpatient treatment—antimicrobials
- Importance of increasing fluid intake
- Percussion and postural drainage (teach significant other)
- Supplemental oxygen if necessary—safety factors
- Obtaining adequate rest
- Proper disposal of soiled tissues
- Proper hand-washing technique
- Prevention through vaccination
- Medications used and side effects (see Pharmacotherapeutics)

Referral

To MD if NP does not have hospital privileges or if treatment fails

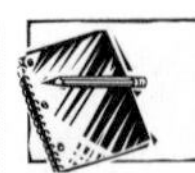

EVALUATION

Outcome

In otherwise healthy individuals, resolves without sequelae

Possible Complications

- Pulmonary abscess
- Adult respiratory distress syndrome
- Superinfection
- Pleural effusion
- Empyema

Follow-up

- Telephone contact in 24 hours; return to clinic in 3 to 4 days; then in 2 to 3 weeks
- Repeat chest film in 4 to 6 weeks, especially if patient >40 years or a smoker

FOR YOUR INFORMATION

Life Span

Pediatric: High morbidity and mortality in children <1 year

Geriatric: High morbidity and mortality if >70 years

Pregnancy: Consider hospitalization and consultation with a specialist

Miscellaneous

All patients with chronic illnesses and those over 65 years of age should receive pneumococcal vaccine.

References

Bartlett JG: *Pocket book of infectious disease therapy,* ed 7, Baltimore, 1996, Williams & Wilkins, pp 112-113, 266-271.

Koster FT, Barker LR: Respiratory tract infections. In Barker LR, Burton JR, Zieve PD, editors: *Principles of ambulatory medicine,* ed 4, Baltimore, 1995, Williams & Wilkins, pp 342-347.

US Department of Health and Human Services, Public Health Service: *Clinician's handbook of preventive services: put prevention into practice,* Washington, DC, US Government Printing Office, pp 263-265.

PHARMACOTHERAPEUTICS

Drug of Choice	Mechanism of Action	Prescribing Information	Side Effects
For patients <60 years of age and without comorbidity:			
Erythromycin (E-Mycin), 500 mg PO bid to qid × 7-14 days; children, 30-50 mg/kg/day PO in divided doses q6h	Inhibits protein synthesis	***Contraindication:*** Hypersensitivity ***Cost:*** 500-mg tab, 4/day × 10 days: \$10-\$20 ***Pregnancy category:*** B	Nausea, vomiting, diarrhea, abdominal pain, anorexia, rash, urticaria, pseudomembranous colitis—rarely
If patient is unable to tolerate E-Mycin or is a smoker:			
Clarithromycin (Biaxin), 500 mg PO bid × 7-14 days; children >6 months, 15 mg/kg/day PO in divided doses q12h	Inhibits protein synthesis	***Contraindication:*** Hypersensitivity ***Cost:*** 500-mg tab, 60 tabs: \$185 ***Pregnancy category:*** C	Nausea, vomiting, diarrhea, abdominal pain, anorexia, rash, urticaria, pseudomembranous colitis—rarely
If patient is intolerant of macrolides:			
Doxycycline (Doryx), 100 mg PO bid × 7-14 days; children >8 years, 4.4 mg/kg/day PO in divided doses q12h × 7-14 days	Tetracycline; inhibits protein synthesis	***Contraindications:*** Hypersensitivity; children <8 years ***Cost:*** 100-mg tab, 20 tabs: \$5 ***Pregnancy category:*** D	Eosinophilia, neutropenia, thrombocytopenia, hemolytic anemia, dysphagia, glossitis, nausea, abdominal pain, vomiting, diarrhea, anorexia, hepatotoxicity, flatulence, abdominal cramps, gastritis, pericarditis, rash, urticaria, exfoliative dermatitis, angioedema
For patients with comorbidity and/or >60 years of age, use one of the following:			
Cefuroxime axetil (Ceftin), 500 mg PO bid × 7-14 days; children <2 years, 125 mg PO bid × 7-14 days	Cephalosporin; inhibits cell wall synthesis	***Contraindication:*** Hypersensitivity ***Cost:*** 500-mg tab, 20 tabs: \$128 ***Pregnancy category:*** B	Headache, dizziness, nausea, vomiting, diarrhea, anorexia, glossitis, pseudomembranous colitis, proteinuria, vaginitis, nephrotoxicity, renal failure, leukopenia, thrombocytopenia, agranulocytosis, eosinophilia, lymphocytosis, rash, urticaria, anaphylaxis
Trimethoprim/sulfamethoxazole (TMP/SMZ), DS (Bactrim DS), 1 DS tab PO bid; children, 8 mg/kg TMP and 40 mg/kg SMZ qd in 2 divided doses	Blocks 2 consecutive steps in bacterial synthesis of nucleic acids and protein	***Contraindications:*** Hypersensitivity to trimethoprim or sulfonamides; term pregnancy; lactation; megaloblastic anemia; infants <2 months; creatinine clearance <15 ml/min ***Cost:*** DS tab × 14 days: \$2 ***Pregnancy category:*** C	Anaphylaxis, hypersensitivity, Stevens-Johnson syndrome, allergic myocarditis, nausea, vomiting, abdominal pain, hepatitis, enterocolitis, renal failure, toxic nephrosis, leukopenia, thrombocytopenia, hemolytic anemia
For prevention:			
Pneumococcal vaccine (Pnu-Imune 23); adults and children, 0.5 ml IM or SQ; most authorities recommend that all persons >65 years should receive vaccine at least once; also recommended for vaccination: adults and children with chronic illnesses or immunocompromised individuals (including patients with HIV) and residents of special environments with increased risk; much debate about revaccination; generally, revaccinate at 6 or more years	Causes production of antibodies against 23 capsular types	***Contraindications:*** Hypersensitivity; patients with Hodgkin's disease treated with certain therapy (see manufacturer's prescribing information) ***Cost:*** 2.5 ml: \$71 ***Pregnancy category:*** C	Injection site soreness, erythema, swelling, rash, urticaria, arthritis, malaise, myalgia, headache, fever; rarely—Guillain-Barré and anaphylaxis

Pneumonia, Mycoplasmal

OVERVIEW

Mycoplasmal pneumonia is an acute infection of the lungs (particularly the lower lobes) and the bronchi. It is more commonly seen in the summer and fall.

Pathogenesis
Cause—*Mycoplasma pneumoniae*

Patient Profile
- Males > Females
- Can occur at any age, but more common in children and young adults

Signs and Symptoms
- Low-grade fever; dry, nonproductive cough
- Sore throat
- Bullous myringitis
- Headache
- Myalgias
- Arthralgias
- Wheezing
- Nasal congestion
- Blood-streaked sputum

Differential Diagnosis
Other causes of pneumonia:
- Viral
- Bacterial
- Fungal
- *Chlamydia, Pneumocystis carinii*
- *Legionella*

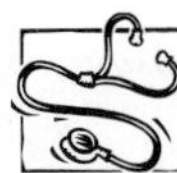

ASSESSMENT

History
Inquire about:
- Onset and duration of symptoms
- Other members of household affected (this is frequently the case)
- Underlying conditions
- Current medications

Physical Findings
- Fever
- Throat—erythematous
- Ears—bullous myringitis (fluid-filled vesicles on tympanic membrane)
- Lungs—decreased breath sounds, inspiratory rales, wheezes, pleural friction rub
- Heart—possibly tachycardia

Initial Workup
Laboratory
- CBC with differential—normal
- Erythrocyte sedimentation rate (ESR)—elevated
- Complement fixation—elevated
- Cold agglutinins—positive if 1:258 or greater
- Sputum culture—mycobacterium very slow growing

Radiology: Chest—PA and lateral—diffuse interstitial infiltrates; small, bilateral pleural effusion

Further Workup
None indicated

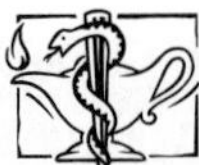

INTERVENTIONS

Office Treatment
None indicated

Lifestyle Modifications
- Smoking cessation
- Adequate rest
- Proper hand washing

Patient Education
Teach patient about:
- Condition and treatment:
  - Hospitalization if severely ill
  - Outpatient treatment with antimicrobials
- Importance of increased fluid intake and adequate rest
- Proper hand-washing technique
- Proper disposal of soiled tissues
- Medications used and side effects (see Pharmacotherapeutics)

Referral
To MD if hospitalization required and NP does not have privileges

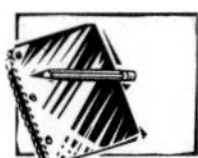

EVALUATION

Outcome
Resolves without sequelae in about 2 weeks

Possible Complications
- Reactive airway disease
- Hemolytic anemia
- Erythema multiforme
- Stevens-Johnson syndrome
- Pericarditis
- Myocarditis
- Polyneuritis
- Polyarthritis
- Respiratory distress syndrome

Follow-up
- Telephone contact in 48 hours; return to clinic in 2 weeks
- Repeat chest film if patient >40 years or a smoker

FOR YOUR INFORMATION

Life Span
Pediatric: Common in this age group
Geriatric: Rare in this age group
Pregnancy: Should consult a specialist regarding antibiotic use

Miscellaneous
N/A

References

Koster FT, Barker LR: Respiratory tract infections. In Barker LR, Burton JR, Zieve PD, editors: *Principles of ambulatory medicine,* ed 4, Baltimore, 1995, Williams & Wilkins, pp 342-347.

Stauffer JL: Lung. In Tierney LM Jr, McPhee SJ, Papadakis MA, editors: *Current medical diagnosis and treatment,* ed 34, Norwalk, Conn, 1995, Appleton & Lange, pp 225-232.

NOTES

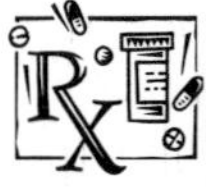

PHARMACOTHERAPEUTICS

Drug of Choice	Mechanism of Action	Prescribing Information	Side Effects
Erythromycin (E-Mycin), 500 mg PO qid × 10-14 days; children, 30-50 mg/kg/day PO divided q6h × 10-14 days	Inhibits protein synthesis	***Contraindication:*** Hypersensitivity ***Cost:*** 500-mg tab, 4/day × 10 days: $10-$20, 4/day × 10 days: $4 ***Pregnancy category:*** B	Nausea, vomiting, diarrhea, abdominal pain, anorexia, rash, urticaria, pseudomembranous colitis—rarely
Tetracycline (Achromycin), 250-500 mg PO q6h; children >8 years, 25-50 mg/kg/day PO in 4 divided doses	Inhibits protein synthesis and phosphorylation in microorganisms	***Contraindications:*** Hypersensitivity; children <8 years; lactation ***Cost:*** 500-mg tab, 40 tabs: $4-$15 ***Pregnancy category:*** D	Eosinophilia, neutropenia, thrombocytopenia, leukocytosis, hemolytic anemia, dysphagia, glossitis, oral candidiasis, nausea, abdominal pain, vomiting, diarrhea, hepatotoxicity, flatulence, abdominal cramps, rash, urticaria, photosensitivity, exfoliative dermatitis, angioedema

Pneumonia, *Pneumocystis carinii* (PCP)

OVERVIEW

Pneumocystis carinii pneumonia (PCP) is an opportunistic infection of the lungs that is seen in immunocompromised persons, particularly patients with HIV infection. It rarely causes symptoms.

Pathogenesis
Cause—*P. carinii*

Patient Profile
- Males > Females
- Any age if immunocompromised

Signs and Symptoms
- Insidious onset of dyspnea
- Cough—nonproductive or productive of clear, white sputum
- Fever and chills
- Weakness
- Fatigue
- Malaise

Differential Diagnosis
- Other causes of pneumonia—viral, fungal, bacterial
- Tuberculosis
- *Mycobacterium avium-intracellulare*

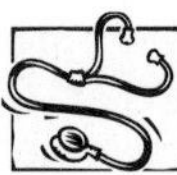

ASSESSMENT

History
Inquire about:
- Onset and duration of symptoms
- HIV status
- Underlying conditions
- Current medications

Physical Findings
- Fever
- Tachypnea
- Lungs—rales, rhonchi, wheezing, decreased breath sounds
- Heart—tachycardia

Initial Workup
Laboratory
- CBC with differential—may be normal or leukopenic, anemia, thrombocytopenia
- If HIV status unknown, ELISA; if positive, confirm with Western Blot
- CD4 count <200
- Arterial blood gases—hypoxemia
- Chemistry panel to include electrolytes, liver function studies (LDH level frequently elevated), renal function

Radiology
- Chest film—PA and lateral—75% show bilateral interstitial or peripheral infiltrate
- May also be normal or have unilateral disease, pleural effusions, abscesses, cavitation, pneumothorax, or lobar consolidation

Further Workup
Bronchoscopy

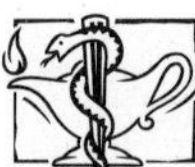

INTERVENTIONS

Office Treatment
None indicated

Lifestyle Modifications
- Smoking cessation
- Well-balanced diet

Patient Education
Teach patient about:
- Condition and treatment:
  - Hospitalization if severely ill, otherwise outpatient
  - Antimicrobial therapy—AIDS patient will require lifelong prophylaxis
- Using oxygen and safety considerations
- Medications used and side effects (see Pharmacotherapeutics)

Referrals
- Consult with MD on treatment
- Refer to MD for hospitalization if NP does not have privileges
- Consider referral to specialist

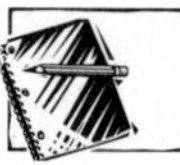

EVALUATION

Outcome
10% to 15% mortality rate

Possible Complications
- Respiratory failure
- Pneumothorax
- Extrapulmonary pneumocystis

Follow-up
Every 2 weeks until stable

FOR YOUR INFORMATION

Life Span
Pediatric: PCP prophylaxis should be given to HIV-positive children
Geriatric: High mortality rate
Pregnancy: To specialist

Miscellaneous
N/A

References

Koster FT, Barker LR: Respiratory tract infections. In Barker LR, Burton JR, Zieve PD, editors: *Principles of ambulatory medicine,* ed 4, Baltimore, 1995, Williams & Wilkins, pp 342-347.

Stauffer JL: Lung. In Tierney LM Jr, McPhee SJ, Papadakis MA, editors: *Current medical diagnosis and treatment,* ed 34, Norwalk, Conn, 1995, Appleton & Lange, pp 225-232.

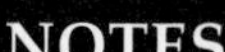

NOTES

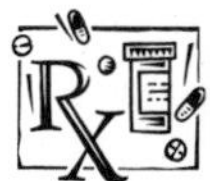

PHARMACOTHERAPEUTICS

Drug of Choice	Mechanism of Action	Prescribing Information	Side Effects
Trimethoprim/sulfamethoxazole (Septra, Bactrim), 10-20 mg/kg/day of trimethoprim PO or IV in divided doses q6h × 21 days; 1 DS tab contains 160 mg of trimethoprim; also used for prophylaxis	Blocks two consecutive steps in bacterial synthesis of nucleic acids and protein	***Contraindications:*** Hypersensitivity to trimethoprim or sulfonamides; term pregnancy; lactation; megaloblastic anemia; infants <2 months; creatinine clearance <15 ml/min ***Cost:*** DS tab × 14 days: $2 ***Pregnancy category:*** C	Anaphylaxis, hypersensitivity, Stevens-Johnson syndrome, allergic myocarditis, nausea, vomiting, abdominal pain, hepatitis, enterocolitis, renal failure, toxic nephrosis, leukopenia, thrombocytopenia, hemolytic anemia
Pentamidine (Pentam 300), 4 mg/kg/day IM or IV × 21 days; may also be used in a nebulizer for prophylaxis—safety in children not established	Interferes with DNA/RNA synthesis in protozoa	***Contraindication:*** Hypersensitivity ***Cost:*** 300 mg/ml, 1 ml: $114 ***Pregnancy category:*** C	Severe hypotension, hypoglycemia, acute pancreatitis, cardiac arrhythmias, acute renal failure, renal toxicity, nausea, vomiting, diarrhea, disorientation, dizziness, confusion, cough, bronchospasm (with aerosol), fatigue, chills, night sweats

In addition to the medications listed here, several others may be used. However, they are beyond the scope of this book.

Pneumonia, Viral

OVERVIEW

Viral pneumonia is an infection of the lungs caused by a virus.

Pathogenesis
Causes:
- Influenza A and B
- Parainfluenza 1, 2, 3, and 4
- Respiratory syncytial virus
- Adenovirus
- Cytomegalovirus
- Herpes simplex
- Varicella

Patient Profile
- Males = Females
- Any age

Signs and Symptoms
- Fever
- Chills
- Productive cough
- Dyspnea
- Headache
- Recent history of upper respiratory tract infection
- Pleurisy

Differential Diagnosis
- Other types of pneumonia
- Pulmonary edema
- Cystic fibrosis
- Pneumothorax

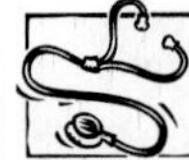

ASSESSMENT

History
Inquire about:
- Onset and duration of symptoms
- Recent upper respiratory tract infection
- Underlying conditions
- Current medications

Physical Findings
- Fever
- Lungs—rales, rhonchi, pleural friction rub
- Heart—tachycardia
- Cervical adenopathy

Initial Workup
Laboratory
- CBC with differential—leukocyte count normal to slightly decreased
- Viral culture if indicated

Radiology: Chest film—PA and lateral—interstitial pneumonia, peribronchial thickening, pleural effusion

Further Workup
Bronchoscopy with bronchoalveolar lavage

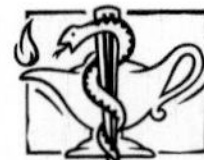

INTERVENTIONS

Office Treatment
None indicated

Lifestyle Modifications
- Smoking cessation
- Adequate rest
- Increased fluid intake

Patient Education
Teach patient about:
- Condition and treatment—antiviral therapy for herpes, varicella, and cytomegalovirus
- Importance of adequate rest
- Importance of increased fluid intake
- Proper hand-washing technique
- Proper disposal of soiled tissues
- Chest percussion and postural drainage (teach significant other)
- Medications used and side effects (see Pharmacotherapeutics)

Referral
To MD for treatment failure or if hospitalization required and NP does not have privileges

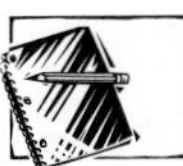

EVALUATION

Outcomes

- Usually resolves without sequelae
- Death can occur in very young with adenovirus or in elderly with influenza

Possible Complications

- Superimposed bacterial infection
- Respiratory distress
- Adult respiratory distress syndrome

Follow-up

In 1 week; repeat chest film in 2-3 weeks

FOR YOUR INFORMATION

Life Span

Pediatric: Infants <4 months old with pneumonia should be hospitalized
Geriatric: High morbidity and mortality
Pregnancy: To specialist

Miscellaneous

N/A

References

Koster FT, Barker LR: Respiratory tract infections. In Barker LR, Burton JR, Zieve PD, editors: *Principles of ambulatory medicine,* ed 4, Baltimore, 1995, Williams & Wilkins, pp 342-347.

Stauffer JL: Lung. In Tierney LM Jr, McPhee SJ, Papadakis MA, editors: *Current medical diagnosis and treatment,* ed 34, Norwalk, Conn, 1995, Appleton & Lange, pp 225-232.

NOTES

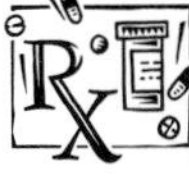

PHARMACOTHERAPEUTICS

Drug of Choice	Mechanism of Action	Prescribing Information	Side Effects
Amantadine, (Symmetrel); adults and children >9 years, 100 mg PO bid; children 1-9 years, 4.4-8.8 mg/kg/day PO divided bid to tid, not to exceed 200 mg/day × 3-5 days; only for influenza A—only effective if administered within first 48 hours	Prevents penetration of virus to host by preventing uncoating of nucleic acid in viral cell	***Contraindications:*** Hypersensitivity; children <1 year; lactation ***Cost:*** 100-mg tab, 100 tabs: $19-$62 ***Pregnancy category:*** C	Headache, dizziness, fatigue, anxiety, hallucinations, convulsions, orthostatic hypotension, congestive heart failure (CHF), photosensitivity, blurred vision, leukopenia, nausea, vomiting, constipation, urinary frequency, urinary retention
For herpes simplex, herpes zoster, or varicella:			
Acyclovir (Zovirax); adults, 5 mg/kg IV q8h; children, 250 mg/m^2 IV q8h × 10 days	Interferes with DNA synthesis, decreasing viral replication	***Contraindication:*** Hypersensitivity ***Cost:*** 500 mg/10 ml, 10 vials: $509 ***Pregnancy category:*** C	Tremors, confusion, lethargy, convulsions, dizziness, headache, nausea, vomiting, oliguria, proteinuria, hematuria, acute renal failure, glomerulonephritis, gingival hyperplasia, rash, urticaria, joint pain, leg pain, muscle cramps
For cytomegalovirus:			
Ganciclovir (Cytovene), 5 mg/kg IV q12h—safety in children not established	Inhibits replication of virus	***Contraindication:*** Hypersensitivity to ganciclovir or acyclovir ***Cost:*** 500-mg vial, 25 vials: $870 ***Pregnancy category:*** C	Granulocytopenia, thrombocytopenia, anemia, eosinophilia, increased liver function tests, anorexia, diarrhea, rash, alopecia, fever, chills, coma, confusion, headache, psychosis, hematuria, increased BUN and creatinine

Pneumothorax

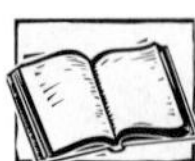

OVERVIEW

Pneumothorax is the accumulation of air in the pleural space of the lung, resulting in collapse of the lung. A pneumothorax is usually classified as either spontaneous or traumatic. A spontaneous pneumothorax may be primary or secondary. In primary pneumothorax there is no underlying cause, whereas in secondary pneumothorax there is an underlying pulmonary pathologic condition.

Pathogenesis

- Primary spontaneous pneumothorax—rupture of a bleb due to high negative intrapleural pressures
- Secondary spontaneous pneumothorax—complication of chronic obstructive pulmonary disease (COPD), asthma, cystic fibrosis, tuberculosis, *Pneumocystis carinii* pneumonia (PCP)
- Traumatic pneumothorax—penetrating or nonpenetrating trauma; may be iatrogenic following procedures such as central line placement, thoracentesis, etc.

Patient Profile

- Males > Females
- Primary spontaneous pneumothorax—most common age group: 20 to 40 years; mainly affects tall, thin men
- Secondary spontaneous pneumothorax—most commonly >40 years
- Traumatic—any age

Signs and Symptoms

- Sharp chest pain—worse with breathing, coughing, moving
- Asymmetric chest movements
- Dyspnea
- Occasionally cyanosis
- Moderate to profound respiratory distress
- May develop tension pneumothorax—with pallor; neck vein distention; weak, thready pulse; anxiety; tracheal deviation
- Shock
- Circulatory collapse

Differential Diagnosis

- Pulmonary embolism
- Pleurisy
- Myocardial infarction
- Pericarditis
- Dissecting aortic aneurysm
- Diaphragmatic hernia

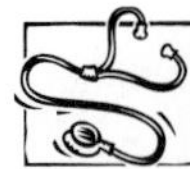

ASSESSMENT

History

Inquire about:

- Onset and duration of symptoms
- Smoking history
- Being at high altitude (flying)
- Vigorous stretching or exercises
- Severe coughing
- Recent trauma
- Underlying conditions
- Current medications

Physical Findings

- Asymmetric chest movement
- Anxiety
- Lungs—decreased breath sounds
- Assess for tracheal deviation, weak, rapid pulse, neck vein distention—all signs of tension pneumothorax—a medical emergency!

Initial Workup

Laboratory: Arterial blood gases if lung collapse >30%—PO_2 decreased, PCO_2 increased

Radiology: Chest film—PA and lateral—to determine amount of lung collapse

Further Workup

None indicated

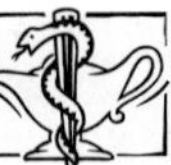

INTERVENTIONS

Office Treatment

Tension pneumothorax—immediate transport to emergency room

Lifestyle Modifications

- Smoking cessation
- Avoidance of high altitudes, unpressurized aircraft, scuba diving

Patient Education

Teach patient about:

- Condition and treatment—hospitalization—if small, may resolve spontaneously; if large, chest tube insertion, serial chest films to monitor for progression (some authorities feel a small pneumothorax can be managed in outpatient setting)
- Importance of bed rest
- Tips for smoking cessation
- Importance of avoiding high altitudes, unpressurized aircraft, scuba diving
- Recurrent pneumothorax—may require thoracotomy or chemical pleurodesis
- Medications are not used except for chemical pleurodesis, which is beyond the scope of this book

Referrals

- To MD for hospitalization if NP does not have privileges
- To pulmonologist for management of recurrent pneumothorax

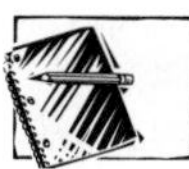

EVALUATION

Outcome
Resolves without sequelae

Possible Complications
- Tension pneumothorax
- Reexpansion pulmonary edema
- Recurrent pneumothorax

Follow-up
1 week after hospitalization

FOR YOUR INFORMATION

Life Span
Pediatric: Usually due to trauma
Geriatric: Usually secondary spontaneous; higher morbidity and mortality
Pregnancy: To specialist

Miscellaneous
N/A

References
Smith PL, Britt EJ, Terry PB: Common pulmonary problems: cough, hemoptysis, dyspnea, chest pain, and the abnormal chest x-ray. In Barker LR, Burton JR, Zieve PD, editors: *Principles of ambulatory medicine,* ed 4, Baltimore, 1995, Williams & Wilkins, pp 648-649.

Stauffer JL: Lung. In Tierney LM Jr, McPhee SJ, Papadakis MA, editors: *Current medical diagnosis and treatment,* ed 34, Norwalk, Conn, 1995, Appleton & Lange, pp 278-279.

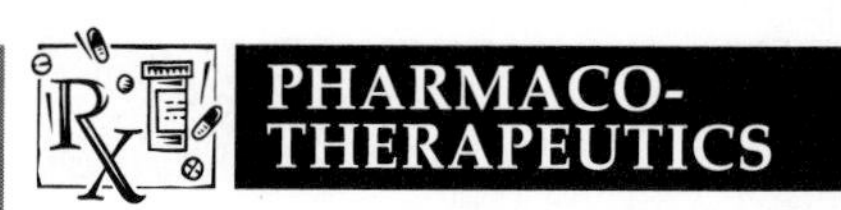

PHARMACOTHERAPEUTICS

Medications are not used except for chemical pleurodesis, which is beyond the scope of this book.

Polyarteritis Nodosa

OVERVIEW

Polyarteritis nodosa is a collagen vascular disease characterized by inflammation of the media of small and medium-sized arteries. It may affect any organ or organ system. It varies in severity from mild, self-limited skin lesions to severe, systemic multiorgan dysfunction and death.

Pathogenesis
- Cause—unclear
- 50% of patients have evidence of hepatitis B or C
- Suggestive evidence of immunologic involvement

Patient Profile
- Males > Females
- Any age

Signs and Symptoms
Depends on organ system involved:
- General—fever, weakness, weight loss, malaise, myalgia, headache, abdominal pain
- Renal system—hypertension, hematuria, progressive renal failure
- Musculoskeletal system—myalgia, migratory arthralgia, arthritis
- Skin—purpura, urticaria, subcutaneous hemorrhages, rashes, subcutaneous nodules
- Gastrointestinal system—abdominal pain, recurrent and severe hepatomegaly, nausea, vomiting, bleeding
- Respiratory system—hilar adenopathy, patchy infiltrates
- Central nervous system—seizures, cerebrovascular accident, headache, altered mental status
- Cardiovascular system—pericarditis, congestive heart failure, hypertension, myocardial infarction

Differential Diagnosis
- Systemic lupus erythematosus
- Trichinosis
- Subacute endocarditis

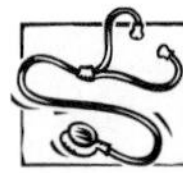

ASSESSMENT

History
Inquire about:
- Onset and duration of symptoms
- Past history of hepatitis B or C
- Past history of IV drug abuse
- Underlying conditions
- Current medications

Physical Findings
- Fever
- Weight loss
- Livedo reticularis
- Purpura
- Hypertension with renal or cardiac involvement
- Abdominal examination—pain, hepatomegaly
- Other physical findings based on organ system involved

Initial Workup
Laboratory
- None specifically diagnostic
- CBC with differential—leukocytosis; anemia; rare—eosinophilia
- Urinalysis—proteinuria, hematuria, RBC casts
- Erythrocyte sedimentation rate—increased
- Serum gamma globulin—elevated
- Hepatitis B and C—positive (30% to 50% of the time)

Radiology: Angiography—visceral

Further Workup
Biopsy of involved organs

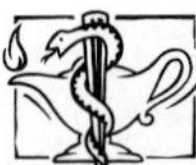

INTERVENTIONS

Office Treatment
None indicated

Lifestyle Modifications
- Smoking cessation
- Low-salt and low-protein diet for renal involvement
- Learning to cope with a chronic, terminal illness

Patient Education
Teach patient about:
- Condition and treatment—steroids and cytotoxic agents
- Signs and symptoms of infection and to report immediately
- Tips for smoking cessation
- Renal diet and fluid restriction if indicated
- Medications used and side effects (see Pharmacotherapeutics)

Referral
To specialist—nephrologist, rheumatologist, or oncologist

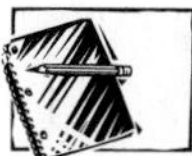

EVALUATION

Outcomes
- Untreated—may be rapidly fatal
- With treatment—5-year survival = 50%

Possible Complications
- Glomerulonephritis
- Thrombosis
- Infarction
- Tissue/organ necrosis

Follow-up
Weekly follow-up during acute phase

FOR YOUR INFORMATION

Life Span
Pediatric: Treatment is the same
Geriatric: Shorter survival rate
Pregnancy: Must be followed by specialist; attain remission before becoming pregnant

Miscellaneous
The patient will need a great deal of support to deal with this devastating illness.

References

Hellman DB: Arthritis and musculoskeletal disorders. In Tierney LM Jr, McPhee SJ, Papadakis MA, editors: *Current medical diagnosis and treatment,* ed 34, Norwalk, Conn, 1995, Appleton & Lange, pp 725-726.

Woolliscroft JO: *Current diagnosis and treatment: a quick guide for the general practitioner,* Philadelphia, 1996, Current Medicine, pp 416-417.

NOTES

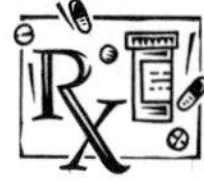

PHARMACOTHERAPEUTICS

Drug of Choice	Mechanism of Action	Prescribing Information	Side Effects
Prednisone (Deltasone); up to 60 mg PO qd until fever and inflammation controlled; taper dose to withdraw	Corticosteroid; antiinflammatory	***Contraindications:*** Hypersensitivity; psychosis; idiopathic thrombocytopenia; acute glomerulonephritis; amebiasis; nonasthmatic bronchial disease; AIDS; TB; children <2 years old ***Cost:*** 15-mg tab, 100 tabs: $14-$35 ***Pregnancy category:*** C	Hypertension, circulatory collapse, thrombophlebitis, embolism, tachycardia, fungal infections, increased intraocular pressure, diarrhea, nausea, GI hemorrhage, thrombocytopenia, acne, poor wound healing, fractures, osteoporosis, weakness
Cyclophosphamide (Cytoxan), 1-5 mg/kg/day; use in addition to prednisone; dosage will be decided by specialist; should be prescribed by someone familiar with its use	Nitrogen mustard; alkylated DNA and RNA; inhibits enzymes that allow synthesis of amino acids in proteins	***Contraindications:*** Hypersensitivity; lactation ***Cost:*** 25-mg tab, 100 tabs: $152 ***Pregnancy category:*** D	Cardiotoxicity, thrombocytopenia, leukopenia, pancytopenia, mylosuppression, nausea, vomiting, diarrhea, weight loss, hepatotoxicity, hemorrhagic cystitis, hematuria, amenorrhea, sterility, alopecia, dermatitis, fibrosis, syndrome of inappropriate antidiuretic hormone

OVERVIEW

Polycythemia vera is a myeloproliferative, malignant disorder in which there are excessive erythroid, myeloid, and megakaryocytic elements in the bone marrow.

Pathogenesis

Cause—unknown; may be result of chromosomal mutation

Patient Profile

- Males > Females
- More common in middle to late adulthood, but can occur at any age

Signs and Symptoms

- Early stage may be asymptomatic
- Headaches
- Tinnitus
- Vertigo
- Dizziness
- Visual disturbances
- Intermittent claudication
- Pruritis
- Petechiae
- Epistaxis
- Ecchymoses
- GI bleeding
- Hepatomegaly
- Splenomegaly
- Peptic ulcer disease
- Ruddy complexion (plethora)
- Bone pain
- Secondary gout
- Sweating
- Weight loss

Differential Diagnosis

- Secondary polycythemia
- Hemoglobinopathy

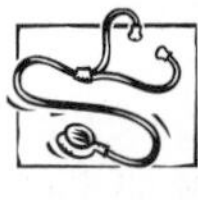

ASSESSMENT

History

Inquire about:

- Onset and duration of symptoms
- Frequent nosebleeds
- Weight loss
- Easy bruising
- Family history
- Underlying conditions
- Current medications

Physical Findings

- Bruises
- Weight loss
- May have increased BP
- Ruddy complexion on face, hands, feet
- Abdominal examination—hepatomegaly and/or splenomegaly

Initial Workup

Laboratory

- CBC with differential—increased hemoglobin and hematocrit, increased RBC count, increased WBC count, increased platelet count, basophilia
- Leukocyte alkaline phosphatase—increased
- Uric acid—increased
- Vitamin B_{12} levels—increased

Radiology: CT scan of abdomen—evaluate splenomegaly/hepatomegaly

Further Workup

Bone marrow biopsy

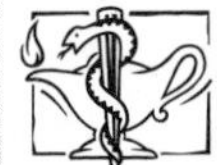

INTERVENTIONS

Office Treatment

None indicated

Lifestyle Modifications

- Adjustment to living with a chronic illness
- Safety measures to prevent injuries that could result in hemorrhage

Patient Education

Teach patient about:

- Condition and treatment:
  - Phlebotomy—mainstay of therapy; may need to be performed every 2 to 3 days initially to decrease hematocrit to 45%; 250 to 500 ml removed each time; will need lifelong phlebotomy for maintenance
  - Chemotherapy for myelosuppression
- Signs and symptoms of hemorrhage and importance of seeking care immediately
- Importance of wearing medical alert tag and carrying identification
- Importance of adequate hydration
- Signs and symptoms of gout and to take medication as directed to prevent gout attack
- Medications used and side effects (see Pharmacotherapeutics)

Referral

To oncologist or hematologist for myelosuppressive therapy

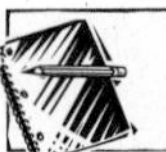

EVALUATION

Outcome

Prognosis difficult to predict—without treatment, median survival—6-18 months; with treatment, median survival—10 years or more

Possible Complications

- Uric acid stones
- Gout
- Vascular thrombosis
- Peptic ulcer
- Hemorrhage
- Conversion to leukemia

Follow-up

Initially every 2 to 3 days; once hematocrit decreased to 45%, weekly hematocrit determinations and phlebotomy as needed

FOR YOUR INFORMATION

Life Span

Pediatric: Very rare
Geriatric: Occurs most commonly in this age group; for patients >70 years, phlebotomy needs to be done slowly, and amount removed each time should be less
Pregnancy: Phlebotomy is only treatment option

Miscellaneous

Some patients live symptom-free for 20 years or more.

References

Whedon MB: Nursing role in management: hematologic problems. In Lewis SM, Collier IC, Heitkemper MM, editors: *Medical-surgical nursing: assessment and management of clinical problems,* ed 4, St Louis, 1996, Mosby, pp 792-794.

Woolliscroft JO: *Current diagnosis and treatment: a quick reference for the general practitioner,* Philadelphia, 1996, Current Medicine, pp 268-269.

PHARMACOTHERAPEUTICS

Drug of Choice	Mechanism of Action	Prescribing Information	Side Effects
For hyperuricemia:			
Allopurinol (Zyloprim), 300 mg PO qd—usually not recommended for children	Inhibits xanthine oxidase, which reduces uric acid synthesis	***Contraindication:*** Hypersensitivity ***Cost:*** 300-mg tab, 100 tabs: $11-$45 ***Pregnancy category:*** B	Agranulocytosis, thrombocytopenia, aplastic anemia, bone marrow depression, headache, drowsiness, nausea, vomiting, anorexia, malaise, myopathy, arthralgia, cholestatic jaundice, renal failure, retinopathy, fever, chills, dermatitis, pruritus, alopecia
For pruritus:			
Cyproheptadine (Periactin), 4 mg PO tid-qid prn; children 2-6 years, 2 mg bid or tid; children 7-14 years, 4 mg bid or tid	Competes with histamine for H_1 receptor sites	***Contraindications:*** Hypersensitivity; acute asthma attack ***Cost:*** 4-mg tab, 100 tabs: $2-$18 ***Pregnancy category:*** B	Dizziness, drowsiness, poor coordination, fatigue, anxiety, euphoria, hypotension, palpitations, wheezing, chest tightness, constipation, dry mouth, nausea, vomiting, anorexia, rash, urticaria, photosensitivity, urinary retention, dysuria, blurred vision, dilated pupils, nasal stuffiness, dry nose and throat
For GI hyperacidity: Famotidine or cimetidine (Pepcid or Tagamet): • Pepcid, 20 mg PO bid—not for children • Tagamet, 300 mg PO with meals and at bedtime—not for children <16 years	Inhibits histamine at H_2 receptor sites	***Contraindication:*** Hypersensitivity ***Cost:*** Pepcid, 20-mg tab, 30 tabs: $45; Tagamet, 300-mg tab, 100 tabs: $45 ***Pregnancy category:*** B	Confusion, headache, depression, dizziness, convulsions, diarrhea, abdominal cramps, paralytic ileus, jaundice, gynecomastia, galactorrhea, increased BUN and creatinine, agranulocytosis, thrombocytopenia, neutropenia, aplastic anemia, urticaria, exfoliative dermatitis

Myelosuppressive agents, including bisulfan, hydroxyurea, and nalphalan, may also be used. These should be administered by a professional familiar with their use.

Posttraumatic Stress Disorder (PTSD)

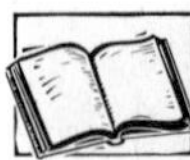

OVERVIEW

Posttraumatic stress syndrome (PTSD) is an anxiety disorder in which the patient suffers severe anxiety attacks in response to the memory of some severe past trauma.

Pathogenesis

Severe catastrophic event outside of realm of normal experience—rape, combat, assault, domestic abuse, etc.

Patient Profile

- Males = Females
- Any age

Signs and Symptoms

- History of traumatic event
- Intrusive thoughts
- Disturbing dreams
- Flashbacks to event
- Psychologic and physical distress when reminded of event
- Sleep problems
- Irritability
- Trouble concentrating
- Impaired functioning in daily activities
- Hypervigilence
- Startle response
- Chest pain
- Depression

Differential Diagnosis

- Psychotic disorders
- Dementia
- Impulsive behavior
- Irritable behavior
- Aggressive behavior
- Substance abuse
- Panic attacks
- Adjustment disorder
- Hypoglycemia
- Acute hypoxia
- Pheochromocytoma
- Seizure disorder
- Thyroid disorder

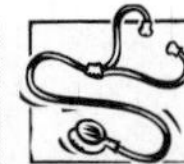

ASSESSMENT

History

Inquire about:

- Onset and duration of symptoms
- Previous exposure to traumatic event
- Substance abuse
- Depression
- Underlying conditions
- Current medications

Physical Findings

- May be none if between attacks
- If patient is anxious:
  - Increased heart and respiratory rate
  - Increased blood pressure
  - Restlessness
  - Looks worried
  - Cold, clammy hands
  - Shakiness

Initial Workup

Laboratory

- Chemistry profile—should be normal
- Thyroid function—should be normal

Radiology: None indicated

Further Workup

ECG—should be normal

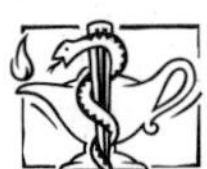

INTERVENTIONS

Office Treatment

- Provide supportive environment
- Attempt to calm patient if having an attack

Lifestyle Modifications

- Cessation of substance abuse, if present
- If precipitating factors in everyday life, may need major lifestyle changes, such as new job, change in home situation, etc.

Patient Education

Teach patient about:

- Condition and treatment:
  - Antidepressants
  - Buspirone
  - Crisis counseling
  - Psychotherapy
  - Relaxation techniques
  - Biofeedback
  - Meditation
- Available support groups
- Medications used and side effects (see Pharmacotherapeutics)

Referral

To counselor, psychiatric NP or CNS, psychiatrist, or psychologist, as indicated

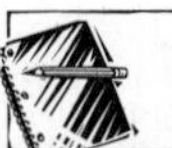

EVALUATION

Outcomes

- Depends on length of time since trauma
- If crisis intervention performed immediately, prognosis good
- If symptoms last over 3 months, chronic PTSD develops—prognosis poor

Follow-up

- Done by specialist
- Initially needs psychotherapy weekly

FOR YOUR INFORMATION

Life Span

Pediatric: May act out traumatic event during play; nightmares, but unable to describe; may fail to grow and progress developmentally

Geriatric: Fewer social supports; medications should be started at lower doses

Pregnancy: Need to avoid medications, especially in first trimester

Miscellaneous

Because of the increasing violence present in society, the health care professional may begin seeing more cases of PTSD. It is estimated that 30% of victims of disasters develop PTSD.

References

Goldberg RJ: *Practical guide to the care of the psychiatric patient,* St Louis, 1995, Mosby, pp 103-104.

Roca PD: Anxiety. In Barker LR, Burton JR, Zieve PD, editors: *Principles of ambulatory medicine,* ed 4, Baltimore, 1995, Williams & Wilkins, pp 147-152.

PHARMACOTHERAPEUTICS

Drug of Choice	Mechanism of Action	Prescribing Information	Side Effects
Buspirone (BuSpar), 5 mg PO tid; maximum 20 mg PO tid; no information on children <18 years	Unknown; anxiolytic	***Contraindications:*** Hypersensitivity; do not use if patient is taking MAOIs ***Cost:*** 5-mg tabs, 1 month: $50 ***Pregnancy category:*** B	Dizziness, insomnia, nervousness, drowsiness, lightheadedness, nausea, vomiting, headache, fatigue
Selective serotonin reuptake inhibitors (SSRIs): • Fluoxetine (Prozac), 10 mg/day PO; maximum 80 mg/day PO; above 20 mg, give bid • Sertraline (Zoloft), 50 mg/day PO; maximum 200 mg/day PO • Paroxetine (Paxil), 10 mg/day PO; maximum 50 mg/day PO • Safety not established for children	Block reuptake of serotonin	***Contraindications:*** With or within 14 days of MAOIs; with drugs metabolized by P450 system ***Cost:*** Prozac, 20-mg tabs, 1 month: $63; Zoloft, 50-mg tabs, 1 month: $56; Paxil, 20-mg tabs, 1 month: $52 ***Pregnancy category:*** B	Dry mouth, constipation, sleepiness, nausea, weight loss, headache, palpitations, postural hypertension, rash, sweating, dizziness, ejaculatory disturbance
Tricyclic antidepressants: • Amitriptyline (Elavil); adults, 75 mg/day PO in divided doses; maximum 150 mg/day; children >12 years and elderly, 10 mg PO tid and 20 mg PO hs • Nortriptyline (Pamelor), 25 mg PO tid or qid; maximum 150 mg/day; children >12 years and elderly, 30-50 mg/day PO in divided doses • Trimipramine (Surmontil), 75 mg/day in divided doses PO; maximum 200 mg/day PO; children >12 years and elderly, 50 mg/day PO in divided doses—not recommended for children <12 years	Unknown	***Contraindications:*** With or within 14 days of MAOIs; with antiarrhythmics ***Cost:*** Elavil, 50-mg tab, 1/day × 90 days: $2; Pamelor, 25-mg tabs, 3/day for 90 days: $188; Surmontil, 25-mg tabs, 3/day × 90 days: $52 ***Pregnancy category:*** Inconclusive	Dry mouth, dizziness, headache, nausea, weakness, weight gain, unpleasant taste, hypoglycemia
Monoamine oxidase inhibitors (MAOIs): • Tranylcypromine (Parnate), 20 mg/day PO in divided doses; maximum 60 mg/day • Phenelzine (Nardil), 15 mg PO tid; maximum 90 mg/day in divided doses • Isocarboxazid (Marplan), 30 mg/day PO; maximum 30 mg/day PO; reduce to 10-20 mg/day when improvement observed • Do not use in children • Use only when tricyclics fail!	Block metabolism of biogenic amines, which increases synaptic concentration; suppress REM sleep	***Contraindications:*** Known sensitivity; pheochromocytoma; sympathomimetics—amphetamines, cocaine, epinephrine, etc. decongestants; meperidine ***Cost:*** Parnate 10-mg tabs, 3/day × 90 days: $117; Nardil, 15-mg tabs, 3/day × 90 days: $99; Marplan, 10-mg tabs, 2/day × 90 days: $99 ***Pregnancy category:*** C	Dangerous drugs, hypertensive crisis, hepatotoxicity, excessive CNS stimulation, orthostatic hypotension, must avoid foods high in tyramine or dopamine such as pickled herring, liver, dry sausage, cheese, yogurt, beer, wine, yeast extract, excessive amounts of chocolate and caffeine

Premenstrual Syndrome (PMS)

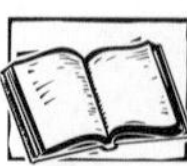

OVERVIEW

Premenstrual syndrome (PMS) is a group of symptoms that generally occur in the late luteal phase of the female menstrual cycle. The symptoms usually abate within 1 to 2 days of the onset of menses.

Pathogenesis

- Cause—unknown; several etiologies proposed—hormone imbalance, nutritional deficiencies (especially vitamin B_6), endocrine imbalance, psychiatric hypotheses
- Lifestyle factors (increased caffeine, nicotine, alcohol, red meat) may contribute to symptoms

Patient Profile

- Females
- Menarche to menopause

Signs and Symptoms

- Depression
- Crying spells
- Irritability
- Mood swing
- Changes in libido
- Sleep disturbance
- Anxiety
- Breast tenderness
- Bloating
- Acne
- Increased appetite
- Weight gain

Differential Diagnosis

- Cyclothymic disorder
- Depression
- Marital discord
- Drug/alcohol abuse
- Endocrine abnormalities
- Eating disorder

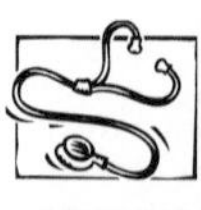

ASSESSMENT

History

Inquire about:

- Onset and duration of symptoms
- Time in cycle when symptoms are most severe
- Menarche, last menstrual period, and type of birth control
- Variation of symptoms from cycle to cycle
- Treatments tried and results
- Underlying conditions
- Current medications

Physical Findings

Physical examination, including pelvic—within normal limits

Initial Workup

Laboratory: Only done if history indicates possibility of underlying cause
Radiology: None indicated

Further Workup

None indicated

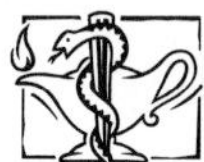

INTERVENTIONS

Office Treatment

Provide a supportive environment

Lifestyle Modifications

- Smoking and alcohol cessation
- Regular exercise program
- Low-salt/low-sugar diet
- Decreased caffeine and red meat consumption
- Stress reduction

Patient Education

Teach patient about:

- Syndrome and treatment options—NSAIDs, vitamin supplements, oral contraceptives, other medications
- Keeping a diary for 2 months to record occurrence of symptoms and severity
- Tips for smoking and alcohol cessation
- Tips for starting an exercise program (aerobic program is best)
- Low-salt/low-sugar diet to decrease water retention
- Decreasing caffeine consumption gradually to avoid headache
- Stress reduction—biofeedback, relaxation techniques, yoga
- Medications used and side effects (see Pharmacotherapeutics)

Referral

To support group, counselor, or psychologist if treatment fails

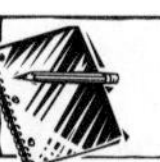

EVALUATION

Outcome

Patient's symptoms become controllable, and patient experiences minimal disruption in lifestyle

Possible Complication

Major lifestyle disruption

Follow-up

In 2 months to review diary; then every 3 months

FOR YOUR INFORMATION

Life Span

Pediatric: May begin within 6 months of menarche, but rare
Geriatric: N/A
Pregnancy: N/A

Miscellaneous

It is estimated that 20% to 90% of women suffer some form of PMS. About 20% have symptoms severe enough to interfere with their lifestyle.

References

Baker S: Menstruation and related problems and concerns. In Youngkin EQ, Davis MS, editors: *Women's health: a primary care clinical guide,* Norwalk, Conn, 1994, Appleton & Lange, pp. 92-98.

Parker PD: Premenstrual syndrome, *Am Fam Physician* 50(6):1309-1317, 1994.

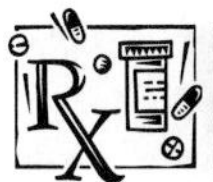

PHARMACOTHERAPEUTICS

Vitamin supplementation has been found to be helpful in some patients. Caution the patient on overuse of vitamins.

Drug of Choice	Mechanism of Action	Prescribing Information	Side Effects
Naproxen sodium (Anaprox DS), 550 mg PO stat, then 275 mg q6-12h; children, 10 mg/kg in 2 divided doses	Nonsteroidal antiinflammatory; inhibits synthesis of prostaglandin to decrease pain	***Contraindications:*** Hypersensitivity; asthma; severe renal disease; severe hepatic disease; ulcer ***Cost:*** 275-mg tab, 100 tabs: $60-$90 ***Pregnancy category:*** B	Nausea, anorexia, vomiting, diarrhea, cholestatic hepatitis, constipation, GI ulceration, GI perforation, dizziness, drowsiness, tachycardia, peripheral edema, nephrotoxicity, azotemia, blood dyscrasias, tinnitus, hearing loss
Mefenamic acid (Ponstel), 500 mg PO tid × 3 days; adults and children >14 years	Nonsteroidal antiinflammatory; inhibits prostaglandin synthesis	***Contraindications:*** Hypersensitivity; asthma; severe renal disease; severe hepatic disease; ulcer disease ***Cost:*** 250-mg tab, 100 tabs: $92 ***Pregnancy category:*** C	Nausea, anorexia, vomiting, diarrhea, cholestatic hepatitis, constipation, flatulence, dizziness, drowsiness, fatigue, tremors, tachycardia, peripheral edema, palpitations, nephrotoxicity, blood dyscrasias, tinnitus, hearing loss
Vitamin E, 400 IU/day PO	Fat-soluble vitamin	***Contraindication:*** Hypersensitivity ***Cost:*** OTC ***Pregnancy category:*** A	Weakness, headache, fatigue, nausea, cramps, diarrhea, gonadal dysfunction, blurred vision, contact dermatitis
Pyridoxine (vitamin B_6), 50 mg PO qd	Water-soluble vitamin	***Contraindication:*** Hypersensitivity ***Cost:*** OTC ***Pregnancy category:*** A	Paresthesia, flushing, warmth, lethargy
To decrease breast engorgement 2-3 days before menses:			
Hydrochlorothiazide (HCTZ), 25-50 mg PO qd; children 0.5-1 mg/lb in 2 divided doses	Thiazide diuretic; acts on distal tubule and ascending limb of loop of Henle	***Contraindications:*** Hypersensitivity to thiazides or sulfonamines; anuria; renal decompensation; hypomagnesemia ***Cost:*** 25-mg tab, 80 tabs: $3 ***Pregnancy category:*** B	Uremia, glucosuria, drowsiness, paresthesia, dizziness, weakness, hepatitis, rash, hyperglycemia, hyperuricemia, aplastic anemia, hemolytic anemia, leukopenia, thrombocytopenia, orthostatic hypotension, irregular pulse, electrolyte imbalance
For more severe symptoms:			
Danazol (Danocrine), 100-200 mg PO qd × 3 months—not recommended for children	Decreases FSH and LH; results in amenorrhea/anovulation	***Contraindications:*** Hypersensitivity; severe renal, cardiac, or hepatic disease; pregnancy; abnormal genital bleeding ***Cost:*** 200-mg tab, 60 tabs: $200 ***Pregnancy category:*** C	Rash, acneiform lesions, oily hair, flushing, sweating, dizziness, headache, fatigue, tremors, paresthesias, anxiety, cramps, muscle spasms, increased blood pressure, hematuria, atrophic vaginitis, decreased libido, decreased breast size, clitoral hypertrophy, nausea, vomiting, weight gain, cholestatic jaundice, nasal congestion
Bromocriptine (Parlodel), 2.5 mg PO bid × 3 months—not recommended for children <15 years	Inhibits prolactin release	***Contraindications:*** Hypersensitivity to ergot; severe ischemic disease; severe peripheral vascular disease ***Cost:*** 2.5-mg tab, 30 tabs: $44 ***Pregnancy category:*** D	Blurred vision, headache, depression, restlessness, nervousness, convulsions, hallucinations, anxiety, dizziness, fatigue, urinary frequency and retention, cramps, rash, alopecia, orthostatic hypotension, shock, dysrhythmias
Combination oral contraceptives (many brands available); dosage and instructions vary for different types; see individual package insert for directions	Prevent ovulation by suppressing FSH and LH	***Contraindications:*** Hypersensitivity; breast cancer; thromboembolic disorders; reproductive cancer; undiagnosed vaginal bleeding; pregnancy; hepatic tumor/disease; women 40 and over; cerebrovascular accident (CVA) ***Cost:*** Varies by brand, $20-$30 ***Pregnancy category:*** X	Dizziness, headache, migraines, depression, hypotension, thrombophlebitis, pulmonary embolism, myocardial infarction (MI), cholestatic jaundice, weight gain, diplopia, amenorrhea, cervical erosion, breakthrough bleeding, dysmenorrhea, vaginal candidiasis, spontaneous abortion, rash, urticaria, acne, hirsutism

OVERVIEW

Priapism is a painful, prolonged, penile erection. It is not related to sexual arousal.

Pathogenesis

- Vascular congestion occurs in corpora cavernosa, not in corpus spongiosum
- Associated with venous obstruction
- Cause—60% idiopathic; 40% associated with underlying condition:
  - Sickle cell anemia
  - Spinal cord trauma
  - Leukemia
  - Pelvic tumors
  - Intracavernous infection
  - Therapy for impotence
  - Prolonged sexual activity
  - Injury to penis
  - Urinary tract infections
  - Medications (chlorpromazine, prazosin, trazodone, anticoagulants, antihypertensives)

Patient Profile

- Males
- Young adult most common age

Signs and Symptoms

Painful, prolonged, penile erection

Differential Diagnosis

Peyronie's disease

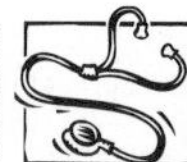

ASSESSMENT

History

Inquire about:

- Onset and duration of symptoms
- Underlying conditions
- Current medications

Physical Findings

Erect penis tender to palpation; may have findings consistent with underlying disease

Initial Workup

Laboratory: No test diagnostic for priapism; may need tests based on underlying cause

Radiology: None indicated

Further Workup

None indicated

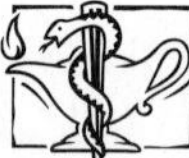

INTERVENTIONS

Office Treatment

Urologic emergency—refer to local emergency department

Lifestyle Modification

Follow treatment plan for underlying condition

Patient Education

Teach patient about:

- Condition and cause if known
- Need for immediate emergency treatment
- Avoiding dehydration if sickle cell anemia underlying cause
- Avoiding excessive sexual stimulation
- Avoiding causative drugs if possible
- Conservative treatment—iced saline enemas, Ketamine (rapid-acting general anesthetic) administration
- Spinal anesthesia

Referral

To urologist

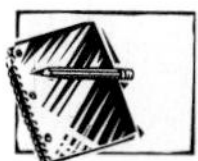

EVALUATION

Outcome
Resolution with preservation of erectile function

Possible Complication
Impotence

Follow-up
By urologist

FOR YOUR INFORMATION

Life Span
Pediatric: Adolescents—inquire about illicit drug use for sexual gratification
Geriatric: Much less likely to be able to preserve erectile function
Pregnancy: N/A

Miscellaneous
Other treatment may include needle aspiration of blood from the corpus spongiosum or creation of a vascular shunt.

References
Driscoll CE: The genitourinary system. In Driscoll CE et al, editors: *The family practice desk reference,* ed 3, St Louis, 1996, Mosby, p 423.

Robinson KM, McCance KL, Gray DP: Alterations of the reproductive system. In McCance KL, Huether SE, editors: *Pathophysiology: the biologic basis for disease in adults and children,* ed 2, St Louis, 1994, Mosby, pp 770-771.

Waterbury L: Anemia. In Barker LR, Burton JR, Zieve PD, editors: *Principles of ambulatory medicine,* ed 4, Baltimore, 1995, Williams & Wilkins, pp 604-605.

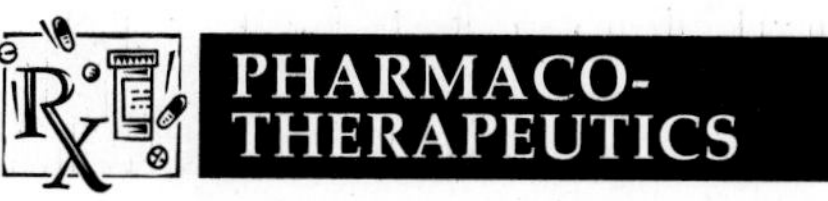

PHARMACOTHERAPEUTICS

No medications are used by the NP to treat this condition.

OVERVIEW

Proctitis is inflammation of the rectum and anus. The condition may be acute or chronic.

Pathogenesis

- Many causes:
  - Most common—*Neisseria gonorrhoeae, Chlamydia trachomatis,* herpes simplex
  - Other causes—amebiasis, papilloma virus, syphilis, candidiasis
- Nonspecific sexually transmitted infection

Patient Profile

- Males > Females
- Young adult most common age
- Idiopathic—major risk factor: rectal intercourse

Signs and Symptoms

- Anorectal pain
- Mucopurulent or bloody discharge
- Tenesmus
- Perianal excoriation
- Constipation
- Mucopurulent rectal mucosa

Differential Diagnosis

- Traumatic proctitis
- Ulcerative colitis
- Crohn's disease
- Shigellosis
- Amebiasis

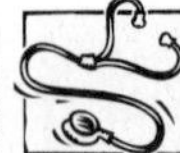

ASSESSMENT

History

Inquire about:

- Onset and duration of symptoms
- Sexual practices
- History of trauma
- Underlying conditions
- Current medications

Physical Findings

- Pain on rectal examination
- Rectal discharge—mucoid, mucopurulent, bloody

Initial Workup

Laboratory

- Stool cultures
- Rapid plasma reagin (RPR)
- Serologic test for amoeba
- Cultures for gonorrhea and chlamydial infection

Radiology: None indicated

Further Workup

None usually; if uncertain of diagnosis—flexible sigmoidoscopy, biopsy

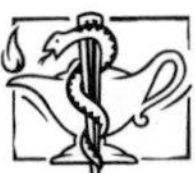

INTERVENTIONS

Office Treatment

None indicated

Lifestyle Modification

Practice safe sex

Patient Education

Teach patient about:

- Disease cause and treatment options—depends on causative agent
- Safe sex practices
- Risk of HIV infection
- Sitz baths
- Medications used and side effects (see Pharmacotherapeutics)

Referrals

Ulcerative proctitis and other cases refractory to standard treatment to physician

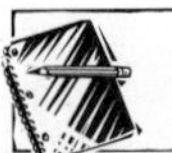

EVALUATION

Outcome

Resolves without sequelae

Possible Complications

- Chronic ulcerative colitis
- Fistula/abscess
- Perforation

Follow-up

In 4-7 days for gonococcal reculture; others in 2 weeks to assess treatment

FOR YOUR INFORMATION

Life Span

Pediatric: Consider sexual abuse
Geriatric: More commonly, ulcerative proctitis—slower to heal
Pregnancy: Cautious use of medications

Miscellaneous

N/A

References

Bartlett JG: *Pocket book of infectious disease therapy,* ed 7, Baltimore, 1996, Williams & Wilkins, pp 304, 306, 313.

Smith GW: Benign conditions of the anus and rectum. In Barker LR, Burton JR, Zieve PD, editors: *Principles of ambulatory medicine,* ed 4, Baltimore, 1995, Williams & Wilkins, pp 1359-1361.

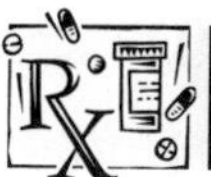

PHARMACOTHERAPEUTICS

All drugs and dosages are CDC recommendations.

Drug of Choice	Mechanism of Action	Prescribing Information	Side Effects
For gonorrhea:			
Ceftriaxone (Rocephin), 125 mg IM × 1 dose; children, 50-75 mg/kg IM × 1 dose, plus regimen for chlamydial infection	Cephalosporin; broad-spectrum bactericidal; inhibits cell wall synthesis	***Contraindications:*** Hypersensitivity; use caution in patients sensitive to penicillin ***Cost:*** 1-g vial: $33 ***Pregnancy category:*** B	Headache, dizziness, weakness, nausea, vomiting, diarrhea, anorexia, pain, glossitis, pseudomembranous colitis, nephrotoxicity, renal failure, leukopenia, thrombocytopenia, neutropenia, lymphocytosis, pancytopenia, rash, anaphylaxis
Ciprofloxacin (Cipro), 500 mg PO × 1 dose, plus regimen for chlamydial infection—not for children	Fluoroquinolone; broad-spectrum; interferes with conversion of intermediate DNA into high molecular weight DNA	***Contraindication:*** Hypersensitivity ***Cost:*** 500-mg tab, 100 tabs: $303 ***Pregnancy category:*** C	Headache, dizziness, fatigue, insomnia, nausea, diarrhea, increased ALT and AST, flatulence, rash, pruritus, flushing, blurred vision, tinnitus
For chlamydial infection:			
Doxycycline (Doryx), 100 mg PO bid × 7 days; children >8 years, 4.4 mg/kg/day in 2 divided doses × 7 days	Tetracycline; bacteriostatic	***Contraindications:*** Hypersensitivity; children <8 years; pregnancy ***Cost:*** 100-mg tab, 20 tabs: $5 ***Pregnancy category:*** D	Fever, eosinophilia, neutropenia, thrombocytopenia, hemolytic anemia, dysphagia, glossitis, decreased calcification of deciduous teeth, nausea, abdominal pain, diarrhea, anorexia, hepatotoxicity, pericarditis, rash, urticaria, photosensitivity, exfoliative dermatitis, angioedema
Azithromycin (Zithromax), 1 g PO × 1 dose; for children, consult package insert	Macrolide; binds to 50S ribosomal subunit and suppresses protein synthesis	***Contraindication:*** Hypersensitivity to azithromycin or erythromycin ***Cost:*** 250-mg tab, 18 tabs: $146 ***Pregnancy category:*** B	Rash, urticaria, pruritus, photosensitivity, palpitations, chest pain, dizziness, headache, nausea, vomiting, diarrhea, hepatotoxicity, abdominal pain, stomatitis, flatulence, cholestatic jaundice
For herpes:			
Acyclovir (Zovirax); first episode, 800 mg PO tid × 7 days; for subsequent episodes, 400 mg PO tid × 5 days	Antiviral; interferes with DNA synthesis	***Contraindication:*** Hypersensitivity ***Cost:*** 800-mg tab, 35 tabs: $124 ***Pregnancy category:*** C	Tremors, confusion, lethargy, hallucinations, convulsions, dizziness, headache, nausea, vomiting, diarrhea, oliguria, proteinuria, hematuria, glomerulonephritis, acute renal failure, gingival hyperplasia, rash, urticaria, pruritus, joint pain, muscle cramps

Prostate Cancer

OVERVIEW

Prostate cancer is a malignant neoplasm of the prostate gland.

Pathogenesis

- Androgen-dependent, slow-growing adenocarcinoma
- Usually starts in posterior or lateral section of prostate
- Metastatic spread through direct extension, lymphatics, bloodstream
- Cause—unknown

Patient Profile

- Males
- Age >60 years
- Risk factors:
  - Family history
  - Environmental factors—high-fat diet, sexually transmitted diseases (STDs)

Signs and Symptoms

- Many asymptomatic
- Symptoms of benign prostatic hypertrophy—urinary frequency, dribbling, nocturia, retention, dysuria, hematuria
- Bone pain (lumbosacral area)
- Weight loss
- Anemia
- Shortness of breath
- Lymphedema

Differential Diagnosis

- Benign prostatic hypertrophy
- Prostate stones
- Bladder cancer

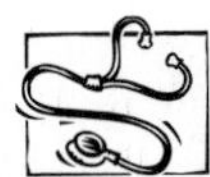

ASSESSMENT

History

Inquire about:

- Onset and duration of symptoms
- Family history
- History of STDs
- Underlying conditions
- Current medications

Physical Findings

Prostate examination:

- Rock-hard nodule or mass
- Prostate may be asymmetric

Initial Workup

Laboratory

- CBC—anemia with metastatic disease
- Prostate-specific antigen (PSA)—elevated
- Acid phosphatase and alkaline phosphatase—elevated with metastases

Radiology

- Transrectal ultrasound if suspect metastases—bone scan
- Skeletal survey
- MRI

Further Workup

Needle biopsy

TABLE 13 ***Whitmore-Jewett Staging of Prostate Cancer***

Stage	Characteristics	Treatment
A	Clinically unrecognized	Medical follow-up; observation; transurethral resection of prostate (TURP) or total prostatectomy
A1	<5% of prostatic tissue neoplastic	Medical follow-up; observation; TURP or total prostatectomy
A2	>5% of prostatic tissue neoplastic; all high-grade tumor	Medical follow-up; observation; TURP or total prostatectomy
B	Clinically intracapsular	Stage B—TURP or total prostatectomy with or without lymphadenectomy; radiation
B1	Nodule <2 cm and palpable normal tissue around it	TURP or total prostatectomy with or without lymphadenectomy
B2	Nodule >2 cm or multiple nodules	TURP or total prostatectomy with or without lymphadenectomy; radiation
C	Clinically extracapsular; localized to periprostatic area	Stage C—radical prostate resection; hormone manipulation; luteinizing hormone–releasing hormone analogs; orchiectomy; external-beam radiation therapy
C1	Minimal extracapsular extension	Radical prostate resection; hormone manipulation; luteinizing hormone–releasing hormone analogs; orchiectomy; external-beam radiation therapy
C2	Large tumors—involves seminal vesicles and/or adjacent structures	Radical prostate resection; hormone manipulation; luteinizing hormone–releasing hormone analogs; orchiectomy; external-beam radiation therapy
D	Metastatic disease	Hormone therapy; radiation to metastatic bone areas; chemotherapy
D1	Pelvic lymph node metastases or urethral obstruction causing hydronephrosis	Hormone therapy; radiation to metastatic bone areas; chemotherapy
D2	Distant metastases to bone, viscera, or other soft tissue structures	Hormone therapy; radiation to metastatic bone areas; chemotherapy

Data from Meredith C: Nursing role in management: male genitourinary problems. In Lewis SM, Collier IC, Heitkemper MM, editors: *Medical-surgical nursing: assessment and management of clinical problems,* ed 4, St Louis, 1996, Mosby, pp 1636-1637.

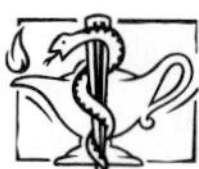

INTERVENTIONS

Office Treatment
None indicated

Lifestyle Modifications
Depends on stage:
- Early stages—cure with preservation of erectile function
- Later stages with metastases—learning to live with chronic terminal illness and preparing for death

Patient Education
Teach patient about:
- Disease process and treatment
- Stages of prostate cancer (Table 13)
- Need for referral to urologist
- Medications that may be used and side effects (see Pharmacotherapeutics)

Referral
To urologist

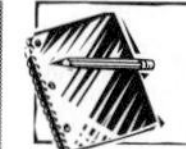

EVALUATION

Outcomes
- Early stages—high cure rate
- Stage D—prognosis poor

Possible Complications
- Impotency—from either surgery or medications
- Pathologic fractures—from metastases
- Pain
- Death

Follow-up
By urologist or oncologist

FOR YOUR INFORMATION

Life Span
Pediatric: N/A
Geriatric: Most commonly affects this population
Pregnancy: N/A

Miscellaneous
The primary responsibility of the NP in treatment of prostate cancer is early diagnosis through yearly prostate examinations and PSA testing for men 50 to 70 years of age. This is however, controversial, and the pros and cons of testing should be discussed with the patient.

References

Meredith C: Nursing role in management: male genitourinary problems. In Lewis SM, Collier IC, Heitkemper MM, editors: *Medical-surgical nursing: assessment and management of clinical problems,* ed 4, St Louis, 1996, Mosby, pp 1636-1637.

Stutzman RE: Bladder outlet obstruction. In Barker LR, Burton JR, Zieve PD, editors: *Principles of ambulatory medicine,* ed 4, Baltimore, 1995, Williams & Wilkins, pp 582-583, 586-588.

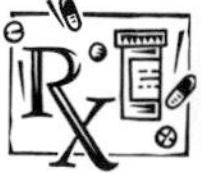

PHARMACOTHERAPEUTICS

Drug of Choice	Mechanism of Action	Prescribing Information	Side Effects
Flutamide (Eulexin), 250 mg PO tid	Antiandrogen; arrests tumor growth in androgen-sensitive tumors by blocking testosterone uptake	***Contraindication:*** Hypersensitivity ***Cost:*** 125-mg tab, 100 tabs: $160 ***Pregnancy category:*** D	Hot flushes, drowsiness, confusion, depression, decreased libido, impotence, gynecomastia, diarrhea, nausea, vomiting, hepatitis, anorexia, rash, photosensitivity, edema, hypertension
Leuprolide (Lupron), 1 mg SQ daily or leuprolide; use in conjunction with flutamide depot, 7.5 mg IM monthly	Potent inhibitor of gonadotropin secretion; initially increases luteinizing hormone and follicle-stimulating hormone, producing transient increase in testosterone; continued use results in decreased levels of all hormones listed above, resulting in medical castration	***Contraindications:*** Hypersensitivity; thromboembolic disorders ***Cost:*** 1 mg/0.2 ml, 2.8 ml: $257 ***Pregnancy category:*** X	Edema, hot flushes, impotence, decreased libido, gynecomastia, initial worsening of bone pain and urinary tract obstruction

Prostatitis

OVERVIEW

Prostatitis is an inflammatory and/or infective condition of the prostate gland. It may be acute or chronic, bacterial or nonbacterial.

Pathogenesis

Causes:

- Acute and chronic bacterial prostatitis:
    - Ascending urethral infection
    - Reflux of infected urine into prostate ducts
    - Direct extension or lymphatic spread from rectal infection
    - Hematogenous spread of organisms—*Escherichia coli, Enterobacter, Klebsiella, Proteus, Pseudomonas, Streptococcus, Staphylococcus*
- Nonbacterial prostatitis—cause unknown; may be *Gardnerella, Ureaplasma, Chlamydia,* or *Mycoplasma*

Patient Profile

- Males
- Acute bacterial and nonbacterial prostatitis—sexually active 30- to 50-year-olds
- Chronic and acute bacterial prostatitis—over age 50 years

Signs and Symptoms

ACUTE BACTERIAL PROSTATITIS

- Fever, chills, malaise
- Dysuria
- Low-back pain
- Perineal pain
- Urinary frequency
- Nocturia
- Acute urinary retention
- Pain on defecation
- Dyspareunia
- Hematuria

CHRONIC BACTERIAL AND NONBACTERIAL PROSTATITIS

- No systemic symptoms
- Dysuria
- Dribbling
- Hesitancy
- Painful ejaculation
- Mild perineal pain
- Mild lower abdominal pain
- Scrotal pain
- Hematospermia
- Recurrent urinary tract infections (UTIs)

Differential Diagnosis

- Benign prostatic hypertrophy
- Urethral stricture
- Cystitis
- Pyelonephritis
- Bladder cancer
- Obstructive calculus

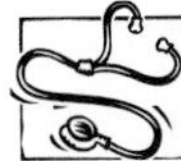

ASSESSMENT

History

Inquire about:

- Onset and duration of symptoms
- Previous history of UTIs
- Sexual history, including number of partners or recent new partner
- Underlying conditions
- Current medications

Physical Findings

ACUTE BACTERIAL PROSTATITIS

- Fever
- Tense, boggy, warm, very tender prostate

CHRONIC BACTERIAL AND NONBACTERIAL PROSTATITIS

- Prostate may feel normal or irregular and mildly tender
- No systemic findings
- Do *not* vigorously massage prostate—can disseminate bacteria into bloodstream

Initial Workup

Laboratory

- Segmented urine cultures and expressed prostatic secretions (EPS):
    - Have patient collect first 5 to 10 ml of voided urine (VB_1)
    - Patient should continue voiding but stop midstream and collect 50 ml of urine (VB_2)
    - Massage prostate and milk urethra—collect EPS on swab, slide, or cup (if suspect acute bacterial prostatitis, do not massage prostate)
    - Have patient void again and collect another 5 to 10 ml of urine (VB_3)
    - Send all specimens for cultures
    - Examine EPS microscopically: >10 WBC/high-power field—suspect some type of prostatitis
    - Interpretation—positive for bacteria in VB_1 and VB_2, negative for bacteria in VB_3 and EPS—cystitis; tenfold increase in VB_3 and EPS—bacterial prostatitis; negative for bacteria in VB_3 and EPS—nonbacterial prostatitis
- For chronic bacterial prostatitis—CBC, BUN, creatinine

Radiology: Chronic bacterial prostatitis—intravenous pyelogram or transrectal ultrasound

Further Workup

May need needle biopsy

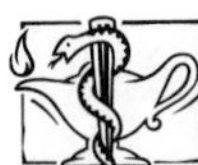

INTERVENTIONS

Office Treatment

None indicated

Lifestyle Modifications

- Increase fluid intake
- Avoid OTC medications with anticholinergic properties

Patient Education

Teach patient about:

- Condition and treatment:
    - Acute and chronic prostatitis—antimicrobials, lengthy treatment
    - Nonbacterial prostatitis—antimicrobials (controversial), antiinflammatory drugs, prostatic massage (controversial)
    - Sitz baths 2 to 3 times daily to relieve pain
    - Possible need for bed rest
    - Increased fluid intake
- Need to stop use of OTC medication with anticholinergic properties (antihistamines/decongestants)
- Medications used and side effects (see Pharmacotherapeutics)

Referral

To urologist for cases resistant to treatment

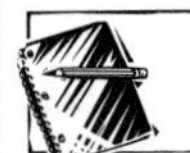

EVALUATION

Outcomes

- May take several months to cure chronic prostatitis
- Acute prostatitis resolves in 4 to 6 weeks

Possible Complications

- Abscess
- Sepsis
- Urine retention

Follow-up

Monthly until cultures negative

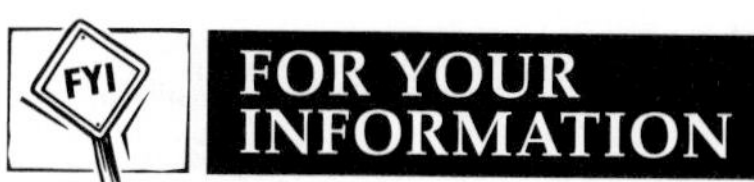

FOR YOUR INFORMATION

Life Span

Pediatric: N/A
Geriatric: Must rule out benign prostatic hypertrophy and prostate cancer
Pregnancy: N/A

Miscellaneous

N/A

References

Criste G, Gray D, Gallo B: Prostatitis: a review of diagnosis and management, *Nurse Pract* 19(7):32-32, 37-38, 1994.

Denman SJ: Genitourinary infections. In Barker LR, Burton JR, Zieve PD, editors: *Principles of ambulatory medicine,* ed 4, Baltimore, 1995, Williams & Wilkins, pp 324-325.

PHARMACOTHERAPEUTICS

Drug of Choice	Mechanism of Action	Prescribing Information	Side Effects
For acute bacterial or chronic prostatitis, use one of the following:			
Trimethoprim (TMP)/sulfamethoxazole (SMZ) (Bactrim DS/Septra DS), 1 DS tab PO bid × 30 days for acute prostatitis; × 6-24 weeks for chronic prostatitis	SMZ interferes with biosynthesis of proteins; TMP blocks synthesis of tetrahydrofolic acid	***Contraindications:*** Hypersensitivity; megaloblastic anemia; creatinine clearance <15 ml/min ***Cost:*** 1-DS tab, 20 tabs: $3-$4 ***Pregnancy category:*** C	Headache, insomnia, hallucinations, depression, vertigo, allergic myocarditis, nausea, vomiting, abdominal pain, stomatitis, hepatitis, enterocolitis, renal failure, toxic nephrosis, leukopenia, neutropenia, thrombocytopenia, agranulocytosis, hemolytic anemia, Stevens-Johnson syndrome, erythema, photosensitivity, anaphylaxis
Norfloxacin (Noroxin), 400 mg PO bid × 30 days for acute prostatitis; × 6-24 weeks for chronic prostatitis	Fluoroquinilone; interferes with conversion of intermediate DNA fragments into high molecular weight DNA	***Contraindication:*** Hypersensitivity ***Cost:*** 400-mg tab, 100 tabs: $365 ***Pregnancy category:*** C	Headache, dizziness, fatigue, insomnia, depression, seizures, confusion, nausea, diarrhea, increased ALT and AST, flatulence, heartburn, oral candidiasis, rash, pruritus, urticaria, photosensitivity, blurred vision
Ciprofloxacin (Cipro), 500 mg PO bid × 30 days for acute prostatitis; × 6-24 weeks for chronic prostatitis	Fluoroquinilone; interferes with conversion of intermediate DNA fragments into high molecular weight DNA	***Contraindication:*** Hypersensitivity ***Cost:*** 500-mg tab, 100 tabs: $365 ***Pregnancy category:*** C	Headache, dizziness, fatigue, insomnia, depression, seizures, confusion, nausea, diarrhea, increased ALT and AST, flatulence, heartburn, oral candidiasis, rash, pruritus, urticaria, photosensitivity, blurred vision
For nonbacterial prostatitis, use one of the following:			
Doxycycline (Doryx), 100 mg PO bid × 14 days; controversial therapy	Tetracycline; inhibits protein synthesis	***Contraindication:*** Hypersensitivity ***Cost:*** 100-mg tab, 20 tabs: $5 ***Pregnancy category:*** D	Eosinophilia, neutropenia, thrombocytopenia, hemolytic anemia, dysphagia, glossitis, nausea, abdominal pain, vomiting, diarrhea, anorexia, hepatotoxicity, flatulence, abdominal cramps, gastritis, pericarditis, rash, urticaria, exfoliative dermatitis, angioedema
Erythromycin (E-Mycin), 250 mg PO qid × 2 weeks	Macrolide; suppresses protein synthesis	***Contraindication:*** Hypersensitivity ***Cost:*** 500-mg tab, 100 tabs: $17 ***Pregnancy category:*** B	Rash, urticaria, pruritus, nausea, vomiting, diarrhea, hepatotoxicity, abdominal pain, stomatitis, heartburn
Nonsteroidal antiinflammatory drugs (NSAIDs); many different types currently marketed; consult manufacturer's package insert for specific dosing and prescribing information	Exact action unknown; may result from inhibition of synthesis of prostaglandins and arachidonic acid	***Contraindications:*** Hypersensitivity to NSAIDs, aspirin; severe hepatic failure; asthma ***Cost:*** Varies with type ***Pregnancy category:*** Depends on product	Stomach distress, flatulence, nausea, abdominal pain, constipation or diarrhea, dizziness, sedation, rash, urticaria, angioedema, anorexia, urinary frequency, increased blood pressure, insomnia, anxiety, visual disturbances, increased thirst, alopecia, peptic ulcer

Pruritus Ani

OVERVIEW

Pruritus ani is an intense, chronic itching in the anal and perianal area.

Pathogenesis

- Often idiopathic
- May be caused by:
  - Oral antibiotics
  - Colchicine
  - Laxatives
  - Psoriasis
  - Atopic dermatitis
  - Contact dermatitis
  - Venereal warts
  - Herpes simplex
  - Tumors
  - Diarrhea
  - Pinworms
  - Scabies
  - Fissures
  - Fistulas
  - Poor hygiene
  - Diabetes mellitus
  - Chronic liver disease
  - Rectal prolapse
  - Obesity and excessive sweating

Patient Profile

- Males > Females
- Any age

Signs and Symptoms

- Anal and perianal itching
- Anal and perianal erythema
- Maceration
- Excoriation
- Lichenification

Differential Diagnosis

Any of the causes listed under Pathogenesis

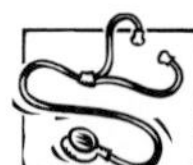

ASSESSMENT

History

Inquire about:

- Onset and duration of symptoms
- Dietary history
- Household contacts with similar symptoms (scabies, pinworms)
- Underlying conditions
- Current medications

Physical Findings

- Red, irritated anal and perianal skin, excoriation, maceration, and/or lichenification
- Digital rectal examination should be done for fissures

Initial Workup

Laboratory: Done to rule out causes:

- CBC—increased WBC count indicates infection
- Glucose—elevated level indicates diabetes mellitus
- Stool for ova and parasites
- Cellophane tape examination for pinworms

Radiology: None indicated

Further Workup

Anoscopy—to rule out fissure, fistula, neoplasm, if indicated

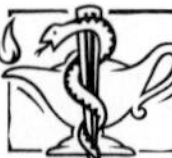

INTERVENTIONS

Office Treatment

None indicated

Lifestyle Modifications

- Depends on cause
- For all, meticulous attention to hygiene

Patient Education

Teach patient about:

- Condition and treatment options—depends on cause
- General measures—tepid sitz bath, particularly at bedtime
- Cleaning anal area—use mild soap, tepid water; ensure all soap is removed
- Diet—eliminate the following as a trial: coffee, beer, cola, vitamin C tabs, spices, citrus fruits
- Wearing cotton underwear
- Using plain talcum powder after cleaning
- Avoiding polyester clothing or prolonged sitting on synthetic material
- Using 0.5 to 1.0% hydrocortisone cream (avoid overusage)
- Acidifying stool with *Lactobacillus acidophilus*
- Medications used and side effects (see Pharmacotherapeutics)

Referral

To gastroenterologist if above measures fail

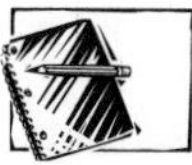

EVALUATION

Outcomes
- Depends on causative factors
- Usually resolves with conservative treatment
- May recur

Possible Complications
- Secondary bacterial infection
- Severe excoriation or lichenification

Follow-up
In 2 weeks to evaluate treatment

FOR YOUR INFORMATION

Life Span
Pediatric: Usually secondary to pinworms or other worms, scabies
Geriatric: Common—may be due to patient having difficulty with personal hygiene
Pregnancy: N/A

Miscellaneous
N/A

Reference
Smith GW: Benign conditions of the anus and rectum. In Barker LR, Burton JR, Zieve PD, editors: *Principles of ambulatory medicine,* ed 4, Baltimore, 1995, Williams & Wilkins, pp 1348-1350.

NOTES

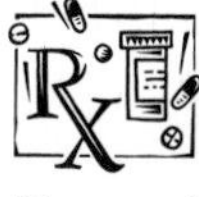

PHARMACOTHERAPEUTICS

Drug of Choice	Mechanism of Action	Prescribing Information	Side Effects
Hydrocortisone cream 0.5%-1% (Cort-aid); apply thin film nightly or bid-tid if severe; discontinue as soon as itching stops	Antiinflammatory; antipruritic	***Contraindications:*** Hypersensitivity; fungal infections ***Cost:*** OTC ***Pregnancy category:*** C	Burning, dryness, irritation, atrophy, telangiectasias, folliculitis, secondary infection
Lactobacillus acidophilus, 1-2 caps PO tid	Produces lactic acid, which makes pH of stool acidic	***Contraindication:*** Hypersensitivity to milk products ***Cost:*** OTC ***Pregnancy category:*** Not categorized	Nausea, GI upset, diarrhea, usually minimal side effects

Pruritis Vulvae

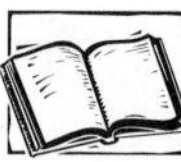

OVERVIEW

Pruritis vulvae is defined as intense itching of the vulva. In the vast majority of patients, pruritis vulvae is a symptom of an underlying disease. It may also be a primary diagnosis, which is the topic of this section.

Pathogenesis

Causes—many:

- As primary diagnosis—idiopathic
- Most common secondary cause—yeast infection with *Candida albicans*
- Other secondary causes:
  - Urinary tract infection
  - Inflammation of vulvar vestibular glands
  - Human papilloma virus
  - Postmenopause estrogen deprivation
  - Malignancy
  - Anal incontinence
  - Excessive heat
  - Soaps
  - Perfumes
  - Nylon panties and panty hose
  - Dietary irritants

Patient Profile

- Females
- Any age

Signs and Symptoms

- Itching of vulva
- Burning of vulva
- Depending on cause, may have vaginal discharge

Differential Diagnosis

Any of the causes listed under Pathogenesis

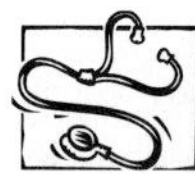

ASSESSMENT

History

Inquire about:

- Onset and duration of symptoms
- Vaginal discharge
- Use of perfumes, soaps
- Dietary irritants, such as methylxanthines (coffee, colas)
- Underlying conditions
- Current medications

Physical Findings

- Depends on cause
- For primary diagnosis—redness of vulva, excoriation from scratching

Initial Workup

Laboratory: Done to rule out specific causes:

- Wet mount
- Urinalysis
- Luteinizing hormone and follicle-stimulating hormone for patient with menopausal symptoms
- Pap smear

Radiology: None indicated

Further Workup

Biopsy if concerned about malignancy

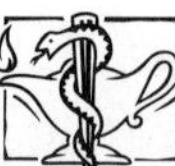

INTERVENTIONS

Office Treatment

None indicated

Lifestyle Modification

Avoidance of irritants (environmental and dietary)

Patient Education

Teach patient about:

- Condition and cause if known
- Treatment of underlying condition if found
- For idiopathic primary pruritis vulvae—lukewarm sitz baths
- Avoidance of environmental irritants, such as soaps, perfumes, bubble baths
- Wearing only cotton underwear
- Avoiding tight-fitting clothing and nylon pantyhose
- Avoiding foods such as coffee, chocolate, tomatoes, peanuts, soda pop
- Avoiding frequent douching
- Medications used and side effects (see Pharmacotherapeutics)

Referral

To MD if conservative measures fail

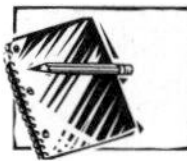

EVALUATION

Outcome
Control of itching

Possible Complication
Severe excoriation with secondary bacterial infection

Follow-up
- In 2 weeks to assess treatment response; then in 3 months
- Monitor closely for premalignant or malignant changes in area of itching

FOR YOUR INFORMATION

Life Span
Pediatric: Same treatment as for adults; most commonly caused by an infection; be alert to possibility of child abuse
Geriatric: Common postmenopausal problem due to decreased estrogen
Pregnancy: Usually have generalized pruritis

Miscellaneous
N/A

Reference
Cullins VE, Huggins GR: Nonmalignant vulvovaginal and cervical disorders. In Barker LR, Burton JR, Zieve PD, editors: *Principles of ambulatory medicine,* ed 4, Baltimore, 1995, Williams & Wilkins, pp 1378-1385.

NOTES

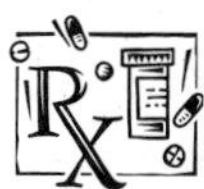

PHARMACOTHERAPEUTICS

Treat the underlying cause if found; for idiopathic primary pruritis vulvae, use topical steroids.

Drug of Choice	Mechanism of Action	Prescribing Information	Side Effects
Hydrocortisone 0.5%, 1%, 2.5%; use lowest effective dosage; apply to area up to qid; many different brand names; start with OTC preparations; if unsuccessful, try prescription topical steroids; stop use as soon as itching subsides	Antipruritic; antiinflammatory	***Contraindications:*** Hypersensitivity; fungal infections ***Cost:*** OTC ***Pregnancy category:*** C	Burning, dryness, irritation, folliculitis, hypopigmentation, secondary infection

Pseudofolliculitis Barbae (PFB)

OVERVIEW

Pseudofolliculitis barbae (PFB) is an inflammatory response to an ingrown hair. It usually occurs on the face, but it may occur anywhere that hair is shaved or plucked, such as the axilla, legs, and scalp.

Pathogenesis
Cause—shaved, curly hair turns inward and grows back into the skin, causing an ingrown hair; results in inflammatory foreign body reaction

Patient Profile
- Males > Females
- African-Americans > Caucasians
- Common in African-Americans—up to 45% of males
- Usual age—postpubertal and middle age (40s to 70s)

Signs and Symptoms
- Papules and/or pustules seen at site of ingrown hair
- Painful with shaving
- Exudate may be present

Differential Diagnosis
Bacterial folliculitis

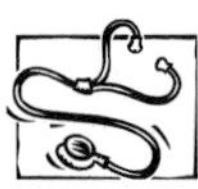

ASSESSMENT

History
Inquire about:
- Onset and duration of symptoms
- Shaving history, particularly number of times per day
- Underlying conditions
- Current medications

Physical Findings
Papules/pustules in beard area, axilla, legs, or any other place where hair has been shaved

Initial Workup
Laboratory: Culture of pustules—usually sterile
Radiology: None indicated

Further Workup
None indicated

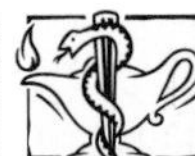

INTERVENTIONS

Office Treatment
Dislodge embedded hair with sterile needle

Lifestyle Modification
Discontinuance of shaving until papules and pustules resolve (minimum 3 to 4 weeks)

Patient Education
Teach patient about:
- Condition and treatment
- Need to stop shaving
- Massaging area with a rough washcloth several times daily
- Preventive measures:
  - Mild cases—remove ingrown hair with small plastic hook before shaving; avoid close shaves; shave in direction of hair growth; do not stretch skin when shaving; use shaving cream or gel, 5% benzoyl peroxide after shaving, and 1% hydrocortisone cream at bedtime
  - Moderate cases—use 0.05% tretinoin liquid or cream after shaving; consider chemical depilatories as alternative to shaving; use oral or topical antibiotics
  - Severe cases—avoid shaving altogether (consider using electrolysis to destroy remaining hair follicles); use oral antibiotics followed by topical antibiotics
- Medications used and side effects (see Pharmacotherapeutics)

Referral
To dermatologist for severe cases

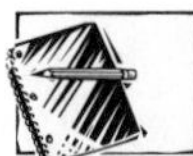

EVALUATION

Outcome
Resolves without sequelae

Possible Complications
- Secondary bacterial infection
- Scarring
- Foreign body granuloma formation
- Disfiguring postinflammatory hyperpigmentation
- Impetigo

Follow-up
Every 2 weeks until resolution

FOR YOUR INFORMATION

Life Span
Pediatric: May start in adolescence
Geriatric: Uncommon after age 70 years
Pregnancy: Most medications should not be used

Miscellaneous
If preventive measures are not followed, the condition will recur. The prognosis is poor if the patient develops progressive scarring and foreign-body granuloma formation is present.

Reference
Habif TP: *Clinical dermatology: a color guide to diagnosis and therapy,* ed 3, St Louis, 1996, Mosby, pp 248-250.

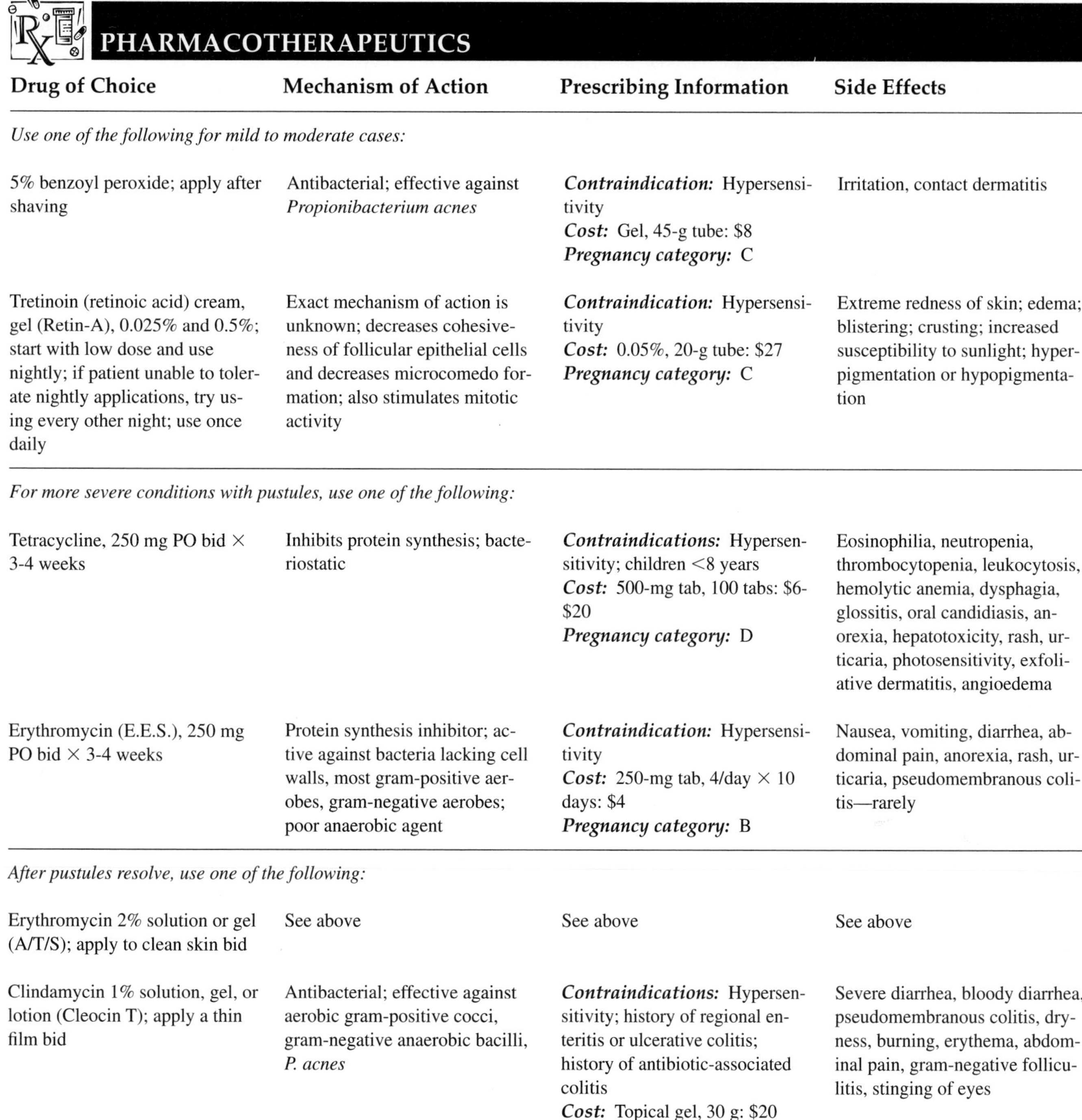

PHARMACOTHERAPEUTICS

Drug of Choice	Mechanism of Action	Prescribing Information	Side Effects
Use one of the following for mild to moderate cases:			
5% benzoyl peroxide; apply after shaving	Antibacterial; effective against *Propionibacterium acnes*	***Contraindication:*** Hypersensitivity ***Cost:*** Gel, 45-g tube: $8 ***Pregnancy category:*** C	Irritation, contact dermatitis
Tretinoin (retinoic acid) cream, gel (Retin-A), 0.025% and 0.5%; start with low dose and use nightly; if patient unable to tolerate nightly applications, try using every other night; use once daily	Exact mechanism of action is unknown; decreases cohesiveness of follicular epithelial cells and decreases microcomedo formation; also stimulates mitotic activity	***Contraindication:*** Hypersensitivity ***Cost:*** 0.05%, 20-g tube: $27 ***Pregnancy category:*** C	Extreme redness of skin; edema; blistering; crusting; increased susceptibility to sunlight; hyperpigmentation or hypopigmentation
For more severe conditions with pustules, use one of the following:			
Tetracycline, 250 mg PO bid × 3-4 weeks	Inhibits protein synthesis; bacteriostatic	***Contraindications:*** Hypersensitivity; children <8 years ***Cost:*** 500-mg tab, 100 tabs: $6-$20 ***Pregnancy category:*** D	Eosinophilia, neutropenia, thrombocytopenia, leukocytosis, hemolytic anemia, dysphagia, glossitis, oral candidiasis, anorexia, hepatotoxicity, rash, urticaria, photosensitivity, exfoliative dermatitis, angioedema
Erythromycin (E.E.S.), 250 mg PO bid × 3-4 weeks	Protein synthesis inhibitor; active against bacteria lacking cell walls, most gram-positive aerobes, gram-negative aerobes; poor anaerobic agent	***Contraindication:*** Hypersensitivity ***Cost:*** 250-mg tab, 4/day × 10 days: $4 ***Pregnancy category:*** B	Nausea, vomiting, diarrhea, abdominal pain, anorexia, rash, urticaria, pseudomembranous colitis—rarely
After pustules resolve, use one of the following:			
Erythromycin 2% solution or gel (A/T/S); apply to clean skin bid	See above	See above	See above
Clindamycin 1% solution, gel, or lotion (Cleocin T); apply a thin film bid	Antibacterial; effective against aerobic gram-positive cocci, gram-negative anaerobic bacilli, *P. acnes*	***Contraindications:*** Hypersensitivity; history of regional enteritis or ulcerative colitis; history of antibiotic-associated colitis ***Cost:*** Topical gel, 30 g: $20 ***Pregnancy category:*** B	Severe diarrhea, bloody diarrhea, pseudomembranous colitis, dryness, burning, erythema, abdominal pain, gram-negative folliculitis, stinging of eyes

Pseudogout/Chondrocalcinosis

OVERVIEW

Pseudogout is an acute, inflammatory condition that resembles gout. It usually involves large (rather than small) joints and is due to deposition of calcium pyrophosphate crystals. It is frequently associated with metabolic disorders, such as hyperparathyroidism, diabetes, hemochromatosis, and hypothyroidism.

Pathogenesis

Cause—calcium pyrophosphate dihydrate crystals deposited in synovial cavity

Patient Profile

- Males > Females
- Most common age >60 years

Signs and Symptoms

- Acute pain and swelling of joint (most commonly knee, then ankle, wrist, shoulder)
- Inflammation
- Joint effusion
- Decreased range of motion
- Fever in 50% of cases

Differential Diagnosis

- Gout
- Septic arthritis
- Trauma
- Rheumatoid arthritis
- Lyme disease
- Reiter's syndrome

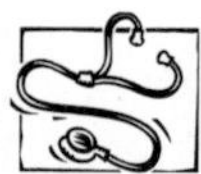

ASSESSMENT

History

Inquire about:

- Onset and duration of symptoms
- Previous similar attacks
- Family history of pseudogout
- Underlying conditions (hyperparathyroidism, hemochromatosis, diabetes mellitus, hypothyroidism)
- Current medications

Physical Findings

- Inflammation of joint
- Decreased range of motion
- Pain on palpation
- Presence of effusion
- Fever (50% of cases)

Initial Workup

Laboratory

- CBC with differential—leukocytosis with mild left shift
- Erythrocyte sedimentation rate (ESR)—increased
- Consider chemistry panel—to include calcium, phosphorus, creatinine, BUN, alkaline phosphatase, glucose, magnesium, uric acid
- Test for ferritin level
- Thyroid function tests (done to rule out metabolic causes)

Radiology: Plain films—calcification of cartilage may be seen

Further Workup

Joint aspiration with fluid analysis

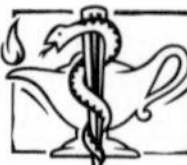

INTERVENTIONS

Office Treatment

None indicated

Lifestyle Modification

Non–weight bearing on affected joint until pain and inflammation subside—patient may need assistance in home

Patient Education

Teach patient about:

- Condition and treatment
- Using a walker or crutches—no weight bearing on affected joint
- Isometric exercises to maintain muscle strength
- Help that is available if patient is living alone
- Range-of-motion exercises once inflammation and pain have subsided
- Medications used and side effects (see Pharmacotherapeutics)

Referrals

- To orthopedist for joint aspiration and/or cortisone injection if resistant to conservative treatment
- To home health agency

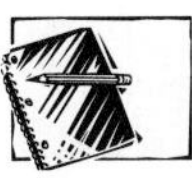

EVALUATION

Outcome
Acute attack usually resolves in 7 to 10 days; prognosis good

Possible Complications
- Destructive arthritis
- Recurrence of pseudogout

Follow-up
In 48 to 72 hours; then in 1 week

FOR YOUR INFORMATION

Life Span
Pediatric: Condition not seen in children
Geriatric: Most commonly seen in this age group
Pregnancy: Not seen

Miscellaneous
N/A

References
Hellman DB: Arthritis and musculoskeletal disorders. In Tierney LM Jr, McPhee SJ, Papadakis MA, editors: *Current medical diagnosis and treatment,* ed 34, Norwalk, Conn, 1995, Appleton & Lange, pp 702-703.

Mercier LR: *Practical orthopedics,* ed 4, St Louis, 1995, Mosby, pp 283-284.

NOTES

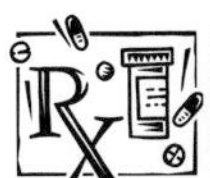

PHARMACOTHERAPEUTICS

Drug of Choice	Mechanism of Action	Prescribing Information	Side Effects
Nonsteroidal antiinflammatory drugs (NSAIDs): ibuprofen (Motrin), 600-800 mg PO tid or qid; any of the other NSAIDs may also be used	Not well understood; may be related to inhibition of prostaglandin synthesis	***Contraindications:*** Aspirin allergy; hypersensitivity; asthma; last trimester of pregnancy; gastric ulcer; bleeding disorders ***Cost:*** 400-mg tab, 4/day × 5 days: $3 ***Pregnancy category:*** Not categorized but not recommended	Nausea, heartburn, diarrhea, GI upset and bleeding, dizziness, headache, rash, tinnitus, edema, acute renal failure

Pseudomembranous Colitis

OVERVIEW

Pseudomembranous colitis is an inflammation of the colon in which pseudomembranes appear. These pseudomembranes consist of fibrin, mucin, and leukocytes produced by bacterial toxin.

Pathogenesis

Cause—antibiotics (most common—clindamycin, lincomycin, ampicillin, cephalosporins; also erythromycin, sulfa-trimethoprim, chloramphenicol, tetracycline); cause proliferation of *Clostridium difficile* and the toxins it produces

Patient Profile

- Males = Females
- Adults 40 to 75 years

Signs and Symptoms

- Abdominal cramps
- Severe diarrhea (may be bloody)
- Lower abdominal tenderness
- Fever

Differential Diagnosis

- Inflammatory bowel disease
- *Salmonella*
- *Shigella*
- *Campylobacter*
- *Yersinia*

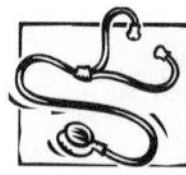

ASSESSMENT

History

Inquire about:

- Onset and duration of symptoms
- Recent antibiotic use
- Underlying conditions
- Current medications

Physical Findings

- Lower abdominal tenderness on palpation
- Fever

Initial Workup

Laboratory

- Stool sample for fecal leukocytes
- CBC—leukocytosis
- ELISA for *C. difficile* toxin—positive

Radiology

- Flat plate of abdomen—distorted haustral markings, colon distention
- CT scan of abdomen—colon wall thick or edematous

Further Workup

Endoscopy

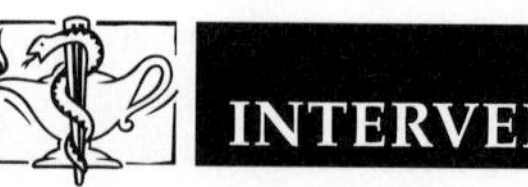

INTERVENTIONS

Office Treatment

None indicated

Lifestyle Modifications

- Use of *Lactobacillus acidophilus* when taking antibiotics
- Increased fluids

Patient Education

Teach patient about:

- Condition and treatment options:
    - Stopping antibiotic
    - For severe cases, hospitalization
    - Increased fluid intake
    - Possible need to be NPO for 24 hours, then bland diet
- Prevention with use of *Lactobacillus acidophilus*
- Medications used and side effects (see Pharmacotherapeutics)

Referral

To MD for severe cases

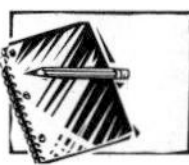

EVALUATION

Outcome
Resolves without sequelae

Possible Complications
- Dehydration
- Hypoalbuminemia
- Shock
- Perforation
- Toxic megacolon
- Death

Follow-up
Every week × 2

FOR YOUR INFORMATION

Life Span
Pediatric: Unusual in children
Geriatric: More difficult recovery
Pregnancy: Can have serious complications

Miscellaneous
Judicious use of antibiotics and keeping the course of antibiotics as short as possible can help prevent this disease.

Reference
Cheskin LJ: Constipation and diarrhea. In Barker LR, Burton JR, Zieve PD, editors: *Principles of ambulatory medicine,* ed 4, Baltimore, 1995, Williams & Wilkins, pp 482-484, 489-490.

NOTES

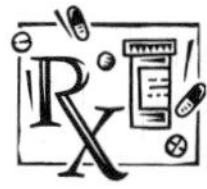

PHARMACOTHERAPEUTICS

Drug of Choice	Mechanism of Action	Prescribing Information	Side Effects
Metronidazole (Flagyl), 250 mg PO tid × 10-14 days; children, 5 mg/kg PO tid × 10-14 days	Direct-acting amebicide/trichomonacide	***Contraindications:*** Hypersensitivity; renal disease; hepatic disease; contracted visual or color fields; blood dyscrasias; pregnancy 1st trimester; lactation; CNS disorders ***Cost:*** 250-mg tab, 100 tabs: $5-$60 ***Pregnancy category:*** B (2nd and 3rd trimesters)	Flat T-waves, headache, dizziness, confusion, irritability, restlessness, depression, fatigue, drowsiness, insomnia, convulsions, blurred vision, sore throat, dry mouth, retinal edema, metallic taste, nausea, vomiting, diarrhea, anorexia, constipation, abdominal cramps, darkened urine, albuminuria, neurotoxicity, leukopenia, bone marrow depression, aplasia, rash, pruritus, urticaria
For severe disease:			
Vancomycin (Vancocin), 125 mg PO q6h × 10-14 days; children, 40 mg/kg/day PO divided q6h × 10-14 days	Inhibits bacterial cell wall synthesis	***Contraindications:*** Hypersensitivity; decreased hearing ***Cost:*** 125-mg tab, 20 tabs: $95 ***Pregnancy category:*** C	Cardiac arrest, vascular collapse, ototoxicity, permanent deafness, leukopenia, eosinophilia, neutropenia, nausea, anaphylaxis, nephrotoxicity, fatal uremia, chills, fever, rash
Cholestyramine (Questran), 4-g packet mixed into water or juice tid	Bile acid sequestrant; may effectively bind *C. difficile* toxin	***Contraindications:*** Hypersensitivity; biliary obstruction ***Cost:*** 4-g packet, 60 packets: $80 ***Pregnancy category:*** C	Headache, dizziness, drowsiness, vertigo, muscle/joint pain, constipation, abdominal pain, nausea, fecal impaction, flatulence, vomiting, peptic ulcer, rash, irritation of perianal area

OVERVIEW

Psoriasis is a papulosquamous skin disease. It is a chronic, recurring condition with exacerbations and remissions. It is a disease of the epidermis.

Pathogenesis

- Cause—unknown
- Genetically transmitted
- May need a combination of environmental factors to trigger onset of disease, such as stress, local trauma, local irritation, infection (such as streptococcal throat infection), alcohol use, or sudden withdrawal of systemic and/or potent topical steroids

Patient Profile

- Males = Females
- Genetic predisposition
- Caucasians > Noncaucasians
- Usually appears between 10 and 30 years of age, but may appear at any age

Signs and Symptoms

- Silvery scales on red plaque
- Usual distribution—knees, elbows, scalp
- Pruritis
- Arthritis
- Nails—pitting, thickening, may separate
- Positive Auspitz sign—pinpoint areas of bleeding under silvery scale
- Several clinical presentations:
  - Discoid or plaque psoriasis—most common; knees, elbows, scalp have plaques; nails have pitting and thickening
  - Guttate psoriasis—occurs most frequently in children; small, numerous papules covering wide area of skin, usually trunk
  - Pustular psoriasis—small pustules over body; may be confined to one area
  - Inverse flexural psoriasis—common in the elderly; affects flexural areas instead of extensor areas; lesions moist without scale; erythroderma (red man syndrome)—skin turns red

Differential Diagnosis

- Seborrheic dermatitis
- Intertrigo
- Candidiasis
- Onychomycosis
- Pityriasis rosea
- Pityriasis rubra
- Tinea corporis
- Squamous cell carcinoma
- Secondary and tertiary syphilis
- Cutaneous lupus erythematosus
- Eczema

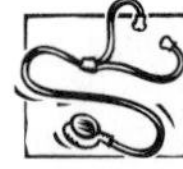

ASSESSMENT

History

Inquire about:

- Onset and duration of symptoms
- Local trauma
- Local irritation
- Infection (recent streptococcal throat infection)
- Stress
- Use of systemic or topical steroids
- Alcohol use
- Family history of psoriasis
- Underlying conditions
- Current medications

Physical Findings

- Most common—silvery scales on red plaque, located on extensor surface of knees and elbows, also on scalp
- Nails—pitting, thickening, separating
- Positive Auspitz sign—pinpoint bleeding when silvery scale removed
- Depending on type, may find small pustules, lesions in flexural areas that are moist, with scale absent
- In children, small papules

Initial Workup

Laboratory: None specifically diagnostic
Radiology: None indicated

Further Workup

None indicated

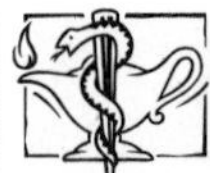

INTERVENTIONS

Office Treatment

If available, ultraviolet light treatment

Lifestyle Modifications

- Stress reduction techniques
- Sun exposure in limited amounts is beneficial; need to avoid overexposure
- If possible, relocation to a desert climate may be beneficial
- Cessation of alcohol use

Patient Education

Teach patient about:

- Disease process and chronicity
- Disease not being contagious
- Stress reduction techniques—biofeedback, relaxation therapy, yoga
- Treatment options:
  - Sun exposure, avoiding overexposure
  - Use of ultraviolet light, oatmeal baths for itching, emollients to soften scale and soft brush to remove scale, topical corticosteroids, tar compounds, keratolytic agents, methotrexate, calcipotriol, psoralen plus ultraviolet light (PUVA)
- Psoriasis being difficult to treat and fact that many therapies may need to be tried
- Medications used and side effects (see Pharmacotherapeutics)

Referral

To dermatologist who specializes in treatment of psoriasis for severe cases or those refractory to treatment

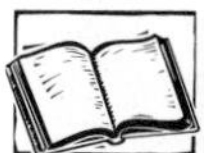

OVERVIEW

Outcome
Initial plaques controlled

Possible Complications
- Pustular psoriasis
- Exfoliative erythrodermatitis
- Rebound of psoriatic process after withdrawal of corticosteroids

Follow-up
- Patient needs continuous supportive care
- Initially, follow-up in 2 weeks
- Some medications require close monitoring

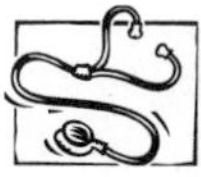

ASSESSMENT

Life Span
Pediatric: In children, onset typically occurs between 3 and 10 years of age
Geriatric: Important to obtain detailed drug history, since many drugs can exacerbate condition
Pregnancy: Some authorities say pregnancy improves symptoms; others report worsening of symptoms

Miscellaneous
Psoriasis can be a devastating disease because of its cosmetic effects. Patients need a great deal of support and reassurance to cope with this disease. With a sudden, severe onset of psoriasis or rapid worsening of existing psoriasis, consider HIV infection.

References
Habif TP: *Clinical dermatology: a color guide to diagnosis and therapy,* ed 3, St Louis, 1996, Mosby, pp 190-211.

Whitmore E: Common problems of the skin. In Barker LR, Burton JR, Zieve PD, editors: *Principles of ambulatory medicine,* ed 4, Baltimore, 1996, Williams & Wilkins, pp 1461-1463.

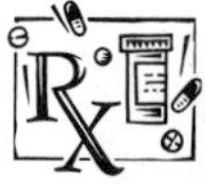

PHARMACOTHERAPEUTICS

There are numerous types of drugs used for treating psoriasis, as reported under Patient Education. To go into detail about each of these drugs is beyond the scope of this book; consult a dermatology text for more detailed information. This section lists only the most common drugs used for mild to moderate psoriasis.

Drug of Choice	Mechanism of Action	Prescribing Information	Side Effects
Topical corticosteroids: Hydrocortisone 1% cream (Cortaid 1%); apply to affected area tid to qid; in adults, may need to prescribe one of the more potent topical steroids, such as Elocon cream or Diprolene cream; use of topical steroids for long periods of time may render them ineffective; overnight occlusion may hasten resolution	Antiinflammatory, antipruritic, and vasoconstrictive	***Contraindication:*** Hypersensitivity ***Cost:*** 1%, 30 g: $12; several available OTC; mometasone 0.1%, 45 g: $29; triamcinolone 0.025%, 30 g: $2-$5; betamethasone 0.05%, 15 g: $3-$16 ***Pregnancy category:*** C	Burning, dryness, itching, irritation acne, folliculitis, hypertrichosis, hypopigmentation, atrophy, striae, perioral dermatitis, secondary infection; if used on large area for extended periods of time, can have systemic side effects
Calcipotriene 0.005% (Dovonex); apply to affected area bid up to 100 g/week × 6-8 weeks	Vitamin D3 analog; inhibits epidermal cell proliferation and enhances cell differentiation	***Contraindications:*** Hypersensitivity; hypercalcemia; vitamin D toxicity; do not use on face ***Cost:*** 30 g: $37 ***Pregnancy category:*** C	Burning, itching, irritation, dry skin, erythema, peeling, rash, dermatitis, skin atrophy, hypercalcemia, folliculitis
Anthralin (Anthra-Derm); begin with lowest concentration 0.1% and increase as patient can tolerate; several different regimens used; most common is short-contact therapy; patient applies anthralin and leaves on for 20 minutes, then washes off—do not apply to face, genitalia, or intertriginous areas	Exact mechanism unknown; thought to bind DNA	***Contraindications:*** Hypersensitivity; acute psoriasis with inflammation ***Cost:*** 0.1%, 50 g: $21 ***Pregnancy category:*** C	May stain skin, hair, and fabric; irritation of normal skin

The above medications may be used alone or in conjunction with ultraviolet light therapy. Tar compounds (Psoriderm, Zetar) are the other preparations that are used in conjunction with ultraviolet light therapy.

Psoriatic Arthritis

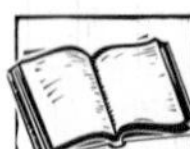

OVERVIEW

Psoriatic arthritis is arthropathy associated with the skin condition known as psoriasis. In 80% of cases, the skin disease precedes the arthritis. Those patients with psoriatic nail disease are more likely to develop arthritis.

Pathogenesis

Cause—unknown; probable genetic predisposition

Patient Profile

- Females > Males
- Common age of onset—30 to 35 years

Signs and Symptoms

- Joint swelling, tenderness, warmth (most common joint—distal interphalangeal joint of fingers and toes; also sacroiliac joint)
- Nails—pitting, onycholysis, transverse ridging, keratosis, yellowing, destruction of entire nail
- Fever
- Malaise
- Decreased range of motion
- Characteristic psoriatic skin lesions (although may be cleared when patient seeks treatment)

Differential Diagnosis

- Rheumatoid arthritis
- Osteoarthritis
- Gout
- Reiter's syndrome

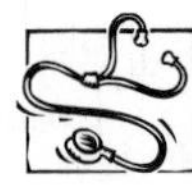

ASSESSMENT

History

Inquire about:

- Onset and duration of symptoms
- History of psoriasis or of undiagnosed skin lesions
- Underlying conditions
- Current medications

Physical Findings

- Joint swelling, tenderness, warmth, decreased range of motion
- Nail pitting, transverse ridges, onycholysis, yellowing
- Sausage-shaped fingers
- Psoriatic skin lesions (may or may not be present)

Initial Workup

Laboratory

- CBC—anemia
- Rheumatoid factor—negative
- Erythrocyte sedimentation rate (ESR)—elevated
- Serum uric acid—elevated

Radiology: Plain films of joints—major or minor destructive changes

Further Workup

None indicated

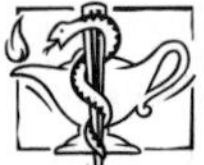

INTERVENTIONS

Office Treatment

Intraarticular steroid injections, if NP trained to do

Lifestyle Modification

Moderate exercise program—swimming is best

Patient Education

Teach patient about:

- Condition and treatment:
  - Heat therapy—may provide comfort and improve mobility
  - Sun exposure—regular, moderate exposure helpful
- Protecting the joints during acute attacks
- Starting exercise program—swimming best; less stressful on joints
- Medications used and side effects (see Pharmacotherapeutics)

Referral

To rheumatologist or orthopedist if conservative treatment fails

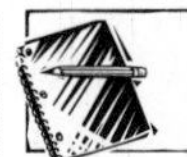

EVALUATION

Outcomes

- Control of skin lesions often improves arthritic symptoms
- Course usually acute and intermittent

Possible Complications

- Arthritis multilans
- Sacroiliitis with spinal involvement

Follow-up

Initially every 2 weeks until stable; then every 3 months

FOR YOUR INFORMATION

Life Span

Pediatric: Condition not seen in this age group
Geriatric: Arthritic symptoms may be worse; start with lower doses of medication
Pregnancy: Cautious use of medications; should be followed by a specialist

Miscellaneous

N/A

References

Hellman DB: Arthritis and musculoskeletal disorders. In Tierney LM Jr, McPhee SJ, Papadakis MA, editors: *Current medical diagnosis and treatment,* ed 34, Norwalk, Conn, 1995, Appleton & Lange, pp 730-731.

Mercier LR: *Practical orthopedics,* ed 4, St Louis, 1995, Mosby, p 288.

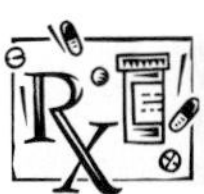

PHARMACOTHERAPEUTICS

Drug of Choice	Mechanism of Action	Prescribing Information	Side Effects
Most authorities recommend starting with one of the following:			
Aspirin, enteric coated, 1 g PO tid or qid; may increase by 300-600 mg/day each week until maximal response seen or toxicity occurs (tinnitus usually 1st symptom); if toxicity occurs, decrease by 600-900 mg/day every 3 days until symptoms resolve; can exacerbate psoriatic skin lesions	Antiinflammatory action may result from inhibition of synthesis and release of prostaglandins	***Contraindications:*** Hypersensitivity; GI bleeding; bleeding disorders ***Cost:*** OTC ***Pregnancy category:*** Should not be used in 3rd trimester	Dyspepsia, thirst, nausea, vomiting, GI bleeding/ulceration, tinnitus, vertigo, reversible hearing loss, prolongation of bleeding time, leukopenia, thrombocytopenia, purpura, urticaria, angioedema, pruritus, asthma, anaphylaxis, mental confusion, drowsiness, dizziness, headache, fever
Nonsteroidal antiinflammatory drugs (NSAIDs): many different types currently marketed; consult manufacturer's package insert for specific dosing and prescribing information; NSAIDs can exacerbate psoriatic skin lesions	Exact action unknown; may result from inhibition of synthesis of prostaglandins and arachidonic acid	***Contraindications:*** Hypersensitivity to NSAIDs, aspirin; severe hepatic failure; asthma ***Cost:*** Varies with type ***Pregnancy category:*** Depends on product	Stomach distress, flatulence, nausea, abdominal pain, constipation or diarrhea, dizziness, sedation, rash, urticaria, angioedema, anorexia, urinary frequency, increased blood pressure, insomnia, anxiety, visual disturbances, increased thirst, alopecia
Prednisone, 5-15 mg PO qd; use for as short a time as possible—until symptoms abate	Corticosteroid; antiinflammatory	***Contraindications:*** Hypersensitivity; psychosis; idiopathic thrombocytopenia; acute glomerulonephritis; amebiasis; nonasthmatic bronchial disease; AIDS; TB; children <2 years old ***Cost:*** 15-mg tab, 100 tabs: $14-$35 ***Pregnancy category:*** C	Hypertension, circulatory collapse, thrombophlebitis, embolism, tachycardia, fungal infections, increased intraocular pressure, diarrhea, nausea, GI hemorrhage, thrombocytopenia, acne, poor wound healing, fractures, osteoporosis, weakness
For persistent, active disease, use one of the following remission-inducing agents:			
Hydroxychloroquine (Plaquenil), 400 mg PO hs × 2-3 months, then 200 mg PO hs × 3 months as a trial	Antimalarial; mechanism of action in psoriatic arthritis unknown	***Contraindications:*** Hypersensitivity; retinal field changes; long-term use in children ***Cost:*** 200-mg tab, 100 tabs: $105 ***Pregnancy category:*** C	Irritability, nervousness, emotional changes, nightmares, psychosis, headache, dizziness, vertigo, nystagmus, muscle weakness, visual disturbances, blurred vision, alopecia, pruritus, skin eruptions, aplastic anemia, agranulocytosis, leukopenia, thrombocytopenia, anorexia, nausea, vomiting, weight loss
Auranofin (Ridaura), 6-10 mg/day PO; reevaluate after 4-6 months	Gold compound; antiinflammatory action unknown	***Contraindications:*** Hypersensitivity to gold; necrotizing enterocolitis; bone marrow aplasia; exfoliative dermatitis; pulmonary fibrosis; blood dyscrasias; recent radiation therapy ***Cost:*** 3-mg tab, 60 tabs: $69 ***Pregnancy category:*** C	Thrombocytopenia, agranulocytosis, aplastic anemia, leukopenia, eosinophilia, rash, pruritus, dermatitis, exfoliative dermatitis, urticaria, dizziness, confusion, hallucinations, seizures, diarrhea, abdominal cramps, stomatitis, nausea, vomiting, enterocolitis, anorexia, flatulence, glossitis, proteinuria, hematuria, iritis, corneal ulcers, interstitial pneumonitis, fibrosis, cough, dyspnea

Other drugs that may be used include sulfasalazine, D-penicillamine, and methotrexate.

Pyelonephritis, Acute

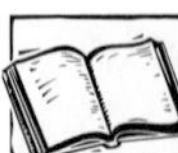

OVERVIEW

Acute pyelonephritis is a bacterial infection of the renal parenchyma and collecting system. Bacteriuria and bacteremia can progress to septic shock and death.

Pathogenesis

Cause:

- Most commonly gram-negative bacteria: *Escherichia coli, Proteus, Klebsiella, Enterobacter, Pseudomonas*
- May also be caused by *Enterococcus, Staphylococcus, Leptospira, Streptococcus*

Patient Profile

- Females > Males
- Any age

Signs and Symptoms

- Fever
- Flank pain
- Shaking chills
- Urinary urgency, frequency, dysuria
- Malaise
- Myalgia
- Anorexia
- Nausea
- Vomiting
- Diarrhea
- Headache
- Suprapubic pain

Differential Diagnosis

- Appendicitis
- Cholecystitis
- Pancreatitis
- Diverticulitis
- Acute glomerulonephritis
- Acute hepatitis
- Renal infarction
- Aortic dissection
- Pelvic inflammatory disease

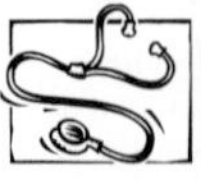

ASSESSMENT

History

Inquire about:

- Onset and duration of symptoms
- Previous genitourinary problems
- Last menstrual period and birth control (use of diaphragm is risk factor)
- Vaginal or urethral discharge
- Underlying conditions
- Current medications

Physical Findings

- Fever
- Tachycardia
- Costovertebral angle—tenderness with palpation
- Abdomen—suprapubic tenderness

Initial Workup

Laboratory

- Urinalysis—hematuria, proteinuria; leukocyte esterase test (positive); nitrites (positive); microscopic examination—WBC casts
- CBC with differential—leukocytosis with left shift
- Urine culture—heavy growth (>100,000 CFU/ml) of offending organism

Radiology: Consider renal ultrasound

Further Workup

Consider renal biopsy in complicated cases

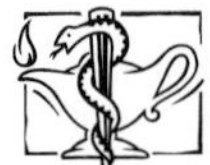

INTERVENTIONS

Office Treatment

None indicated

Lifestyle Modification

Increased fluid intake

Patient Education

Teach patient about:

- Condition and treatment:
  - If severe, hospitalization and IV antibiotics
  - Outpatient care for mild to moderate symptoms, oral antibiotics
- Importance of increased fluids
- Importance of emptying bladder at regular intervals
- Voiding after intercourse (women)
- Using other type of birth control if currently using diaphragm
- Medications used and side effects (see Pharmacotherapeutics)

Referral

Consider referral to nephrologist

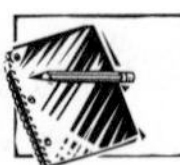

EVALUATION

Outcome

Resolves without sequelae; significant improvement in symptoms in 48 hours

Possible Complications

- Septic shock
- Death
- Chronic renal insufficiency

Follow-up

- If outpatient, phone contact in 24 to 48 hours; return to clinic in 2 weeks
- For inpatient or outpatient—repeat urine culture at 2, 6, and 12 weeks

FOR YOUR INFORMATION

Life Span

Pediatric: Usually require hospitalization
Geriatric: Atypical presentation—may present with confusion
Pregnancy: Requires hospitalization—can result in low-birth-weight baby, premature birth, growth retardation, maternal hypertension, or perinatal fetal death

Miscellaneous

N/A

References

Denman SJ, Murphy PA: Genitourinary infections. In Barker LR, Burton JR, Zieve PD, editors: *Principles of ambulatory medicine,* ed 4, Baltimore, 1995, Williams & Wilkins, pp 327-328.

Hamilton EM: Management of upper and lower urinary tract infections in pregnant women, *J Am Acad Nurse Pract* 8(12):559-563, 1996.

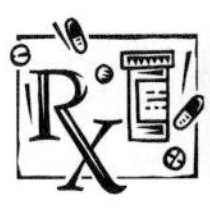

PHARMACOTHERAPEUTICS

Drug of Choice	Mechanism of Action	Prescribing Information	Side Effects
For hospitalized patient, use both of the following:			
Gentamicin (Garamycin), 1 mg/kg IV q8h; children, 2-2.5 mg/kg/day IV in divided doses q8h	Aminoglycoside; interferes with protein synthesis	***Contraindications:*** Hypersensitivity; severe renal failure ***Cost:*** 100 mg/50 ml, 50 ml: $10 ***Pregnancy category:*** C	Oliguria, hematuria, renal damage, renal failure, nephrotoxicity, confusion, convulsions, neurotoxicity, dizziness, ototoxicity, deafness, agranulocytosis, thrombocytopenia, leukopenia, nausea, vomiting, anorexia, hepatic necrosis, hypotension, rash, burning, alopecia
Ampicillin (Omnipen), 1 g IV q6h; children, 100-200 mg/kg/day in divided doses q6h	Penicillin; interferes with cell wall replication	***Contraindication:*** Hypersensitivity ***Cost:*** 125 mg vial, 10 vials: $14-$20 ***Pregnancy category:*** B	Rash, urticaria, anemia, bone marrow depression, granulocytopenia, nausea, vomiting, diarrhea, oliguria, proteinuria, vaginitis, moniliasis, glomerulonephritis, lethargy, anxiety, coma, convulsions
For outpatient, use one of the following:			
Trimethoprim (TMP)/sulfamethoxazole (SMZ) (Septra, Bactrim), 1 DS tab PO bid × 14 days; children, 8 mg/kg TMP/40 mg/kg SMZ PO in 2 divided doses q12h	SMZ interferes with biosynthesis of proteins; TMP blocks synthesis of tetrahydrofolic acid	***Contraindications:*** Hypersensitivity; pregnancy at term; megaloblastic anemia; infants <2 months; creatinine clearance <15 ml/min; lactation ***Cost:*** 1 DS tab, 20 tabs: $3-$4 ***Pregnancy category:*** C	Headache, insomnia, hallucinations, depression, vertigo, allergic myocarditis, nausea, vomiting, abdominal pain, stomatitis, hepatitis, enterocolitis, renal failure, toxic nephrosis, leukopenia, neutropenia, thrombocytopenia, agranulocytosis, hemolytic anemia, Stevens-Johnson syndrome, erythema, photosensitivity, anaphylaxis
Ciprofloxacin (Cipro), 500 mg tab PO bid × 14 days—not dosed for children	Fluoroquinilone; interferes with conversion of intermediate DNA fragments into high molecular weight DNA	***Contraindication:*** Hypersensitivity ***Cost:*** 500-mg tab, 100 tabs: $365 ***Pregnancy category:*** C	Headache, dizziness, fatigue, insomnia, depression, seizures, confusion, nausea, diarrhea, increased ALT and AST, flatulence, heartburn, oral candidiasis, rash, pruritus, urticaria, photosensitivity, blurred vision

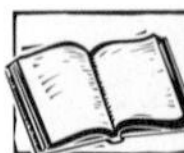

OVERVIEW

Rabies is an acute viral infection of the central nervous system (CNS). Once symptoms develop, the disease is usually fatal. Infection can be prevented with proper, prompt treatment after exposure has occurred.

Pathogenesis

- Passed to humans through bite of infected animal—usually wild animal, but may be domestic animal
- Cause—rabies virus
- Most common reservoirs of virus—skunks, bats, foxes, raccoons, dogs

Patient Profile

- Females = Males
- Any age

Signs and Symptoms

- Incubation period:
  - Lasts 5 days to 5 years
  - Only symptom is animal bite
- Prodrome:
  - Lasts 2 to 10 days
  - Fever
  - Headache
  - Can mimic any number of common infections
- Acute neurologic period:
  - Lasts 2 to 10 days
  - Hyperactivity
  - Hydrophobia
  - Acrophobia
  - Hyperventilation
  - Hypersalivation
  - Paralysis (possibly)
- Coma—evolves over a few days
- Death—occurs within 3 weeks of onset

Differential Diagnosis

Any cause of encephalitis

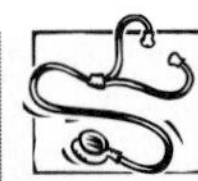

ASSESSMENT

History

Since rabies is a fatal disease, the remainder of this section is directed toward prevention. Inquire about:

- When and how bite occurred
- Whether bite was from domestic or wild animal
- Whether animal was vaccinated against rabies
- Where animal is located and whether it is confined
- How animal was behaving (Did it act ill?)
- When bite occurred
- Tetanus and rabies immunizations
- Underlying conditions
- Current medications

Physical Findings

- Bite wound—assess neurovascular status and motor function distal to wound
- Assess for signs and symptoms of infection

Initial Workup

Laboratory

- CBC with differential—increased WBC count if infection present
- If concerned about rabies disease, test cerebrospinal fluid (CSF):
  - WBC count normal or pleocytosis
  - Protein—normal or moderately elevated
- Rabies antibody titer on serum and CSF (available only at state and federal reference laboratories)

Radiology: Order x-ray studies if suspect injury or foreign body

Further Workup

None indicated

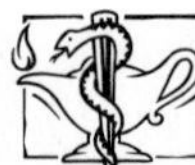

INTERVENTIONS

Office Treatment

- Thorough wound cleaning with copious amounts of saline and 1% povidone-iodine
- Irrigate under pressure
- Scrub surrounding area
- Trim jagged edges
- Debride as needed

Lifestyle Modification

Avoidance of animal bites

Patient Education

Teach patient about:

- Keeping wound clean
- Signs and symptoms of infection
- Signs and symptoms of rabies
- Staying away from wild animals
- Avoiding animals that appear ill
- Medications used and side effects (see Pharmacotherapeutics)

Referrals

- To MD if suspect rabies
- Bites of ears, face, genitalia, hands, and feet—consult or refer

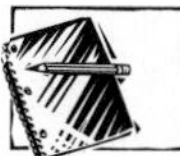

EVALUATION

Outcomes

- With proper postexposure treatment, patient does not develop rabies
- No failures with proper treatment have been reported

Possible Complication

Development of rabies, leading to death

Follow-up

Reevaluate wound and change dressing in 2 days

FOR YOUR INFORMATION

Life Span

Pediatric: Treatment the same
Geriatric: Treatment the same
Pregnancy: Do not give live vaccine

Miscellaneous

N/A

References

Bartlett JG: *Pocket book of infectious disease therapy,* Baltimore, 1996, Williams & Wilkins, pp 110-111.

Pierce NF: Bacterial infections of the skin. In Barker LR, Burton JR, Zieve PD, editors: *Principles of ambulatory medicine,* ed 4, Baltimore, 1995, Williams & Wilkins, pp 305-306, 397.

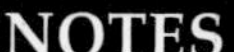

NOTES

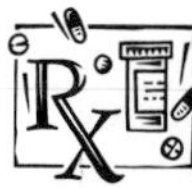

PHARMACOTHERAPEUTICS

For patients not previously immunized, give both human rabies immune globulin and either of the vaccines listed here. For patients previously vaccinated, give either vaccine but do *not* give immune globulin.

Drug of Choice	Mechanism of Action	Prescribing Information	Side Effects
Human rabies immune globulin, 20 IU/kg body weight; half of total dose should be infiltrated around wound if possible; using different syringe, give other half of dosage IM—do not give to patients previously immunized	Provides passive immunity	***Contraindication:*** Hypersensitivity to immune globulin or thimerosal ***Cost:*** 150 IU/ml, 2 ml: $85-$120 ***Pregnancy category:*** C	Pain at injection site, rash, pruritus, arthralgia, lymphadenopathy, anaphylaxis, headache, fatigue, malaise, abdominal pain
Human diploid cell rabies vaccine or rabies vaccine adsorbed: • For patients not previously vaccinated: 1 ml IM in deltoid—not in same site as immune globulin; 1 dose on days 0, 3, 7, 14, and 28 • For patients previously vaccinated: 1 ml IM in deltoid on days 0 and 3	Provides active immunity	***Contraindications:*** None known ***Cost:*** 1 ml: $120 ***Pregnancy category:*** C	Pain; erythema, swelling, and itching at injection site; headache; nausea; abdominal pain; muscle aches; dizziness

Rape Crisis Syndrome

OVERVIEW

Rape crisis syndrome is a syndrome that is suffered by anyone who has been raped. Rape is the act of sexual penetration against a person's will. It is a physically, psychologically, and socially traumatic event.

Pathogenesis
Sexual penetration using force or coercion against a person's will

Patient Profile
- Females > Males
- Most are in teens and early 20s
- Increasing number of males seeking treatment

Signs and Symptoms
- Fear
- Shaking
- Sullen
- Blunted affect
- Physical trauma—may be anywhere on body, but especially on genitalia

Differential Diagnosis
Consenting sex among adults

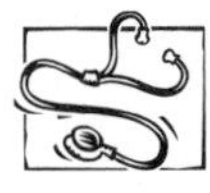

ASSESSMENT

History
Careful history must be taken; inquire about:
- When and where rape occurred
- Type of sexual penetration
- Other injuries sustained
- Description of attacker
- Weapons used
- Whether victim showered or bathed before seeking treatment
- Whether victim changed clothes
- Gynecologic history—last menstrual period; pregnancies and births
- History of sexually transmitted diseases (STDs)
- HIV status
- Gynecologic surgeries
- Birth control
- Underlying conditions
- Current medications

Physical Findings
- Head-to-toe assessment for evidence of physical trauma—document all signs of trauma
- Woods lamp to detect semen on clothes and skin
- Increased heart rate, respiratory rate, and blood pressure
- Gynecologic and rectal examination—lacerations, bruises, vaginal and/or rectal bleeding, bite marks
- Use care obtaining specimens—no lubricant on speculum

Initial Workup
Laboratory
- Wet mount—presence or absence of sperm and whether or not motile; look for trichomonads
- Cultures for gonorrhea and chlamydial infection
- Urine or serum pregnancy test
- HIV screen
- Pap smears from vagina and rectum
- Rapid plasma reagin (RPR) or VDRL
- Hepatitis B

Radiology: None unless possible fracture from physical trauma

Further Workup
- Repeat pregnancy test if next menses missed
- Repeat HIV test and hepatitis B in 3 months

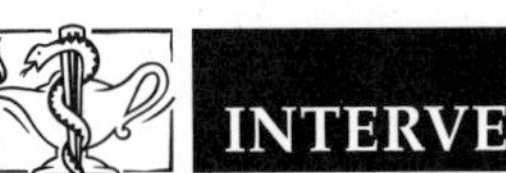

INTERVENTIONS

Office Treatment
- Notify authorities
- Provide supportive environment
- Obtain appropriate specimens

Lifestyle Modifications
- May feel need to move, change jobs
- Relationship with spouse or other partners may change
- May live in fear of repeat attack

Patient Education
Teach patient about:
- Rape being traumatic event—victim not to blame
- Support services available
- Counseling services
- Importance of using counseling and support services
- Importance of involving partner in counseling
- Needing treatment of possible STDs
- Using anxiolytics as necessary
- Needing repeat HIV testing
- Medications used and side effects (see Pharmacotherapeutics)

Referral
To person trained in helping rape victims

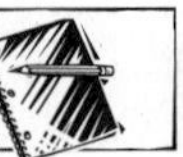

EVALUATION

Outcome
Patient is able to resume normal lifestyle

Possible Complications
- Pregnancy
- Chronic posttraumatic stress disorder
- STDs
- Permanent physical and psychologic scars

Follow-up
- With counselor for therapy
- With NP in 10 to 14 days for pregnancy test, assessment for vaginitis, and repeat cultures for gonorrhea and chlamydial infection
- Repeat RPR in 6 to 8 weeks
- Repeat HIV test in 3 months

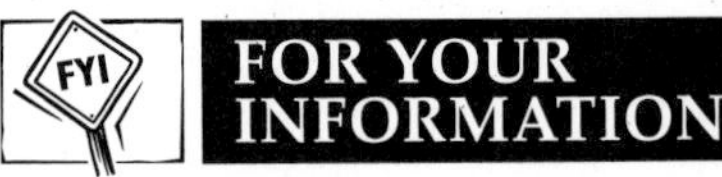

FOR YOUR INFORMATION

Life Span
Pediatric: May require more intense therapy

Geriatric: More likely to suffer severe physical injuries such as fractures

Pregnancy: Close observation for onset of preterm labor

Miscellaneous
Every clinic should have a protocol available for the treatment of rape victims. This will help ensure that all state laws and requirements are met during the examination.

References

Barr NK: Emergency care environment. In Phipps WJ et al, editors: *Medical-surgical nursing: concepts and clinical practice,* ed 5, St Louis, 1995, Mosby, pp 734-737.

Patterson KA, Carngo L: Nursing role in management—female reproductive problems. In Lewis SM, Collier IC, Heitkemper MM, editors: *Medical-surgical nursing: assessment and management of clinical problems,* ed 4, St Louis, 1996, Mosby, pp 1601-1603.

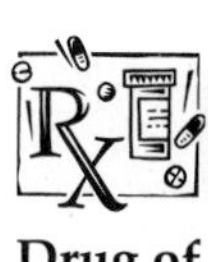

PHARMACOTHERAPEUTICS

Drug of Choice	Mechanism of Action	Prescribing Information	Side Effects
For anxiety, use one of the following:			
Buspirone (BuSpar), 5 mg PO bid-tid, maximum 60 mg daily; used for generalized anxiety disorder—not recommended for children <18 years—do not administer with MAOIs	Unknown; anxiolytic	***Contraindication:*** Hypersensitivity ***Cost:*** 5-mg tab, 100 tabs: \$60-\$65 ***Pregnancy category:*** B	Dizziness, insomnia, nervousness, drowsiness and lightheadedness, nausea, vomiting, headache, fatigue
Benzodiazepine (alprazolam, lorazepam, or diazepam); dosage depends on drug used: • Alprazolam (Xanax), 0.5 mg PO bid-tid—not recommended for children <18 years • Lorazepam (Ativan), 1-3 mg PO bid-tid—not recommended for children <12 years • Diazepam (Valium), 2-10 mg PO tid-qid; children, 1-2.5 mg PO tid-qid; controlled substances, Schedule IV	Antianxiety; anticonvulsant; hypnotic effects; muscle relaxant	***Contraindications:*** Hypersensitivity; narrow-angle glaucoma; psychosis ***Cost:*** Alprazolam: 0.5-mg tab, 100 tabs: \$7-\$72; lorazepam: 1-mg tab, 100 tabs: \$23; diazepam: 2-mg tab, 100 tabs: \$2-\$43 ***Pregnancy category:*** D	Drowsiness, hiccups, dizziness, loss of dexterity, constipation, confusion, nausea, decreased libido, vertigo, sleep disturbances, headaches, abdominal cramping, unsteadiness, blurred vision, addiction—all have high abuse potential
For gonorrhea, use one of the following:			
Ceftriaxone (Rocephin), 250 mg IM × 1; children, 50-75 mg/kg/day IM × 1	Cephalosporin; broad-spectrum antibiotic—bactericidal; inhibits cell wall synthesis	***Contraindication:*** Hypersensitivity to cephalosporins, penicillins ***Cost:*** 1-g vial: \$130 ***Pregnancy category:*** B	Pseudomembranous colitis, pain at injection site, rash, eosinophilia, thrombocytosis, leukopenia, diarrhea, nausea, vomiting
Ciprofloxacin (Cipro), 500 mg PO, 1 dose—not recommended for children	Fluoroquinolone; broad-spectrum antibiotic—bactericidal; interferes with DNA synthesis	***Contraindication:*** Hypersensitivity to quinolones or to ciprofloxacin ***Cost:*** 250-mg tabs, 2/day: \$6 ***Pregnancy category:*** C	Pseudomembranous colitis, nausea, vomiting, diarrhea, abdominal pain/discomfort, headache, restlessness, rash; many other side effects may occur
For chlamydial infection, use one of the following:			
Azithromycin (Zithromax), 1 g PO, 1 dose	Azalide—subclass of macrolides; interferes with protein synthesis	***Contraindication:*** Hypersensitivity to azithromycin or other macrolides ***Cost:*** 250-mg tabs, 4/day: \$32 ***Pregnancy category:*** B	Pseudomembranous colitis, nausea, vomiting, diarrhea, abdominal pain, angioedema, cholestatic jaundice, palpitations, chest pain, monilia, vaginitis, dizziness, headache, fatigue, rash
Doxycycline (Doryx), 100 mg PO bid × 7 days; child >8 years, 4.4 mg/kg/day PO divided q12h × 7 days	Tetracycline, bacteriostatic; inhibits protein synthesis	***Contraindications:*** Hypersensitivity to tetracyclines; last half of pregnancy and children <8 years ***Cost:*** 100-mg tabs, 2/day × 7 days: \$5 ***Pregnancy category:*** D	Anorexia, nausea, vomiting, diarrhea, glossitis, dysphagia, enterocolitis, hepatotoxicity, rash, photosensitivity, anaphylaxis, renal toxicity, pericarditis

Raynaud's Phenomenon or Disease

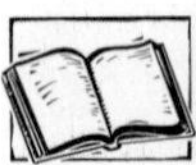

OVERVIEW

Raynaud's phenomenon or disease occurs as a result of vasospasm of the vessels of the digits in response to cold or stress.

Pathogenesis

- Raynaud's phenomenon (50% of cases)—occurs in presence of scleroderma or other connective tissue diseases
- Raynaud's disease (50% of cases)—occurs in absence of other diseases
- Cause—unknown; several theories have implicated adrenergic receptors and serotonin

Patient Profile

- Males = Females—Raynaud's phenomenon
- Females > Males—Raynaud's disease
- Most common age—15 to 45 years

Signs and Symptoms

- With cold exposure, fingertips turn white, then cyanotic; fingertips turn red and are painful with warming
- Severe cases—ulceration of finger pads; progresses to autoamputation

Differential Diagnosis

- Rheumatoid arthritis
- Scleroderma
- Systemic lupus erythematosus
- Carpal tunnel syndrome
- Thoracic outlet syndrome
- Cryoglobulinemias
- Waldenstrom's macroglobulinemia
- Acrocyanosis
- Polycythemia
- Occupational injury
- Drugs (beta-blockers, clonidine, ergotamine, methysergide, amphetamines, bromocriptine, bleomycin, vinblastine, cisplatin, cyclosporine)

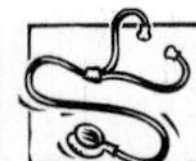

ASSESSMENT

History

Inquire about:

- Onset and duration of symptoms
- Drug history
- Smoking history
- Employment history (working outdoors and/or using vibrating tools are risk factors)
- Treatments tried and results
- Underlying conditions
- Current medications

Physical Findings

- Raynaud's phenomenon—may have early signs of scleroderma or other connective tissue disease
- Raynaud's disease—normal physical examination if between attacks
- Both phenomenon and disease during an attack—pallor followed by cyanosis of fingers (rarely affects toes)
- During recovery—fingers may throb and have slight swelling, paresthesia, and intense rubor
- Raynaud's phenomenon—may be unilateral and only affect 1 or 2 fingers
- Raynaud's disease—tends to be progressive and involve fingers of both hands
- If either phenomenon or disease is severe—ulceration of finger pads, which may progress to autoamputation

Initial Workup

Laboratory: Test for underlying secondary causes—CBC, erythrocyte sedimentation rate (ESR), rheumatoid factor, antinuclear antibody, immunoelectrophoresis

Radiology: None indicated

Further Workup

- Cold challenge test—to elicit color changes in digits
- Nail fold capillaroscopy—look for enlarged, irregular capillary loops as found in other connective tissue diseases

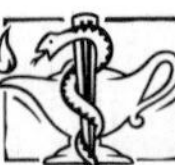

INTERVENTIONS

Office Treatment

None indicated

Lifestyle Modifications

- Smoking cessation
- Avoidance of cold and vibrating tools—could necessitate a change in occupation if possible
- Avoidance of trauma to fingers

Patient Education

Teach patient about:

- Disease process and treatment
- Any underlying conditions
- Treatment with calcium channel blockers to prevent vasospasm
- Dressing warmly and wearing gloves
- Tips for quiting smoking
- Safety precautions to take to avoid trauma to fingers
- Biofeedback techniques to increase hand temperature
- Stress reduction techniques
- Immediately seeking treatment if ulceration occurs
- Medications used and side effects (see Pharmacotherapeutics)

Referral

If underlying disease present, refer to specialist in that field

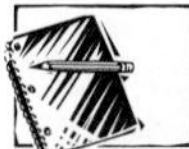

EVALUATION

Outcome

Long disease course requiring much emotional support

Possible Complications

- Gangrene
- Autoamputation

Follow-up

- Every 2 weeks × 2; then monthly × 2; then every 3 months
- Monitor for signs and symptoms of associated diseases

FOR YOUR INFORMATION

Life Span

Pediatric: In children, usually associated with systemic lupus erythematosus or scleroderma
Geriatric: Almost always associated with underlying condition
Pregnancy: To specialist

Miscellaneous

Continuous monitoring for associated diseases is required, since it has been found that Raynaud's phenomenon or disease can precede other diseases by an average of 11 years.

References

Habif TP: *Clinical dermatology: A color guide to diagnosis and therapy,* ed 3, St Louis, 1996, Mosby, pp 556-557.

Hellman D: Nonarticular rheumatic disorders. In Barker LR, Burton JR, Zieve PD, editors: *Principles of ambulatory medicine,* ed 4, Baltimore, 1995, Williams & Wilkins, pp 892-895.

NOTES

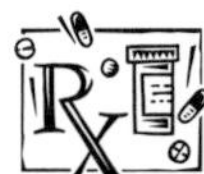

PHARMACOTHERAPEUTICS

Drug of Choice	Mechanism of Action	Prescribing Information	Side Effects
Nifedipine (Procardia XL), 30-90 mg/day; may only need to take during winter months	Calcium channel blocker—prevents vasospasm	***Contraindication:*** Hypersensitivity ***Cost:*** 30-mg tab, 100 tabs: $95 ***Pregnancy category:*** C	Headache, fatigue, drowsiness, dizziness, anxiety, depression, weakness, insomnia, tinnitus, dysrhythmias, edema, congestive heart failure (CHF), hypotension, pulmonary edema, nausea, vomiting, diarrhea, constipation, nocturia, polyuria, rash, pruritus, photosensitivity, flushing, sexual difficulties, fever, chills

Rectal Prolapse

OVERVIEW

Rectal prolapse is protrusion of the rectum through the anus

Pathogenesis

Exact cause unknown; multifactorial:

- Weak muscles in perirectal area
- Weak anal sphincter
- Weak muscles in pelvic diaphragm
- Constipation with resultant straining
- Weak fascial attachments
- Congenital fascial defects

Patient Profile

- Females > Males
- Predominant age—60 to 70 years in adults; 2 years or less in children

Signs and Symptoms

- Pain
- Protruding mass
- Rectal bleeding
- Sensation of incomplete evacuation
- Incontinence—fecal and possibly urinary

Differential Diagnosis

- Tumor
- Rectal polyps
- Intussusception
- Hemorrhoids

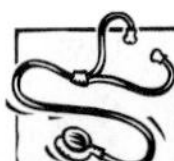

ASSESSMENT

History

Inquire about:

- Onset and duration of symptoms
- Incontinence
- Constipation
- Diet
- Underlying conditions
- Current medications

Physical Findings

- Can be visualized with patient in squatting position and straining (anticipate fecal incontinence)—radial folds seen with mucosal prolapse and concentric folds seen with prolapse of entire rectal wall
- Digital examination—relaxed anal sphincter

Initial Workup

Laboratory: None indicated

Radiology: Possibly barium enema for recurrent prolapses

Further Workup

Possibly sigmoidoscopy for recurrent prolapse to rule out tumor

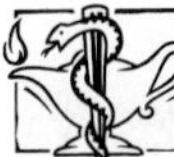

INTERVENTIONS

Office Treatment

If small and only mucosal, attempt reduction

Lifestyle Modification

High-fiber diet with increased fluids to prevent constipation

Patient Education

Teach patient about:

- Condition and treatment options—manual reduction
- Prevention of constipation (high-fiber diet, increased fluids, medication)
- Need to see surgeon if prolapse progresses or is large
- Medications used and side effects (see Pharmacotherapeutics)

Referral

To surgeon if necessary

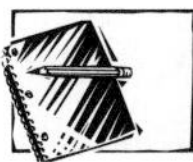

EVALUATION

Outcomes

- Children—spontaneous resolution
- Adults—good outcome with treatment

Possible Complications

- Mucosal ulceration
- Necrosis
- Postoperative complications
- Fecal impaction
- Stricture
- Presacral hemorrhage
- Pelvic abscess
- Intestinal obstruction

Follow-up

- Monthly until resolution or surgery
- Within 1 week of surgery

FOR YOUR INFORMATION

Life Span

Pediatric: Common in children 2 years or less—resolve spontaneously
Geriatric: Common in the elderly; incontinence can create major social barrier
Pregnancy: Rectocele more common postpartum

Miscellaneous

There are several different surgical procedures that may be performed. The NP should encourage and help the patient to evaluate these options so that appropriate treatment is provided.

Reference

Smith GW: Benign conditions of the anus and rectum. In Barker LR, Burton JR, Zieve PD, editors: *Principles of ambulatory medicine,* ed 4, Baltimore, 1995, Williams & Wilkins, pp 1358-1359.

NOTES

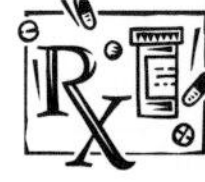

PHARMACOTHERAPEUTICS

Drug of Choice	Mechanism of Action	Prescribing Information	Side Effects
Mineral oil; adults, 15-30 ml PO hs; children, 6-12 years, 5-15 ml PO hs; children 2-5 years, 2.5-5 ml PO hs	Eases stool passage as a result of increased water in feces	***Contraindications:*** Hypersensitivity; intestinal obstruction; abdominal pain ***Cost:*** OTC ***Pregnancy category:*** C	Nausea, vomiting, anorexia, diarrhea, pruritus ani, hypoprothrombinemia
Stool softener: docusate sodium (Colace); adults, 50-200 mg/day PO; children 6-12 years, 40-120 mg/day PO; children 3-6 years, 60 mg/day PO; children <3 years, 10-40 mg/day PO	Surface-active agent—helps keep stool soft	***Contraindications:*** None ***Cost:*** Varies—OTC ***Pregnancy category:*** Not categorized	Bitter taste, throat irritation, nausea

Renal Calculi/Kidney Stones/Nephrolithiasis

OVERVIEW

Renal calculi are stones that form in the urinary tract system. They initially form in the proximal urinary tract and move distally. There are five basic types of stones: calcium phosphate, calcium oxalate, uric acid, cystine, and struvite.

Pathogenesis

Causes:

- Multifactorial—metabolic, dietary, genetic, climatic, lifestyle, occupational influences
- Many theories—crystals in supersaturated urine precipitate and form stones
- Urinary pH:
    - High pH—calcium and phosphate less soluble
    - Low pH—uric acid and cystine less soluble
- Calcium stones—hypercalciuria
- Uric acid stones—overproduction of uric acid; decreased urine volume
- Cystine stones—inborn error in amino acid transport
- Struvite stones—usually secondary to infection with urea-splitting organism

Patient Profile

- Males > Females for all stones except struvite; Females > Males for struvite stones
- Most common age group—20 to 55 years

Signs and Symptoms

- May be asymptomatic
- Excruciating flank pain
- Pain may radiate to groin, testicles, suprapubic area, labia
- Hematuria
- Dysuria
- Urinary frequency
- Diaphoresis
- Tachycardia
- Tachypnea
- Nausea
- Vomiting
- Abdominal distention
- Chills and fever if infection present

Differential Diagnosis

- Gastroenteritis
- Acute peritonitis
- Acute appendicitis
- Diverticulitis
- Salpingitis
- Cholecystitis
- Peptic ulcer disease

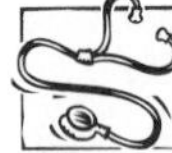

ASSESSMENT

History

Inquire about:

- Onset and duration of symptoms
- Past history of renal stones
- Family history of renal stones
- Underlying conditions
- Current medications

Physical Findings

- General—patient appears anxious, pale; may be unable to sit still if pain is severe
- Fever if infection present
- Increased blood pressure due to pain
- Heart—tachycardia
- Lungs—tachypnea
- Abdomen—distended, increased or decreased bowel sounds
- Costovertebral angle—tenderness

Initial Workup

Laboratory

- CBC with differential—leukocytosis with left shift if infection present
- Urinalysis—acidic or alkalotic pH, hematuria, bacteriuria; microscopic: crystals
- Serum calcium, phosphorus, and uric acid
- Serum BUN and creatinine—should be normal

Radiology

- Plain abdominal films
- Intravenous urography if indicated

Further Workup

Consider 24-hour urine collection to test for calcium, uric acid, magnesium, oxalate, citrate, and creatinine

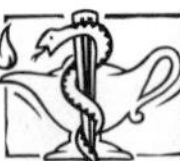

INTERVENTIONS

Office Treatment

Pain medication

Lifestyle Modifications

- Increased fluid intake
- Dietary restrictions dependent on type of stone

Patient Education

Teach patient about:

- Condition and treatment:
    - May require hospitalization for infection, severe nausea and vomiting, large stones
    - Outpatient—increased fluid intake
- Straining urine and saving stones retrieved
- Dietary restrictions—oxalates restricted for calcium oxalate stones; purines restricted for uric acid stones
- Importance of avoiding dehydration
- Possible surgery that may be used to remove stones
- Medications used and side effects (see Pharmacotherapeutics)

Referral

To urologist if indicated

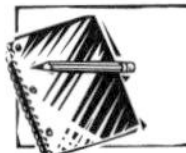

EVALUATION

Outcomes

- Usually stone passes without difficulty
- Recurrence in 5 years in 50% of patients

Possible Complications

- Complete obstruction
- Hydronephrosis
- Kidney failure

Follow-up

- Telephone contact in 24 to 48 hours to assess pain and reinforce need to increase fluids
- Return to clinic in 1 week—send retrieved stone(s) for analysis; repeat plain abdominal films

FOR YOUR INFORMATION

Life Span

Pediatric: Rare in this age group
Geriatric: Higher morbidity and mortality
Pregnancy: Cautious use of medication; frequently confused with false labor

Miscellaneous

Conditions associated with renal calculi include hyperparathyroidism, gout, cystinuria, hyperuricemia, sarcoidosis, and immobilization.

References

Bates P, Lewis SM: Nursing role in management: renal and urologic problems. In Lewis SM, Collier IC, Heitkemper MM, editors: *Medical-surgical nursing: assessment and management of clinical problems,* ed 4, St Louis, 1996, Mosby, pp 1347-1352.

Presti JC, Stoller ML, Carroll PR: Urology. In Tierney LM Jr, McPhee SJ, Papadakis MA, editors: *Current medical diagnosis and treatment,* ed 34, Norwalk, Conn, 1995, Appleton & Lange, pp 802-806.

NOTES

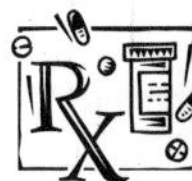

PHARMACOTHERAPEUTICS

Drug of Choice	Mechanism of Action	Prescribing Information	Side Effects
For moderate pain, use one of the following:			
Tramadol hydrochloride (Ultram), 50-100 g PO q4-6h, not to exceed 400 mg/day—not dosed for children <16 years	Centrally acting analgesic; exact mechanism of action unknown	***Contraindications:*** Hypersensitivity; acute intoxication with alcohol, hypnotics, centrally acting analgesics, opioids, psychotropic drugs ***Cost:*** 50-mg tab, 100 tabs: $60 ***Pregnancy category:*** C	Dependence, dizziness, vertigo, nausea, vomiting, constipation, headache, somnolence, pruritus, CNS stimulation, sweating, dyspepsia, dry mouth, hypotension, tachycardia, anxiety, confusion, coordination disturbance, nervousness, sleep disorder, flatulence, abdominal pain, rash
Morphine, 10-15 mg PO or IM q3-4h; children, 0.1-0.2 mg/kg SQ	Centrally acting analgesic	***Contraindications:*** Hypersensitivity; respiratory depression; acute or severe bronchial asthma; paralytic ileus ***Cost:*** 15-mg tab, 100 tabs: $64-$77 ***Pregnancy category:*** C	Respiratory depression, apnea, circulatory depression, respiratory arrest, shock, cardiac arrest, constipation, lightheadedness, dizziness, sedation, nausea, vomiting, sweating, dysphoria, euphoria, weakness, headache, agitation, tremor, seizures, uncoordinated muscle movement, dry mouth, anorexia, diarrhea, cramps, tachycardia, facial flushing, palpitations, syncope, urinary retention, pruritus, rash, edema, blurred vision
For calcium stones resulting from hypercalciuria:			
Hydrochlorothiazide, 50 mg PO bid—safety in children not established	Thiazide diuretic; acts on distal tubule and ascending limb of loop of Henle	***Contraindications:*** Hypersensitivity to thiazides or sulfonamides; anuria; renal decompensation; hypomagnesemia ***Cost:*** 25-mg tab, 100 tabs: $2-$12 ***Pregnancy category:*** B	Uremia, glucosuria, drowsiness, dizziness, fatigue, weakness, nausea, vomiting, anorexia, constipation, hepatitis, rash, urticaria, hyperglycemia, aplastic anemia, hemolytic anemia, leukopenia, agranulocytosis, thrombocytopenia, neutropenia, hypokalemia, orthostatic hypotension, hyponatremia, volume depletion
For calcium oxalate stones or uric acid stones caused by hyperuricosuria:			
Allopurinol (Zyloprim), 100 mg PO tid; children, 150-300 mg/day PO in divided doses	Reduces uric acid synthesis by inhibiting xanthine oxidase	***Contraindications:*** Hypersensitivity to thiazides or sulfonamides; anuria; renal decompensation; hypomagnesemia ***Cost:*** 25-mg tab, 100 tabs: $2-$12 ***Pregnancy category:*** B	Agranulocytosis, thrombocytopenia, aplastic anemia, pancytopenia, bone marrow depression, headache, drowsiness, nausea, vomiting, anorexia, malaise, metallic taste, cramps, myopathy, cholestatic jaundice, renal failure, retinopathy, fever, chills, dermatitis, purpura, alopecia

Renal Failure, Chronic (CRF)

OVERVIEW

Chronic renal failure occurs when the kidneys are unable to function effectively enough to remove waste products, concentrate urine, and conserve electrolytes. It is a deterioration that may occur over months or years.

Pathogenesis

Many causes—most common:

- Hypertensive nephrosclerosis
- Diabetic nephropathy
- Glomerulonephritis
- Interstitial nephritis
- Polycystic kidney disease
- Systemic lupus erythematosus
- Heavy metals
- Nephrotoxic drugs
- Multiple myeloma
- Connective tissue disease

Patient Profile

- Males = Females
- Any age; more common in adults

Signs and Symptoms

- Anemia
- Fatigue
- Anorexia
- Encephalopathy
- Endocrine dysfunction
- Hypertension
- Edema
- Weight gain
- Insomnia
- Intractable hiccups
- Muscle cramps
- Nausea and vomiting
- Pruritus
- Dry skin
- Metallic taste in mouth

Differential Diagnosis

See causes

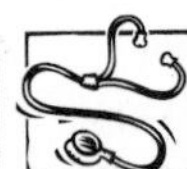

ASSESSMENT

History

Inquire about:

- Onset and duration of symptoms
- Use of NSAIDs and other nephrotoxic agents
- Recent x-ray studies involving radio contrast dye
- Family history of renal failure
- Underlying conditions such as diabetes, hypertension
- Current medications

Physical Findings

- Increased BP
- Dry skin
- Edema
- Pallor
- Complete physical examination to search for underlying cause

Initial Workup

Laboratory

- CBC with differential—anemia, thrombocytopenia
- Chemistry profile:
  - Increased BUN, creatinine, triglycerides, potassium, phosphorus, and uric acid
  - Decreased calcium
- Urinalysis:
  - Proteinuria
  - Microscopic—casts
  - 24-hour urine creatinine clearance and quantitative protein

Radiology: Renal ultrasound

Further Workup

Renal biopsy

INTERVENTIONS

Office Treatment

None indicated

Lifestyle Modifications

- Smoking cessation
- Living with a chronic illness and following the treatment plan

Patient Education

Teach patient about:

- Condition, restrictions, and treatment—vigorous treatment of underlying cause to attempt to slow progression and delay need for dialysis
- Avoiding nephrotoxic drugs
- Dietary protein restriction
- Dialysis—hemodialysis or peritoneal dialysis—several modalities to choose from
- Transplantation
- Dietary restrictions—fluids, potassium, protein, phosphorus, sodium—will depend on type of dialysis
- Medications used and side effects (see Pharmacotherapeutics)

Referral

To nephrologist

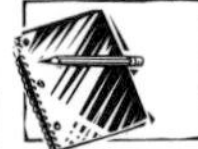

EVALUATION

Outcome

Progressive disease—renal replacement therapy will continue for life unless transplantation occurs

Possible Complications

- Anemia
- Renal osteodystrophy
- Lipid disorders
- Uremia
- Gout
- Infections
- Infertility
- Spontaneous abortions
- Hypothyroidism
- Fractures
- Seizures
- Bleeding

Follow-up

- Follow chemistries monthly
- If stabilized, every 3 months
- Monthly if on dialysis

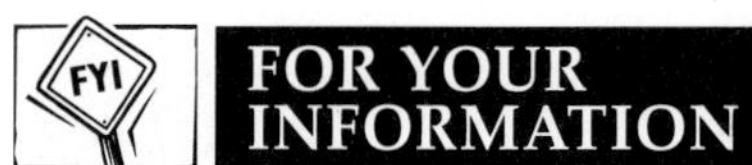

FOR YOUR INFORMATION

Life Span

Pediatric: Growth retardation is a major complication
Geriatric: Higher incidence of morbidity and mortality
Pregnancy: Difficult to carry pregnancy to term—must be handled by a specialist

Miscellaneous

N/A

References

Briefel GR: Chronic renal insufficiency. In Barker LR, Burton JR, Zieve PD, editors: *Principles of ambulatory medicine,* ed 4, Baltimore, 1995, Williams & Wilkins, pp 554-578.

Levine DZ, editor: *Care of the renal patient,* ed 2, Philadelphia, 1991, WB Saunders.

NOTES

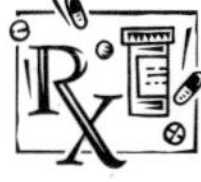

PHARMACOTHERAPEUTICS

Many medications are used in the treatment of chronic renal failure that are beyond the scope of this book. The following table presents some of the more commonly used medications.

Drug of Choice	Mechanism of Action	Prescribing Information	Side Effects
For hypertension, use angiotensin-converting enzyme inhibitor; may slow progression, particularly in diabetic patients.			
Quinapril (Accupril), 10-80 mg PO qd—not dosed for children; others: captopril, enalapril, fosinopril, lisinopril, benazepril	Prevents conversion of angiotensin I to angiotensin II, producing arterial dilation	***Contraindication:*** Hypersensitivity ***Cost:*** 10-mg tab, 100 tabs: $90 ***Pregnancy category:*** 1st trimester—C; 2nd and 3rd trimesters—D	Cough, hypotension, postural hypotension, syncope, decreased libido, impotence, increased BUN and creatinine, thrombocytopenia, agranulocytosis, angioedema, rash, sweating, photosensitivity, hyperkalemia, nausea, vomiting, gastritis, headache, dizziness, fatigue, somnolence, depression, malaise, back pain, arthralgias, arthritis
For anemia:			
Epoetin alfa (Epogen), 50-100 U SQ or IV 3 times weekly; adjust according to hematocrit	Replaces erythropoietin that is no longer produced by kidneys	***Contraindication:*** Hypersensitivity ***Cost:*** 10,000 units/ml, 10 ml: $1200 ***Pregnancy category:*** C	Hypertension, hypertensive encephalopathy, seizures, sweating, bone pain, coldness
For elevated phosphorus and calcium supplement:			
Calcium carbonate (Tums), 2-4 tabs PO qid with meals and hs	Neutralizes gastric acidity; calcium supplement; binds phosphorus	***Contraindications:*** Hypersensitivity; hyperparathyroidism; bone tumors ***Cost:*** OTC ***Pregnancy category:*** C	Constipation, anorexia, obstruction, nausea, vomiting, flatulence, diarrhea, renal stones, renal dysfunction, hypercalcemia

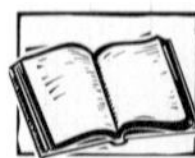

OVERVIEW

Retinopathy is a noninflammatory condition of the retina that occurs as a result of changes in the retinal blood vessels. There are 3 types of retinopathy: background retinopathy, preproliferative retinopathy, and proliferative retinopathy.

Pathogenesis

- Found in patients with insulin- and non–insulin-dependent diabetes mellitus (IDDM and NIDDM)
- Cause—excessive glucose causing damage to retinal capillary periocytes, which, in turn, cause damage to blood vessels

Patient Profile

- Males = Females
- IDDM—after 15 years with disease, 50% have retinopathy
- NIDDM—retinopathy occurs 5 to 7 years *before* diagnosis in many cases
- Number of cases of blindness per year due to diabetes—5800

Signs and Symptoms

- Persistent visual disturbances—blurred vision
- Inability to read
- Inability to see distances

Differential Diagnosis

Visual changes due to erratic blood glucose levels, change in refractive error, astigmatism, radiation retinopathy

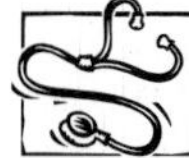

ASSESSMENT

History

Inquire about:

- Onset and duration of symptoms
- Length of time diabetic
- Length of time since last eye examination
- Underlying conditions
- Current medications

Physical Findings

- Decreased visual acuity
- Fundoscopic examination demonstrates:
  - Background retinopathy—microaneurysms >10; hard exudates (deposits of leaked lipids); closed capillaries, resulting in ischemia or soft exudates; macular edema
  - Preproliferative retinopathy—many soft exudates, extensive hemorrhages, intraretinal microvascular anomalies, and venous bleeding from enlarged dilated retinal veins
  - Proliferative retinopathy—neovascularization due to retinal hypoxia; these “new” vessels are on retina, not in retina; are friable and easily broken; cause cobwebs, floaters, or even unilateral blindness; create conditions for retinal detachment and hemorrhage into vitreous

Initial Workup

Laboratory: None indicated
Radiology: None indicated

Further Workup

Done by ophthalmologist

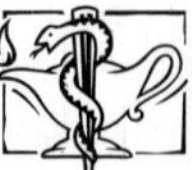

INTERVENTIONS

Office Treatment

None indicated

Lifestyle Modifications

Depends on severity; may need to prepare for eventual blindness

Patient Education

Teach patient about:

- Disease process and treatment options—surgical (photocoagulation or vitrectomy)
- If hypertension present, good control needed to prevent retinal hemorrhages
- Avoiding high altitudes
- Avoiding jarring exercise and lifting of heavy objects to prevent retinal hemorrhages
- Good glucose control (does not slow progression but can delay onset in IDDM)

Referral

To ophthalmologist specializing in retinopathy

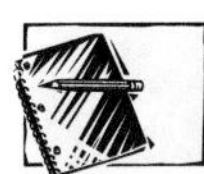

EVALUATION

Outcome
Prevention of total blindness

Possible Complication
Total blindness

Follow-up
By ophthalmologist

FOR YOUR INFORMATION

Life Span
Pediatric: Rarely develops before puberty
Geriatric: Can be especially disabling in this age group
Pregnancy: Can exacerbate retinopathy; needs assessment in first trimester and every 3 months until delivery

Miscellaneous
All diabetic patients need to be evaluated by an ophthalmologist on a yearly basis.

References
Gregerman RI: Diabetes mellitus. In Barker LR, Burton JR, Zieve PD, editors: *Principles of ambulatory medicine,* ed 4, Baltimore, 1995, Williams & Wilkins, pp 1013-1015.

Schwartz SL, Schwartz JT: *Management of diabetic mellitus,* ed 3, Durant, Okla, 1993, Essential Medical Information Systems, pp 168-173.

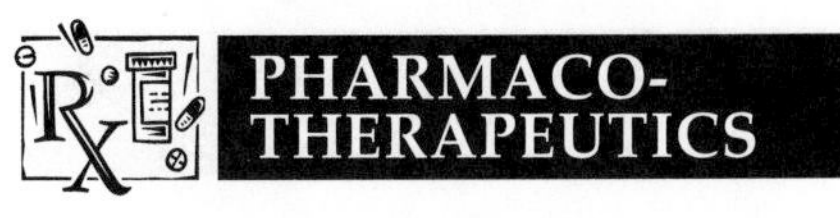

PHARMACOTHERAPEUTICS

No medications are used for this condition.

Reye's Syndrome

OVERVIEW

Reye's syndrome is a rare, potentially fatal encephalopathy that is a complication of influenza and other viral infections. There appears to be a link between aspirin use during the viral illness and development of Reye's syndrome.

Pathogenesis
Cause—unknown; several suggested:
- Viral—varicella, influenza A and B, Echovirus, coxsackie A virus
- Toxins—insecticides, herbicides
- Drugs—salicylates
- Metabolic defects

Patient Profile
- Males = Females
- Children—most commonly 5 to 10 years of age, but does occur in adolescents

Signs and Symptoms
- Vomiting
- Drowsiness
- Lethargy
- Delirium
- Stupor
- Coma
- Confusion
- Irritability
- Combativeness
- Irregular respirations

Differential Diagnosis
- Hepatic coma
- Fulminant hepatitis
- Drug poisoning
- Acute toxic encephalopathy

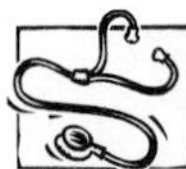

ASSESSMENT

History
Inquire about:
- Onset and duration of symptoms
- Previous viral infection
- Use of aspirin/salicylates, exposure to toxins
- Underlying conditions
- Current medications

Physical Findings
- Vomiting
- Lethargy
- Drowsiness
- Irritability
- Combativeness
- Abdominal pain in right upper quadrant
- Pallor

Initial Workup
Laboratory: To be done in hospital:
- CBC
- Chemistry profile to include glucose, electrolytes, liver function tests, creatinine, and BUN
- Prothrombin time

Radiology: None indicated

Further Workup
Liver biopsy

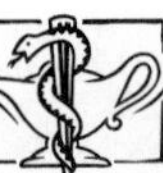

INTERVENTIONS

Office Treatment
To emergency room or direct hospital admission immediately (this is a medical emergency)

Lifestyle Modifications
Depends on residual effects; may require extensive rehabilitation

Patient Education
- Teach parents not to use aspirin in children to prevent Reye's syndrome
- Other teaching done in hospital

Referral
To physician for hospital care

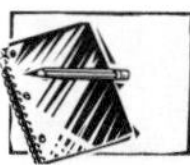

EVALUATION

Outcomes
- Early diagnosis—good prognosis
- Prognosis depends on amount of cerebral edema
- May have difficulty with attention, concentration, speech, language, fine and gross motor skills

Possible Complications
- Aspiration pneumonia
- Respiratory failure
- Cardiac dysrhythmia
- Cerebral edema
- Death

Follow-up
Within 1 week of hospital discharge

FOR YOUR INFORMATION

Life Span
Pediatric: This is the age group affected
Geriatric: N/A
Pregnancy: N/A

Miscellaneous
The incidence of Reye's syndrome has dramatically decreased in the past 10 years.

Reference
Gill EP, Shander WX: Infectious diseases: viral and rickettsial. In Tierney LM Jr, McPhee SJ, Papadakis MA, editors: *Current medical diagnosis and treatment,* ed 34, Norwalk, Conn, 1995, Appleton & Lange, p. 1151.

NOTES

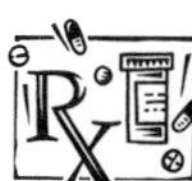

PHARMACOTHERAPEUTICS

Drug of Choice	Mechanism of Action	Prescribing Information	Side Effects
Neomycin (Mycifradin), 100 mg/kg/day PO or IM	Bactericidal; interferes with protein synthesis	***Contraindications:*** Bowel obstruction; severe renal disease; hypersensitivity ***Cost:*** Sol, 87.5 mg/5 ml, 480 ml: $30 ***Pregnancy category:*** C	Oliguria, hematuria, renal damage, proteinemia, renal failure, nephrotoxicity, ototoxicity, deafness, agranulocytopenia, nausea, vomiting, anorexia, hepatic necrosis, hypotension, rash, burning, urticaria
Vitamin K (AquaMEPHYTON), 5 mg/day IM	Replaces vitamin K in body	***Contraindication:*** Hypersensitivity ***Cost:*** 1 mg/0.5 ml, 5 ml: $27 ***Pregnancy category:*** C	Headache, brain damage, nausea, hemolytic anemia, hemoglobinemia, hyperbilirubinemia, rash, urticaria

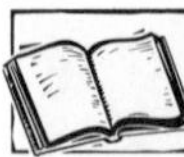

OVERVIEW

Rheumatic fever is a multisystem inflammatory disease that follows group A streptococcal pharyngitis.

Pathogenesis

- Cause—autoimmune mechanism
- Prerequisite—upper respiratory tract infection with group A streptococcus

Patient Profile

- Males = Females
- Most common age—5 to 15 years
- Can see recurrence in adulthood, but first attacks of acute rheumatic fever in adults are rare

Signs and Symptoms

- Fever 101° to 104° F (38.3° to 40° C)
- Chorea
- Abdominal pain
- Carditis (mild or severe with murmurs)—may include pericarditis, myocarditis, or valvular insufficiency
- Arthralgias and/or arthritis, usually involving medium to large joints
- Subcutaneous nodules on extensor surfaces
- Weight loss
- Fatigue
- Irritability
- Prolonged P-R interval on ECG
- Erythema marginatum
- Jones criteria for diagnosis of rheumatic fever:

Major manifestations	Minor manifestations
Carditis	Clinical—arthralgias
Polyarthritis	Previous acute rheumatic fever or evidence of preexisting rheumatic heart disease
Chorea	Laboratory—leukocytosis
Erythema marginatum	Increased erythrocyte sedimentation rate (ESR)
Subcutaneous nodules	Abnormal C-reactive protein
	Prolonged P-R interval or other ECG changes

PLUS: Supporting evidence of preceding streptococcal infection. Two major manifestations or 1 major and 2 minor manifestations are required to make diagnosis.

Differential Diagnosis

- Lupus erythematosus
- Rheumatoid arthritis
- Viral myocarditis
- Innocent murmurs
- Tourette's syndrome

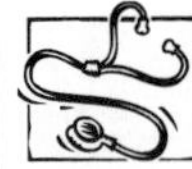

ASSESSMENT

History

Inquire about:

- Onset and duration of symptoms
- Pharyngitis within previous 6 months
- Past history of heart murmur or previous cardiac disease
- Family history of rheumatic fever
- Underlying conditions
- Current medications

Physical Findings

- Chorea—purposeless, involuntary movements
- Erythema marginatum—red macular lesions with pale centers
- Subcutaneous nodules—painless, movable nodules on extensor surfaces
- Cardiac examination—new or changed murmur, pericardial friction rub, pericardial effusion, heart enlargement
- Fever 101° to 104° F (38.3° to 40° C)

Initial Workup

Laboratory

- ESR—increased
- C-reactive protein—abnormal
- Antistreptolysin O titer, Streptozyme, or antideoxyribonuclease B—evidence of group A streptococcal infection

Radiology

- Chest film—PA and lateral
- Echocardiogram

Further Workup

ECG

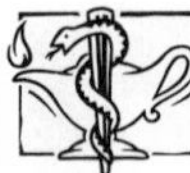

INTERVENTIONS

Office Treatment

None indicated

Lifestyle Modifications

- Initial bed rest, increasing activity as tolerated
- Need for prophylaxis for at least 5 years and possibly longer

Patient Education

Teach patient about:

- Condition and treatment:
  - Antimicrobials
  - If carditis present—prednisone
  - If no carditis—aspirin
- Importance of bed rest initially and gradually increasing activity
- Carditis—low-sodium diet
- Importance of long-term prophylaxis to prevent recurrence
- Valvular damage—dental and high-risk prophylaxis for life
- Medications used and side effects (see Pharmacotherapeutics)

Referral

Consultation with physician for carditis

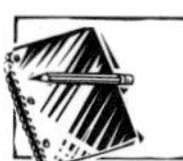

EVALUATION

Outcome
Depends on severity of acute attack

Possible Complications
- Subsequent attacks following streptococcal infections
- Carditis
- Mitral stenosis
- Congestive heart failure

Follow-up
Initially weekly × 4; then every 4 weeks × 3; then every 3 to 6 months

FOR YOUR INFORMATION

Life Span
Pediatric: Most common age group affected by acute rheumatic fever
Geriatric: Development of mitral stenosis
Pregnancy: May exacerbate valvular disease

Miscellaneous
N/A

References
Koster FT, Barker LR: Respiratory tract infections. In Barker LR, Burton JR, Zieve PD, editors: *Principles of ambulatory medicine,* ed 4, Baltimore, 1995, Williams & Wilkins, pp 335-336.

Massie BM: Heart. In Tierney LM Jr, McPhee SJ, Papadakis MA, editors: *Current medical diagnosis and treatment,* ed 34, Norwalk, Conn, Appleton & Lange, pp 362-363.

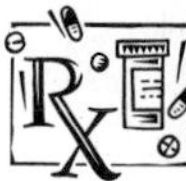

PHARMACOTHERAPEUTICS

Drug of Choice	Mechanism of Action	Prescribing Information	Side Effects
To treat acute rheumatic fever:			
Penicillin, benzathine, 1.2 mil units IM × 1 dose; children >27 kg, 900,000 units IM × 1 dose; children <27 kg, 50,000 units/kg × 1 dose; for prophylaxis, 1.2 mil units IM monthly for at least 5 years; consult with MD if patient allergic to penicillin	Interferes with cell wall replication	***Contraindication:*** Hypersensitivity ***Cost:*** 600,000 units/ml, 10 ml: $68 ***Pregnancy category:*** B	Anemia, bone marrow depression, granulocytopenia, nausea, vomiting, diarrhea, increased AST and ALT, oliguria, proteinuria, hematuria, vaginitis, moniliasis, glomerulonephritis, lethargy, coma, convulsions, local pain and tenderness at injection site, rash, anaphylaxis
For acute rheumatic fever without cardiomegaly:			
Aspirin, 60 mg/kg/day PO in divided doses for 4-6 weeks	Inhibits synthesis and release of prostaglandins	***Contraindications:*** Hypersensitivity to aspirin or nonsteroidal antiinflammatory agents; recent GI bleed or bleeding disorder ***Cost:*** OTC ***Pregnancy category:*** D	Thrombocytopenia, agranulocytosis, leukopenia, hemolytic anemia, increased bleeding time, stimulation, drowsiness, dizziness, confusion, convulsions, hallucinations, nausea, vomiting, GI bleeding, hepatitis, rash, tinnitus, hearing loss, pulmonary edema, anaphylaxis
If response to salicylates inadequate or cardiomegaly present:			
Prednisone, 2 mg/kg/day (max 60 mg) PO daily × 2 weeks, then taper over 2 weeks; start aspirin at beginning of taper and continue for 6 weeks	Corticosteroid; antiinflammatory	***Contraindications:*** Hypersensitivity; psychosis; idiopathic thrombocytopenia; acute glomerulonephritis; amebiasis; nonasthmatic bronchial disease; AIDS; TB; children <2 years old ***Cost:*** 15-mg tab, 100 tabs: $14-$35 ***Pregnancy category:*** C	Hypertension, circulatory collapse, thrombophlebitis, embolism, tachycardia, fungal infections, increased intraocular pressure, diarrhea, nausea, GI hemorrhage, thrombocytopenia, acne, poor wound healing, fractures, osteoporosis, weakness

Rheumatoid Arthritis (RA)

OVERVIEW

Rheumatoid arthritis (RA) is a chronic inflammatory disease that predominantly affects the peripheral joints. RA may also be accompanied by extraarticular manifestations, such as arteritis, rheumatoid nodules, neuropathy, scleritis, lymphadenopathy, splenomegaly, or pericarditis.

Pathogenesis
Cause—unknown; most commonly believed etiology—autoimmunity

Patient Profile
- Females > Males
- Most common age—25 to 45 years

Signs and Symptoms
- Insidious onset—fatigue, anorexia, weight loss, generalized stiffness
- Proceeds to symmetric joint swelling and warmth of hands, feet, wrists, knees, hips
- Joint stiffness after waking and after periods of inactivity
- Deformities due to inflammation and fibrosis of joint capsule—ulnar drift, swan neck, boutonniere deformity
- Rheumatoid nodules
- Entrapment neuropathies
- Lymphadenopathy
- Splenomegaly
- Ocular disease

Differential Diagnosis
- Systemic lupus erythematosus
- Osteoarthritis
- Polymyositis
- Gout
- Pseudogout
- Scleroderma
- Chronic infection

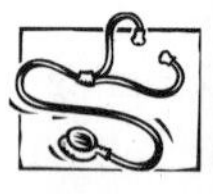

ASSESSMENT

History
Inquire about:
- Onset and duration of symptoms
- Distribution of involved joints
- Severity of pain
- Treatment tried and results
- Ability to perform activities of daily living (ADLs)
- Family history of RA
- Underlying conditions
- Current medications

Physical Findings
- Weight loss
- Painful, swollen, erythematous joints—most commonly proximal interphalangeal and metacarpophalangeal joints of fingers, wrists, knees, ankles, toes
- May have limited range of motion
- Rheumatoid nodules—commonly bony prominences
- Lymphadenopathy
- Splenomegaly on abdominal examination
- May find entrapment neuropathies, such as carpal tunnel syndrome

Initial Workup
Laboratory
- CBC—mild anemia
- Erythrocyte sedimentation rate (ESR)—usually elevated
- Rheumatoid factor >1:80 titer
- Synovial fluid—decreased viscosity
- WBC count—increased

Radiology: May be useful in following progression of disease

Further Workup
American College of Rheumatology criteria for diagnosis of RA (4 of the 7 must be present for diagnosis):
- Morning stiffness for over 1 hour for at least 6 weeks
- Arthritis with swelling in at least 3 joints for at least 6 weeks
- Arthritis involving hand joints with swelling for at least 6 weeks
- Symmetric arthritis for at least 6 weeks
- Subcutaneous nodules
- Positive rheumatoid factor test
- Radiographic changes typical for diagnosis of RA

INTERVENTIONS

Office Treatment
None indicated

Lifestyle Modifications
- Adjustment to living with a chronic disease
- Maintaining previous lifestyle for as long as possible
- Smoking cessation

Patient Education
Teach patient about:
- Disease and treatment aim: relief of symptoms and prevention of disability
- Importance of good nutrition
- Starting a moderate exercise program
- Avoiding heavy work and vigorous exercise during active phases
- Living with a chronic illness
- Importance of discussing fears and concerns with family and NP
- Using splints to help avoid deformity
- Using warm, moist heat for relief of stiffness
- Using ice packs during active periods
- Products available to assist patient with ADLs
- Medications used and side effects (see Pharmacotherapeutics)

Referrals
- To rheumatologist if available
- To physical therapist
- To occupational therapist

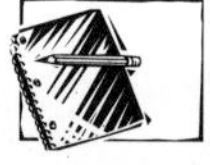

EVALUATION

Outcomes
- Patient will maintain previous lifestyle with minimal disability for as long as possible
- Disease is usually progressive

Possible Complications
- Skin vasculitis
- Pericarditis
- Intracardiac rheumatoid nodules
- Joint destruction
- Sjögren's syndrome
- Treatment-induced complications

Follow-up
- In 2 weeks × 2; then monthly × 2; then every 3 months
- Will depend on treatment

FOR YOUR INFORMATION

Life Span
Pediatric: Affected by juvenile rheumatoid arthritis

Geriatric: Onset less common; start with lower doses of medications

Pregnancy: Significant percentage show improvement during pregnancy; cautious use of medications

Miscellaneous
RA can be a devastating disease. The patient needs a great deal of psychologic support and encouragement.

References

Hellman DB: Arthritis and musculoskeletal disorders. In Tierney LM Jr, McPhee SJ, Papadakis MA, editors: *Current medical diagnosis and treatment,* ed 34, Norwalk, Conn, Appleton & Lange, pp 711-716.

Mercier LR: *Practical orthopedics,* ed 4, St Louis, 1995, Mosby, pp 284-285.

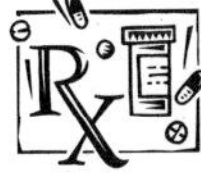

PHARMACOTHERAPEUTICS

There are many medications that may be used to treat RA. The following table lists only those most commonly prescribed by the NP.

Drug of Choice	Mechanism of Action	Prescribing Information	Side Effects
Most authorities recommend starting with aspirin or a nonsteroidal antiinflammatory drug (NSAID).			
Aspirin, enteric coated, 1 g PO tid or qid; may increase by 300-600 mg/day each week until maximal response seen or toxicity occurs (tinnitus usually 1st symptom); if toxicity occurs, decrease by 600-900 mg/day every 3 days until symptoms resolve	Antiinflammatory action may result from inhibition of synthesis and release of prostaglandins	***Contraindications:*** Hypersensitivity; GI bleeding; bleeding disorders ***Cost:*** OTC ***Pregnancy category:*** Should not be used in 3rd trimester	Dyspepsia, thirst, nausea, vomiting, GI bleeding/ulceration, tinnitus, vertigo, reversible hearing loss, prolongation of bleeding time, leukopenia, thrombocytopenia, purpura, urticaria, angioedema, pruritus, asthma, anaphylaxis, mental confusion, drowsiness, dizziness, headache, fever
NSAIDs: many different types currently marketed; consult manufacturer's package insert for specific dosing and prescribing information	Exact action unknown; may result from inhibition of synthesis of prostaglandins and arachidonic acid	***Contraindications:*** Hypersensitivity to NSAIDs, aspirin; severe hepatic failure; asthma ***Cost:*** Varies with type ***Pregnancy category:*** Depends on product	Stomach distress, flatulence, nausea, abdominal pain, constipation or diarrhea, dizziness, sedation, rash, urticaria, angioedema, anorexia, urinary frequency, increased blood pressure, insomnia, anxiety, visual disturbances, increased thirst, alopecia
For severe RA:			
Prednisone, 5-15 mg PO qd; use for as short a time as possible—until symptoms abate	Corticosteroid; antiinflammatory	***Contraindications:*** Hypersensitivity; psychosis; idiopathic thrombocytopenia; acute glomerulonephritis; amebiasis; nonasthmatic bronchial disease; AIDS; TB; children <2 years old ***Cost:*** 15-mg tab, 100 tabs: $14-$35 ***Pregnancy category:*** C	Hypertension, circulatory collapse, thrombophlebitis, embolism, tachycardia, fungal infections, increased intraocular pressure, diarrhea, nausea, GI hemorrhage, thrombocytopenia, acne, poor wound healing, fractures, osteoporosis, weakness
For persistent active disease, use one of the following remission-inducing agents:			
Hydroxychloroquine (Plaquenil), 400 mg PO hs × 2-3 months, then 200 mg PO hs × 3 months as a trial	Antimalarial; mechanism of action in RA unknown	***Contraindications:*** Hypersensitivity; retinal field changes; long-term use in children ***Cost:*** 200-mg tab, 100 tabs: $105 ***Pregnancy category:*** C	Irritability, nervousness, emotional changes, nightmares, psychosis, headache, dizziness, vertigo, nystagmus, muscle weakness, visual disturbances, blurred vision, alopecia, pruritus, skin eruptions, aplastic anemia, agranulocytosis, leukopenia, thrombocytopenia, anorexia, nausea, vomiting, weight loss
Auranofin (Ridaura), 6-10 mg/day PO; reevaluate after 4-6 months	Gold compound; antiinflammatory action unknown	***Contraindications:*** Hypersensitivity to gold; necrotizing enterocolitis; bone marrow aplasia; exfoliative dermatitis; pulmonary fibrosis; blood dyscrasias; recent radiation therapy ***Cost:*** 3-mg tab, 60 tabs: $69 ***Pregnancy category:*** C	Thrombocytopenia, agranulocytosis, aplastic anemia, leukopenia, eosinophilia, rash, pruritus, dermatitis, exfoliative dermatitis, urticaria, dizziness, confusion, hallucinations, seizures, diarrhea, abdominal cramps, stomatitis, nausea, vomiting, enterocolitis, anorexia, flatulence, glossitis, proteinuria, hematuria, iritis, corneal ulcers, interstitial pneumonitis, fibrosis, cough, dyspnea

Other drugs that may be used include sulfasalazine, D-penicillamine, and methotrexate.

Rocky Mountain Spotted Fever

OVERVIEW

Rocky mountain spotted fever is an acute systemic rickettsial infection transmitted to humans by the bite of an infected tick.

Pathogenesis

- Cause—*Rickettsia rickettsii,* transmitted by tick bite; tick must attach and feed for 4 to 6 hours for infection to be spread to human
- No human-to-human transmission
- Organism directly invades endothelial cells

Patient Profile

- Males > Females
- Any age

Signs and Symptoms

Manifestations 3 to 10 days after bite:

- Malaise
- Anorexia
- Nausea
- Headache
- Sore throat
- Chills
- Fever
- Myalgia and arthralgia
- Abdominal pain
- Rash—macular, maculopapular, petechial
- Delirium
- Lethargy
- Seizures
- Stupor
- Coma
- Splenomegaly
- Hepatomegaly
- Cough

Differential Diagnosis

- Measles
- Typhoid
- Meningoencephalitis
- Lyme disease
- Infectious mononucleosis

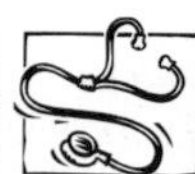

ASSESSMENT

History

Inquire about:

- Onset and duration of symptoms
- Known tick bite, recent camping trip or outdoor activities
- Underlying conditions
- Current medications

Physical Findings

- Fever
- Observe general appearance for signs of distress/lethargy
- Inspect skin for rash/lesions/petechiae
- Throat—red with edematous tonsils
- Lung examination for pneumonitis
- Complete neurological examination

Initial Workup

Laboratory

- CBC with differential—increased WBC count, decreased platelet count, slightly decreased hemoglobin
- Serum electrolytes—hyponatremia
- Urinalysis—proteinuria, hematuria
- Serum proteus OX-19 antibody—fourfold increase
- Serum complement fixation antibody—fourfold increase

Radiology: Chest film—PA and lateral—nonspecific pneumonic infiltrates

Further Workup

None indicated

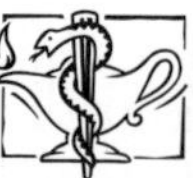

INTERVENTIONS

Office Treatment

None indicated

Lifestyle Modification

Proper measures to avoid tick bites

Patient Education

Teach patient about:

- Disease and treatment:
    - Moderately ill—hospitalization
    - Mild illness—outpatient treatment with antimicrobials
    - Bed rest until symptoms subside
- Importance of keeping follow-up appointments
- Danger signs signaling need for immediate treatment—altered mental status, stiff neck, severe headache, prolonged nausea and vomiting, shortness of breath, high fever, decreased urine output
- Avoiding future tick bites—wear light-colored clothing, long-sleeved shirts; tuck pants into socks and shirt into pants; wear hat; avoid overhanging brush and grass; use insect repellent containing *N,N*-diethyl-*m*-toluamide—apply every 1 to 2 hours; remove clothing promptly, and wash and dry on hot temperature setting; if tick is found, remove promptly using tweezers
- Medications used and side effects (see Pharmacotherapeutics)

Referral

To physician for moderate illness if NP does not have admitting privileges

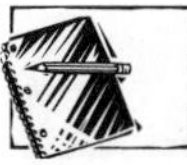

EVALUATION

Outcome
Usually resolves without sequelae with prompt treatment

Possible Complications
- Encephalopathy
- Seizures
- Renal insufficiency
- Hepatitis
- Congestive heart failure
- Respiratory failure

Follow-up
- If patient taking chloramphenicol, follow every 2 to 3 days for CBC with differential
- With other antimicrobials, return to clinic 48 hours after starting therapy and after completion of therapy

FOR YOUR INFORMATION

Life Span
Pediatric: Avoid use of tetracyclines in children <8 years of age
Geriatric: Higher risk of morbidity and mortality
Pregnancy: Consult with specialist

Miscellaneous
Treatment should not be delayed for serologic test confirmation.

References
Bartlett JG: *Pocket book of infectious disease therapy,* Baltimore, 1996, Williams & Wilkins, p 37.

Gill EP, Shandera WX: Infectious diseases: viral and rickettsial. In Tierney LM Jr, McPhee SJ, Papadakis MA, editors: *Current medical diagnosis and treatment,* ed 34, Norwalk, Conn, 1995, Appleton & Lange, pp. 1158-1159.

NOTES

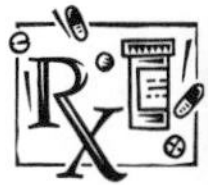

PHARMACOTHERAPEUTICS

Drug of Choice	Mechanism of Action	Prescribing Information	Side Effects
Doxycycline (Doryx), 100 mg PO bid × 7 days; children >8 years, 2.2-2.4 mg/kg/day PO in divided doses × 7 days	Tetracycline; inhibits protein synthesis	***Contraindications:*** Hypersensitivity; children <8 years ***Cost:*** 100-mg tab, 20 tabs: $5 ***Pregnancy category:*** D	Eosinophilia, neutropenia, thrombocytopenia, hemolytic anemia, dysphagia, glossitis, nausea, abdominal pain, vomiting, diarrhea, anorexia, hepatotoxicity, flatulence, abdominal cramps, gastritis, pericarditis, rash, urticaria, exfoliative dermatitis, angioedema
Chloramphenicol (Chloromycetin); adults and children, 50 mg/kg/day PO divided into 4 doses at 6-hour intervals; not to exceed 4 g/day	Interference or inhibition of protein synthesis	***Contraindications:*** Hypersensitivity; severe renal or hepatic disease; minor infections ***Cost:*** 250-mg tab, 100 tabs: $25-$125 ***Pregnancy category:*** C	Anemia, thrombocytopenia, aplastic anemia, granulocytopenia, optic neuritis, nausea, vomiting, diarrhea, abdominal pain, glossitis, colitis, itching, rash, gray syndrome in newborns, headache, depression, confusion

OVERVIEW

Roseola is an acute illness characterized by a high fever followed by a macular rash that closely resembles measles.

Pathogenesis
- Cause—newest research indicates human herpesvirus 6
- Incubation period—5 to 15 days.

Patient Profile
- Males = Females
- Very young—6 months to 3 years
- Majority of cases involve 2-year-olds
- More likely in spring and fall

Signs and Symptoms
- Sudden onset of fever (103° to 105° F [39.4° to 40.6° C])
- May have single episode of vomiting, a runny nose, or cough, but generally appears well
- Often playful with good appetite, even with high fever (with other viral exanthems, child is lethargic)
- Slight anorexia
- Irritability
- Fever subsides in about 4 days
- Rash appears—numerous pale pink macules on trunk, arms, and neck
- Rash blanches with pressure
- Rash subsides in a few hours to 2 days
- Cervical and posterior auricular lymphadenopathy throughout course

Differential Diagnosis
- Sepsis
- Urinary tract infection
- Measles
- Otitis media
- Meningitis
- Drug eruption

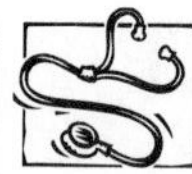

ASSESSMENT

History
Inquire about:
- Onset and duration of symptoms
- Exposure to child with similar symptoms
- Treatments tried and results
- Underlying conditions
- Current medications

Physical Findings
- Initially fever may be only finding
- Later—numerous pale pink macules on trunk, arms, and neck

Initial Workup
Laboratory
- CBC—leukopenia with lymphocytosis
- Urinalysis—should be normal

Radiology: Chest film—negative

Further Workup
None indicated

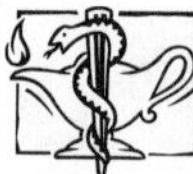

INTERVENTIONS

Office Treatment
Reduce fever

Lifestyle Modifications
- Keeping child home
- Adequate rest until fever breaks
- Tap water baths to keep fever down

Patient Education
Teach parent about:
- Disease being self-limiting
- High fever possibly causing seizures—need to keep calm, protect child from injury; seizures will not cause brain damage
- Keeping child well hydrated
- Using acetaminophen or ibuprofen and tap water baths for fever (see Pharmacotherapeutics)

Referrals
None indicated

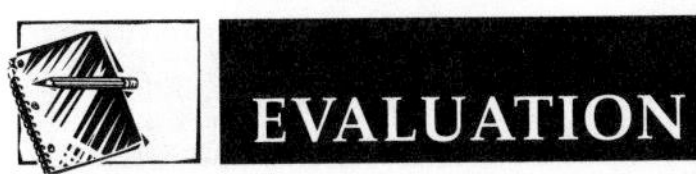

EVALUATION

Outcome
Resolves without sequelae in about 7 days

Possible Complications
- Febrile seizures
- Encephalitis (rare)

Follow-up
None after rash appears

FOR YOUR INFORMATION

Lifestyle
Pediatric: Common in this age group
Geriatric: Not seen in this age group
Pregnancy: N/A

Miscellaneous
A single attack of roseola confers permanent immunity to the individual.

Reference
Habif TP: *Clinical dermatology: a color guide to diagnosis and therapy,* ed 3, St Louis, 1996, Mosby, p 421.

NOTES

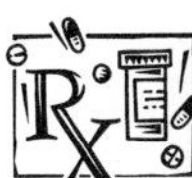

PHARMACOTHERAPEUTICS

The medications listed here are for fever and myalgia

Drug of Choice	Mechanism of Action	Prescribing Information	Side Effects
Acetaminophen (Tylenol), 10-15 mg/kg q4h PO	Decreases fever through action on hypothalamic heat-regulating center of brain; produces analgesia by elevating pain threshold	***Contraindication:*** Hypersensitivity ***Cost:*** OTC ***Pregnancy category:*** Not categorized	Anaphylaxis, leukopenia, neutropenia, drowsiness, nausea, vomiting, hepatotoxicity, rash, angioedema, urticaria, toxicity
Ibuprofen (Motrin), 400 mg qid PO; children 6 months to 12 years, 5 mg/kg if temperature <102.5° F (39.2° C); 10 mg/kg if temperature >102.5° F q6h	Not well understood; may be related to inhibition of prostaglandin synthesis	***Contraindications:*** Aspirin allergy; hypersensitivity; asthma; last trimester of pregnancy; gastric ulcer; bleeding disorders ***Cost:*** 400-mg tab, 4/day × 5 days: $3 ***Pregnancy category:*** Not recommended	Nausea, heartburn, diarrhea, GI upset and bleeding, dizziness, headache, rash, tinnitus, edema, acute renal failure

Roundworms (Ascariasis)

OVERVIEW

Ascariasis is an intestinal infestation with *Ascaris lumbricoides,* a large roundworm.

Pathogenesis
Ingestion of eggs from soil, food, or water contaminated by human feces

Patient Profile
- Males = Females
- Any age

Signs and Symptoms
- May be asymptomatic
- Nausea and vomiting
- Anorexia
- Weight loss
- Fever
- Irritability
- Diarrhea
- Abdominal cramping
- With lung invasion:
    - Cough
    - Blood-tinged sputum
    - Wheezing
    - Rales
    - Dyspnea
    - Eosinophilia

Differential Diagnosis
- Infection with other parasites
- Asthma
- Pneumonia
- Malnutrition
- Other causes of pancreatitis
- Duodenitis
- Esophagitis
- Cholecystitis

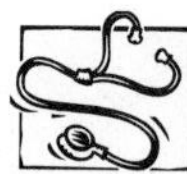

ASSESSMENT

History
Inquire about:
- Onset and duration of symptoms
- Cough, fever
- Whether worm seen in stool
- Underlying conditions and current medications

Physical Findings
- Weight loss
- Tenderness on abdominal palpation
- Rectal examination—stool for occult blood; may see worm

Initial Workup
Laboratory
- CBC with differential—eosinophilia
- Stool for ova and parasites
- If worms visualized, no tests needed

Radiology: None indicated

Further Workup
None indicated

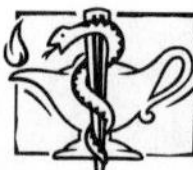

INTERVENTIONS

Office Treatment
None indicated

Lifestyle Modifications
- Good hand washing
- Avoidance of fecally contaminated soil, food, or water

Patient Education
Teach patient about:
- Condition and how contracted
- Proper hand-washing technique
- Proper sanitation
- Medications used and side effects (see Pharmacotherapeutics)

Referrals
None needed

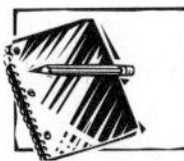

EVALUATION

Outcome

Resolves without sequelae

Possible Complications

Worms migrate, causing cholangitis, pancreatitis, appendicitis, diverticulitis, liver abscess, intestinal obstruction

Follow-up

May wish to recheck stools in 2 weeks

FOR YOUR INFORMATION

Life Span

Pediatric: Second most common infection after pinworms
Geriatric: Symptoms may be more severe
Pregnancy: Cautious use of medications

Miscellaneous

N/A

Reference

Goldsmith RS: Infectious diseases: helminthic. In Tierney LM Jr, McPhee SJ, Papadakis MA, editors: *Current medical diagnosis and treatment,* ed 34, Norwalk, Conn, Appleton & Lange, pp 1260-1261.

NOTES

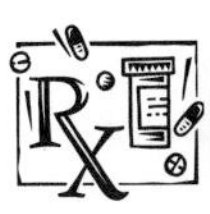

PHARMACOTHERAPEUTICS

Drug of Choice	Mechanism of Action	Prescribing Information	Side Effects
Mebendazole (Vermox); adults and children >2 years, 100 mg PO bid × 3 days	Anthelmintic; inhibits formation of worm's microtubules and depletes its glucose	***Contraindication:*** Hypersensitivity ***Cost:*** 100-mg tab, 12 tabs: $55 ***Pregnancy category:*** C	Dizziness, fever, transient diarrhea, abdominal pain, rash, urticaria, angioedema
Pyrantel pamoate (Antiminth); adults and children >2 years, 11 mg/kg PO as single dose, not to exceed 1 g; repeat in 2 weeks	Paralyzes worm; worm is then expelled by normal peristalsis	***Contraindication:*** Hypersensitivity ***Cost:*** 250 mg/5 ml: $5-$15 ***Pregnancy category:*** C	Rash, dizziness, headache, drowsiness, insomnia, fever, nausea, vomiting, anorexia, diarrhea, distention

OVERVIEW

Sarcoidosis is a multisystem disease frequently characterized by granulomatous inflammation of the lungs and hilar adenopathy. Ocular and skin lesions may be present, and other organs may also be involved (spleen, liver, heart, lymphatic system, central nervous system).

Pathogenesis
Cause—unknown

Patient Profile
- Females > Males
- Most common age group—20 to 60 years
- Highest incidence in African-Americans and Northern European whites

Signs and Symptoms
- May be asymptomatic
- Malaise
- Fever
- Dyspnea
- Fatigue
- Skin rashes
- Erythema nodosum
- Parotid gland enlargement
- Lymphadenopathy
- Hepatomegaly
- Splenomegaly
- Pain or irritation of eyes

Differential Diagnosis
- Tuberculosis
- Lymphoma
- Malignancy
- Fungal infection

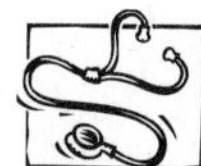

ASSESSMENT

History
Inquire about:
- Onset and duration of symptoms
- Underlying conditions
- Current medications

Physical Findings
- Fever
- Skin lesions or rashes
- Lungs—may or may not find adventitious sounds
- Lymphadenopathy
- Parotid gland enlargement
- Hepatomegaly
- Splenomegaly

Initial Workup
Laboratory
- CBC with differential—leukopenia, eosinophilia
- Erythrocyte sedimentation rate (ESR)—elevated
- Chemistry panel to include liver function studies and calcium—alkaline phosphatase increased; calcium possibly increased
- Serum angiotensin–converting enzyme (ACE)—elevated

Radiology: Chest film—PA and lateral:
- Stage 0—normal
- Stage I—hilar adenopathy alone
- Stage II—hilar adenopathy plus parenchymal infiltrates
- Stage III—parenchymal infiltrates alone

Further Workup
Biopsy of accessible skin lesions or lymph nodes

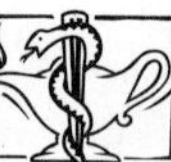

INTERVENTIONS

Office Treatment
None indicated

Lifestyle Modifications
- Smoking cessation
- Avoidance of high-calcium foods

Patient Education
Teach patient about:
- Condition and treatment
- Benign nature of condition and that it is not contagious
- Tips for smoking cessation
- Foods high in calcium and to avoid these
- Medications used and side effects (see Pharmacotherapeutics)

Referral
To MD if treatment fails or for severe cases

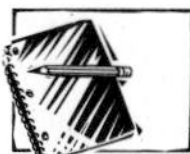

EVALUATION

Outcomes

- 80% have resolution in 2 years
- 10% have significant fibrosis, but no worsening of disease
- 10% develop chronic disease

Possible Complications

- Cor pulmonale
- Significant involvement of other organs
- Chronic disease

Follow-up

- Monthly if patient taking prednisone to monitor for side effects
- If patient not taking prednisone, every 3 months to assess for progression of disease

FOR YOUR INFORMATION

Life Span

Pediatric: Rare in this age group
Geriatric: Rare for onset to occur in this age group
Pregnancy: Should be handled by a specialist

Miscellaneous

N/A

References

Phipps WJ, Brucia JJ: Management of persons with problems of the lower airway. In Phipps WJ et al, editors: *Medical-surgical nursing: concepts and clinical practice,* ed 5, St Louis, 1995, Mosby, p 1091.

Stauffer JL: Lung. In Tierney LM Jr, McPhee SJ, Papadakis MA, editors: *Current medical diagnosis and treatment,* ed 34, Norwalk, Conn, 1995, Appleton & Lange, pp 249-250.

NOTES

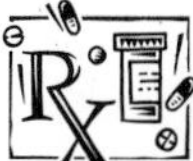

PHARMACOTHERAPEUTICS

Drug of Choice	Mechanism of Action	Prescribing Information	Side Effects
Prednisone, 60 mg PO qd × 2 months; then 40 mg PO qd × 2 months; then use tapering dose over next year to 18 months	Corticosteroid; decreases inflammation	***Contraindications:*** Hypersensitivity; psychosis; idiopathic thrombocytopenia; acute glomerulonephritis; amebiasis; nonasthmatic bronchial disease; AIDS; TB; children <2 years old ***Cost:*** 15-mg tab, 100 tabs: $14-$35 ***Pregnancy category:*** C	Hypertension, circulatory collapse, thrombophlebitis, embolism, tachycardia, fungal infections, increased intraocular pressure, diarrhea, nausea, GI hemorrhage, thrombocytopenia, acne, poor wound healing, fractures, osteoporosis, weakness

Scabies

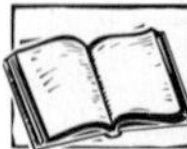

OVERVIEW

Scabies is a common skin disease caused by infestation with a mite. It is usually acquired by close contact, such as sleeping with an infested individual or sleeping on the bed linens of an infested individual.

Pathogenesis

- Cause—mite: *Sarcoptes scabiei*
- Female mite burrows into outermost layer of skin and deposits fertilized eggs and feces
- Larvae hatch and in about 14 days are ready to replicate
- Pruritis caused by hypersensitivity reaction
- Incubation period 4 to 6 weeks

Patient Profile

- Males = Females
- Children and young adults more commonly infested
- Institutionalized more commonly infested

Signs and Symptoms

- Generalized pruritis with increased intensity at night
- Burrows, gray or skin-colored ridges, may be evident in finger webs, wrists, hands, feet, axillae, waistline, penis, scrotum
- Vesicles—isolated, pinpoint, and filled with serous fluid
- Papules—hypersensitivity reaction, small and isolated
- Chronic cases—secondary lesions with erythema and scaling
- Infants and elderly—Norwegian scabies—penetration of underlying epidermis by hundreds of mites causes generalized urticarial rash

Differential Diagnosis

- Pediculosis
- Atopic dermatitis
- Eczema
- Insect bites
- Pityriasis rosea
- Seborrheic dermatitis
- Syphilis

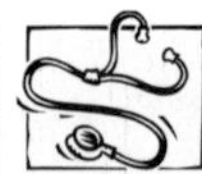

ASSESSMENT

History

Inquire about:

- Onset and duration of symptoms
- Pruritis and whether problem is worse at night
- Similar symptoms in friends and family members
- Treatments tried and results
- Underlying conditions
- Current medications

Physical Findings

- Gray or skin-colored burrows, which appear as ridges up to a few centimeters long
- Isolated tiny vesicles or papules
- Common sites—webs of fingers, waistline, axillae, hands, feet, scrotum, penis, buttocks

Initial Workup

Laboratory

- If burrows found, take 25 gauge needle and insert it into black dot at end of burrow; mite, ova, or feces will stick to needle; transfer to slide or, using sterile scalpel blade held parallel to skin, slice off whole burrow and transfer to slide
- Add drop of emersion oil and coverslip, and examine under microscope
- No burrows—no diagnostic tests

Radiology: None indicated

Further Workup

None indicated

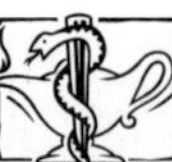

INTERVENTIONS

Office Treatment

None indicated

Lifestyle Modification

Good personal hygiene on daily basis

Patient Education

Teach patient about:

- Need to treat all household members at same time
- Laundering all clothing in hot water and drying in hot dryer (clothes that cannot be laundered should be dry cleaned and sealed in plastic storage bags for 2 weeks)
- Fact that pruritis may continue for up to 2 weeks after treatment
- Showering and drying skin thoroughly before applying scabicide
- Medications used and side effects (see Pharmacotherapeutics)

Referrals

None needed unless treatment fails or complications arise; then to dermatologist

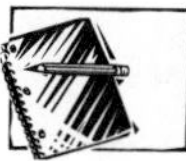

EVALUATION

Outcomes
- Resolves without sequelae
- Itching and dermatitis may continue for 7 to 14 days after treatment

Possible Complications
- Eczema
- Pyoderma
- Nodular scabies

Follow-up
In 2 weeks to assess response to therapy

FOR YOUR INFORMATION

Life Span
Pediatric: Infants usually have more widespread involvement
Geriatric: Treatment is the same
Pregnancy: Use lindane cautiously and not more than twice because of its potential to cause neurotoxicity

Miscellaneous
N/A

Reference
Whitmore E: Common problems of the skin. In Barker LR, Burton JR, Zieve PD, editors: *Principles of ambulatory medicine,* ed 4, Baltimore, 1995, Williams & Wilkins, pp 1471-1472.

NOTES

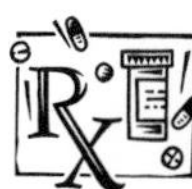

PHARMACOTHERAPEUTICS

Drug of Choice	Mechanism of Action	Prescribing Information	Side Effects
Lindane (Kwell) shampoo or lotion; shampoo for scalp—apply to dry hair and work in thoroughly, leave on for 10 minutes, rinse thoroughly; lotion for body and pubic area—apply cream from neck down, leave on 8-12 hours, wash off thoroughly	Parasiticidal and ovacidal	***Contraindications:*** Hypersensitivity; premature neonates; seizure disorder ***Cost:*** Lotion, 60 ml: $2-$6; shampoo, 2 oz: $3-$6 ***Pregnancy category:*** B	CNS stimulation ranging from dizziness to convulsions; skin irritation; hypersensitivity reaction; nausea, vomiting; diarrhea; liver damage
Permethrin 5% (Elimite); apply from neck down; leave on 8-14 hours and rinse off; apply second application 48 hours later	Pediculicidal and ovacidal	***Contraindications:*** Hypersensitivity to pyrethroid, pyrethrine, or chrysanthemums ***Cost:*** 60 g: $17 ***Pregnancy category:*** B	Pruritus, burning, stinging, tingling, numbness, rash

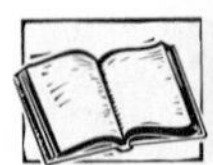

OVERVIEW

Schizophrenia is a major psychotic disorder. It consists of active symptoms, prodromal symptoms, and residual symptoms. Active symptoms must last at least 1 week, and there must be some continual disturbance for 6 months.

Pathogenesis

Cause—unknown; probably combination of inherited and environmental factors

Patient Profile

- Males = Females
- Onset before age 45 years
- More common in lower socioeconomic classes

Signs and Symptoms

- Active symptoms—two of the following must be present:
  - Delusions, hallucinations, incoherence, or loosening of association
  - Catatonic behavior
  - Flat or grossly inappropriate affect
  - Marked negative effect on functioning
- Prodromal/residual symptoms:
  - Social withdrawal or isolation
  - Impaired role functioning
  - Peculiar behavior
  - Impaired self-care
  - Blunted or inappropriate affect
  - Speech content abnormality
  - Odd beliefs
  - Unusual perceptual experiences
  - Loss of initiative and energy

Differential Diagnosis

- Organic mental disorder due to trauma
- Infection
- Tumor
- Metabolic and/or endocrine disturbances
- Intoxication
- Neurologic disorders
- Substance use/abuse
- Mood disorders

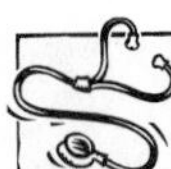

ASSESSMENT

History

Inquire about:

- Onset and duration of symptoms—may be difficult to obtain an adequate history if patient in active phase
- Drug and/or alcohol use
- Work and social functioning
- Underlying conditions
- Current medications

Physical Findings

- Unkempt appearance
- Abnormal thought processes
- Unusual or bizarre verbal behavior
- Abnormal motor movements
- Abnormal affect
- Abnormal perception
- Abnormal ego function (lack of self-control, lack of reality testing)

Initial Workup

Laboratory: Done to rule out organic disorders:

- Blood chemistries
- Thyroid function
- Urinalysis
- Tests for B_{12}, folate, thiamine
- Blood and urine for drugs and alcohol

Radiology: CT scan and/or MRI of brain to rule out organic disease

Further Workup

None indicated

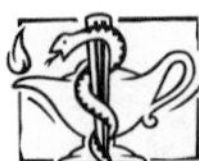

INTERVENTIONS

Office Treatment

- Will probably need admission to inpatient psychiatric unit
- Can treat as outpatient if not harmful to self and others
- Consult with collaborative physician regarding referral to psychiatrist

Lifestyle Modifications

- Lifestyle may be in total disarray because of disease process
- May quit or lose job because of inability to function
- Family relations may be strained
- Once controlled, need to resume some "normal" functioning

Patient Education

Teach patient about:

- Disease process
- Including family in educational process
- Need for treatment by a professional trained in this area
- Neuroleptic medication and importance of taking medication as directed
- NP following patient once stabilized, along with psychiatrist
- Support groups available
- Medications and side effects (see Pharmacotherapeutics)

Referral

To psychiatrist; NP's responsibility is to ensure that patient obtains appropriate care

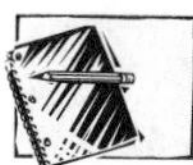

EVALUATION

Outcome

Good outcome associated with:

- Family history of affective disorders
- Good premorbid functioning
- Acute onset in midlife
- Presence of affective component
- Intact family function

Possible Complications

- Suicide
- Side effects of neuroleptic medications—can be serious

Follow-up

- By psychiatrist
- NP may see patient for other medical problems

FOR YOUR INFORMATION

Life Span

Pediatric: Unusual before puberty
Geriatric: More likely to require institutionalization.
Pregnancy: Complications of taking neuroleptic medication

Miscellaneous

N/A

Reference

Goldberg RJ: *Practical guide to the care of the psychiatric patient,* St Louis, 1995, Mosby, pp 135-147.

NOTES

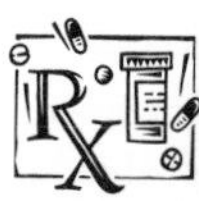

PHARMACOTHERAPEUTICS

The following are some of the more commonly used medications for schizophrenia. It is important for the NP to remember that these drugs can have serious side effects and interact with numerous other medications. The listing here is intended only as a guide.

Drug of Choice	Mechanism of Action	Prescribing Information	Side Effects
Neuroleptics: haloperidol (Haldol), loxapine (Loxitane), thiothixene (Navane), chlorpromazine (Thorazine); dosages not included, since they vary widely, depending on symptoms	All block postsynaptic dopamine receptors	***Contraindications:*** Hypersensitivity; comatose state; Parkinson's disease; interact with many drugs—antihypertensives, antacids, epinephrine, anticholinergics, anticonvulsants, tricyclics, SSRIs, lithium, nicotine ***Cost:*** Haldol, 0.5-mg tab, 100 tabs: $2; Loxitane, 5-mg tab, 100 tabs: $36; Navane, 1-mg tab, 100 tabs: $12; Thorazine, 10-mg tab, 100 tabs: $3 ***Pregnancy category:*** Use only if absolutely necessary	Dystonia, acute dystonia, akinesia, akathisia, tardive dyskinesia, sedation, anticholinergic activity, orthostatic hypotension, jaundice, increased prolactin, lower seizure threshold, weight gain, neuroleptic malignant syndrome, retinitis pigmentosa
Clozapine (Clozaril), 25 mg ½ tab bid PO, maximum 300 mg tid PO; used when patient fails to respond to 2 other neuroleptics	Differs from other neuroleptics; low affinity for D_2 receptors; high affinity for D_1 and D_4 receptors	***Contraindications:*** Previous granulocytopenia; severe hepatic or renal impairment; pregnancy; history of poor compliance ***Cost:*** 100 mg, 3/day × 1 year: $3800 ***Pregnancy category:*** Should *only* be used if absolutely necessary	Significant risk of agranulocytosis—must monitor CBC weekly; seizures, orthostatic hypotension, respiratory or cardiac arrest, neuroleptic malignant syndrome, fever, sedation, drowsiness
Risperidone (Risperdal), 1 mg PO bid, maximum 16 mg/day in divided doses	Combined serotonin-dopamine antagonist	***Contraindication:*** Hypersensitivity ***Cost:*** 1 mg, 3/day for 1 month: $182 ***Pregnancy category:*** C	Neuroleptic malignant syndrome, tardive dyskinesia, orthostatic hypotension, seizures, dizziness, somnolence, nausea, headache, rhinitis, coughing, sinusitis, rash, tachycardia

Seborrheic Dermatitis

OVERVIEW

Seborrheic dermatitis is a chronic, inflammatory condition. It affects parts of the body with hair, most commonly the scalp, eyebrows, and face. It can affect the axillae, inframammary folds, groin, and umbilicus.

Pathogenesis

Cause—probably a yeast, *Pityrosporum ovale*

Patient Profile

- Males = Females
- Infancy through adulthood

Signs and Symptoms

- Infants:
  - Cradle cap—greasy scaling scalp
  - May have mild erythema
- Adolescents and adults:
  - Scaling rash that is red and greasy
  - Consists of patches and plaques with distinct margins
  - Located in hairy areas such as scalp and scalp margins, eyebrows and eyelid margins, and nasolabial folds
  - Has periods of remission and recurrence

Differential Diagnosis

- Dandruff
- Atopic dermatitis
- Psoriasis
- *Candidal* infection
- Tinea cruris or capitis
- Eczema
- Rosacea
- Discoid lupus erythematosus

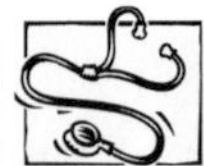

ASSESSMENT

History

Inquire about:

- Onset and duration of symptoms
- Previous episodes of similar symptoms
- Treatments tried and results
- Underlying conditions—Parkinson's disease, AIDS, emotional stress—may be risk factors
- Current medications

Physical Findings

- Infants:
  - Cradle cap—greasy scaling scalp
  - May have mild erythema
- Adolescents and adults:
  - Scaling rash that is red and greasy
  - Consists of patches and plaques with distinct margins
  - Located in hairy areas such as scalp and scalp margins, eyebrows and eyelid margins, and nasolabial folds

Initial Workup

Laboratory: None indicated
Radiology: None indicated

Further Workup

None indicated

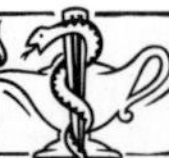

INTERVENTIONS

Office Treatment

None indicated

Lifestyle Modifications

- Shampoo hair on a daily basis
- Stress reduction techniques

Patient Education

Teach patient about:

- Disease process, chronicity, and treatment:
  - For infants—parents should shampoo scalp frequently with salicylic and sulfur shampoos and apply 1% hydrocortisone lotion—for thick scale, apply warm olive oil or mineral oil—wash off several hours later with mild dishwashing liquid
  - For adults—shampoo with antiseborrheic shampoo daily (can be purchased OTC)—for thick scale, apply coal tar at bedtime and then wash out with mild detergent the next morning
  - For other areas of the body, apply 1% hydrocortisone cream; for mild to moderate facial and chest involvement, use ketoconazole 2%
- Medications used and side effects (see Pharmacotherapeutics)

Referrals

None, unless treatment fails; then to dermatologist

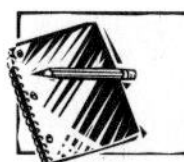

EVALUATION

Outcomes

- Infants—resolution occurs in 6 to 8 months
- Adults—control of disease is expected outcome, since disease is of chronic nature

Possible Complications

- Usually related to treatment:
  - Skin atrophy
  - Glaucoma—from fluorinated corticosteroids
- Secondary bacterial infections

Follow-up

- Every 2 weeks until controlled
- Consult with physician if no improvement in 1 month

FOR YOUR INFORMATION

Life Span

Pediatric: Commonly referred to as cradle cap in infants

Geriatric: Treatment is the same

Pregnancy: Ketoconazole cream should not be used—could result in enough systemic absorption to cause problems, particularly if used on large area

Miscellaneous

Because of the chronicity of the disease and its cosmetic effects, patients may require a great deal of emotional support to cope with the disease.

Reference

Habif TP: *Clinical dermatology: a color guide to diagnosis and therapy,* ed 3, St Louis, 1996; Mosby, pp 214-217.

NOTES

PHARMACOTHERAPEUTICS

Drug of Choice	Mechanism of Action	Prescribing Information	Side Effects
Selenium sulfide 2.5%; shampoo; shampoo daily	Has a cytostatic effect on cells of epidermis	***Contraindication:*** Hypersensitivity ***Cost:*** 4 oz: $3-$12 ***Pregnancy category:*** C	Do not use if acute inflammation or exudate present; skin irritation; discoloration, oiliness, or dryness of hair
Topical corticosteroid: hydrocortisone 1% cream (Cortaid 1%); apply to affected area bid to qid; effective in 90% of cases; may need to prescribe one of the more potent topical steroids, such as mometasone (Elocon) cream or betamethasone (Diprolene) cream	Antiinflammatory, antipruritic, and vasoconstrictive	***Contraindication:*** Hypersensitivity ***Cost:*** 1%, 30 g: $12; several available OTC; mometasone 0.1%, 45 g: $29; betamethasone 0.05%, 15 g: $3-$16 ***Pregnancy category:*** C	Burning, dryness, itching, irritation acne, folliculitis, hypertrichosis, hypopigmentation, atrophy, striae, peripheral dermatitis, secondary infection; if used on large area for extended periods of time, can have systemic side effects
Ketoconazole 2% cream (Nizoral); apply to affected area bid × 4-6 weeks—safety in children not established	Broad-spectrum antifungal	***Contraindication:*** Hypersensitivity ***Cost:*** 15 g: $13 ***Pregnancy category:*** C	Severe irritation, pruritus, stinging, allergic reaction

Seizure Disorder

OVERVIEW

Seizure disorder is a disorder in which there is hyperexcitation of the neurons in the brain. It is a paroxysmal disturbance in consciousness, behavior, or motor activity. Epilepsy is a chronic neurologic condition that produces recurrent seizures.

Pathogenesis

Most are idiopathic; other etiologies are based on age:

- Neonatal seizures—birth trauma or congenital malformation
- Infancy or early childhood—fever, metabolic disorders, CNS infections
- Children—idiopathic epilepsy, CNS infections
- Adolescence to early adulthood—idiopathic epilepsy, trauma, alcohol and drug abuse
- Adults and seniors—idiopathic epilepsy, trauma, neoplasm, or stroke

Patient Profile

- Males = Females
- All ages

Signs and Symptoms

Varies with type of seizure—based on mode of onset and spread; 2 main types—partial seizures and generalized seizures:

- Partial seizures:
  - Simple symptoms—no loss of consciousness, motor symptoms (start in single muscle group and spread to one side of body), somatosensory symptoms (paresthesias), autonomic symptoms (loss of bowel and bladder function), psychic symptoms (hallucinations)
  - Complex symptoms—same symptoms as above, but consciousness is impaired either at onset or progressively
- Generalized seizures:
  - Absence (petit mal) seizures—sudden stopping of motor activity, blank stare
  - Myoclonic seizures—brief, sudden, shocklike contractions of large muscles
  - Tonic-clonic (grand mal) seizures—aura (possibly), tonic contractions, loss of consciousness, clonic contractions, loss of bladder and bowel function (possibly), postictal period

Differential Diagnosis

- Vasovagal faint
- Psychomimetic drug use
- Migraine
- Transient ischemic attacks (TIAs)
- Syncope
- Vertigo
- Schizophrenia
- Hypoglycemia
- Narcolepsy
- Renal failure

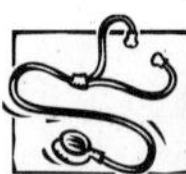

ASSESSMENT

History

Inquire about:

- Onset and duration of symptoms
- Family members or witnesses to seizure activity (have them describe activity)
- Precipitating factors
- Loss of consciousness or incontinence
- Aura and postictal period
- History of trauma, drug or alcohol withdrawal, barbiturates or benzodiazepines
- Exposure to toxins
- Family history of seizures
- Underlying conditions
- Current medications

Physical Findings

- Between seizures—physical examination may be normal
- Systemic disease may be found
- Asymmetry of hands, feet, and face
- Abnormality in one cerebral hemisphere
- Clumsiness, hyperreflexia, marked impairment
- Head trauma or trauma to mouth may be present

Initial Workup

Laboratory

- CBC with differential
- Chemistry panel to include electrolytes, liver function tests, glucose, BUN, creatinine
- Urinalysis
- Drug screen—if a concern.

Radiology: CT scan or MRI of head for intractable seizures, focal neurologic abnormalities, first seizure in adult

Further Workup

EEG

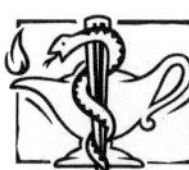

INTERVENTIONS

Office Treatment

- During seizure—maintain airway, prevent injury, give oxygen if cyanotic, record events
- Status epilepticus (seizure >10 minutes)—prompt transport to emergency room

Lifestyle Modifications

- Healthy lifestyle
- Smoking cessation
- Alcohol withdrawal
- Nutritious diet
- Exercise plan
- Avoidance of precipitating events
- May need to make transportation arrangements
- May need change of employment

Patient Education

Teach patient and family about:

- Condition and treatment options—medications to control seizures
- Emergency management of seizure
- Need for medical alert tag
- State law concerning driving
- For well-controlled seizures, minimum restrictions—swim with buddy; wear helmet for sports, video games (may trigger seizures)
- Avoidance of precipitating events
- Possible need for counseling to cope with diagnosis
- Importance of adequate rest and healthy lifestyle to prevent infection
- Medications used and side effects (see Pharmacotherapeutics)

Referral

Consult with MD on when treatment should be started and with what medication; may refer to neurologist for evaluation and initiation of medication

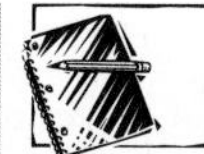

EVALUATION

Outcome

Seizures controlled; minimal side effects from medication

Possible Complications

- Status epilepticus
- Severe injury from seizure
- Drug toxicity

Follow-up

Every 2 weeks × 3; then monthly follow-up based on medication used; may be followed by neurologist

FOR YOUR INFORMATION

Life Span

Pediatric: More prone to febrile seizures or idiopathic; no medication needed for febrile seizures

Geriatric: First seizure—investigate for underlying cause

Pregnancy: Increased risk of congenital abnormalities in infants born to mothers taking anticonvulsant medications

Miscellaneous

The newly diagnosed patient with seizures will need a great deal of support from the NP. This diagnosis can create a great deal of stress and anxiety for the patient because of the social stigma attached to it.

References

Kaplan PW, Fisher RS: Seizure disorders. In Barker LR, Burton JR, Zieve PD, editors: *Principles of ambulatory medicine,* ed 4, Baltimore, 1995, Williams & Wilkins, pp 1178-1197.

Parks BR, Dostrow VG, Noble SL: Drug therapy for epilepsy, *Am Fam Physician* 50(3):639-648, 1994.

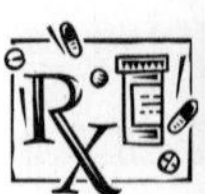

PHARMACOTHERAPEUTICS

Careful consideration must be given to starting drug therapy in the patient with new onset of seizures. If the seizure was provoked, can the provoking factor be corrected? If the answer is yes, no therapy is necessary; otherwise, consider therapy. If the seizure was unprovoked, estimate the recurrence risk and consequences. The benefits of therapy must outweigh the risks. In a child with unprovoked seizures, no treatment is given unless the consequences are grave. It is also important to have an accurate diagnosis of the type of seizure, since medications are prescribed based on type.

Drug of Choice	Mechanism of Action	Prescribing Information	Side Effects
For generalized tonic-clonic and partial complex seizures:			
Primidone (Mysoline); adults and children >8 years, 250 mg PO qd; increase by 250 mg each week, maximum dose 2 g/day in divided doses qid; children <8 years, 125 mg PO qd, increase by 125 mg/week, maximum dose 1 g/day in divided doses qid	Raises seizure threshold by conversion of drug to phenobarbital	***Contraindications:*** Hypersensitivity; porphyria; pregnancy ***Cost:*** 250-mg tab, 100 tabs: \$15-\$45 ***Pregnancy category:*** D ***Laboratory tests:*** Drug level, CBC every 6 months	Thrombocytopenia, leukopenia, neutropenia, eosinophilia, megaloblastic anemia, lymphadenopathy, stimulation, drowsiness, dizziness, confusion, sedation, headache, hallucinations, nausea, vomiting, anorexia, rash, edema, alopecia, diplopia, nystagmus, impotence
For absence, myoclonic, tonic-clonic, and partial seizures:			
Valproate (Depakene); adults and children, 15 mg/kg/day PO divided in 2-3 doses; increase by 5-10 mg/kg/day PO every week; maximum dose, 30 mg/kg/day PO	Increases levels of gamma-aminobutyric acid (GABA) in brain, which decreases seizure activity	***Contraindications:*** Hypersensitivity; pregnancy ***Cost:*** 250-mg tab, 100 tabs: \$15-\$45 ***Pregnancy category:*** D ***Laboratory tests:*** Baseline liver function tests, then every 2-3 months × 2; long-term therapy—CBC, folate, prothrombin time	Thrombocytopenia, leukopenia, lymphocytosis, increased prothrombin time, sedation, dizziness, drowsiness, headache, depression, hallucinations, nausea, vomiting, constipation, diarrhea, heartburn, hepatic failure, pancreatitis, toxic hepatitis, rash, alopecia, enuresis, irregular menses

Drug of Choice	Mechanism of Action	Prescribing Information	Side Effects
For tonic-clonic and partial seizures, use one of the following:			
Carbamazepine (Tegretol); adults and children >12 years, 200 mg PO bid, increase by 200 mg/day; maximum dose, 1200 mg/day; children <12 years, 10-20 mg/kg/day PO bid or tid	Inhibits nerve impulses by limiting influx of sodium ions across cell membranes in motor cortex	***Contraindications:*** Hypersensitivity to carbamazepine or tricyclic antidepressant; bone marrow depression; concomitant use of MAOIs ***Cost:*** 200-mg tab, 100 tabs: $10-$35 ***Pregnancy category:*** C ***Laboratory tests:*** CBC; liver function tests every 2-3 weeks for first 2 months, then every 3 months	Thrombocytopenia, agranulocytosis, leukocytosis, neutropenia, aplastic anemia, eosinophilia, drowsiness, dizziness, confusion, paralysis, headache, hallucinations, nausea, constipation, diarrhea, anorexia, vomiting, abdominal pain, hepatitis, Stevens-Johnson syndrome, tinnitus, dry mouth, hypertension, congestive heart failure (CHF), pulmonary hypertension, albuminuria, glycosuria, impotence
Phenytoin (Dilantin); adult loading dose 900 mg-1.5 g PO tid, then 300 mg/day; child loading dose 15 mg/kg PO q8-12h, then 5-7 mg/kg q12h	Inhibits spread of seizure activity in motor cortex by altering ion transport	***Contraindications:*** Hypersensitivity; psychiatric conditions; pregnancy; bradycardia; sinoatrial (SA) and atrioventricular (AV) block; Stokes-Adams syndrome ***Cost:*** 100-mg tab, 100 tabs: $7-$20 ***Pregnancy category:*** D	Drowsiness, dizziness, insomnia, paresthesias, depression, suicidal tendencies, hypotension, ventricular fibrillation, nystagmus, diplopia, nausea, vomiting, constipation, anorexia, hepatitis, nephritis, agranulocytosis, leukopenia, aplastic anemia, thrombocytopenia, megaloblastic anemia, lupus erythematosus, Stevens-Johnson syndrome, hypocalcemia
Adjunct treatment for partial seizures:			
Gabapentin (Neurontin), 300 mg PO day 1; 300 mg PO bid day 2; 300 mg PO tid day 3; maximum dose 1800 mg/day	Unknown	***Contraindication:*** Hypersensitivity ***Cost:*** 300-mg tab, 50 tabs: $54 ***Pregnancy category:*** C	Dizziness, fatigue, anxiety, somnolence, ataxia, amnesia, abnormal gait, vasodilation, dry mouth, blurred vision, constipation, increased appetite, impotence, leukopenia, pruritus, myalgia, rhinitis, coughing

Sexual Dysfunction in Women

OVERVIEW

Sexual dysfunction in women can include a disorder of desire, a disorder of arousal, dyspareunia or vaginismus, or orgasmic disorders. Any or all of the above conditions may exist. A disorder of desire exists when a woman has no desire for sexual activity, fails to have sexual dreams or fantasies, or becomes frustrated by lack of sexual activity. A disorder of arousal occurs when the woman fails to attain or maintain vaginal lubrication or sexual excitement during the sexual encounter. Dyspareunia is painful sexual intercourse. Vaginismus is involuntary, spastic, sometimes painful contractions of the vaginal muscles that occur with attempted penetration. Orgasmic disorder can be primary (the patient has never achieved orgasm) or secondary (the patient has achieved orgasm in the past, but not with the current partner).

Pathogenesis

DISORDER OF DESIRE

Cause—unknown; may be stress related

DISORDER OF AROUSAL

Cause—unknown; strong psychiatric basis

DYSPAREUNIA

Many causes:

- Sexually transmitted diseases (STDs)
- Diabetes
- Bladder disease
- Decreased estrogen production
- Soaps
- Perfumes
- Psychologic basis

VAGINISMUS

Causes—varied:

- Sexual trauma
- Strong, conservative religious beliefs
- Hostile feelings toward partner

ORGASMIC DISORDERS

Causes:

- Primary causes:
  - Restrictive home environment
  - Cultural conditioning
  - Unrealistic expectations
  - Interrelational difficulties
- Secondary causes:
  - Diabetes
  - Psychoactive drugs
  - Dyspareunia
  - Thyroid disease
  - Oophorectomy
  - Spinal cord damage

Patient Profile

Most commonly in late 20s to early 30s

Signs and Symptoms

- Complaint to NP
- May have rather vague symptoms—NP needs to ask if patient is having sexual problems
- Infertility
- Marital conflict
- Family dysfunction

Differential Diagnosis

- Must differentiate type of dysfunction
- Anatomic or congenital disorders

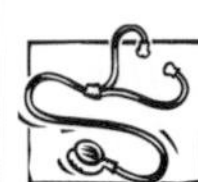

ASSESSMENT

History

Inquire about:

- Onset and duration of symptoms
- Menstrual and obstetric history
- Age of first coitus
- History of STDs
- Desire for sex
- Dyspareunia or vaginismus
- Ability to become aroused
- Ability to attain orgasm currently and in the past
- Relationship with partner
- Current stressors at home and at work
- Past sexual abuse or trauma
- Underlying conditions (diabetes, thyroid disease, etc.)
- Current medications

Physical Findings

Complete physical examination, including pelvic examination—may all be within normal limits

Initial Workup

Laboratory: Done to rule out organic causes:

- CBC
- Chemistry panel
- Thyroid panel
- Liver function studies
- If indicated, cultures for gonorrhea and chlamydial infection
- Rapid plasma reagin (RPR)
- HIV screen

Radiology: None unless indicated by history and physical examination

Further Workup

None unless indicated by history and physical examination

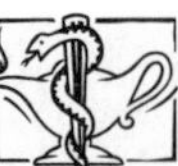

INTERVENTIONS

Office Treatment

Provide supportive environment

Lifestyle Modifications

- Smoking and alcohol cessation
- Weight reduction if problematic

Patient Education

Teach patient about:

- Condition and cause if known
- Treatment—depends on cause
- Prescription medication thought to be cause—change medication if possible
- Sexual feelings and give patient permission to have these feelings and desires
- Areas of concern, giving specific facts to questions patient may have
- Specific behaviors that may alleviate problems, such as use of water-soluble lubricants for vaginal dryness or change in sexual positions
- Vaginal dilation for vaginismus
- Counseling with sex therapist if above measures fail
- Estrogen therapy if needed (see Pharmacotherapeutics)

Referral

To sex therapist for intensive treatment

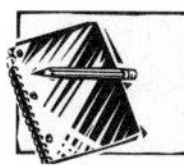

EVALUATION

Outcome
Patient is able to enjoy a happy, healthy, sexual relationship

Possible Complications
- Marital discord
- Clinical depression

Follow-up
Every 2 weeks × 2; then monthly; may be followed by sex therapist

FOR YOUR INFORMATION

Life Span
Pediatric: Peer pressures may create anxiety for adolescent
Geriatric: Vaginal dryness due to normal aging process may be causative factor; may be less willing to discuss sexuality
Pregnancy: May have difficulty because of unwarranted fear of harming fetus

Miscellaneous
It is important for the NP to provide an open environment in which the patient can feel free to discuss her problems. Often the NP will need to initiate a discussion about sexuality in order to put the patient at ease.

Reference
Fogel CI: Women and sexuality. In Youngkin EQ, Davis MS, editors: *Women's health: a primary care clinical guide,* Norwalk, Conn, Appleton & Lange, pp 66-72.

NOTES

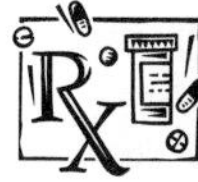

PHARMACOTHERAPEUTICS

Drug of Choice	Mechanism of Action	Prescribing Information	Side Effects
For postmenopausal patient:			
Estrogen (Premarin), 0.625 mg PO 1 tab daily; estrogen is available in pills, as a transdermal patch, or as a vaginal cream; method of administration should be decided on by NP and patient together by determining which method best meets patient's needs	Affects release of pituitary gonadotropins; inhibits ovulation	***Contraindications:*** Hypersensitivity; breast cancer; thromboembolic disorders; reproductive cancer; undiagnosed vaginal bleeding; pregnancy ***Cost:*** 0.625-mg tab, 100 tabs: $50; transdermal or topical estrogen per year: $107 ***Pregnancy category:*** X	Dizziness, headache, migraines, depression, hypotension, thrombophlebitis, thromboembolism, pulmonary embolism, myocardial infarction (MI), nausea, vomiting, cholestatic jaundice, weight gain, diplopia, amenorrhea, cervical erosion, breakthrough bleeding, dysmenorrhea, vaginal candidiasis, spontaneous abortion, rash, urticaria, acne, hirsutism, photosensitivity
If patient has intact uterus, add:			
Medroxyprogesterone acetate (Provera), 10 mg PO on days 1-12 or days 13-25; or can give 2.5 mg PO daily; estrogen and medroxyprogesterone acetate are now available in 1 tablet sold under trade name Prempro	Inhibits secretion of pituitary gonadotropins; stimulates growth of mammary tissue	***Contraindications:*** Hypersensitivity; breast cancer; thromboembolic disorders; reproductive cancer; undiagnosed vaginal bleeding; pregnancy ***Cost:*** 5-mg tab, 30 tabs: $16 ***Pregnancy category:*** X	Dizziness, headache, migraines, depression, hypotension, thrombophlebitis, thromboembolism, pulmonary embolism, MI, nausea, vomiting, cholestatic jaundice, weight gain, diplopia, amenorrhea, cervical erosion, breakthrough bleeding, dysmenorrhea, vaginal candidiasis, spontaneous abortion, rash, urticaria, acne, hirsutism, photosensitivity

OVERVIEW

Silicosis is a chronic fibrotic lung disease that is caused by inhaling silica dust. It is found in metal miners, foundry workers, pottery makers, and any workers involved with cutting, polishing, or shearing rock. There are several different types: chronic simple, chronic complicated, subacute, and acute. Patients with chronic silicosis have an increased incidence of tuberculosis.

Pathogenesis

- Cause—exposure and inhalation of silica dust
- Chronic simple type—seen after 10 to 12 years of exposure
- Chronic complicated type—seen after >20 years of exposure
- Subacute type—seen after 3 to 6 years of heavy exposure
- Acute type—seen after <2 years of massive exposure

Patient Profile

- Males > Females
- Acute type—any age
- Other types—most common age group—40 to 75 years

Signs and Symptoms

CHRONIC SIMPLE TYPE

- Asymptomatic
- Cough
- Mild dyspnea

CHRONIC COMPLICATED AND SUBACUTE TYPES

- Chest tightness
- Cough with sputum production
- Dyspnea
- Right-sided heart failure

ACUTE TYPE

- Fever
- Dry cough
- Severe dyspnea

Differential Diagnosis

- Sarcoidosis
- Other causes of pneumoconiosis
- Hodgkin's disease
- Tuberculosis
- Fungal pneumonia
- Neoplasm

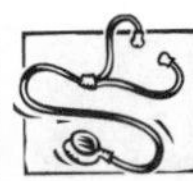

ASSESSMENT

History

Inquire about:

- Onset and duration of symptoms
- Occupational history
- Smoking history
- Underlying conditions
- Current medications

Physical Findings

- Dyspnea
- Pursed-lip breathing
- Lungs—wheezes, rales, rhonchi, decreased breath sounds
- Right-sided heart failure—weight gain, edema, heart murmur, jugular venous distention, hepatomegaly

Initial Workup

Laboratory

- Arterial blood gases—decreased PO_2 and increased PCO_2
- CBC—may see polycythemia
- TB skin test—significant number will be positive

Radiology: Chest film—PA and lateral:

- Chronic simple type—egg shell calcifications in hilar lymph nodes
- Other types—large conglomerate densities in upper lobes
- Opacities >1 cm; may cavitate

Further Workup

Pulmonary function tests:

- Chronic simple type—normal
- Chronic complicated type—obstructive and restrictive dysfunction

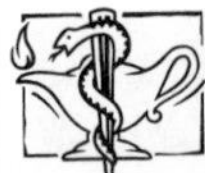

INTERVENTIONS

Office Treatment

None indicated

Lifestyle Modifications

- Smoking cessation
- Chronic simple type—consider occupational change; stop exposure

Patient Education

Teach patient about:

- Condition and treatment:
    - Chronic simple type—nonprogressive once exposure stops
    - Chronic complicated type—no effective treatment; stopping exposure will not stop progression
- Chest percussion and postural drainage (teach significant other)
- Signs and symptoms of infection and to report promptly
- Using cool-mist vaporizer
- Maintaining regular exercise program
- Pulmonary rehabilitation
- Increasing fluids
- TB skin test—if positive, patient needs prophylaxis for 1 year
- Medications used and side effects (see Pharmacotherapeutics)

Referral

To pulmonologist

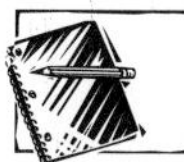

EVALUATION

Outcomes

- Chronic simple type—nonprogressive if exposure stopped
- Chronic complicated type—pulmonary fibrosis progresses, leads to cor pulmonale and right-sided heart failure; may need lung transplant

Possible Complications

- Massive fibrosis
- Cor pulmonale
- Right-sided heart failure
- Mycobacterial or fungal infections
- Respiratory failure
- Death

Follow-up

Initially, every 2 weeks; then, if stable, every 2 to 3 months

FOR YOUR INFORMATION

Life Span

Pediatric: Extremely rare
Geriatric: Higher morbidity and mortality
Pregnancy: Should be handled by a specialist

Miscellaneous

N/A

References

Mitchell JT: Nursing role in management: lower respiratory problems. In Lewis SM, Collier IC, Heitkemper MM, editors: *Medical-surgical nursing: assessment and management of clinical problems,* ed 4, St Louis, 1996, Mosby, pp 654-656.

Stauffer JL: Lung. In Tierney LM Jr, McPhee SJ, Papadakis MA, editors: *Current medical diagnosis and treatment,* ed 34, Norwalk, Conn, 1995, Appleton & Lange.

NOTES

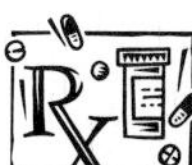

PHARMACOTHERAPEUTICS

Drug of Choice	Mechanism of Action	Prescribing Information	Side Effects
For patient with positive PPD:			
Isoniazid (INH), 300 mg PO qd × 6-12 months; children, 10 mg/kg/day PO × 12 months	Bactericidal; interferes with lipid and nucleic acid biosynthesis	***Contraindications:*** Hypersensitivity; optic neuritis ***Cost:*** 300-mg tab, 100 tabs: $2-$12 ***Pregnancy category:*** C	Fever, rash, peripheral neuropathy, toxic encephalopathy, convulsions, blurred vision, agraunlocytosis, hemolytic anemia, aplastic anemia, thrombocytopenia, eosinophilia, dyspnea, vitamin B_6 deficiency, hyperglycemia, metabolic acidosis, gynecomastia, nausea, vomiting, jaundice, fatal hepatitis

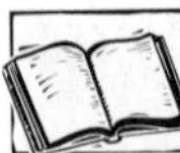

OVERVIEW

Sinusitis is an inflammation and/or infection of the mucous membranes that line the paranasal sinuses. The condition may be acute or chronic.

Pathogenesis

ACUTE SINUSITIS

- Edema of nasal mucosa blocks small sinus ostia
- Bacterial pathogens—*Streptococcus pneumoniae, Hemophilus influenzae, Moraxhella catarrhalis, Chlamydia pneumoniae, Streptococcus pyrogenes*

CHRONIC SINUSITIS

- Anatomic abnormality of osteomeatal unit
- Interferes with mucociliary clearance mechanism
- Bacterial pathogens—anaerobic bacteria, *Staphylococcus aureus*

Patient Profile

- Males = Females
- All ages

Signs and Symptoms

ACUTE SINUSITIS

- Yellow or green nasal drainage;
- Fever
- Nasal congestion
- Sore throat
- Facial pain
- Toothache
- Headache—worse when bending over
- Periorbital edema
- Malaise

CHRONIC SINUSITIS

- Cough
- Nasal congestion
- Nasal drainage (yellow or green–may be streaked with red) lasting >30 days
- Dull ache or pressure across face or headache
- Popping ears
- Halitosis
- Chronic cough

Differential Diagnosis

- Viral rhinitis
- Allergic rhinitis
- Dental abscess
- Headaches—cluster or migraine
- Nasal polyp
- Tumor
- Foreign body
- Vasomotor rhinitis

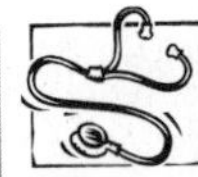

ASSESSMENT

History

Inquire about:

- Onset and duration of symptoms
- Prior history and treatment
- Fever, cough, and color of nasal drainage
- Pain and its location
- Eye puffiness in the morning
- Headaches
- History of allergies
- Underlying conditions
- Current medications, including OTC sinus medications

Physical Findings

- Fever
- Periorbital edema
- Allergic shiners
- Nasal mucosa—erythematous, edematous, yellow/green discharge
- Will be unable to transilluminate sinuses
- Pain on percussion of frontal and maxillary sinuses
- Lymphadenopathy
- Throat—erythematous with yellow or green postnasal drip
- Nasal polyps

Initial Workup

Laboratory

- For classic presentation—none indicated
- CBC—elevated WBC count
- Culture of nasal drainage

Radiology: Sinus films for recurrent or chronic cases—cloudiness, air fluid levels, thick mucosa in affected sinuses

Further Workup

CT scan or MRI if necessary to look for causes of chronic sinusitis

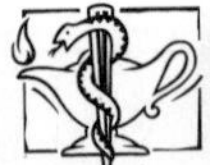

INTERVENTIONS

Office Treatment

None indicated

Lifestyle Modifications

- Smoking cessation
- Avoidance of environmental pollutants
- Humidification of air

Patient Education

Teach patient about:

- Disease process and treatment options—antibiotics, decongestants, nasal inhalers
- Tips for smoking cessation
- Humidification of air
- Warm compresses to face
- Increased fluid intake
- Avoiding swimming, diving, and airplane travel—may worsen condition
- Returning if symptoms not improved or worsen within 48 to 72 hours
- Possible complications
- How to take medications and side effects (see Pharmacotherapeutics)

Referral

To ear, nose, and throat specialist for chronic cases unresponsive to treatment

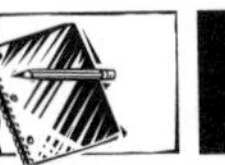

EVALUATION

Outcome

Resolves without sequelae

Possible Complications

- Meningitis
- Osteomyelitis
- Orbital infection
- Septic cavernous thrombosis

Follow-up

In 48 to 72 hours if no improvement or worsening of symptoms; otherwise, in 2 weeks

FOR YOUR INFORMATION

Life Span

Pediatric: Increases in latter part of childhood; chronic sinusitis—look for cause
Geriatric: May be more difficult to treat
Pregnancy: Cautious use of medications

Miscellaneous

Air travel with an upper respiratory tract infection can trigger acute sinusitis.

References

Smith CW Jr: The ears, nose, and throat. In Driscoll CE et al, editors: *The family practice desk reference,* ed 3, St Louis, 1996, Mosby, pp 97-98.

Wilder B: Pearls for practice: management of sinusitis. *J Am Acad Nurse Pract* 8(11):525-529, 1996.

PHARMACOTHERAPEUTICS

Drug of Choice	Mechanism of Action	Prescribing Information	Side Effects
Amoxicillin and clavulanate (Augmentin), 500-875 mg PO bid for 14-21 days; children, 25-45 mg/kg/day PO in 2 divided doses × 14-21 days	Bactericidal; cell wall inhibitor; effective against beta-lactamase–producing organisms	***Contraindication:*** Hypersensitivity ***Cost:*** 500-mg tab, 30 tabs: $82 ***Pregnancy category:*** B	Diarrhea, nausea, vomiting, stomatitis, black hairy tongue, pseudomembranous colitis, candidiasis, rash, urticaria, angioedema, anaphylaxis, arthralgia, myalgia, anemia, thrombocytopenia, leukopenia, anxiety, insomnia, confusion
Sulfamethoxazole/trimethoprim DS (Bactrim DS), 1 tab q12h × 14 days; children, 8 mg/kg trimethoprim and 40 mg/kg sulfamethoxazole/day in divided doses q12h × 14 days; for acute or chronic conditions—may extend to 21 days	Blocks 2 consecutive steps in bacterial synthesis of nucleic acids and protein	***Contraindications:*** Hypersensitivity to trimethoprim or sulfonamides; term pregnancy; lactation; megaloblastic anemia; infants <2 months; creatinine clearance <15 ml/min ***Cost:*** DS tab × 14 days: $2 ***Pregnancy category:*** C	Anaphylaxis, hypersensitivity, Stevens-Johnson syndrome, allergic myocarditis, nausea, vomiting, abdominal pain, hepatitis, enterocolitis, renal failure, toxic nephrosis, leukopenia, thrombocytopenia, hemolytic anemia
Topical decongestant: oxymetazoline (Afrin, Neo-Synephrine); children 6 years and up, 2 sprays each nostril bid—do not use >3-4 days or exceed dosing—rebound congestion may occur	Sympathomimetic; causes vasoconstriction, which decreases congestion	***Contraindications:*** Hypersensitivity; hypertension; diabetes; heart disease; thyroid disease; difficulty urinating because of enlarged prostate ***Cost:*** OTC: $3-$5 ***Pregnancy category:*** C	Habituation, stinging of nasal mucosa, dry membranes
Oral decongestants: 130 different products listed in *PDR* for nonprescription drugs; many in combination with an antihistamine; most contain pseudoephedrine, phenylephrine, or phenylpropanolamine; see labels for dosage—do not exceed dosage	Sympathomimetics; cause nasal vasoconstriction, producing decongestion	***Contraindications:*** Hypersensitivity; hypertension (controversial); diabetes; heart or thyroid disease; prostate enlargement ***Cost:*** Varies with product ***Pregnancy category:*** Pseudoephedrine—B; phenylephrine and phenylpropanolamine—C	Drowsiness, dry mouth, insomnia, headache, nervousness, fatigue, irritability, disorientation, rash, palpitations, sore throat, cough
Topical steroids: • Beclomethasone (Beconase AQ), 2 sprays each nostril bid; children 6-12 years, 1 spray each nostril daily—not for children <6 years • Flunisolide (Nasalide), 2 inhalations each nostril bid; children >6 years, 2 inhalations each nostril bid—do not use for those <6 years • Triamcinolone (Nasacort), 2 inhalations each nostril daily—may increase to 2 inhalations bid—for use in patients 12 years and older	Potent glucocorticoids; antiinflammatory—mechanism for this property is unknown	***Contraindication:*** Hypersensitivity ***Cost:*** Beconase AQ, 21 g: $31; Nasalide, 25 ml: $27; Nasacort, 10 g: $38 ***Pregnancy category:*** C	Use caution if patient is being transferred from oral steroids—could show signs of adrenal insufficiency; headache, nasal irritation, dry mucous membranes, throat discomfort

OVERVIEW

Obstructive sleep apnea occurs when there is upper airway obstruction during sleep that interferes with normal respiration. Oxygen desaturation commonly occurs. Repeated periods of apnea will lead to excessive daytime drowsiness.

Pathogenesis

Cause—upper airway narrowing due to:

- Enlarged tonsils
- Enlarged adenoids
- Enlarged uvula
- Low soft palate
- Loss of pharyngeal muscle tone, allowing pharynx to collapse during inspiration
- Large or posteriorly located tongue

Patient Profile

- Males > Females
- Middle age
- Risk factors:
    - Obesity
    - Smoking
    - Nasal obstruction
    - Hypothyroidism
    - Acromegaly

Signs and Symptoms

- Excessive daytime sleepiness
- Loud snoring
- Frequent awakenings with feeling of shortness of breath
- Significant other reports observing periods of apnea
- Poor concentration
- Memory problems
- Irritability
- Personality changes
- Headaches

Differential Diagnosis

- Narcolepsy
- Asthma
- Chronic obstructive pulmonary disease (COPD)
- Congestive heart failure (CHF)
- Panic attacks causing awakenings
- Gastroesophageal reflux

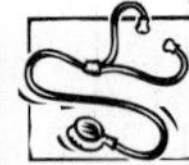

ASSESSMENT

History

Inquire about:

- Onset and duration of symptoms
- Significant other's observations
- Alcohol use
- Excessive daytime sleepiness
- Smoking history
- Number of awakenings
- Underlying conditions
- Current medications

Physical Findings

- May be normal
- General—obesity
- Narrowing of upper airway due to tonsillar hypertrophy, enlarged adenoids or uvula
- Retrognathia
- Nose—polyps
- Findings compatible with hypothyroidism

Initial Workup

Laboratory

- CBC—may find polycythemia
- Thyroid function studies—to rule out hypothyroidism

Radiology: None diagnostic

Further Workup

Polysomnogram—gives definitive diagnosis

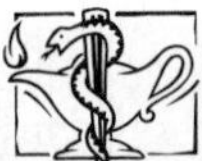

INTERVENTIONS

Office Treatment

None indicated

Lifestyle Modifications

- Smoking cessation
- Reduction in alcohol intake
- Weight loss
- Avoidance of sleeping in supine position

Patient Education

Teach patient about:

- Condition and treatment
- Tips for smoking cessation
- Reducing alcohol intake, particularly before bed
- Avoiding sedative medication, which may worsen problem
- Weight reduction diet and exercise program
- Avoiding supine sleeping position—sew tennis ball in back of nightshirt to keep from lying on back
- Surgery to correct upper airway narrowing
- Using continuous positive airway pressure machine
- Medications used and side effects (see Pharmacotherapeutics)

Referral

To specialist if treatment fails or surgery required

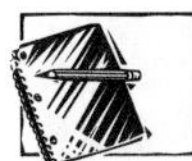

EVALUATION

Outcome

If treatment program followed, excessive daytime drowsiness should improve dramatically

Possible Complications

- Pulmonary hypertension
- Cardiac arrhythmias
- Cor pulmonale
- CHF

Follow-up

- Every 2 weeks initially to encourage compliance and assess response
- When stable, every 3-6 months

FOR YOUR INFORMATION

Life Span

Pediatric: Uncommon, if present, usually because of tonsillar hypertrophy; tonsillectomy corrects condition
Geriatric: Common in this age group
Pregnancy: Uncommon

Miscellaneous

Failure to follow the treatment plan is the primary cause of treatment failure. The NP needs to encourage and work with the patient to make the treatment work.

References

Stauffer JL: Lung. In Tierney LM Jr, McPhee SJ, Papadakis MA, editors: *Current medical diagnosis and treatment,* ed 34, Norwalk, Conn, Appleton & Lange, pp 268-269.

Wooliscroft JO: *Current diagnosis and treatment: a quick reference for the general practitioner,* Philadelphia, 1996, Current Medicine, pp 368-369.

NOTES

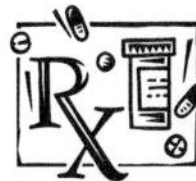

PHARMACOTHERAPEUTICS

Drug of Choice	Mechanism of Action	Prescribing Information	Side Effects
The following drug may be useful in improving excessive daytime drowsiness:			
Protriptyline (Vivactil), 10-30 mg PO qd in divided doses	Tricyclic antidepressant; blocks reuptake of norepinephrine and serotonin	***Contraindications:*** Hypersensitivity; recovery phase of myocardial infarction (MI) ***Cost:*** 10-mg tab, 100 tabs: $67 ***Pregnancy category:*** C	Agranulocytosis, thrombocytopenia, eosinophilia, leukopenia, dizziness, drowsiness, confusion, headache, anxiety, tremors, weakness, insomnia, diarrhea, dry mouth, paralytic ileus, hepatitis, acute renal failure, urinary retention, rash, urticaria, orthostatic hypotension, tachycardia, hypertension, blurred vision, tinnitus

Smoking Cessation/Tobacco Dependence

OVERVIEW

Tobacco dependence can be defined as continuous use of tobacco products with unsuccessful attempts to stop or reduce use, withdrawal symptoms occurring with cessation, or continued smoking despite illness.

Pathogenesis

Cause—multifactorial:

- Physical dependence due to nicotine in cigarettes
- Psychologic dependence—pleasurable sensations
- Social or behavioral dependence—habit that becomes part of daily activities

Patient Profile

- Males > Females
- Any age

Signs and Symptoms

Nicotine withdrawal:

- Anxiety
- Mood disturbances
- Hunger
- Cravings
- Restlessness
- Sleep disturbances
- Sweating
- Dizziness
- Headache
- Tremors
- Irritability

Differential Diagnosis

Type of tobacco used:

- Cigarettes
- Cigars
- Pipe
- Chewing tobacco
- Snuff

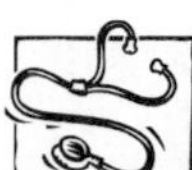

ASSESSMENT

History

Inquire about:

- Amount smoked and for how long
- How long after awakening before tobacco is first used
- Whether patient has ever tried to quit, how successful, and for how long
- Cough, shortness of breath, frequent upper and lower respiratory tract infections
- Family history of heart disease, pulmonary disease, and cancer
- Underlying conditions
- Current medications

Physical Findings

- Nose and mouth—inflammation from tobacco
- Lungs—crackles that clear with cough
- Heart—tachycardia (if recently used tobacco); otherwise, heart rate is normal or slow

Initial Workup

Laboratory

- Consider CBC with differential—may show polycythemia
- Chemistry panel to include cholesterol level—need to evaluate for other risk factors

Radiology: Consider chest film—PA and lateral—routine screening not recommended

Further Workup

Consider pulmonary function studies

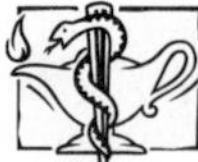

INTERVENTIONS

Office Treatment

Counseling and support

Lifestyle Modifications

- Smoking cessation
- Avoidance of precipitants to extent possible

Patient Education

Teach patient about:

- Benefits of smoking cessation, such as:
  - Improved health and well-being
  - Decreased number of respiratory tract infections
  - Improved oral hygiene
  - Improved odor in home, car, and on clothes
- Tips for smoking cessation, such as:
  - Picking a quit date
  - Keeping a smoking diary to become aware of triggers
  - Having low-calorie snacks available
  - Telling people about quit date and eliciting their support
  - Starting an exercise program
  - Getting rid of ashtrays in the house
  - Deep breathing and relaxation techniques
  - Drinking increased amount of water
  - Making a contract to stop smoking
- Using nicotine gum or nicotine patch (see Pharmacotherapeutics)

Referral

To smoking cessation program

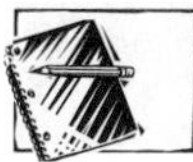

EVALUATION

Outcome
Patient permanently stops smoking

Possible Complications
Any number of smoking-related illnesses

Follow-up
1 week after quit date; then in 1 month—continue to provide support and encouragement

FOR YOUR INFORMATION

Life Span
Pediatric: Educate children on hazards of smoking and not to start
Geriatric: May have major health problems
Pregnancy: Increased rate of spontaneous abortion, low birth weight, and fetal death in smokers

Miscellaneous
Carefully explain to the patient the hazards of smoking when using nicotine replacement therapy.

References
Bigelow GE, Haines CS: Tobacco use and dependence. In Barker LR, Burton JR, Zieve PD, editors: *Principles of ambulatory medicine,* ed 4, Baltimore, 1995, Williams & Wilkins, pp 212-220.

Fiore MC et al: *Smoking cessation,* Clinical Practice Guideline No 18, AHCPR Pub No 96-0692, Rockville, Md, 1996, US Department of Health and Human Services, Public Health Service, Agency for Health Care Policy and Research.

NOTES

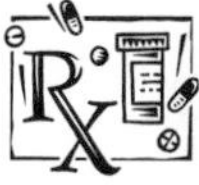

PHARMACOTHERAPEUTICS

Drug of Choice	Mechanism of Action	Prescribing Information	Side Effects
Nicotine gum (Nicorette), 2- or 4-mg pieces of gum, chew slowly for 30 minutes, maximum of 30 pieces/day—do not use for longer than 6 months	Nicotine receptor agonist	***Contraindications:*** Hypersensitivity; immediately after myocardial infarction (MI); severe angina ***Cost:*** OTC, 96 pieces per package: $35-$80 ***Pregnancy category:*** X	Dyspnea, cough, wheezing, irritation of buccal cavity, dizziness, vertigo, insomnia, headache, nausea, vomiting, anorexia, indigestion, tachycardia, arrhythmias, palpitations, edema, flushing
Nicotine transdermal system (Nicoderm, Nicotrol, Habitrol); available in varying strengths; use stronger doses for heavy smokers; apply to upper arm or thigh; some brands remain on 24 hours, others are removed after 16 hours; read package insert; assist patient in choosing right type	Nicotine receptor agonist	***Contraindications:*** Hypersensitivity; immediately after MI; severe angina ***Cost:*** OTC: $27-$100 ***Pregnancy category:*** D	Cough, pharyngitis, sinusitis, back pain, chest pain, skin irritation, pruritus, sweating, rash, diarrhea, dyspepsia, nausea, abdominal pain, dry mouth, insomnia, nervousness, headache, dizziness, tachycardia

Sprains and Strains

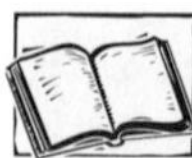

OVERVIEW

A sprain is an injury to the ligament, whereas a strain is an injury to either the muscle or tendon. With either type of injury, there may be complete or partial disruption of the involved tissue. Sprains are classified according to grades:

- Grade I—Pain or tenderness at joint; no laxity in ligament
- Grade II—Pain or tenderness at joint; ecchymosis; ligaments lax but joint intact
- Grade III—Pain or tenderness/swelling at joint; ecchymosis; no end point when joint stressed

Pathogenesis

- Strains—overuse injury
- Sprains—Usually due to trauma, falls

Patient Profile

- Males > Females
- Any age

Signs and Symptoms

- Pain
- Swelling
- Ecchymosis
- Erythema
- Decreased range of motion

Differential Diagnosis

- Fracture
- Tendonitis
- Bursitis

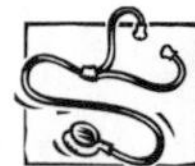

ASSESSMENT

History

Inquire about:

- Onset and duration of symptoms
- Recent trauma with twisting motion
- Situations that may produce overuse of joint, such as repetitive movements at work or play, or recently starting an exercise program
- Underlying conditions
- Current medications

Physical Findings

- Swelling at joint
- Ecchymosis
- Pain at rest and with movement
- Decreased range of motion
- Check stability of joint

Initial Workup

Laboratory: None indicated

Radiology: Plain films of joint—rule out fracture

Further Workup

Consider CT scan or MRI if patient continues to have severe pain and swelling after treatment

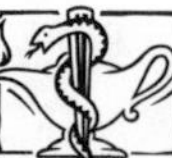

INTERVENTIONS

Office Treatment

Application of Ace wrap, splint, or cast, depending on severity

Lifestyle Modifications

- Disruption of usual lifestyle until healing occurs
- Off school or work
- If lower extremity involved, immobility

Patient Education

Teach patient about:

- Injury and treatment
- RICE therapy:
  - **R**est
  - **I**ce
  - **C**ompression
  - **E**levation
- Applying an Ace wrap
- Cast care if applicable
- Using crutches
- Medications used and side effects (see Pharmacotherapeutics)

Referrals

- To orthopedist if treatment fails or if severe enough to require surgery
- Physical therapy

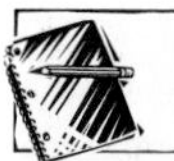

EVALUATION

Outcome
Resolves without sequelae if treatment plan followed

Possible Complications
- Arthritis
- Chronic joint instability

Follow-up
In 1 week; then in 3 weeks

FOR YOUR INFORMATION

Life Span
Pediatric: Common in children, particularly if participating in sports
Geriatric: Evaluate carefully for fracture
Pregnancy: Could have an adverse effect on natural delivery

Miscellaneous
N/A

References
Mercier LR: *Practical orthopedics,* ed 4, St Louis, 1995, Mosby, pp 4, 20, 213-217, 238-240.

Ruda S: Nursing role in management: musculoskeletal problems. In Lewis SM, Collier IC, Heitkemper MM, editors: *Medical-surgical nursing: assessment and management of clinical problems,* ed 4, St Louis, 1996, Mosby, pp 1839-1841.

NOTES

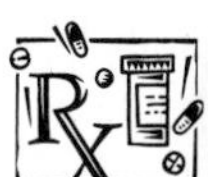

PHARMACOTHERAPEUTICS

Drug of Choice	Mechanism of Action	Prescribing Information	Side Effects
Nonsteroidal antiinflammatory drugs (NSAIDs): many different types currently marketed; consult manufacturer's package insert for specific dosing and prescribing information	Exact action unknown; may result from inhibition of synthesis of prostaglandins and arachidonic acid	***Contraindications:*** Hypersensitivity to NSAIDs, aspirin; severe hepatic failure; asthma ***Cost:*** Varies with type ***Pregnancy category:*** Depends on product	Stomach distress, flatulence, nausea, abdominal pain, constipation or diarrhea, dizziness, sedation, rash, urticaria, angioedema, anorexia, urinary frequency, increased BP, insomnia, anxiety, visual disturbances, increased thirst, alopecia

Squamous Cell Carcinoma, Cutaneous

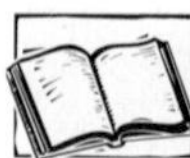

OVERVIEW

Cutaneous squamous cell carcinoma is a malignant tumor of the epithelium. It is the second most common type of skin cancer and occurs when atypical squamous cells develop in the epidermis from keratinocytes. These atypical cells penetrate the epidermal membrane and proliferate into the dermis

Pathogenesis

- Cause—unknown, but ultraviolet B radiation plays a major role in development
- Arises in skin damaged by thermal burns or inflammation; can be metastatic, depending on where the lesion is—areas that have previously had radiation or thermal injury, chronic draining sinuses, or chronic ulcers have high frequency of metastases
- If lesion originates in actinically damaged areas, less likely to metastasize

Patient Profile

- Males > Females
- Incidence increases with age
- Highest incidence in the elderly
- Occurs in sun-exposed areas of body
- High incidence of lip squamous cell cancer in smokers

Signs and Symptoms

- Tumors may have thick, adherent scale; have friable surface; be soft and movable, have erythematous base
- Or tumors may be firm, movable, and elevated, with well-defined border

Differential Diagnosis

- Keratoacanthoma
- Basal cell carcinoma
- Actinic keratosis
- Malignant melanoma

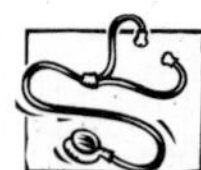

ASSESSMENT

History

Inquire about:

- Onset and duration of symptoms
- Changes in previous nevi
- Length of time lesion has been present
- History of sun exposure
- History of prior radiation, thermal injury, or cigarette smoking
- Underlying conditions
- Current medications

Physical Findings

- Raised lesion on sun-exposed surface, particularly on scalp, backs of hands, superior surface of pinna, lips
- May be scaly, soft or hard, movable, with friable surface
- Bleeding may be present
- Color—red, red-brown, tan, white in moist areas

Initial Workup

Laboratory: Biopsy for precise diagnosis
Radiology: None indicated

Further Workup

None indicated

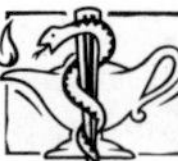

INTERVENTIONS

Office Treatment

None

Lifestyle Modifications

- Smoking cessation
- Sunscreen
- Long sleeves when outdoors
- Hat to shade face and head

Patient Education

Teach patient about:

- Condition and treatment
- Treatment options:
  - Surgical excision (most common)
  - Electrodesiccation and curettage
  - If many lesions and metastases present—surgical excision along with chemotherapy, radiation therapy
  - Risk factors for developing disease
  - Using sunscreen daily, particularly on backs of hands, scalp, and pinnae.

Referral

To dermatologist for definitive diagnosis and treatment of all suspicious lesions

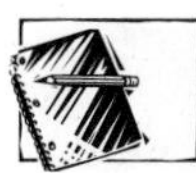

EVALUATION

Outcome

Lesion removed; site heals without sequelae

Possible Complications

- Recurrence
- Metastatic disease

Follow-up

After treatment, skin examination monthly × 3 months; then every 6 months × 1; then yearly

FOR YOUR INFORMATION

Life Span

Pediatric: Not seen in this age group
Geriatric: More commonly seen in this age group
Pregnancy: If metastases present, may need to make decision regarding termination of pregnancy

Miscellaneous

Lesions that are equal to or greater than 2 cm have a greater risk of recurrence than smaller lesions.

References

Habif TP: *Clinical dermatology: a color guide to diagnosis and therapy,* ed 3, St Louis, 1996, Mosby, pp 666-668.

Kuflik AS, Schwartz RA: Actinic keratosis and squamous cell carcinoma, *Am Fam Physician* 49(4):817-820, 1994.

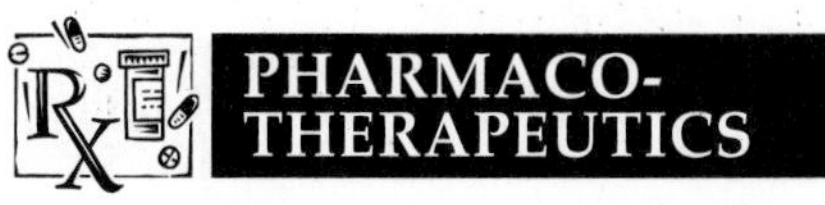

PHARMACOTHERAPEUTICS

There are no specific pharmacotherapeutics for the treatment of cutaneous squamous cell carcinoma. If metastasis occurs, then chemotherapy or radiation may be used.

Stevens-Johnson Syndrome

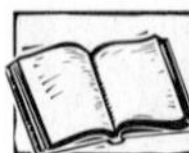

OVERVIEW

Stevens-Johnson syndrome has long been considered a severe form of erythema multiforme. However, a new classification system has now separated the two diseases. Stevens-Johnson syndrome is a severe vesiculobullous disease that involves the skin, mouth, eyes, and genitals. It is usually a severe, drug-induced reaction.

Pathogenesis

Causes:

- Drug hypersensitivity reaction, particularly to phenytoin, phenobarbital, sulfonamides, penicillins
- Also hypersensitivity reactions to viral infections, bacterial infections, protozoan infections, collagen vascular disease, malignancy, pregnancy, premenstrual hormonal changes, consumption of beer, Reiter's syndrome, sarcoidosis, *Mycoplasma pneumoniae*

Patient Profile

- Males > Females
- More common in children and young adults

Signs and Symptoms

- Prodrome of upper respiratory tract infection
- Widespread, flat macules
- Vesicles
- Bullae
- Mucous membranes—vesicles and ulcers
- Fever
- Myalgia
- Arthralgias
- Rhinitis
- Cough
- Conjunctivitis
- Corneal ulcerations
- Vulvovaginitis or balanitis—erosive
- Hematuria
- Albuminuria
- Arrhythmias
- Pericarditis
- Congestive heart failure
- Seizures
- Coma
- Sepsis
- Entire skin surface may appear burned

Differential Diagnosis

- Bullous impetigo
- Pemphigus vulgaris
- Pemphigold
- Septicemia
- Serum sickness
- Hand-foot-mouth disease
- Collagen vascular disease
- Meningococcemia
- Staphylococcal scalded skin syndrome

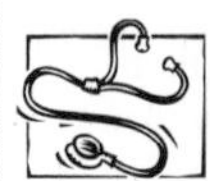

ASSESSMENT

History

Inquire about:

- Onset and duration of symptoms
- Prodrome of upper respiratory tract infection
- History of fever
- Previous history of erythema multiforme or Stevens-Johnson syndrome
- Underlying conditions
- Medication used and current medications

Physical Findings

Flat, macular rash with vesicles and bullae present on conjunctivae and mucous membranes of nares, mouth, anorectal region, vulvovaginal regions, and urethral meatus.

Initial Workup

Laboratory: Skin biopsy
Radiology: Chest—patchy changes indicate pulmonary involvement

Further Workup

Workup will be dictated by extent of disease

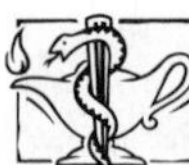

INTERVENTIONS

Office Treatment

None indicated

Lifestyle Modification

Avoidance of causative agent if known

Patient Education

Teach patient about:

- Condition and treatment:
  - Hospitalization
  - Oral steroids
- Importance of determining causative agent if possible and wearing medical alert tag at all times
- Using cool Burow's compresses to treat blisters and importance of meticulous skin care
- Switching to either a liquid or soft diet and the use of viscous lidocaine to relieve oral pain
- Medications used and side effects (see Pharmacotherapeutics)

Referral

To MD immediately

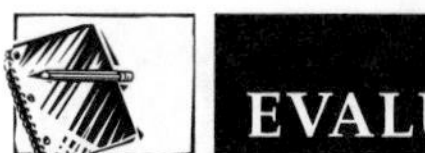

EVALUATION

Outcomes

- Complete resolution in 4 to 6 weeks
- Scarring may occur
- Blindness or corneal opacities may occur
- Risk of recurrence

Possible Complications

- Secondary infections
- Sepsis
- Pneumonia
- Electrolyte disturbances
- Acute tubular necrosis
- Arrhythmias
- Death

Follow-up

Within 1 week of hospitalization

FOR YOUR INFORMATION

Life Span

Pediatric: More common in this age group
Geriatric: Rare in this age group
Pregnancy: Possible causative agent; may need to make decision regarding termination of pregnancy

Miscellaneous

If the disease develops as a result of a reaction to a drug, it will generally take 7-14 days after the first exposure to the drug for the symptoms of Stevens-Johnson syndrome to begin. Subsequent exposure to the same drug may result in the syndrome developing much more quickly.

Reference

Habif TP: *Clinical dermatology: a color guide to diagnosis and therapy,* ed 3, St Louis, 1996, Mosby, pp 570-571.

NOTES

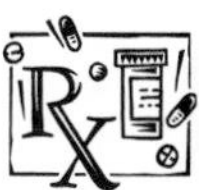

PHARMACOTHERAPEUTICS

There is some controversy over the use of steroids in the treatment of Stevens-Johnson syndrome. However, most authorities still recommend their use. Topical steroids *should not* be applied to the skin lesions. The use of antibiotics should be avoided except in the case of established secondary bacterial infections.

Drug of Choice	Mechanism of Action	Prescribing Information	Side Effects
Prednisone, 1-2 mg/kg/day PO; once control of disease has occurred, taper dosage	Synthetic analog of glucocorticoid; antiinflammatory	***Contraindication:*** Hypersensitivity ***Cost:*** 15-mg tab, 100 tabs: $14-$35 ***Pregnancy category:*** C	May mask signs of infection; increased stress may need increased dose; drug-induced secondary adrenocortical insufficiency; gradual reduction in dose; psychic derangement

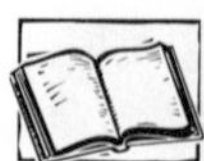

OVERVIEW

Stomatitis is an inflammation of the oral mucosa. It may have many different causes.

Pathogenesis

Causes:

- Nutritional deficiencies—vitamin B_{12}, folate, iron
- Systemic disease—syphilis, leukemia
- Allergies—foods, drugs
- Virus—herpes simplex I or II, coxsackie A
- Trauma
    - Chemical injury—smoking, chewing tobacco, mouthwash
    - Mechanical injury—cheek biting, dentures
    - Thermal injury—hot foods
- Unknown—aphthous stomatitis, Behçet's disease, Vincent's stomatitis, angular stomatitis

Patient Profile

- Males = Females
- Most common in children and young adults

Signs and Symptoms

- Depends on etiology
- May have minimal to severe pain
- May have few to many intraoral ulcers
- May have fever, malaise, and headache
- Nutritional deficiencies—smooth, fiery red, and painful (pellagra)
- Systemic disease—mucous patches (syphilis); strawberry and Koplik's spots (measles)
- Allergic type—itching, dryness, burning, shiny erythema
- Viral type:
    - Primary herpes—usually children; initial vesicle becomes ulcer in 2 to 3 days with yellow-gray membrane on erythematous base; confined to pharynx, tonsils, soft palate; high fever; lymphadenopathy
    - Secondary herpes—adults and young adults; burning sensation—vesicles evolve into ulcers; heal in 4 to 10 days
    - Herpangina—children; high fever, anorexia, dysphagia 1 to 4 days before lesions erupt; multiple lesions—papular, vesicular, and ulcerative—on tonsillar pillars, soft palate, tonsils, pharynx, posterior buccal mucosa
- Aphthous stomatitis (canker sores)—usually single indurated papule that progresses to ulcer; lesions never vesiculate; located on vestibular and buccal mucosa, tongue, soft palate, fauces, and floor of mouth; no fever or lymphadenopathy
- Vincent's stomatitis—adolescents and adults; ulcers on gingivae with purulent, gray exudate

Differential Diagnosis

- Must differentiate between causes
- Oral cancer
- Stevens-Johnson syndrome
- Acute necrotizing ulcerative gingivitis

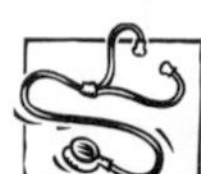

ASSESSMENT

History

Inquire about:

- Onset and duration of symptoms
- Fever, headache, malaise
- Diet
- Smoking history, including pipes, cigars, chewing tobacco
- Underlying conditions
- Current medications

Physical Findings

- Fever (possibly)
- Mouth lesions or ulcers; may be vesicular or papular
- Mouth and throat—erythema, edema
- Lymphadenopathy (see Signs and Symptoms for findings specific to various causes)

Initial Workup

Laboratory

- Base workup on history and physical findings—none may be indicated
- CBC—anemia may be present
- Folate, vitamin B_{12}, iron levels if suspect nutritional deficiencies
- Tzanck smear if suspect herpes
- Rapid plasma reagin (RPR) for syphilis

Radiology: None indicated

Further Workup

None indicated

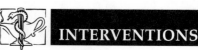

INTERVENTIONS

Office Treatment

None indicated

Lifestyle Modifications

- Smoking cessation
- No chewing tobacco
- No hot or spicy foods

Patient Education

Teach patient about:

- Cause of stomatitis and treatment options—usually symptomatic: mouth rinses (3% hydrogen peroxide and water, 1:1, gargle), topical anesthetic
- Usually resolves without further treatment
- Vincent's stomatitis—symptomatic treatment and antibiotics
- Herpetic stomatitis—symptomatic and acyclovir (possibly)
- Smoking cessation
- Medications used and side effects (see Pharmacotherapeutics)

Referrals

- Usually none
- To MD if not healed in 2 to 3 weeks

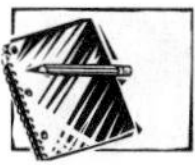

EVALUATION

Outcome
Usually resolves without sequelae; most have 9- to 14-day course

Possible Complications
- Depends on cause
- Behçet's syndrome may result in visual loss, pneumonia, colitis, vasculitis, thrombophlebitis, or encephalitis
- Gangrenous stomatitis—may lead to death
- Herpetic stomatitis—ocular or CNS involvement

Follow-up
Severe cases—in 48 to 72 hours; otherwise in 2 to 3 weeks

FOR YOUR INFORMATION

Life Span
Pediatric: Primary herpes and herpangina most common in this age group
Geriatric: Dentures most common cause in this group
Pregnancy: May bring on recurrence

Miscellaneous
In patients with AIDS, the lesions may be very severe and difficult to treat.

References

Bull TR: *Color atlas of E.N.T. diagnosis,* ed 3, London, 1995, Mosby-Wolfe, pp 160-164.

Jackler RK, Kaplan MJ: Ear, nose, throat. In Tierney LM Jr, McPhee SJ, Papadakis MA, editors: *Current medical diagnosis and treatment,* ed 34, Norwalk, Conn, 1995, Appleton & Lange, pp 190-191.

NOTES

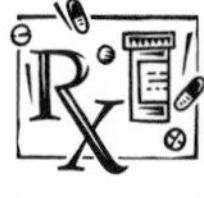

PHARMACOTHERAPEUTICS

Drug of Choice	Mechanism of Action	Prescribing Information	Side Effects
2% viscous lidocaine (Xylocaine), 15 ml swish and swallow or spit q3h; children <3 years, ¼ tsp applied directly to area q3h	Stabilizes neuronal membrane by inhibiting ion fluxes	***Contraindication:*** Hypersensitivity ***Cost:*** 100 ml: $4 ***Pregnancy category:*** B	CNS depression or excitation, rash, irritation; patient should be cautioned to use at recommended dose to prevent too much systemic absorption
Triamcinolone (Kenalog) in Orabase 0.1% for severe attacks; apply thin film to lesions at bedtime; may need to apply 2-3 times during day—not recommended for children	Topical corticosteroid; antiinflammatory, antipruritic, vasoconstrictive actions	***Contraindication:*** Hypersensitivity ***Cost:*** 5 g: $7 ***Pregnancy category:*** C	Burning, itching, irritation, dryness, acneiform eruptions, hypopigmentation, perioral dermatitis, maceration of skin
Acyclovir (Zovirax); only FDA approved for herpetic stomatitis in immunocompromised patients; recent studies have shown it causes blisters to heal faster and recur less frequently in healthy patients; 400 mg PO bid × 10 days; children, 20 mg/kg PO qid × 5 days	Interferes with DNA synthesis, preventing replication	***Contraindication:*** Hypersensitivity ***Cost:*** 400-mg tab, 20 tabs: $85 ***Pregnancy category:*** C	Nausea, vomiting, rash, hives, anemia, anuria, headache, diaphoresis, anorexia, convulsions, proteinuria, glomerulonephritis, acute renal failure, joint pain, leg pain, muscle cramps
For Vincent's stomatitis:			
• Penicillin (Pen-Vee K), 250-500 mg PO tid or qid × 10 days; children <12 years, 25-50 mg/kg/day PO in divided doses × 10 days • Penicillin G benzathine, 1.2 mil units IM	Bactericidal	***Contraindications:*** Hypersensitivity to penicillin or cephalosporins ***Cost:*** 250-mg tab, 40 tabs, $5 ***Pregnancy category:*** B	Nausea, vomiting, epigastric distress, diarrhea, black hairy tongue, anaphylaxis

Syncope

OVERVIEW

Syncope is a sudden, brief lapse in consciousness.

Pathogenesis

- Cause—anything that decreases cerebral blood flow, such as decreased peripheral vascular resistance, decreased cardiac output, failure of vasoconstrictive reflexes, cerebrovascular occlusion
- Most common causes—vasovagal, situational, orthostatic hypotension, drug-induced condition, organic heart disease, arrhythmias

Patient Profile

- Females > Males
- Any age

Signs and Symptoms

Depends on cause:

- Vasovagal condition (common faint):
  - Cold hands
  - Pallor
  - Dimming vision, sweating, nausea, loss of balance—only occurs when patient is upright
  - Precipitated by fear or anxiety
- Situational condition—sudden loss of consciousness; precipitated by micturition, cough, defecation, swallowing
- Orthostatic hypotension—sudden loss of consciousness when patient stands up; may also be precipitated by warm environment, diuretics, or autonomic blocking agents
- Organic heart disease—generalized weakness, fatigue, pallor; worse when standing, improves when lying down, but may occur in any position

Differential Diagnosis

- Seizures
- Vertigo
- Parkinson's disease
- Migraines
- Cerebellar disease
- Psychologic disorder
- Anemia
- Must differentiate from various causes of syncope

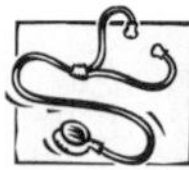

ASSESSMENT

History

Inquire about:

- Onset and duration of symptoms
- Precipitating events
- When the syncope occurs—position of patient
- Past cardiac history
- Number of times syncope has occurred
- Other underlying conditions
- Current medications

Physical Findings

- Orthostatic hypotension
- Cardiac arrthymias
- Carotid bruits
- May have normal physical examination
- No cause found 40% to 50% of the time

Initial Workup

Laboratory

- CBC—anemia
- Chemistry panel—to include electrolytes, glucose, liver function tests, BUN, creatinine
- Urinalysis

Radiology: CT scan or MRI of head if indicated

Further Workup

If indicated by history and physical:

- ECG
- Holter monitor
- Echocardiogram
- Cardiac catherization
- EEG
- Psychiatric evaluation
- Tilt testing
- Electrophysiologic studies

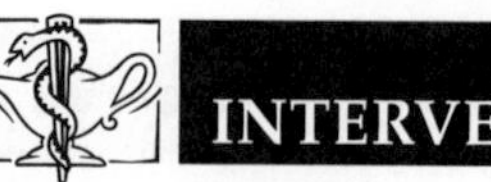

INTERVENTIONS

Office Treatment

None indicated

Lifestyle Modifications

- Depends on underlying cause
- Smoking cessation
- Alcohol withdrawal
- Drug withdrawal

Patient Education

Teach patient about:

- Cause of syncope if found and treatment options:
  - If orthostatic hypotension is cause, changing positions slowly, sleeping with head of bed elevated, avoidance of knee-high stockings, exercising legs before standing, wearing support hose
  - For vasovagal condition, may try beta-blockers or anticholinergics
- Treatment of underlying problems as appropriate
- Medications used and side effects (see Pharmacotherapeutics)

Referrals

Usually none

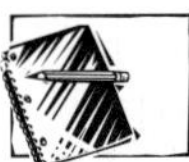

EVALUATION

Outcome
No further syncopal episodes

Possible Complications
- Trauma from falls
- Death if cause is cardiac

Follow-up
- In 2 weeks × 2; frequent follow-up if cause is cardiac
- If on medication for vasovagal syncope, every 3 months for side effects

FOR YOUR INFORMATION

Life Span
Pediatric: Rare
Geriatric: More common; if cause is cardiac, prognosis poor
Pregnancy: May occur as a result of hemodynamic changes of pregnancy

Miscellaneous
Psychologic distress may also cause a syncopal episode. The patient will usually report numbness of fingers and around mouth.

References
Bass EB, Lewis RF: Dizziness, vertigo, motion sickness, near syncope, syncope, and disequilibrium. In Barker LR, Burton JR, Zieve PD, editors: *Principles of ambulatory medicine,* ed 4, Baltimore, 1995, Williams & Wilkins, pp 1207-1214.

Uphold CR, Graham MV: *Clinical guidelines in adult health,* Gainesville, Fla, 1994, Barmarrae Books, pp 304-308.

NOTES

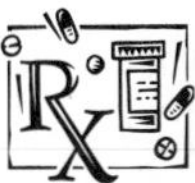

PHARMACOTHERAPEUTICS

Drug of Choice	Mechanism of Action	Prescribing Information	Side Effects
For frequent vasovagal syncopal episodes:			
Beta-blocker: propranolol (Inderal), 20 mg PO bid, maximum 160 mg/day;	Nonselective beta-blocker with negative inotropic, chronotropic, dromotropic properties	***Contraindications:*** Hypersensitivity; cardiac failure; cardiogenic shock; 2nd- or 3rd-degree heart block; bronchospastic disease; sinus bradycardia; congestive heart failure (CHF) ***Cost:*** 20-mg tab, 100 tabs: $3-$20 ***Pregnancy category:*** C	Dyspnea, bronchospasm, bradycardia, hypotension, CHF, atrioventricular (AV) block, peripheral vascular insufficiency, agranulocytosis, thrombocytopenia, nausea, vomiting, diarrhea, colitis, constipation, cramps, impotence, decreased libido, joint pain, facial swelling, depression, hallucinations, sore throat, laryngospasm, blurred vision, hyperglycemia, hypoglycemia
For less-frequent vasovagal syncopal episodes:			
Scopolamine transdermal disk (Transderm-Scop), 1 disk behind ear, leave for 3 days—not for children; use with great caution in elderly	Inhibition of vestibular input to CNS; antagonizes acetylcholine at receptor sites in eyes, smooth muscle, cardiac muscle	***Contraindications:*** Hypersensitivity; glaucoma ***Cost:*** 12 disks: $45 ***Pregnancy category:*** C	Dizziness, drowsiness, confusion, disorientation, blurred vision, dilated pupils, dry mouth, acute narrow-angle glaucoma, rash, erythema

Syphilis

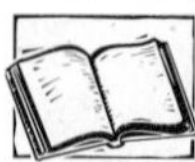

OVERVIEW

Syphilis is a sexually transmitted disease (STD) that can involve many systems of the body. The clinical stages of syphilis are primary, secondary, latent, and tertiary.

Pathogenesis

- Cause—*Treponema pallidum,* a spirochete
- Transmitted by sexual contact
- Organism penetrates skin or mucous membranes
- Organism multiplies and spreads to regional lymph nodes
- Spirochetes enter bloodstream and travel to other organs
- Organism can cross placenta and result in congenital syphilis

Patient Profile

- Males > Females
- Most common age group—15- to 25-year-olds, but may be seen at any age

Signs and Symptoms

PRIMARY SYPHILIS

- Chancre, usually on genitalia
- Regional lymphadenopathy usually present
- Heals spontaneously in 1 to 5 weeks

SECONDARY SYPHILIS

- Occurs 6 to 8 weeks after chancre
- Most contagious stage
- Headache
- Generalized arthralgia
- Malaise
- Fever
- Lymphadenopathy
- Rash—macular, papular, annular, follicular—commonly occurs on palms and soles; mucous patches, and condyloma lata (flat, moist, warty lesions) can occur in mouth, throat, cervix, glans, vulva, perianal area
- Resolves spontaneously

LATENT SYPHILIS

- Asymptomatic
- Not infectious after 1 year
- Varies in length of time in latent period; one third of patients go on to tertiary syphilis

TERTIARY SYPHILIS

- Cardiovascular disease
- Neurologic disease, including dementia
- Gummas
- Orthopedic disease

CONGENITAL SYPHILIS

- Rhinitis
- Lymphadenopathy
- Failure to thrive
- Meningitis
- Hepatosplenomegaly
- Rash similar to secondary syphilis; may be bullous or vesicular

Differential Diagnosis

- Primary syphilis:
  - Genital herpes
  - Lymphogranuloma venereum
  - Chancroid
  - Trauma
- Secondary syphilis—mimics many skin disorders, such as pityriasis rosea or drug eruption
- Tertiary disease—any cardiovascular, neurologic, or orthopedic disease

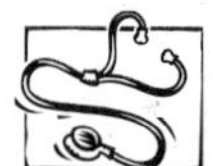

ASSESSMENT

History

Inquire about:

- Onset and duration of symptoms
- History of or presence of chancre
- History of or presence of rash, mucous patches, condyloma lata
- Sexual history, including number of partners, sexual behaviors, use of condoms, known contact with infected individual, previous history of STDs
- Underlying conditions
- Current medications

Physical Findings

Depends on stage:

- Primary syphilis:
  - Chancre on genitalia (most common)
  - Nontender ulcer with hard edge and yellow base
  - Lymphadenopathy
- Secondary syphilis:
  - Rash—particularly on soles and palms, bilateral and symmetric
  - Mucous patches—thin gray smears
  - Condyloma lata—moist, flat, pink lesions
  - Lymphadenopathy
- Tertiary syphilis:
  - Dementia
  - Other neurologic signs
  - Cardiovascular disease—murmurs of aortic valve defect, aneurysms
  - Destructive granulomatous pockets (gummas)
  - Charcot's joints (swelling and hypermobility of joint, overgrowth of bone and crepitus may be palpated)

Initial Workup

Laboratory

- VDRL or rapid plasma reagin (RPR)—if positive, should be confirmed with specific treponemal tests: fluorescent treponemal antibody absorption (FTA-ABS) or micro-hemagglutination treponema pallidum (MHA-TP); patient remains positive for FTA-ABS and MHA-TP for life
- Cerebrospinal fluid (CSF) serologies may be needed for latent syphilis or when neurologic symptoms are present
- Encourage HIV testing

Radiology: Only in tertiary syphilis if osteomyelitis or Charcot's joints are present

Further Workup

Dark-field microscopy

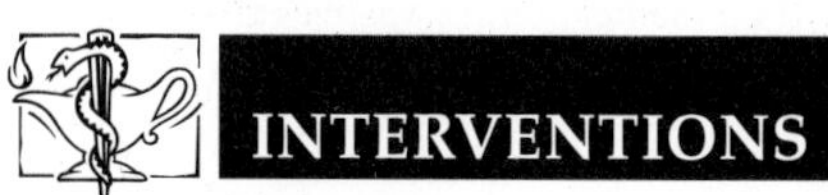

INTERVENTIONS

Office Treatment

None indicated

Lifestyle Modification

Safe sex practices

Patient Education

Teach patient about:

- Disease and treatment—antibiotics
- Importance of tracing and treating all contacts (must be reported to local health department)
- Avoiding sexual intercourse until treatment complete and declared cured
- Safe sex practices—use of condoms, monogamous relationship
- Medications used and side effects (see Pharmacotherapeutics)

Referrals

- To infectious disease specialist for treatment failure
- To pediatrician for infant with congenital syphilis

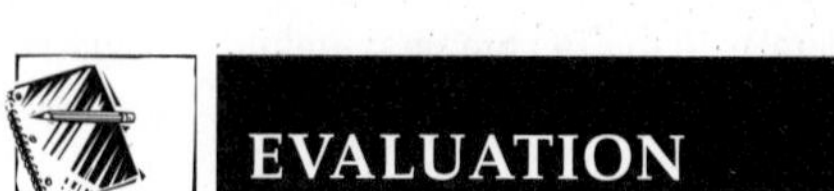

EVALUATION

Outcomes

- Resolves without sequelae in primary, secondary, and latent syphilis
- Tertiary syphilis—may stop progress, but usually does not reverse it

Possible Complications

- Cardiovascular disease
- Irreversible neurologic disease
- Irreversible organ damage
- Death

Follow-up

- Repeat serology at 3 months and 6 months
- If HIV-positive, repeat serology at 1, 2, 3, 6, 9, and 12 months

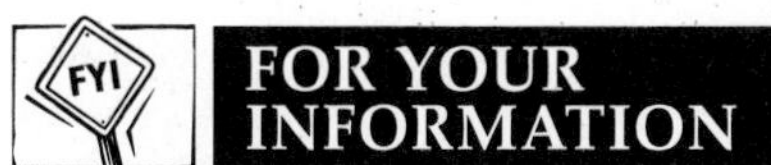

FOR YOUR INFORMATION

Life Span

Pediatric: Congenital syphilis most common; in noncongenital case, consider child abuse

Geriatric: Consider tertiary syphilis in patients with dementia.

Pregnancy: Early detection and treatment to avoid infecting fetus

Miscellaneous

N/A

References

Hook EW III, Ennis DM: Selected spirochetal infections: syphilis and lyme disease. In Barker LR, Burton JR, Zieve PD, editors: *Principles of ambulatory medicine,* ed 4, Baltimore, 1995, Williams & Wilkins, pp 358-366.

Uphold CR, Graham MV: *Clinical guidelines in adult health,* Gainesville, Fla, 1994, Barmarrae Books, pp. 668-672.

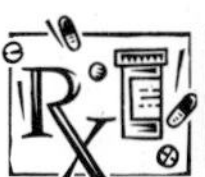

PHARMACOTHERAPEUTICS

Drug of Choice	Mechanism of Action	Prescribing Information	Side Effects
Penicillin G benzathine (Bicillin L-A); for primary, secondary, and early latent disease, 2.4 mil units IM × 1; for late latent and tertiary disease, excluding neurosyphilis, 2.4 mil units IM/week × 3 weeks—same for children	Interferes with cell wall replication	***Contraindications:*** Hypersensitivity; neonates ***Cost:*** 600,000 units/ml, 10 ml: $68 ***Pregnancy category:*** B	Bone marrow depression; granulocytopenia; nausea, vomiting; diarrhea; oliguria; proteinuria; hematuria; vaginitis; moniliasis; glomerulonephritis; lethargy; hallucinations; convulsions; coma; hyperkalemia/hypokalemia; local pain, tenderness, and erythema at injection site; anaphylaxis; hypersensitivity; rash; urticaria
For patients allergic to penicillin:			
Doxycycline (Doryx), 100 mg PO bid × 14 days; used for primary, secondary, and early latent disease; for late latent and tertiary disease, excluding neurosyphilis, 100 mg PO bid × 28 days; children >7 years, 4 mg/kg/day PO in 2 divided doses q12h	Tetracycline; inhibits protein synthesis	***Contraindications:*** Hypersensitivity; children <8 years ***Cost:*** 100-mg tab, 20 tabs: $5 ***Pregnancy category:*** D	Eosinophilia, neutropenia, thrombocytopenia, hemolytic anemia, dysphagia, glossitis, nausea, abdominal pain, vomiting, diarrhea, anorexia, hepatotoxicity, flatulence, abdominal cramps, gastritis, pericarditis, rash, urticaria, exfoliative dermatitis, angioedema
For neurosyphilis, use one of the following:			
Penicillin G sodium (Crystapen), 2-4 mil units IV q4h × 10-14 days	Interferes with cell wall replication	***Contraindications:*** Hypersensitivity; neonates ***Cost:*** 5 mil units/vial, 10 vials: $66 ***Pregnancy category:*** B	Bone marrow depression; granulocytopenia; nausea, vomiting; diarrhea; oliguria; proteinuria; hematuria; vaginitis; moniliasis; glomerulonephritis; lethargy; hallucinations; convulsions; coma; hyperkalemia/hypokalemia; local pain, tenderness, and erythema at injection site; anaphylaxis; hypersensitivity; rash; urticaria
Penicillin G procaine (Wycillin), 2-4 mil units IM daily × 10-14 days	Interferes with cell wall replication	***Contraindication:*** Hypersensitivity to penicillin or procaine ***Cost:*** 600,000 units/ml, 10 ml: $29 ***Pregnancy category:*** B	Same as above for penicillin G sodium
Plus:			
Probenecid (Benemid), 500 mg PO qid × 10-14 days	Inhibits renal tubular secretion of penicillin	***Contraindications:*** Hypersensitivity; severe hepatic disease; blood dyscrasias; severe renal disease; creatinine clearance <50 ml/min; history of uric acid calculus ***Cost:*** 500-mg tab, 100 tabs: $10-$30 ***Pregnancy category:*** B	Drowsiness, headache, bradycardia, nephrotic syndrome, gastric irritation, nausea, vomiting, anorexia, hepatic necrosis, rash, dermatitis, pruritus, acidosis, apnea

For congenital syphillis, consult appropriate pediatric text.

Systemic Lupus Erythematosus (SLE)

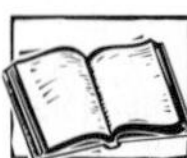

OVERVIEW

Systemic lupus erythematosus (SLE) is a chronic inflammatory disease that affects many systems. It is characterized by remissions and exacerbations and may be mild, having only a few features, to severe, having multiple-system involvement.

Pathogenesis

- Autoimmune disease—altered cellular immunity results in tissue inflammation and injury
- Cause—unknown

Patient Profile

- Females > Males
- Most common age group—20- to 50-year-olds, but may be seen at any age
- Strong genetic component

Signs and Symptoms

- Fever
- Anorexia
- Weight loss
- Skin lesions (butterfly rash)
- Oral ulcers
- Arthritis
- Pallor
- Nausea, vomiting
- Diarrhea
- Aching, stiff, tender muscles
- Headaches
- Photophobia
- Pleurisy
- Pleural effusion
- Bronchopneumonia
- Pneumonitis
- Eye pain
- Visual problems
- Proteinuria
- Glomerulonephritis

Differential Diagnosis

- Rheumatoid arthritis
- Scleroderma
- Mixed connective tissue disease
- Dermatologic disorders

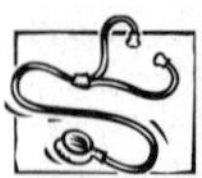

ASSESSMENT

History

Inquire about:

- Onset and duration of symptoms
- Family history of SLE
- Weight loss and fever
- Symptoms in each organ system
- Underlying conditions
- Current medications

Physical Findings

- Vary widely
- Fever
- Weight loss
- Joint pain and stiffness on palpation
- Skin—rash (may be in butterfly form) or lesions
- Oral ulcers
- Lungs—crackles, decreased breath sounds
- May have difficulty reading Snellen eye chart
- Conjunctivitis
- Cotton-wool spots on fundoscopic examination
- Cardiac arrhythmias
- Hepatomegaly
- Splenomegaly

Initial Workup

Laboratory

- Antinuclear antibody—positive
- LE preparation—positive
- VDRL—false positive
- Antibody to native DNA or Sm
- CBC with differential—anemia, leukopenia, lymphopenia, thrombocytopenia
- Serum creatinine—may be increased
- Urinalysis—proteinuria
- Coombs' test—positive

Radiology: Chest—PA and lateral—pulmonary infiltrates, pleural effusion

Further Workup

American Rheumatology Association diagnostic criteria*:

- Malar (butterfly) rash
- Discoid rash
- Photosensitivity
- Oral ulcers
- Arthritis (nonerosive)
- Pleuritis or pericarditis (serositis)
- Renal disease—proteinuria/cellular casts
- Neurologic disorder—seizures and/or psychosis
- Hematologic disorder—hemolytic anemia
- Immunologic disorder—positive LE preparation; antibody to native DNA; antibody to Sm; VDRL—false positive
- Antinuclear antibody (ANA)—positive

*Four or more criteria should be present for diagnosis of SLE.

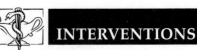

INTERVENTIONS

Office Treatment

None indicated

Lifestyle Modifications

- Maintenance of lifestyle as much as possible
- Protection from ultraviolet (UV) light
- Stress management

Patient Education

Teach patient about:

- Disease and treatment
- Treatment aimed at symptom relief; no curative drug
- Importance of protecting skin from UV light
- Reporting signs and symptoms of infection promptly
- Starting moderate exercise program
- Obtaining adequate rest
- Avoiding stress—biofeedback, relaxation techniques, yoga
- Using hot or cold packs for arthritis
- If kidneys involved—renal diet
- Medications used and side effects (see Pharmacotherapeutics)

Referrals

- To rheumatologist for severe disease
- To nephrologist for renal disease

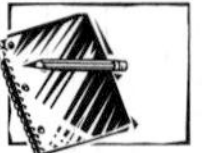

EVALUATION

Outcomes

- Patient is able to maintain lifestyle
- Prognosis—variable, but generally good for long-term survival

Possible Complications

- Renal failure
- Endocarditis
- Peripheral neuropathy
- Infertility
- Seizures
- Avascular necrosis of bone
- Pancreatitis

Follow-up

- Initially and during acute exacerbations may need weekly visits
- During stable periods, every 3 months

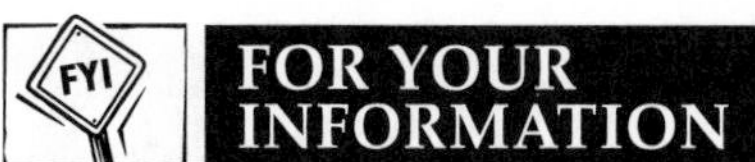

Life Span

Pediatric: Rare in young children, but severe when it occurs
Geriatric: Less likely for onset to occur in this age group; more males affected
Pregnancy: Specialist should handle

Miscellaneous

Patients with renal lupus should be taught about dialysis and renal transplant

References

Casterline GZ: Nursing role in management: arthritis and other rheumatic disorders. In Lewis SM, Collier IC, Heitkemper MM, editors: *Medical-surgical nursing: assessment and management of clinical problems,* ed 4, St Louis, 1996, Mosby, pp 1918-1925.

Hellman DB: Arthritis and musculoskeletal disorders. In Tierney LM Jr, McPhee SJ, Papadakis MA, editors: *Current medical diagnosis and treatment,* ed 34, Norwalk, Conn, 1995, Appleton & Lange, pp 717-720.

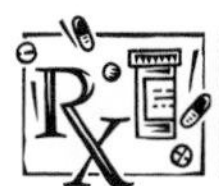

PHARMACOTHERAPEUTICS

Drug of Choice	Mechanism of Action	Prescribing Information	Side Effects
For skin lesions:			
Topical steroids; many types available; start with 1% hydrocortisone and apply to area bid to qid	Antiinflammatory action	***Contraindications:*** Hypersensitivity; fungal infection ***Cost:*** OTC ***Pregnancy category:*** C	Burning, dryness, itching, irritation, acne, hypopigmentation, perioral dermatitis, atrophy, striae, secondary infection
For arthritis:			
Nonsteroidal antiinflammatory drugs (NSAIDs); many different types currently marketed; consult manufacturer's package insert for specific dosing and prescribing information	Exact action unknown; may result from inhibition of synthesis of prostaglandins and arachidonic acid	***Contraindications:*** Hypersensitivity to NSAIDs, aspirin; severe hepatic failure; asthma ***Cost:*** Varies with type ***Pregnancy category:*** Depends on product	Stomach distress, flatulence, nausea, abdominal pain, constipation or diarrhea, dizziness, sedation, rash, urticaria, angioedema, anorexia, urinary frequency, increased blood pressure, insomnia, anxiety, visual disturbances, increased thirst, alopecia
For minor or major inflammatory disease:			
Prednisone, low-dose or high-dose, depending on severity; use for shortest time possible; withdraw, using tapering doses	Corticosteroid; antiinflammatory	***Contraindications:*** Hypersensitivity; psychosis; idiopathic thrombocytopenia; acute glomerulonephritis; amebiasis; nonasthmatic bronchial disease; AIDS; TB; children <2 years old ***Cost:*** 15-mg tab, 100 tabs: $14-$35 ***Pregnancy category:*** C	Hypertension, circulatory collapse, thrombophlebitis, embolism, tachycardia, fungal infections, increased intraocular pressure, diarrhea, nausea, GI hemorrhage, thrombocytopenia, acne, poor wound healing, fractures, osteoporosis, weakness
For more severe arthritis or dermal lupus:			
Hydrochloroquine (Plaquenil), 400 mg PO hs × 2-3 months, then 200 mg PO hs × 2-3 months	Antimalarial; mechanism of action in SLE unknown	***Contraindications:*** Hypersensitivity; retinal field changes; long-term use in children ***Cost:*** 200-mg tab, 100 tabs: $105 ***Pregnancy category:*** C	Irritability, nervousness, emotional changes, nightmares, psychosis, headache, dizziness, vertigo, nystagmus, muscle weakness, visual disturbances, blurred vision, alopecia, pruritus, skin eruptions, aplastic anemia, agranulocytosis, leukopenia, thrombocytopenia, anorexia, nausea, vomiting, weight loss

Temporomandibular Joint (TMJ) Syndrome

OVERVIEW

Temporomandibular joint (TMJ) syndrome is characterized by pain and tenderness in the muscles used for mastication and by pain and popping or clicking in the TMJ.

Pathogenesis

Cause—may be multifactorial:

- Grinding of teeth
- Trauma
- Poorly fitting dentures
- Muscle spasms
- Synovitis of TMJ
- Malocclusion
- Emotional stress
- Whiplash injury

Patient Profile

- Females > Males
- Most common age group—30- to 50-year-olds

Signs and Symptoms

- Facial pain
- Pain in TMJ
- Headache
- Earache
- Neck pain
- Decreased TMJ range of motion
- Popping or clicking of joint

Differential Diagnosis

- Condylar fracture or dislocation
- Neoplasm
- Trigeminal neuralgia
- Dental or periodontal conditions
- Temporal arteritis

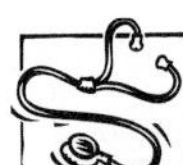

ASSESSMENT

History

Inquire about:

- Onset and duration of symptoms
- Past or recent history of trauma
- History of teeth grinding
- Dentures
- Underlying conditions
- Current medications

Physical Findings

- Subjective complaints of pain on movement of mandible
- May hear popping or clicking of TMJ or feel crepitus
- May see chin shift when opening and closing mouth
- Masseter muscle may be tender on palpation

Initial Workup

Laboratory: None indicated

Radiology: Plain films—may or may not demonstrate an abnormality

Further Workup

Panoramic dental films

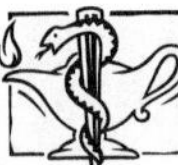

INTERVENTIONS

Office Treatment

None indicated

Lifestyle Modifications

- Soft diet
- Night guard when sleeping
- Stress reduction

Patient Education

Teach patient about:

- Condition and treatment
- Appropriate dental care
- Stress reduction techniques—biofeedback, yoga, relaxation techniques
- Eliminating jaw clinching with above techniques
- Using local heat therapy
- Resting jaw as much as possible
- Medications used and side effects (see Pharmacotherapeutics)

Referral

To oral surgeon

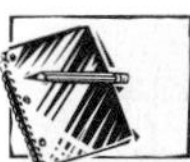

EVALUATION

Outcome
Most cases resolve without sequelae

Possible Complications
- Chronic pain
- Loss of range of motion
- Secondary degenerative joint disease

Follow-up
In 2 weeks; then monthly until resolution

FOR YOUR INFORMATION

Life Span
Pediatric: Rare in this age group; if occurs, trauma from child abuse frequent cause
Geriatric: Most commonly due to poorly fitting dentures
Pregnancy: Cautious use of medication

Miscellaneous
N/A

References

Aminoff MJ: Nervous system. In Tierney LM Jr, McPhee SJ, Papadakis MA, editors: *Current medical diagnosis and treatment,* ed 34, Norwalk, Conn, 1995, Appleton & Lange, p 832.

MacLeod DK: Common problems of the teeth and oral cavity. In Barker LR, Burton JR, Zieve PD, editors: *Principles of ambulatory medicine,* ed 4, Baltimore, 1995, Williams & Wilkins, pp 1483-1484.

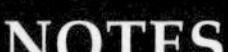

NOTES

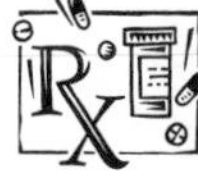

PHARMACOTHERAPEUTICS

Drug of Choice	Mechanism of Action	Prescribing Information	Side Effects
Aspirin, enteric coated, 1 g PO tid or qid; may increase by 300-600 mg/day each week until maximal response seen or toxicity occurs (tinnitus usually 1st symptom); if toxicity occurs, decrease by 600-900 mg/day every 3 days until symptoms resolve	Antiinflammatory action may result from inhibition of synthesis and release of prostaglandins	***Contraindications:*** Hypersensitivity; GI bleeding; bleeding disorders ***Cost:*** OTC ***Pregnancy category:*** Should not be used in 3rd trimester	Dyspepsia, thirst, nausea, vomiting, GI bleeding/ulceration, tinnitus, vertigo, reversible hearing loss, prolongation of bleeding time, leukopenia, thrombocytopenia, purpura, urticaria, angioedema, pruritus, asthma, anaphylaxis, mental confusion, drowsiness, dizziness, headache, fever
Nonsteroidal antiinflammatory drugs (NSAIDs), many different types currently marketed, consult manufacturer's package insert for specific dosing and prescribing information	Exact action unknown; may result from inhibition of synthesis of prostaglandins and arachidonic acid	***Contraindications:*** Hypersensitivity; GI bleeding; bleeding disorders ***Cost:*** OTC ***Pregnancy category:*** Should not be used in 3rd trimester	Stomach distress, flatulence, nausea, abdominal pain, constipation or diarrhea, dizziness, sedation, rash, urticaria, angioedema, anorexia, urinary frequency, increased blood pressure, insomnia, anxiety, visual disturbances, increased thirst, alopecia

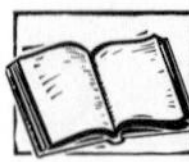

OVERVIEW

Tendinitis is inflammation of a tendon. It usually occurs at the point of insertion into the bone or at the point of muscle origin.

Pathogenesis

Cause—repetitive movement or trauma

Patient Profile

- Males > Females
- Any age

Signs and Symptoms

- Pain and tenderness over affected tendon
- Overlying skin—erythema and warmth
- Pain with movement

Differential Diagnosis

- Bursitis
- Infectious tenosynovitis
- Arthritis
- Tendon avulsion
- Stress fracture
- Compartment syndrome

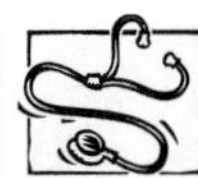

ASSESSMENT

History

Inquire about:

- Onset and duration of symptoms
- Occupation
- Sports participated in
- Underlying conditions
- Current medications

Physical Findings

- Erythema and warmth of overlying skin
- Pain and tenderness with movement and palpation

Initial Workup

Laboratory: None diagnostic
Radiology: CT scan or MRI—can demonstrate tendon integrity; usually not necessary

Further Workup

Real-time sonogram—can observe dynamics of tendon during contraction; usually not necessary

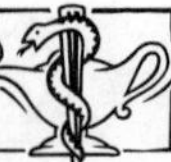

INTERVENTIONS

Office Treatment

Application of sling, Ace wrap, splint, or even cast may be necessary

Lifestyle Modification

Alteration in normal activities because of limited mobility or range of motion.

Patient Education

Teach patient about:

- Condition and treatment:
  - Rest and immobilization until pain resolves
  - Nonsteroidal antiinflammatory drugs
- Using sling, cane, crutches
- Cast care if applicable
- Applying ice
- Physical therapy once pain resolves
- Medications used and side effects (see Pharmacotherapeutics)

Referral

To orthopedist for steroid injection if conservative treatment fails

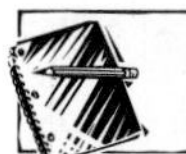

EVALUATION

Outcome
Resolves without sequelae

Possible Complications
- Tendon rupture
- Avulsion fracture
- Repeated pain

Follow-up
In 72 hours to 1 week; then in 2 weeks

FOR YOUR INFORMATION

Life Span
Pediatric: Osgood-Schlatter disease (patellar tendinitis) seen in adolescents
Geriatric: May need assistance with activities of daily living; longer healing time
Pregnancy: Conservative treatment without medication

Miscellaneous
It is important for the NP to ensure that the well-conditioned athlete understands the importance of resting the injured tendon.

Reference
Mercier LR: *Practical orthopedics,* ed 4, St Louis, 1995, Mosby, pp 57-59, 227, 240, 245, 303.

NOTES

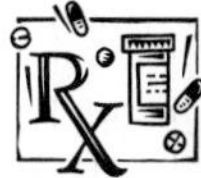

PHARMACOTHERAPEUTICS

Drug of Choice	Mechanism of Action	Prescribing Information	Side Effects
Nonsteroidal antiinflammatory drugs (NSAIDs); many different types currently marketed; consult manufacturer's package insert for specific dosing and prescribing information	Exact action unknown; may result from inhibition of synthesis of prostaglandins and arachidonic acid	***Contraindications:*** Hypersensitivity; GI bleeding; bleeding disorders ***Cost:*** Varies with type ***Pregnancy category:*** Should not be used in 3rd trimester	Stomach distress, flatulence, nausea, abdominal pain, constipation or diarrhea, dizziness, sedation, rash, urticaria, angioedema, anorexia, urinary frequency, increased blood pressure, insomnia, anxiety, visual disturbances, increased thirst, alopecia

Testicular Cancer

OVERVIEW

Testicular cancer is a malignant neoplasm of the testis. The tumors are classified as either germinal (most common; 90% to 95% of all tumors) or nongerminal. Germinal tumors are further classified as either seminomatous or nonseminomatous (embryonal, teratoma, choriocarcinomas, yolk sac).

Pathogenesis
Cause—unknown

Patient Profile
- Males
- Most common age—20 to 40 years, but can occur at any age
- Risk factors—Caucasian race; higher social status; unmarried; residing in rural area; history of cryptorchidism (even if repaired)

Signs and Symptoms
- Scrotal nodule, mass, or swelling, usually painless
- Does *not* transilluminate
- Feeling of heaviness in scrotum
- Hydrocele
- Gynecomastia
- Signs and symptoms of metastases—neck mass, respiratory problems, low-back pain, abdominal mass

Differential Diagnosis
- Hydrocele (transilluminates)
- Hernia
- Hematoma
- Spermatocele
- Varicocele

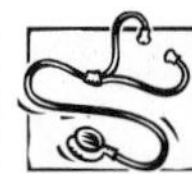

ASSESSMENT

History
Inquire about:
- Onset and duration of symptoms
- History of cryptorchism (undescended testicle)
- Social history
- Underlying conditions
- Current medications

Physical Findings
- Firm, nontender mass on testicle
- May have enlarged inguinal lymph nodes

Initial Workup
Laboratory
- Alpha-fetoprotein—increased in embryonal carcinoma, teratocarcinoma, yolk sac tumor
- Beta–human chorionic gonadotropin—increased in choriocarcinoma, embryonal carcinoma
- Placental alkaline phosphatase—increased in seminomas

Radiology
- Scrotal ultrasound
- Chest film—PA and lateral
- CT scan of chest and abdomen

Further Workup
Biopsy

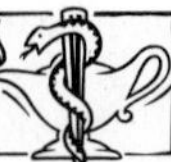

INTERVENTIONS

Office Treatment
None indicated

Lifestyle Modifications
- Adjustment to probable sterility
- Smoking cessation

Patient Education
Teach patient about:
- Disease and treatment options:
  - Treatment will depend on stage—all require radical orchiectomy
  - May require radiation and/or chemotherapy
- Early detection through monthly testicular examination
- Importance of follow-up treatment

Referral
To surgeon

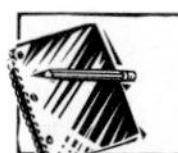

EVALUATION

Outcomes
- If disease is caught early—complete cure
- With advanced disease—70% to 80% have complete cure

Possible Complications
- Metastases to lung, abdomen
- Postoperative complications—wound infection, urinary retention
- Radiation or chemotherapy side effects or complications

Follow-up
To be done by surgeon or oncologist

FOR YOUR INFORMATION

Life Span
Pediatric: Increased incidence in boys 0 to 10 years of age
Geriatric: Increased incidence in patients over 60 years of age
Pregnancy: N/A

Miscellaneous
How to perform testicular examination:
- Perform when scrotum is warm; good time is during shower or bath
- Palpate scrotal contents—roll testicle between thumb and fingers
- Testicles will feel round and soft, like hard-boiled egg; check for lumps, irregularities, dragging sensation; epididymis not as smooth; spermatic cord firm, smooth, cordlike
- Examine monthly and report any abnormalities to provider immediately

Reference
Meredith C: Nursing role in management: male genitourinary problems. In Lewis SM, Collier IC, Heitkemper MM, editors: *Medical-surgical nursing: assessment and management of clinical problems,* ed 4, St Louis, 1996, Mosby, pp 1641-1642.

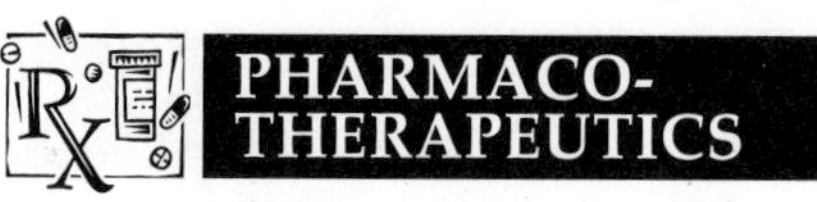

PHARMACOTHERAPEUTICS

Chemotherapeutic agents may be used. These are beyond the scope of this book.

Testicular Torsion

OVERVIEW

Testicular torsion is a twisting of the testis and spermatic cord. This twisting results in compromised blood flow to the testis, resulting in acute ischemia.

Pathogenesis

- Testis has inadequate, incomplete, or absent fixation in scrotum (is free floating); allows testis to rotate on spermatic cord
- Cause—usually idiopathic; may occur after trauma, exercise, cold, or sexual stimulation

Patient Profile

- Males
- Any age
- Peak incidence in adolescence

Signs and Symptoms

- Pain—usually acute, but may have gradual onset
- Nausea and vomiting
- Scrotum enlarged, red, edematous
- Testis may be high in scrotum
- Fever (rare)

Differential Diagnosis

- Epididymitis
- Orchitis
- Incarcerated and/or strangulated inguinal hernia
- Acute hydrocele
- Acute varicocele
- Vasculitis
- Tumor
- Scrotal abscess

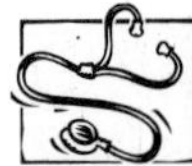

ASSESSMENT

History

Testicular torsion is an emergent condition—obtain history quickly; inquire about:

- Onset and duration of symptoms
- Nausea, vomiting, fever, dysuria, urethral discharge
- Trauma or excessive physical activity just before symptoms
- Underlying conditions
- Current medications

Physical Findings

- Scrotum—enlarged, red, edematous
- Testis—high in scrotum; painful on palpation
- Cremasteric reflex—absent
- Elevating scrotum *increases* pain

Initial Workup

Laboratory: Urinalysis—within normal limits

Radiology

- CT scan or ultrasound of scrotal contents
- Radionuclide scrotal imaging—decreased blood flow
- These tests rarely needed

Further Workup

None needed

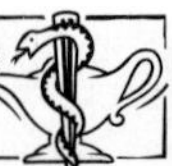

INTERVENTIONS

Office Treatment

None indicated

Lifestyle Modifications

None needed

Patient Education

Teach patient about:

- Condition and treatment:
  - Needs immediate referral for surgery or manual reduction
  - No medications useful in treatment
- Possibility of testicular atrophy and decreased sperm count or loss of testicle

Referral

To urologist or emergency department

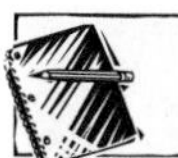

EVALUATION

Outcome
Testicle is saved—directly related to length of time torsion exists—85% to 97% saved if torsion exists <6 hours; <10% saved if torsion exists >24 hours

Possible Complications
- Testicular atrophy
- Infertility

Follow-up
Done by surgeon

FOR YOUR INFORMATION

Life Span
Pediatric: Most common in 14-year-olds
Geriatric: Rarely seen in this age group
Pregnancy: N/A

Miscellaneous
N/A

References
Driscoll CE: The genitourinary system. In Driscoll CE et al, editors: *The family practice desk reference,* ed 3, St Louis, 1996, Mosby, p 422.

Pesti JC, Stoller ML, Carroll PR: Urology. In Tierney LM Jr, McPhee SJ, Papadakis MA, editors: *Current medical diagnosis and treatment,* ed 34, Norwalk, Conn, 1995, Appleton & Lange, pp 793-794.

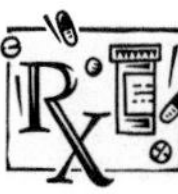

PHARMACOTHERAPEUTICS

No specific medications are used for this condition.

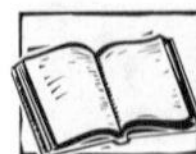

OVERVIEW

Tetanus is a systemic bacterial infection that occurs as a result of a contaminated wound in an unvaccinated individual.

Pathogenesis

- Cause—*Clostridium tetani*
- Releases toxin, which causes tentanospasm, which leads to interference with neurotransmission
- Spores ubiquitous in soil
- Incubation period 5 days to 15 weeks, usually 8 to 12 days

Patient Profile

- Females = Males
- Any age

Signs and Symptoms

- Jaw stiffness
- Jaw muscle spasms
- Neck stiffness
- Dysphagia
- Irritability
- Hyperreflexia
- Spasms of abdomen, neck, and back
- Spasms of glottis and respiratory muscles
- Temperature normal to slightly elevated
- Tonic convulsions

Differential Diagnosis

- Side effect of phenothiazines
- Strychnine poisoning

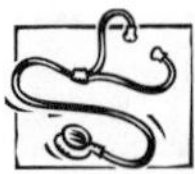

ASSESSMENT

History

Inquire about:

- Onset and duration of symptoms
- History of recent dirty wound
- Tetanus immunization
- Underlying conditions
- Current medications

Physical Findings

- Jaw and neck stiffness
- Irritability
- Muscle spasms may occur with minor stimuli
- Tonic convulsions may occur with minor stimuli

Initial Workup

Laboratory: None indicated—diagnosis made by history and physical; may do wound culture, but not always positive for *C. tetani*
Radiology: None indicated

Further Workup

None indicated

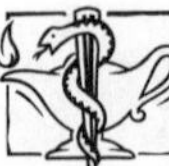

INTERVENTIONS

Office Treatment

Direct hospital admission

Lifestyle Modification

Regular health care with immunizations for primary prevention

Patient Education

Teach patient about:

- Condition and treatment:
  - Hospitalization
  - Bed rest
  - Quiet environment
  - May require sedation or paralysis
- Immunizations
- Medications used and side effects (see Pharmacotherapeutics and Table 14)

Referral

To MD if NP does not have hospital privileges

TABLE 14 ***Tetanus Prophylaxis***

	Clean minor wounds		Other†	
History of tetanus toxoid	Td	TiG	Td	TiG
Unknown or <3 doses	Yes	No	Yes	Yes
≥3 doses*	No, unless >10 years since last dose	No	No, unless >5 years since last dose	No

Td, Tetanus toxoid; *TiG,* tetanus immune globulin.
*If patient only had 3 doses, give fourth dose regardless of when other doses were given.
†Wounds contaminated with dirt, stool, saliva, etc.; puncture wounds; avulsions; crushing; burns; frostbite; from missiles.

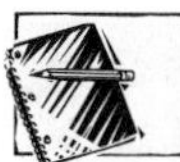

EVALUATION

Outcomes
- 40% mortality rate
- Otherwise, full recovery

Possible Complications
- Respiratory arrest
- Cardiac failure
- Pulmonary emboli
- Vertebral fractures
- Urinary retention
- Constipation
- Rhabdomyolysis
- Death

Follow-up
1 week after hospitalization

FOR YOUR INFORMATION

Life Span
Pediatric: Mortality high in very young
Geriatric: Mortality high
Pregnancy: To specialist

Miscellaneous
N/A

Reference
Chambers HF: Infectious diseases: bacterial and chlamydial. In Tierney LM Jr, McPhee SJ, Papadakis MA, editors: *Current medical diagnosis and treatment,* ed 34, Norwalk, Conn, 1995, Appleton & Lange, pp 1169-1171.

NOTES

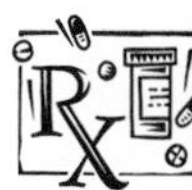

PHARMACOTHERAPEUTICS

There are many medications that are used in the acute care setting. However, they are beyond the scope of this book. Consult an acute care text.

Drug of Choice	Mechanism of Action	Prescribing Information	Side Effects
Tetanus immune globulin (human), 3000-6000 units IM; infiltrate half around wound; use separate syringe to give other half IM	Provides antibodies against tetanus	***Contraindication:*** Hypersensitivity ***Cost:*** 250-unit vial, 10 vials: $118 ***Pregnancy category:*** C	Local tenderness, stiffness, rash, anaphylaxis
Tetanus toxoid, 0.5 ml IM × 1 dose if patient previously immunized; if not previously immunized, give basic course, 0.5 ml at 0, 1 month, and 6-12 months	Causes body to produce antibodies to *Clostridium tetani*	***Contraindications:*** Acute respiratory tract infection; hypersensitivity ***Cost:*** 0.5 ml-vial, 10 vials: $13 ***Pregnancy category:*** C	Nausea, vomiting, anorexia, skin abscess, urticaria, itching, tachycardia, hypotension, lymphadenitis, anaphylaxis, crying, fretfulness, fever

Thalassemia

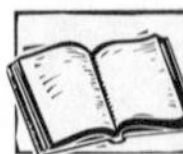

OVERVIEW

The thalassemias are a group of disorders that affect the synthesis of either the beta-globin or alpha-globin chains in hemoglobin. Thalassemia is usually named for the affected globin chain (beta-thalassemia or alpha-thalassemia). This defective synthesis results in microcytic anemia. There are 3 types of thalassemia: beta-thalassemia major, thalassemia intermedia, and thalassemia trait (alpha or beta).

Pathogenesis

Cause—genetic defect that affects hemoglobin synthesis; autosomal recessive

Patient Profile

- Males = Females
- Symptoms start at 3 to 6 months of age
- Ethnic groups from Mediterranean region, Middle East, and Southeast Asia most commonly affected

Signs and Symptoms

- Pallor
- Fatigue
- Shortness of breath
- Poor growth
- Splenomegaly
- Jaundice
- Pathologic fractures
- Beta-thalassemia major—symptoms severe
- Thalassemia intermedia—milder symptoms
- Thalassemia trait—usually asymptomatic with mild anemia

Differential Diagnosis

- Iron deficiency anemia
- Sickle cell anemia
- Other hemoglobinopathies
- Other hemolytic anemias

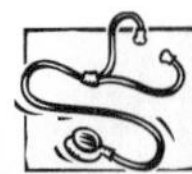

ASSESSMENT

History

Inquire about:

- Onset and duration of symptoms
- Family history of thalassemia
- Underlying conditions
- Current medications

Physical Findings

- Pallor
- Bone deformities
- Growth retardation when compared with growth charts
- Shortness of breath (may note extreme shortness of breath when child is nursing)
- Jaundice
- Abdominal examination—splenomegaly

Initial Workup

Laboratory

- CBC with differential—mild to severe anemia, microcytosis, decreased mean corpuscular volume (MCV), anisocytosis, increased target cells
- Reticulocyte count—increased
- Hemoglobin electrophoresis:
  - Thalassemia trait—Hb A_2 levels increased
  - Thalassemia intermedia—Hb A_1 decreased; Hb A_2 increased; HbF increased
  - Beta-thalassemia major—Hb A_1 absent; Hb A_2 increased; HbF increased

Radiology: Not necessary for diagnosis

Further Workup

Bone marrow aspiration

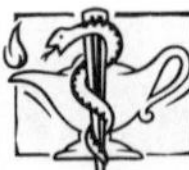

INTERVENTIONS

Office Treatment

None indicated

Lifestyle Modifications

- Depends on severity
- Avoidance of strenuous activity
- Avoidance of iron-rich foods

Patient Education

Teach patient and family about:

- Disease, how transmitted, and treatment:
  - Thalassemia trait—no treatment required
  - Thalassemia intermedia—normally no treatment; if hemoglobin falls dangerously low—transfusions
  - Beta-thalassemia major—regular transfusions every 3 to 5 weeks, iron chelation therapy, folate supplementation, possible splenectomy at 4 to 6 years of age, bone marrow transplant
- Signs and symptoms of infection and to report promptly—need prompt antimicrobial therapy
- Importance of avoiding strenuous activity and contact sports
- Avoiding foods high in iron
- Signs of iron overload (drinking tea may help reduce iron)
- Genetic counseling
- Medications used and side effects (see Pharmacotherapeutics)

Referral

To specialist

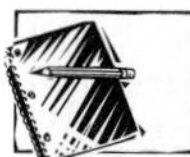

EVALUATION

Outcomes

- Beta-thalassemia major—life span to late teens or early 20s
- Thalassemia intermedia and trait—normal life span

Possible Complications

- Depends on severity
- Increased susceptibility to infections after splenectomy
- Pathologic bone fractures
- Growth retardation
- Cardiac disease from iron overload
- Hepatic siderosis

Follow-up

Depends on severity; should be followed by specialist if patient has thalassemia intermedia or beta-thalassemia major

FOR YOUR INFORMATION

Life Span

Pediatric: Pediatric disorder
Geriatric: N/A
Pregnancy: Genetic counseling before pregnancy

Miscellaneous

N/A

References

Linker CA: Blood. In Tierney LM Jr, McPhee SJ, Papadakis MA, editors: *Current medical diagnosis and treatment,* ed 34, Norwalk, Conn, 1995, Appleton & Lange, pp 426-428.

Whedon MB: Nursing role in management: hemolytic problems. In Lewis SM, Collier IC, Heitkemper MM, editors: *Medical-surgical nursing: assessment and management of clinical problems,* ed 4, St Louis, 1996, Mosby, pp 783.

NOTES

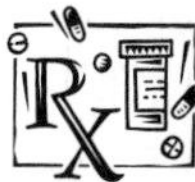

PHARMACOTHERAPEUTICS

Drug of Choice	Mechanism of Action	Prescribing Information	Side Effects
Folic acid supplement (Folate); adults and children, up to 1 mg PO qd	Folic acid supplement necessary for normal erythropoiesis	***Contraindication:*** Hypersensitivity ***Cost:*** 1-mg tab, 30 tabs: $2 ***Pregnancy category:*** A	Allergic reaction has been reported
Deferoxamine (Desferal); 40 mg/kg/day over 10 hours SQ using infusion pump	Binds iron to form water-soluble complex excreted by kidneys	***Contraindications:*** Hypersensitivity; severe renal disease ***Cost:*** 500-mg vial, 4 vials: $40 ***Pregnancy category:*** C	Generalized erythema, urticaria, anaphylactic reaction, tachycardia, hypotension, shock, abdominal pain, diarrhea, ocular and auditory disturbances, dysuria, leg cramps, fever, localized irritation and pain, swelling and induration

Thrombophlebitis, Superficial

OVERVIEW

Superficial thrombophlebitis is an inflammation with secondary thrombosis of the vein. It may occur in the upper or lower extremities.

Pathogenesis

- Inflammatory process of superficial vein
- Causes:
  - Spontaneous process—secondary to pregnancy, postpartum period, varicose veins, thromboangiitis obliterans
  - Trauma—blow to leg or arm; IV therapy with irritating solutions

Patient Profile

- Males = Females
- Any age

Signs and Symptoms

- Dull pain
- Localized induration, redness, tenderness
- Firm venous cord
- Chills and fever if septic

Differential Diagnosis

- Deep vein thrombosis
- Cellulitis
- Erythema nodosum
- Erythema induratum
- Sarcoidosis
- Fibrositis

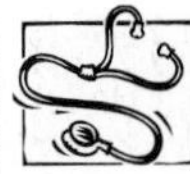

ASSESSMENT

History

Inquire about:

- Onset and duration of symptoms
- Pregnancy or recent pregnancy
- Trauma to area
- Use of IV drugs
- Recent hospitalization and IV medications
- Underlying conditions
- Current medications

Physical Findings

- Localized pain, erythema, tenderness along course of vein
- Firm venous cord
- Suppurative drainage if septic

Initial Workup

Laboratory

- If septic—culture of drainage
- CBC with differential—leukocytosis, left shift

Radiology: Usually none needed for localized, superficial thrombophlebitis

Further Workup

Depends on extent; ultrasound of veins may be indicated

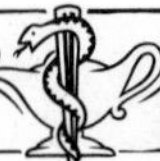

INTERVENTIONS

Office Treatment

If septic—direct hospital admission

Lifestyle Modifications

- Smoking cessation
- Bed rest with limb elevated until resolution

Patient Education

Teach patient about:

- Condition and treatment:
  - If aseptic—limb elevation, warm compresses, nonsteroidal antiinflammatory drugs (NSAIDs), vein ligation if extensive and progressing toward saphenofemoral junction
  - If septic—hospitalization for IV antibiotic therapy
- Medications used and side effects (see Pharmacotherapeutics)

Referral

To MD for hospitalization if NP does not have privileges

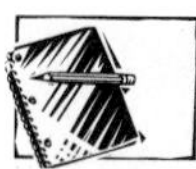

EVALUATION

Outcomes

- Usually resolves without sequelae, dependent on underlying cause
- Septic thrombophlebitis—if untreated, mortality high

Possible Complications

- Aseptic thrombophlebitis—deep vein thrombosis
- Septic thrombophlebitis—systemic sepsis, pneumonia, septic pulmonary emboli

Follow-up

In 1 week for outpatient or 1 week after hospitalization

FOR YOUR INFORMATION

Life Span

Pediatric: May develop long-bone abscess as complication
Geriatric: Higher morbidity and mortality rate
Pregnancy: Increased risk, especially with increased age, parity, and hypertension

Miscellaneous

N/A

References

Rudolphi D, Doyle J: Nursing role in management: vascular disorders. In Lewis SM, Collier IC, Heitkemper MM, editors: *Medical-surgical nursing: assessment and management of clinical problems,* ed 4, St Louis, 1996, Mosby, pp 1054-1060.

Tierney LM Jr: Blood vessels and lymphatics. In Tierney LM Jr, McPhee SJ, Papadakis MA, editors: *Current medical diagnosis and treatment,* ed 34, Norwalk, Conn, 1995, Appleton & Lange, pp 413-414.

NOTES

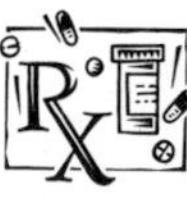

PHARMACOTHERAPEUTICS

For inpatient IV antibiotic therapy, consult an acute care text.

Drug of Choice	Mechanism of Action	Prescribing Information	Side Effects
Nonsteroidal antiinflammatory drugs (NSAIDs); many different types currently marketed; consult manufacturer's package insert for specific dosing and prescribing information	Exact action unknown; may result from inhibition of synthesis of prostaglandins and arachidonic acid	***Contraindications:*** Hypersensitivity to NSAIDs, aspirin; severe hepatic failure; asthma ***Cost:*** Varies with type ***Pregnancy category:*** Depends on product	Stomach distress, flatulence, nausea, abdominal pain, constipation or diarrhea, dizziness, sedation, rash, urticaria, angioedema, anorexia, urinary frequency, increased blood pressure, insomnia, anxiety, visual disturbances, increased thirst, alopecia
Anticoagulant therapy (rarely needed unless condition extends to deep vein system):			
Warfarin (Coumadin); usually start with 10-15 mg PO qd, then titrate to maintain prothrombin time INR between 2 and 3	Depresses synthesis of coagulation factors that are dependent on vitamin K (II, VII, IX, X)	***Contraindications:*** Hypersensitivity; hemophilia; peptic ulcer disease; thrombocytopenic purpura; severe hepatic disease; severe hypertension; subacute bacterial endocarditis; acute nephritis; blood dyscrasias; pregnancy ***Cost:*** 5-mg tab, 100 tabs: $30-$50 ***Pregnancy category:*** D	Diarrhea, nausea, vomiting, anorexia, stomatitis, cramps, hepatitis, hematuria, rash, dermatitis, fever, hemorrhage, agranulocytosis, leukopenia, eosinophilia

Thrombosis, Deep Vein (DVT)

OVERVIEW

Deep vein thrombosis (DVT) is the development of a blood clot or blood clots of the deep veins. Most commonly, it begins in the calf, although it may begin in the femoral or iliac veins. Usually there is accompanying inflammation of the vessel wall.

Pathogenesis

Development of thrombus in deep veins due to:

- Venous stasis secondary to bed rest, major surgical procedures, etc.
- Injury to vessel wall
- Hypercoagulable states, such as occurs with use of oral contraceptive (particularly in those who smoke), carcinoma, or polycythemia vera

Patient Profile

- Females > Males
- Most common age—usually over 40 years

Signs and Symptoms

- Limb pain and swelling
- Positive Homan's sign
- May have warmth and erythema over area, fever, swelling of superficial veins
- Increased extremity diameter
- Edema of extremity

Differential Diagnosis

- Cellulitis
- Muscle strain or contusion
- Ruptured Baker's cyst
- Tumor compressing vein

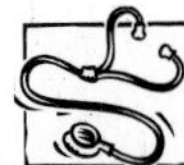

ASSESSMENT

History

Inquire about:

- Onset and duration of symptoms
- Fever
- History of DVT, recent surgery, bed rest
- Recent trauma
- Underlying conditions
- Current medications

Physical Findings

- Calf tenderness, warmth, swelling
- Positive Homan's sign
- Increased extremity diameter

Initial Workup

Laboratory: None specific for diagnosis

Radiology

- Doppler studies
- Plethysmography

Further Workup

None indicated

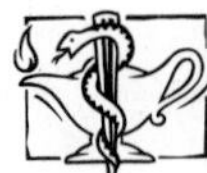

INTERVENTIONS

Office Treatment

None indicated

Lifestyle Modifications

- Smoking cessation
- Avoidance of prolonged immobility
- Alternative form of birth control if taking oral contraceptives

Patient Education

Teach patient about:

- Condition and treatment:
  - Hospitalization
  - Intravenous anticoagulation; then oral anticoagulant; bed rest until resolution
- Preventing future DVTs
- Avoiding prolonged immobility if possible
- Using support hose
- Avoiding constrictive clothing
- Options for birth control
- Avoiding prolonged sitting or standing
- Importance of regular follow-up and laboratory tests to monitor anticoagulant therapy
- Importance of immediately reporting any abnormal bleeding
- Medications used and side effects (see Pharmacotherapeutics)

Referral

To MD for hospitalization if NP does not have privileges

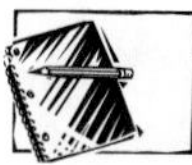

EVALUATION

Outcome
Prognosis is usually good with appropriate treatment

Possible Complications
- Pulmonary embolism
- Chronic venous insufficiency
- Hemorrhage from anticoagulant therapy

Follow-up
Weekly for prothrombin time until stable; then monthly as long as patient is receiving anticoagulant therapy—3 to 6 months for first episode, 12 months if prior attack

FOR YOUR INFORMATION

Life Span
Pediatric: Rare—look for congenital condition
Geriatric: More commonly seen in this age group
Pregnancy: Coumadin contraindicated in pregnancy—should be followed by a specialist

Miscellaneous
N/A

References
Tierney LM Jr: Blood vessels and lymphatics. In Tierney LM Jr, McPhee SJ, Papadakis MA, editors: *Current medical diagnosis and treatment,* ed 34, Norwalk, Conn, 1995, Appleton & Lange, pp 411-413.

Uphold CR, Graham MV: *Clinical guidelines in adult health,* Gainesville, Fla, 1994, Barmarrae Books, pp 311-312.

NOTES

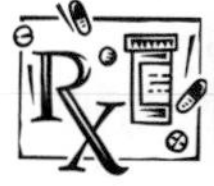

PHARMACOTHERAPEUTICS

Drug of Choice	Mechanism of Action	Prescribing Information	Side Effects
Heparin, 5000-10,000 units IV bolus; then 1000 units/hr to achieve activated partial thromboplastin time (APTT) 2 × normal	Prevents conversion of fibrinogen to fibrin and prothrombin to thrombin	***Contraindications:*** Hypersensitivity; severe active bleeding; severe hepatic or renal disease; recent neurosurgical procedure; peptic ulcer disease; blood dyscrasias ***Cost:*** 10,000 units/ml, 5 ml: $11 ***Pregnancy category:*** C	Fever, chills, diarrhea, nausea, vomiting, anorexia, stomatitis, hepatitis, hematuria, hemorrhage, thrombocytopenia, rash, dermatitis, urticaria, alopecia, pruritus
Warfarin (Coumadin), 5-10 mg PO qd; start 1-5 days after heparin; monitor with prothrombin times—INR 2.0-3.0	Depresses synthesis of coagulation factors that are dependent on vitamin K (II, VII, IX, X)	***Contraindications:*** Hypersensitivity; hemophilia; peptic ulcer disease; thrombocytopenic purpura; severe hepatic disease; severe hypertension; subacute bacterial endocarditis; acute nephritis; blood dyscrasias; pregnancy ***Cost:*** 5-mg tab, 100 tabs: $30-$50 ***Pregnancy category:*** D	Diarrhea, nausea, vomiting, anorexia, stomatitis, cramps, hepatitis, hematuria, rash, dermatitis, fever, hemorrhage, agranulocytosis, leukopenia, eosinophilia

Thyroiditis

OVERVIEW

Thyroiditis can be any one of a variety of disorders that cause inflammation of the thyroid. It can cause either enlargement or atrophy of the thyroid and may lead to either hypothyroidism or hyperthyroidism. There are 2 types of thyroiditis—lymphocytic and granulomatous.

Pathogenesis

LYMPHOCYTIC THYROIDITIS

- Hashimoto's thyroiditis:
  - Autoimmune disease
  - Most common form
  - Thyroid tissue replaced by lymphocytes and fibrous tissue
  - Leads to hypothyroidism
- Silent thyroiditis:
  - Autoimmune process
  - One form occurs postpartum and another form is similar to granulomatous thyroiditis without pain

GRANULOMATOUS THYROIDITIS

- Acute thyroiditis:
  - Due to bacterial or fungal infection
  - Also called suppurative thyroiditis
- Subacute granulomatous thyroiditis (de Quervain's thyroiditis):
  - Chronic inflammatory response to thyroid tissue
  - Probably related to viral infection

Patient Profile

- Females > Males
- All ages, but primarily postpuberty
- Lymphocytic thyroiditis—familial tendency

Signs and Symptoms

- Lymphocytic thyroiditis (Hashimoto's and silent thyroiditis)—slow onset of goiter, hypothyroidism with associated symptoms; may be associated with other autoimmune diseases
- Granulomatous thyroiditis (acute and subacute thyroiditis)—pain, tenderness, enlargement of one or both thyroid lobes, malaise, fever; may have symptoms of hyperthyroidism, history of recent respiratory tract infection

Differential Diagnosis

- Lymphocytic thyroiditis—simple goiter, iodine-deficient goiter, early Graves' disease, lithium-induced goiter
- Granulomatous thyroiditis—infection of oropharynx and trachea, hemorrhage into thyroid cyst, subacute systemic illness, suppurative thyroiditis

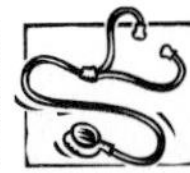

ASSESSMENT

History

Inquire about:

- Onset and duration of symptoms
- Family history of thyroid problems
- Underlying conditions
- Current medications

Physical Findings

LYMPHOCYTIC THYROIDITIS

- Physical findings of hypothyroidism—dry, coarse skin; dull facial expression; periorbital puffiness
- Bradycardia
- Decreased systolic blood pressure with increased diastolic blood pressure
- Delayed relaxation of deep tendon reflexes
- Reduced body and scalp hair

GRANULOMATOUS THYROIDITIS

- Pain on palpation of thyroid
- Thyroid enlargement on palpation of either one or both lobes
- Fever
- May have physical findings of hyperthyroidism—nervousness, sweating, tachycardia, ophthalmopathy, warm and moist skin

Initial Workup

Laboratory

- Thyroid panel—can be normal, or with granulomatous thyroiditis: T_3 and T_4 elevated and TSH decreased; with lymphocytic thyroiditis: T_3 and T_4 decreased and TSH elevated
- Free thyroxine index—with granulomatous thyroiditis: >12; with lymphocytic thyroiditis: <5
- Erythrocyte sedimentation rate (ESR)—elevated in granulomatous thyroiditis
- CBC with differential—WBC count may be elevated

Radiology

- Thyroid scan if granulomatous thyroiditis suspected
- May also need thyroid ultrasound

Further Workup

Antithyroid antibodies—elevated in lymphocytic thyroiditis

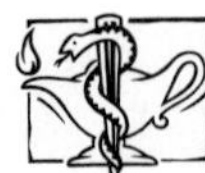

INTERVENTIONS

Office Treatment

None indicated

Lifestyle Modifications

- Diet to meet daily calorie output—if hypothyroid, need reduced calories; if hyperthyroid, need increased calories
- Smoking cessation
- If Hashimoto's thyroiditis present, will need to adjust to living with chronic illness
- May also have other autoimmune disease
- Stress management techniques

Patient Education

Teach patient about:

- Disease process and treatment options:
  - Lymphocytic (Hashimoto's) thyroiditis—will need thyroid hormone replacement for life
  - Granulomatous thyroiditis—treat symptoms; if acute, will need antibiotics or antifungals, possibly surgical drainage; if subacute, will need nonsteroidal antiinflammatory drugs (if no response in 48 hours, use corticosteroids); treat symptoms of hyperthyroidism (with propranolol or may need antithyroid medication—propylthiouracil or methimazole) or hypothyroidism (with thyroid hormone)
- Stress management techniques—biofeedback, relaxation techniques (increased stress can aggravate autoimmune disease)
- Proper caloric intake
- Foods that are goitrogens and to avoid—turnips, rutabagas, soybeans, skins of peanuts, seafood, green leafy vegetables, peanuts, peaches, peas, strawberries, carrots, cabbage, mustard seed, radishes
- Medications used and side effects (see Pharmacotherapeutics)

Referral

To endocrinologist if possible

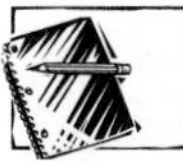

EVALUATION

Outcomes

- Lymphocytic (Hashimoto's) thyroiditis—will need thyroid hormone for life
- Granulomatous thyroiditis—usually returns to normal in weeks to months

Possible Complication

Treatment-induced hypothyroidism or hyperthyroidism

Follow-up

- Granulomatous thyroiditis—weekly × 2 until symptoms controlled; recheck thyroid function every 3 weeks
- Lymphocytic thyroiditis—recheck thyroid every 6 to 8 weeks

FOR YOUR INFORMATION

Life Span

Pediatric: Rare in this age group
Geriatric: Signs and symptoms may be more subtle
Pregnancy: Needs to be followed by a specialist

Miscellaneous

Patients with lymphocytic thyroiditis need to be screened for other autoimmune diseases, such as diabetes, primary adrenal insufficiency, or ovarian failure.

References

Gregerman RI: Thyroid disorders. In Barker LR, Burton JR, Zieve PD, editors: *Principles of ambulatory medicine,* ed 4, Baltimore, 1995, Williams & Wilkins, pp 1045-1046.

Haas L: Endocrine problems. In Lewis SM, Collier IC, Heitkemper MM, editors: *Medical-surgical nursing: assessment and management of clinical problems,* ed 4, St Louis, 1996, Mosby, pp 1495-1496.

NOTES

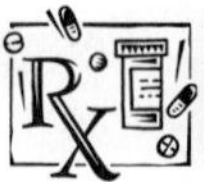

PHARMACOTHERAPEUTICS

Antibiotics and antifungals used in the treatment of acute thyroiditis are not covered here because of the rarity of the condition. Consult a text specific to that condition.

Drug of Choice	Mechanism of Action	Prescribing Information	Side Effects
For granulomatous (subacute) thyroiditis to relieve pain and inflammation:			
Ibuprofen (Motrin, Advil); dose varies with type of drug; many other NSAIDs are available	Not well understood, but may be related to inhibition of prostaglandin synthesis	***Contraindications:*** Aspirin allergy; hypersensitivity; asthma; last trimester of pregnancy; gastric ulcer; bleeding disorders ***Cost:*** 400-mg tab, 4/day × 5 days: $3 ***Pregnancy category:*** Not recommended	Nausea, heartburn, diarrhea, GI upset and bleeding, dizziness, headache, rash, tinnitus, edema, acute renal failure
If no response to NSAIDs, consider:			
Prednisone 60-120 mg PO qd, then taper over several days	Corticosteroid; decreases inflammation	***Contraindications:*** Hypersensitivity; psychosis; idiopathic thrombocytopenia; acute glomerulone- phritis; amebiasis; nonasthmatic bronchial disease; AIDS; TB; children <2 years old ***Cost:*** 15-mg tab, 100 tabs: $14-$35 ***Pregnancy category:*** C	Hypertension, circulatory collapse, thrombophlebitis, embolism, tachycardia, fungal infections, increased intraocular pressure, diarrhea, nausea, GI hemorrhage, thrombocytopenia, acne, poor wound healing, fractures, osteoporosis, weakness
For hypothyroidism:			
Levothyroxine (Synthroid, Levothroid, etc.), 50-100 μg/day; increase by 25-μg increments until TSH is normal	Replacement of decreased thyroid hormone; thyroid hormone increases metabolic rate of tissue	***Contraindications:*** Untreated thyrotoxicosis; hypersensitivity; uncorrected adrenal insufficiency ***Cost:*** 50-μg tab, 100 tabs: $4-$21 ***Pregnancy category:*** A	Thyrotoxicosis caused by overdose, rash, urticaria, hair loss, pseudotumor cerebri—can occur in pediatric patients

Drug of Choice	Mechanism of Action	Prescribing Information	Side Effects
For granulomatous disease if symptoms of hyperthyroidism are present:			
Propranolol (Inderal), 40-240 mg/day;	Blocks beta-adrenergic receptors that are increased because of increased thyroid hormones	***Contraindications:*** Hypersensitivity; cardiac failure; cardiogenic shock; 2nd- or 3rd-degree heart block; bronchospastic disease; sinus bradycardia; congestive heart failure (CHF) ***Cost:*** 40-mg tab, 100 tabs: $2-$40 ***Pregnancy category:*** C	Headache, fatigue, drowsiness, dizziness, anxiety, depression, weakness, insomnia, tinnitus, dysrhythmias, edema, CHF, hypotension, pulmonary edema, nausea, vomiting, diarrhea, constipation, nocturia, polyuria, rash, pruritus, photosensitivity, flushing, sexual difficulties, fever, chills
For hyperthyroidism, use one of the following:			
Propylthiouracil (PTU); initially 100 mg PO tid; increase as needed to obtain euthyroid state; check laboratory values every 6 weeks; maintenance dose usually 100-150 mg PO qd; children >10 years, start with 150-300 mg PO in three divided doses; preferred drug in pregnancy, elderly, and patients with cardiac disease	Inhibits synthesis of thyroid hormones	***Contraindications:*** Hypersensitivity; lactating mothers ***Cost:*** 50-mg tab, 100 tabs: $5-$10 ***Pregnancy category:*** D	Agranulocytosis most serious side effect; leukopenia, thrombocytopenia, aplastic anemia, drug fever, lupuslike syndrome, hepatitis, periarteritis, nephritis, interstitial pneumonitis, erythema nodosum, skin rash, urticaria, nausea, vomiting, hair loss, pruritus, drowsiness, edema
Methimazole (Tapazole), 15-60 mg PO qd in 3 doses separated by 8 hours; maintenance dose 5-15 mg PO qd; children, 0.4 mg/kg/day PO in 3 divided doses at 8-hour intervals; maintenance dose about half initial dose	Inhibits synthesis of thyroid hormone	***Contraindications:*** Hypersensitivity; nursing mothers ***Cost:*** 5-mg tab, 100 tabs: $13 ***Pregnancy category:*** D	Agranulocytosis most serious side effect; leukopenia, thrombocytopenia, aplastic anemia, drug fever, lupuslike syndrome, hepatitis, periarteritis, nephritis, interstitial pneumonitis, erythema nodosum, skin rash, urticaria, nausea, vomiting, hair loss, pruritus, drowsiness, edema

Tinea Capitis

OVERVIEW

Tinea capitis is a fungal infection of the scalp. It is commonly referred to as "ringworm." It is spread by direct contact with another infected human or animal.

Pathogenesis

Cause—fungus of genus *Trichophyton* (*T. tonsurans*—90%) or *Microsporum* (*M. canis, M. audouinii,* or *M. gypseum*)

Patient Profile

- Males = Females
- Most common in children
- Risk factors—day care centers and schools; living in confined quarters; poor hygiene; immunosuppression

Signs and Symptoms

- Round patches of scale on scalp; erythema
- Characteristic "black dot" pattern—patches of broken hair
- Severe inflammation leading to kerion formation—a pustular, exudative nodule

Differential Diagnosis

- Psoriasis
- Seborrheic dermatitis
- Pyoderma
- Alopecia areata
- Trichotillomania

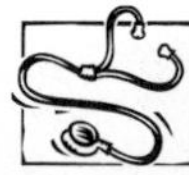

ASSESSMENT

History

Inquire about:

- Onset and duration of symptoms
- Length of time lesions have been present
- Contact with individuals or animals with similar lesions
- Treatments tried
- Underlying conditions
- Current medications

Physical Findings

- Patches of hair loss ("black dot pattern")
- Scaly areas with erythema on scalp
- May find indurated area that feels boggy (kerion)

Initial Workup

Laboratory

- Skin scraping for potassium hydroxide (KOH) preparation (scrape edge of lesion with No. 15 scapel moistened with tap water; transfer to slide with small drop of water; add 1 to 2 drops KOH; cover with coverslip; warm for 15 to 30 seconds)—spores and/or hyphae present
- Fungal culture
- Liver function tests before institution of therapy

Radiology: None indicated

Further Workup

None indicated

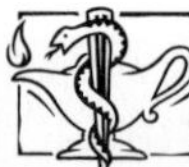

INTERVENTIONS

Office Treatment

None indicated

Lifestyle Modifications

- Good personal hygiene
- If infection is from pet, need to get pet treated
- Need for laundering of towels, clothing, and headgear—no sharing of headgear

Patient Education

Teach patient about:

- Disease and how spread
- Proper hand washing
- Importance of laundering towels, clothing, and headgear to prevent spread
- Treatment with oral antifungals being lengthy (6-8 weeks) and need to complete all medication
- Shampooing hair with 1% selenium sulfide shampoo (OTC preparation) twice weekly
- Medications used and side effects (see Pharmacotherapeutics)

Referrals

- Usually none
- To dermatologist if infection is severe, with kerion formation

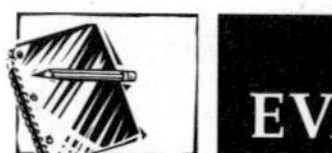

EVALUATION

Outcome
Resolves without sequelae

Possible Complications
Permanent scarring and hair loss

Follow-up
In 2 weeks × 3

FOR YOUR INFORMATION

Life Span
Pediatric: Most common in this age group
Geriatric: May be found in nursing home population
Pregnancy: Oral antifungal agents contraindicated

Miscellaneous
Selenium sulfide shampoo is an important adjunct to oral antifungal therapy. Givens, Murray, and Baker (1995) found that using 1% selenium sulfide shampoo was just as effective at stopping spore shedding as 2.5% selenium sulfide shampoo. This is an important issue for cost containment, since 1% shampoo is available OTC and costs significantly less than the 2.5% prescription shampoo.

References
Givens TG et al: Comparison of 1% and 2.5% selenium sulfide in the treatment of tinea capitis, *Arch Pediatr Adolesc Med* 149(7):808-811, 1995.

Habif TP: *Clinical dermatology: a color guide to diagnosis and therapy,* ed 3, St Louis, Mosby, pp 380-385.

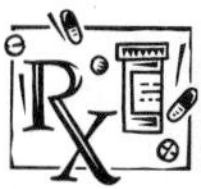

PHARMACOTHERAPEUTICS

Drug of Choice	Mechanism of Action	Prescribing Information	Side Effects
Griseofulvin (Fulvicin), 500 mg PO as single or divided dose × 6-8 weeks; children 30-50 lb, 125-250 mg PO qd; children >50 lb: 250-500 mg PO qd × 6-8 weeks; increased absorption when taken with fatty meal; perform baseline liver function tests and repeat every 3 months if treatment lengthy; may potentiate alcohol	Fungistatic	***Contraindications:*** Hypersensitivity; patients with porphyria, hepatocellular failure; pregnancy or contemplated pregnancy ***Cost:*** 125-mg tab, 100 tabs: $28 ***Pregnancy category:*** Contraindicated	Porphyria, hepatocellular failure, leukopenia, persistent anemia, skin rash, urticaria, paresthesias of hands and feet, nausea, vomiting, diarrhea, headache, epigastric distress, dizziness
Ketoconazole (Nizoral), 200 mg PO qd; may increase to 400 mg PO qd in severe cases; children >2 years, 3.3-6.6 mg/kg/day PO × 6-8 weeks; baseline liver function tests should be obtained; monitor every 3 months; for children, potential benefit must outweigh risks	Antifungal agent	***Contraindications:*** Hypersensitivity; coadministration of terfenadine, astemizole, and cisapride ***Cost:*** 200-mg tab, 100 tabs: $271 ***Pregnancy category:*** C	Hepatotoxicity, anaphylaxis, nausea, vomiting, abdominal pain, headache, dizziness, somnolence, fever, photophobia, diarrhea, gynecomastia, impotence, thrombocytopenia, leukopenia, neuropsychiatric disturbances
1% or 1.5% selenium sulfide shampoo (Selsun); shampoo daily	Has a cytostatic effect on cells of epidermis	***Contraindication:*** Hypersensitivity ***Cost:*** 1% OTC 2.5%, 4 oz: $3-$12 ***Pregnancy category:*** C	Do not use if acute inflammation or exudate present; skin irritation; discoloration, oiliness, or dryness of hair

Tinea Corporis

OVERVIEW

Tinea corporis is a fungal infection of the face, trunk, and extremities. It is commonly referred to as "ringworm." It is spread by direct contact with an infected human or animal.

Pathogenesis

Cause—fungus of genus *Trichophyton (T. tonsurans, T. rubrum,* or *T. verrucosum)* or *Microsporum (M. canis, M. audouinii,* or *M. gypseum)*

Patient Profile

- Male = Female
- Affects all ages

Signs and Symptoms

- Flat, scaly, circular spots
- Bright red
- Raised border develops
- Border spreads outward, and center becomes hypopigmented
- Border may have papules and vesicles
- Intense itching

Differential Diagnosis

- Pityriasis rosea
- Eczema
- Contact dermatitis
- Syphilis
- Psoriasis

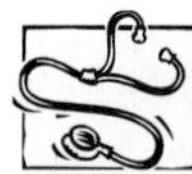

ASSESSMENT

History

Inquire about:

- Onset and duration of symptoms
- Contact with individuals or animals with similar lesions
- Treatments tried
- Underlying conditions
- Current medications

Physical Findings

- Red, scaly, circular macules with raised borders on trunk, face (excluding beard area), and extremities
- Border may have papules and vesicles

Initial Workup

Laboratory

- Skin scraping for potassium hydroxide (KOH) preparation (scrape edge of lesion with No. 15 scapel moistened with tap water; transfer to slide with small drop of water; add 1 to 2 drops KOH; cover with coverslip; warm for 15 to 30 seconds)—look for hyphae and/or spores
- Tinea corporis does not fluoresce with Wood's light
- If oral agents used—liver function studies

Radiology: None indicated

Further Workup

None indicated

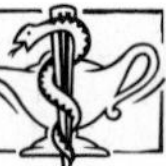

INTERVENTIONS

Office Treatment

None indicated.

Lifestyle Modifications

- Good personal hygiene
- If infection is from animal, need to get animal treated
- Need for laundering of towels, clothing

Patient Education

Teach patient about:

- Disease and how spread
- Proper hand washing
- Importance of laundering towels, clothing to prevent spread
- Need for treatment to continue for at least 1 week after resolution of lesions, with either topical or oral antifungal agents
- Medication used and side effects (see Pharmacotherapeutics)

Referrals

None, unless resistant to treatment; then to dermatologist

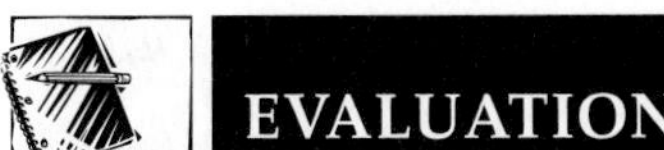

EVALUATION

Outcome
Lesions resolve without sequelae

Possible Complication
Bacterial superinfection

Follow-up
Every 2 weeks until resolution occurs

FOR YOUR INFORMATION

Life Span
Pediatric: Treatment is the same
Geriatric: Treatment is the same
Pregnancy: Oral antifungals contraindicated; best handled by a specialist

Miscellaneous
N/A

References

Bergus GR, Johnson JS: Superficial tinea infections, *Am Fam Physician* 48(2):259-268, 1996.

Habif TP: *Clinical dermatology: a color guide to diagnosis and therapy,* ed 3, St Louis, 1996, Mosby, pp 374-376.

PHARMACOTHERAPEUTICS

Drug of Choice	Mechanism of Action	Prescribing Information	Side Effects
Clotrimazole 1% (Lotrimin); adults and children, topical; apply to lesions bid until resolution of lesions and for 1 week after resolution	Broad-spectrum antifungal; fungistatic and fungicidal	***Contraindication:*** Hypersensitivity ***Cost:*** 15-g tube: $8-$9 ***Pregnancy category:*** B	Hypersensitivity, irritation, stinging, erythema, edema, burning
Ketoconazole 2% (Nizoral), topical; apply to lesions daily until resolution of lesions and for 1 week after resolution	Broad-spectrum antifungal	***Contraindication:*** Hypersensitivity ***Cost:*** 15-g tube: $13 ***Pregnancy category:*** C	Severe irritation, pruritus, stinging
Terbinafine 1% (Lamisil), topical; apply to lesion twice daily until lesions resolve and for 1 week after resolution—safety not established in children	Fungicidal; synthetic allylamine derivative	***Contraindication:*** Hypersensitivity ***Cost:*** 15-g tube: $26 ***Pregnancy category:*** B	Irritation, stinging, erythema, burning, itching

There are many other topical antifungal agents available. All agents have approximately equal efficacy. If the patient has extensive infestation, an oral agent should be used, such as one of the following:

Drug of Choice	Mechanism of Action	Prescribing Information	Side Effects
Griseofulvin (Fulvicin), 500 mg PO in 1 or 2 doses; treat for 4 weeks; children 30-50 lb, 125-250 mg PO qd; children >50 lb, 250-500 mg PO qd; increased absorption when taken with fatty meal; perform baseline liver function tests and repeat every 3 months if treatment lengthy	Fungistatic	***Contraindications:*** Hypersensitivity; patients with porphyria, hepatocellular failure; pregnancy or contemplated pregnancy ***Cost:*** 125-mg tab, 100 tabs: $28 ***Pregnancy category:*** Contraindicated	Porphyria, hepatocellular failure, leukopenia, persistent anemia, skin rash, urticaria, paresthesias of hands and feet, nausea, vomiting, diarrhea, headache, epigastric distress, dizziness
Ketoconazole (Nizoral), 3.3-6.6 mg/kg/day PO up to 200 mg/day for 4 weeks; children >2 years, 3.3-6.6 mg/kg/day PO; baseline liver function tests should be obtained; monitor every 3 months; for children potential benefit must outweigh risks	Antifungal agent	***Contraindications:*** Hypersensitivity; coadministration of terfenadine, astemizole, and cisapride ***Cost:*** 200-mg tab, 100 tabs: $271 ***Pregnancy category:*** C	Hepatotoxicity, anaphylaxis, nausea, vomiting, abdominal pain, headache, dizziness, somnolence, fever, photophobia, diarrhea, gynecomastia, impotence, thrombocytopenia, leukopenia, neuropsychiatric disturbances

Tinea Cruris

OVERVIEW

Tinea cruris is a fungal infection of the groin. It is commonly referred to as "ringworm" or "jock itch."

Pathogenesis

Cause—fungus of genus *Trichophyton, Microsporum,* or *Epidermophyton*

Patient Profile

- Males > Females
- Rare before puberty
- Common condition
- Risk factors—hot, humid climate; wearing wet clothing; wearing multiple layers of clothing; obesity; immunosuppression

Signs and Symptoms

- Pruritis
- Half-moon–shaped plaque in groin, with well-defined scaly border that advances out onto thigh
- May have vesicles around border
- May involve buttock and gluteal cleft
- Scrotum usually not involved

Differential Diagnosis

- Intertrigo
- Erythrasma
- Seborrheic dermatitis
- Psoriasis
- Candidiasis

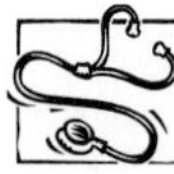

ASSESSMENT

History

Inquire about:

- Onset and duration of symptoms
- Treatments tried and results
- Underlying conditions
- Current medications

Physical Findings

- Half-moon–shaped plaque with well-defined scaly border in groin
- May involve buttocks and gluteal cleft
- Usually does not involve scrotum, as *Candida* does

Initial Workup

Laboratory

- Skin scraping for potassium hydroxide (KOH) preparation (scrape edge of lesion with No. 15 scapel moistened with tap water; transfer to slide with small drop of water; add 1 to 2 drops KOH; cover with coverslip; warm for 15 to 30 seconds)—spores and/or hyphae present
- Fungal culture

Radiology: None indicated

Further Workup

None indicated

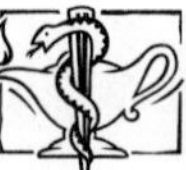

INTERVENTIONS

Office Treatment

None indicated

Lifestyle Modifications

- Avoidance of wet clothing
- Need to keep area as dry as possible
- Avoidance of constrictive clothing
- Weight loss

Patient Education

Teach patient about:

- Disease process
- Treatment—topical antifungals; may take 4 weeks
- Keeping area dry—use of absorbent powders may be beneficial
- Benefits of weight loss
- Not using steroid preparations
- Medications used and side effects (see Pharmacotherapeutics)

Referrals

None needed

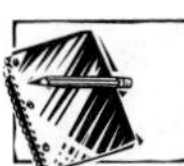

EVALUATION

Outcome
Resolves without sequelae

Possible Complication
Secondary bacterial infection

Follow-up
Every 2 weeks until resolution

FOR YOUR INFORMATION

Life Span
Pediatric: Rare before puberty
Geriatric: Treatment is the same
Pregnancy: Rare

Miscellaneous
Tinea incognito is a condition that arises as a result of a tinea infection being treated with steroid cream. The rash may be much more extensive, involving the scrotum, and red papules may be present at the borders and in the center of the lesion. A careful history is needed to make the appropriate diagnosis.

References
Bergus GR, Johnson JS: Superficial tinea infections, *Am Fam Physician* 48(2):259-268, 1996.
Habif TP: *Clinical dermatology: a color guide to diagnosis and therapy,* ed 3, St Louis, 1996, Mosby, pp 371-373.

NOTES

PHARMACOTHERAPEUTICS

Drug of Choice	Mechanism of Action	Prescribing Information	Side Effects
Clotrimazole 1% (Lotrimin); adults and children, topical; apply to lesions bid until resolution of lesions and for 1 week after resolution	Broad-spectrum antifungal; fungistatic and fungicidal	***Contraindication:*** Hypersensitivity ***Cost:*** 15-g tube: $8-$9 ***Pregnancy category:*** B	Hypersensitivity, irritation, stinging, erythema, edema, burning
Ketoconazole 2% (Nizoral), topical; apply to lesions daily until resolution of lesions and for 1 week after resolution	Broad-spectrum antifungal	***Contraindication:*** Hypersensitivity ***Cost:*** 15-g tube: $13 ***Pregnancy category:*** C	Severe irritation, pruritus, stinging
Terbinafine 1% (Lamisil), topical; apply to lesion twice daily until lesions resolve and for 1 week after resolution—safety not established in children	Fungicidal; synthetic allylamine derivative	***Contraindication:*** Hypersensitivity ***Cost:*** 15-g tube: $26 ***Pregnancy category:*** B	Irritation, stinging, erythema, burning, itching

Tinea Pedis

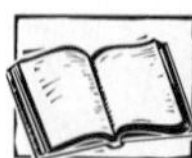

OVERVIEW

Tinea pedis is a fungal infection of the foot. It is commonly referred to as "ringworm" or "athlete's foot."

Pathogenesis

Cause—dermatophyte of genus *Trichophyton* or *Epidermophyton*

Patient Profile

- Males = Females
- All ages, but more common in teens and young adults
- Risk factors:
  - Hot, humid weather
  - Occlusive footwear (tennis shoes)
  - Immunosuppression
  - Prolonged application of steroids

Signs and Symptoms

- Pruritis
- Scaling
- Maceration
- Vesicles
- Usually located between toes, but may be on sole and arch

Differential Diagnosis

- Interdigital psoriasis
- Intertrigo
- Hyperkeratosis
- Contact dermatitis
- Eczema
- Dyshidrosis
- Pustular psoriasis

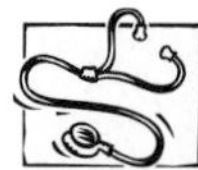

ASSESSMENT

History

Inquire about:

- Onset and duration of symptoms
- Pruritis
- Type of footwear worn
- Type of socks worn
- Treatments tried and results
- Underlying conditions
- Current medications

Physical Findings

Three forms of presentation:

- Interdigital presentation—areas of maceration, scaling, vesicles; may have classic pattern of circular erythema with scaly border
- Diffuse plantar scaling—dry skin and scaling of plantar surface
- Vesiculopapular presentation—vesicles and papules on instep of foot

Initial Workup

Laboratory

- Skin scraping for potassium hydroxide (KOH) preparation (scrape edge of lesion with No. 15 scapel moistened with tap water; transfer to slide with small drop of water; add 1 to 2 drops KOH; cover with coverslip; warm for 15 to 30 seconds)
- Fungal culture

Radiology: None indicated

Further Workup

None indicated

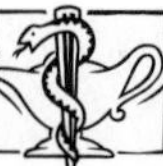

INTERVENTIONS

Office Treatment

None indicated

Lifestyle Modifications

- Avoidance of occlusive footwear
- Wearing cotton socks and changing them frequently
- Keeping feet dry; absorbent powder may help (Tinactin)

Patient Education

Teach patient about:

- Disease and cause
- Treatment—topical antifungals
- Keeping feet dry, cotton socks, foot powder
- Removing dead tissue after bathing
- Wearing rubber or wooden sandals in community showers to prevent infection
- Thoroughly drying between toes after bathing
- Medications used and side effects (see Pharmacotherapeutics)

Referrals

Usually none needed

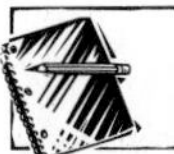

EVALUATION

Outcome
Resolves without sequelae

Possible Complications
- Secondary bacterial infection
- Eczematoid changes

Follow-up
In 2 weeks

FOR YOUR INFORMATION

Life Span
Pediatric: Most commonly seen in adolescents
Geriatric: Elderly people are more susceptible to infection because of peripheral vascular disease causing changes in tissues of feet—poor circulation makes tissue more prone to infection
Pregnancy: Treatment is the same

Miscellaneous
N/A

Reference
Habif TP: *Clinical dermatology: a color guide to diagnosis and therapy,* ed 3, St Louis, 1996, Mosby, pp 366-369.

NOTES

PHARMACOTHERAPEUTICS

Drug of Choice	Mechanism of Action	Prescribing Information	Side Effects
Clotrimazole 1% (Lotrimin); adults and children, topical; apply to lesions bid until resolution of lesions and for 1 week after resolution	Broad-spectrum antifungal; fungistatic and fungicidal	***Contraindication:*** Hypersensitivity ***Cost:*** 15-g tube: $8-$9 ***Pregnancy category:*** B	Hypersensitivity, irritation, stinging, erythema, edema, burning
Ketoconazole 2% (Nizoral), topical; apply to lesions daily until resolution of lesions and for 1 week after resolution	Broad-spectrum antifungal	***Contraindication:*** Hypersensitivity ***Cost:*** 15-g tube: $13 ***Pregnancy category:*** C	Severe irritation, pruritus, stinging
Terbinafine 1% (Lamisil), topical; apply to lesions twice daily until lesions resolve and for 1 week after resolution—safety not established in children	Fungicidal; synthetic allylamine derivative	***Contraindication:*** Hypersensitivity ***Cost:*** 15-g tube: $26 ***Pregnancy category:*** B	Irritation, stinging, erythema, burning, itching

OVERVIEW

Tinea versicolor is a fungal infection of the skin.

Pathogenesis

- Cause—lipophilic yeast—*Pityrosporum obiculare* and *Pityrosporum ovale;* some authors believe these are the same organism with different presentations (*P. obiculare* = round lesions; *P. ovale* = oval lesions)
- Most commonly occurs in summer

Patient Profile

- Males = Females
- Most common in teenagers and young adults
- Risk factors—high heat and humidity; excessive sweating

Signs and Symptoms

- Onset—small, round macules of various colors (white, pink, tan, or brown)
- Progression—lesions will increase in size; may also have papules and patches, mild scaling
- Upper trunk most common site; may spread to upper arms, neck, abdomen

Differential Diagnosis

- Vitiligo
- Pityriasis alba
- Seborrheic dermatitis
- Secondary syphilis
- Pityriasis rosea

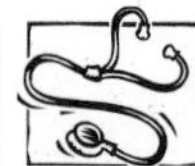

ASSESSMENT

History

Inquire about:

- Onset and duration of symptoms
- Treatment tried and results
- Prior history of similar lesions
- Underlying conditions
- Current medications

Physical Findings

Multiple small, round macules of various colors (white, pink, tan, or brown) with mild scaling

Initial Workup

Laboratory: Skin scraping for potassium hydroxide (KOH) preparation (scrape edge of lesion with No. 15 scalpel moistened with tap water; transfer to slide with small drop of water; add 1 to 2 drops KOH; cover with coverslip; warm for 15 to 30 seconds)—short, curved hyphae and clusters of round yeast cells "spaghetti-and-meatball" appearance

Radiology: None indicated

Further Workup

None indicated

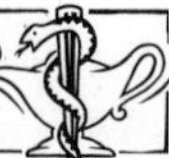

INTERVENTIONS

Office Treatment

None indicated

Lifestyle Modification

Avoidance of tanning—will accentuate condition

Patient Education

Teach patient about:

- Disease process and probability of recurrence
- Applying medication to affected areas with cotton ball
- Possibly needing to repeat treatment each year before tanning
- Medications used and side effects (see Pharmacotherapeutics)

Referrals

- Usually none
- To dermatologist if resistant to treatment

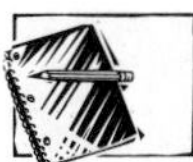

EVALUATION

Outcome
- Resolves without sequelae
- Recurrences common

Possible Complications
None expected

Follow-up
Return to clinic if condition does not resolve with treatment

FOR YOUR INFORMATION

Life Span
Pediatric: Usually occurs after adolescence
Geriatric: Rare
Pregnancy: Treatment is the same

Miscellaneous
Warn patients that whiteness in areas of lesions will remain for many months in Caucasians. In African-Americans there may be hyperpigmentation that may last for many months.

References
Habif TP: *Clinical dermatology: a color guide to diagnosis and therapy,* ed 3, St Louis, 1996, Mosby, pp 402-405.
Uphold CR, Graham MV: *Clinical guidelines in adult health,* Gainesville, Fla, 1994, Barmarrae Books, pp 162-163.

NOTES

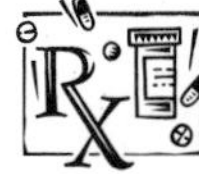

PHARMACOTHERAPEUTICS

Drug of Choice	Mechanism of Action	Prescribing Information	Side Effects
2.5% selenium sulfide shampoo; apply daily, allowing to dry for 20 minutes and shower off for 1 week or apply to lesions and leave on for 24 hours; shower off and repeat 1 time/week for 4 weeks	Has a cytostatic effect on cells of epidermis	***Contraindication:*** Hypersensitivity ***Cost:*** 4 oz: $3-$12 ***Pregnancy category:*** C	Do not use if acute inflammation or exudate present; skin irritation; discoloration, oiliness, or dryness of hair
Clotrimazole 1% (Lotrimin), topical; apply to lesions bid until resolution of lesions—2-4 weeks	Broad-spectrum antifungal; fungistatic and fungicidal	***Contraindication:*** Hypersensitivity ***Cost:*** 15-g tube: $8-$9 ***Pregnancy category:*** B	Hypersensitivity, irritation, stinging, erythema, edema, burning
Ketoconazole 2% (Nizoral), topical; apply to lesions daily until resolution of lesions—2-4 weeks	Broad-spectrum antifungal	***Contraindication:*** Hypersensitivity ***Cost:*** 15-g tube: $13 ***Pregnancy category:*** C	Severe irritation, pruritus, stinging

Transient Ischemic Attacks (TIAs)

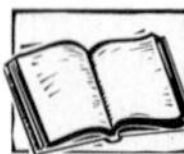

OVERVIEW

A transient ischemic attack (TIA) occurs when there is an episode of acute cerebral insufficiency, causing neurologic disturbance. The attack lasts less than 24 hours, and there is complete recovery of function.

Pathogenesis

Causes—most common:

- Ischemia or microemboli breaking off from atherosclerotic plaque
- Cardiac embolism
- Myocardial infarction
- Cardiac arrhythmia
- Atrial fibrillation

Patient Profile

- Males > Females
- Risk increases in patients > 45 years of age
- Most common age—70s and 80s.

Signs and Symptoms

- Depends on type of event
- Occlusion—anterior circulation (carotid artery syndrome)—hemiparesis, aphasia, neglect of one side of body, blindness in one eye, cognitive and behavioral abnormalities
- Occlusion—posterior circulation (vertebrobasilar)—diplopia, vertigo, ataxia, facial paresis, motor and sensory deficits on both sides of body, dysphagia, nystagmus, extraocular movement (EOM) dysfunction
- Repeat attacks usually have same symptoms

Differential Diagnosis

- Reversible ischemic neurologic deficit (lasts >24 hours, but resolves within 3 weeks)
- Completed cerebrovascular accident (CVA)
- Migraine
- Focal seizure
- Hypoglycemia
- Tumors
- Dissecting aortic aneurysm
- Multiple sclerosis
- Bell's Palsy

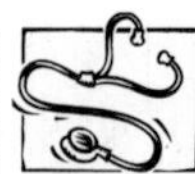

ASSESSMENT

History

Inquire about:

- Onset and duration of symptoms
- Frequency of attacks
- Smoking history
- Family history
- Past medical history—hypertension, diabetes, cardiac disease
- Other underlying conditions
- Current medications

Physical Findings

- Depends on type—if between TIAs, physical examination will be within normal limits
- Fundoscopic—ocular plaques, hemorrhages (hypertension)
- Elevated blood pressure
- Carotid arteries—bruits
- Cardiac arrhythmias
- Various neurologic deficits may be present

Initial Workup

Laboratory

- CBC
- Chemistry panel—glucose, electrolytes, liver function tests, creatinine, BUN, lipid studies
- Rapid plasma reagin (RPR)

Radiology: CT scan or MRI of head

Further Workup

- ECG
- Holter Monitor
- Carotid Doppler studies
- Cerebral angiography (high risk of morbidity and mortality), as indicated

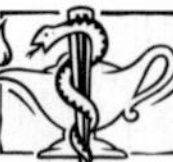

INTERVENTIONS

Office Treatment

If patient presents during acute attack, consider transfer to emergency room

Lifestyle Modifications

- Smoking cessation
- Control of hypertension
- Low-fat, low-salt diet
- Weight loss

Patient Education

Teach patient about:

- Disease process (one third of patients with TIAs have completed CVA within 5 years) and treatment options—antiplatelet therapy, antiarrhythmic medications, antihypertensive therapy, carotid endarterectomy if candidate
- Tips for smoking cessation
- Low-fat, low-salt diet
- Weight reduction
- Medications used and side effects (see Pharmacotherapeutics)

Referral

To neurologist, neurosurgeon, or vascular surgeon if indicated

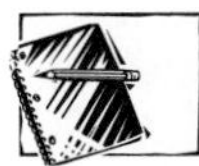

EVALUATION

Outcome
Prevention of further TIAs

Possible Complications
- Completed CVA
- Trauma from falls
- Death from cardiac source

Follow-up
In 2 weeks × 2; then, if stable, every 3 months

FOR YOUR INFORMATION

Life Span
Pediatric: Rare—usually cardiac source
Geriatric: Atrial fibrillation frequent cause
Pregnancy: Increased vascular volume and hypercoagulability during pregnancy

Miscellaneous
In adults <45 years of age, a full cardiac workup should be done. Cardiac events are the most common cause.

References
Mumma CM: Nursing role in management: stroke patient. In Lewis SM, Collier IC, Heitkemper MM, editors: *Medical-surgical nursing: assessment and management of clinical problems,* ed 4, St Louis, 1996, Mosby, pp 1725-1727.

Woolliscroft JO: *Current diagnosis and treatment: a quick reference for the general practitioner,* Philadelphia, 1996, Current Medicine, pp 398-399.

NOTES

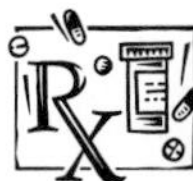

PHARMACOTHERAPEUTICS

Treatment is based on the cause of the TIA. The following two medications are the mainstay of treatment. Use one of these.

Drug of Choice	Mechanism of Action	Prescribing Information	Side Effects
Aspirin, enteric-coated, 650 mg, 1 PO bid	Decreases platelet aggregation	***Contraindications:*** Hypersensitivity to salicylates, tartrazine; GI bleeding; bleeding disorders; children <12 years; pregnancy; lactation; vitamin K deficiency; peptic ulcer ***Cost:*** OTC ***Pregnancy category:*** D	Thrombocytopenia, agranulocytosis, leukopenia, hemolytic anemia, convulsion, confusion, dizziness, nausea, vomiting, GI bleeding, hepatitis, anorexia, rash, tinnitus, rapid pulse, pulmonary edema, wheezing, hypoglycemia, hyponatremia, hypokalemia
Ticlopidine (Ticlid), 250 mg PO bid—not recommended for children <18 years	Inhibits platelet aggregation	***Contraindications:*** Hypersensitivity; active liver disease; blood dyscrasias ***Cost:*** 250-mg tab, 30 tabs: $41 ***Pregnancy category:*** B	Rash, pruritus, nausea, vomiting, diarrhea, cholestatic jaundice, hepatitis, bleeding, agranulocytosis, neutropenia, thrombocytopenia

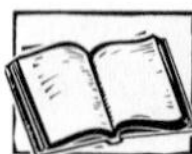

OVERVIEW

Trichinosis is a parasitic disease that infects humans who have consumed meat that contains the encysted larvae stage of the parasite. The larvae may be found in improperly cooked pork, bear, walrus, horse, or other game.

Pathogenesis

- Cause—*Trichinella spiralis*
- Occurs in 3 phases:
  - Phase 1, intestinal phase—encysted larvae, liberated by gastric juices, mature and mate; female burrows into intestinal mucosa—discharges larvae
  - Phase 2, larval migration—larvae travel to different sites via lymphatic and blood systems; muscle invasion occurs
  - Phase 3, muscle encystment—larvae that reach striated muscle encyst
- Infection ranges from asymptomatic to severe multisystem disease
- Incubation period—12 hours to 28 days

Patient Profile

- Males = Females
- Any age

Signs and Symptoms

- Phase 1:
  - Diarrhea
  - Abdominal cramps
  - Malaise
  - Nausea and vomiting
  - Chills
  - Fever
- Phase 2:
  - Periorbital edema
  - Muscle soreness
  - Joint pain
  - Edema
  - Muscle spasm
  - Sweating
  - Photophobia
  - Conjunctivitis
  - Rash
  - May develop meningitis
  - Encephalitis
  - Myocarditis
  - Nephritis
  - Bronchopneumonia
- Phase 3:
  - Malaise
  - Hoarseness
  - Dyspnea
  - Prostration

Differential Diagnosis

- Encephalitis
- Rheumatic fever
- Gastroenteritis
- Meningitis
- Pneumonia
- Polyarteritis nodosa
- Typhoid fever
- Tuberculosis

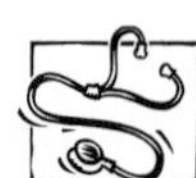

ASSESSMENT

History

Inquire about:

- Onset and duration of symptoms
- Eating improperly cooked pork or game
- Whether anyone else has similar symptoms
- Underlying conditions
- Current medications

Physical Findings

Depends on phase of disease:

- Phase 1:
  - Abdominal pain on palpation
  - Fever
- Phase 2:
  - Joint and muscle pain on palpation
  - Periorbital edema
  - Injected conjunctivae
  - Lungs—adventitious sounds, shortness of breath
  - Nuchal rigidity
  - Mental status—confusion
  - Heart—extra heart sound, murmurs
  - Generalized edema
- Phase 3:
  - Hoarseness
  - Shortness of breath

Initial Workup

Laboratory

- CBC with differential—leukocytosis, eosinophilia (up to 90%)
- Creatine kinase and lactate dehydrogenase—elevated
- Serologic tests—bentonite flocculation—positive titer >1:5
- Immunofluorescence—positive titer >16
- Albumin/globulin ratio—reversed with marked hyperglobinemia
- Stool—adult worms (rarely found)

Radiology: Chest—patchy infiltrates

Further Workup

Muscle biopsy

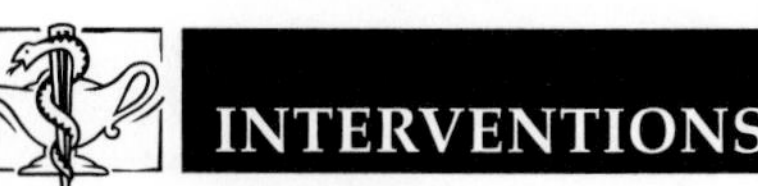

INTERVENTIONS

Office Treatment

None indicated

Lifestyle Modification

Proper cooking, storage, and disposal of suspect foods

Patient Education

Teach patient about

- Condition and treatment:
  - Antihelminthic agents
  - If severe, may require hospitalization
  - Bed rest may relieve muscle pain
- Proper cooking, storage, and disposal of pork and game
- Medications used and side effects (see Pharmacotherapeutics)

Referral

Consult with MD regarding treatment for phase 3

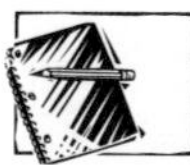

EVALUATION

Outcome
Prognosis good in most cases—resolves without sequelae

Possible Complications
- Meningitis
- Encephalitis
- Myocarditis
- Nephritis
- Sinusitis
- Glomerulonephritis
- Cardiac failure

Follow-up
In 48 hours; then weekly × 2

FOR YOUR INFORMATION

Life Span
Pediatric: Children have less severe infections
Geriatric: Higher morbidity and mortality
Pregnancy: Refer to specialist

Miscellaneous
Trichinosis is a relatively rare disease in the United States, but periodic outbreaks occur.

Reference
Goldsmith RS: Infectious diseases: helminthic. In Tierney LM Jr, McPhee SJ, Papadakis MA, editors: *Current medical diagnosis and treatment*, ed 34, Norwalk, Conn, 1995, Appleton & Lange, pp 1271-1273.

NOTES

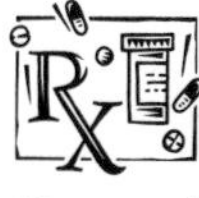

PHARMACOTHERAPEUTICS

Drug of Choice	Mechanism of Action	Prescribing Information	Side Effects
Mebendazole (Vermox); adults and children, 200-400 mg PO tid × 3 days; then 400-500 mg PO tid × 10 days	Anthelmintic	***Contraindication:*** Hypersensitivity ***Cost:*** 100-mg tab, 12 tabs: $52 ***Pregnancy category:*** C	Dizziness, fever, abdominal pain, transient diarrhea
Thiabendazole (Mintezol); 30 lb, 250 mg PO bid; 50 lb, 500 mg PO bid; 75 lb, 750 mg PO bid; 100 lb, 1000 mg PO bid; 125 lb, 1250 mg PO bid; 150 lb and over, 1500 mg PO bid × 5-7 days	Anthelmintic	***Contraindication:*** Hypersensitivity ***Cost:*** 500-mg tab, 36 tabs: $36 ***Pregnancy category:*** C	Anaphylaxis, hematuria, nephrotoxicity, erythema, Stevens-Johnson syndrome, dizziness, headache, drowsiness, convulsions, tinnitus, blurred vision, nausea, vomiting, anorexia, diarrhea, jaundice, liver damage, hypotension
For severe symptoms, add to one of the above medications:			
Prednisone, 60-120 mg PO qd, then taper over several days	Corticosteroid; decreases inflammation	***Contraindications:*** Hypersensitivity; psychosis; idiopathic thrombocytopenia; acute glomerulonephritis; amebiasis; nonasthmatic bronchial disease; AIDS; TB; children <2 years old ***Cost:*** 15-mg tab, 100 tabs: $14-$35 ***Pregnancy category:*** C	Hypertension, circulatory collapse, thrombophlebitis, embolism, tachycardia, fungal infections, increased intraocular pressure, diarrhea, nausea, GI hemorrhage, thrombocytopenia, acne, poor wound healing, fractures, osteoporosis, weakness

Trichomoniasis

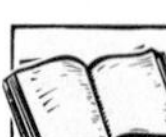

OVERVIEW

Trichomoniasis is a common sexually transmitted disease (STD).

Pathogenesis

Cause—*Trichomonas vaginalis,* a flagellated protozoa

Patient Profile

- Males = Females
- Any age after onset of sexual activity

Signs and Symptoms

- Males:
  - Asymptomatic carriers
  - Urethral discharge
  - Dysuria
  - Rarely epididymitis
- Females:
  - May be asymptomatic
  - Vaginal discharge (foul, fishy smelling, yellow-green, frothy)
  - Dysuria
  - Vulvovaginal irritation

Differential Diagnosis

- Males—chlamydial urethritis
- Females:
  - Bacterial vaginosis
  - Candidiasis
  - Chlamydial infections
  - Gonorrhea

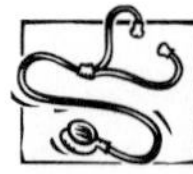

ASSESSMENT

History

Inquire about:

- Onset and duration of symptoms
- Dysuria
- Sexual history and behaviors
- Recent change in partner
- Previous history of STDs
- Underlying conditions
- Current medications

Physical Findings

- Males—physical examination within normal limits
- Females:
  - Yellow-green, frothy discharge
  - Speculum examination: vagina—erythema, edema; cervix—red with punctate lesions (strawberry cervix)
  - Foul, fishy odor

Initial Workup

Laboratory

- Males—collect 20 ml of first morning urine specimen and examine under microscope for trichomonads
- Females:
  - Wet mount—trichomonads present—flagellated, motile organisms; increased number of polymorphonuclear leukocytes
  - Vaginal secretions—pH >4.5
  - Trichomonads may be identified on Pap smears
- ELISA and direct antibody tests can be done (usually not necessary)
- Consider rapid plasma reagin (RPR)
- Cultures for gonorrhea and chlamydial infection
- HIV screen

Radiology: None indicated

Further Workup

None indicated

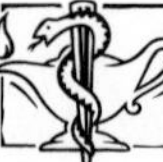

INTERVENTIONS

Office Treatment

None indicated

Lifestyle Modification

Safe sex practices

Patient Education

Teach patient about:

- Condition and treatment—trichomonacide
- Importance of partner receiving treatment
- Safe sex practices, use of condoms
- No sexual intercourse until treatment completed and partner treated
- Medications used and side effects (see Pharmacotherapeutics)

Referrals

None needed

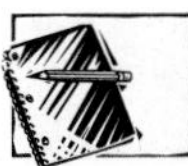

EVALUATION

Outcome
Usually resolves without sequelae

Possible Complication
Recurrent infection

Follow-up
None needed if symptoms resolve

FOR YOUR INFORMATION

Life Span
Pediatric: Should suspect child abuse if found in prepubertal child
Geriatric: Treatment is the same
Pregnancy: Do not use metronidazole in first trimester.

Miscellaneous
N/A

References
Bartlett JG: *Pocket book of infectious disease therapy,* ed 7, Baltimore, 1996, Williams & Wilkins, p 315.

Bennett EC: Vaginitis and sexually transmitted diseases. In Youngkin EQ, Davis MS, editors: *Women's health: a primary care clinical guide,* Norwalk, Conn, 1994, Appleton & Lange, pp 237-238.

NOTES

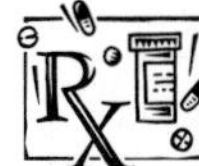

PHARMACOTHERAPEUTICS

Drug of Choice	Mechanism of Action	Prescribing Information	Side Effects
Metronidazole (Flagyl), 2 g PO × 1 dose or 500 mg PO bid × 7 days; if treatment fails on single-dose therapy, treat with 500 mg PO bid × 7 days; advise patient to avoid alcohol while taking metronidazole; partner should be treated the same way; children, 40 mg/kg PO × 1 dose or 15 mg/kg/day PO divided q8h × 7 days	Direct-acting amebicide/trichomonacide	***Contraindications:*** Hypersensitivity; 1st-trimester pregnancy; CNS disorders ***Cost:*** 500-mg tab, 14 tabs: $3 ***Pregnancy category:*** B (2nd and 3rd trimesters)	Flat T-waves, headache, confusion, irritability, depression, fatigue, insomnia, convulsions, blurred vision, sore throat, retinal edema, nausea, vomiting, diarrhea, anorexia, abdominal cramps, pseudomembranous colitis, dark urine, albuminuria, dysuria, neurotoxicity, leukopenia, bone marrow depression, aplasia, rash, pruritus, flushing

Trigeminal Neuralgia

OVERVIEW

Trigeminal neuralgia is a neurologic condition of the fifth cranial nerve (trigeminal nerve). It may affect all three branches of the nerve or only one.

Pathogenesis

- Cause—either degeneration of nerve or compression on nerve
- No specific cause identified

Patient Profile

- Males > Females (slightly)
- Age over 40 years

Signs and Symptoms

- Unilateral
- Symptoms vary with branch affected:
  - First branch—severe, excruciating pain around eyes, over forehead
  - Second branch—severe, excruciating pain in upper lip, nose, cheek
  - Third branch—severe, excruciating pain on side of tongue, in lower lip; wincing, flushing, tearing, salivation, pain elicited by tickle or touch
- Pain bursts for several seconds, then remits

Differential Diagnosis

- Migraine
- Chronic meningitis
- Acute polyneuropathy
- Neoplasm

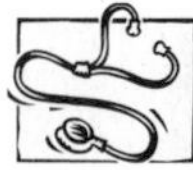

ASSESSMENT

History

Inquire about:

- Onset and duration of symptoms
- What elicits pain
- Underlying conditions
- Current medications

Physical Findings

- Grimacing
- Flushing
- Tearing
- Increased BP due to pain

Initial Workup

Laboratory: None indicated
Radiology: CT scan or MRI of head to rule out neoplasm

Further Workup

None indicated

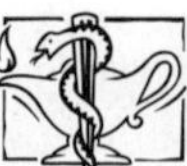

INTERVENTIONS

Office Treatment

None indicated

Lifestyle Modification

Avoidance of precipitating factors such as air, heat, or cold

Patient Education

Teach patient about:

- Condition and possible cause
- Treatment options—medications (anticonvulsants); if no response, invasive treatment
- Medications used and side effects (see Pharmacotherapeutics)

Referral

To neurosurgeon if medication fails

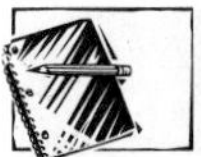

EVALUATION

Outcomes
- Controlled with medications
- Exacerbations usually occur in fall and spring

Possible Complications
Side effects of medication

Follow-up
Every 2 weeks × 3 for liver function tests and CBC; then every 3 months

FOR YOUR INFORMATION

Life Span
Pediatric: Rare
Geriatric: Most commonly seen in this age group
Pregnancy: Uncommon

Miscellaneous
N/A

References
Johnson CJ: Headaches and facial pain. In Barker LR, Burton JR, Zieve PD, editors: *Principles of ambulatory medicine,* ed 4, Baltimore, 1995, Williams & Wilkins, p 1176.

Woolliscroft JO: *Current diagnosis and treatment: a quick reference for the general practitioner,* Philadelphia, 1996, Current Medicine, pp 278-279.

NOTES

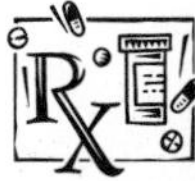

PHARMACOTHERAPEUTICS

Drug of Choice	Mechanism of Action	Prescribing Information	Side Effects
Carbamazepine (Tegretol); adults and children >12 years; 1000 mg PO bid, increase in 3 days to tid; maximum dose 1200 mg/day	Inhibits nerve impulses by limiting influx of sodium ions across cell membranes in motor cortex	***Contraindications:*** Hypersensitivity to carbamazepine or tricyclic antidepressant; bone marrow depression; concomitant use of MAOIs ***Cost:*** 200-mg tab, 100 tabs: \$10-\$35 ***Pregnancy category:*** C	Thrombocytopenia, agranulocytosis, leukocytosis, neutropenia, aplastic anemia, eosinophilia, drowsiness, dizziness, confusion, paralysis, headache, hallucinations, nausea, constipation, diarrhea, anorexia, vomiting, abdominal pain, hepatitis, Stevens-Johnson syndrome, tinnitus, dry mouth, hypertension, congestive heart failure (CHF), pulmonary hypertension, albuminuria, glycosuria, impotence

Tuberculosis (TB)

OVERVIEW

Tuberculosis (TB) is primarily a lung infection caused by inhalation of the tubercle bacilli. Other areas of the body may also be involved. The incubation period is 2 to 10 weeks.

Pathogenesis

- Cause—mycobacterium tuberculosis
- Bacilli inhaled—multiply and cause lung inflammation
- Macrophages engulf bacilli and form a granulomatous lesion (tubercle)
- Infected tissue in tubercle dies, causing caseation necrosis
- Scar tissue grows around tubercle, isolating bacilli
- May remain dormant or become active if immune system impaired

Patient Profile

- Males > Females
- Any age

Signs and Symptoms

- Fever
- Night sweats
- Cough
- Hemoptysis
- Weight loss
- Malaise and fatigue
- Pleuritic pain
- Adenopathy

Differential Diagnosis

- Pneumonia from any cause
- Lymphoma
- Fungal infection
- Malignancy
- Silicosis

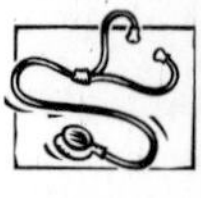

ASSESSMENT

History

Inquire about:

- Onset and duration of symptoms
- History of exposure to TB
- Previous TB skin test or chest film results
- Travel to countries where TB is endemic
- Presence of risk factors, such as alcoholism, steroid use, HIV infection
- Residence—institutionalized, homeless, correctional facilities—increased incidence
- Underlying conditions
- Current medications

Physical Findings

- Pallor
- Lymphadenopathy
- Lungs—rales in upper posterior chest, whispered pectoriloquy, bronchovesicular breath sounds

Initial Workup

Laboratory

- CBC with differential—anemia, monocytosis, thrombocytosis
- Sputum culture and acid-fast smear—should be done 3 times; culture takes 3 to 6 weeks
- Liver enzymes, bilirubin, BUN, and creatinine should be checked before instituting therapy and every 3 months during therapy
- Purified Protein Derivative (PPD) skin test or Mantoux test—should be read in 48 to 72 hours; interpretation (REMEMBER: Absence of a reaction does not exclude diagnosis):

Induration	Positive if meets criteria
≥5 mm	Close contact with person with active TB; HIV-positive or risk factors for HIV; fibrotic chest film consistent with healed TB
≥10 mm	IV drug users; persons with other medical conditions that increase risk of progressing from latent to active TB, such as diabetes, diseases requiring high-dose steroids or immunosuppressive therapy, chronic renal failure, malignancies, weight loss ≥10% of ideal body weight, silicosis, gastrectomy; residents and employees of prisons, nursing homes, health care facilities, homeless shelters; foreign-born persons from countries with high prevalence and residing in United States 5 years or less; medically underserved, low-income populations; high-risk minority populations; children <4 years or infants, children, and adolescents exposed to adults in high-risk categories
≥15 mm	All other persons

Radiology: Chest—PA and lateral—infiltrate with or without effusion, cavitary lesions, hilar adenopathy

Further Workup

Fluorescent staining and DNA probes for rapid diagnosis

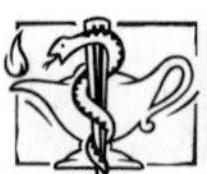

INTERVENTIONS

Office Treatment

Direct observation therapy—if compliance is a concern, patient comes to clinic 2 to 3 times per week and medication is administered

Lifestyle Modifications

- Smoking cessation
- Cover mouth and nose when coughing
- Proper disposal of tissues
- Proper hand-washing technique

Patient Education

Teach patient about:

- Condition, treatment, and mode of transmission:
  - If PPD positive with no evidence of disease—isoniazid treatment for 6 to 12 months
  - Active disease—combination drug therapy
- Importance of taking medication as directed and for proper length of time
- Importance of keeping follow-up appointments
- Proper hand-washing technique
- Proper disposal of soiled tissue
- Covering mouth and nose when coughing
- Importance of notifying all contacts
- Direct observation therapy—will need to come to clinic 2 to 3 times weekly for duration of therapy
- Telling future health care providers of positive PPD test
- Medications used and side effects (see Pharmacotherapeutics)

Referral

To TB specialist if treatment fails after 3 months

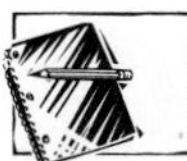

EVALUATION

Outcome

Complete resolution if treatment plan followed

Possible Complications

- Secondary bacterial infection of cavitary lesions
- Spread of disease
- Drug resistance

Follow-up

- Direct observation therapy—2 to 3 times weekly
- Others—initially every 2 weeks × 2; then monthly × 2
- After 3 months repeat chest film, acid-fast smear, and culture
- Then every month if stable

FOR YOUR INFORMATION

Life Span

Pediatric: Primary infection more common in infants and adolescents
Geriatric: PPD before entering a nursing home; may have more side effects from isoniazid
Pregnancy: To specialist

Miscellaneous

There has been an increased incidence of TB infections since 1986. Once the diagnosis is confirmed, it must be reported to the local health department. BCG vaccination is *not* recommended for adults in the United States.

References

Murphy PA: Tuberculosis in the ambulatory patient. In Barker LR, Burton JR, Zieve PD, editors: *Principles of ambulatory medicine,* ed 4, Baltimore, 1995, Williams & Wilkins, pp 348-357.

US Department of Health and Human Services, Public Health Service: *Clinician's handbook of preventive services: put prevention into practice,* Washington DC, 1994, US Government Printing Office, pp 227-232.

Walsh K: Guidelines for the prevention and control of tuberculosis in the elderly, *Nurse Pract* 19(11):79-85, 1994.

NOTES

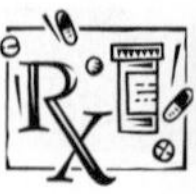

PHARMACOTHERAPEUTICS

Drug of Choice	Mechanism of Action	Prescribing Information	Side Effects
Isoniazid (INH): • For prophylaxis—adults, 300 mg PO qd × 9-12 months; children, 10 mg/kg/day PO × 9 months; maximum dose 300 mg/day • For active disease—adults, 300 mg PO qd; children, 10-20 mg/kg PO qd; or adults, 15 mg/kg PO 2 times weekly; children, 20-40 mg/kg PO 2-3 times weekly; maximum dose 900 mg	Antitubercular; bactericidal	***Contraindications:*** Hypersensitivity; optic neuritis ***Cost:*** 300-mg tab, 100 tabs: $2-$14 ***Pregnancy category:*** C	Fever, rash, peripheral neuropathy, toxic encephalopathy, convulsions, blurred vision, agranulocytosis, hemolytic anemia, aplastic anemia, thrombocytopenia, eosinophilia, dyspnea, vitamin B_6 deficiency, hyperglycemia, metabolic acidosis, gynecomastia, nausea, vomiting, jaundice, fatal hepatitis
Rifampin (Rifadin); adults, 600 mg PO qd; children, 10-20 mg/kg PO qd, maximum dose 600 mg PO qd; or 10 mg/kg PO 2-3 times weekly, maximum dose 600 mg	Antitubercular; decreases replication of bacilli	***Contraindication:*** Hypersensitivity ***Cost:*** 300-mg tab, 60 tabs: $89-$126 ***Pregnancy category:*** C	Rash, pruritus, visual disturbances, flulike syndrome, nausea, vomiting, anorexia, diarrhea, pseudomembranous colitis, heartburn, pancreatitis, hematuria, acute renal failure, hemoglobinuria, headache, fatigue, hemolytic anemia, eosinophilia, thrombocytopenia, leukopenia; urine, stool, saliva, sputum, sweat, and tears may be red-orange color
Pyrazinamide; adults and children, 15-30 mg/kg PO in divided doses, maximum dose 2 g; or 50-70 mg/kg PO 2-3 times weekly, maximum dose 4 g 2 times/week, 3 g 3 times/week	Antitubercular; bactericidal	***Contraindication:*** Hypersensitivity ***Cost:*** 500-mg tab, 100 tabs: $87-$116 ***Pregnancy category:*** C	Photosensitivity, headache, hepatotoxicity, peptic ulcer, urinary difficulty, hemolytic anemia
Streptomycin, 15 mg/kg IM daily, maximum dose 1 g; or 25-30 mg/kg IM, 2-3 times weekly, maximum dose 1.5 g 2 times/week, 1 g 3 times/week	Antiinfective/antitubercular; interferes with protein synthesis, causing cell death	***Contraindications:*** Hypersensitivity; severe renal disease ***Cost:*** 1 g/vial, 1 vial: $4 ***Pregnancy category:*** B	Oliguria; hematuria; renal damage; azotemia; renal failure; nephrotoxicity; confusion; depression; convulsions; neurotoxicity; ototoxicity; deafness; agranulocytosis; thrombocytopenia; leukopenia; eosinophilia; anemia; nausea, vomiting; anorexia; increased AST, ALT, and bilirubin; hepatic necrosis; hypotension; rash; dermatitis; alopecia

Drug of Choice	Mechanism of Action	Prescribing Information	Side Effects
Ethambutol (Myambutol); adults and children >13 years, 15-25 mg/kg PO qd; or 50 mg/kg PO 2 times/week or 25-30 mg/kg PO 3 times/week, maximum dose 2.5 g	Antitubercular; inhibits RNA synthesis, decreasing bacilli replication	***Contraindications:*** Hypersensitivity; optic neuritis; children <13 years ***Cost:*** 100-mg tab, 100 tabs: $48 ***Pregnancy category:*** D	Abdominal distress, anorexia, nausea, vomiting, dermatitis, headache, confusion, fever, malaise, dizziness, blurred vision, optic neuritis, photophobia, acute gout, thrombocytopenia, joint pain

Four treatment options are available. Options 1 to 3 are for TB without HIV infection; option 4 is for TB with HIV infection.

Option 1

Use daily administration of isoniazid, rifampin, and pyrazinamide for 8 weeks, followed by daily or 2-times-per-week administration of isoniazid and rifampin for 16 weeks in areas where the isoniazid resistance rate is not <4%. Ethambutol or streptomycin should be included in the initial regimen until susceptibility testing is back. Treat for 6 months—3 months beyond the culture conversion. Consult an expert if the patient is symptomatic or the smear or culture is positive after 3 months.

Option 2

Use daily administration of isoniazid, rifampin, pyrazinamide, and ethambutol or streptomycin for 2 weeks, followed by 2-times-per-week administration of the same drugs by direct-observation therapy for 6 weeks, followed by 2-times-per-week administration of isoniazid and rifampin by direct-observation therapy for 16 weeks. Consult an expert if the patient is symptomatic or the smear or culture is positive after 3 months.

Option 3

Use 3-times-per-week administration of isoniazid, rifampin, pyrazinamide, and ethambutol or streptomycin by direct-observation therapy for 6 months. Consult an expert if the patient is symptomatic or the smear or culture is positive after 3 months.

Option 4

With HIV infection, use options 1, 2, or 3, but continue treatment for 9 months—at least 6 months after the culture conversion.

Typhoid Fever

OVERVIEW

Typhoid fever is an acute systemic bacterial infection. It is a type of enteric fever caused by the genus *Salmonella.*

Pathogenesis
- Cause—*Salmonella typhi*
- Most commonly transmitted through ingestion of contaminated food, milk, or water
- Incubation period—5 to 14 days

Patient Profile
- Males = Females
- Any age
- Endemic in underdeveloped countries

Signs and Symptoms
- Insidious onset
- Headache
- Malaise
- Cough
- Sore throat
- Abdominal pain
- Constipation
- Fever that increases over 7 to 10 days
- Abdominal distention
- Severe constipation
- Confusion
- Lethargy
- Splenomegaly
- Hepatomegaly
- Cervical adenopathy

Differential Diagnosis
- Enteric fever from other cause
- Hepatitis
- Q fever
- Infectious mononucleosis
- Subacute bacterial endocarditis
- Tuberculosis
- Brucellosis

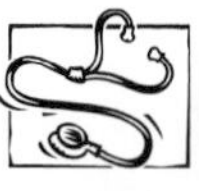

ASSESSMENT

History
Inquire about:
- Onset and duration of symptoms
- Travel to third-world country
- Ingestion of known contaminated food, milk, or water
- Underlying conditions
- Current medications

Physical Findings
- General appearance—exhausted and prostrated
- Abdomen—distended; hypoactive bowel sounds; pain on palpation; splenomegaly; hepatomegaly
- Lungs—clear
- Heart—bradycardia

Initial Workup
Laboratory
- Blood cultures—*S. typhi* isolated
- Liver enzymes—may be elevated
- CBC with differential—anemia, leukopenia, thrombocytopenia

Radiology: Abdominal films—check for intestinal perforation

Further Workup
None needed

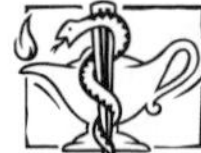

INTERVENTIONS

Office Treatment
None indicated

Lifestyle Modifications
- Bed rest, possible hospitalization
- Avoidance of contaminated food, milk, or water

Patient Education
Teach patient about:
- Disease—how contracted and treatment
    - Antimicrobials
    - Increased fluid intake
    - Bed rest initially or hospitalization
- Possibility of relapse—seeding can occur in biliary tract
- Possible cholecystectomy—for chronic carriers, relapse, intolerance to antimicrobials
- Avoidance of contaminated food, water, milk
- Vaccine for frequent travelers
- Proper hand-washing technique
- Medications used and side effects (see Pharmacotherapeutics)

Referral
Possibly to infectious disease specialist

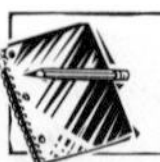

EVALUATION

Outcome
Resolves without sequelae

Possible Complications
- Intestinal hemorrhage and perforation
- Becomes chronic carrier
- Osteomyelitis
- Meningitis
- Endocarditis

Follow-up
Weekly if treating as outpatient—serial abdominal x-ray films to monitor for perforation

FOR YOUR INFORMATION

Life Span
Pediatric: Onset may be abrupt
Geriatric: Higher rate of morbidity and mortality
Pregnancy: Consult with specialist

Miscellaneous
N/A

References

Bartlett JG: *Pocket book of infectious disease therapy,* Baltimore, 1996, Williams & Wilkins, pp 37 and 289.

Chambers HF: Infectious diseases: bacterial and chlamydial. In Tierney LM Jr, McPhee SJ, Papadakis MA, editors: *Current medical diagnosis and treatment,* ed 34, Norwalk, Conn, 1995, Appleton & Lange, pp 1178-1179.

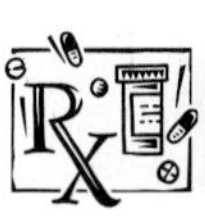

PHARMACOTHERAPEUTICS

Drug of Choice	Mechanism of Action	Prescribing Information	Side Effects
For active disease, use one of the following:			
Chloramphenicol (Chloromycetin); adults and children, 50 mg/kg/day PO in 4 divided doses × 10-14 days	Interference or inhibition of protein synthesis	***Contraindications:*** Hypersensitivity; severe renal or hepatic disease; minor infections ***Cost:*** 250-mg tab, 100 tabs: \$25-\$125 ***Pregnancy category:*** C	Anemia, thrombocytopenia, aplastic anemia, granulocytopenia, optic neuritis, nausea, vomiting, diarrhea, abdominal pain, glossitis, colitis, itching, rash, gray syndrome in newborns, headache, depression, confusion
Sulfamethazole (SMZ)/trimethoprim (TMP), 1-2 DS tabs PO bid × 10-14 days; children, 8 mg/kg TMP and 40 mg/kg SMZ per day PO in 2 divided doses q12h	Blocks 2 consecutive steps in bacterial synthesis of nucleic acids and protein	***Contraindications:*** Hypersensitivity to TMP or SMZ; term pregnancy; lactation; megaloblastic anemia; infants <2 months; creatinine clearance <15 ml/min ***Cost:*** DS tab × 14 days: \$2 ***Pregnancy category:*** C	Anaphylaxis, hypersensitivity, Stevens-Johnson syndrome, allergic myocarditis, nausea, vomiting, abdominal pain, hepatitis, enterocolitis, renal failure, toxic nephrosis, leukopenia, thrombocytopenia, hemolytic anemia
Ciprofloxacin (Cipro), 500 mg PO bid × 10-14 days; may be used for carrier state—500-750 mg PO bid × 6 weeks—not dosed for children	Fluoroquinolone; interferes with conversion of intermediate DNA fragments into high molecular weight DNA	***Contraindication:*** Hypersensitivity ***Cost:*** 500-mg tab, 100 tabs: \$365 ***Pregnancy category:*** C	Headache, dizziness, fatigue, insomnia, depression, seizures, confusion, nausea, diarrhea, increased ALT and AST, flatulence, heartburn, oral candidiasis, rash, pruritus, urticaria, photosensitivity, blurred vision
For carrier state, use both of the following:			
Amoxicillin, 6 g/day PO in 3 divided doses × 6 weeks; children, 100 mg/kg/day PO in 3 divided doses q8h	Bactericidal; broad-spectrum; not effective against beta-lactamase–producing pathogens	***Contraindications:*** Hypersensitivity to penicillins; use caution if allergic to cephalosporins ***Cost:*** 500-mg tabs, 3/day × 10 days: \$4 ***Pregnancy category:*** B	Anaphylactoid reaction, nausea, vomiting, diarrhea, rashes, Stevens-Johnson syndrome, pseudomembranous colitis
Probenecid (Benemid), 2 g/day PO in divided doses × 6 weeks; children, initial dose 25 mg/kg PO, then 40 mg/kg/day PO in 4 divided doses	Inhibits renal tubular secretion of penicillin	***Contraindications:*** Hypersensitivity; severe hepatic disease; blood dyscrasias; severe renal disease; creatinine clearance <50 ml/min; history of uric acid calculus ***Cost:*** 500-mg tab, 100 tabs: \$10-\$30 ***Pregnancy category:*** B	Drowsiness, headache, bradycardia, nephrotic syndrome, gastric irritation, nausea, vomiting, anorexia, hepatic necrosis, rash, dermatitis, pruritus, acidosis, apnea
Typhoid vaccine, live; oral, 1 capsule PO 1 hour before a meal on days 1, 3, 5, and 7, or 0.5 ml SQ × 2, 4 or more weeks apart; children <10 years, 0.25 ml SQ on same schedule as above	Protection against *Salmonella typhi*	***Contraindications:*** Hypersensitivity; immunodeficient states; acute active infections ***Cost:*** Oral, 4 tabs: \$33; 8 units/ml, 5 ml: \$12 ***Pregnancy category:*** C	Abdominal pain, diarrhea, vomiting, fever, headache, rash, malaise, myalgia; all side effects usually mild

Ulcerative Colitis

OVERVIEW

Ulcerative colitis is an inflammatory disease of the colon and rectum, similar to Crohn's disease. In ulcerative colitis, the inflammation spreads in a continuous fashion, whereas in Crohn's disease, the inflammation is patchy with segments of healthy tissue between the patches. Crohn's disease may occur in any part of the gastrointestinal tract from the mouth to the anus, whereas ulcerative colitis is generally limited to the colon and rectum.

Pathogenesis
Cause—unknown; appears multifactorial, with genetic, infectious, immunologic, and psychologic factors

Patient Profile
- Males = Females
- Peak incidence—15 to 35 years of age; second peak occurs in 60s

Signs and Symptoms
- Bloody diarrhea
- Lower abdominal cramps and urgency
- Anemia
- Weight loss
- Fever
- Arthralgia and arthritis
- Tenesmus
- Tachycardia

Differential Diagnosis
- Crohn's disease
- Infectious process such as occurs with *Salmonella, Shigella, Escherichia coli,* giardiasis
- "Gay bowel" syndrome
- Pseudomembranous colitis
- Hemorrhoids
- Tumor
- Diverticulitis

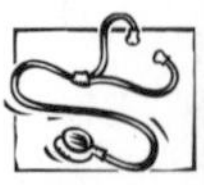

ASSESSMENT

History
Inquire about:
- Onset and duration of symptoms
- Weight loss
- Frequency
- Amount and consistency of stool
- Underlying conditions and current medications

Physical Findings
- Tachycardia
- Weight loss
- Pain on palpation of lower abdomen
- Orthostatic hypotension (possibly)
- Rectal examination—may find bright red blood

Initial Workup
Laboratory
- CBC—anemia and leukocytosis
- Erythrocyte sedimentation rate (ESR)—elevated
- Chemistry profile—hypokalemia, hypoalbuminemia

Radiology: Air-contrast barium enema

Further Workup
Colonoscopy/sigmoidoscopy, usually with biopsy

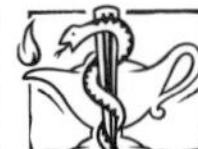

INTERVENTIONS

Office Treatment
None indicated

Lifestyle Modifications
- Learning to live with a chronic illness
- May require hospitalization during acute attack if severe
- Stress reduction

Patient Education
Teach patient about:
- Disease process and treatment options:
  - For severe disease—possible hospitalization for fluid replacement and nutritional support or surgery
  - For milder cases—medication to decrease inflammation
- Increased fluid intake, particularly fluids with electrolytes (Gatorade)
- Nutritionally balanced diet
- Living with a chronic illness (patient will need much support)
- Stress reduction techniques—biofeedback, relaxation, yoga
- Medications used and side effects (see Pharmacotherapeutics)

Referral
To gastroenterologist

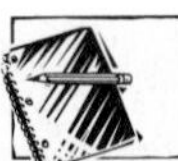

EVALUATION

Outcomes
Prognosis extremely variable; high risk of colon cancer; good prognosis with (L)-sided colitis and proctitis

Possible Complications
- Perforation
- Toxic megacolon
- Liver disease
- Stricture
- Colon cancer

Follow-up
By gastroenterologist

FOR YOUR INFORMATION

Life Span
Pediatric: Approximately 20% are younger than 21 years of age at time of diagnosis
Geriatric: May have more difficult recovery from acute attack
Pregnancy: Encourage patient to delay pregnancy until disease is inactive

Miscellaneous
In severe or refractory disease, a colectomy may need to be performed. This is usually curative, but it often results in a permanent colostomy.

References

McQuaid LR: Alimentary tract. In Tierney LM Jr, McPhee SI, Papadakis MA, editors: *Current medical diagnosis and treatment,* ed 34, Norwalk, Conn, Appleton & Lange, pp 535-539.

Woolliscroft JO: *Current diagnosis & treatment: a quick reference for the general practitioner,* Philadelphia, 1996, Current Medicine, pp 408-409.

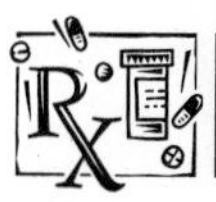

PHARMACOTHERAPEUTICS

Drug of Choice	Mechanism of Action	Prescribing Information	Side Effects
For rectum and left-sided disease:			
Mesalamine (Rowasa); adults, enema, 4 g/60 ml PR hs, retain 8 hours, × 3-6 weeks; suppository, 500 mg 1 PR bid × 3-6 weeks; tabs, 800 mg PO tid × 6 weeks—safety in children not established	5-Aminosalicylic acid (S-ASA); decreases inflammation by blocking cyclooxygenase; inhibits prostaglandin production in colon	***Contraindication:*** Hypersensitivity to this drug or salicylates ***Cost:*** Enema, 4 g/60 ml × 7: $62; suppository, 500 mg/supp × 12: $34; tabs, 400-mg tab, 100 tabs: $57 ***Pregnancy category:*** B	Pericarditis, myocarditis, cramps, gas, nausea, diarrhea, headache, fever, dizziness, insomnia, rash, itching, flu, malaise, back pain, peripheral edema, leg and joint pain, sore throat, cough, pharyngitis
Prednisone, 20-60 mg PO qd, taper gradually after 4-6 weeks; children's dosage same	Decreases inflammation by suppression of migration of polymorphonuclear leukocytes, fibroblasts; reversal to increase capillary permeability; and lysosomal stabilization	***Contraindications:*** Psychosis; hypersensitivity; idiopathic thrombocytopenia; acute glomerulonephritis; amebiasis; fungal infections; nonasthmatic bronchial disease; children <2 years; AIDS; TB ***Cost:*** 20-mg tab, 100 tabs: $7-$18 ***Pregnancy category:*** C	Depression, flushing, sweating, headache, mood change, hypertension, circulatory collapse, thrombophlebitis, embolism, tachycardia, fungal infections, increased intraocular pressure, blurred vision, diarrhea, nausea, abdominal distention, GI hemorrhage, increased appetite, pancreatitis, thrombocytopenia, acne, poor wound healing, fractures, osteoporosis, weakness
Sulfasalazine (Azulfidine), 0.5 g PO bid, increase q4d until reaching 1 g qid; children >2 years, 40-60 mg/kg/day PO in 4-6 divided doses, maximum 2 g/day	Prodrug to deliver sulfapyridine and 5-aminosalicylic acid	***Contraindication:*** Hypersensitivity to sulfonamides or salicylates; pregnancy at term; children <2 years; intestinal/urinary obstruction ***Cost:*** 500-mg tab, 100 tabs: $10-$22 ***Pregnancy category:*** C	Anaphylaxis, nausea, vomiting, abdominal pain, stomatitis, hepatitis, glossitis, pancreatitis, headache, confusion, insomnia, hallucinations, convulsions, leukopenia, neutropenia, thrombocytopenia, agranulocytosis, hemolytic anemia, rash, dermatitis, Stevens-Johnson syndrome, renal failure, toxic nephrosis, increased BUN, creatinine, allergic myocarditis

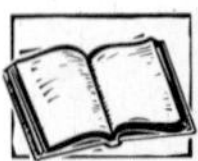

OVERVIEW

Urethritis is inflammation of the urethra characterized by painful urination. It is usually caused by a sexually transmitted disease (STD).

Pathogenesis

Causes—many:

- *Neisseria gonorrhoeae*
- *Chlamydia trachomatis*
- *Trichomonas vaginalis*
- *Ureaplasma urealyticum*
- Many other bacteria

Patient Profile

- Males > Females
- Most common in 15- to 25-year-olds who are sexually active; may occur at any age

Signs and Symptoms

- Males:
  - Gonorrhea—yellow, purulent discharge
  - Nongonococcal urethritis—clear to white discharge, dysuria, suprapubic discomfort, urethral itching, dyspareunia; may be asymptomatic
- Females:
  - Gonorrhea—yellow, purulent vaginal discharge
  - Nongonococcal urethritis—dysuria, urethral itching and/or tenderness, dyspareunia, cystitis, suprapubic discomfort
  - Will usually have some type of vaginal discharge

Differential Diagnosis

- Postgonococcal urethritis
- Allergic reaction (soaps, perfumes, douches)
- Cystitis
- Epididymitis
- Prostatitis
- Atrophy
- Trauma

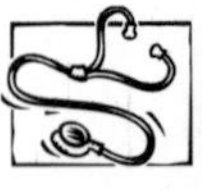

ASSESSMENT

History

Inquire about:

- Onset and duration of symptoms
- Sexual history, including age of first coitus, partners with symptoms, number of partners
- Use of condoms
- Past history of STDs
- Underlying conditions
- Current medications

Physical Findings

- Males:
  - Irritation and tenderness of urethra
  - Discharge—yellow, purulent, or clear to white; or no discharge
- Females:
  - Edema, inflammation, tenderness of urethral meatus
  - Speculum examination—yellow, purulent discharge in vaginal vault, or clear to white discharge; or no discharge; check cervix for friability and cervical motion tenderness
  - Bimanual examination—should be within normal limits

Initial Workup

Laboratory

- Wet mount—look for *Trichomonas*
- Gram stain of discharge:
  - Presence of polymorphonuclear neutrophils and intracellular gram-negative diplococci—strongly suggests gonorrhea
  - Polymorphic neutrophils without organisms—nongonococcal urethritis
  - Few or no polymorphic neutrophils—other cause
- Cultures of discharge for gonorrhea or chlamydial infection
- Urinalysis—within normal limits
- Urine culture—within normal limits
- Serology for HIV and syphilis if indicated

Radiology: None indicated

Further Workup

None indicated

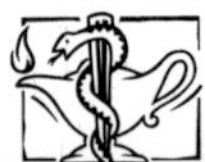

INTERVENTIONS

Office Treatment

None indicated

Lifestyle Modifications

- Safe sex practices
- No sexual intercourse until treatment complete

Patient Education

Teach patient about:

- Condition and cause if known
- Treatment with antibiotics
- Safe sex practices—use of condoms; limiting number of partners
- Increasing fluid intake
- Need to avoid perineal deodorant sprays
- Need to avoid perfumes and perfumed tampons or pads
- Partner's need for treatment
- Medications used and side effects (see Pharmacotherapeutics)

Referrals

Usually none indicated

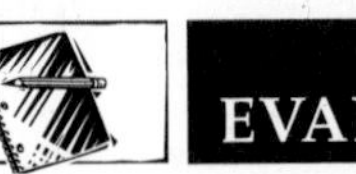

EVALUATION

Outcome

Resolves without sequelae

Possible Complications

- Urethral stricture formation
- Untreated—females can develop pelvic inflammatory disease (PID); males can develop prostatitis; infertility can occur in both males and females

Follow-up

- In 1 week
- May wish to reculture

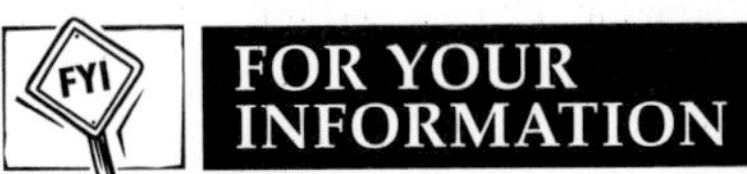

FOR YOUR INFORMATION

Life Span

Pediatric: With positive cultures for an STD, consider child abuse

Geriatric: Treatment is the same

Pregnancy: Cautious use of medications

Miscellaneous

Females with gonorrhea or other infections that cause simple urethritis in males will usually have a vaginal discharge.

References

Bates P, Lewis SL: Nursing role in management: renal and urologic problems. In Lewis SM, Collier IC, Heitkemper MM, editors: *Medical-surgical nursing: assessment and management of clinical problems,* ed 4, St Louis, 1996, Mosby, pp 1336-1337.

Uphold CR, Graham MV: *Clinical guidelines in adult health,* Gainesville, Fla, 1994, Barmarrae Books, pp 431, 662-664.

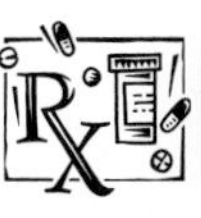

PHARMACOTHERAPEUTICS

Drug of Choice	Mechanism of Action	Prescribing Information	Side Effects
For gonorrhea, use one of the following:			
Ceftriaxone (Rocephen), 125 mg IM × 1 dose; children, 50-75 mg/kg IM × 1 dose	Cephalosporin; inhibits bacterial cell wall synthesis	***Contraindication:*** Hypersensitivity to cephalosporins ***Cost:*** 250-mg vial, 1 vial: $11 ***Pregnancy category:*** C	Headache; dizziness; weakness; paresthesias; nausea; vomiting, diarrhea; anorexia; increased AST, ALT, bilirubin, LDH, and alkaline phosphatase; pseudomembranous colitis; proteinuria; nephrotoxicity; leukopenia; thrombocytopenia; agranulocytosis; neutropenia; hemolytic anemia; rash; urticaria; anaphylaxis
Ciprofloxacin (Cipro), 500 mg PO × 1 dose—not dosed for children	Fluoroquinolone; interferes with conversion of intermediate DNA fragments into high molecular weight DNA	***Contraindication:*** Hypersensitivity ***Cost:*** 500-mg tab, 100 tabs: $365 ***Pregnancy category:*** C	Headache, dizziness, fatigue, insomnia, depression, seizures, confusion, nausea, diarrhea, increased ALT and AST, flatulence, heartburn, oral candidiasis, rash, pruritus, urticaria, photosensitivity, blurred vision
Ofloxacin (Floxin), 400 mg PO × 1 dose—not dosed for children	Fluoroquinolone; interferes with conversion of intermediate DNA fragments into high molecular weight DNA	***Contraindication:*** Hypersensitivity ***Cost:*** 400-mg tab, 100 tabs: $365 ***Pregnancy category:*** C	Headache, dizziness, fatigue, insomnia, depression, seizures, confusion, nausea, diarrhea, increased ALT and AST, flatulence, heartburn, oral candidiasis, rash, pruritus, urticaria, photosensitivity, blurred vision
For chlamydial infection, use one of the following:			
Doxycycline (Doryx), 100 mg PO bid × 7 days; children >8 years, 4.4 mg/kg/day divided q12h	Tetracycline; inhibits protein synthesis	***Contraindications:*** Hypersensitivity; children <8 years ***Cost:*** 100-mg tab, 20 tabs: $5 ***Pregnancy category:*** D	Eosinophilia, neutropenia, thrombocytopenia, hemolytic anemia, dysphagia, glossitis, nausea, abdominal pain, vomiting, diarrhea, anorexia, hepatotoxicity, flatulence, abdominal cramps, gastritis, pericarditis, rash, urticaria, exfoliative dermatitis, angioedema
Azithromycin (Zithromax), 1 g PO × 1 dose	Macrolide; suppresses protein synthesis	***Contraindication:*** Hypersensitivity ***Cost:*** 250-mg tab, 18 tabs: $147 ***Pregnancy category:*** B	Rash, urticaria, pruritus, dizziness, headache, vertigo, diarrhea, hepatotoxicity, abdominal pain, cholestatic jaundice, flatulence, vaginitis, moniliasis
Erythromycin (E-Base), 500 mg PO qid × 7 days; children, 30-50 mg/kg/day in divided doses q12h	Macrolide; suppresses protein synthesis	***Contraindication:*** Hypersensitivity ***Cost:*** 500-mg tab, 100 tabs: $17 ***Pregnancy category:*** B	Rash, urticaria, pruritus, nausea, vomiting, diarrhea, hepatotoxicity, abdominal pain, stomatitis, heartburn, vaginitis, moniliasis
For trichomoniasis:			
Metronidazole (Flagyl), 2 g PO × 1 dose or 500 mg PO bid × 7 days; if treatment fails with single-dose therapy, treat with 500 mg PO bid × 7 days; advise patient to avoid alcohol while taking metronidazole; children, 40 mg/kg PO × 1 dose or 15 mg/kg/day PO divided q8h × 7 days	Direct-acting amebicide/trichomonacide	***Contraindications:*** Hypersensitivity; 1st-trimester pregnancy; CNS disorders ***Cost:*** 500-mg tab, 14 tabs: $3 ***Pregnancy category:*** B (2nd and 3rd trimesters)	Flat T-waves, headache, confusion, irritability, depression, fatigue, insomnia, convulsions, blurred vision, sore throat, retinal edema, nausea, vomiting, diarrhea, anorexia, abdominal cramps, pseudomembranous colitis, dark urine, albuminuria, dysuria, neurotoxicity, leukopenia, bone marrow depression, aplasia, rash, pruritus, flushing

OVERVIEW

Urinary incontinence is the involuntary loss of urine. The types of incontinence that can occur are transient, stress, urge, overflow, and functional.

Pathogenesis

Cause varies by type (see Table 15)

Patient Profile

- Females > Males
- Incidence increases with age

Signs and Symptoms

- Subjective complaint of involuntary loss of urine
- Urinary urgency
- Burning with urination
- Perineal irritation

Differential Diagnosis

- Must differentiate different types and causes
- Urinary tract infection
- Bladder prolapse

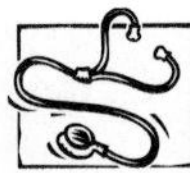

ASSESSMENT

History

Inquire about:

- Onset and duration of symptoms
- Characteristics such as stress, urge, dribbling
- Precipitating events—cough, surgery, new medications
- Dysuria, hesitancy, hematuria, nocturia
- Fluid intake—amount and type
- Depression and mental status changes
- Use of protective devices
- Access to toileting facilities
- Underlying conditions
- Current medications

Physical Findings

- Males:
  - Abdominal examination for masses
  - Genital and perineal examination for irritation
  - Rectal examination to examine prostate and check for fecal impaction
  - All may be within normal limits
- Females:
  - Abdominal examination for masses
  - Examination of genitalia and perineum for irritation
  - Pelvic examination for cystocele, rectocele, uterine prolapse, vaginal muscle tone
  - Rectal examination for fecal impaction
  - All may be within normal limits
- Males and females:
  - Neurologic examination
  - Mini–mental state examination
  - Musculoskeletal examination to assess ambulation
  - Measurement of postvoid residual volume: <50 ml, adequate voiding; >200 ml, inadequate voiding
  - Have patient cough vigorously and observe urethra for urine loss

Initial Workup

Laboratory

- Urinalysis—to check for urinary tract infection (UTI)
- Urine culture if infection present
- CBC
- Chemistry profile to include BUN and creatinine

Radiology

- Intravenous pyelogram
- Renal ultrasound
- Pelvic ultrasound
- Transrectal ultrasound—done if indicated by history and physical examination

Further Workup

Voiding cystourethrogram

TABLE 15 *Types of Urinary Incontinence*

Type	Definition	Cause
Transient	Reversible, temporary condition	Urinary tract infections (UTIs), atrophic urethitis, congestive heart failure (CHF), restricted mobility, depression, stool impaction
Stress	Urine leaks when abdominal pressure increased	Females—pelvic floor muscle weakness, urethal sphincter weakness; males—prostate gland problems, urethral stricture, neurologic problems, detrusor failure
Urge	Inability to delay urination	Lower urinary tract cancer or obstruction, CNS disorders such as stroke, multiple sclerosis, or Parkinson's disease
Overflow	Overdistention of bladder	Detrusor muscle underactivity or acontractility from drugs, fecal impaction, diabetic neuropathy, low spinal cord injury; bladder outlet or urethral obstruction from prostatic hypertrophy, prostate cancer, or urethral stricture; females—cystocele or uterine prolapse
Functional	Inability to toilet properly	Dementia or immobility; may have mixed types of incontinence

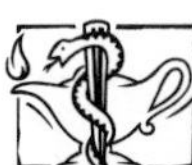

INTERVENTIONS

Office Treatment
None indicated

Lifestyle Modifications
- Smoking cessation
- Decreased intake of caffeine- and alcohol-containing products
- Use of absorbent pads
- Encourage patient to maintain active lifestyle

Patient Education
Teach patient about:
- Condition and cause if known
- Treatment—treat any underlying problems
- Bladder retraining
- Kegel exercises to strengthen pelvic muscles
- Biofeedback
- Obtaining grab bars and elevated toilet seat, urinal, or commode; mobility aids
- Decreasing alcohol and caffeine intake
- Increasing fiber in diet to prevent constipation
- Using absorbent pads
- Need for intermittent catherization, indwelling catheters, penile clamps, pessaries in selected patients; need for surgical intervention for bladder or urethral obstruction, detrusor overactivity, intrinsic and sphincter deficiency, urethral hypermobility in selected patients
- Medications used and side effects (see Pharmacotherapeutics)

Referral
To urologist or surgeon, if indicated

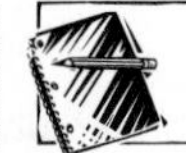

EVALUATION

Outcome
Patient will continue to lead a full, active lifestyle

Possible Complications
- Urinary tract infection
- Perineal irritation with resultant decubitus formation
- Total disruption of lifestyle
- Hydronephrosis
- Renal failure

Follow-up
- Weekly telephone contact
- Every 2 weeks

FOR YOUR INFORMATION

Life Span
Pediatric: In children, condition referred to as enuresis
Geriatric: Most common age group for this problem
Pregnancy: Can have stress incontinence during pregnancy, which can cause decrease in pelvic muscle tone

Miscellaneous
Urinary incontinence can have a major impact on the patient. It is imperative that the NP provide as much support and assistance as possible.

References
Finucane TE, Burton JR: Geriatric medicine: special considerations. In Barker LR, Burton JR, Zieve PD, editors: *Principles of ambulatory medicine,* ed 4, Baltimore, 1995, Williams & Wilkins, pp 78-85.

Urinary Incontinence Panel: *Urinary incontinence in adults: a patient's guide,* Clinical Practice Guideline, AHCPR Pub No 92-0040, Rockville, Md, 1992, US Department of Health and Human Services, Public Health Service, Agency for Health Care Policy and Research.

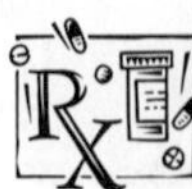

PHARMACOTHERAPEUTICS

Drug of Choice	Mechanism of Action	Prescribing Information	Side Effects
For atrophic vaginitis:			
Estrogen (Premarin), 0.625 mg PO 1 daily or estrogen cream trial of 1 month	Affects release of pituitary gonadotropins; inhibits ovulation	***Contraindications:*** Hypersensitivity; breast cancer; thromboembolic disorders; reproductive cancer; undiagnosed vaginal bleeding; pregnancy ***Cost:*** 0.625-mg tab, 100 tabs: $50; topical estrogen per year: $107 ***Pregnancy category:*** X	Dizziness, headache, migraines, depression, hypotension, thrombophlebitis, thromboembolism, pulmonary embolism, myocardial infarction (MI), nausea, vomiting, cholestatic jaundice, weight gain, diplopia, amenorrhea, cervical erosion, breakthrough bleeding, dysmenorrhea, vaginal candidiasis, spontaneous abortion, rash, urticaria, acne, hirsutism, photosensitivity
If successful, and uterus is intact, add:			
Medroxyprogesterone (Provera), 10 mg PO 1 daily, days 1-12 or days 13-25, or 2.5 mg PO 1 daily continuously	Inhibits secretion of pituitary gonadotropins; stimulates growth of mammary tissue	***Contraindications:*** Hypersensitivity; breast cancer; thromboembolic disorders; reproductive cancer; undiagnosed vaginal bleeding; pregnancy ***Cost:*** 5-mg tab, 30 tabs: $16 ***Pregnancy category:*** X	Dizziness, headache, migraines, depression, hypotension, thrombophlebitis, thromboembolism, pulmonary embolism, MI, nausea, vomiting, cholestatic jaundice, weight gain, diplopia, amenorrhea, cervical erosion, breakthrough bleeding, dysmenorrhea, vaginal candidiasis, spontaneous abortion, rash, urticaria, acne, hirsutism, photosensitivity

Drug of Choice	Mechanism of Action	Prescribing Information	Side Effects
For urge incontinence, use one of the following:			
Propantheline (Pro-Banthine), 7.5-30 mg PO tid	Inhibits muscarinic actions of acetylcholine at postganglionic parasympathetic neuroeffector sites	***Contraindications:*** Hypersensitivity; narrow-angle glaucoma; GI obstruction; myasthenia gravis; paralytic ileus; GI atony; toxic megacolon ***Cost:*** 15-mg tab, 100 tabs: $5-$20 ***Pregnancy category:*** C	Confusion, stimulation in elderly, headache, insomnia, dizziness, drowsiness, dry mouth, paralytic ileus, heartburn, nausea, vomiting, dysphagia, urinary hesitancy and/or retention, palpitations, tachycardia, blurred vision, photophobia, mydriasis, urticaria, rash, pruritus, allergic reaction
Oxybutynin (Ditropan), 2.5-5.0 mg PO tid/qid, maximum 5 mg qid	Relaxes smooth muscles of urinary tract	***Contraindications:*** Hypersensitivity; GI obstruction; GI hemorrhage; glaucoma; severe colitis; myasthenia gravis; urinary tract obstruction ***Cost:*** 5-mg tab, 100 tabs: $13-$44 ***Pregnancy category:*** C	Leukopenia, eosinophilia, anxiety, restlessness, dizziness, convulsions, palpitations, sinus tachycardia, nausea, vomiting, anorexia, abdominal pain, dysuria, urinary retention, urticaria, blurred vision, dry mouth, increased intraocular tension
For urge and stress incontinence:			
Imipramine (Tofranil), 10-25 mg PO tid, maximum dose 100 mg PO tid	Blocks reuptake of neuroepinephrine and serotonin, increasing action of norepinephrine and serotonin	***Contraindications:*** Hypersensitivity to tricyclic antidepressants; recovery phase of MI; convulsive disorders; prostatic hypertrophy ***Cost:*** 10-mg tab, 100 tabs: $2-$25 ***Pregnancy category:*** C	Agranulocytosis, thrombocytopenia, eosinophilia, leukopenia, dizziness, drowsiness, confusion, headache, anxiety, tremors, stimulation, diarrhea, dry mouth, nausea, vomiting, paralytic ileus, increased appetite, hepatitis, urinary retention, acute renal failure, rash, urticaria, orthostatic hypotension, ECG changes, tachycardia, hypertension
For stress incontinence:			
Pseudoephedrine (Novafed, Sudafed), 30-60 mg PO tid	Alpha-adrenergic antagonist	***Contraindications:*** Hypersensitivity; narrow-angle glaucoma ***Cost:*** Sudafed, OTC; Novafed, 60-mg tab, 100 tabs: $4-$25 ***Pregnancy category:*** C	Tremors, anxiety, insomnia, headache, dizziness, seizures, dry nose, palpitations, tachycardia, hypertension, chest pain, dysrhythmias, anorexia, nausea, vomiting, dysuria

Urinary Tract Infection (UTI, Cystitis) in Men

OVERVIEW

Cystitis is inflammation and infection of the bladder. It is considered a lower urinary tract infection (UTI). In young men, cystitis suggests the presence of a structural abnormality, bacterial prostatitis, or a sexually transmitted disease (STD).

Pathogenesis

Cause—usually a single gram negative bacterium; common causative organisms—*Escherichia coli, Klebsiella, Enterobacter, Proteus, Pseudomonas, Serratia*

Patient Profile

- Males
- Usually >50 years of age; uncommon in men <50 years of age
- Risk factors:
    - Homosexuality
    - Benign prostatic hypertrophy
    - Fecal or urinary incontinence
    - Anal intercourse
    - HIV infection
    - Urinary tract instrumentation
    - Prostate infection
    - Recent urologic surgery

Signs and Symptoms

- Dysuria
- Urinary frequency and/or urgency
- Nocturia
- Suprapubic discomfort
- Low-back pain

Differential Diagnosis

- Gonococcal or nongonococcal urethritis
- Prostatitis
- Epididymitis
- Genitourinary tract tumors
- Benign prostatic hypertrophy
- Renal calculi

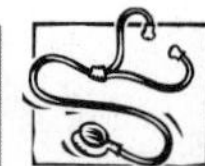

ASSESSMENT

History

Inquire about:

- Onset and duration of symptoms
- Urethral discharge
- Prior history of UTIs
- Strength and character of urine stream
- Known exposure to STDs
- Underlying conditions
- Current medications

Physical Findings

- Abdominal examination—suprapubic tenderness
- Palpation of costovertebral angle for tenderness—should not be tender
- Rectal and prostate examination—should not have prostate tenderness
- Inspection and palpation of genitalia—should be within normal limits

Initial Workup

Laboratory

- Urinalysis:
    - Positive for leukocyte esterase and nitrites
    - Urine culture and sensitivity
    - Segmented urine and expressed prostatic secretions (EPS)—collect first 5 to 10 ml of voided urine (VB_1); patient should void but stop midstream and collect 50 ml of urine (VB_2); massage prostate and milk urethra; collect EPS on swab, slide, or cup (if suspect acute bacterial prostatitis, do not massage prostate); have patient void and collect another 5 to 10 ml of urine (VB_3); send all specimens for cultures and examine EPS microscopically: >10 WBCs/high-power field, suspect some type of prostatitis
    - Interpretation: positive for bacteria in VB_1 and VB_2, negative for bacteria in VB_3 and EPS—cystitis; tenfold increase in VB_3 and EPS—bacterial prostatitis; negative for bacteria in VB_3 and EPS—non-bacterial prostatitis
- In young men, consider STD—cultures for gonorrhea and chlamydial infection, rapid plasma reagin (RPR), and HIV screen

Radiology

- Intravenous pyelogram
- Cystoscopy
- Ultrasound

Further Workup

Urologic workup

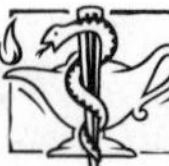

INTERVENTIONS

Office Treatment

None indicated

Lifestyle Modifications

- Increased water intake
- No sexual activity until cured if STD present

Patient Education

Teach patient about:

- Condition and treatment—antibiotics
- Avoiding full bladder
- Drinking cranberry juice or taking cranberry tablets
- Avoiding sexual activity until cured
- Importance of completing all medications
- Medications used and side effects (see Pharmacotherapeutics)

Referral

To urologist (young men)

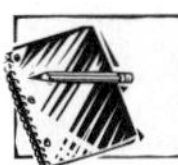

EVALUATION

Outcome
Resolves without sequelae

Possible Complications
- Recurrent infections
- Pyelonephritis

Follow-up
In 2 weeks for repeat urinalysis and urine culture

FOR YOUR INFORMATION

Life Span
Pediatric: Usually have congenital abnormality that obstructs normal urine flow
Geriatric: Common in this age group of men; may be asymptomatic
Pregnancy: N/A

Miscellaneous
Indwelling Foley catheters are a major source of infection for men. Catheters should only be used if absolutely necessary and must be inserted using strict aseptic technique.

Reference
Denman SJ, Murphy PA: Genitourinary infections. In Barker LR, Burton JR, Zieve PD, editors: *Principles of ambulatory medicine,* ed 4, Baltimore, 1995, Williams & Wilkins, pp 324-325.

NOTES

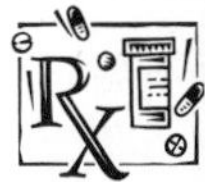

PHARMACOTHERAPEUTICS

Drug of Choice	Mechanism of Action	Prescribing Information	Side Effects
Trimethoprim (TMP)/Sulfamethoxazole (SMZ) (Septra DS, Bactrim DS), 1 DS tab PO bid × 7-10 days; for complicated or recurrent cases, 14-21 days; children, 8 mg/kg TMP, 40 mg/kg SMZ PO q12h × 7-10 days	SMZ interferes with biosynthesis of proteins; TMP blocks synthesis of tetrahydrofolic acid	***Contraindications:*** Hypersensitivity; megaloblastic anemia; infants <2 months; creatinine clearance <15 ml/min ***Cost:*** 1 DS tab, 20 tabs: $3-$4 ***Pregnancy category:*** C	Headache, insomnia, hallucinations, depression, vertigo, allergic myocarditis, nausea, vomiting, abdominal pain, stomatitis, hepatitis, enterocolitis, renal failure, toxic nephrosis, leukopenia, neutropenia, thrombocytopenia, agranulocytosis, hemolytic anemia, Stevens-Johnson syndrome, erythema, photosensitivity, anaphylaxis
Ciprofloxacin (Cipro), 500 mg PO bid × 7-10 days; for complicated or recurrent cases, 14-21 days—not dosed for children; any fluoroquinolone may be used	Fluoroquinolone; interferes with conversion of intermediate DNA fragments into high molecular weight DNA	***Contraindication:*** Hypersensitivity ***Cost:*** 500-mg tab, 100 tabs: $365 ***Pregnancy category:*** C	Headache, dizziness, fatigue, insomnia, depression, seizures, confusion, nausea, diarrhea, increased ALT and AST, flatulence, heartburn, oral candidiasis, rash, pruritus, urticaria, photosensitivity, blurred vision

Urinary Tract Infection (UTI, Cystitis) in Women

OVERVIEW

Cystitis is inflammation and infection of the bladder. It is considered a lower urinary tract infection (UTI).

Pathogenesis
Cause—usually a single gram-negative bacterium; common causative organisms—*Escherichia coli, Klebsiella, Enterobacter, Proteus, Pseudomonas, Serratia*

Patient Profile
- Females
- Any age

Signs and Symptoms
- Dysuria
- Burning on urination
- Urgency
- Suprapubic pain
- Low-back pain
- Sensation of incomplete bladder emptying

Differential Diagnosis
- Vulvovaginitis
- Vaginitis
- Cervicitis
- Bladder outlet obstruction
- Renal calculi
- Sexually transmitted disease (STD)

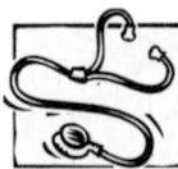

ASSESSMENT

History
Inquire about:
- Onset and duration of symptoms
- Vaginal discharge
- Menstrual history, including menarche, length of cycle, last menstrual period
- Method of birth control (diaphragm—increased risk)
- Prior history of UTIs and treatment success
- Underlying conditions
- Current medications

Physical Findings
- Abdominal examination—may have suprapubic tenderness
- Costovertebral angle for tenderness—should not be tender
- Pelvic examination—should be within normal limits

Initial Workup
Laboratory
- Urinalysis:
  - Positive for leukocyte esterase and nitrites
  - Urine culture and sensitivity
- If suspect STD—cultures for gonorrhea and chlamydial infection, rapid plasma reagin (RPR), and HIV screen

Radiology: For recurrent infections and infants:
- Voiding cystourethrogram
- Cystoscopy
- Ultrasound

Further Workup
Usually none indicated

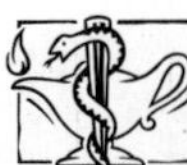

INTERVENTIONS

Office Treatment
None indicated

Lifestyle Modifications
- Increased water intake
- Postcoital voiding
- Proper hygiene

Patient Education
Teach patient about:
- Condition and treatment—antibiotics
- Importance of voiding immediately after coitus
- Increasing water intake and use of cranberry juice or cranberry tablets
- Avoiding use of diaphragm for contraception—increased risk of UTI
- Avoiding sexual intercourse until treatment completed if suspect STD
- Medications used and side effects (see Pharmacotherapeutics)

Referrals
- Usually none
- To urologist for frequent recurrent infections or suspected anatomic abnormality

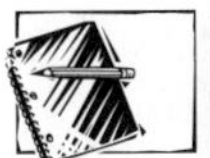

EVALUATION

Outcome

Resolves without sequelae

Possible Complications

- Recurrent infections
- Pyelonephritis
- Renal abscess

Follow-up

- If first UTI and not pregnant—no follow-up if symptoms resolve
- For all others, repeat urinalysis and culture following treatment

FOR YOUR INFORMATION

Life Span

Pediatric: Young children are at higher risk of pyelonephritis
Geriatric: May be asymptomatic; look for urinary tract abnormality
Pregnancy: Usually requires 10 to 14 days of treatment; always repeat urinalysis and urine culture following treatment; cautious use of medication; amoxicillin is preferred treatment

Miscellaneous

For patients with frequent intercourse-related UTIs, postcoital, single-dose antibiotic therapy may be beneficial.

References

Hamilton EM: Management of upper and lower urinary tract infections in pregnant women, *J Am Acad Nurse Pract* 8(12):559-563, 1996.

Hancock LC, Selig PM: Medical problems in primary care. In Youngkin EQ, Davis MS, editors: *Women's health: a primary care clinical guide,* Norwalk, Conn, 1994, Appleton & Lange, pp 643-652.

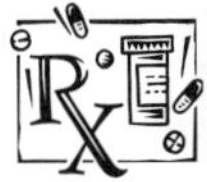

PHARMACOTHERAPEUTICS

Drug of Choice	Mechanism of Action	Prescribing Information	Side Effects
Trimethoprim (TMP)/Sulfamethoxazole (SMZ) (Septra DS, Bactrim DS), 1 DS tab PO bid × 3 days or 1 DS tab PO bid × 7 days or 1 DS tab PO bid × 10-14 days, depending on severity of infection; for postcoital prophylaxis, 1 DS tab PO postcoital; children, 8 mg/kg TMP, 40 mg/kg SMZ PO bid × 3-14 days, depending on severity of infection	SMZ interferes with biosynthesis of proteins; TMP blocks synthesis of tetrahydrofolic acid	***Contraindications:*** Hypersensitivity; pregnancy at term; megaloblastic anemia; infants <2 months; creatinine clearance <15 ml/min; lactation ***Cost:*** 1 DS tab, 20 tabs: $3-$4 ***Pregnancy category:*** C	Headache, insomnia, hallucinations, depression, vertigo, allergic myocarditis, nausea, vomiting, abdominal pain, stomatitis, hepatitis, enterocolitis, renal failure, toxic nephrosis, leukopenia, neutropenia, thrombocytopenia, agranulocytosis, hemolytic anemia, Stevens-Johnson syndrome, erythema, photosensitivity, anaphylaxis
Ciprofloxacin (Cipro), 250 mg PO bid × 3 days or 250 mg 1 tab PO bid × 7 days or 250 mg PO bid × 10-14 days, depending on severity of infection—not dosed for children; any fluoroquinolone may be used	Fluoroquinolone; interferes with conversion of intermediate DNA fragments into high molecular weight DNA	***Contraindication:*** Hypersensitivity ***Cost:*** 250-mg tab, 100 tabs: $225 ***Pregnancy category:*** C	Headache, dizziness, fatigue, insomnia, depression, seizures, confusion, nausea, diarrhea, increased ALT and AST, flatulence, heartburn, oral candidiasis, rash, pruritus, urticaria, photosensitivity, blurred vision
In pregnancy:			
Amoxicillin (Amoxil), 500 mg 1 tab PO tid × 10-14 days; children, 20-40 mg/kg/day PO in 3 divided doses × 7-10 days	Interferes with cell wall replication	***Contraindication:*** Hypersensitivity to penicillins ***Cost:*** 500-mg tab, 30 tabs: $5-$10 ***Pregnancy category:*** B	Bone marrow depression, granulocytopenia, nausea, vomiting, diarrhea, pseudomembranous colitis, anaphylaxis, respiratory distress, increased AST and ALT, abdominal pain, glossitis

OVERVIEW

Uveitis is inflammation of the uveal tract of the eye. The uveal tract consists of the iris, ciliary body, and choroid. Uveitis is classified as anterior, intermediate, or posterior.

Pathogenesis

Causes:

- Anterior uveitis:
  - Ankylosing spondylitis
  - Ulcerative colitis
  - Crohn's disease
  - Juvenile rheumatoid arthritis
  - Syphilis
  - Tuberculosis
  - Herpes simplex and zoster
  - Kawasaki disease
- Intermediate uveitis—cause unknown
- Posterior uveitis:
  - Toxoplasmosis
  - Cytomegalovirus
  - AIDS
  - Tuberculosis

Patient Profile

- Males > Females
- Occurs primarily in adults, rarely in children

Signs and Symptoms

- Anterior, intermediate, and posterior uveitis—signs and symptoms overlap; may be asymptomatic
- Deep aching eye pain—acute onset
- Photophobia
- Blurred vision
- Numerous floaters (particularly with posterior uveitis)
- Constricted or irregularly shaped pupil
- Injection of bulbar conjunctiva

Differential Diagnosis

- Conjunctivitis
- Glaucoma
- Cataracts
- Retinitis pigmentosa
- Foreign body

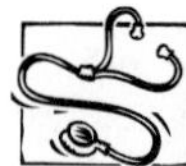

ASSESSMENT

History

Inquire about:

- Onset and duration of symptoms
- Visual acuity, tearing, photophobia
- Past history of eye problems and treatment
- Past medical history
- Past sexual history
- Underlying conditions
- Current medications

Physical Findings

- Constricted or irregularly shaped pupil
- Injected bulbar conjunctiva
- Fundoscopic examination—cloudy vitreous, yellow-white retinal patches
- Complete physical examination to search for underlying cause

Initial Workup

Laboratory

- No specific test for uveitis—search for underlying cause as indicated by history and physical examination
- CBC
- Chemistry panel to include BUN and creatinine—interstitial nephritis
- HLA-B27 typing—ankylosing spondylitis
- Antinuclear antibody and erythrocyte sedimentation rate (ESR)—systemic lupus erythematosus
- VDRL and FTA—syphilis
- Purified protein derivative (PPD)—tuberculosis

Radiology

- Chest film—tuberculosis, sarcoidosis, histoplasmosis, lymphoma
- Sacroiliac film—ankylosing spondylitis

Further Workup

By ophthalmologist

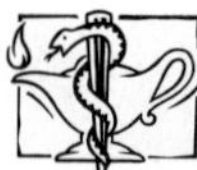

INTERVENTIONS

Office Treatment

None indicated

Lifestyle Modifications

- Depends on causative factor
- May need to prepare for loss of vision

Patient Education

Teach patient about:

- Disease process and treatment options—immediate referral to ophthalmologist; will probably treat with cycloplegic agent and antiinflammatory agent
- How to instill eye drops
- Need to wear dark glasses for photophobia

Referrals

- Immediately to ophthalmologist
- Possibly to primary care physician for treatment of underlying condition after resolution of uveitis

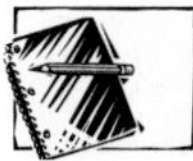

EVALUATION

Outcomes

- Depends on causative factors—with infections, usually resolves once infection is treated
- With other systemic diseases, may resolve but has tendency to recur

Possible Complication

Loss of vision

Follow-up

By ophthalmologist

FOR YOUR INFORMATION

Life Span

Pediatric: Most common cause in this age group is infection
Geriatric: More likely to suffer from a systemic disease that is causative factor
Pregnancy: Cautious use of medications

Miscellaneous

There are many synonyms for this disease, most of which refer to the anatomic location of the problem (e.g., iritis, iridocyclitis, choroiditis, retinochoroiditis, anterior uveitis, posterior uveitis).

References

Astle B, Allen M: Management of persons with problems of the eye. In Phipps WJ et al, editors: *Medical-surgical nursing: concepts and clinical practice,* ed 5, St Louis, 1995, Mosby, pp 2087-2088.

Riordan-Eva P, Vaughn DG: Eye. In Tierney LM Jr, McPhee SJ, Papadakis MA, editors: *Current medical diagnosis and treatment,* ed 34, Norwalk, Conn, 1995, Appleton & Lange, pp 154-155.

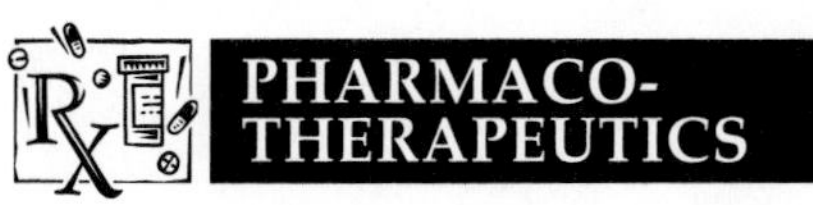

PHARMACOTHERAPEUTICS

Medication will be prescribed and monitored by the ophthalmologist.

Vaginismus

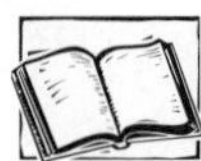

OVERVIEW

Vaginismus is a disorder in which the patient has involuntary painful contractions of the muscles of the lower third of the vagina and introitus.

Pathogenesis

Causes:

- Sexual trauma, especially incest or rape
- Strong, conservative religious values
- Vaginal infections
- Skin disorders of vulva
- Scarring following episiotomy or vaginal repair operations
- Decreased lubrication after menopause

Patient Profile

- Females
- Any age after puberty

Signs and Symptoms

- Painful vaginal intercourse due to muscle contractions
- Infertility
- Avoidance of pelvic examinations
- Inability to insert tampon
- Generally occurs with first attempt at intercourse

Differential Diagnosis

Differentiate psychologic causes from organic causes

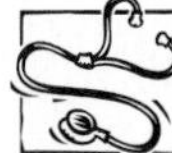

ASSESSMENT

History

Inquire about:

- Onset and duration of symptoms
- Menstrual and obstetric history
- Age at first coitus
- Prior history of sexual abuse or trauma
- Whether symptoms have occurred with previous partners
- Previous pelvic examinations
- Use of tampons
- Underlying conditions
- Current medications

Physical Findings

- Inability to perform pelvic examination because of muscle spasms
- Rigid hymen
- Small, nondistensible vaginal opening

Initial Workup

Laboratory: Only needed if infection suspected

Radiology: Only if anatomic abnormality suspected

Further Workup

Psychologic testing

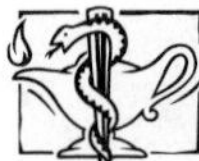

INTERVENTIONS

Office Treatment

Provide a supportive, nonjudgmental environment

Lifestyle Modifications

Smoking and alcohol cessation

Patient Education

Teach patient about:

- Condition and cause if known
- Treatment:
  - May consist of psychologic counseling
  - Rigid hymen—surgical removal
  - Small vaginal opening—progressive dilation by inserting progressively larger objects into vagina
  - Insufficient lubrication—use water-based lubricant
- No specific medications used for treatment

Referral

To specialist in sexual counseling

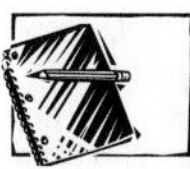

EVALUATION

Outcome
Patient will be able to enjoy a happy, healthy sex life

Possible Complications
- Major psychiatric illness
- Inability to have intimate relationship

Follow-up
Done by sex counselor

FOR YOUR INFORMATION

Life Span
Pediatric: Generally occurs with first attempt at sexual intercourse, which may be in adolescence
Geriatric: N/A
Pregnancy: N/A

Miscellaneous
N/A

Reference
Fogel CA: Women and sexuality. In Youngkin EQ, Davis MS, editors: *Women's health: a primary care clinical guide,* Norwalk, Conn, 1994, Appleton & Lange, pp 67-68, 259.

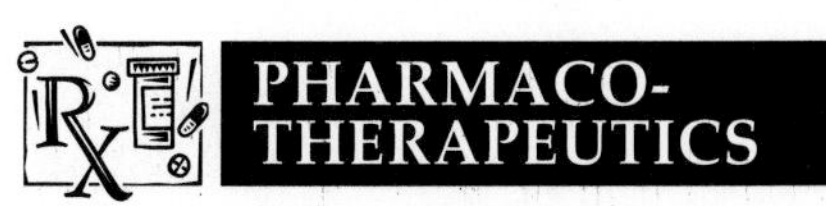

PHARMACOTHERAPEUTICS

There are no specific medications used for treatment of vaginismus. Medications may be needed to treat the underlying cause.

OVERVIEW

Varicose veins are dilated, tortuous, superficial veins with incompetent valves.

Pathogenesis

- Either defective valves or weak venous walls cause dilation of veins; then venous reflux occurs, leading to further dilation and valve failure
- High venous pressure due to prolonged standing, heavy lifting, pregnancy, obesity, wearing constrictive garments

Patient Profile

- Females > Males
- Most commonly seen in middle age

Signs and Symptoms

- Affects greater saphenous vein and its tributaries
- Dull, aching pain
- Heaviness
- Burning sensation
- Mild edema

Differential Diagnosis

- Venous insufficiency
- Arterial insufficiency
- Arthritis
- Peripheral neuritis

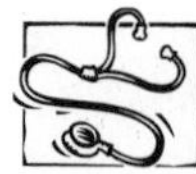

ASSESSMENT

History

Inquire about:

- Onset and duration of symptoms
- Family history of varicose veins
- Type of job performed
- What treatment has been tried
- Underlying conditions
- Current medications

Physical Findings

Dilated, tortuous veins of medial and anterior ankle, calf, and thigh

Initial Workup

Laboratory: None diagnostic
Radiology: None indicated

Further Workup

None indicated

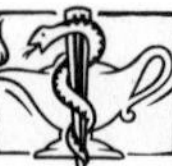

INTERVENTIONS

Office Treatment

None indicated

Lifestyle Modifications

- Smoking cessation
- Weight reduction

Patient Education

Teach patient about:

- Condition and treatment
- Avoiding prolonged standing/sitting (walk around for 5 minutes every hour)
- Sitting with legs elevated
- Using support hose
- Avoiding constrictive garments such as girdles, garters, knee-high stockings
- Weight loss diet if obese
- Surgical options available (sclerotherapy, vein stripping) and the possibility of redevelopment of varicosities
- No medications available

Referral

To vascular surgeon for surgical treatment

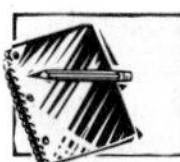

EVALUATION

Outcome
Has chronic course

Possible Complications
- Chronic edema
- Superimposed infection
- Varicose ulcers
- Recurrence after surgery

Follow-up
In 1 month to assess effectiveness of treatment

FOR YOUR INFORMATION

Life Span
Pediatric: N/A
Geriatric: Most common in this age group
Pregnancy: Frequently occur as a result of pregnancy

Miscellaneous
N/A

References
Tierney LM Jr: Blood vessels and lymphatics. In Tierney LM Jr, McPhee SJ, Papadakis MA, editors: *Current medical diagnosis and treatment,* ed 34, Norwalk, Conn, 1995, Appleton & Lange, pp 409-410.

Walsh ME: Management of persons with vascular problems. In Phipps WJ et al, editors: *Medical-surgical nursing: concepts and clinical practice,* ed 5, St Louis, 1995, Mosby, pp 912-913.

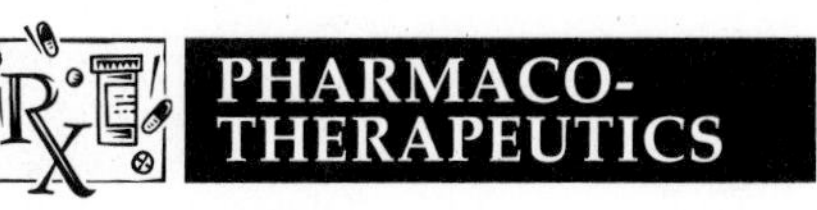

PHARMACOTHERAPEUTICS

There are no specific medications used for treatment of varicose veins.

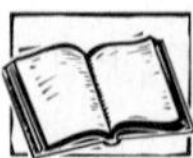

OVERVIEW

Vertigo is an abnormal sensation of movement of either the body or the surroundings. It is a sensation of either the world turning around the patient or the patient turning around in place.

Pathogenesis

Disturbance of either peripheral or central vestibular system:

- Peripheral causes (external, middle, or inner ear; eighth cranial nerve):
  - Middle or inner ear infection
  - Impacted cerumen
  - Acute labyrinthitis
  - Cholesteatoma
  - Postural vertigo
  - Motion sickness
  - Meniere's disease
  - Posttraumatic vertigo—middle ear hemorrhage
  - Lesions in vestibular vessels
  - Vestibulotoxic drugs—salicylates, diuretics, aminoglycoside antibiotics
  - Acoustic neuroma
- Central causes (brain, spinal tract, or nuclear lesion):
  - CNS infection
  - Transient ischemic attacks (TIAs)
  - Trauma
  - Tumor
  - Subclavian steal syndrome
  - Multiple sclerosis
  - Infarct of brainstem or cerebellum
  - Secondary or tertiary syphilis

Patient Profile

- Males = Females
- Any age—more common in adults and elderly

Signs and Symptoms

- Subjective complaint of vertigo; must differentiate from dizziness and syncope (dizziness—sensation of faintness or loss of balance; syncope—brief loss of consciousness)
- May be accompanied by nystagmus (benign positional vertigo), worsening with position change and following upper respiratory tract or GI infections (peripheral vestibulopathy), hearing loss, tinnitus (Meniere's disease, acoustic neuroma), ataxia, visual disturbances, or dysarthria (vertibrobasilar disease)

Differential Diagnosis

- Must differentiate different causes
- Multiple sensory defects
- Parkinson's disease

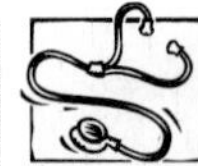

ASSESSMENT

History

Inquire about:

- Onset and duration of symptoms
- Sensation patient feels—must differentiate vertigo, dizziness, and syncope
- Previous upper respiratory tract or GI infection
- Unsteadiness in gait
- Falling
- Ear infections
- Trauma
- Underlying conditions
- Current medications and medications used in preceding 2 to 3 months

Physical Findings

- Assessment for orthostatic hypotension—should not be present
- Ear examination:
  - Tympanic membrane may be injected, bulging, retracted; may have impacted cerumen, landmarks obscured, cholesteatoma
  - Rinne and Weber tests—may indicate hearing loss
- Presence of nystagmus in 5 positions of gaze and with Bárány maneuver
- Assessment of carotid artery for bruits
- Neurologic examination to rule out central lesions
- Cardiovascular examination—should be within normal limits

Initial Workup

Laboratory

- CBC—anemia
- Elevated WBC count with bacterial infection
- Chemistry panel—electrolyte imbalances, abnormal glucose
- Thyroid panel
- Rapid plasma reagin (RPR), VDRL, or FTA-ABS for syphilis

Radiology: CT scan or MRI of head or cerebral angiography to rule out central lesions

Further Workup

- Audiometry
- Caloric testing
- Electronystagmography

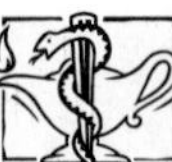

INTERVENTIONS

Office Treatment

If due to cerumen impaction—cerumen removal: soften with Ceruminex, 1:1 hydrogen peroxide and water, or liquid docusate sodium (Colace)—irrigate with syringe with butterfly tubing attached or with Water Pik

Lifestyle Modifications

- Smoking cessation
- Protection from injury—if elderly or living alone, may need assistance

Patient Education

Teach patient about:

- Condition, cause, and treatment options—usually symptomatic treatment
- For benign positional vertigo—exercise program to promote vestibular compensation (repeat any head or body movements that produce vertigo; hold position until vertigo resolves; repeat exercise 5 to 6 times daily
- Using caution when changing positions
- Tips for smoking cessation
- Medications used and side effects (see Pharmacotherapeutics)

Referral

To otolaryngologist if symptoms worsen or do not resolve in 3 to 6 weeks or to neurologist if neurologic deficits present

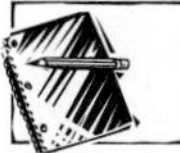

EVALUATION

Outcome
Resolves spontaneously in 3 to 6 weeks without sequelae

Possible Complications
- Severe neurologic deficits
- Hearing loss

Follow-up
Every 2 weeks until resolution

FOR YOUR INFORMATION

Life Span
Pediatric: Uncommon—usually due to ear infection
Geriatric: Benign positional vertigo common in this age group; must also rule out central lesion
Pregnancy: Usually have syncope related to hemodynamic changes—important to differentiate whether patient is experiencing vertigo or syncope

Miscellaneous
Use extra caution when performing assessment tests to prevent patient from injuring self.

Reference
Bass EB, Lewis RF: Dizziness, vertigo, motion sickness, near syncope, syncope, and disequilibrium. In Barker LR, Burton JR, Zieve PD, editors: *Principles of ambulatory medicine,* ed 4, Baltimore, 1995, Williams & Wilkins, pp 1198-1206.

NOTES

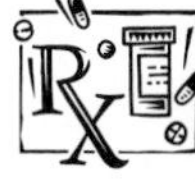

PHARMACOTHERAPEUTICS

Drug of Choice	Mechanism of Action	Prescribing Information	Side Effects
Prochlorperazine suppositories (Compazine), 25 mg PR bid; children, 2.5 mg bid-tid; for vomiting—do not use in children <2 years	Phenothiazine; centrally blocks chemoreceptor trigger zone, which acts on vomiting center	***Contraindications:*** Hypersensitivity; coma; seizures; encephalopathy; bone marrow depression ***Cost:*** 25-mg suppository 12 suppositories: $22 ***Pregnancy category:*** C	Euphoria, depression, extrapyramidal symptoms, restlessness, dizziness, nausea, vomiting, anorexia, dry mouth, diarrhea, constipation, weight loss, circulatory failure, tachycardia, respiratory depression
Meclizine (Antivert), 25 mg PO tid-qid—not recommended for children <12 years; for vertigo	Antihistamine	***Contraindications:*** Hypersensitivity; shock; lactation ***Cost:*** 25-mg tab, 30 tabs: $6 ***Pregnancy category:*** B	Drowsiness, fatigue, restlessness, headache, insomnia, nausea, anorexia, dry mouth, blurred vision
Dimenhydrinate (Dramamine), 50 mg PO q4h; rectal, 100 mg qd or bid; children, 5 mg/kg in 4 equal divided doses	Decreases vestibular stimulation	***Contraindications:*** Hypersensitivity; shock ***Cost:*** 50-mg tab, 100 tabs: $7 ***Pregnancy category:*** B	Drowsiness, restlessness, confusion, convulsions in young children, nausea, anorexia, diarrhea, dry mouth, blurred vision, rash, urticaria
Scopolamine transdermal disk (Transderm-Scop), 1 disk behind ear, leave for 3 days—not for children; use with great caution in elderly	Inhibition of vestibular input to CNS; antagonizes acetylcholine at receptor sites in eyes, smooth muscle, cardiac muscle	***Contraindications:*** Hypersensitivity; glaucoma ***Cost:*** 12 disks: $45 ***Pregnancy category:*** C	Dizziness, drowsiness, confusion, disorientation, blurred vision, dilated pupils, dry mouth, acute narrow-angle glaucoma, rash, erythema

OVERVIEW

Vitiligo is caused by an absence of melanocytes, which results in depigmentation of the skin. There are 2 types. Type A vitiligo, which constitutes 75% of cases, is nondermatomal and widespread, and continues to spread throughout the individual's life. Type B vitiligo, which accounts for the remaining 25% of cases, is dermatomal, lies along dermatomes, and rapidly spreads for 1 year.

Pathogenesis

Cause—absence of epidermal melanocytes; why absent is unknown; may be autoimmune disease

Patient Profile

- Males = Females
- All ages, but 50% begin before 20 years of age
- Positive family history in 30%

Signs and Symptoms

- Loss of skin pigment
- Increased sunburning at site of pigment loss
- Pruritis
- Premature graying of hair
- Koebner's phenomenon—vitiligo at sites of previous trauma, such as previously sunburned skin

Differential Diagnosis

- Pityriasis alba
- Tinea versicolor
- Leprosy
- Lupus erythematosus
- Atopic dermatitis
- Alopecia areata
- Chemical exposure
- Steroid exposure
- Hypopituitarism
- Hypothyroidism
- Addison's disease

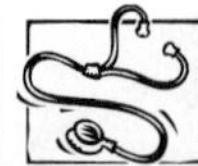

ASSESSMENT

History

Inquire about:

- Onset and duration of symptoms
- Family history of vitiligo
- History of autoimmune disorder
- Treatments tried and results
- Underlying conditions
- Current medications

Physical Findings

- Loss of skin pigment
- Increased sunburning
- Premature hair graying
- Accentuated hypopigmented areas on Woods lamp examination

Initial Workup

Laboratory

- CBC
- Screen for autoimmune diseases—thyroid function, antinuclear antibody (ANA), lupus erythematosus (LE) prep, rheumatoid arthritis (RA) factor, etc.

Radiology: None indicated

Further Workup

Skin biopsy—absence of melanocytes

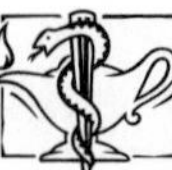

INTERVENTIONS

Office Treatment

None indicated

Lifestyle Modifications

- Need to use caution when in the sun (areas of vitiligo will burn easily—need adequate sunscreen)
- May be other lifestyle modifications if patient has underlying autoimmune disorder

Patient Education

Teach patient about:

- Disease process
- Using cosmetics and skin dyes (Covermark and Dermablend)
- Coping mechanisms—vitiligo has a major psychologic impact on patients
- Treatment options:
  - In light-skinned individuals, no treatment may be needed
  - Cosmetics and skin dyes
  - Topical steroids and psoralens
  - PUVA
  - Surgical grafting and transplantation
  - Systemic steroids
  - Depigmentation of the remaining skin
- Vitiligo not being contagious and not life-threatening
- Medications used and side effects (see Pharmacotherapeutics)

Referrals

- To dermatologist for extensive cases
- May need referral to psychologist for psychologic manifestations

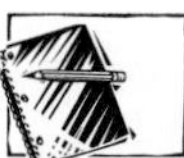

EVALUATION

Outcomes

- Only 5% will have spontaneous repigmentation
- Best result with PUVA, but even that is only 70% repigmentation of head and neck area, with less in other areas of body

Possible Complications

- Phototoxic reactions with PUVA
- Skin atrophy and telangiectasias with topical steroids
- Contact dermatitis with cosmetics

Follow-up

- Every 2 weeks to assess psychologic ramifications of disease and provide counseling
- If patient is receiving PUVA, will need CBC, liver and renal function tests, and ANA test every 6 months

FOR YOUR INFORMATION

Life Span

Pediatric: High incidence of autoimmune and endocrine diseases
Geriatric: Usually not seen in this age group
Pregnancy: Cautious use of medications

Miscellaneous

For most NPs, treatment of vitiligo will be confined to use of topical steroids and cosmetics. If the patient requires PUVA, psoralens, or surgical grafting, a referral should be made to a dermatologist. The NP may need to provide the emotional support the patient with vitiligo requires. This condition can be devastating to the patient psychologically.

Reference

Habif TP: *Clinical dermatology: a color guide to diagnosis and therapy,* ed 3, St Louis, 1996, Mosby, pp 616-620.

NOTES

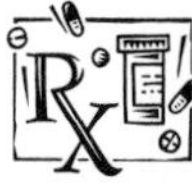

PHARMACOTHERAPEUTICS

Drug of Choice	Mechanism of Action	Prescribing Information	Side Effects
Topical corticosteroid 1% hydrocortisone (Cortaid 1%) cream; apply to affected area tid to qid; in adults may need to prescribe one of the more potent topical steroids, such as mometasone (Elocon) cream or betamethasone dipropionate (Diprolene) cream; use of topical steroids for long periods of time may render them ineffective	Antiinflammatory; antipruritic	***Contraindication:*** Hypersensitivity ***Cost:*** 1%, 30 g: $12; several available OTC; mometasone 0.1%, 45 g: $29; betamethasone 0.05%, 15 g: $3-$16 ***Pregnancy category:*** C	Burning, dryness, itching, irritation, acne, folliculitis, hypertrichosis, hypopigmentation, atrophy, striae, perioral dermatitis, secondary infection; if used on large area for extended periods of time, can have systemic side effects
Trioxsalen (Trisoralen) 5-mg tab; use in conjunction with sunlight: take 2 tabs 2-4 hours before sun exposure; 1st exposure—15 min; 2nd exposure—20 min; 3rd exposure—25 min; 4th exposure—30 min; gradually increase exposure time based on erythema and tenderness—use for adults and children >12 years; potent drug—should only be used by those experienced with its use	Exact mechanism of action unknown, but causes melanogenesis	***Contraindications:*** In diseases associated with photosensitivity such as porphyria; do not use with any photosensitizing agents ***Cost:*** 5-mg tab, 28 tabs: $67 ***Pregnancy category:*** Not categorized	Severe sunburn, gastric discomfort

Vulvovaginal Candidiasis

OVERVIEW

Vulvovaginal candidiasis is an infection of the vulva and vagina that produces an abnormal vaginal discharge and vulvar irritation.

Pathogenesis

Cause: *Candida albicans,* a common yeast; upset in homeostatic balance leads to overgrowth of *Candida* organisms and infection

Patient Profile

- Females
- Menarche to menopause

Signs and Symptoms

- Vulvar pruritis
- Vulvar erythema
- Vulvar edema and excoriation
- Vaginal discharge (white, consistency of cottage cheese)

Differential Diagnosis

- Bacterial vaginosis
- Trichomoniasis
- Gonorrhea
- Chlamydial infection

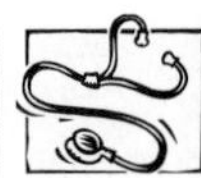

ASSESSMENT

History

Inquire about:

- Onset and duration of symptoms
- Past history of yeast infections and treatment results
- Predisposing factors—pregnancy, recent antibiotics, estrogen therapy, diabetes, HIV status
- Underlying conditions
- Current medications

Physical Findings

- Pelvic examination—vulvar erythema, excoriation, edema
- Speculum examination—white patches or plaques in vagina; *no* odor

Initial Workup

Laboratory

- pH of vaginal secretions <4.5
- Place vaginal secretions on slide and mix with 10% potassium hydroxide (KOH); microscopic findings—yeast and pseudohyphae

Radiology: None indicated

Further Workup

None indicated

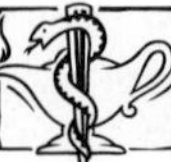

INTERVENTIONS

Office Treatment

None indicated

Lifestyle Modifications

- Weight loss diet if overweight
- Keeping perineal area clean and dry
- Avoiding frequent douching
- Chronic candidiasis—learning to cope with chronic infection

Patient Education

Teach patient about:

- Condition and treatment—intravaginal or oral antifungals
- Keeping perineal area clean (use mild soap and water)
- Wearing cotton underwear
- Avoiding clothing made from nonventilated material
- Avoiding frequent douching—destroys normal protective flora
- Avoiding broad-spectrum antibiotics when possible
- Tips for weight loss
- Limiting intake of sweets and alcohol
- Avoiding hot tubs and sitting around in wet bathing suits
- Sexual partner not needing treatment—candidiasis is not sexually transmitted
- Possibility of oil-based vaginal creams weakening latex condoms and diaphragms
- Medications used and side effects (see Pharmacotherapeutics)

Referrals

- Usually none
- To physician if patient has frequent infections (>3 per year)

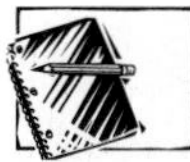

EVALUATION

Outcome
Resolves without sequelae

Possible Complication
Secondary bacterial infection

Follow-up
None needed if symptoms resolve

FOR YOUR INFORMATION

Life Span
Pediatric: Rare before puberty
Geriatric: Postmenopausal; vagina and vulva are more prone to infection because of normal physiologic changes
Pregnancy: Pregnancy increases risk of candidiasis; only topical therapy should be used (and should be used for 7 days)

Miscellaneous
N/A

References
Bennett EC: Vaginitis and sexually transmitted diseases. In Youngkin EQ, Davis MS, editors: *Women's health: a primary care clinical guide,* Norwalk, Conn, 1994, Appleton & Lange, pp 210-212.

Reed BD, Eyler A: Vaginal infections: diagnosis and management, *Am Fam Physician* 47(8):1805-1816, 1993.

NOTES

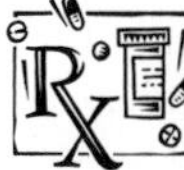

PHARMACOTHERAPEUTICS

Drug of Choice	Mechanism of Action	Prescribing Information	Side Effects
Fluconazole (Diflucan), 150 mg PO × 1 dose—not dosed for children for this condition	Antifungal; inhibits ergosterol biosynthesis; directly damages phospholipid membrane	***Contraindication:*** Hypersensitivity ***Cost:*** 150-mg tab, 12 tabs: $128 ***Pregnancy category:*** B	Nausea, vomiting, diarrhea, cramping, flatus, hepatotoxicity, Stevens-Johnson syndrome, headache
Clotrimazole (Gyne-Lotrimin) 1% cream; adults and children, 5 g intravaginally × 7-14 days; or 100-mg vaginal tab, 1 per vagina × 7 days; or 100-mg vaginal tab—2 per vagina × 3 days; or 500-mg vaginal tab, 1 per vagina × 1 dose	Topical antifungal fungicidal	***Contraindication:*** Hypersensitivity ***Cost:*** Cream and 100-mg tab: OTC; 500-mg tab, 1 tab: $13 ***Pregnancy category:*** B	Rash, urticaria, stinging, burning, peeling, blistering, skin fissures, abdominal cramps, bloating, urinary frequency, dyspareunia
Butoconazole 2% (Femstat), 5 g intravaginally hs × 3 days—safety in children not established	Antifungal	***Contraindication:*** Hypersensitivity ***Cost:*** 3 applicators: $20 ***Pregnancy category:*** C	Rash, stinging, burning, itching, soreness, swelling, discharge, itching of fingers
Miconazole (Monistat), 2% cream; adults and children, 5 g intravaginally × 7 days; or 200-mg vaginal suppository, 1 suppository × 3 days; or 100-mg suppository, 1 suppository × 7 days	Antifungal	***Contraindication:*** Hypersensitivity ***Cost:*** Cream and 100-mg suppository: OTC; 200-mg suppository, 3 suppositories: $23 ***Pregnancy category:*** B	Vulvovaginal burning, itching, cramps, rash, urticaria, stinging, burning, contact dermatitis

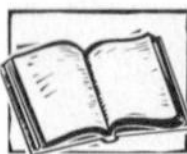

OVERVIEW

Estrogen-deficient vulvovaginitis or atrophic vaginitis results in thinning and atrophy of the vaginal and vulvar epithelium.

Pathogenesis

Cause—decreased estrogen production due to natural or surgically induced menopause

Patient Profile

- Females
- Any age if postmenopausal

Signs and Symptoms

- Vaginal atrophy
- Vaginal dryness
- Dyspareunia
- Bleeding after intercourse
- Vulvar pruritus
- Vaginal discharge
- Infection

Differential Diagnosis

- Malignancies
- Vaginal infections—*Candida albicans*
- Bacterial vaginosis
- Trichomoniasis
- Gonorrhea
- Chlamydial infection

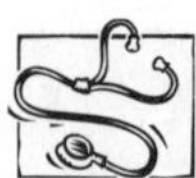

ASSESSMENT

History

Inquire about:

- Onset and duration of symptoms
- Menstrual history, including menarche, last menstrual period
- Vasomotor symptoms—hot flushes, paresthesias, dizziness
- Sexual history and behaviors
- Underlying conditions
- Current medications

Physical Findings

Pelvic examination:

- Vaginal epithelium: thin and pale
- Disappearance of rugae
- Brittle pubic hair

Initial Workup

Laboratory

- Serum follicle-stimulating hormone >40 mIU/ml = menopause
- Pap smear—maturation index
- Wet mount
- Cultures for gonorrhea and chlamydial infection

Radiology: None indicated

Further Workup

None indicated

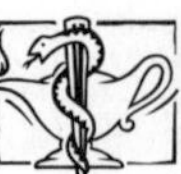

INTERVENTIONS

Office Treatment

None indicated

Lifestyle Modifications

- Adapting to normal physiologic changes
- Smoking cessation

Patient Education

Teach patient about:

- Condition and treatment:
  - Hormone replacement therapy
  - Use of water-soluble lubricants
  - Kegel exercises to help strengthen pelvic muscles
- Possibility that regular sexual activity may help decrease problems from atrophic changes
- Possible benefit of tepid sitz baths, yogurt douches, and tablets containing *Lactobacilus acidophilus*
- Medications used and side effects (see Pharmacotherapeutics)

Referrals

Usually none needed

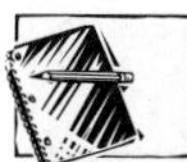

EVALUATION

Outcome
Patient will be able to enjoy a happy, healthy sexual relationship

Possible Complication
From estrogen therapy

Follow-up
In 1 month if patient is receiving estrogen therapy; then every 3 to 6 months to monitor for side effects

FOR YOUR INFORMATION

Life Span
Pediatric: N/A
Geriatric: Common in this age group because of normal physiologic changes
Pregnancy: N/A

Miscellaneous
A woman who is breast-feeding is in a hypoestrogen state and may need to use a water-based lubricant before sexual intercourse

References
Garner CH: The climacteric, menopause, and the process of aging. In Youngkin EQ, Davis MS, editors: *Women's health: a primary care clinical guide,* Norwalk, Conn, 1994, Appleton & Lange, pp 317-318.

Uphold CR, Graham MV: *Clinical guidelines in adult health,* Gainesville, Fla, 1994, Barmarrae Books, pp 474-476.

NOTES

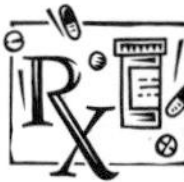

PHARMACOTHERAPEUTICS

Drug of Choice	Mechanism of Action	Prescribing Information	Side Effects
Estrogen (Premarin), 0.625 mg PO 1 tab daily; estrogen is available in pills, as transdermal patch, or as vaginal cream; method of administration should be decided on by NP and patient together by determining which method best meets patient's needs	Affects release of pituitary gonadotropins; inhibits ovulation	***Contraindications:*** Hypersensitivity; breast cancer; thromboembolic disorders; reproductive cancer; undiagnosed vaginal bleeding; pregnancy ***Cost:*** 0.625-mg tab, 100 tabs: $50; transdermal or topical estrogen per year: $107 ***Pregnancy category:*** X	Dizziness, headache, migraines, depression, hypotension, thrombophlebitis, thromboembolism, pulmonary embolism, myocardial infarction (MI), nausea, vomiting, cholestatic jaundice, weight gain, diplopia, amenorrhea, cervical erosion, breakthrough bleeding, dysmenorrhea, vaginal candidiasis, spontaneous abortion, rash, urticaria, acne, hirsutism, photosensitivity
If patient has intact uterus, add:			
Medroxyprogesterone acetate (Provera), 10 mg PO on days 1-12 or days 13-25; or can give 2.5 mg PO daily; estrogen and medroxyprogesterone acetate are now available in 1 tab sold under trade name Prempro	Inhibits secretion of pituitary gonadotropins; stimulates growth of mammary tissue	***Contraindications:*** Hypersensitivity; breast cancer; thromboembolic disorders; reproductive cancer; undiagnosed vaginal bleeding; pregnancy ***Cost:*** 5-mg tab, 30 tabs: $16 ***Pregnancy category:*** X	Dizziness, headache, migraines, depression, hypotension, thrombophlebitis, thromboembolism, pulmonary embolism, MI, nausea, vomiting, cholestatic jaundice, weight gain, diplopia, amenorrhea, cervical erosion, breakthrough bleeding, dysmenorrhea, vaginal candidiasis, spontaneous abortion, rash, urticaria, acne, hirsutism, photosensitivity

OVERVIEW

Warts are benign skin lesions. There are several different types of warts: common wart (verruca vulgaris), plantar wart (verruca plantaris), flat wart (verruca plana), venereal wart (condyloma acuminatum; for detailed information, see section on condyloma acuminata/genital warts), filiform wart, and digitate wart. Warts are transmitted through direct contact. Most will resolve spontaneously in weeks or months; others may last for years.

Pathogenesis

Cause—viral infection of keratinocytes; human papillomavirus (HPV) is causative agent

Patient Profile

- Females > Males
- Most common age groups—young adults and children

Signs and Symptoms

- Common warts—smooth, flesh-colored papules; become dome-shaped, gray-brown growths with black dots
- Plantar warts—thick, painful callous formation on plantar surface of foot
- Flat warts—slightly elevated, flat-topped papules; pink, light brown, or light yellow in color
- Venereal warts—thin, flexible, tall, flesh-colored papules
- Filiform and digitate warts—fingerlike, skin-colored projections protruding from a narrow or broad base

Differential Diagnosis

- Corns
- Scar tissue
- Molluscum contagiosum
- Condyloma lata
- Seborrheic keratoses

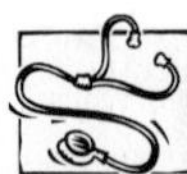

ASSESSMENT

History

Inquire about:

- Onset and duration of symptoms
- Treatments tried and results
- History of atopic dermatitis
- Use of locker rooms
- Underlying conditions
- Current medications

Physical Findings

- Common warts:
  - Smooth, flesh-colored papules that become dome-shaped growths
  - Interrupt the normal skin lines
  - Gray-brown in color with black dots
  - Most common site is hands, but may be anywhere
- Plantar warts—thick, painful callous formation on plantar surface of foot
- Flat warts:
  - Slightly elevated, flat-topped papules, commonly in lineal arrangement
  - Pink, light brown, or light yellow in color
  - Commonly occur on forehead, around mouth, on backs of hands, and in shaved areas
- Venereal warts:
  - Thin, flexible, tall, flesh-colored papules
  - Found on genitalia
- Filiform and digitate warts:
  - Fingerlike, skin-colored projections protruding from a narrow or broad base
  - Commonly located around mouth, eyes, and beard area

Initial Workup

Laboratory: None indicated
Radiology: None indicated

Further Workup

None indicated

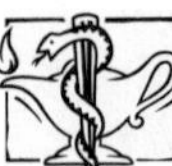

INTERVENTIONS

Office Treatment

- If treatment is with topical agent, wart should be pared as closely as possible
- Cryotherapy can be used for all warts
- Filiform and digitate warts can be removed with a curette, using one smooth stroke across base of wart
- Excision with electrocautery or laser ablation can also be done

Lifestyle Modifications

- Covering feet with rubber or wooden sandals when using public showers and locker rooms
- Plantar warts can cause significant discomfort—may need to alter activity level

Patient Education

Teach patient about:

- Cause of warts and that they can be spread from individual to individual
- Treatment options:
  - Cryotherapy—usually less scar formation
  - Surgical excision with electrocautery, laser ablation, curettage
  - Various salicylic acid preparations
  - Topical retinoids for flat warts—long treatment time
  - Easiest and safest treatment is as follows: cover with waterproof tape and leave in place for 1 week; remove for 12 hours; if wart still present, repeat treatment—works best with warts on fingers and toes
  - Soaking area in warm water before applying medication
- Medications used and side effects (see Pharmacotherapeutics)

Referrals

None, unless extensive and resistant to above treatments

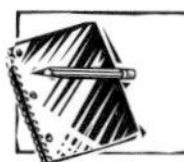

EVALUATION

Outcome
Warts resolve with minimal or no scarring

Possible Complications
- Autoinoculation
- Scar formation
- Chronic pain after removal of plantar wart
- Nail deformity

Follow-up
- Depends on treatment—weekly if cryotherapy performed; may take several treatments
- If treatment done at home, return to clinic every 2 weeks

FOR YOUR INFORMATION

Life Span
Pediatric: Generally more common in children
Geriatric: Treatment is the same
Pregnancy: Cautious use of medications

Miscellaneous
Information on condyloma acuminata, or genital warts, is presented in a separate section on condyloma acuminata/genital warts.

Reference
Habif TP: *Clinical dermatology: a color guide to diagnosis and therapy,* ed 3, St Louis, 1996, Mosby, pp 325-333.

NOTES

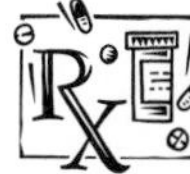

PHARMACOTHERAPEUTICS

Drug of Choice	Mechanism of Action	Prescribing Information	Side Effects
Salicylic acid (Keralyt); apply to affected area and occlude at night	Desquamation of horny layer of skin	***Contraindications:*** Hypersensitivity; children <2 years old ***Cost:*** 1 oz: $16 ***Pregnancy category:*** C	Excessive erythema, scaling
Retinoic acid cream, gel (Retin-A), 0.025% and 0.5%; apply bid; works best on flat warts—lengthy treatment	Exact mechanism of action is unknown; decreases cohesiveness of follicular epithelial cells and decreases microcomedo formation; also stimulates mitotic activity	***Contraindication:*** Hypersensitivity ***Cost:*** 0.05%, 20-g tube, 1 tube: $27 ***Pregnancy category:*** C	Extreme redness of skin, edema, blistering, crusting, increased susceptibility to sunlight, hyperpigmentation or hypopigmentation

PART TWO

Patient History

Collecting a health history can present a challenge to even the most experienced practitioner. The history needs to be collected in a succinct, precise, and timely manner and yet needs to convey to the reader a complete picture of the patient's current and past health status.

The process of collecting the health history is the first step in the patient-practitioner encounter. It is a time when first impressions are easily formed, and care must be taken by the practitioner to present a professional, yet cordial, demeanor to the patient. This is a time for the practitioner and patient to get to know each other; collecting the history allows the practitioner time to put the patient at ease. Much of the information needed for the history is of a very personal nature. A patient who does not feel comfortable with the practitioner may be less likely to answer the questions truthfully or to provide complete information.

The practitioner must be skillful at keeping the conversation focused on the task at hand. Often it may be necessary to redirect the conversation in order to keep the process moving along. Therefore it is necessary to have the main topics of the history firmly committed to memory.

CULTURE

Culture can be a major barrier in collecting a health history. The practitioner must be familiar with the patient population being served (Table 16). Many cultures use various types of nontraditional remedies to treat an illness. Although it would be ideal if the provider were familiar with these treatments, in reality it is often difficult for a practitioner from a different culture to obtain information on nontraditional treatments the patient has received. The practitioner should ask the patient what the treatment consists of and what, if any, types of herbs or medicines are being used. Cultural awareness and sensitivity are key to forming a good patient-practitioner relationship.

COMPONENTS OF THE HEALTH HISTORY

The components of a complete health history are delineated in the following paragraphs. Whether the practitioner chooses to include all of the components described here depends in large part on the practice setting and the reason for the visit. The following health history is designed for the practitioner in the primary care setting. Every practitioner must develop his or her own system for obtaining a health history. Many clinics and offices have developed history forms for patients to fill out while they are waiting. These forms can be a valuable asset and can save a great deal of time. However, it is imperative that the practitioner review the form with the patient and have the patient elaborate on any positive findings. The following is a list of topics that should be included in the health history: (1) biographical data, (2) chief complaint or reason for visit, (3) past medical history, (4) family history, (5) social history, (6) functional assessment, and (7) review of systems. In the following paragraphs each topic is discussed in depth, with examples given of information that should be included under that topic.

Biographical Data

Biographical data should include the patient's name, address, phone number, age, date of birth, sex, marital status, and ethnic origin. A statement should be made about who the informant is and whether or not the informant seems reliable.

Chief Complaint or Reason for Visit

Many practitioners prefer not to use the term *chief complaint (CC)* because they believe that it labels the patient as a complainer. However, there are still many who do use this term. One reason for doing so is that *CC* is an easy, short, and generally well known abbreviation. Perhaps in the future more

Text continued on p. 626

TABLE 16 ***Cultural Characteristics Related to Health Care***

Cultural group	Health beliefs	Health practices
Asian-Americans		
Chinese	A healthy body viewed as gift from parents and ancestors and must be cared for Health is one of the results of balance between the forces of *yin* (cold) and *yang* (hot), energy forces that rule the world Illness caused by imbalance Believe blood is source of life and is not regenerated *Chi* is innate energy Lack of *chi* and blood results in deficiency that produces fatigue, poor constitution, and long illness	Goal of therapy is to restore balance of *yin* and *yang* Acupuncturist applies needles to appropriate meridians identified in terms of *yin* and *yang* Acupressure and *tai chi* replacing acupuncture in some areas Moxibustion is application of heat to skin over specific meridians Wide use of medicinal herbs procured and applied in prescribed ways Folk healers are herbalist, spiritual healer, temple healer, fortune healer Meals may or may not be planned to balance hot and cold Milk intolerance relatively common Use of condiments (e.g., monosodium glutamate and soy sauce) may create difficulty with some diet regimens (e.g., low-salt diets)
Japanese	Three major belief systems: *Shinto* religious influence Humans inherently good Evil caused by outside spirits Illness caused by contact with polluting agents (e.g., blood, corpses, skin diseases) Chinese and Korean influence Health achieved through harmony and balance between self and society Disease caused by disharmony with society and not caring for body Portuguese influence Upholds germ theory of disease	Believe evil removed by purification Energy restored by means of acupuncture, acupressure, massage, and moxibustion along affected meridians *Kampō* medicine—use of natural herbs Believe in removal of diseased parts Trend is to use both Western and Oriental healing methods Care of disabled viewed as family's responsibility Take pride in child's good health Seek preventive care, medical care for illness May avoid some food combinations (e.g., milk and cherries, watermelon and crab) and believe pickled plums to have special properties
Vietnamese	Good health considered to be balance between *yin* (cold) and *yang* (hot) Believe person's life has been predisposed toward certain phenomena by cosmic forces Health believed to be result of harmony with existing universal order; harmony attained by pleasing good spirits and avoiding evil ones Belief in *am duc,* the amount of good deeds accumulated by ancestors Many use rituals to prevent illness Practice some restrictions to prevent incurring wrath of evil spirits	Family uses all means possible before using outside agencies for health care Fortune-tellers determine event that caused disturbance May visit temple to procure divine instruction Use astrologer to calculate cyclical changes and forces Regard health as family responsibility; outside aid sought when resources run out Certain illnesses considered only temporary (such as pustules, open wounds) and ignored Seek generalist health healers May use special diets to prevent illness and promote health Lactose intolerance prevalent
Filipinos	Believe God's will and supernatural forces govern universe Illness, accidents, and other misfortunes are God's punishment for violations of His will Widely accept "hot" and "cold" balance and imbalance as cause of health and illness	Some use amulets as a shield from witchcraft or as good luck pieces Catholics substitute religious medals and other items

From Wong DL: *Whaley and Wong's essentials of pediatric nursing,* ed 5, St Louis, 1997, Mosby.

Family relationships	Communication	Comments
Extended family pattern common Strong concept of loyalty of young to old Respect for elders taught at early age—acceptance without questioning or talking back Children's behavior a reflection on family Family and individual honor and "face" important Self-reliance and self-restraint highly valued; self-expression repressed Males valued more highly than females; women submissive to men in family	Open expression of emotions unacceptable Often smile when do not comprehend	Do not react well to painful diagnostic workup; are especially upset by drawing of blood Deep respect for their bodies and believe it best to die with bodies intact; therefore may refuse surgery Believe in reincarnation Older members fear hospitals; often believe hospital is a place to go to die Children sometimes breast-fed for up to 4 or 5 years*
Close intergenerational relationships Family provides anchor Family tends to keep problems to self Value self-control and self-sufficiency Concept of *haji* (shame) imposes strong control; unacceptable behavior of children reflects on family Many adopt practices of contemporary middle class Concern for child's missing school may result in sending to school before fully recovered from illness	*Issei*—born in Japan; usually speak Japanese only *Nisei, Sansei,* and *Yonsei* have few language difficulties New immigrants able to read and write English better than able to speak or understand it Make significant use of nonverbal communication with subtle gestures and facial expression Tend to suppress emotions Will often wait silently	Generational categories: *Issei*—1st generation to live in United States *Nisei*—2nd generation *Sansei*—3rd generation *Yonsei*—4th generation *Issei* and *Nissei*—tolerant and permissive childrearing until 5 or 6, then emphasis on emotional reserve and control Cleanliness highly valued Time considered valuable and used wisely Tendency to practice emotional control may make assessment of pain more difficult
Family is revered institution Multigenerational families Family is chief social network Children highly valued Individual needs and interests are subordinate to those of family group Father is main decision maker Women taught submission to men Parents expect respect and obedience from children	Many immigrants are not proficient in speaking and understanding English May hesitate to ask questions Questioning authority is sign of disrespect; asking questions considered impolite Use indirectness rather than forthrightness in expressing disagreement May avoid eye contact with health professionals as a sign of respect	Consider status more important than money Children taught emotional control Time concept more relaxed—consider punctuality less significant than other values (i.e., propriety) Place high value on social harmony
Family is highly valued, with strong family ties Multigenerational family structure common, often with collateral members as well Personal interests are subordinated to family interests and needs Members avoid any behavior that would bring shame on the family	Immigrants and older persons may not be able to speak or understand English	Tend to have a fatalistic outlook on life Believe time and providence will solve all

*Most Asian cultures consider the child 1 year old at the time of birth. Traditional Chinese custom adds 1 year on January 1 regardless of the birthday—a child born in December is 2 years old the next January.

Continued

TABLE 16 ***Cultural Characteristics Related to Health Care—cont'd***

Cultural group	Health beliefs	Health practices
American Blacks	Illness classified as: Natural—affected by forces of nature without adequate protection (e.g., cold air, pollution, food and water) Unnatural—evil influences (e.g., witchcraft, voodoo, hoodoo, hex, fix, rootwork); symptoms often associated with eating Believe serious illness sent by God as punishment (e.g., parents punished by illness or death of child) Believe serious illness can be avoided May resist health care because illness is "will of God"	Self-care and folk medicine very prevalent Folk therapies usually religious in origin Attempt home remedies first; poorer people do not seek help until illness serious Usually seek help from: "Old lady"—woman in community with a common knowledge of herbs; consulted regarding pediatric care Spiritualist—has received gift from God for healing incurable diseases or solving personal problems; strongly based in Christianity Priest (voodoo priest/priestess)—most powerful healer Root doctor—meets need for herbs, oils, candles, and ointments Prayer is common means for prevention and treatment
Haitians*	Illnesses have a supernatural or natural origin Supernatural illnesses are caused by angry voodoo spirits, enemies, or the dead, especially deceased ancestors Natural illnesses are based on conceptions of natural causation: Irregularities of blood volume, flow, purity, viscosity, color and/or temperature (hot/cold) Gas *(gaz)* Movement and consistency of mother's milk Hot/cold imbalance in the body Bone displacement Movement of diseases Health is maintained by good dietary and hygienic habits	Health is a personal responsibility Foods have properties of "hot"/"cold" and "light"/"heavy" and must be in harmony with one's life cycle and bodily states Natural illnesses are treated by home remedies first Supernatural illness treated by healers: voodoo priest *(houngan)* or priestess *(mambo),* midwife *(fam saj),* and herbalist or leaf doctor *(dokte fey)* Amulets and prayer used to protect against illness due to curses or willed by evil people
Hispanic Americans		
Mexican-Americans (Latinos, Chicanos, Raza-Latinos)	Health beliefs have strong religious association Believe in body imbalance as a cause of illness, especially imbalance between *caliente* (hot) and *frio* (cold) or "wet" and "dry" Some maintain good health is a result of "good luck"—a reward for good behavior Illness prevented by performing properly, eating proper foods, and working proper amount of time; accomplished through prayer, wearing religious medals or amulets, and sleeping with relics at home Illness is a punishment from God for wrongdoing, forces of nature, and the supernatural	Seek help from *curandero* or *curandera,* especially in rural areas Curandero(a) receives his/her position by birth, apprenticeship, or a "calling" via dream or vision Treatments involve use of herbs, rituals, and religious artifacts Practice for severe illness—make promises, visit shrines, offer medals and candles, offer prayers Adhere to "hot" and "cold" food prescriptions and prohibitions for prevention and treatment of illness
Puerto Ricans	Subscribe to the "hot-cold" theory of causation of illness Believe some illnesses caused by evil spirits and forces	Infrequent use of health care systems Seek folk healers—use of herbs, rituals Consult spiritualist medium for mental disorders *Santeria* is system and practitioners are called *santero* Treatments classified as "hot" or "cold"

*This section was written by Lydia DeSantis, PhD, RN.

Family relationships	Communication	Comments
Strong kinship bonds in extended family; members come to aid of others in crisis Less likely to view illness as a burden Augmented families common (unrelated persons living in same household) Place strong emphasis on work and ambition Sex-role sharing among parents Elderly members respected	Alert to any evidence of discrimination Place importance on nonverbal behavior May use nonstandard English or "black English" Use "testing" behaviors to assess personnel in health care situations before seeking active care Best to use simple, direct, but caring approach	High level of caution and distrust of majority group Social anxiety related to tradition of humiliation, oppression, and loss of dignity Will elect to retain dignity rather than seek care if values are compromised Strong sense of peoplehood High incidence of poverty Black minister a strong influence in black community Visits by family minister are sought, expected, and valued in helping to cope with illness and suffering
Maintenance of family reputation is paramount Lineal authority supreme; children in a subordinate position in family hierarchy Children valued for parental social security in old age and expected to contribute to family welfare at an early age Children viewed as "gifts from god" and treated with indulgence and affection	Recent immigrants and older persons may speak only Haitian creole May prefer family/friends to act as translators and confidants Often smile and nod in agreement when do not understand Quiet and gentle communication style and lack of assertiveness lead health care providers to falsely believe they comprehend health teaching and are compliant Will not ask questions if health care provider is busy or rushed	Will use biomedical and ethnomedical (folk) systems simultaneously Resistant to dietary and work restrictions Adherence to prescribed treatments directly related to perceived severity of illness
Traditionally men considered breadwinners and key decision makers in matters outside the home; women considered homemakers Males considered big and strong *(macho)* Strong kinship; extended families include *compadres* (godparents) established by ritual kinship Children valued highly and desired, taken everywhere with family Many homes contain shrines with statues and pictures of saints Elderly treated with respect	May use nonstandard English Most bilingual; many only speak Spanish May have a strong preference for native language and revert to it in times of stress May shake hands or engage in introductory embrace Interpret prolonged eye contact as disrespectful	High degree of modesty—often a deterrent to seeking medical care and open discussions of sex Youngsters often reluctant to share communal showers in schools Relaxed concept of time—may be late for appointments More concerned with present than with future and therefore may focus on immediate solutions rather than long-term goals Magicoreligious practices common May view hospital as place to go to die
Family usually large and home centered—the core of existence Father has complete authority in family—family provider and decision maker Wife and children subordinate to father Children valued—seen as a gift from God Children taught to obey and respect parents; corporal punishment to ensure obedience	May use nonstandard English Spanish speaking or bilingual Strong sense of family privacy—may view questions regarding family as impudent	Relaxed sense of time Pay little attention to *exact* time of day Suspicious and fearful of hospitals

Continued

TABLE 16 ***Cultural Characteristics Related to Health Care—cont'd***

Cultural group	Health beliefs	Health practices
Cuban-Americans*	Prevention and good nutrition are related to good health	Diligent users of the medical model, in part because of aggressive public health practices on the island before and after the revolution Eclectic health-seeking practices, including preventive measures, extensive use of the medical model, and, in some instances, folk medicine of both religious and nonreligious origins; home remedies; in many instances seek assistance of ***santeros*** (Afro-Cuban healers) and spiritualists to complement medical treatment Nutrition is important; parents show overconcern with eating habits of their children and spend a considerable part of the budget on food; traditional Cuban diet is rich in meat and starch; consumption of fresh vegetables added in United States
Native Americans (Numerous Tribes)	Believe health is state of harmony with nature and universe Respect of bodies through proper management All disorders believed to have aspects of supernatural Violation of a restriction or prohibition thought to cause illness Fear of witchcraft May carry objects believed to guard against witchcraft Theology and medicine strongly interwoven	Medicine persons: Altruistic persons who must use powers in purely positive ways Persons capable of both good and evil—perform negative acts against enemies Diviner-diagnosticians—diagnose but do not have powers or skill to implement medical treatment Specialists—use herbs and curative but nonsacred medical procedures Medicine persons—use herbs and ritual Singers—cure by the power of their song obtained from supernatural beings; effect cures by laying on of hands

*This section was written by Mercedes Sandaval, PhD.

practitioners will write *RFV* (reason for visit). The RFV should be a short statement of why the patient has come to see the practitioner. Generally, this is just a one-line sentence in the patient's own words. For example:

"I have a cold."
"I'm out of my medicine."
"I need a physical for work."
"I'm here for a follow-up visit."

In many organizations this information is obtained by the practitioner's assistant.

History of Present Illness

The history of present illness (HPI) includes all of the pertinent information concerning the present illness. If the patient is getting a physical examination for work or school, it is important to write a statement about the patient's health at the present time and a statement about the type of work the patient does. If the examination is required for a school or sport, a statement concerning the school that the examination is for or the sport that the patient is participating in is appropriate. For example:

"Patient here for work physical. Works as nursing assistant at a local nursing home. Feeling well today."

"Patient here for sports physical. Attends Highland High School and participates in football. Feeling well today."

If the patient is being seen for an illness, the following information needs to be included in this section:

1. Signs and symptoms
2. Onset of symptoms (When did the illness start?)
3. Duration of symptoms (How long has the patient had the symptoms? If the patient has had a symptom for an extended period of time, ask why the patient decided to come in now.)
4. Frequency or timing of symptoms (Are the symptoms intermittent or constant? Do they occur with food? Without food?)
5. Severity of symptoms (How do the symptoms rate on a scale of 1 to 10 [1 being no symptoms and 10 being the worst the symptoms have ever been]?)
6. Where and what (What was the patient doing, and where was the patient when the symptoms began?)
7. Better or worse (What makes the symptoms better or worse? This is also a good time to find out what the patient has been taking or doing to try to relieve the symptoms. Particularly, ask about over-the-counter or home remedies that might have been used or alternative healers who may have been consulted.)
8. Association with other symptoms (Is the primary symptom associated with any other symptom? For example, is the chest pain associated with shortness of breath?)

Family relationships	Communication	Comments
Strong family ties with mother and father kinships Children supported and assisted by parents long after becoming adults Elderly cared for at home	Most are bilingual (English/Spanish) except for segments of the senior population	In less than 30 years Cubans have been able to obtain a higher standard of living than other Hispanic groups in United States Have been able to retain many of their former social institutions: bilingual and private schools, clinics, social clubs, the family as an extended network of support, etc. Many do not feel discriminated against nor harbor feelings of inferiority with respect to Anglo-Americans or "main-stream" population
Extended family structure—usually includes relatives from both sides of family Elder members assume leadership roles	Most continue to speak their Indian language, as well as English Nonverbal communication	Time orientation—present Respect for age Going to hospital associated with illness or disease; therefore may not seek prenatal care, since pregnancy viewed as natural process Tend to take time to form an opinion of professionals

Past Medical History

The past medical history (PMI) includes information concerning the patient's prior or continuing medical problems. Normally, the place to start is with questions concerning childhood illnesses. It is important to list the specific illness and the year it occurred, since some illnesses, such as measles, were common 20 years ago but are uncommon today. Also ask if the patient has or has ever been told that he or she has any chronic illnesses, such as diabetes, hypertension, heart disease, lung disease, kidney disease, mental illness, lupus erythematosus, sickle cell anemia, seizures, or cancer. If the patient answers any of these questions in the affirmative, find out if the patient is currently being treated for the condition and, if so, with what. Next, ask if the patient is currently taking any medication, including over-the-counter medication, on a regular or as-needed basis. Does the patient have any allergies to medications, foods, or the environment? If allergies exist, attempt to find out the type of reaction that the patient has when coming in contact with the offending agent.

Another important component of the past medical history is information regarding any hospitalizations. Find out when, where, the health care provider, and what the hospitalization was for. Determine if the hospitalization was an inpatient stay or a visit to the emergency room (ER) or outpatient clinic. Next, find out about past surgical procedures. Be sure to ask the patient about any outpatient surgery. Again, it is necessary to know where the surgery was done, why it was done, who did it, and what exactly was done. Information concerning whether the patient suffered any complications of the procedure can also provide valuable insight into the patient's health status. Has the patient been involved in any serious accidents or suffered any serious injuries? This information should include any history of fractures, head injuries, motor vehicle accidents, or gunshot or stab wounds. It is appropriate to find out the patient's immunization history. However, in the adult this may be difficult.

Family History

The family history can provide insight into any illnesses or diseases that the patient might be more prone to acquire and may be used in designing a preventive program for the patient. Ask about the patient's spouse, children, mother, father, and siblings. Obtain information about any history of strokes, blood disorders, high blood pressure, diabetes, cancer, arthritis, obesity, heart disease, lung disease, alcoholism, mental illness, seizures, or kidney disease.

Once patients reach their 60s, family history becomes less important, and a very brief summary may be listed. With younger patients it may be easier to do a genogram of the patient's family history. This can be a quick, efficient method of

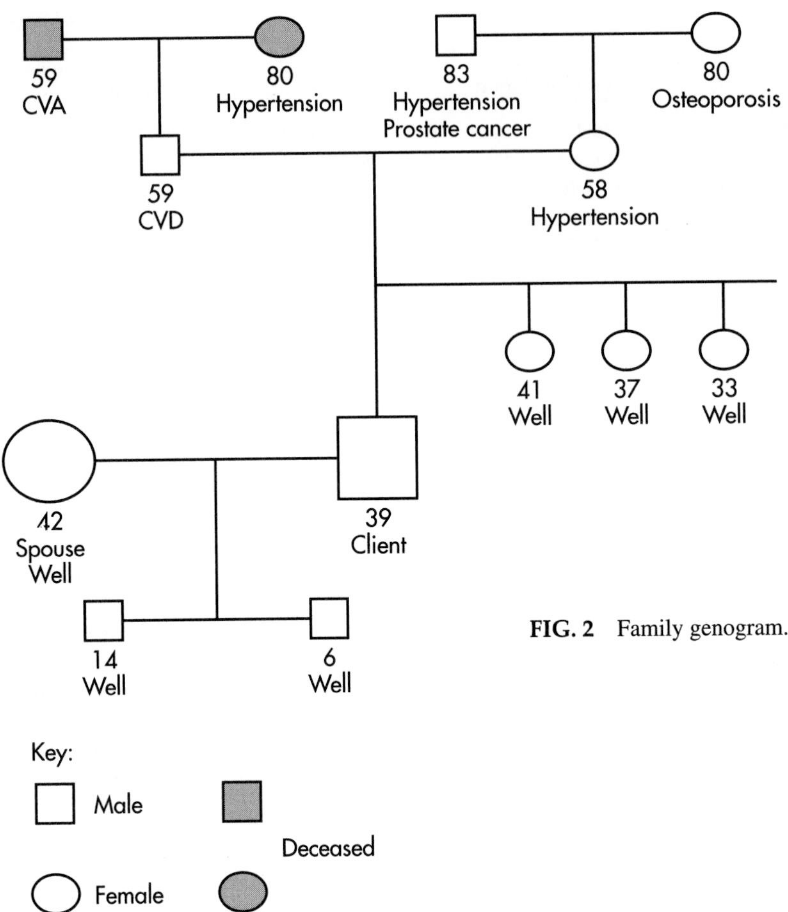

FIG. 2 Family genogram.

providing the information. For an example of a genogram, see Fig. 2.

Social History

The social history provides a more complete picture of the patient and should include information on whether the patient is married, single, or divorced, and with whom the patient lives. Do not be tempted to state, "Married, lives with spouse" just because the patient has stated that he or she is married. The best way to ascertain whom the patient lives with is to ask, "Who lives with you in your home or apartment?" This is also a good time to ask about smoking (number of packs per day and number of years), alcohol, and illicit drug use. Other questions to include regarding the patient's living situation are: "How safe is your home and neighborhood? Are environmental hazards present, such as air pollution, unsanitary conditions, or street violence?" When performing a physical examination for sports, be sure to ask about the use of anabolic steroids. Discussing these issues later in the encounter may put the patient more at ease and make him or her more willing to divulge this information.

Functional Assessment

The functional assessment should address the patient's ability to care for himself or herself. Although many practitioners believe that the functional assessment is only appropriate for the geriatric patient, it is also important to do a functional assessment on those patients who may have a physical or mental disability that may affect whether or not they are able to become or remain independent. Can the patient perform the necessary activities of daily living alone or with assistance? What is his or her diet like? How much sleep does the patient get each night? Does the patient take naps? If so, how long are they? Is exercise a routine part of the patient's daily activities? What type of exercise, and for how long? What is the patient's spiritual belief system, and how important is it to his or her daily life?

Review of Systems

The review of systems is the final step in history taking. This section of the history includes systematic questioning of the patient regarding the various body systems. Hopefully, in this section areas that may have been missed previously will be discovered. Keep in mind that the questions need to be asked in terms that the patient can understand.

Skin, hair, and nails. Ask about skin color, texture, moisture, rashes, pruritus, bruising, and any lesions. Ask about hair color, texture, growth, loss, and distribution. Find out about nail color, brittleness, ridging, and configuration.

Head and neck. Start by asking if the patient has unusually severe or frequent headaches, dizziness, syncope, severe head injury, loss of consciousness, or vertigo.

Eyes. Has the patient had any blurring of vision, double vision, sensitivity to light, or pain? How is his or her vision, and when was the last vision examination? Is there any history of trauma, glaucoma, or excessive tearing or discharge? Does the patient use eye drops? If so, what kind, and why?

Ears. Has the patient noticed any decrease in hearing? Any pain, discharge, or ringing in the ears? Any dizziness? Is there a past history of ear infections?

Nose. Ask the patient about his or her sense of smell. How often does the patient get a cold? Does the patient have any obstruction or discharge from the nose, suffer from nosebleeds, have any sinus tenderness, or suffer from allergies or hay fever?

Throat and mouth. Ask about any hoarseness or change in the voice. Inquire about the frequency of sore throats, bleeding or swelling of the gums, or any lesions of the mouth. Does the patient have any toothaches, and when was his or her last dental checkup? Does the patient have any soreness of the tongue, ulcers, or disturbance of taste?

Neck. Ask the patient about any pain, lumps, or swelling. Is there any enlargement or tenderness of the lymph nodes? Has the patient ever been told that he or she has a goiter?

Respiratory system. Ask the patient about any pain related to respiration, shortness of breath, cyanosis, or orthopnea. Ask about any cough, sputum, or hemoptysis. Does the patient have night sweats or been exposed to tuberculosis? Has the patient ever been exposed to any toxins, such as coal dust or asbestos?

Cardiovascular system. Ask the patient about any chest pain or palpitations. Does the patient have any cyanosis, shortness of breath on exertion, nocturia, or edema? If the patient complains about dyspnea on exertion, find out what type of exertion produces the dyspnea. Be sure to quantify the answer. Is there any history of murmurs, hypertension, or coronary artery disease? To determine the presence of nocturnal dyspnea, ask the patient how many pillows he or she sleeps on.

Gastrointestinal system. Ask about the patient's appetite and about indigestion, heartburn, nausea, vomiting, and any food intolerances. Ask about constipation or diarrhea. What is the patient's usual bowel pattern? Has the patient noticed any change in consistency or color of the stool? Has the patient noticed any blood in his or her stool? Has the patient been experiencing an unusual amount of flatulence? Does the patient have any history of hemorrhoids, hepatitis, bowel surgery, gallstones, ulcer, or tumors? Has the patient ever had any bowel examinations?

Genitourinary system

Urinary system. Ask if the patient suffers from dysuria, flank pain, urgency, frequency, nocturia, or incontinence. Has the patient noticed any hematuria or difficulty starting or stopping the stream? Does the patient have a history of kidney stones or any other type of kidney problems?

Genitalia. Has the patient ever been told that he or she has a sexually transmitted disease? If so, what kind, and how was it treated? For female patients, ask about the age of menarche or menopause, regularity of menses, amount of flow, and when her last menstrual period was. Does the patient have any vaginal discharge, itching, or bleeding between periods? Ask the patient if he or she is sexually active and the patient's age at first intercourse. Ask if the patient has any pain with intercourse, any sexual difficulties, or problems with infertility. Obtain pregnancy information, such as gravida, para, spontaneous abortions, or mechanical abortions. Inquire about difficulties with pregnancies and use of birth control. When was the patient's last Pap smear and breast examination? Does the patient perform breast self-examinations, and has she noticed any unusual lumps, masses, dimpling, nipple discharge, or pain? Has the patient ever had a mammogram?

For male patients, ask about the onset of puberty and about any difficulty with erections, emissions, or libido. Ask about any testicular pain. Does the patient perform testicular self-examinations? If so, how often? It is important to also ask male patients about their breasts and whether they have noticed any pain, lumps, masses, or nipple discharge.

Musculoskeletal system. Does the patient have any difficulty with joint stiffness, pain, restriction of movement, swelling, redness, heat, or bone deformity? If the patient answers yes to any of these questions, ask if the patient is taking any over-the-counter preparations for pain relief.

Neurologic system. Does the patient have syncope, seizures, numbness or tingling in extremities, paralysis, weakness, decreased sensation, poor coordination, tremors, or loss of memory?

Psychiatric history. Does the patient feel depressed, have difficulty concentrating, or difficulty sleeping? Is the patient under a great deal of stress? Has the patient ever thought about suicide? Has the patient noticed any mood changes, nervousness, or irritability?

• • •

At the end of the history-taking session, ask the patient if there is anything else that he or she would like to talk about or that has not been covered. If the patient has many problems, it might be appropriate to ask the patient which problem he or she would like to work on first. Be careful to explain to the patient that it is not always possible to handle all the problems at one time and that the other problems will be addressed on subsequent visits.

Taking a good history can be a long, arduous task, but it is well worth the effort. Many problems can be solved just by taking a thorough history. Countless time and money for expensive tests can be saved as a direct result of a comprehensive history.

Mnemonics

Even the most advanced practitioner may find mnemonics useful for remembering some of the important points when obtaining a health history. The following are some of the more common mnemonics currently in use. The first three mnemonics are used to evaluate a patient's symptom of pain. However, they can easily be applied to other symptoms as well. The remaining mnemonics are used to help remember symptoms of various conditions.

PQRST

P *Provocation. Palliative factors*—What causes the pain/symptom? What helps the pain/symptom?

Q *Quality.* What does the pain/symptom feel like? Most patients will describe the quality as one of the following:

1. Pricking, sharp, cutting, knifelike
2. Burning, hot, stinging
3. Deep, aching, boring, pounding, heavy, constricting

Generally speaking, qualities 1 and 2 indicate superficial pain, and quality 3 is deep pain that is more difficult to localize.

R *Region/radiation.* Where is the pain/symptom located, and does it travel to any other portion of the body?

S *Severity.* How severe is the pain/symptom? Ask the patient to compare the pain/symptom with something that he or she has had in the past. Sometimes it is helpful to have the patient rate the severity on a scale of 1 to 10, with 1 being no pain/symptom and 10 being the worst that the patient has ever experienced.

T *Temporal characteristics.* This relates to the timing of the pain/symptom. Is the pain constant or intermittent? How long has the patient had the pain/symptom?

Modified from DeGowin RL: *DeGowin and DeGowin's diagnostic examination,* ed 6, New York, 1994, McGraw-Hill.

COLDERRA

C *Character.* What is the character of the pain/symptom? Is it burning, stabbing, shooting, etc.?

O *Onset.* When did it start? What was the patient doing when it started?

L *Location.* Where is the pain/symptom located?

D *Duration.* How long has the patient had the pain/symptom?

E *Exacerbation.* What makes the pain/symptom worse?

R *Relief.* What provides some relief from the pain/symptom?

R *Radiation.* Does the pain/symptom radiate? If so, where?

A *Association.* Is the pain/symptom associated with any other signs or symptoms?

Modified from Winningham ML, Preusser BA: *Critical thinking in medical-surgical settings: a case study approach,* St Louis, 1996, Mosby.

CARLID BMW

C *Character.* What is the character of the pain? Is it burning, sharp, stabbing, shooting, etc?
A *Associated symptoms.* What symptoms are associated with the main symptom?
R *Radiation.* Does the pain/symptom radiate to other parts of the body? If so, where?
L *Location.* Where is the pain/symptom located?
I *Intensity.* How intense is the pain/symptom? It would be appropriate to have the patient rate the pain/symptom on a scale of 1 to 10.
D *Duration.* How long has the patient had the pain/symptom?
B *Better.* What makes the pain/symptom better?
M *Medications.* What medications, including over-the-counter medications, has the patient taken?
W *Worse.* What makes the pain/symptom worse?

Courtesy Pam Cacchione.

A B C D *Rule for malignant melanoma*

A *Asymmetry.* Are some areas of the lesion flat while others are raised?
B *Border.* Is there irregularity of the border?
C *Color.* Is the lesion variegated in color, such as blue, black, and brown?
D *Diameter.* Is the diameter increasing?

Modified from Habif TP: *Clinical dermatology: a color guide to diagnosis and therapy,* ed 3, St Louis, 1996, Mosby.

P A L S *For enlarged lymph nodes*

P *Primary site.* Make sure that a thorough assessment is done of the area where the enlarged node was found.
A *All associated nodes.* All nodes within the chain of the primary node need to be carefully assessed.
L *Liver.* A thorough assessment of the liver needs to be performed.
S *Spleen.* A thorough assessment of the spleen needs to be performed.

Modified from Shipman JJ: *Mnemonics and tactics in surgery and medicine,* London, 1984, Lloyd-Luke.

FIVE DS *For nipple assessment*

D *Discharge.* Does the patient have a discharge? If so, what color is it?
D *Depression.* This characteristic is also commonly referred to as inversion. If the nipples are depressed, is the depression unilateral or bilateral? Is the depression recent, or has the patient always had depressed nipples?
D *Discoloration.* With pregnancy, discoloration can be a normal variation.
D *Dermatologic changes.* Are there any changes in the skin of the breast or nipple?
D *Deviation.* Compare one nipple with the other.

Modified from Seidel HM et al: *Mosby's guide to physical examination,* ed 3, St Louis, 1995, Mosby.

NINE FS *Of abdominal distention*

F *Fat*
F *Fetus*
F *Full bladder*
F *Fluid*
F *Flatus*
F *False pregnancy*
F *Feces*
F *Fibroid*
F *Fatal tumor*

From Seidel HM et al: *Mosby's guide to physical examination,* ed 3, St Louis, 1995, Mosby.

PERITONITIS

P *Pain (may be in front, back, sides, or shoulders)*
E *Electrolytes fall and shock ensues*
R *Rigidity or rebound of anterior abdominal wall*
I *Immobile abdomen and patient*
T *Tenderness (rebound)*
O *Obstruction*
N *Nausea and vomiting*
I *Increasing pulse, decreasing blood pressure*
T *Temperature falls, then rises*
I *Increasing abdominal girth*
S *Silent abdomen (no bowel sounds)*

From Shipman JJ: *Mnemonics and tactics in surgery and medicine,* London, 1984, Lloyd-Luke.

CONSTIPATED

C *Congenital: Hirschsprung's disease*
O *Obstruction*
N *Neoplasms*
S *Stricture of colon*
T *Topical: painful hemorrhoids or fissure*
I *Impacted feces*
P *Prolapse of rectum*
A *Anorexia and depression*
T *Temperature high, dehydration results*
E *Endocrine: hypothyroidism*
D *Diet, diverticulitis, and drugs*

From Shipman JJ: *Mnemonics and tactics in surgery and medicine,* London, 1984, Lloyd-Luke.

CRANIAL NERVES: *On Old Olympus Towering Tops A Fin And German Viewed Some Hops.*

O *Olfactory*
O *Optic*
O *Oculomotor*
T *Trochlear*
T *Trigeminal*
A *Abducens*
F *Facial*
A *Acoustic*
G *Glossopharyngeal*
V *Vagal*
S *Spinal accessory*
H *Hypoglossal*

From Seidel HM et al: *Mosby's guide to physical examination,* ed 3, St Louis, 1995, Mosby.

DELIRIUM

D *Drugs; ethanol, bromism*
E *Electrolyte imbalance*
L *Low* Po_2
I *Injury to brain*
R *Relapsing fever*
I *Infection*
U *Uremia*
M *Metabolic*

From Shipman JJ: *Mnemonics and tactics in surgery and medicine,* London, 1984, Lloyd-Luke.

DEMENTIA

D *Drugs or toxins*
E *Endocrine*
M *Metabolic and mechanical*
E *Epilepsy*
N *Nutritional status and nervous system*
T *Tumor or trauma*
I *Infection*
A *Arterial insufficiency*

From Shipman JJ: *Mnemonics and tactics in surgery and medicine,* London, 1984, Lloyd-Luke.

Causes of incontinence: D R I P

D *Delirium*
R *Restricted mobility or retention*
I *Infection, inflammation, or impaction*
P *Pharmaceutical or polyuria*

Modified from Driscoll CE: The genitourinary system. In Driscoll CE et al, editors: *The family practice desk reference,* ed 3, St Louis, 1996, Mosby.

D I A P P E R S *For incontinence*

D *Delirium*
I *Infection*
A *Atrophic urethritis or vaginitis*
P *Pharmaceuticals*
P *Psychologic*
E *Endocrine*
R *Restricted mobility*
S *Stool impaction*

Modified from Driscoll CE: The genitourinary system. In Driscoll CE et al, editors: *The family practice desk reference,* ed 3, St Louis, 1996, Mosby.

S O U P *For incontinence*

S *Stress*
O *Overflow*
U *Urge*
P *Psychologic*

Modified from Driscoll CE: The genitourinary system. In Driscoll CE et al, editors: *The family practice desk reference,* ed 3, St Louis, 1996, Mosby.

CHILD HEALTH HISTORY QUESTIONNAIRE (SAMPLE)

CONFIDENTIAL

Child's Name ______________ Age ______________ Sex M F Date of Birth ______________
(circle)

PREGNANCY AND BIRTH

Please complete this section if your child is under age 2 years.

	Yes	No
Was this pregnancy planned?	☐	☐
Did the mother smoke during pregnancy?	☐	☐
Did the mother drink alcohol during pregnancy (beer, wine or mixed drinks)?	☐	☐
Did the mother take any medications during pregnancy? Please list ______________	☐	☐
Did the mother take any other drugs during pregnancy? Please list ______________	☐	☐

Please circle any problems during pregnancy:

Bleeding	Edema	High blood pressure
Kidney infection	Diabetes	Vaginal infection

Birthweight _____ lb. _____ oz.
Was birth ☐ on time ☐ late ☐ early?
Was delivery ☐ vaginal ☐ C-section?
Did the mother have any problems during or after labor and delivery? ☐ Yes ☐ No

Please circle any problems your baby had in the hospital:

Yellow jaundice	Turned blue	Seizures	Vomiting
Breathing trouble	Infection	Constipation	

DEVELOPMENT

Please complete this section if your child is under age 2 years. Please list the age in months when your child did each of these:

Smiled	______________	Crawled	______________
Transferred objects from one hand to the other	______________	Walked alone	______________
		Said 2 words	______________
Turned head to voice	______________	Fed him/herself	______________
Sat alone	______________	Said 10 words	______________

FAMILY HISTORY

Please complete this section for any-age child.

Mother's name ______________ Age ______________ Living at home? ☐ Yes ☐ No
Mother's health ______________ Occupation ______________
Father's name ______________ Age ______________ Living at home? ☐ Yes ☐ No
Father's health ______________ Occupation ______________
Brothers and sisters:

Names	Birth Dates	Health Problems	Shots up-to-date? Yes	No
______	______	______	☐	☐
______	______	______	☐	☐
______	______	______	☐	☐

Please circle any of these diseases that your child's grandparents, parents, aunts, uncles, brothers, or sisters have or have had:

Asthma	Hay fever	Eczema	Tuberculosis	Kidney trouble	Depression
High cholesterol	Diabetes	Seizures	Stroke	Heart attack	Hearing loss
SIDS	Heart murmurs	Alcoholism	Cancer	Drug addiction	Other ______

Courtesy Methodist Hospital of Indiana, Inc.

Continued

CHILD HEALTH HISTORY QUESTIONNAIRE (SAMPLE)—cont'd

SAFETY

Please answer for any-age child.

	Yes	No
Does anyone smoke at home?	☐	☐
Do you have a smoke detector at home?	☐	☐
Do you have any guns in your home?	☐	☐
If your child is under age 5, do you have ipecac syrup and the Poison Control phone # posted in your home?	☐	☐
Is your hot water heater turned down to 120°?	☐	☐
If your child rides a bicycle, does he/she wear a helmet?	☐	☐
Do you know how to do the Heimlich maneuver for children?	☐	☐
Do you use a #15 (or higher) sunscreen on your child?	☐	☐

DENTAL

Please answer for any-age child.

	Yes	No
Do you have well water in your home?	☐	☐

Please answer if child is 2 years or older.

	Yes	No
Does your child brush his/her teeth daily?	☐	☐
Does your child see a dentist regularly?	☐	☐

SCHOOL

Please answer if child has started school.

	Yes	No
Has your child failed any grades?	☐	☐
Has your child had any learning problems?	☐	☐
Has your child been absent from school more than 10 days a year?	☐	☐

SOCIAL

Please check if any of these concerns are troubling your family.

________ Hospital bills ________ Housing/rent/heat
________ Occupation ________ Emotional problems/nerves
________ Transportation ________ Community agencies
________ Legal ________ Other money matters
________ Marriage ________ Other stresses ________

NUTRITION

Please answer for any-age child.

	Yes	No
Does your child have any eating problems?	☐	☐

Please answer if child is over age 1 year.

	Yes	No
Do you limit sweets, fats, and junk food?	☐	☐
Does your child eat foods from each of the 4 Food Groups (fruits and vegetables, breads and cereals, dairy products, meats) daily?	☐	☐
Does your child skip meals?	☐	☐
Does your child eat paint chips or chew on window sills?	☐	☐
Is your child in the WIC program?	☐	☐

BEHAVIOR

Please answer if child is age 1 year or older by checking any behavior problems that your child has.

________ Temper tantrums ________ Steals
________ Whines ________ Lies
________ Cries easily ________ Hyperactive
________ Hits or bites ________ Short attention span
________ Shyness ________ Disobedient
________ Sleep problems ________ Talks back

HABITS

Please answer if child is 1 year or older.

	Yes	No
Does your child watch more than 1 or 2 hours of TV daily?	☐	☐
Does your child always use a car seat or seat belt?	☐	☐
Does your child exercise regularly?	☐	☐
Does your child have a regular bedtime?	☐	☐

CHILD HEALTH HISTORY QUESTIONNAIRE (SAMPLE)—cont'd

PAST ILLNESSES

Please check any illnesses or problems that your child has had.

_____ Asthma
_____ Hay fever
_____ Eczema
_____ Kidney trouble
_____ Heart murmur
_____ Seizures
_____ High cholesterol
_____ Hearing loss
_____ Chickenpox
_____ Pneumonia
_____ Frequent sore throats
_____ Frequent headaches
_____ Speech problems
_____ Bed-wetting
_____ Constipation
_____ Kidney or bladder infection
_____ Frequent ear infections
_____ Other _____

IMMUNIZATIONS/TB TESTS

Please list the month and year of any shots or TB tests your child has had.

	Dates				
DPT/DT	_____	_____	_____	_____	_____
Polio	_____	_____	_____	_____	_____
HIB	_____	_____	_____	_____	
Measles	_____	_____			
Rubella	_____	_____			
Mumps	_____	_____			
TB tests	_____	_____	_____	_____	_____

SURGERY

Please check any surgery that your child has had.

_____ Tubes in ears
_____ Tonsils/adenoids
_____ Hernia
_____ Appendix
_____ Other _____

ALLERGIES

Please check any allergies that your child has had and write down the reactions.

	Reaction
_____ Penicillin	_____
_____ Amoxicillin	_____
_____ Sulfa (Bactrim or Septra)	_____
_____ Erythromycin	_____
_____ Cefaclor (Ceclor)	_____
_____ Aspirin	_____
_____ Codeine	_____
_____ Insect sting	_____
_____ Foods: (list)	_____
_____ _____	_____
_____ _____	_____
_____ Other	
_____ _____	_____

MEDICINES

Please list any medicines that your child takes every day, including prescription and over-the-counter medicines.

_____
_____
_____

INJURIES

Please list the date and type of any serious injuries your child has had.

Date	Type of Injury
_____	_____
_____	_____

HOSPITALIZATIONS

Please list the date and reasons if your child has ever been in the hospital.

Date	Reason
_____	_____
_____	_____
_____	_____
_____	_____

ADOLESCENT HEALTH HISTORY QUESTIONNAIRE (SAMPLE)

CONFIDENTIAL

Name ______________________ Age ______________ Date ______________

PAST ILLNESSES

Please check any illnesses you have had.

_______ Asthma
_______ Hay fever
_______ Eczema
_______ Tuberculosis
_______ Kidney trouble
_______ Heart murmur
_______ High cholesterol
_______ Rheumatic fever
_______ Seizures
_______ Hepatitis
_______ Hearing loss
_______ Urinary tract infection
_______ Chickenpox
_______ Mumps
_______ Pneumonia
_______ Other ______________________

ALLERGIES

Please check any allergies that you have had and write down the reactions.

		Reaction
_____ Penicillin		_______
_____ Amoxicillin		_______
_____ Sulfa		_______
_____ Aspirin		_______
_____ Codeine		_______
_____ Insect sting		_______
_____ Foods: (list)		_______
_______	_______	_______
_______	_______	_______
_____ Other		
_______	_______	_______

FEMALES ONLY

Age at 1st menstrual period _______
Have you ever had sex? ☐ Yes ☐ No

If the answer is "yes," please answer these questions:

Number of times pregnant _______
Number of living children _______
Date of last Pap smear _______
Birth control method: (circle)

none	pills	condoms	IUD
diaphragm	sponge	rhythm	

Do you consider yourself to be:
☐ heterosexual (straight)
☐ lesbian
☐ bisexual

MALES ONLY

Have you ever had sex? ☐ Yes ☐ No

If the answer is "yes," please answer these questions:

Do you use condoms (rubbers)? ☐ Yes ☐ No
Do you consider yourself to be:
☐ heterosexual (straight)
☐ gay
☐ bisexual

SURGERY

Please check any surgery that you have had.

_______ Appendix
_______ Tonsils/adenoids
_______ Tubes in ear
_______ Hernia
_______ Other ______________________

Courtesy Methodist Hospital of Indiana, Inc.

ADOLESCENT HEALTH HISTORY QUESTIONNAIRE (SAMPLE)—cont'd

IMMUNIZATIONS

Please write down the month and year of any shots you have had.

	Dates				
DPT/DT	____	____	____	____	____
Polio	____	____	____	____	____
HIB	____	____	____	____	
Measles	____	____			
Rubella	____	____			
Mumps	____	____			

INJURIES

Please list the date and type of any serious injuries you have had.

Date	Type of Injury
____	____
____	____
____	____

PRESENT MEDICATIONS

Please list any medicines that you take every day including prescription and over-the-counter medicines.

____
____
____
____

HOSPITALIZATIONS

Please list date and reasons for all hospitalizations.

Date	Reason
____	____
	____
____	____
	____

FAMILY HISTORY

Mother's name ____ Age ____ Living at home? ☐ Yes ☐ No
Mother's health ____ Occupation ____
Father's name ____ Age ____ Living at home? ☐ Yes ☐ No
Father's heatlh ____ Occupation ____

Brothers and sisters:

Names	Birth Dates	Health Problems
____	____	____
____	____	____
____	____	____

Please circle any of these diseases that your child's grandparents, parents, aunts, uncles, brothers, or sisters have or have had:

Asthma	Hay fever	Stroke	Kidney trouble	Depression
High cholesterol	Diabetes	Seizures	Heart attack	Other ____
Familial polyposis	High blood pressure	Alcholism	Cancer	

Continued

ADOLESCENT HEALTH HISTORY QUESTIONNAIRE (SAMPLE)—cont'd

PERSONAL HISTORY

	Check Yes	No
Do you have any trouble reading?	☐	☐
Do you have any special interests or hobbies?	☐	☐
Please list ______		
Do you get regular dental checkups?	☐	☐
Do you exercise at least 3 times a week?	☐	☐
Do you limit sweets, fats, and junk food in your diet?	☐	☐
Do you always wear your seat belt?	☐	☐
Do you wear a helmet when you ride a bicycle or motorcycle?	☐	☐
Do you limit sun exposure or use sunscreens (#15 or higher) when tanning?	☐	☐
Have you ever been physically or sexually abused?	☐	☐
Do you smoke cigarettes?	☐	☐
Packs per day ______ Years ______		
Do you chew tobacco?	☐	☐
Do you smoke pot?	☐	☐
Have you ever taken steroids?	☐	☐
Do you ever use alcohol or drugs to feel better?	☐	☐
Do your friends get drunk or high at parties?	☐	☐
Do you get drunk or high at parties?	☐	☐
Have you been drunk more than 10 times?	☐	☐
Have your grades gone down recently?	☐	☐
Have you ever been arrested?	☐	☐

Below are some common concerns of teenagers. Please check "yes" or "no" to let us know if you have any of these concerns.

	Yes	No
Feeling "bummed out," down, or depressed	☐	☐
Trouble sleeping	☐	☐
Tired during the day	☐	☐
Pain with menstrual periods	☐	☐
Dizzy spells	☐	☐
Frequent headaches	☐	☐
Stomach pains	☐	☐
Worried about school	☐	☐
Worried about sex	☐	☐
Worried about my height	☐	☐
Worried about my weight	☐	☐
Worried about my parents' relationship	☐	☐
Other concerns ______		

The rest of these questions are for you to see if you might be at risk to get AIDS. **You do not have to write down your answers,** but if any answers are "yes," you could be at risk for AIDS, and you should talk to your doctor about it.

	Yes	No
Have you had more than one sexual partner in the past year?	☐	☐
Has your partner had sex with anyone other than you since you have been partners?	☐	☐
Have you or your sexual partners ever used IV drugs?	☐	☐
Have any of your sexual partners had AIDS or a positive HIV test?	☐	☐
Have you ever had a venereal disease (VD)?	☐	☐
Did you have a blood transfusion between 1979 and 1985?	☐	☐
Have you had sex without using condoms when unsure of your sexual partners?	☐	☐
FOR MALES:		
Have you ever had sexual contact with a male?	☐	☐
FOR FEMALES:		
Have any of your sexual partners been bisexual males, or have they had sex with other males?	☐	☐

ADULT HEALTH HISTORY QUESTIONNAIRE (SAMPLE)

CONFIDENTIAL

Name ______________________ Date ______________ Occupation ______________

PAST ILLNESSES

Please check any illnesses you have had.

_____ Asthma
_____ Hay fever
_____ Emphysema
_____ TB
_____ Kidney trouble
_____ High blood pressure
_____ Heart trouble
_____ High cholesterol
_____ Rheumatic fever
_____ Diabetes
_____ Stroke
_____ Cancer ______________ (type)
_____ Anemia
_____ Arthritis
_____ Gout
_____ Abnormal Pap smear
_____ Stomach ulcer
_____ Mental illness
_____ Seizures
_____ Depression
_____ Back trouble
_____ Bowel trouble
_____ Thyroid disease
_____ Glaucoma
_____ Gallstones
_____ Hepatitis
_____ Liver problems
_____ Bleeding problems
_____ Skin problems
_____ Alcohol problem
_____ Drug addiction
_____ Hearing loss
_____ Polyps of bowel
_____ Sexually transmitted disease (VD)
_____ Other ______________

IMMUNIZATIONS

Please check any immunizations you have had and write down the year.

		Year
_____	Rubella	_____
_____	Measles	_____
_____	Tetanus	_____
_____	Pneumovax	_____
_____	Hepatitis B	_____

ALLERGIES

Please check any allergies that you have had and write down the reactions.

		Reactions
_____	Penicillin	_____
_____	Sulfa	_____
_____	Aspirin	_____
_____	Codeine	_____
_____	Bee stings	_____
_____	Foods: _____	_____
	_____	_____
_____	Other: _____	_____

SURGERY

Please check any surgery you have had.

_____ Appendix
_____ Tonsils
_____ Hernia
_____ Gall bladder

Women only

_____ Uterus
_____ Ovaries
_____ Breast
_____ D & C
_____ Tubal ligation
_____ Other ______________

Men only

_____ Testes
_____ Prostate
_____ Vasectomy
_____ Other ______________

HOSPITALIZATIONS

Please list dates and reasons for all hospitalizations.

Date	Reason
_____	______________
	______________
_____	______________
	______________

MEDICATIONS

Please list any medicines that you take, including prescription and over-the-counter medicines.

____
____
____
____
____
____

WOMEN ONLY

Age at 1st menstrual period _____
# of times pregnant _____
# of living children _____
Date of last Pap smear _____
Age when periods stopped _____
Birth control method: (circle)
pills condoms IUD sponge tubal
rhythm diaphragm vasectomy none

MEN AND WOMEN

Do you consider yourself to be:
☐ heterosexual (straight)
☐ gay
☐ bisexual

FAMILY HISTORY

Please check the diseases that your parents, grandparents, aunts, uncles, brothers, or sisters have or have had.

_____ Diabetes
_____ Asthma
_____ Stroke
_____ Cancer ______________ (type)
_____ Alcoholism
_____ Seizures
_____ Mental illness
_____ Heart attack
_____ High blood pressure
_____ Familial polyposis
_____ Other ______________

Courtesy Methodist Hospital of Indiana, Inc.

Continued

ADULT HEALTH HISTORY QUESTIONNAIRE (SAMPLE)—cont'd

PERSONAL HISTORY

	Check Yes	No
Do you have any trouble reading?	☐	☐
# years of school completed ______		
Do you have any special interests or hobbies?	☐	☐
Please list ______		
Do you have any personal concerns which are troubling you?	☐	☐

If "yes," please check those concerns:

☐ Hospital bills	☐ Family	☐ Housing/rent/heat
☐ Social Security	☐ Marriage	☐ Other money matters (food, clothing, etc.)
☐ Occupation	☐ Sex	☐ Community agencies (Welfare, etc.)
☐ Transportation	☐ Loneliness	☐ Emotional problems/nerves
☐ Legal	☐ Death	☐ Other ______

	Yes	No
Would you like to talk with our chaplain/counselor or social worker?	☐	☐
Would you like to talk with our nutritionist?	☐	☐
Do you get regular dental checkups?	☐	☐
Do you exercise at least 3 times a week?	☐	☐
Are you satisfied with your sex life?	☐	☐
Do you always wear your seat belt?	☐	☐
Do you keep a gun in your home?	☐	☐
Do you have smoke detectors in your home?	☐	☐
Do you limit sun exposure or use sunscreens (#15 or higher) when tanning?	☐	☐
Have you ever been physically or sexually abused?	☐	☐
Did you ever receive x-ray treatment to your upper body?	☐	☐
Do you smoke cigarettes?	☐	☐
Packs per day ______ Years ______		
Do you smoke cigars?	☐	☐
Do you use snuff or chewing tobacco?	☐	☐
Do you drink alcohol (beer, wine or mixed drinks)?	☐	☐
# drinks per day ______		
If you have 2 or more drinks a day, please answer these four questions:		
Have you ever felt a need to cut down on your drinking?	☐	☐
Have you ever been annoyed by criticism of your drinking?	☐	☐
Have you ever had guilty feelings about your drinking?	☐	☐
Do you ever drink a morning eye-opener?	☐	☐
Do you smoke pot?	☐	☐
Do you use other drugs?	☐	☐

The rest of these questions are for you to see if you might be at risk to get AIDS. **You do not have to write down your answers,** but if any answers are "yes," you could be at risk for AIDS, and you should talk to your doctor about it.

	Yes	No
Have you had more than one sexual partner in the past year?	☐	☐
Has your partner had sex with anyone other than you since you have been partners?	☐	☐
Have you or your sexual partners ever used IV drugs?	☐	☐
Have any of your sexual partners had AIDS or a positive HIV test?	☐	☐
Have you ever had a venereal disease (VD)?	☐	☐
Did you have a blood transfusion between 1979 and 1985?	☐	☐
Have you had sex without using condoms when unsure of your sexual partners?	☐	☐
FOR MEN:		
Have you had sexual contact with a man in the past 10 years?	☐	☐
FOR WOMEN:		
Have any of your sexual partners been bisexual men, or have they had sex with other men?	☐	☐

REFERENCES

DeGowin RL: *DeGowin and DeGowin's diagnostic examination,* ed 6, New York, 1994, McGraw-Hill.

Driscoll CE: The genitourinary system. In Driscoll CE et al, editors: *The family practice desk reference,* St Louis, 1996, Mosby.

Habif TP: *Clinical dermatology: a color guide to diagnosis and therapy,* ed 3, St Louis, 1996, Mosby.

Jarvis C: *Physical examination and health assessment,* Philadelphia, 1992, WB Saunders.

Osdol WV, Johnston PE: *Quality medical records for primary care centers,* Indianapolis, 1989, Methodist Hospital of Indiana.

Seidel HM et al: *Mosby's guide to physical examination,* ed 3, St Louis, 1995, Mosby.

Shipman JJ: *Mnemonics and tactics in surgery and medicine,* London, 1984, Lloyd-Luke.

Winningham ML, Preusser BA: *Critical thinking in medical-surgical settings,* St Louis, 1996, Mosby.

PART THREE

Physical Examination

This part presents a review of the physical examination. Some of the more common pieces of equipment used during a physical examination are discussed, as well as the skills needed to perform a complete physical examination and the order in which to perform the examination.

EQUIPMENT

Having the proper equipment and knowing how to use it are of utmost importance when performing a physical examination. The most valuable pieces of "equipment" are the practitioner's own eyes, ears, and hands. Even in the most dismal situation, these are available. The following is a discussion of some of the more common pieces of equipment used in clinics today.

Basic Requirements

First it is necessary to have adequate space and lighting. There should be a table for the patient to sit or lie on and enough room for the practitioner to walk around the table. Lighting should be indirect (should not cast shadows). A freestanding lamp that can be directed toward areas needing more illumination is helpful. The temperature in the room should be warm enough that the patient feels comfortable dressed in a paper gown, but not so warm that the patient perspires. There should be some way for the examiner to wash his or her hands; there needs to be a sink with soap and water available or a germicidal hand-washing solution that does not require the use of water. Gloves must also be available. REMEMBER: Wearing gloves does not mean that you do not have to wash your hands. Hand washing is still the most effective method of preventing the spread of infection.

Scale

There should be a scale with a height attachment, a thermometer, and a sphygmomanometer. These items are necessary for measuring the patient's height, weight, and vital signs.

Stethoscope

The stethoscope should be a personal item of the practitioner.

Tongue Blades

Tongue blades are necessary to aid in the inspection of the mouth, tongue, and pharynx.

Snellen Chart

The Snellen chart is used to assess far vision. The chart consists of various letters in various sizes. Each line of letters has a set of standardized numbers at the end of the line. The numbers indicate the patient's visual acuity when read from a distance of 20 feet. There is also a Snellen chart that consists of the letter E in different positions. This version is for use with children or adults who are unable to read. Instead of reading the letters, the patient states which way the legs of the E are facing.

Specially designed charts, such as the Rosenbaum or Jaeger, can be used to test near vision. If these charts are unavailable, simply use newsprint.

Ophthalmoscope

The ophthalmoscope is used to visualize the interior structures of the eyes. It consists of mirrors, lenses, and a light source with aperture. The lens can be adjusted from −20 to +40 diopters. These variously powered lenses allow the examiner to bring into focus the structures of the internal eye. Start with the lens set on 0 and adjust accordingly. The aperture can be adjusted depending on what is being visualized. The large aperture, the one most commonly used, casts a large, round beam of light. The small aperture is for use with small pupils. The red-free filter produces a green beam for the examination of the optic disc for pallor and minute vessel changes. The red-free filter also changes the appearance of blood to black, permitting recognition of retinal hemorrhages. The slit aperture allows examination of the anterior eye. The grid aperture allows the examiner to approximate the size of fundal lesions.

To perform the fundoscopic examination, start with the lens set at 0. When examining the patient's left eye, use your left eye. When examining the patient's right eye, use your right eye. Darken the room, and start with the ophthalmoscope about 12 inches from the patient's eye and locate the red reflex. Once the red reflex is located, move the ophthalmoscope closer to the patient to visualize the internal structures, vessels, cup, and disc. Adjust the lens to the appropriate setting to focus on the structures. It is important to tell the patient not to look at the light, but to focus on a spot on the wall. The last area to assess is the macula. This is the site of central vision and is usually 2 disc diameters temporally from the disc. It may be difficult to examine this area without the pupil being dilated with a mydriatic. Light in this area causes intense pupillary constriction and may cause tearing. It may be helpful to ask the patient to look directly at the light to help bring this area into your field of vision.

Tuning Fork

Tuning forks are used for screening the patient's hearing ability and for vibratory sensation. To activate the tuning fork, gently squeeze the prongs while holding the base. The tuning fork can also be activated by gently striking the prongs on the heel of the hand while holding the base. The tuning fork is also used to perform the Weber and Rinne tests (see Assessment Tests at the end of this chapter).

Otoscope

The otoscope is used to visualize the ear canal, tympanic membrane, and underlying structures. A speculum, the size of which is based on the size of the patient's external canal, is attached to the end of the otoscope. A glass plate acts as the viewing window and magnifies the structures. Most otoscopes have a pneumatic attachment that allows for insufflation of air onto the tympanic membrane to assess for mobility. If this attachment is not available, having the patient perform Valsalva's maneuver (holding the nose and blowing) will provide the same information.

When performing the examination, hold the otoscope between the thumb and index finger with the otoscope supported by the middle finger. Place the ulnar side of the hand holding the otoscope against the patient's cheek or head. This helps to stabilize the patient's head. Use the left hand for the left ear and the right hand for the right ear. Gently tilt the patient's head toward the opposite shoulder and pull the auricle up and back to better visualize the membrane. For infants and young children, it is necessary to pull the auricle down. Gently insert the speculum into the canal about 1 to 1.5 cm. Avoid inserting the speculum too far, since doing so can be painful. Inspect the external auditory canal and the tympanic membrane.

The otoscope can also be used as a nasal speculum, or a separate instrument (a nasal speculum) can be used to inspect the nasal cavity. When inspecting the nares, be sure to insert the speculum slowly and avoid touching the nasal septum, since touching the septum causes pain.

Percussion (Reflex) Hammer

The percussion hammer is used to test deep tendon reflexes. The hammer should be held between the thumb and index finger. Movement of the hammer should come from the wrist, not the arm, so that the hammer swings loosely. The hammer should strike the tendon quickly and smoothly and should not come to rest on the tendon.

The percussion hammer consists of a flat side and a pointed side. The flat side is more useful for striking the patient directly. Use the pointed side when striking your own thumb, such as in testing the brachial reflex.

Vaginal Speculum

The vaginal speculum is used to visualize the internal female genitalia. The instrument consists of two blades and a handle. Vaginal specula come in a variety of sizes and are either plastic or metal. The metal speculum has two positioning devices located on the handle. The plastic speculum has one positioning device, which is a ratchet-type mechanism. To become comfortable with their use, it is important to practice with both types of specula.

To insert the speculum, place two fingers just inside the vaginal opening and apply downward pressure. Next, take the speculum in the opposite hand and, with the blades closed, insert the tip of the blades in the vertical position. Remove your fingers while advancing the speculum at a 45-degree angle, rotating it to the horizontal position. Once the speculum is completely inserted, open the blades. Then sweep the speculum slowly upward to visualize the cervix.

Tape Measure

A tape measure is used to measure circumference, length, and diameter. It is helpful if the tape measure has markings for both inches and metric units. Tape measures can be found in a variety of materials.

Penlight

The penlight can be used as a direct light source for such things as checking pupillary response or examining the nares. The penlight may also come in handy when performing suture removal or assessing a small skin lesion.

VITAL SIGNS

Vital signs are an important part of the physical examination. They can give the practitioner a baseline from which to begin the assessment and an overview of the patient's health status. Vital signs may be checked by the practitioner's assistant or by the practitioner. Checking the vital signs may be done at the beginning of the patient encounter, before taking the patient history, or during the examination.

The vital signs consist of temperature, respirations, pulse, and blood pressure.

Temperature

The patient's temperature can give the practitioner some insight into the severity of the patient's illness. The temperature can be measured orally, rectally, at the axilla, or using the tympanic membrane. Most institutions are now using digital/electronic thermometers, which have substantially decreased the amount of time necessary to take the temperature. For measuring the temperature using the tympanic membrane, a special tympanic thermometer must be used. Regardless of the method used, some type of disposable cover must be placed over the end of the probe.

Respirations

Respirations are defined as the number of times the patient inhales and exhales in a minute. Observe the rise and fall of the patient's chest for 1 minute to count the number of respirations. It may be helpful to place one hand on the patient's chest to feel the movement. While observing this rise and fall, also note the effort required for breathing and the use of accessory muscles.

Pulse Rate

The pulse rate is obtained by counting the number of times the patient's heart beats in 1 minute. The pulse can be obtained at any pulse site. However, the most common sites are the radial and the apical pulses.

To take a radial pulse, place the pads of two fingers over the radial pulse and count the number of pulsations. The pulsations can be counted for 15 seconds and the number multiplied by 4 to obtain the pulse rate for 1 minute. While counting the pulse, note the rate, rhythm, force, and elasticity. If the rhythm is irregular, count the pulse for 1 full minute.

To take the apical pulse, place a stethoscope over the point of maximal impulse (PMI) and count the heartbeats. Again this can be done for 15 seconds and multiplied by 4. However, if the pulse is irregular, it must be counted for 1 full minute.

Blood Pressure

Blood pressure is the force of the blood pushing on the vessel walls. The systolic pressure is the force exerted during systole or left ventricular contraction and is the maximum pressure exerted on the vessel walls. The diastolic pressure is the pressure exerted during relaxation of the ventricle.

The blood pressure is usually measured using a stethoscope and a sphygmomanometer. Electronic cuffs, which do not require the use of a stethoscope, are also available. The sphygmomanometer consists of a cuff with a rubber bladder, a pressure gauge, and a rubber bulb with a valve for inflating and deflating the rubber bladder. The width of the bladder should be one third to one half the circumference of the extremity. When taking the blood pressure, make sure you have the proper-size cuff. If the cuff bladder is too narrow, an erroneously high reading may be obtained.

The most common site for obtaining the blood pressure measurement is at the brachial pulse. The cuff is placed approximately 2 to 3 cm above the antecubital crease, with the bladder centered over the brachial artery. Palpate the brachial artery and inflate the cuff until the brachial artery is no longer palpable, and continue inflating 20 to 30 mm Hg above this point. Place the stethoscope over the brachial artery and begin releasing the air from the cuff at the rate of about 2 mm Hg per beat. Listen for the first two consecutive beats; this is the systolic pressure, or phase 1 of Korotkoff sounds. Next, note the point when the sounds become muffled; this is phase 4 of Korotkoff sounds and is also the first diastolic sound. Next, note the point at which the sounds disappear; this is the second diastolic sound, or phase 5 of the Korotkoff sounds. Most authorities, including the American Heart Association, recommend recording all three readings for the blood pressure (e.g., 128/88/84). It is important to note the difference between the systolic and diastolic pressures. This number is known as the pulse pressure and is normally between 30 and 40 mm Hg. Widened pulse pressure may occur normally in patients with hypertension or may be an abnormal sign found in aortic regurgitation, thyrotoxicosis, coarctation of the aorta, or stress/anxiety states. A narrowed pulse pressure can occur in tachycardia, severe aortic stenosis, constrictive pericarditis, pericardial effusion, or ascites.

HEIGHT AND WEIGHT

The patient's height and weight should also be obtained. For adults, height and weight are usually measured using a platform scale with a height attachment. Before weighing the patient, make sure the scale is properly calibrated. This is done by placing the weights all the way to the left. The balance beam should center itself. Have the patient stand on the platform facing the height attachment, and move the weights until the balance beam is balanced. Read the weight off of the scale on the balance beam. To measure the patient's height, have the patient face away from the height attachment. Pull the height attachment up and then position the headpiece at the patient's crown. The height of the patient is listed in feet and inches on the height attachment.

SUBJECTIVE AND OBJECTIVE DATA

Subjective data for the patient encounter are provided through the health history described in Part Two. The physical assessment or examination provides the objective data for the patient encounter. To perform an adequate physical assessment, the practitioner needs to be proficient in the four skills used during the assessment. These skills and the order in which they should be performed are inspection, palpation, percussion, and auscultation. This is the order used in all areas of the body with the exception of the abdomen. The order for the abdominal assessment is inspection, auscultation, palpation, and percussion, because performing palpation before auscultation will cause an increase in peristalsis, yielding an inaccurate evaluation of bowel sounds.

Inspection

To perform an adequate inspection, the practitioner needs to develop the art of observation. Inspection is performed by "looking at" the patient. It is important to remember to look at both sides of the patient and compare the right with the left and the front with the back. Inspection begins when the practitioner first meets the patient and continues through the history-taking process and the physical examination. When performing the inspection, remember to use your nose, as well as your eyes. Unusual odors can alert the skilled practitioner to underlying disease processes. When inspecting a patient, do not hurry. If something unusual is observed, do not be afraid to question the patient about the finding. Often, the patient is very aware of the deviation and can provide valuable information about it. Remember, you can learn a great deal by listening to what the patient has to say.

Palpation

Palpation uses the sense of touch to assess and gather information regarding the patient's health. Different areas of the hand are used to provide different types of information. For instance, the dorsal surface of the hand is best used to discriminate temperature. This measurement is a rather crude one; however, it is useful in differentiating temperature differences when comparing two areas of the body. The palmer surface of the fingers and the finger pads are more sensitive than the fingertips. These areas are used when determining position, texture, size, consistency, crepitus, masses, and fluid. Palpation can be either light or deep. Whether it is considered light or deep depends on the amount of pressure exerted. Usually, during light palpation the skin is depressed no more than 1 cm, and during deep palpation the skin is depressed up to about 4 cm. Light palpation should precede deep palpation. If the patient has indicated in his or her history that an area to be palpated is painful, palpate that area last.

Percussion

Percussion requires striking one object with another to produce a sound. The type of sound produced is dependent on the density of the underlying tissue. The sounds are commonly described as tympanic, hyperresonant, resonant, dull, and flat. Tympany is loud and high pitched with a drumlike quality. Hyperresonance is very loud and low pitched with a boomlike quality. Resonance is loud and low pitched with a hollow quality. A dull sound is soft to moderately loud with a moderate to high pitch and a thudlike quality. A flat sound is soft and high pitched with a dull or dead quality.

Percussion can be performed either directly or indirectly. Most practitioners find that the indirect method is the most beneficial and least threatening to the patient. In the indirect method the practitioner uses one or two fingers of the nondominant hand as the striking plate and the fingertips of one or two fingers on the opposite hand as the striker. The fingers used as the striking plate must be placed firmly against the skin to produce the desired sound. Snap the wrist of the other hand sharply, allowing the fingertips of either the middle finger or the middle and first finger to strike the interphalangeal joints of the striking plate. This skill takes some practice to master. Many new practitioners want to use the elbow or shoulder to provide the movement, but wrist action is what is required.

The direct method of percussion is done by tapping directly on the patient's body. Fist percussion is commonly used to elicit tenderness over the gallbladder or kidney. This can be done by applying a blow directly to the area or by hitting the stationary hand with the fist. Another type of direct percussion is done by using the percussion hammer (e.g., to elicit deep tendon reflexes).

Auscultation

Auscultation is the art of listening to sounds that are produced by the body. Some body sounds can be heard with the naked ear. However, the majority of body sounds require a stethoscope in order to be heard. It is imperative that the practitioner find a stethoscope that is a "perfect fit." The earpieces should fit snugly, but not so snug that they cause pain. The tubing on the stethoscope should be short enough that the sound does not get lost in the tubing. Ideally, the tubing should be a single tube no longer than 12 to 15 inches.

The stethoscope should have both a bell and a diaphragm. The bell is a hollow cone that has a rubber or plastic rim as its base. The bell is most beneficial for listening to low-pitched sounds in the chest, such as the murmur of mitral stenosis. When using the bell, place it lightly on the chest wall. Applying too much pressure will stretch the skin over the bell's circumference so that the skin acts like a diaphragm and excludes low-pitched sounds.

The diaphragm is a flat saucer that is covered with a thin membrane that serves as a filter to filter out low-pitched sounds. As a result of filtering out low-pitched sounds, high-pitched sounds seem to be amplified. The diaphragm is used for such high-pitched sounds as the murmur of aortic regurgitation and breath sounds. The diaphragm should be placed firmly against the skin surface to block out extraneous noise.

Auscultation needs to be performed in a quiet room without distractions or interruptions. It is important to isolate each sound that is being heard and to concentrate on the sound. Sometimes, closing your eyes while auscultating will help with concentration and differentiation of the sounds heard. Warn the patient that it takes time to adequately evaluate his or her heart and chest sounds and that the fact that you are listening for a long time does not mean that there is anything wrong. It is also important to auscultate the heart with the patient in different positions, such as sitting, standing, left lateral position, and even squatting. These positions may help demonstrate heart murmurs that may otherwise go undetected.

EXAMINATION PROCESS

Every practitioner must develop his or her own method of performing the physical examination. The following order is described by many as the head-to-toe examination. Some practitioners may find it more beneficial to perform the examination by systems or may find it beneficial to perform a modified head-to-toe examination in which the system of the body causing the patient's symptoms is left for last. Whatever method is used, a thorough examination includes all of the following areas:

1. *Skin, hair, and nails.* Examine these areas, noting the texture, temperature, color, distribution, and presence of any lesions.
2. *Head.* Note the configuration of the head. Palpate the scalp for any tenderness, masses, or lesions.
3. *Eyes.* Perform a visual acuity test (Snellen chart). Check extraocular movements by having the patient focus on an object held at eye level. Move the object from side to side, top to bottom, and corner to corner. Instruct the patient to follow the object only with his or her eyes. Assess visual fields for gross defects. This can be done using the confrontation method, which is described as follows: Have the patient cover his or her right eye. Place your face in front of the patient at eye level and about 40 inches away. Have the patient fix constantly on your eyes. Close your left eye. With a finger or penlight bring the target toward the midline. Have the patient indicate when the target is seen. Test vertical, oblique, and nasal fields the same way. Inspect the conjunctivae and sclerae for color and clarity. Inspect the eye from the front and side, noting any protrusion or recession of the globe. Check pupillary reaction to light and accommodation. Perform the fundoscopic examination of the lens, discs, and retinal vessels.
4. *Ears.* Test auditory acuity using the whisper, Weber, and Rinne tests. Perform otoscopic examination of the ear canals and the tympanic membrane. The tympanic membrane is normally a pearly gray color and moves with insufflation.
5. *Nose.* Inspect the nares. Assess the turbinates for color and size.
6. *Mouth.* Inspect the lips, teeth and gingiva, buccal mucosa, and tongue. Assess the pharynx and tonsillar tissue for erythema, edema, or exudate.
7. *Neck.* Note the configuration of the neck. Palpate the thyroid gland and the carotid arteries. The thyroid gland may be palpated from either the front or the back. To palpate from behind, stand behind the patient and have the patient rest his or her head against his or her body. Place your thumbs behind the patient's neck and curl your fingers around the front of the neck to explore the trachea. Then gently shift the trachea to the side to palpate the gland, first with the right and then with the left hand. Have the patient swallow to assess movement of any masses noted. To palpate the thyroid gland from the front, stand or sit in front of the patient. Use one thumb to gently shift the trachea to the opposite side while palpating the gland with the other thumb and forefinger. Again, have the patient swallow to assess movement of any masses. Auscultate the thyroid gland and carotid arteries for any bruits. Palpate the cervical, clavicular, axillary, and epitrochlear lymph nodes for enlargement.
8. *Hands and arms.* Note the muscles and joints of the shoulders, arms, and hands. Assess muscle strength and joint mobility. Palpate the radial pulses. Percuss the deep tendon reflexes of the upper extremities (biceps, triceps, and brachioradial).
9. *Thorax.* Note the configuration of the chest and breasts. Assess the duration of inspiration and expiration. Note the configuration of the spine. Palpate the ribs, breasts, and spine. Palpate the precordium for character and location of the PMI. Percuss the lung fields, diaphragm, and apex of the heart. Auscultate the lungs and the heart. When auscultating the heart, note the rate and rhythm, as well as rubs, clicks, or murmurs. When auscultating the lungs, listen for adventitious breath sounds.
10. *Abdomen.* Inspect the abdomen's configuration. Note any scars or herniae. Auscultate for bowel sounds or bruits. Palpate, using light and deep palpation, for any organomegaly. Percuss the liver and spleen. Palpate for enlarged inguinal lymph nodes. Palpate the femoral arteries for equality and strength. Auscultate the femoral arteries for the presence of bruits.
11. *Legs and feet.* Inspect the skin, muscles, and joints. Assess muscle strength and joint movement. Inspect and palpate for temperature and edema. Palpate the dorsalis pedis and posterior tibial pulses. Percuss the patellar, ankle, and plantar reflexes.
12. *Genitalia—male.* Inspect and palpate the genitalia, searching for abnormal lesions or masses. Perform an inguinal hernia examination (see Fig 1 in Part One, section on hernias). Inspect the rectum for hemorrhoids. Perform a digital examination of the rectum and prostate. Test the stool for occult blood.

    Genitalia—female. Inspect and palpate the external genitalia, including the rectum, for masses, lesions, or, in the case of the rectum, hemorrhoids. Inspect the internal genitalia with a speculum and obtain specimens for a Pap smear or cultures as necessary. Perform a bimanual examination by placing two fingers in the patient's vagina. Place the other hand on the patient's lower abdomen. Apply gentle, but firm, downward pressure to the abdomen to make the uterus and adnexa accessible to the intravaginal fingers. With the intravaginal fingers assess for any tenderness, lesions, or masses. Perform a rectovaginal examination. Test the stool for occult blood.

Assessment Tests

Name of test	How to perform	Interpretation
Adson's test	Have patient sit with arms pronated, chin raised high and pointed toward side being examined. Have patient inspire and hold his or her breath. Check radial pulse to see if it is still present. If present, is it diminished?	If radial pulse is absent or diminished, test is positive—indicates subclavian compression or scalenus anticus syndrome.
Allen's test	Have patient sit with arms supinated. Occlude both radial arteries with your fingers and have patient pump his or her hands 3 times. Have patient open his or her hands with radial artery still compressed. Observe color of patient's palm. Repeat test, occluding ulnar arteries.	If palms are not a normal pink color but are white or very pale pink, this indicates that either radial or ulnar artery is occluded.
Anvil test	Raise limb of supine patient from table with knee in extension; strike calcaneus with fist, using a moderate blow in direction of hip.	This maneuver causes pain in early hip joint disease.
Babinski's reflex	Using a blunt object, stroke along lateral side of foot from heel to ball, and across ball of foot to medial side.	Dorsiflexion of big toe with extension fanning of other toes is a positive reflex. This reflex is normal in infants and abnormal in children and adults—indicates pyramidal tract disease.
Bárány's test (caloric test)	Alternately irrigate ears with warm water or air and cold water or air. Warm irrigation produces rotary nystagmus toward irrigated side, and cold irrigation produces rotary nystagmus away from irrigated side.	If ear is diseased, less nystagmus is produced.
Barre's pyramidal sign	With patient in recumbent position, watch lateral or vertical movement of one leg.	If opposite leg makes a similar movement, this sign is positive, indicating a prefrontal brain lesion.
Brodie-Trendelenburg test	With patient supine, elevate leg vertically until veins are empty. Patient then stands, and examiner observes filling of veins.	If valves are incompetent, veins fill from above. If valves are normal, veins fill from bottom. Incompetent valves are seen in varicose veins.
Brudzinski's sign	With patient supine, passively flex neck to chin while holding down thorax	Involuntary hip flexion occurs with nuchal rigidity.
CAGE questionnaire*	**C** Feels need to *cut* down on drinking **A** Is *annoyed* by criticism **G** Feels *guilty* **E** Has an *eye-opener*	Any positive answer indicates that alcoholism is possible.
Chaddock's reflex	Firmly stroke ulnar surface of forearm.	Flexion of wrist and extension of fingers in a fanlike position is a positive reflex. This reflex is abnormal and is seen in hemiplegia.
Chadwick's sign	Perform internal examination of female genitalia.	If cervix is bluish purple, this sign is positive; Chadwick's sign is a presumptive sign of pregnancy.
Charcot's triad	Assess for intention tremors, nystagmus, and scanning speech.	Presence of Charcot's triad is a sign of brainstem involvement in multiple sclerosis.
Chvostek's sign	Tap facial nerve against bone just anterior to ear.	Ipsilateral contraction of facial muscle is a positive sign of tetany, as in parathyroid deficit; may indicate calcium or magnesium deficit.
Costovertebral tenderness	Strike with heel of palm between spine and twelfth rib.	Tenderness indicates inflammation of kidney.
Cranial nerves	I—olfactory II—optic III—oculomotor	Test smell. Test vision (fundoscopic examination). Test eye movement (pupillary reflex and size, shape, and equality of pupils).

Name of test	How to perform	Interpretation
	IV—trochlear	Test eye movement (ability to follow moving objects).
	V—trigeminal	Test head and face movement and sensation to pain, touch, and temperature.
	VI—abducens	Test lateral rectus muscle.
	VII—facial	Test muscles of face, scalp, and auricula.
	VIII—acoustic	Test hearing and for nystagmus.
	IX—glossopharyngeal	Test with vagus nerve.
	X—vagus	Test uvula elevation, gag reflex, and swallow reflex.
	XI—accessory	Test resistance of trapezii; turn head against resistance.
	XII—hypoglossal	Test tongue muscle strength.
Crossed-leg raise	Have patient with low-back pain lie supine and raise unaffected leg with knee extended.	Pain in affected leg and sciatic pain in unaffected leg indicate herniated disc.
Drawer's sign	With patient supine, have patient flex affected knee at right angle. Sit on patient's foot. With both hands grasp upper part of legs with fingers in popliteal fossa and pull head of tibia toward you.	Movement more than 1 cm is positive sign—indicates rupture of anterior cruciate ligament.
Finger-to-nose test	With arms extended and eyes open, ask patient to quickly bring his or her finger in a wide arc to nose.	In cerebellar disease, this motion is accompanied by an action tremor.
Goodell's sign	Assess during bimanual female examination.	Softening of cervix is a probable sign of pregnancy.
Graenslen's test	With patient supine, have him or her hold knee of affected side with both hands, flexing knee and hip to fix lumbar spine to table; hyperextend other thigh by pushing it over end of table.	An affected sacroiliac joint will emit pain.
Hegar's sign	Assess during bimanual female examination.	Softening of lower uterine segment is a probable sign of pregnancy.
Homans' sign	Assess dorsiflexion of foot.	Pain produced in calf of same leg indicates thrombophlebitis or thrombosis.
Hoover's sign	Have patient in supine position. Stand at foot and take each heel in one of your palms, and rest your hands on table. Have patient attempt to raise affected limb.	This test is used to differentiate hysterical paralysis from organic paralysis. In organic disease, the movement causes unaffected heel to press downward. In hysteria, it does not.
Kernig's sign	With patient supine, passively flex hip, with knee flexed at 90 degrees. Keep hip flexed and attempt to straighten knee.	This reliable sign of meningeal irritation can occur with herniated disc or tumor of cauda equina. Resistance to knee extension is a positive sign.
McBurney's sign	Palpate McBurney's point, which is a point in right lower quadrant of abdomen. It is about 2 inches from right anterosuperior iliac spine, in a line between spine and umbilicus.	Severe pain and tenderness are found in appendicitis.
McMurray's test	Have patient supine or standing on affected side. Place one hand on foot and one on knee. Flex knee until heel nearly touches buttocks. Rotate foot laterally and extend knee to 90 degrees.	Click indicates torn medial meniscus.
Murphy's sign	Palpate subhepatic area deeply.	Inspiratory arrest secondary to extreme tenderness indicates cholecystitis.
Naffziger's sign	Compress external jugular vein.	If maneuver produces nerve root irritation, it is diagnostic for sciatica or herniated nucleus pulposus.

Continued

Assessment Tests—cont'd

Name of test	How to perform	Interpretation
Ortolani's sign	Place infant on his or her back on examining table, flex hips and knees at right angles, and abduct until lateral aspect of knees touch table. Examiner's hands should be around infant's thighs and knees. Attempt internal and external rotation.	Click or popping sound indicates joint instability.
Patrick's test	With patient supine, flex knee and place foot on opposite patella. Pull flexed knee lateralward as far as possible.	No pain means test is negative and excludes hip joint disease.
Phalen's maneuver	Flex both wrists to 90 degrees with dorsal surfaces in opposition for 60 seconds.	Tingling, pain, or numbness indicates carpal tunnel syndrome. Extension brings relief.
Pulse deficit	Two examiners are needed. One counts radial pulse, and other counts apical pulse	If radial pulse is less than apical pulse, there is a lack of peripheral perfusion.
Rebound tenderness	In region of abdomen remote to suspect area, push deeply and then withdraw abruptly.	Pain experienced in affected area is sign of peritoneal irritation (e.g., peritonitis or appendicitis).
Rinne test	Hold vibrating tuning fork on mastoid process; when sound is no longer heard, hold fork in air next to ear.	AC > BC is positive test (normal); BC > AC is negative test.
Romberg's test	Have patient standing with legs together and arms at sides, first with eyes open and then with eyes closed.	Loss of balance is positive test—indicates cerebellar ataxia or vestibular dysfunction.
Simmonds' test	With patient prone and with feet off table, squeeze calf muscle transversely.	Plantar flexion indicates normal or incomplete rupture of Achilles tendon. There is no motion with complete rupture.
Straight-leg raises (SLRs)	With patient supine, elevate each leg passively with knee extended.	Radicular pain at 30 to 60 degrees is positive test.

Name of test	How to perform	Interpretation
Tinel's sign	Light percussion on radial side of palmaris longus tendon.	Tingling sensation indicates carpal tunnel syndrome.
Trendelenburg's sign	Have patient stand on one foot unsupported.	In normal hip, buttock rises and falls; in dislocation of hip, there is weakness of gluteal muscle or paralysis.
Trousseau's sign	Occlude brachial artery for 3 minutes with a BP cuff.	No response is normal. Carpal spasm indicates latent tetany, as seen in hypocalcemia or hypomagnesemia.
2-minute orthopedic examination†	Stand facing examiner.	Assess acromioclavicular joints and general habitus.
	Look at ceiling, floor, over both shoulders; touch ears to shoulders.	Assess cervical spine motion.
	Shrug shoulders (examiner resists).	Assess trapezius strength.
	Abduct shoulders 90 degrees (examiner resists at 90 degrees).	Assess deltoid strength.
	Perform full external rotation of arms.	Assess shoulder motion.
	Flex and extend elbows.	Assess elbow motion.
	With arms at sides and elbows 90 degrees flexed, pronate and supinate wrists.	Assess elbow and wrist motion.
	Spread fingers; make fist.	Assess hand or finger motion and deformities.
	Tighten quadriceps; relax quadriceps.	Assess symmetry and knee effusion, as well as ankle effusion.
	Duck walk 4 steps (away from examiner with buttocks on heels).	Assess hip, knee, and ankle motion.
	Turn back to examiner.	Assess for symmetry. Back is asymmetric in scoliosis.
	With knees straight, touch toes.	Assess for scoliosis, hip motion, and hamstring tightness.
	Rise up on toes; raise heels.	Assess for calf symmetry and leg strength.
Weber test	Place vibrating tuning fork in midline of skull.	In normal hearing, sound is heard the same in both ears. In conductive loss, sound lateralizes to bad ear. In sensorineural loss, sound lateralizes to good ear.

*From Ewing JA: CAGE questionnaire, *JAMA* 252:1908, 1984.
†From Committee on Sports Medicine and Fitness: The two-minute orthopedic exam. In *Sports medicine: health care for young athletes,* Elk Grove, Ill., 1991, American Academy of Pediatrics.

Prevention

Prevention and early detection of disease processes should be a major part of any nurse practitioner's practice (Fig. 3).

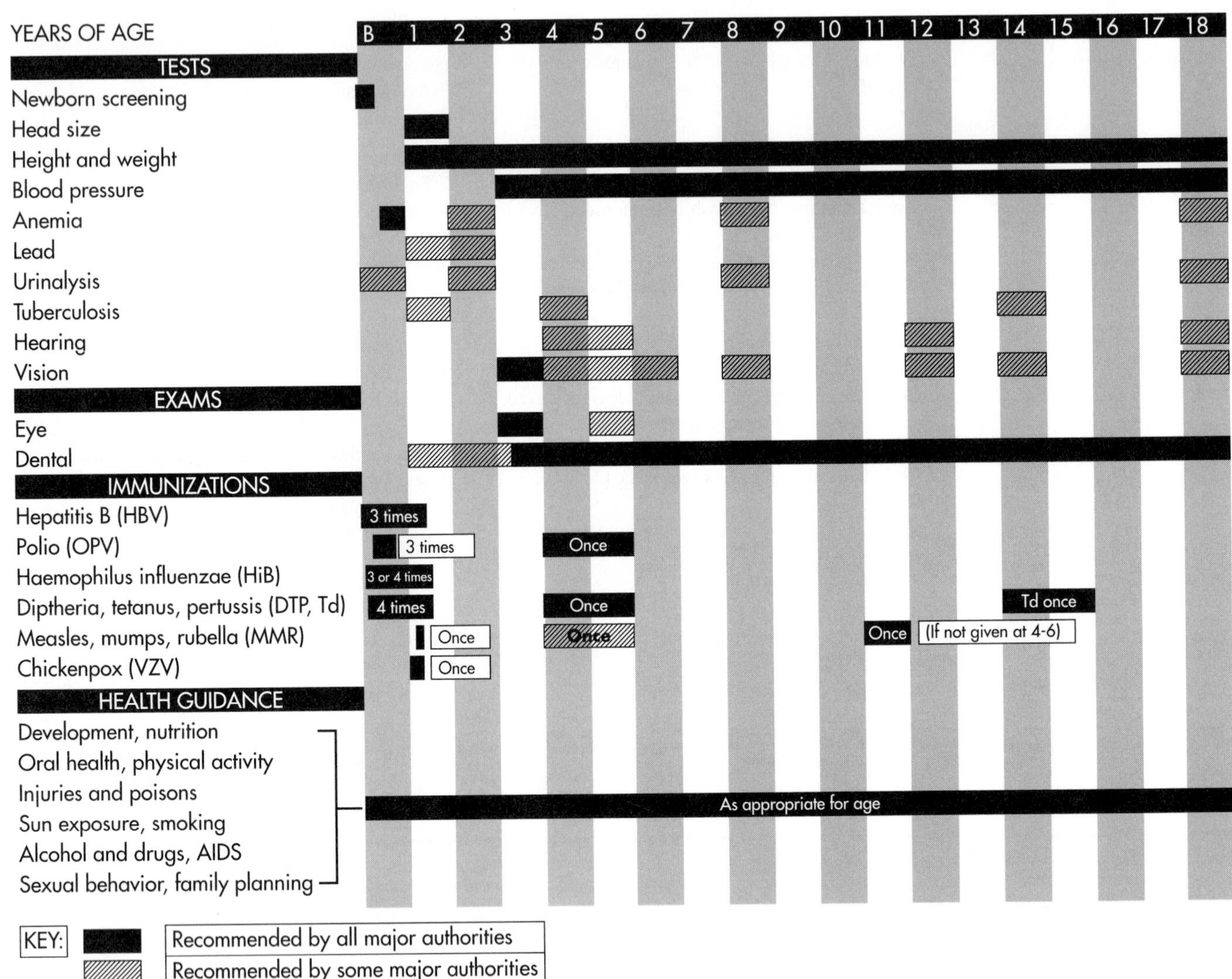

FIG. 3 Major preventive services that should be offered throughout the life span. (From US Department of Health and Human Services, Public Health Service: *Clinician's handbook of preventive services: put prevention into practice,* Washington DC, 1994, US Government Printing Office.)

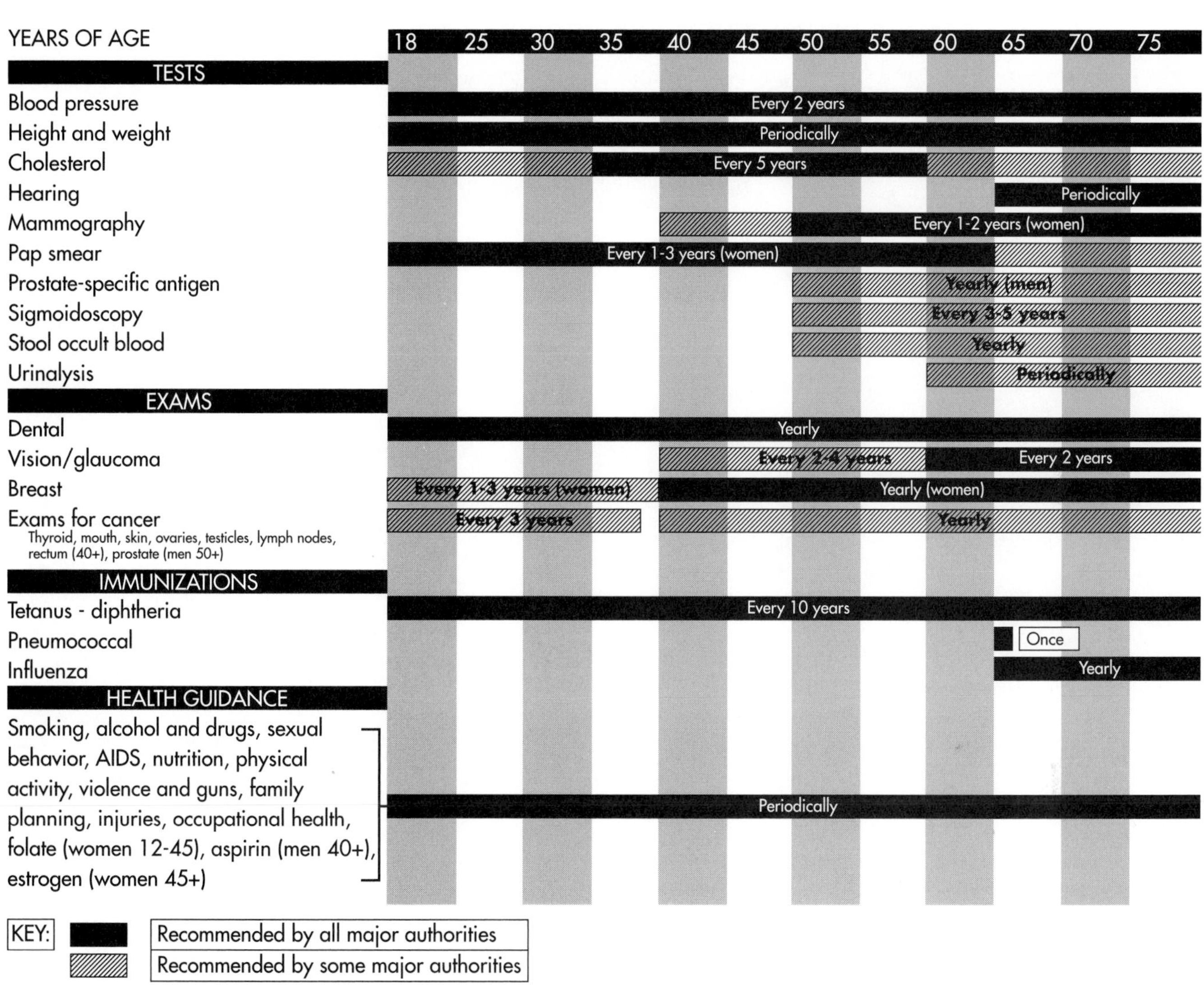

FIG. 3, cont'd For legend see opposite page.

REFERENCES

American Academy of Pediatrics, Committee on Sports Medicine and Fitness: *Sports medicine: health care for young athletes,* ed 2, Elk Grove Village, Ill, 1991, American Academy of Pediatrics.

DeGowin RL: *DeGowin and DeGowin's diagnostic examination,* ed 6, New York, 1994, McGraw-Hill.

Ewing JA: Detecting alcoholism, the CAGE questionnaire, *JAMA* 252:1905-1907, 1984.

Habif TP: *Clinical dermatology: a color guide to diagnosis and therapy,* ed 3, St Louis, 1996, Mosby.

Jarvis C: *Physical examination and health assessment,* Philadelphia, 1992, WB Saunders.

Mercier LR: *Practical orthopedics,* ed 4, St Louis, 1995, Mosby.

Seidel HM et al: *Mosby's guide to physical examination,* ed 3, St Louis, 1995, Mosby.

US Department of Health and Human Services, Public Health Service: *Clinician's handbook of preventive services: put prevention into practice,* Washington, DC, 1994, US Government Printing Office.

Bibliography

Acute Pain Management Guideline Panel: *Acute pain management: operative or medical procedures and trauma,* Clinical Practice Guideline 1, AHCPR Pub No 92-0032, Rockville, Md, 1992, US Department of Health and Human Services, Public Health Service, Agency for Health Care Policy and Research.

Alemi F et al: A review of factors affecting treatment outcomes: expected treatment outcome scale, *Am J Drug Alcohol Abuse* 21(4):483-509, 1995.

Allison OC, Porter ME, Briggs GC: Chronic constipation: assessment and management in the elderly, *J Am Acad Nurse Pract* 6(7):311-317, 1994.

Aloi JA: Evaluation of amenorrhea, *Compr Ther* 21(10):575-576, 1995.

American Academy of Dermatology: *Pityriasis rosea,* Schaumburg, Ill, 1993, American Acad of Dermatology.

American Academy of Pediatrics, Committee on Sports Medicine and Fitness: *Sports medicine: health care for young athletes,* ed 2, Elk Grove Village, Ill, 1991, American Academy of Pediatrics.

American Health Consultants: Potent new AIDS drugs underscore promise of combination therapy, *AIDS Alert* 11(1):1-12, 1996.

Anderson KN, Anderson LE, Glanze WD, editors: *Mosby's medical, nursing, and allied health dictionary,* ed 5, St Louis, 1998, Mosby.

Bahadori RS, Bohne BA: Adverse effects of noise on hearing, *Am Fam Physician* 47(5):1219-1226, 1993.

Barach EM: Asthma in ambulatory care: use of objective diagnostic criteria, *J Fam Pract* 38(2):161-165, 1994.

Barker LR, Burton JR, Zieve PD, editors: *Principles of ambulatory medicine,* ed 4, Baltimore, 1995, Williams & Wilkins.

Bartlett JG: *Pocket book of infectious disease therapy,* ed 7, Baltimore, 1996, Williams & Wilkins.

Baughman OL III: Rapid diagnosis and treatment of anxiety and depression in primary care: the somatizing patient, *J Fam Pract* 39(4):373-377, 1994.

Belmonte K: Carpal tunnel syndrome, *J Am Acad Nurse Pract* 8(11):511-517, 1996.

Bemben DA et al: Thyroid disease in the elderly. I. Prevalence of undiagnosed hypothyroidism, *J Fam Pract* 38(6):577-581, 1994.

Bemben DA et al: Thyroid disease in the elderly. II. Predictability of subclinical hypothyroidism, *J Fam Pract* 38(6):583-588, 1994.

Bergus GR, Johnson JS: Superficial tinea infections, *Am Fam Physician* 48(2):259-268, 1993.

Bienkowski J: An overview of the progression of diabetic retinopathy with treatment recommendations, *Nurse Pract* 19(7):50-58, 1994.

Blake GH: Primary hypertension: the role of individualized therapy, *Am Fam Physician* 50(1):138-146, 1994.

Bratton RL, Nesse RE: St. Anthony's fire: diagnosis and management of erysipelas, *Am Fam Physician* 51(2):401-404, 1995.

Braunwald E et al: *Diagnosing and managing unstable angina,* Quick Reference Guide for Clinicians No 10, AHCPR Pub No 94-0603, Rockville, Md, 1994, US Department of Health and Human Services, Public Health Service, Agency for Health Care Policy and Research and National Heart, Lung, and Blood Institute.

Bull TR: *Color atlas of E.N.T. diagnosis,* ed 3, London, 1995, Mosby-Wolfe.

Bundred NJ et al: Breast abscesses and cigarette smoking, *Br J Surg* 79(1):58-59, 1992.

Carnevali DL, Patrick M, editors: *Nursing management for the elderly,* ed 3, Philadelphia, 1993, JB Lippincott.

Cataract Management Guideline Panel: *Cataract in adults: management of functional impairment,* Clinical Practice Guideline No 4, AHCPR Pub No 93-0542, Rockville, Md, 1993, US Department of Health and Human Services, Public Health Service, Agency for Health Care Policy and Research.

Caulker-Burnett I: Primary care screening for substance abuse, *Nurse Pract* 19(6):42-48, 1994.

Clinical Guidelines: Cancer detection by physical examination: breast and pelvic organ examination, *Nurse Pract* 19(10):20-24, 1994.

Clinical Guidelines: Papanicolaou smear, *Nurse Pract* 19(12):74-77, 1994.

Conry C: Evaluation of a breast complaint: is it cancer? *Am Fam Physician* 49(2):445-450, 1994.

Coons TA: MRI's role in assessing and managing breast disease, *Radiol Technol* 67(4):311-336, 1996.

Craig C: Clinical recognition and management of adult attention deficit hyperactivity disorder, *Nurse Pract* 21(11):101-108, 1996.

Criste G, Gray D, Gallo B: Prostatitis: a review of diagnosis and management, *Nurse Pract* 19(7):32-33, 37-38, 1994.

Cunningham MA: Non–insulin-dependent diabetes: getting the attention it deserves, *Clin Excel Nurse Pract* 1(2):95-104, 1997.

Dale DC, Federman DD: *Scientific American: medicine,* vols 1 to 3, New York, 1976-1996, Scientific American.

Dalton CB, Drossman DA: Calming the irritable bowel: close-up on new diagnostic criteria, *Adv Nurse Pract* 4(12):30-34, 1996.

Danton WG et al: Nondrug treatment of anxiety, *Am Fam Physician* 49(1):161-166, 1994.

Davis AE: Primary care management of chronic musculoskeletal pain, *Nurse Pract* 21(8):72, 75, 79-82, 1996.

DeGowin RL: *DeGowin and DeGowin's diagnostic examination,* ed 6, New York, 1994, McGraw-Hill.

DeGruy F: Management of mixed anxiety and depression, *Am Fam Physician* 49(4):860-865, 1994.

Depression Guideline Panel: *Depression in primary care,* vol 1, *Detection and diagnosis,* Clinical Practice Guideline. No 5, AHCPR Pub No 93-0550, Rockville, Md, 1993, US Department of Health and Human Services, Public Health Service, Agency for Health Care Policy and Research.

Depression Guideline Panel: *Depression in primary care,* vol 2, *Treatment of major depression,* Clinical Practice Guideline No 5, AHCPR Pub No 93-0551, Rockville, Md, 1993, US Department of Health and Human Services, Public Health Service, Agency for Health Care Policy and Research.

Dettenmeier PA: *Radiographic assessment for nurses,* St Louis, 1995, Mosby.

The Diabetes Control and Complications Trial Research Group: The effect of intensive treatment of diabetes on the development and progression of long-term complications in insulin-dependent diabetes mellitus, *N Engl J Med* 329(14):977-986, 1993.

Diamond S: *Clinical symposia: head pain,* vol 46, No 3, Summit, NJ, 1994, Ciba-Geigy.

Dirksen SR, Lewis SM, Collier IC: *Clinical companion to medical-surgical nursing,* St Louis, 1996, Mosby.

Dracup K: Heart failure secondary to left ventricular systolic dysfunction, *Nurse Pract* 21(9):56, 58, 61, 65-68, 1996.

Driscoll CE et al, editors: *The family practice desk reference,* ed 3, St Louis, 1996, Mosby.

Edwards S: Balanitis and balanoposthitis: a review, *Genitourinary Med* 72(3):155-159, 1996.

El-Sadr W et al: *Evaluation and management of early HIV infection,* Clinical Practice Guideline No 7, AHCPR Pub No 94-0572, Rockville, Md, 1994, US Department of Health and Human Services, Public Health Service, Agency for Health Care Policy and Research.

Ewing JA: Detecting alcoholism: the CAGE questionnaire, *JAMA* 252:1905-1907, 1984.

Fay M, Jaffe PE: Diagnostic and treatment guidelines for *Helicobacter pylori, Nurse Pract* 21(7):28-34, 1996.

Fiore MC et al: *Smoking cessation,* Clinical Practice Guideline No 18, AHCPR Pub No 96-0692, Rockville, Md, 1996, US Department of Health and Human Services, Public Health Service, Agency for Health Care Policy and Research.

Fraser H: Ambylopia—or lazy eye, *Austr Fam Physician* 24(6):1021-1023, 1995.

Frohlich ED: The JNC-V: consensus recommendations for the treatment of hypertension, *Physician Assist* 10:45-46, 50-61, 1993.

Frymoyer CL: Practical therapeutics: preventing spread of viral hepatitis, *Am Fam Physician* 48(8):1479-1486, 1993.

Givens TG et al: Comparison of 1% and 2.5% selenium sulfide in the treatment of tinea capitis, *Arch Pediatr Adolesc Med* 149(7):808-811, 1995.

Goens JL, Schwartz RA, DeWolf K: Mucocutaneous manifestations of chancroid, lymphogranuloma venereum, and granuloma inguinale, *Am Fam Physician* 49(2):415-418, 423-425, 1994.

Goldberg RJ: *Practical guide to the care of the psychiatric patient,* St Louis, 1995, Mosby.

Golden R: Dementia and Alzheimer's disease indications, diagnosis, and treatment, *Minn Med* 78(1):25-29, 1995.

Griffith CJ: Allergic rhinitis: practical guide to diagnosis and management, *Physician Assist,* pp 19-21, 24-26, 29-30, 32-36, July 1994.

Guidelines Sub-Committee: 1993 guidelines for the management of mild hypertension: memorandum from a World Health Organization/International Society of hypertension meeting, *J Hypertens* 11(9):905-916, 1993.

Habif TP: *Clinical dermatology: a color guide to diagnosis and therapy,* ed 3, St Louis, 1996, Mosby.

Hall-Jordan R: Intensive insulin therapy in diabetes, *Physician Assist,* pp 17, 21-24, 27-28, 30, June 1994.

Hamilton EM: Management of upper and lower urinary tract infections in pregnant women, *J Am Acad Nurse Pract* 8(12):559-563, 1996.

Hanson MJS: Acute otitis media in children, *Nurse Pract* 21(5):72, 74, 80, 1996.

Haque R et al: Rapid diagnosis of *Entomoeba* infection by using *Entamoeba* and *Entamoeba histolytica* stool antigen detection kits, *J Clin Microbiol* 33(10):2558-2561, 1995.

Heck JE, Cohen MB: Traveler's diarrhea, *Am Fam Physician* 48(5):793-800, 1993.

Heiligenstein E, Keeling RP: Presentation of unrecognized attention deficit hyperactivity disorder in college students, *J Am Coll Health* 43(5):226-228, 1995.

Hilding DA: Literature review: the common cold, *Ear Nose Throat J* 73:639-643, 646-647, 1994.

Hoffert MJ: Treatment of migraine: a new era, *Am Fam Physician* 49(3):633-638, 1994.

ICD-9-CM: International classification of diseases, 9th revision, clinical modification, ed 4, Los Angeles, 1996, Practice Management Information.

Jacox A et al: *Management of cancer pain,* Clinical Practice Guideline No 9, AHCPR Pub No 94-0592, Rockville, Md, 1994, US Department of Health and Human Services, Public Health Service, Agency for Health Care Policy and Research.

Jarvis C: *Physical examination and health assessment,* Philadelphia, 1992, WB Saunders.

Johannsen JM: Chronic obstructive pulmonary disease: current comprehensive care for emphysema and bronchitis, *Nurse Pract* 19(1):59-67, 1994.

Johnson JR: Urinary tract infection: selecting the optimal agent, *Physician Assist,* pp 155-158, 163-164, Feb 1992.

Jones JM, Dupree-Jones K: What's happening: pearls and perils of the perimenopause, *J Am Acad Nurse Pract* 8(11):531-535, 1996.

Jones JM: The scorn of Horton's demon: understanding cluster headache, *Physician Assist* 18(8):38-41, 44-46, 48-50, 1994.

Katz RT: Carpal tunnel syndrome: a practical review, *Am Fam Physician* 49(6):1371-1379, 1994.

Kauvar D, Brandt LJ: Treatment of common GI disorders in the elderly, *Physician Assist,* pp 105-111, Feb 1992.

Kessenich CR: Update on pharmacologic therapies for osteoporosis, *Nurse Pract* 21(8):19-20, 22-24, 1996.

Kimble-Haas S: Primary care treatment approach to nongenital verruca, *Nurse Pract* 21(10):29-36, 1996.

Kiselica D: Group a beta-hemolytic streptococcal pharyngitis: current clinical concepts, *Am Fam Physician* 49(5):1147-1153, 1994.

Klaus MV, Wieselthier JS: Contact dermatitis, *Am Fam Physician* 48(4):629-632, 1993.

Konstam M et al: *Heart failure: management of patients with left-ventricular systolic dysfunction,* Quick Reference Guide for Clinicians No 11, AHCPR Pub No 94-0613, Rockville, Md, 1994, US Department of Health and Human Services, Public Health Service, Agency for Health Care Policy and Research.

Kowdley KV: Update on therapy for hepatobiliary diseases, *Nurse Pract* 21(7):78-88, 1996.

Kuflik AS, Schwartz RA: Actinic keratosis and squamous cell carcinoma, *Am Fam Physician* 49(4):817-820, 1994.

Kupeca D: Alprostadil for the treatment of erectile dysfunction, *Nurse Pract* 21(5):143-145, 1996.

Leiner S: Acute bronchitis in adults: commonly diagnosed but poorly defined, *Nurse Pract* 22(1):104, 107-108, 113-114, 1997.

Lesseig DZ: Primary care diagnosis and pharmacologic treatment of depression in adults, *Nurse Pract* 21(10):72, 75-76, 78, 81-85, 1996.

Levine DZ, editor: *Care of the renal patient,* ed 2, Philadelphia, 1991, WB Saunders.

Lewis SM, Collier IC, Heitkemper MM: *Medical-surgical nursing: assessment and management of clinical problems,* ed 4, St Louis, 1996, Mosby.

Lindsay R: *Osteoporosis: a guide to diagnosis, prevention, and treatment,* New York, 1992, Raven Press.

Marghoob AA et al: Basal cell and squamous cell carcinomas are important risk factors for cutaneous malignant melanoma: screening implications, *Cancer* 75:707-714, 1995.

McCance KL, Huether SE: *Pathophysiology: the biological basis for disease in adults and children,* ed 2, St Louis, 1994, Mosby.

McConnell JD et al: *Benign prostatic hyperplasia: diagnosis and treatment,* Clinical Practice Guideline No 8, AHCPR Pub No 94-0582, Rockville, Md, 1994, US Department of Health and Human Services, Public Health Service, Agency for Health Care Policy and Research.

McFarlane J, Parker B, Soeken K: Abuse during pregnancy: associations with maternal health and infant birth weight, *Nurs Res* 45(1):37-42, 1996.

McKenry LM, Salerno E: *Mosby's pharmacology in nursing,* ed 19, St Louis, 1995, Mosby.

Mercier LR: *Practical orthopedics,* ed 4, St Louis, 1995, Mosby.

Meyers DG: Auscultatory findings in heart disease, *Hosp Med,* pp 23-24, 26-28, 32-33, 37-38, Nov 1993.

Miller JL: Clinical evaluation and treatment of osteoporosis, *Physician Assist,* pp 23-24, 26, 28, 30, 32-33, March 1994.

Millikan LE: Recognizing drug-related skin eruptions, *Physician Assist,* pp 44, 49, 53-57, July 1994.

Millonig VL: *Adult nurse practitioner certification review guide,* ed 2, Potomac, Md, 1994, Health Leadership Associates.

Mladenovic J: *Primary care secrets,* Philadelphia, 1995, Hanley & Belfus.

Mosby's GenRx, ed 8, St Louis, 1998, Mosby.

Moser M: Treatment of hypertension in the elderly, *Physician Assist,* pp 135-140, 152-153, Feb 1992.

Muglia JJ, McDonald CJ: Skin cancer screening, *Physician Assist,* pp 21-24, 29-32, Jan 1994.

Nelson JD: *Pocket book of pediatric antimicrobial therapy,* ed 12, Baltimore, 1996, Williams & Wilkins.

Nelson JK et al: *Mayo Clinic diet manual: a handbook of dietary practices,* ed 7, St Louis, 1994, Mosby.

Newmann RE, Nishimoto PW: 1996 human immunodeficiency virus update for the primary care provider, *Nurse Pract Forum* 7(1):16-22, 1996.

Nguyen QH, Kim YA, Schwartz RA: Management of acne vulgaris, *Am Fam Physician* 50(1):89-95, 1994.

Noel H, Dempster JS: Continuing education forum: essential hypertension: evaluation and treatment, *J Am Acad Nurse Pract* 6(9):421-435, 1994.

Noel H, Dempster JS: Continuing education forum: essential hypertension: pathophysiology, *J Am Acad Nurse Pract* 6(7):322-333, 1994.

Noel H, Dempster JS: Continuing education forum: hypertension: complications and problems, *J Am Acad Nurse Pract* 6(11):540-548, 1994.

Osdol WV, Johnston PE: *Quality medical records for primary care centers,* Indianapolis, 1989, Methodist Hospital of Indiana.

Otitis Media Guideline Panel, US Department of Health and Human Services, Public Health Service, Agency for Health Care Policy and Research: *Quick reference guide for clinicians:* managing otitis media with effusion in young children, *J Am Acad Nurse Pract* 6(10):493-500, 1995.

Pagana KD, Pagana TJ: *Mosby's diagnostic and laboratory test reference,* ed 3, St Louis, 1997, Mosby.

Panel on the Prediction and Prevention of Pressure Ulcers in Adults: *Pressure ulcers in adults: prediction and prevention,* Quick Reference Guide for Clinicians, AHCPR Pub No 92-0050, Rockville, Md, 1992, US Department of Health and Human Services, Public Health Service, Agency for Health Care Policy and Research.

Parker PD: Premenstrual syndrome, *Am Fam Physician* 50(6):1309-1317, 1994.

Parks BR, Dostrow VG, Noble SL: Drug therapy for epilepsy, *Am Fam Phys* 50(3):639-648, 1994.

Perna WC: Pearls for practice: mastalgia: diagnosis and treatment, *J Am Acad Nurse Pract* 8(12):579-584, 1996.

Peters S: Hitting the bull's eye: practical diagnosis and treatment of lyme disease, *Adv Nurse Pract* 4(11):14-17, 49, 57, 1996.

Peters S: Osteoarthritis options: new guidelines for primary care, *Adv Nurse Pract* 4(12):41-42, 50, 1996.

Petersen MJ, Baughman RA: Recurrent aphthous stomatitis: primary care management, *Nurse Pract* 21(5):36, 38-40, 42, 1996.

Phipps WJ et al, editors: *Medical-surgical nursing: concepts and clinical practice,* ed 5, St Louis, 1995, Mosby.

Physicians' desk reference: for nonprescription drugs, ed 16, Montvale, NJ, 1995, Medical Economics Data.

Ramsey PG, Larson EB: *Medical therapeutics,* ed 2, Philadelphia, 1993, WB Saunders.

Raspa RF, Wilson CC: Calcium channel blockers in the treatment of hypertension, *Am Fam Physician* 48(3):461-470, 1993.

Reed BD, Eyler A: Practical therapeutics: vaginal infections: diagnosis and management, *Am Fam Physician* 47(8):1805-1816, 1993.

Religo WM, Johnson CD: Prostatic-specific antigen: not a specific answer to a specific question, *Physician Assist,* pp 23-24, 27, 30, 32, April 1994.

Riley KE, Schumann L: Continuing education forum: evaluation and management of primary nocturnal enuresis, *J Am Acad Nurse Pract* 9(1):33-39, 1997.

Rosenfeld JA: Update on continuous estrogen-progestin replacement therapy, *Am Fam Physician* 50(7):1519-1523, 1994.

Runkle GP, Zaloznik AJ: Malignant melanoma, *Am Fam Physician* 49(1):91-98, 1994.

Ruppert SD: Differential diagnosis of pediatric conjunctivitis (red eye), *Nurse Pract* 21(7):12, 15-18, 24, 26, 1996.

Sandroni P, Young RR: Tremor: classification, diagnosis and management, *Am Fam Physician* 50(7):1505-1512, 1994.

Scharbo-DeHaan M: Hormone replacement therapy, part 2, *Nurse Pract* 21(12):1-13, 1996.

Schwartz SL, Schwartz JT: *Management of diabetes mellitus,* ed 3, Durant, Okla, 1993, Essential Medical Information Systems.

Seidel HM et al: *Mosby's guide to physical examination,* ed 3, St Louis, 1995, Mosby.

Shipman JJ: *Mnemonics and tactics in surgery and medicine,* London, 1984, Lloyd-Luke.

Short Communications: Info & research exchange: new guidelines on thyroid disease to improve diagnosis, *Nurse Pract* 21(8):8, 10, 1996.

Sickle Cell Disease Guideline Panel: *Sickle cell disease: screening, diagnosis, management, and counseling in newborns and infants,* Clinical Practice Guideline No 6, AHCPR Pub No 93-0562, Rockville, Md, 1993, US Department of Health and Human Services, Public Health Service, Agency for Health Care Policy and Research.

Skidmore-Roth L: *Mosby's 1997 nursing drug reference,* ed 10, St Louis, 1996, Mosby.

Sokoloff F: Identification and management of pediculosis, *Nurse Pract* 19(8):62-64, 1994.

Stein JH et al, editors: *Internal medicine,* ed 4, St Louis, 1994, Mosby.

Sullivan CA, Samuelson WM: Gastroesophageal reflux: a common exacerbating factor in adult asthma, *Nurse Pract* 21(11):82-84, 93-94, 96, 1996.

Swain SE: Multiple sclerosis: primary health care implications, *Nurse Pract* 21(7):40, 43, 47-50, 53-54, 1996.

Talley NJ: Nonulcer dyspepsia: current approaches to diagnosis and management, *Am Fam Physician* 47(6):1407-1415, 1993.

Thiboutot DM: Acne rosacea, *Am Fam Physician* 50(8):1691-1697, 1994.

Tierney LM Jr, McPhee SJ, Papadakis MA: *Current medical diagnosis and treatment,* ed 34, Norwalk, Conn, 1995, Appleton & Lange.

Tucker JB: Practical therapeutics: screening for open-angle glaucoma, *Am Fam Physician* 48(1):75-80, 1993.

Turner C, Fitzgerald M: Pharmacologic highlights: hormone replacement therapy: its use in the management of acute menopausal symptoms, *J Am Acad Nurse Pract* 6(7):318-320, 1994.

US Department of Health and Human Services, Public Health Service: *Clinician's handbook of preventive services: put prevention into practice,* Washington, DC, 1994, US Government Printing Office.

US Department of Health and Human Services, Public Health Service: Put prevention into practice: blood pressure screening in adults, *Am Fam Physician* 50(8):1729-1732, 1994.

US Department of Health and Human Services, Public Health Service: Put prevention into practice: counseling to prevent unintended pregnancy, *Am Fam Physician* 50(5):971-974, 1994.

US Department of Health and Human Services, Public Health Service: Put prevention into practice: thyroid function, *J Am Acad Nurse Pract* 8(10):495-496, 1996.

US Department of Health and Human Services, Public Health Service: Put prevention into practice: urinalysis, *Am Fam Physician* 50(2):351-353, 1994.

US Department of Health and Human Services, Public Health Service, Agency for Health Care Policy and Research: Quick Reference Guide for Clinicians: managing otitis media with effusion in young children, *J Am Acad Nurse Pract* 6(10):493-500, 1994.

Ungvarski PJ: Update on HIV infection, *Am J Nurs* 97(1):44-51, 1997.

Uphold CR, Graham MV: *Clinical guidelines in adult health,* Gainesville, Fla, 1994, Barmarrae Books.

Urinary Incontinence Guideline Panel: *Urinary incontinence in adults: a patient's guide,* Clinical Practice Guideline, AHCPR Pub No 92-0040, Rockville, Md, 1992, US Department of Health and Human Services, Public Health Service, Agency for Health Care Policy and Research.

Valente SM: Diagnosis and treatment of panic disorder and generalized anxiety in primary care, *Nurse Pract* 21(8):26, 32-34, 37-38, 41-44, 1996.

Walsh K: Guidelines for the prevention and control of tuberculosis in the elderly, *Nurse Pract* 19(11):79-85, 1994.

Walthall J, Goldman M, Hopkins-Hutti M: What's happening: new and developing methods of contraception, *J Am Acad Nurse Pract* 6(5):217-223, 1994.

Wasson J et al: *The common symptom guide: a guide to the evaluation of common adult and pediatric symptoms,* ed 4, New York, 1997, McGraw-Hill.

Webster DC, Brennan T: Use and effectiveness of physical self-care strategies for interstitial cystitis, *Nurse Pract* 19(10):55-61, 1994.

Wenger NK et al: *Cardiac rehabilitation,* Clinical Practice Guideline No 17, AHCPR Pub No 96-0672, Rockville, Md, 1995, US Department of Health and Human Services, Public Health Service, Agency for Health Care Policy and Research and the National Heart, Lung, and Blood Institute.

Wilder B: Pearls for practice: management of sinusitis, *J Am Acad Nurse Pract* 8(11):525-529, 1996.

Wilens TE et al: Pharmacotherapy of adult attention deficit/hyperactivity disorder: a review, *J Clin Psychopharmacol* 15(14):270-279, 1995.

Winningham ML, Preusser BA: *Critical thinking in medical-surgical settings,* St Louis, 1996, Mosby.

Wispert C: Urinary incontinence: guidelines for the primary care PA, *Physician Assist,* pp 27-28, 31-32, 37, Aug 1994.

Woodhead GA: The management of cholesterol in coronary heart disease risk reduction, *Nurse Pract* 21(9):45, 48, 51, 53, 1996.

Woolliscroft JO: *Current diagnosis and treatment: a quick reference for the general practitioner,* Philadelphia, 1996, Current Medicine.

Youngkin EQ, Davis MS, editors: *Women's health: a primary care clinical guide,* Norwalk, Conn, 1994, Appleton & Lange.

Zaldel LB: Guidelines on thyroid disease to improve diagnosis, *Nurse Pract* 21(8):8, 1996.

APPENDIX A

Computer Health Information

The following information is presented to provide access to the wealth of medical reference information available. The addresses were functional at the time of this printing; however, because of the dynamic nature of the Information Highway, some addresses and Web sites may have changed.

INFORMATION SITES

MedWeb is located at Emory University and offers an informational database that is easily searched with text entries. The address is:

http://www.cc.emory.edu/WHSCL/medweb.html

Medworld is another information database located at Stanford University and provides research and journal articles in a searchable format. The address is:

http://www-med.stanford.edu/medworld

The *Merck Manual* is presented in its entirety and can be searched for any condition. The address is:

http://www.merck.com/!!sSiWnOSiWsSiWnOSiW/pubs/mmanual/

Grateful Med is another database that allows the user to search for information from the National Library of Medicine. The address is:

http://igm.nlm.nih.gov

Health Information Resource provides toll-free numbers for various organizations, such as Cleft Palate Foundation, Alzheimer's Disease Education and Referral Center, etc. The address is:

http://nhic-nt.health.org/

The grant seeker's page provides free advice on how to get a project funded, tips on writing grants, and links to the Federal Register and other sources of grants. The address is:

http://www.idimagic.com

Medical Links gives the reader information on alternative health care and information on health insurance. The address is:

http://ccme-mac4.bsd.uchicago.edu

Nightingale is a Web site presented by the University of Tennessee, Knoxville—College of Nursing. It has information on nursing informatics and technology, geriatric nursing, and nursing theory. The address is:

http://nightingale.con.utk.edu/

Nurse Practitioner Resources by the University of California, San Francisco, provides easy links to many valuable Internet sites. The address is:

http://nurseweb.ucsf.edu

Go to Learning Resource Center and click on Computing.

PHARMACEUTICAL INFORMATION SITES

Mosby's GenR$_x$ on the Internet is offered by Mosby and provides on-line reference material for drugs and prescribing information. The address is:

http://www.genrx.com

PharmWeb is another database Web site with information on drugs and prescribing information. The address is:

http://www.pharmweb.net/

GOVERNMENT INFORMATION SITES

Centers for Disease Control and Prevention, located at:

http://www.cdc.gov/cdc.html

U.S. Department of Health and Human Services, located at:

http://www.usddhs.gov/

National Institutes of Health, located at:

http://www.nih.gov/

Agency for Health Care Policy and Research (AHCPR), located at:

http://www.ahcpr.gov/

ORGANIZATION INFORMATION SITES

Nurse Practitioner Support Services provides information on listservs and job listings. The address is:

http://www.nurse.net/np

NP Listserv is a Web site where nurse practitioners can share information with other nurse practitioners from across the United States and around the world. To subscribe to this free list, send a message to the following address with the word *subscribe* in the body of the message:

NPINFO-Request@npl.com

AMA–National Specialty Societies gives an extensive list of specialty societies, such as American Academy of Allergy, Asthma, and Immunology; American Academy of Child Adolescent Psychiatry; and American Academy of Dermatology. The address is:

http://www.ama-assn.org/med___link/nation.htm

The following is a list of some of the more common medical organizations that may be accessed on the Internet:

American Academy of Dermatology:

http://www.aad.org/

American Academy of Family Physicians:

http://www.aafp.org/

American Academy of Orthopaedic Surgeons:

http://www.aaos.org/

American Academy of Pediatrics:

http://www.aap.org/

Much more information can be located by using commercial search engines, such as Excite and Yahoo. Commercial online services, such as America Online and Microsoft Internet Explorer, also have reference sections and search engines with their browsers that make retrieving information easy and that provide links to other Web sites too numerous to mention here.

APPENDIX B

Drugs Metabolized by P450 Enzymes

CYP1A2

amitriptyline
caffeine
clomipramine
imipramine
paracetamol
phenacetin
propranolol
theophylline

CYP2C19

citalopram
clomipramine
diazepam
hexobarbital
imipramine
mephobarbital
omeprazole
proguanil
propranolol

CYP2D6

Antiarrhythmics
encainide
flecainide
mexiletine
propafenone

Antipsychotics
clozapine
haloperidol
perphenazine
reduced haloperidol
risperidone
thioridazine
zuclopenthixol

Beta-blockers
alprenolol
burarolol
metoprolol
propranolol
timolol

Miscellaneous
amiflamine
gunaoxan
4-hydro-amphetamine
indoramin
methoxphenamine
perhexiline
phenformin
N-propyl-ajmaline
tomoxetine

Opiates
codeine
dextromethorphan
ethylmorphine

SSRIs
fluoxetine
N-desmethyl-citalopram
norfluoxetine
paroxetine

Tricyclic antidepressants
amitriptyline
clomipramine
desipramine
imipramine
N-desmethyl-clomipramine
nortriptyline
trimipramine

Other antidepressant
venlafaxine

CYP3A3/4

Antiarrhythmics
lidocaine
propafenone
quinidine

Anticonvulsant
carbamazepine

Antidepressant
nefazodone

Benzodiazepines
alprazolam
midazolam
triazolam

Calcium channel blockers
diltiazem
felodipine
nifedipine
verapamil

Miscellaneous
cyclosporine
cortisol
erythromycin
ethinyl estradiol
tamoxifen

From Preskorn SH: Clinically relevant pharmacology of selective serotonin reuptake inhibitors: an overview with emphasis on pharmacokinetics and effects on oxidative drug metabolism, *Clin Pharmacokinet* 32(suppl 1):1-21, 1997.

INDEX

D

E

G

H

I

S

U

V

W

Y

Z